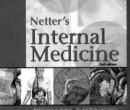
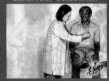
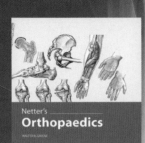
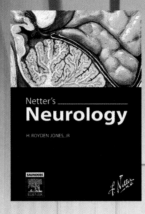
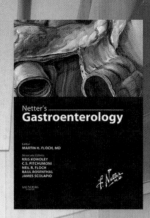
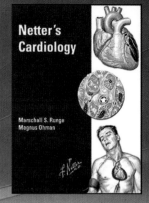
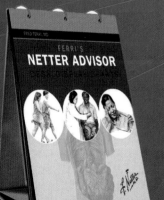
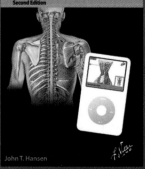
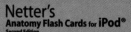

Netter's Obstetrics and Gynecology

Second Edition

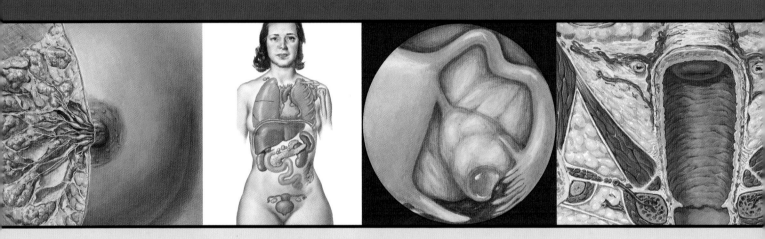

ROGER P. SMITH, MD

University of Missouri–Kansas City

Illustrations by Frank H. Netter, MD

CONTRIBUTING ILLUSTRATORS

Carlos A.G. Machado, MD
John A. Craig, MD
James A. Perkins, MS, MFA
Kristen Wienandt Marzejon
Joe Chovan

SAUNDERS

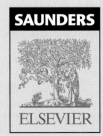

ELSEVIER

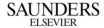

1600 John F. Kennedy Blvd.
Ste 1800
Philadelphia, PA 19103-2899

NETTER'S OBSTETRICS AND GYNECOLOGY,   ISBN: 978-1-4160-5682-9
SECOND EDITION
Copyright © 2008 by Saunders, an imprint of Elsevier Inc.

Notice

Library of Congress Cataloging-in-Publication Data

Smith, Roger P. (Roger Perry), 1949–
Netter's obstetrics and gynecology / Roger P. Smith ; illustrations by Frank H. Netter ; contributing illustrators, Carlos A.G. Machado, John A. Craig, Kristen Wienandt Marzejon. – 2nd ed.
    p. ; cm.
  Rev. ed. of: Netter's obstetrics, gynecology, and women's health / Roger P. Smith. c2002.
  Includes bibliographical references and index.
  ISBN 978-1-4160-5682-9
  1. Gynecology–Handbooks, manuals, etc. 2. Obstetrics–Handbooks, manuals, etc. 3. Women–Diseases–Handbooks, manuals, etc. I. Netter, Frank H. (Frank Henry), 1906–1991. II. Smith, Roger P. (Roger Perry), 1949–. Netter's obstetrics, gynecology, and women's health. III. Title. IV. Title: Obstetrics and gynecology. [DNLM: 1. Genital Diseases, Female–Atlases. 2. Obstetrics–Atlases. WP 17 S658na 2009]
  RG110.S53 2009
  618–dc22

                                                                    2008030671

Acquisitions Editor: Elyse O'Grady
Developmental Editor: Marybeth Thiel
Project Manager: Mary Stermel
Design Direction: Lou Forgione
Illustrations Manager: Karen Giacomucci
Marketing Manager: Jason Oberacker
Editorial Assistant: Julie Goolsby

Printed in China

Last digit is the print number: 9 8 7 6 5 4 3 2 1

This work is dedicated to my father,
who taught me the "art" of medicine
and who first introduced me to the art of Dr. Netter.

Preface

No student of medicine, past or present, is unaware of the extraordinary series of medical illustrations created by Dr. Frank Netter; it is an incredible body of work that has been carried forward by the talented Carlos Machado, MD, and John Craig, MD, since Dr. Netter's passing. Older physicians have looked with envy at these images, wishing they had been available when they were learning; established physicians return to them as comfortable sources of information; young physicians seek them out for the wealth of information they contain and their ability to make clear difficult clinical concepts. This spirit of concise reference and resource is the premise of this text.

This second edition maintains the same consistent format in presenting topics to facilitate rapid access—the same information is in the same location—that was so well received in the first edition. Chapters have been organized to provide a quick, concise resource for the diagnosis and treatment of common conditions encountered by anyone who provides care for women. In producing this second edition, more than 40 new topics have been added, a more intuitive organization has been developed, a new section on commonly encountered procedures has been added, new artwork has been developed, and subtle enhancements (such as indications of the level of evidence provided for references) have been made throughout the work.

It is our hope that this work will be both a useful resource and celebration of the artistic richness that is clinical medicine.

Roger P. Smith, MD

About the Author

Although Roger P. Smith, MD, has spent much of his career in academic medicine, and has a *curriculum vitae* that is appropriately long, he regards himself as a clinician. Dr. Smith received his undergraduate education at Purdue University and his medical education, internship (in General Surgery), and residency at Northwestern University in Chicago. He then spent almost 10 years in a multi-disciplinary group practice at the Carle Clinic in Urbana, Illinois, before moving to the Medical College of Georgia in 1985, where he was Chief of the Section of General Obstetrics and Gynecology. In 1999, Dr. Smith joined the University of Missouri–Kansas City, where he served as Vice Chair and Residency Program Director until 2008.

About the Artists

Frank H. Netter, MD

Frank H. Netter was born in 1906 in New York City. He studied art at the Art Student's League and the National Academy of Design before entering medical school at New York University, where he received his medical degree in 1931. During his student years, Dr. Netter's notebook sketches attracted the attention of the medical faculty and other physicians, allowing him to augment his income by illustrating articles and textbooks. He continued illustrating as a sideline after establishing a surgical practice in 1933, but he ultimately opted to give up his practice in favor of a full-time commitment to art. After service in the United States Army during World War II, Dr. Netter began his long collaboration with the CIBA Pharmaceutical Company (now Novartis Pharmaceuticals). This 45-year partnership resulted in the production of the extraordinary collection of medical art so familiar to physicians and other medical professionals worldwide.

In 2005 Elsevier, Inc. purchased the Netter Collection and all publications from Icon Learning Systems. There are now over 50 publishcations featuring the art of Dr. Netter available through Elsevier, Inc. (in the US: www.us.elsevierhealth.com/Netter and outside the US: www.elsevierhealth.com)

Dr. Netter's works are among the finest examples of the use of illustration in the teaching of medical concepts. The 13-book *Netter Collection of Medical Illustrations*, which includes the greater part of the more than 20,000 paintings created by Dr. Netter, became and remains on eof the most famous medical works ever published. *The Netter Atlas of Human Anatomy*, first published in 1989, presents the anatomical paintings from the Netter Collection. Now translated into 16 languages, it is the anatomy atlas of choice among medical and health professions students the world over.

The Netter illustrations are appreciated not only for their aesthetic qualities, but, more important, for their intellectual content. As Dr. Netter wrote in 1949, ". . . clarification of a subject is the aim and goal of illustration. No matter how beautifully painted, how delicately and subtly rendered a subject may be, it is of little value as a *medical illustration* if it does not serve to make clear some medical point." Dr. Netter's planning, conception, point of view, and approach are what inform his paintings and what make them so intellectually valuable.

Frank H. Netter, MD, physician and artist, died in 1991.

Learn more about the physician-artist whose work has inspired the Netter Reference collection: http://www.netterimages.com/artist/netter.htm

Carlos A.G. Machado, MD

Carlos Machado was chosen by Novartis to be Dr. Netter's successor. He continues to be the main artist who contributes to the Netter collection of medical illustrations.

Self-taught in medical illustration, cardiologist Carlos Machado has contributed meticulous updates to some of Dr. Netter's original plates and has created many paintings of his own in the style of Netter as an extension of the Netter collection. Dr. Machado's photorealistic expertise and his keen insight into the physician/patient relationship informs his vivid and unforgettable visual style. His dedication to researching each topic and subject he paints places him among the premier medical illustrators at work today.

Learn more about his background and see more of his art at: http://www.netterimages.com/artist/machado.htm

Contents

SECTION III
Vulvar Disease

SECTION IV
Vaginal Disease

SECTION V
Cervical Disease

SECTION VI
Uterine Pathology

SECTION XI
Obstetric Conditions and Concerns

PART 3 PROCEDURES

SECTION XII
Procedures

GYNECOLOGY AND WOMEN'S HEALTH

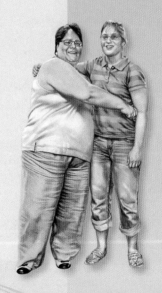

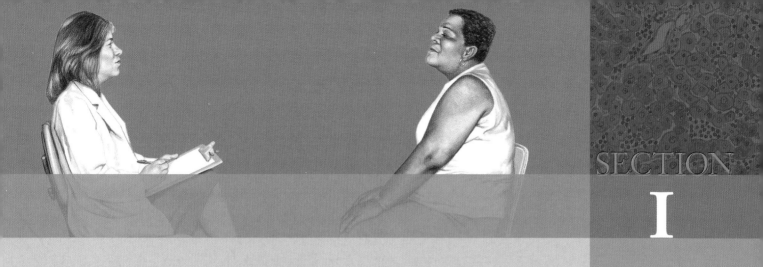

General Health Considerations and Counseling

Puberty: Normal Sequence

THE CHALLENGE

Adolescence with the onset of puberty is a time of great emotional and physical change. By understanding the normal sequence of events and being sensitive to the presence of abnormalities, the caregiver may be able to make the most of opportunities to improve health and well-being.

Scope of the Problem

The variety of decisions, concerns, and changes confronting an adolescent are formidable, not the least of which are health issues raised by rapid growth, sexual maturation, and emerging sexuality. Puberty involves physical, emotional, and sexual changes that mark the transition from childhood to adulthood. Despite the potential need for medical education and care, teenagers have the lowest rate of physician office visits of any group. Embarrassment, inability to pay, lack of familiarity with health care delivery options, and legal obstructions to access all contribute to this lack of care.

Objectives of Management

Understanding the normal sequence of events involved in sexual maturation is important for counseling young women who may be concerned about "being normal." It is also pivotal to the important task of identifying those in whom the progression is not normal so that timely evaluation and intervention may be achieved.

TACTICS

Relevant Pathophysiology

Hormonally, puberty involves a change from negative gonadal feedback to the establishment of circadian and ultradian gonadal rhythms and the positive feedback controls that result in monthly cycles and fertility. It appears that three elements must be present for puberty to progress normally: adequate body mass, adequate sleep, and exposure to light. These factors appear to facilitate or allow the complex hypothalamic, pituitary, and ovarian changes that must occur. As the hypothalamus matures there is a decrease in its sensitivity to estrogen, resulting in an increase in the production and release of gonadotropin-releasing hormone. Consequently, follicle-stimulating hormone levels begin to increase at about the 8th to the 10th year of life, accompanied by an increase in estrogen levels. As the sensitivity of the hypothalamus to negative feedback further decreases, follicle-stimulating hormone and luteinizing hormone levels continue to rise. Eventually these hormones reach a sufficient level that the follicles can respond, initiating cyclic ovulation and menstruation.

Strategies

The changes of puberty generally follow a predictable pattern. A growth spurt and the rounding of body curves generally herald puberty. Breast tissue begins to develop; nipples darken; and fat is laid down in the shoulders, hips, and buttocks and in front of the pubic bone (the mons). Body hair begins to appear because of the influence of androgens made in small amounts by the ovary and adrenal glands. Height increases because of accelerated growth in the long bones of the body, capped off by the closure of the growth centers near the end of puberty. Generally this growth spurt begins approximately 2 years before the start of menstruation itself, with growth slowing about the same time menstruation begins.

Patient Education

American College of Obstetricians and Gynecologists: Growing up (Especially for Teens). ACOG Patient Education Pamphlet AP041.
American College of Obstetricians and Gynecologists: Menstruation. ACOG Patient Education Pamphlet AP049.

IMPLEMENTATION
Special Considerations

The average age of first menstruation (menarche) is 11.6 years, with ages 8 to 16 years being the normal range. These age ranges have been gradually declining over the past few years. Puberty occurs as much as 2 years earlier for girls of African-American descent. Menarche generally occurs after the growth spurt and beginning of breast development, while changes in the pubic hair and labia are still under way. Although there is some variation in the normal progression of events, thelarche is the indication of pubertal change for most, followed by adrenarche, then peak growth velocity, and ending with the onset of menstruation. This sequence generally takes 4½ years to run its course, with a range of 1½ to 6 years.

REFERENCES

Level II
Lee PA: Normal ages of pubertal events among American males and females. J Adolesc Health Care 1980;1:26.
McDowell MA, Brody DJ, Hughes JP: Has age at menarche changed? Results from the National Health and Nutrition Examination Survey (NHANES) 1999–2004. J Adolesc Health 2007;40:227. Epub 2007 Jan 24.
Zacharias L, Rand WM, Wurtman RJ: A prospective study of sexual development and growth in American girls: The statistics of menarche. Obstet Gynecol Surv 1976;31:325.

Level III
American College of Obstetricians and Gynecologists: Breast concerns in the adolescent. ACOG Committee Opinion 350. Washington, DC, ACOG, 2006.
Reindollar RH, McDonough PG: Pubertal aberrancy: Etiology and clinical approach. J Reprod Med 1984;29:391.

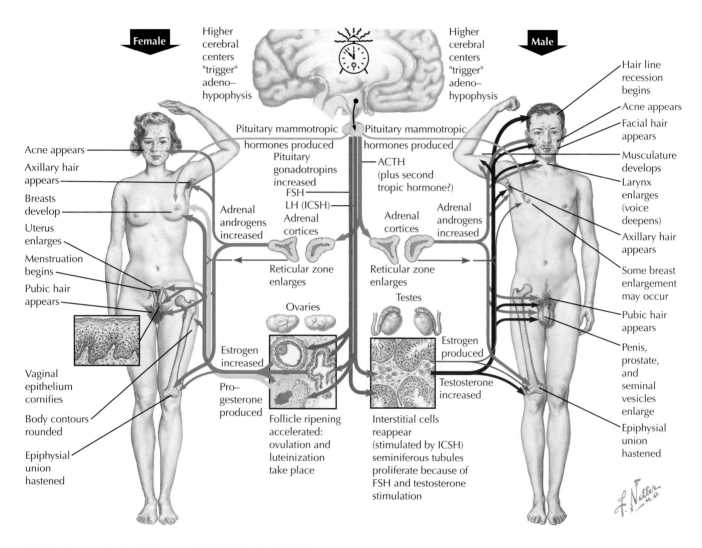

Female

Higher cerebral centers "trigger" adeno–hypophysis

Higher cerebral centers "trigger" adeno–hypophysis

Male

Pituitary mammotropic hormones produced

Pituitary mammotropic hormones produced

Pituitary gonadotropins increased
FSH
LH (ICSH)

ACTH (plus second tropic hormone?)

Acne appears

Axillary hair appears

Breasts develop

Uterus enlarges

Menstruation begins

Pubic hair appears

Adrenal androgens increased

Adrenal cortices

Adrenal cortices

Adrenal androgens increased

Hair line recession begins

Acne appears

Facial hair appears

Musculature develops

Larynx enlarges (voice deepens)

Axillary hair appears

Some breast enlargement may occur

Reticular zone enlarges

Reticular zone enlarges

Ovaries

Testes

Vaginal epithelium cornifies

Body contours rounded

Epiphysial union hastened

Estrogen increased

Pro–gesterone produced

Estrogen produced

Testosterone increased

Pubic hair appears

Penis, prostate, and seminal vesicles enlarge

Epiphysial union hastened

Follicle ripening accelerated: ovulation and luteinization take place

Interstitial cells reappear (stimulated by ICSH) seminiferous tubules proliferate because of FSH and testosterone stimulation

F. Netter M.D.

ACTH, adrenocorticotropic hormone; FSH, follicle-stimulating hormone;
ICSH, interstitial cell stimulating hormone; LH, luteinizing hormone.

IMPORTANT CONSIDERATIONS (PHYSIOLOGIC CHANGES)

The 12- to 18-years age group is notable for the development and consolidation of reproductive capacity, sexual identity, and expressiveness. Changing life roles and self-awareness present both challenges and opportunities for the development of good health practices. The first visit to the obstetrician–gynecologist for screening and the provision of preventive health care services and guidance should generally take place between the ages of 13 and 15 years; however, this visit should not be viewed by anyone involved, patient or caregiver, as the right time for the first internal pelvic examination, unless indicated by the medical history.

Health care for the adolescent should include review of normal menstruation; diet and exercise; healthy sexual decision-making; the development of healthy, safe relationships; immunizations; and injury prevention. (Most of the health problems facing this age group are the result of risk-taking behaviors such as unsafe sexual practices, reckless driving, poor or distorted eating patterns, and substance use such as alcohol and drugs.)

Leading Causes of Death

- Motor vehicle accidents
- Malignant neoplasms
- Homicide
- Suicide
- Congenital anomalies
- Leukemia

Leading Causes of Morbidity:

- Nose, throat, and upper respiratory conditions
- Viral, bacterial, and parasitic infections
- Sexual abuse
- Musculoskeletal and soft tissue injuries
- Acute ear infections
- Digestive system and acute urinary conditions
- Obesity
- Sexually transmitted diseases (STDs)
- Vaginitis

Screening

History

- Reason for visit
- Health status: medical, surgical, family
- Dietary/nutritional assessment
- Physical activity
- Tobacco, alcohol, other drugs (including complementary and alternative medicines) (Data from the 2003 Youth Risk Behavior Surveillance Report indicate that many adolescents will begin engaging in risk-taking behaviors by age 13 years: 27.8% of adolescents report alcohol use before age 13 years.)
- Abuse/neglect (20% to 40% of adults report abuse or sexual victimization before age 18 years)
- Sexual practices

Physical

- Height
- Weight (body mass index)
- Blood pressure
- Secondary sexual characteristics (Tanner staging)
- Pelvic examination (yearly 3 years after becoming sexually active or by age 21 years)
- Skin

Laboratory (only as dictated by the patient's history)

Periodic:

- Pap test (within 3 years of becoming sexually active or by age 21 years and annually thereafter until at least three negative test results, then the interval may be increased. Note: Many patients are unaware of the difference between a Pap test and a pelvic examination for any other reason; this can be a good opportunity to discuss the difference.)
- Cholesterol, high-density lipoprotein cholesterol (every 5 years)

As Indicated by Risk Factors:

- Hemoglobin
- Bacteriuria testing
- STD testing: Chlamydia and gonorrhea (If the patient has had sexual intercourse, screening for STDs is important, but urine-based STD testing, if available, can be an efficient means for doing so without a speculum examination.)
- Human immunodeficiency virus testing
- Genetic testing/counseling
- Rubella titer
- Tuberculosis skin test
- Lipid profile
- Fasting glucose

Imaging

- None indicated as routine care

COUNSELING

It is important to discuss issues of confidentiality with both the patient and her parent or guardian; concerns over confidentiality often are a barrier to the delivery of health care services, especially reproductive health care, for adolescents. To overcome this obstacle, a discussion of this topic at the initial visit, along with advice about relevant state and local statutes, is important. For example, if the patient discloses any evidence or risk of bodily harm to herself or others, confidentiality must be breached. Furthermore, state laws may mandate the reporting of physical or sexual abuse of minors. (Physicians should be familiar with state and local statutes regarding the rights of minors to health care services and the federal and state laws that affect confidentiality.)

The main purpose of the initial reproductive health visit is preventive health, including educational information, rather than problem-focused care. Preventive counseling for parents or other supportive adults can include discussions about physical, sexual, and emotional development; signs and symptoms of common conditions affecting adolescents; and encouragement of lifelong healthy behaviors.

- Sexuality (inclusion of topics such as prevention of pregnancy and STDs is important because more than 85% of adolescent females will have had some form of sexual contact (vaginal, anal, oral, or same-sex) by age 19 years; nearly one third of all 9th graders report having had sexual intercourse, and more than 60% of all 12th graders report having had sexual intercourse.)
- Development
- High-risk behaviors
- Preventing unwanted/unintended pregnancy
  - Postponing sexual involvement
  - Contraceptive options (should also include emergency contraceptive options)
  - STDs
  - Partner selection
  - Barrier protection
- Date rape prevention
- Fitness
- Hygiene (including dental); fluoride supplementation/treatment
- Dietary/nutritional assessment (including eating disorders, calcium intake, and folic acid supplementation of 0.4 mg of folic acid per day)
- Exercise: discussion of program
- Psychosocial evaluation
- Interpersonal/family relationships
- Sexual identity
- Personal goal development
- Behavioral/learning disorders
- Abuse/neglect
- Cardiovascular risk factors
  - Family history
  - Hypertension
  - Dyslipidemia
  - Obesity
  - Diabetes mellitus
- Health/risk behaviors
- Injury prevention
  - Safety belts and helmets
  - Recreational hazards
  - Firearms
  - Hearing damage
  - Sports
  - Skin exposure to ultraviolet rays
  - Suicide: depressive symptoms
  - Tobacco, alcohol, other drugs

COUNSELING RESOURCES

American College of Obstetricians and Gynecologists: Birth control (Especially for Teens). ACOG Patient Education Pamphlet AP112. Washington, DC, ACOG, 2005.

American College of Obstetricians and Gynecologists: Growing up (Especially for Teens). ACOG Patient Education Pamphlet AP041. Washington, DC, ACOG, 1997.

American College of Obstetricians and Gynecologists: You and your sexuality (Especially for Teens). ACOG Patient Education Pamphlet AP042. Washington, DC, ACOG, 1996.

American College of Obstetricians and Gynecologists: Your first ob-gyn visit (Especially for Teens). ACOG Patient Education Pamphlet AP150. Washington, DC, ACOG, 2001.

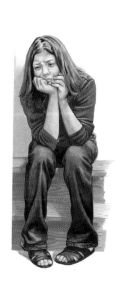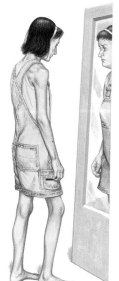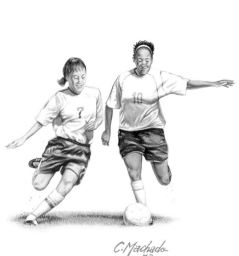

The ages of 12–18 represent a time of extreme changes in body, body image, personality, and personal interactions.

The physician must be aware of these changes, initiate a frank and open dialogue and assure confidentiality except in those cases where safety or bodily harm are involved.

INTERVENTIONS: IMMUNIZATIONS

If not already accomplished, this age group should receive a human papillomavirus and hepatitis B vaccine series.

Meningococcal conjugate vaccine is now recommended. For adolescents who have not received meningococcal conjugate vaccine, the Centers for Disease Control and Prevention now recommend vaccination before entry into high school, at approximately 15 years of age.

Periodic

• Tetanus–diphtheria booster (once between ages 14 and 16)

High-Risk Groups

• Measles, mumps, rubella vaccine
• Hepatitis B vaccine

REFERENCES

Level II

Grunbaum JA, Kann L, Kinchen S, et al: Youth risk behavior surveillance—United States, 2003 MMWR Surveill Summ 2004; 53:1. *Errata* MMWR Morb Mortal Wkly Rep 2004;53:536 and 2005; 54:608.

Mosher WD, Chandra A, Jones J: Sexual behavior and selected health measures: Men and women 15–44 years of age, United States, 2002. Adv Data 2005;362:1.

Level III

American College of Obstetricians and Gynecologists: Cervical cancer screening in adolescents. ACOG Committee Opinion No. 300. Obstet Gynecol 2004;104:885.

American College of Obstetricians and Gynecologists: Confidentiality in adolescent health care. In: Health Care for Adolescents. Washington, DC, ACOG, 2003:25.

American College of Obstetricians and Gynecologists: Guidelines for Women's Health Care, 2nd ed. Washington, DC, ACOG, 2002.

American College of Obstetricians and Gynecologists: Initial reproductive health visit. Committee Opinion No. 335. Washington, DC, ACOG, 2006.

American College of Obstetricians and Gynecologists: Meningococcal vaccination for adolescents. Committee Opinion 314. Washington, DC, ACOG, 2005.

American College of Obstetricians and Gynecologists: Primary and Preventive Care. Clinical Updates in Women's Health Care. 2007;VI(2):1.

American College of Obstetricians and Gynecologists: Primary and preventive health care for female adolescents. In Health Care for Adolescents. Washington, DC, ACOG, 2003, p 1.

American College of Obstetricians and Gynecologists: Routine Cancer Screening. Committee Opinion No. 356. Washington, DC, ACOG, 2006.

American College of Obstetricians and Gynecologists: Tool kit for teen care. Washington, DC, ACOG, 2003.

Lentz GM: History, physical examination, and preventive health care. In Katz VL, Lentz GM, Lobo RA, Gershenson DM: Comprehensive Gynecology, 5th ed. Philadelphia, Mosby/Elsevier, 2007, p 148.

Ornstein RM, Fisher MM: Hormonal contraception in adolescents: special considerations. Paediatr Drugs 2006;8:25.

Zuckerbrot RA, Maxon L, Pagar D, et al: Adolescent depression screening in primary care: Feasibility and acceptability. Pediatrics 2007;119:101.

IMPORTANT CONSIDERATIONS (PHYSIOLOGIC CHANGES)

The 19- to 39-years group is notable for more established menstrual function, punctuated for many by one or more pregnancies. Sexuality and sexual expression patterns have generally become well established and comfortable. Health care is directed toward prevention and health promotion because health is generally good in patients during these years.

Leading Causes of Death

- Malignant neoplasms
- Motor vehicle accidents
- Cardiovascular disease
- Suicide
- Acquired immunodeficiency syndrome
- Homicide
- Cerebrovascular disease
- Diabetes mellitus and its complications

Leading Causes of Morbidity

- Diabetes mellitus
- Nose, throat, and upper respiratory conditions
- Menstrual disorders
- Musculoskeletal and soft tissue including back and upper and lower extremities
- Obesity
- Sexual assault/domestic abuse
- STD

SCREENING

History

- Reason for visit
- Health status: medical, surgical, family
- Dietary/nutritional assessment
- Physical activity
- Tobacco, alcohol, other drugs (including complementary and alternative medicines)
- Abuse/neglect
- Sexual practices

Physical

- Height
- Weight (body mass index)
- Blood pressure
- Neck: adenopathy, thyroid
- Breasts
- Abdomen
- Pelvic examination
- Skin

Laboratory

Periodic

- Pap test (physician and patient discretion after three consecutive normal test results if low risk)
- Cholesterol, high-density lipoprotein cholesterol (every 5 years)

As Indicated by Risk Factors

- Bacteriuria testing
- Fasting glucose test
- Genetic testing/counseling
- Hemoglobin
- Human immunodeficiency virus testing
- Mammography
- Rubella titer
- STD testing
- Thyroid-stimulating hormone test
- Tuberculosis skin test

Imaging

Screening mammography may be started before age 40 years for patients with a strong family history of early-onset breast cancer or heritable cancer syndromes.

COUNSELING

For those considering or at risk for pregnancy, counseling regarding preconception testing, immunization, and nutrition is always appropriate. Health care encounters during this period are also an excellent opportunity to discuss long-term health improvement strategies such as weight control, exercise, and nutrition.

Sexuality

- High-risk behaviors
- Contraceptive options
  - Genetic counseling
  - Prevention of unwanted pregnancy (including emergency contraceptive options)
- STD
  - Partner selection
  - Barrier protection
- Sexual function

Fitness

- Hygiene (including dental)
- Dietary/nutritional assessment (folic acid supplementation for those at risk for or considering pregnancy; 0.4 mg of folic acid per day has been shown to reduce the risk of neural tube defects)
- Exercise: discussion of program

Psychosocial Evaluation

- Interpersonal/family relationships
- Domestic violence (more than 1.5 million cases of domestic violence occur each year; 20% to 40% of adults report abuse or sexual victimization before age 18 years, and 10% to 25% of wives report abuse or sexual victimization)
- Job satisfaction
- Lifestyle/stress
- Sleep disorders

Cardiovascular Risk Factors

- Family history
- Hypertension

- Dyslipidemia
- Obesity/diabetes mellitus
- Lifestyle

Health/Risk Behaviors

- Injury prevention
  - Safety belts and helmets
  - Recreational hazards
  - Firearms
  - Hearing
  - Breast self-examination (Although data on the efficacy of breast self-examination are lacking, the possibility of detecting breast disease makes this recommendation reasonable.)
  - Breast cancer chemoprophylaxis (selective estrogen receptor modulator therapy for women older than age 35 years at high risk)
  - Skin exposure to ultraviolet rays
  - Suicide: depressive symptoms
  - Tobacco, alcohol, other drugs

COUNSELING RESOURCES

American College of Obstetricians and Gynecologists: Breast Self-Exam. ACOG Patient Education Pamphlet AP145. Washington, DC, ACOG, 2001.

American College of Obstetricians and Gynecologists: Cholesterol and your health. ACOG Patient Education Pamphlet AP101. Washington, DC, ACOG, 2004.

American College of Obstetricians and Gynecologists: Eating disorders. ACOG Patient Education Pamphlet BP144. Washington, DC, ACOG, 2000.

American College of Obstetricians and Gynecologists: Good health before pregnancy. ACOG Patient Education Pamphlet AP056. Washington, DC, ACOG, 2007.

American College of Obstetricians and Gynecologists: Staying healthy at all ages. ACOG Patient Education Pamphlet AB006. Washington, DC, ACOG, 2006.

INTERVENTIONS: IMMUNIZATIONS

If not already accomplished, initiate human papillomavirus and hepatitis B vaccine series.

Periodic

- Tetanus–diphtheria booster (every 10 years)

High-Risk Groups

- Measles, mumps, rubella vaccine
- Hepatitis B vaccine

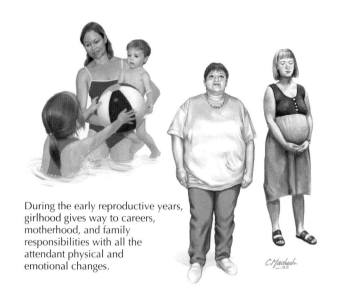

During the early reproductive years, girlhood gives way to careers, motherhood, and family responsibilities with all the attendant physical and emotional changes.

- Influenza vaccine
- Pneumococcal vaccine

REFERENCES

Level II

Hahn KA, Strickland PA, Hamilton JL, et al: Hyperlipidemia guideline adherence and association with patient gender. J Womens Health (Larchmt) 2006;15(9):1009.

Mosher WD, Chandra A, Jones J: Sexual behavior and selected health measures: Men and women 15–44 years of age, United States, 2002. Adv Data 2005;362:1.

Level III

American College of Obstetricians and Gynecologists: Guidelines for Women's Health Care, 2nd ed. Washington, DC, ACOG, 2002.

American College of Obstetricians and Gynecologists: Primary and preventive care. Clinical Updates in Women's Health Care. 2007;VI(2):1.

American College of Obstetricians and Gynecologists: Routine cancer screening. Committee Opinion No. 356. Washington, DC, ACOG, 2006.

American College of Obstetricians and Gynecologists: Selective estrogen receptor modulators. ACOG Practice Bulletin No. 39. Obstet Gynecol 2002;100:835.

Lentz GM: History, physical examination, and preventive health care. In Katz VL, Lentz GM, Lobo RA, Gershenson DM: Comprehensive Gynecology, 5th ed. Philadelphia, Mosby/Elsevier, 2007, p 148.

O'Brien WF: Weight control in women: A challenge to the obstetrician-gynecologist. Obstet Gynecol 1996;88:888.

THE CHALLENGE

Assisting couples in identifying and using the most appropriate method of controlling fertility is an important challenge. Changing patterns of sexual expression, new technologies, increased consumerism, and heightened cost pressures all affect the choices made in the search for fertility control. The very nature of the topic gives contraception personal, religious, and political overtones that often lead to conflict, emotionality, and confusion.

SCOPE OF THE PROBLEM

In the United States, more than half (56%) of all pregnancies are unplanned, despite the fact that 90% of women at risk (fertile, sexually active, and neither pregnant nor seeking pregnancy) are using some form of contraception. The 10% or so of women not using contraception account for more than half of these unintended pregnancies. The remaining unplanned pregnancies occur as a result of either failure of the contraceptive method used or the improper or inconsistent use of the method.

OBJECTIVES OF COUNSELING

No "ideal" contraceptive method exists. Although efficacy and an acceptable risk of side effects are important in the choice of contraceptive methods, these are often not the factors on which the final choice is made. Motivation to use, or continue to use, a contraceptive method is based on education; cultural background; cost; and individual needs, preferences, and prejudices. Factors such as availability, cost, coital dependence, personal acceptability, and the patient's perception of the risk all have a role in the final choice of methods.

TACTICS

Relevant Pathophysiology

Currently available contraceptive methods seek to prevent pregnancy by preventing the sperm and egg from uniting or by preventing implantation and growth. These goals are accomplished by preventing the development and release of the egg (oral and nonoral hormonal contraceptives, long-acting hormonal methods), preventing union of sperm and egg by imposing a mechanical, chemical, or temporal barrier between sperm and egg (condom, diaphragm, foam, intrauterine devices, rhythm, withdrawal, postcoital oral contraception), or altering the likelihood of implantation or growth (RU-486). Relative efficacy (first-year failure, both real and theoretical) is shown in the accompanying table.

Strategies

For a couple to use a method, it must be accessible, immediately available (especially in coitally dependent or "use-oriented" methods), and of reasonable cost. The impact of a method on spontaneity, or the modes of sexual expression preferred by the patient and her partner, may also be important considerations. A decision tree based on these concepts is presented in the accompanying figure.

Patient Education

American College of Obstetricians and Gynecologists: Birth Control. ACOG Patient Education Booklet AP005.

American College of Obstetricians and Gynecologists: Birth Control (Especially for Teens). ACOG Patient Education Booklet AP112.

American College of Obstetricians and Gynecologists: Sterilization for Women and Men. ACOG Patient Education Booklet AP011.

American College of Obstetricians and Gynecologists: The Intrauterine Device. ACOG Patient Education Booklet AP014.

American College of Obstetricians and Gynecologists: Birth Control Pills. ACOG Patient Education Booklet AP021.

American College of Obstetricians and Gynecologists: Barrier Methods of Contraception. ACOG Patient Education Booklet AP022.

American College of Obstetricians and Gynecologists: Natural Family Planning. ACOG Patient Education Booklet AP024.

CONTRACEPTIVE USE AMONG U.S. WOMEN, 2002

Method	Percent of users	Perfect use failure*	Actual use failure*
Oral contraceptives	30.6	0.3	8.0
Sterilization (female)	27.0	0.5	0.5
Condom (male)	18.0	2.0	15.0
Sterilization (male)	9.2	0.1	0.15
Withdrawal	4.0	4.0	27.0
Intrauterine device	2.0	0.1–0.6	0.1–0.8
Periodic abstinence (calendar)	1.2	9.0	25.0
Implant	<1	0.05	0.05
Injectable (1 month)	<1	0.05	3.0
Transdermal patch	<1	0.3	8.0
Diaphragm	<1	6.0	16.0
Other (sponge, cervical cap, female condom, etc.)	<1	5–26	16–32
(No method)	—	85	85

*Percent of women experiencing unintended pregnancy within first year of use.
Data from The Alan Guttmacher Institute. Contraceptive use. Facts in Brief. New York, AGI, 2006. Available at www.guttmacher.org/pubs/fb_contr_use.pdf. Accessed May 20, 2008.

American College of Obstetricians and Gynecologists: Sterilization by Laparoscopy. ACOG Patient Education Booklet AP035.

American College of Obstetricians and Gynecologists: Postpartum Sterilization. ACOG Patient Education Booklet AP052.

American College of Obstetricians and Gynecologists: Emergency Contraception. ACOG Patient Education Booklet AP114.

American College of Obstetricians and Gynecologists: Hormonal Contraception Injections, Rings, and Patches. ACOG Patient Education Booklet AP159.

IMPLEMENTATION

Special Considerations

Adolescent patients require reliable contraception but often have problems with compliance. Careful counseling about options (including abstinence), the risks of pregnancy and STDs, and the need for both contraception and disease protection must be provided. These patients may

be better served by methods that rely less on the user for reliability (intrauterine devices or long-acting hormonal agents such as injections, ring, patches, and implants) than those that depend on consistent use (use-oriented methods and those that are time sensitive such as progestin-only contraceptives).

Contraception for breastfeeding mothers may include oral contraceptives if milk flow is well established. (Long-acting progesterone contraceptives may actually result in a slight increase in breast milk production.) Barrier contraceptives are not contraindicated in these patients. An intrauterine device, copper or hormone containing, may also be placed once the uterus has returned to normal.

Patients older than age 35 years may continue to use low-dose oral contraceptives if they have no other risk factors and do not smoke. Compliance concerns are generally less in these patients, making use-oriented methods more acceptable and reliable. Long-term methods (intrauterine devices, long-acting progesterone contraception, or sterilization) may also be appropriate. Until menopause is confirmed by clinical or laboratory methods, contraception must be continued if pregnancy is not desired.

Ovulation may occur as soon as 2 weeks following abortion (spontaneous or induced). If oral contraceptives are chosen as the contraceptive method, they should be started immediately after the loss.

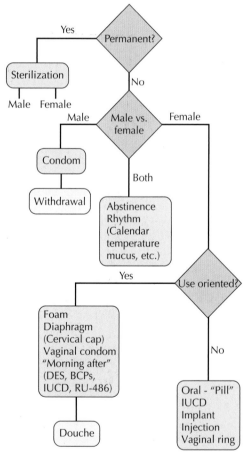

One of many possible decision tree approaches to the choice of contraceptive methods. (Methods shown in blue have the highest failure rate and should not be used if pregnancy prevention is a high priority.) (Modified from Beckman RB, Ling FW, Smith RP, et al. Obstetrics and Gynecology, 5th ed. Baltimore, Williams & Wilkins, 2006, p 244.)

BCP, birth control pill; DES, diethylstilbestrol; IUCD, intrauterine contraceptive device.

REFERENCES

Level III

American College of Obstetricians and Gynecologists: Emergency contraception. ACOG Practice Bulletin 69. Washington, DC, ACOG, 2005.

American College of Obstetricians and Gynecologists: Use of hormonal contraception in women with coexisting medical conditions. ACOG Practice Bulletin 73. Washington, DC, ACOG, 2006.

Benagiano G, Bastianelli C, Farris M: Contraception today. Ann N Y Acad Sci 2006;1092:1.

Deligeoroglou E, Christopoulos P, Creatsas G: Contraception in adolescence. Ann N Y Acad Sci 2006;1092:78.

Draper BH, Morroni C, Hoffman M, et al: Depot medroxyprogesterone versus norethisterone oenanthate for long-acting progestogenic contraception. Cochrane Database Syst Rev 2006;3: CD005214.

Glasier A, Gulmezoglu AM, Schmid GP, et al: Sexual and reproductive health: A matter of life and death. Lancet 2006;368:1595.

Hansen LB, Saseen JJ, Teal SB: Levonorgestrel-only dosing strategies for emergency contraception. Pharmacotherapy 2007;27:278.

Kulier R, Helmerhorst FM, O'Brien P, et al: Copper containing, framed intra-uterine devices for contraception. Cochrane Database Syst Rev 2006;3:CD005347.

Lesnewski R, Prine L: Initiating hormonal contraception. Am Fam Physician 2006;74:105.

Masimasi N, Sivanandy MS, Thacker HL: Update on hormonal contraception. Cleve Clin J Med 2007;74:186, 188, 193 passim. Review.

McNamee K: The vaginal ring and transdermal patch: New methods of contraception. Sex Health 2006;3:135.

Nelson AL: Reversible female contraception: current options and new developments. Expert Rev Med Devices 2007;4:241.

Practice Committee of the American Society for Reproductive Medicine: Hormonal contraception: recent advances and controversies. Fertil Steril 2006;86(5 Suppl):S229.

Smith RP: Gynecology in Primary Care. Baltimore, Williams & Wilkins, 1997, p 209.

Szarewski A: Hormonal contraception: Recent advances. J Fam Health Care 2006;16:35.

The Alan Guttmacher Institute: Contraceptive use. Facts in Brief. New York, AGI, 2006.

IMPORTANT CONSIDERATIONS (PHYSIOLOGIC CHANGES)

The 40- to 64-years age group is notable for the transitions from reproductive function to maturity, from rhythmic menstrual function to menopause, and from robust health to the emergence of age-related health changes.

Leading Causes of Death

- Breast, lung, colorectal, and ovarian cancer
- Coronary artery disease
- Cerebrovascular disease
- Obstructive pulmonary disease
- Accidents
- Diabetes mellitus and its complications

Leading Causes of Morbidity

- Nose, throat, and upper respiratory conditions
- Osteoporosis
- Arthritis
- Hypertension
- Depression
- Orthopedic deformities, including back and upper and lower extremities
- Obesity
- Heart disease
- Hearing and vision impairments

SCREENING

History

- Reason for visit
- Health status: medical, surgical, family
- Dietary/nutritional assessment
- Physical activity
- Tobacco, alcohol, other drugs (including complementary and alternative medicines)
- Abuse/neglect
- Sexual practices
- Urinary and fecal incontinence (These issues become more common with childbearing and age, but patients seldom volunteer these complaints.)

Physical

- Height
- Weight (body mass index)
- Blood pressure
- Oral cavity
- Neck: adenopathy, thyroid
- Breasts
- Abdomen
- Pelvic and rectovaginal examination
- Skin

Laboratory

Periodic

- Pap test (physician and patient discretion after three consecutive normal test results if low risk)
- Cholesterol, high-density lipoprotein cholesterol (every 5 years, starting at age 45 years)
- Fecal occult blood test (Testing requires the collection of two to three samples of stool collected by the patient at home to be valid. A single stool sample collected at the time of digital rectal examination is not sufficient to adequately screen for colon cancer.)
- Sigmoidoscopy (every 3 to 5 years after age 50 years; double-contrast barium enema study may be substituted or a complete colonoscopy may be performed every 10 years)

As Indicated by Risk Factors

- Bacteriuria testing
- Colonoscopy
- Fasting glucose test
- Hemoglobin
- Human immunodeficiency virus testing
- Lipid profile
- Mammography
- STD testing
- Thyroid-stimulating hormone test
- Tuberculosis skin test

Imaging

- Mammography (every 1 to 2 years until age 50 years, yearly beginning at 50)
- Bone density assessment (Testing should be performed on the basis of an individual woman's risk profile and is not indicated unless the results will influence a treatment or management decision. Testing may be recommended to postmenopausal women younger than age 65 years who have risk factors for osteoporosis.)

COUNSELING

Health care encounters during this period are an excellent opportunity to discuss long-term health improvement strategies such as weight control, exercise, and nutrition. As women approach the transition from reproduction to maturity, opportunities for rededication to leading healthy lifestyles and preventing illness and morbidity increase. The increasing importance of surveillance as one ages is also an important message for patients in this age group.

Sexuality

- High-risk behaviors
- Contraceptive options
  - Genetic counseling (for selected women in this age range)
  - Prevention of unwanted pregnancy (including emergency contraceptive options)
- STDs
  - Partner selection
  - Barrier protection
- Sexual function

Fitness

- Hygiene (including dental)
- Dietary/nutritional assessment (1000 to 1200 mg of calcium by diet and/or supplements; folic acid supplementation of 0.4 mg of folic acid per day to age 50 years)
- Exercise: discussion of program and the importance of remaining physically active

Psychosocial Evaluation

- Interpersonal/family relationships
- Domestic violence
- Job/work satisfaction
- Lifestyle/stress
- Retirement planning
- Sleep disorders

Cardiovascular Risk Factors

- Family history
- Hypertension
- Dyslipidemia
- Obesity/diabetes mellitus
- Lifestyle

Health/Risk Behaviors

- Hormone replacement therapy (Recent data suggest that when hormone replacement is begun within 10 years of menopause it is not associated with some of the adverse effects reported in the Women's Health Initiative [WHI] study and may even be associated with reductions in such things as cardiovascular disease.)
- Breast cancer chemoprophylaxis (selective estrogen receptor modulator therapy for women older than age 35 years at high risk)
- Injury prevention
  - Safety belts
  - Recreational hazards
  - Sports involvement
  - Vision and hearing
- Breast self-examination
- Skin exposure to ultraviolet rays
- Suicide: depressive symptoms
- Tobacco, alcohol, other drugs

COUNSELING RESOURCES

American College of Obstetricians and Gynecologists: Cholesterol and your health. ACOG Patient Education Pamphlet AP101. Washington, DC, ACOG, 2004.

American College of Obstetricians and Gynecologists: Eating disorders. ACOG Patient Education Pamphlet BP144. Washington, DC, ACOG, 2000.

American College of Obstetricians and Gynecologists: Midlife transitions: A guide to approaching menopause. ACOG Patient Education Pamphlet AP013. Washington, DC, ACOG, 2003.

Leading Causes of Death and Morbidity in Women Aged 40–64 Years

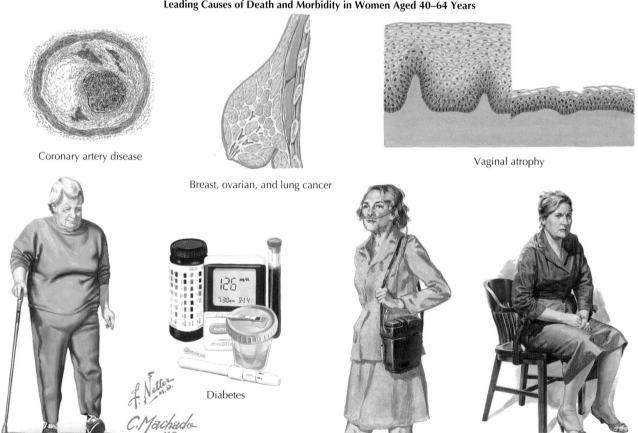

Coronary artery disease

Breast, ovarian, and lung cancer

Vaginal atrophy

Diabetes

Osteoporosis and obesity

Obstructive pulmonary disease

Depression

American College of Obstetricians and Gynecologists: Staying healthy at all ages. ACOG Patient Education Pamphlet AB006. Washington, DC, ACOG, 2006.

American College of Obstetricians and Gynecologists: The menopause years. ACOG Patient Education Pamphlet AP047. Washington, DC, ACOG, 2003.

INTERVENTIONS: IMMUNIZATIONS

Periodic

- Tetanus–diphtheria booster (every 10 years)
- Influenza vaccine (annually beginning at age 50)

High-Risk Groups

- Measles, mumps, rubella vaccine
- Hepatitis A and/or B vaccine
- Influenza vaccine
- Pneumococcal vaccine
- Varicella vaccine

REFERENCES

Level II

Grodstein F, Manson JE, Stampfer MJ: Hormone therapy and coronary heart disease: The role of time since menopause and age at hormone initiation. J Women's Health 2006;15:35.

Rossouw JE, Prentice RL, Manson JE, et al: Postmenopausal hormone therapy and risk of cardiovascular disease by age and years since menopause. JAMA 2007;297:1465.

Level III

American College of Obstetricians and Gynecologists: Guidelines for Women's Health Care, 2nd ed. Washington, DC, ACOG, 2002.

American College of Obstetricians and Gynecologists: Osteoporosis. Clinical management guidelines for obstetricians-gynecologists No. 50. Washington, DC, ACOG, 2004.

American College of Obstetricians and Gynecologists: Primary and preventive care. Clinical Updates in Women's Health Care. 2007;VI(2):1.

American College of Obstetricians and Gynecologists: Routine cancer screening. Committee Opinion No. 356. Washington, DC, ACOG, 2006.

American College of Obstetricians and Gynecologists: Use of botanicals for management of menopausal symptoms. Clinical management guidelines for obstetricians-gynecologists No. 28. Washington, DC, ACOG, 2001.

Hahn KA, Strickland PA, Hamilton JL, et al: Hyperlipidemia guideline adherence and association with patient gender. J Womens Health (Larchmt) 2006;15(9):1009.

Lentz GM: History, physical examination, and preventive health care. In Katz VL, Lentz GM, Lobo RA, Gershenson DM: Comprehensive Gynecology, 5th ed. Philadelphia, Mosby/Elsevier, 2007, p 148.

Manson JE, Hsia J, Johnson KC, et al: Estrogen plus progestin and the risk of coronary heart disease. N Engl J Med 2003;349:523.

O'Brien WF: Weight control in women: A challenge to the obstetrician-gynecologist. Obstet Gynecol 1996;88:888.

Health Maintenance: Ages 65 Years and Older

IMPORTANT CONSIDERATIONS (PHYSIOLOGIC CHANGES)

The 65 years and older age group is notable for maturity, leisure, and age-related health changes. Health care is still directed toward prevention, but it becomes more and more occupied by the management of general medical and age-related illness. Although reproductive health issues no longer are the focus of well-women visits, the women's health care provider is often still the patient's primary entry point for health care.

Leading Causes of Death

- Cardiovascular disease
- Coronary artery disease
- Colorectal, lung, and breast cancer
- Cerebrovascular disease
- Obstructive lung disease
- Alzheimer's disease
- Pneumonia/influenza
- Diabetes mellitus and its complications
- Renal disease
- Accidents

Leading Causes of Morbidity

- Nose, throat, and upper respiratory conditions
- Osteoporosis
- Arthritis
- Hypertension
- Urinary and fecal incontinence
- Heart disease
- Musculoskeletal and soft tissue injuries
- Hearing and vision impairment
- Colon disease (e.g., diverticulitis)

SCREENING

History

- Reason for visit
- Health status: medical, surgical, family
- Dietary/nutritional assessment
- Physical activity and activities of daily life
- Tobacco, alcohol, other drugs (concurrent medications including complementary and alternative medicines)
- Abuse/neglect (two thirds of the victims of elder abuse are women, with almost 90% of abuse cases occurring in the home)
- Sexual practices/activity
- Urinary and fecal incontinence (These issues become more common with childbearing and age, but patients seldom volunteer these complaints.)

Physical

- Height
- Weight (body mass index)
- Blood pressure
- Oral cavity
- Neck: adenopathy, thyroid
- Breasts
- Abdomen
- Pelvic and rectovaginal examination
- Skin
- Hearing and vision screening (including glaucoma testing)

Laboratory

Periodic

- Pap test (physician and patient discretion after three consecutive normal test results if low risk)
- Urinalysis/dipstick
- Cholesterol, high-density lipoprotein cholesterol (every 3 to 5 years)
- Fecal occult blood test (Testing requires the collection of two to three samples of stool collected by the patient at home to be valid. A single stool sample collected at the time of digital rectal examination is not sufficient to adequately screen for colon cancer.)
- Sigmoidoscopy (every 3 to 5 years; double-contrast barium enema study may be substituted or a complete colonoscopy may be performed every 10 years)
- Thyroid-stimulating hormone test (every 3 to 5 years)

As Indicated by Risk Factors

- Hemoglobin
- Fasting glucose test
- STD testing
- Human immunodeficiency virus testing
- Tuberculosis skin test
- Lipid profile

Imaging

- Mammography
- Bone density assessment (Bone mineral density testing should be recommended to all postmenopausal women age 65 years or older. In the absence of new risk factors, densitometry should not be performed more frequently than every 2 years.)

COUNSELING

As function changes as a result of aging, both the patient and the provider must be vigilant in detecting subtle losses of abilities and must be prepared to make accommodations as needed.

Sexuality

- Sexual functioning
- Sexual behaviors
- STDs

Fitness

- Hygiene (general and dental)
- Dietary/nutritional assessment (Women in this age group should take 1200 mg of calcium and 10 µg of vitamin D per day to prevent osteoporosis.)

- Exercise: discussion of program and the importance of remaining physically active

Psychosocial Evaluation

- Neglect/abuse
- Lifestyle/stress
- Depression/sleep disorders (These are particularly prevalent, but often overlooked, as patients age.)
- Family relationships
- Job/work/retirement satisfaction

Cardiovascular Risk Factors

- Hypertension
- Dyslipidemia
- Obesity
- Diabetes mellitus
- Sedentary lifestyle

Health/Risk Behaviors

- Hormone replacement therapy
- Breast cancer chemoprophylaxis (selective estrogen receptor modulator therapy for women at high risk)
- Injury prevention
  - Safety belts and helmets
  - Occupational hazards
  - Recreational hazards
  - Fall prevention

- Hearing and visual acuity/glaucoma screening
- Breast self-examination
- Skin exposure to ultraviolet rays
- Suicide: depressive symptoms
- Tobacco, alcohol, other drugs

COUNSELING RESOURCES

American College of Obstetricians and Gynecologists: A healthy diet. ACOG Patient Education Pamphlet BP151. Washington, DC, ACOG, 2001.

American College of Obstetricians and Gynecologists: Cholesterol and your health. ACOG Patient Education Pamphlet AP101. Washington, DC, ACOG, 2004.

American College of Obstetricians and Gynecologists: Herbal products for menopause. ACOG Patient Education Pamphlet AP158. Washington, DC, ACOG, 2003.

American College of Obstetricians and Gynecologists: Hormone therapy. ACOG Patient Education Pamphlet AP066. Washington, DC, ACOG, 2003.

American College of Obstetricians and Gynecologists: Osteoporosis. ACOG Patient Education Pamphlet AP048. Washington, DC, ACOG, 2003.

American College of Obstetricians and Gynecologists: Staying active. ACOG Patient Education Pamphlet BP153. Washington, DC, ACOG, 2001.

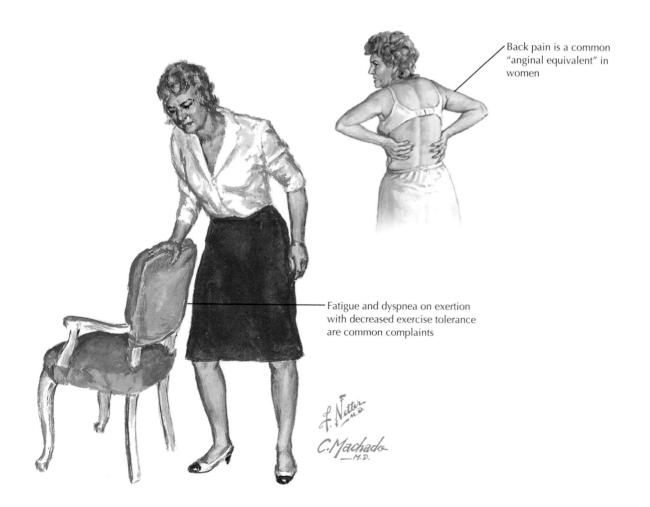

Back pain is a common "anginal equivalent" in women

Fatigue and dyspnea on exertion with decreased exercise tolerance are common complaints

American College of Obstetricians and Gynecologists: Staying healthy (for women ages 65 and older). ACOG Patient Education Pamphlet BP141. Washington, DC, ACOG, 2004.

American College of Obstetricians and Gynecologists: Taking medications. ACOG Patient Education Pamphlet BP152. Washington, DC, ACOG, 2001.

INTERVENTIONS: IMMUNIZATIONS
Periodic

- Tetanus–diphtheria booster (every 10 years)
- Influenza vaccine (annually)
- Pneumococcal vaccine (once)

High-Risk Groups

- Hepatitis B vaccine

REFERENCES
Level II
Bradley CS, Zimmerman MB, Qi Y, et al: Natural history of pelvic organ prolapse in postmenopausal women. Obstet Gynecol 2007; 109:848.

Centers for Disease Control and Prevention: Use of mammograms among women aged ≥40 years—United States, 2000–2005. MMWR Morb Mortal Wkly Rep 200726;56:49.

Huang A, Grady D, Blackwell T, Bauer D Hot flushes, bone mineral density, and fractures in older postmenopausal women. Obstet Gynecol 2007;109:841.

Level III
American College of Obstetricians and Gynecologists: Guidelines for Women's Health Care, 2nd ed. Washington, DC, ACOG, 2002.

American College of Obstetricians and Gynecologists: Primary and preventive care. Clinical Updates in Women's Health Care. 2007; VI(2):1.

American College of Obstetricians and Gynecologists: Routine cancer screening. Committee Opinion No. 356. Washington, DC, ACOG, 2006.

Lentz GM: History, physical examination, and preventive health care. In Katz VL, Lentz GM, Lobo RA, Gershenson DM: Comprehensive Gynecology, 5th ed. Philadelphia, Mosby/Elsevier, 2007, p 148.

Nowalk MP, Zimmerman RK, Cleary SM, Bruehlman RD Missed opportunities to vaccinate older adults in primary care. J Am Board Fam Pract 2005;18:20.

Stenchever MA: Gynogeriatrics: A challenge for the 21st century. Obstet Gynecol (Editorial) 1997;90:632.

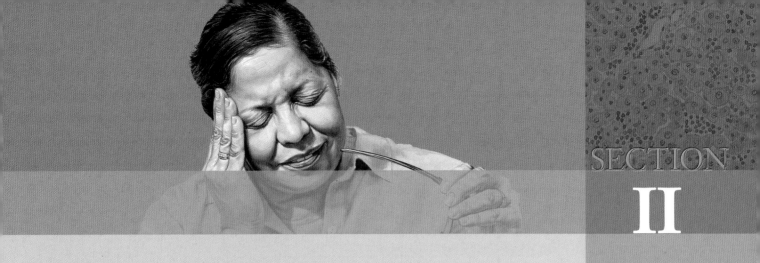

Diseases, Disorders, and Common Problems

Abortion

INTRODUCTION

Description: Abortion is the loss or failure of early pregnancy in several forms: complete, incomplete, inevitable, missed, septic, and threatened. A complete abortion is the termination of a pregnancy before the age of viability, typically defined as occurring at less than 20 weeks from the first day of the last normal menstrual period or involving a fetus of weight less than 500 g. Most complete abortions generally occur before 6 weeks or after 14 weeks of gestation. An incomplete abortion is the spontaneous passage of some, but not all, of the products of conception, associated with uniform pregnancy loss. A pregnancy in which rupture of the membranes and/or cervical dilation takes place during the first half of pregnancy is labeled an inevitable abortion. Uterine contractions typically follow, ending in spontaneous loss of the pregnancy for most patients. A missed abortion is the retention of a failed intrauterine pregnancy for an extended period; however, with ultrasound studies, this can often be detected significantly sooner than it could be on clinical grounds alone. A septic abortion is a variant of an incomplete abortion in which infection of the uterus and its contents has occurred. A threatened abortion is a pregnancy that is at risk for some reason. Most often, this applies to any pregnancy in which vaginal bleeding or uterine cramping takes place but no cervical changes have occurred.

Prevalence: Estimates for the frequency of complete abortions are as high as 50% to 60% of all conceptions and between 10% and 15% of known pregnancies. Of pregnant women hospitalized for bleeding, 60% have an incomplete abortion. Less than 2% of fetal losses are missed abortions. Septic abortions occur in 0.4 to 0.6 of 100,000 spontaneous pregnancy losses. Threatened abortions occur in 30% to 40% of pregnant women.

Predominant Age: Reproductive.

Genetics: Some chromosomal abnormalities are associated with reduced or absent fertility and increased risk of fetal loss (e.g., translocations).

ETIOLOGY AND PATHOGENESIS

Causes: Endocrine abnormalities (25% to 50%)—hyperandrogenism, in utero diethylstilbestrol (DES) exposure, luteal phase defect, thyroid disease. Genetic factors (10% to 70%)—balanced translocation/carrier state, nondisjunction, trisomy (40% to 50%, trisomy 16 most common, any possible except trisomy 1), monosomy X (15% to 25%), triploidy (15%), tetraploidy (5%). Reproductive tract abnormalities (6% to 12%)—abnormality of placentation, bicornuate or unicornuate uterus, incompetent cervix, intrauterine adhesions (Asherman's syndrome), in utero diethylstilbestrol exposure, leiomyomata uteri (submucous), septate uterus. Infection—*Mycoplasma hominis*, syphilis, toxoplasmosis, *Ureaplasma ureolyticus*, possibly chlamydia and herpes. Systemic disease—chronic cardiovascular disease, chronic renal disease, diabetes mellitus, systemic lupus erythematosus/lupus anticoagulant. Environmental factors—alcohol, anesthetic gases, drug use, radiation, smoking, toxins. Other factors—advanced maternal age, delayed fertilization (old egg), trauma.

Risk Factors: Increasing parity, increasing maternal age, increasing paternal age, a short interval between pregnancies, excessive caffeine consumption (≥6 cups of coffee per day). Retention of tissue after pregnancy loss increases the risk of a septic abortion.

CLINICAL CHARACTERISTICS

Signs and Symptoms

- General—vaginal bleeding (may be bright red to dark in color)
  - Abdominal cramping (generally rhythmic, accompanied by pelvic or low back pressure)
  - Passage of tissue (complete and incomplete abortion)
  - Cervical dilation (typical of all types of abortion except missed and threatened)
  - Cervical dilation with tissue visible at the cervical os (diagnostic of either incomplete or inevitable abortion)
- Missed abortion—decreased or minimal uterine growth early in pregnancy
  - Vaginal bleeding that changes to a dark-brown discharge that continues
  - Loss of early symptoms of pregnancy, such as breast fullness or morning sickness
  - Disseminated intravascular coagulopathy (DIC) can occur when an intrauterine fetal demise in the second trimester has been retained beyond 6 weeks after the death of the fetus (rare)
- Septic abortion—severe hemorrhage (vaginal)
  - Midline lower abdominal pain
  - Uterine and perimetric tenderness
  - Bacteremia
  - Septic shock
  - Renal failure
- Threatened abortion—implantation bleeding
  - Cervical polyps, cervicitis
  - Other causes of lower abdominal discomfort (e.g., urinary tract infection, constipation)

DIAGNOSTIC APPROACH

Differential Diagnosis

- Ectopic pregnancy
- Cervical polyps, cervicitis
- Molar pregnancy
- Possibility of trauma, including perforation of the uterus or vagina, when sepsis is present

Associated Conditions: Thirty percent of patients treated by sharp curettage for missed abortion form intrauterine adhesions. Septic abortion is associated with septic shock, ascending infection (myometritis, pelvic inflammatory disease), disseminated intravascular coagulopathy, and renal failure.

Workup and Evaluation

Laboratory: Administer a pregnancy test (if pregnancy has not been confirmed). If serial determinations of quantitative β-human chorionic gonadotropin (β-hCG) do not show at least a 66% increase every 48 hours, the outlook for the pregnancy is poor. Perform complete blood count (if blood loss has been excessive). Serial determinations of serum β-hCG may be used to confirm pregnancy loss but are not required for diagnosis.

Imaging: Ultrasonography of the uterus may be used to confirm loss of intrauterine contents, the absence of a fetal pole, or failure to grow.

Special Tests: None indicated.

Diagnostic Procedures: If significant cervical dilation is identified by speculum and bimanual examination or if tissue is seen at the cervix, the diagnosis of inevitable or incomplete abortion is established.

Pathologic Findings

Products of conception (including chorionic villi); in a missed abortion there is the absence of a fetal pole.

MANAGEMENT AND THERAPY
Nonpharmacologic

General Measures: Support and evaluation are helpful; analgesia if required. Rh-negative mothers should be treated with Rh immune globulin after completion of the abortion. Because ovulation may occur as early as 2 weeks after an abortion, a discussion of contraception is warranted.

Specific Measures: When there is a complete abortion, immediate considerations include control of bleeding, prevention of infection, pain relief (if needed), and emotional support. Ensuring that all the products of the conception have been expelled from the uterus controls bleeding. Although most patients with an incomplete or inevitable abortion spontaneously pass the remaining tissue (complete abortion), bleeding, cramping, and the risk of infection associated with expectant management generally require surgical evacuation. If retained tissue is present or cannot be ruled out, curettage must be performed promptly. When a missed abortion is diagnosed, evacuation of the uterus can be accomplished either through dilation and evacuation or through medical therapies such as prostaglandin suppositories or mifepristone (RU-486), based on the stage of the pregnancy and other considerations. Septic abortion requires immediate and aggressive management. Broad-spectrum parenteral antibiotics, fluid therapy, and prompt evacuation of the uterus are indicated. Emergency evacuation of the uterine contents is mandatory because of the significant threat they represent. When the diagnosis of threatened abortion is made, intervention should be minimal, even when bleeding is accompanied by low abdominal pain and cramping. If there is no evidence of cervical change, the patient can be reassured and encouraged to continue normal activities. If significant pain or bleeding persists, especially bleeding leading to hemodynamic alterations, evacuation of the uterus should be carried out.

Diet: No specific dietary changes are indicated unless immediate surgical therapy is being considered; in that case, nothing should be taken by mouth.

Activity: Generally there is no restriction. When sepsis is present, bed rest is initially required while therapy is instituted. After evacuation is accomplished and fever is reduced, the patient may return to normal activity. Although frequently recommended, a short period of bed rest has no documented benefit for patients with a threatened abortion.

Patient Education: Reassurance; American College of Obstetricians and Gynecologists Patient Education Pamphlet AP038 (Bleeding During Pregnancy), AP090 (Early Pregnancy Loss: Miscarriage, Ectopic Pregnancy, and Molar Pregnancy), AP062 (Dilation and Curettage [D&C]), and AB012 (Planning Your Pregnancy).

Drug(s) of Choice

To hasten the expulsion of tissue and reduce bleeding—oxytocin 10 to 20 units/L IV fluids or methylergonovine maleate (Methergine) 0.2 mg IM may be used.

Septic abortion—aggressive fluid therapy, antibiotic therapy (ampicillin 1 to 2 g IV followed by 500 mg IV every 4 to 6 hours, ampicillin/sulbactam 1.5 to 3 g IV every 6 hours, or clindamycin 600 mg IV or IM every 6 hours and gentamicin 80 mg IM every 8 hours).

Contraindications: Undiagnosed vaginal bleeding.

Precautions: Methergine should be used with care in patients with hypertension.

Interactions: Vasoconstrictors and ergot alkaloids.

Alternative Drugs

Prostaglandin E₂, mifepristone (RU-486). For septic abortion, other broad-spectrum antibiotics, singly or in combination, are available.

FOLLOW-UP

Patient Monitoring: Anticipate normal return of menstrual function in 4 to 6 weeks and offer contraceptive counseling. Patients with septic abortions must be monitored for the possibility of septic shock.

Prevention/Avoidance: None. Septic abortions may be prevented by the prompt evacuation of the uterus for patients with incomplete or inevitable abortions. Data on the risk of sepsis for patients with missed abortions are lacking; therefore, expectant, medical, or surgical managements are all acceptable.

Possible Complications: Infection (myometritis, pelvic inflammatory disease) may occur. Removal of the products of conception, combined with vaginal rest (no tampons, douches, or intercourse), provides adequate protection against infection for most patients.

Expected Outcome: The risk of pregnancy loss subsequent to a spontaneous abortion increases slightly, although much of this increase may be due to selection for those with factors that preclude successful pregnancy. For those with an inevitable abortion who do not spontaneously lose the pregnancy, infection or bleeding often ensue, requiring evacuation of the uterus. Missed abortions may spontaneously abort, progressing through incomplete to complete stages, or they may be evacuated. After the pregnancy has terminated (spontaneous abortion or surgical evacuation of products of conception), normal menses return in 4 to 6 weeks. With aggressive antibiotic treatment and prompt evacuation

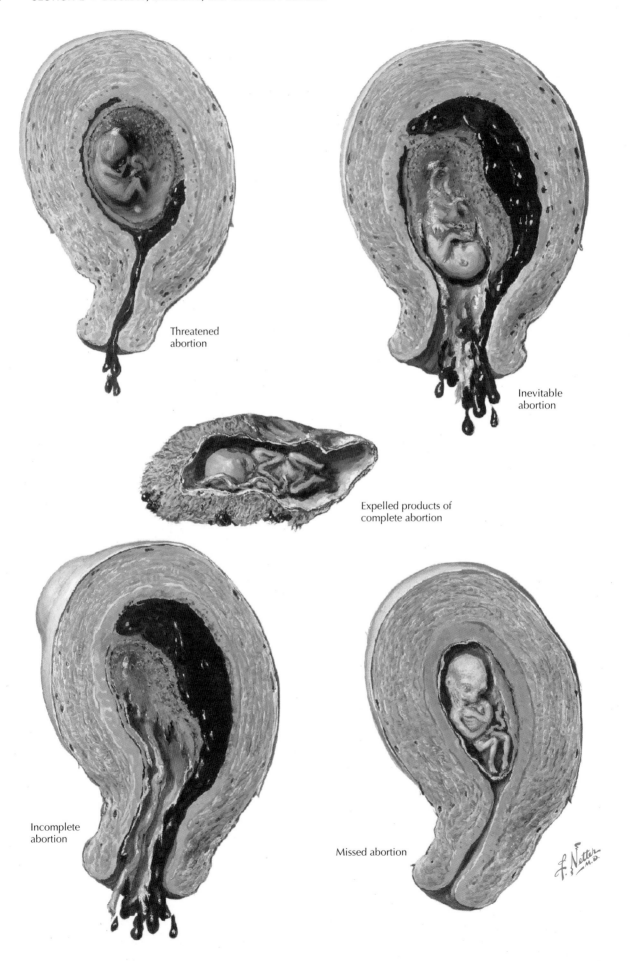

Threatened
abortion

Inevitable
abortion

Expelled products of
complete abortion

Incomplete
abortion

Missed abortion

of the uterus, the outcome should be good for patients with a septic abortion. Among patients with a threatened abortion, one half go on to lose the pregnancy in a spontaneous abortion. (The risk of failure is greater in those who bleed for 3 or more days.) For those who carry the fetus to viability there is a greater risk for preterm delivery and low fetal birth weight and a higher incidence of perinatal mortality. There does not, however, appear to be a higher incidence of congenital malformations in these newborns.

MISCELLANEOUS

Other Notes: When losses are caused by aneuploidy or polyploidy, they tend to happen earlier in gestation (75% before 8 weeks) and are more likely to recur in subsequent pregnancies. Abnormal development, including the zygote, embryo, fetus, or placenta, is common. Expulsion of the pregnancy is almost always preceded by the death of the embryo or fetus. For threatened abortion, intercourse is usually proscribed for 2 to 3 weeks, or longer, although this probably provides more psychological support than medical effect. Progesterone therapy for threatened abortions is of no benefit and may potentially result in virilization of a fetus or a missed abortion. It should not be used. Incomplete abortions are more common after the 10th week of gestation, when fetal and placental tissues tend to be passed separately.

ICD-9-CM Codes: 634.9 (Complete abortion), 637.9 (Incomplete abortion), 634.7 (Inevitable abortion), 632 (Missed abortion), 634.0, 635.0 (Septic abortion following legal termination of pregnancy), 636.0 (Septic abortion following illegal termination of pregnancy), 640.0 (Threatened abortion).

REFERENCES

Level II

Batzofin JH, Fielding WI, Friedman EA: Effect of vaginal bleeding in early pregnancy on outcome. Obstet Gynecol 1984;63:515.

Boklage CE: Survival probability of human conceptions from fertilization to term. Int J Fertil 1990;35:75.

Bromley B, Harlow BL, Laboda LA, Benacerraf BR: Small sac size in the first trimester: a predictor of poor fetal outcome. Radiology 1991;178:375.

Funderburk SJ, Guthrie D, Meldrum D: Outcome of pregnancies complicated by early vaginal bleeding. Br J Obstet Gynecol 1980; 87:100.

Hakim-Elahie E, Tovell HM, Burnhill MS: Complications of first-trimester abortions: a report of 170,000 cases. Obstet Gynecol 1990;76:129.

Johannisson E, Oberholzer M, Swahn ML, Bygdeman M: Vascular changes in the human endometrium following the administration of the progesterone antagonist RU 486. Contraception 1989: 39;103.

Mackenzie WE, Holmes DS, Newton JR: Spontaneous abortion rate in ultrasonographically viable pregnancies. Obstet Gynecol 1988; 71:81.

Schaff EA, Stadalius LS, Eisinger SH, Franks P: Vaginal misoprostol administered at home after mifepristone (RU486) for abortion. J Fam Pract 1997;44:353.

Swahn ML, Bygdeman M: The effect of the antiprogestin RU 486 on uterine contractility and sensitivity to prostaglandin and oxytocin. Br J Obstet Gynaecol 1988:95;126.

Thom DH, Nelson LM, Vaughan TL: Spontaneous abortion and subsequent adverse birth outcomes. Am J Obstet Gynecol 1992; 166:111.

Warburton D, Fraser FC: Spontaneous abortion risks in man: data from reproductive histories collected in a medical genetics unit. Am J Human Genet 1964;16:1.

Level III

American College of Obstetricians and Gynecologists: Medical management of abortion. ACOG Clinical management guidelines for obstetricians and gynecologists, Number 67. Washington, DC: ACOG; 2005.

Chen BA, Creinin MD. Contemporary management of early pregnancy failure. Clin Obstet Gynecol 2007;50:67.

Goldstein SR. Embryonic death in early pregnancy: a new look at the first trimester. Obstet Gynecol 1994;84:294.

Hogue CJR. Impact of abortion on subsequent fecundity. Clin Obstet Gynecol 1986;13:95.

Katz VL. Spontaneous and recurrent abortion, (CH16). In Katz VL, Lentz GM, Lobo RA, et al: Comprehensive Gynecology, 5th ed. Philadelphia, Mosby/Elsevier, 2007, p 359.

Kripke C. Expectant management vs. surgical treatment for miscarriage. Am Fam Physician 2006;74:1125.

Poland BJ, Miller JR, Jones DC, Trimble BK: Reproductive counseling in patients who have had a spontaneous abortion. Am J Obstet Gynecol 1977;127:685.

Smith RP. Gynecology in Primary Care. Baltimore, Williams & Wilkins, 1997, p 99.

Stubblefield PG, Grimes DA. Septic abortion. N Engl J Med 1994;331:310.

Tang OS, Ho PC. Clinical applications of mifepristone. Gynecol Endocrinol 2006;22:655.

INTRODUCTION

Description: Abuse is a pattern of physical trauma that occurs within a continuing relationship. Although the definition of abuse requires only one episode of physical abuse, a pattern of escalating violence is more typical. (In at least one fourth of cases, there have been three or more episodes of violence in the 6 months preceding the report of abuse.) In the United States, women are at greater risk of injury or death at the hands of a domestic partner than from an unrelated attacker. Sexual abuse is a specific form of physical abuse that relates to trauma of a sexual nature or a pattern of coercive sexual activities. Sexual abuse includes, but is not limited to, disrobing, exposure, photography or posing, oral–genital contact, insertion of foreign bodies, and vaginal or rectal intercourse.

Prevalence: More than 1.5 million cases of domestic violence occur each year. It is estimated that between 5% and 25% of women treated for injuries in emergency rooms receive these injuries as a result of domestic violence. Of adults, 20% to 40% report abuse or sexual victimization before age 18 years, and 10% to 25% of wives report one or more episodes of sexual abuse.

Predominant Age: Any, most common teens to 30s.

Genetics: Women are the primary victims of domestic violence, accounting for almost 95% of incidents.

ETIOLOGY AND PATHOGENESIS

Causes: Multiple factors. Alcohol or drugs are often involved, although they are not causative factors.

Risk Factors: Such abuse occurs at a slightly higher rate among those of lower educational or socioeconomic status.

CLINICAL CHARACTERISTICS

Signs and Symptoms

- Physical abuse—Signs and symptoms are highly variable. (In almost 85% of reported cases, the injuries sustained are sufficient to require medical treatment. Between 5% and 25% of women treated for injuries in emergency rooms receive these injuries as a result of domestic violence. The correct diagnosis is rendered in less than 5% of women. The most frequent locations for injuries are the head, neck, chest, abdomen, and breasts. Upper-extremity injuries result from defensive efforts.)
- Sexual abuse—Signs and symptoms are nonspecific.

DIAGNOSTIC APPROACH

Differential Diagnosis

- Depression (may mimic the vague complaints that should raise the suspicion of abuse)
- Coagulopathy (leading to bruising)

Associated Conditions: More than one half of men who abuse their wives abuse their children as well. Between one third and one half of all murders of women occur at the hands of a male partner.

Workup and Evaluation

Laboratory: No evaluation is indicated.

Imaging: No imaging is indicated unless fracture or other injury is suspected.

Special Tests: The five-question Abuse Assessment Screen increases the likelihood of detecting abuse. The longer it has been since an assault or when abuse is ongoing, the more likely it is for the presenting complaints to be unrelated to the underlying acute concerns generated by the attack. Somatic complaints and subtle behavioral changes may suggest the possibility of domestic violence or abuse.

Diagnostic Procedures: History and suspicion. Because one of the pivotal aspects of sexual assault is the loss of control, every effort should be made to allow the patient control over even the most trivial aspects of the physical examination.

Pathologic Findings

In the typical battering relationship three phases are usually present: a tension-building phase that gradually escalates; the battering incident, which may be triggered by almost any event; and a period of contrition during which the batterer apologizes and asks for forgiveness. This cycle tends to repeat and escalate with greater physical harm and risk and less remorse.

MANAGEMENT AND THERAPY

Nonpharmacologic

General Measures: Offer support, contact with social agencies, and assistance with developing means for independence (e.g., money, transportation, destination, child care) should escape become necessary.

Specific Measures: Assess and manage any injuries present. The patient should be given the telephone number of and directions to a shelter or safe house.

Diet: No specific dietary changes are indicated.

Activity: No restriction.

Patient Education: American College of Obstetricians and Gynecologists Patient Education Pamphlet AP083 (The Abused Woman).

Drug(s) of Choice

None indicated. Great care must be used with any antidepressants or other mood-altering drugs given in these situations.

FOLLOW-UP

Patient Monitoring: In many locations, suspected sexual assault must be reported to law enforcement authorities. In all locations, suspected abuse, sexual or otherwise, occurring to a minor must be reported.

Prevention/Avoidance: None. Patients must be told they are not at fault and that their efforts to change the abuser are unlikely to have an effect in reducing the number of future episodes.

Possible Complications: Escalating violence with an increasing risk of severe injury or death.

Sexual Abuse in Girls

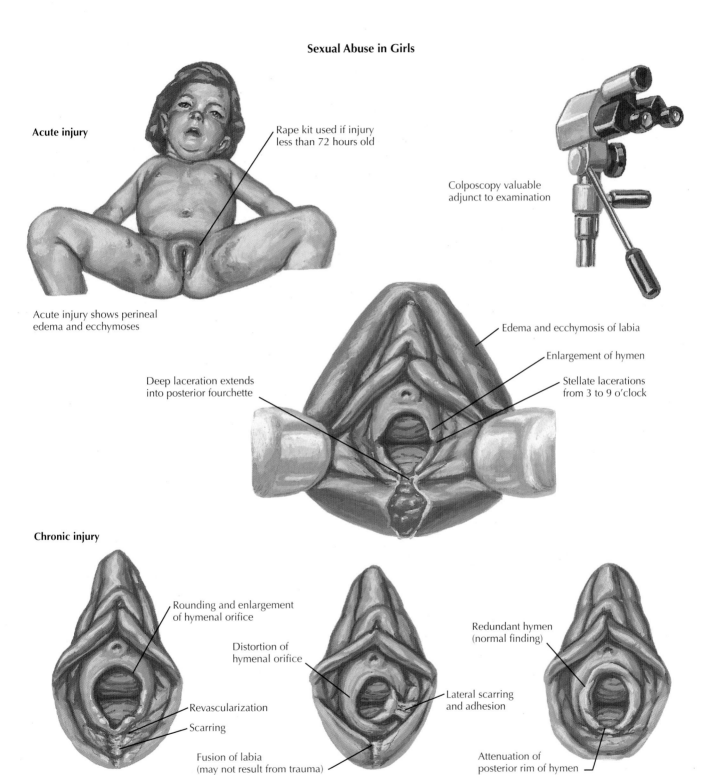

Acute injury

Rape kit used if injury less than 72 hours old

Colposcopy valuable adjunct to examination

Acute injury shows perineal edema and ecchymoses

Edema and ecchymosis of labia

Enlargement of hymen

Stellate lacerations from 3 to 9 o'clock

Deep laceration extends into posterior fourchette

Chronic injury

Rounding and enlargement of hymenal orifice

Distortion of hymenal orifice

Redundant hymen (normal finding)

Revascularization

Lateral scarring and adhesion

Scarring

Fusion of labia (may not result from trauma)

Attenuation of posterior rim of hymen

Abuse: Physical and Sexual

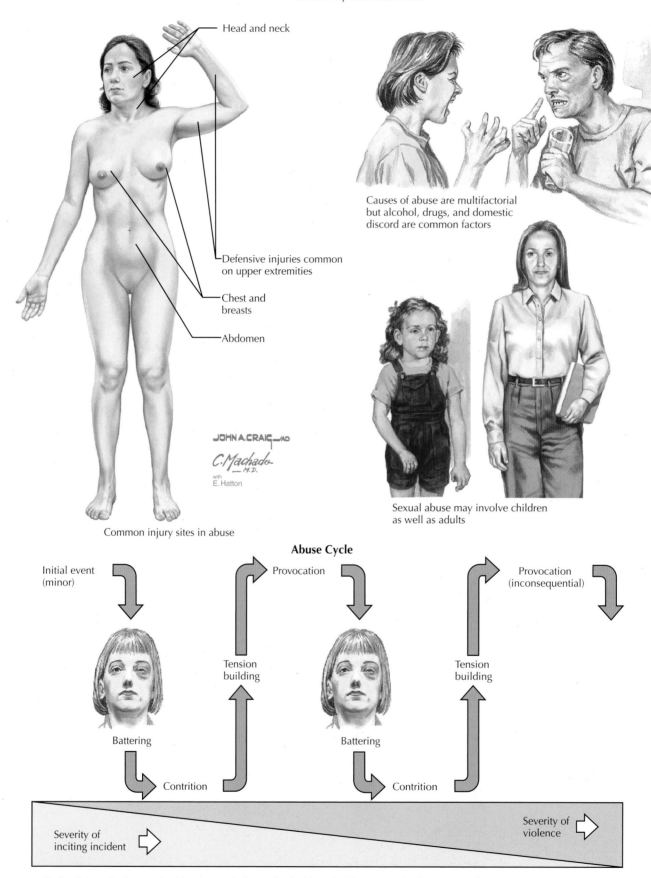

Head and neck

Defensive injuries common on upper extremities

Chest and breasts

Abdomen

JOHN A. CRAIG—MD

C. Machado—M.D.

with
E. Hatton

Common injury sites in abuse

Causes of abuse are multifactorial but alcohol, drugs, and domestic discord are common factors

Sexual abuse may involve children as well as adults

Abuse Cycle

Initial event (minor)

Provocation

Provocation (inconsequential)

Tension building

Tension building

Battering

Battering

Contrition

Contrition

Severity of inciting incident

Severity of violence

Cycle of abuse is characterized by progressively smaller incidents inciting progressively greater violence interspersed with periods of remorse.

Expected Outcome: The pattern of physical or sexual abuse is ongoing. Acute management of trauma is only a part of the larger problem and interpersonal dysfunction. If the abuser receives counseling and treatment, the outcome can be good; without it there is great risk of continued or worsening abuse. Abuse is associated with poorer general and sexual health for the victim. In one study, more than half of women who were abused had experienced common physical complaints during the previous 12 months compared with one third of the nonabused.

MISCELLANEOUS

Pregnancy Considerations: Of pregnant women, 10% to 20% report physical abuse during pregnancy. For these women, injuries to the breast and abdomen are more frequent.
ICD-9-CM Codes: 995.81, 995.85 (Multiple forms).

REFERENCES

Level II

Elliott L, Nerney M, Jones T, Friedmann PD: Barriers to screening for domestic violence. J Gen Intern Med 2002;17:112.

Leserman J: Sexual abuse history: prevalence, health effects, mediators, and psychological treatment. Psychosom Med 2005;67:906.

Rodriquez MA, Bauer HM, McLoughlin E, Grumbach K: Screening and intervention for intimate partner abuse: practices and attitudes of primary care physicians. JAMA 1999;282:468.

Ulla Pikarinen U, Saisto T, Schei B, et al: Experiences of physical and sexual abuse and their implications for current health. Obstet Gynecol 2007;109:1116.

Level III

AMA Council on Scientific Affairs: Violence against women: relevance for medical practitioners. JAMA 1992;267:3184.

American College of Obstetricians and Gynecologists: Health care for homeless women. ACOG Committee Opinion 312. Washington, DC, ACOG, 2005.

American College of Obstetricians and Gynecologists: Psychosocial risk factors: perinatal screening and intervention. ACOG Committee Opinion 343. Washington, DC, ACOG, 2006.

American Medical Association: Diagnostic and Treatment Guidelines on Domestic Violence. Chicago, American Medical Association, 1992.

Chez RA: Woman battering. Am J Obstet Gynecol 1988;158:1.

Chrisler JC, Ferguson S: Violence against women as a public health issue. Ann N Y Acad Sci 2006;1087:235.

Council on Scientific Affairs: Diagnosis and management of family violence. Chicago, American Medical Association, 2005. Available at http://www.ama-assn.org/ama/pub/category/15248. html Accessed May 11, 2007.

Gerber GL, Cherneski L: Sexual aggression toward women: reducing the prevalence. Ann N Y Acad Sci 2006;1087:35.

Hillard PJ: Physical abuse in pregnancy. Obstet Gynecol 1985; 66:185.

Lentz GM: Rape, incest, and domestic violence. In Katz VL, Lentz GM, Lobo RA, Gershenson DM: Comprehensive Gynecology, 5th ed. Philadelphia, Mosby/Elsevier, 2007, p 203.

U.S. Preventive Services Task Force: Screening for family and intimate partner violence: Recommendation statement. March 2004. Rockville, MD, Agency for Healthcare Research and Quality. Available at http://www.ahrq.gov/clinic/3rduspstf/famviolence/famviolrs.htm Accessed May 11, 2007.

Wathen CN, MacMillan HL: Prevention of violence against women: Recommendation statement from the Canadian Task Force on Preventive Health Care. CMAJ 2003;169:582.

INTRODUCTION

Description: Acne is an inflammatory disorder of the sebaceous glands that results in comedones, papules, inflammatory pustules, and scarring. The significance of acne for a woman often exceeds that dictated by medical considerations. It is often a reason to either choose or discontinue the use of oral contraceptives. Acne, or the fear of it, is a major factor in poor compliance with oral contraceptives.

Prevalence: Most adolescents, 15% seek care.

Predominant Age: Early teens to 20s, may persist into 40s.

Genetics: No genetic pattern. Women generally have milder forms of acne than men, although the social consequences are often greater.

ETIOLOGY AND PATHOGENESIS

Causes: Increased turnover of keratin in sebaceous glands under the influence of androgens. This results in a keratin plug (comedone) that obstructs sebum drainage from the gland. Infection by *Propionibacterium acnes* results in inflammation and pustule formation.

Risk Factors: Increased androgen of adolescence, oily cosmetics or moisturizers, virilizing conditions, medications (oral contraceptives, iodides, bromides, lithium, phenytoins, corticosteroids), and poor local hygiene.

CLINICAL CHARACTERISTICS

Signs and Symptoms

- Closed comedones (whiteheads)
- Open comedones (blackheads, black because of oxidation of sebum)
- Nodules and papules
- Pustules and cysts, with or without erythema and edema, may result in scarring
- Most lesions concentrated over the forehead, cheeks, nose, upper back, and chest

DIAGNOSTIC APPROACH

Differential Diagnosis

- Chemical exposure (grease, oils, tars)
- Folliculitis
- Steroid acne
- Virilizing tumors

Concerns about acne may serve as a surrogate for other issues including sexual development, menstruation, and contraception.

Associated Conditions: Social or emotional withdrawal.

Workup and Evaluation

Laboratory: No evaluation indicated.

Imaging: No imaging indicated.

Special Tests: None indicated.

Diagnostic Procedures: History and physical examination.

Pathologic Findings

Increased oiliness of the skin, increased skin thickness with hypertrophic sebaceous glands, perifolliculitis, and scarring.

MANAGEMENT AND THERAPY

Nonpharmacologic

General Measures: General hygiene, nail clipping (to reduce secondary trauma and infections), twice-a-day cleansing with a mild soap, oil-free sunscreens.

Specific Measures: Comedone extraction (with extractor), topical medical therapy. Light-based treatment modalities have also begun to show efficacy.

Diet: No specific dietary changes indicated. (None have been shown to be effective.)

Activity: No restriction.

Patient Education: General hygiene measures, need for long-term treatment. American College of Obstetricians and Gynecologists Patient Education Pamphlet AP014 (Growing Up [Especially for Teens]), AP112 (Birth Control [Especially for Teens]), AP021 (Birth Control Pills).

Drug(s) of Choice

Benzoyl peroxide 5% applied to skin every night

Tretinoin (retinoic acid) 0.025% cream applied to skin every night (applying 1/2 hour after washing reduces side effects)

Topical antibiotics—erythromycin, clindamycin (2%) in water base

Systemic antibiotics—tetracycline 250 mg PO four times daily for 7 to 10 days then tapering to lowest effective dose, erythromycin 250 mg PO four times daily for 7 to 10 days then tapering to lowest effective dose.

Oral contraceptives

Contraindications: Known or suspected allergy, hepatic dysfunction for oral agents, pregnancy (tetracycline and isotretinoin).

Precautions: Tetracycline may cause photosensitivity.

Interactions: Tetracycline should not be given with antacids, dairy products, or iron. Erythromycin should not be given with terfenadine (Seldane) and astemizole because it may cause cardiac abnormalities including arrhythmias and death. Broad-spectrum antibiotics may (theoretically) interfere with oral contraceptive efficacy.

Alternative Drugs

Tretinoin (retinoic acid) 0.025% gel applied on chest or back every night.

Isotretinoin (Accutane) 0.5 to 1 mg/kg/day in two doses for 12 to 16 weeks with a second course possible after an 8-week interval (associated with significant side effects including dry skin, dryness of the mucous membranes, and cheilitis).

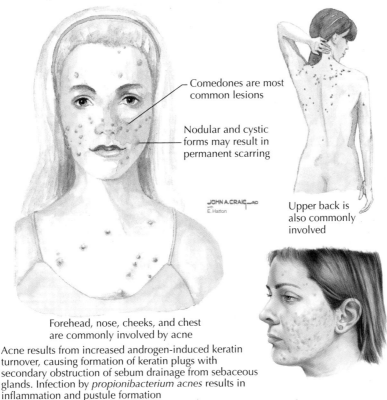

Comedones are most common lesions

Nodular and cystic forms may result in permanent scarring

Upper back is also commonly involved

JOHN A. CRAIG—AD
with
E. Hatton

Forehead, nose, cheeks, and chest are commonly involved by acne

Acne results from increased androgen-induced keratin turnover, causing formation of keratin plugs with secondary obstruction of sebum drainage from sebaceous glands. Infection by *propionibacterium acnes* results in inflammation and pustule formation

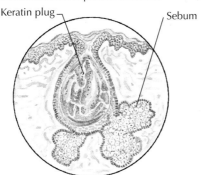

Keratin plug   Sebum

Section of closed comedone (whitehead) showing keratin plug and accumulated sebum in sebaceous glands

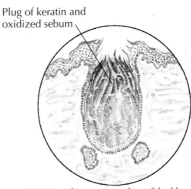

Plug of keratin and oxidized sebum

Section of open comedone (blackhead) showing plug of keratin and oxidized sebum

FOLLOW-UP

Patient Monitoring: Periodic follow-up (monthly) until control is obtained. For patients receiving isotretinoin, liver function, lipid concentrations, and the possibility of pregnancy should be monitored.

Prevention/Avoidance: None.

Possible Complications: Scarring, hypopigmentation or hyperpigmentation, keloidal scarring on the sternum or shoulders.

Expected Outcome: Gradual improvement over time and with therapy.

MISCELLANEOUS

Pregnancy Considerations: Pregnancy may cause a flare-up or remission of acne. Isotretinoin and erythromycin should not be used during pregnancy.

ICD-9-CM Codes: 706.1.

REFERENCES

Level I

Rafiei R, Yaghoobi R: Azithromycin versus tetracycline in the treatment of acne vulgaris. J Dermatol Treat 2006;17:217.

Level II

Santos MA, Belo VG, Santos G: Effectiveness of photodynamic therapy with topical 5-aminolevulinic acid and intense pulsed light versus intense pulsed light alone in the treatment of acne vulgaris: comparative study. Dermatol Surg 2005;31:910.

Level III

Arowojolu AO, Gallo MF, Lopez LM, et al: Combined oral contraceptive pills for treatment of acne. Cochrane Database Syst Rev 200724;CD004425.

Mariwalla K, Rohrer TE: Use of lasers and light-based therapies for treatment of acne vulgaris. Lasers Surg Med 2005;37:333.

Purdy S, de Berker D: Acne. BMJ 2006;333:949.

Strauss JS, Krowchuk DP, Leyden JJ, et al; American Academy of Dermatology/American Academy of Dermatology Association: Guidelines of care for acne vulgaris management. J Am Acad Dermatol 2007;56:651.

Williams C, Layton AM: Persistent acne in women: implications for the patient and for therapy. Am J Clin Dermatol 2006;7:281.

Alzheimer's Disease

INTRODUCTION

Description: Alzheimer's disease is a degenerative organic mental syndrome characterized by progressive intellectual deterioration and dementia—the most common form of dementia.

Prevalence: Five million cases annually, 40% of patients older than 85, seventh leading cause of death (2004).

Predominant Age: Older than age 65.

Genetics: 2-fold to 3-fold more common in women, increased familial risk (50% of patients). Markers have been found on chromosomes 1 and 14 for early onset and 12 and 19 for late onset.

ETIOLOGY AND PATHOGENESIS

Causes: Unknown. Proposed—slow virus, aluminum exposure, accelerated aging, autoimmune process, genetic alteration in amyloid production or metabolism.

Risk Factors: Aging, head trauma, Down syndrome, and family history.

CLINICAL CHARACTERISTICS

Signs and Symptoms

- Loss of mental function (calculation, abstraction, memory, aphasia)
- Social withdrawal (anhedonia, apathy, personality change, anxiety, depression)
- Delusions and confabulation
- Dementia
- Sleep disturbances and restlessness
- Behavioral change (aphasia, disorientation, disinhibition, violence or passivity)

DIAGNOSTIC APPROACH

Differential Diagnosis

- Dementia (vascular, infarct, Parkinson's disease)
- Multiple sclerosis
- Brain tumor (primary or metastatic)
- Alcohol or drug use/abuse
- Drug reaction
- Depression
- Hepatic or renal failure leading to toxicity
- Neurosyphilis
- Hypothyroidism

Associated Conditions: Down syndrome, depression, and insomnia.

Workup and Evaluation

Laboratory: Screening to rule out other causes as indicated.

Imaging: Computed tomography (CT) or magnetic resonance imaging (MRI) may show characteristic changes but are not required to make the diagnosis.

Special Tests: Spinal tap as indicated by the diagnoses being considered. Special paper and pencil tests are available to help with the assessment of cognitive function.

Diagnostic Procedures: History and clinical characteristics.

Pathologic Findings

β-Amyloid deposits in neuritic plaques and on arteriolar walls characterize the disease. Pyramidal cell loss, decreased cholinergic innervation, and neuritic senile plaques are also seen.

MANAGEMENT AND THERAPY

Nonpharmacologic

General Measures: Support, exercise to reduce restlessness and improve sleep, continued cognitive challenge, family support.

Specific Measures: Estrogen replacement is associated with a 50% reduction in risk and a delay in onset of symptoms in some studies, although more recent studies do not confirm these findings. For those with Alzheimer's changes, estrogen replacement near the time of menopause seems to improve function; late replacement (as in the Women's Health Initiative study) does not.

Diet: No specific dietary changes indicated.

Activity: No restriction except those imposed by ability.

Patient Education: Reassurance; extensive educational materials are available from support groups, Internet sites, and the Alzheimer's Association (Chicago).

Drug(s) of Choice

Studies on agents to enhance memory (donepezil [Aricept] 5 to 10 mg daily, galantamine [Razadyne] 4 to 8 mg two times daily, rivastigmine [Exelon] 1.5 to 4.5 mg two times daily) suggest some improvement for 30% to 50% of patients with severe disease. Drugs may be used to improve specific manifestations such as insomnia or depression. Several additional drugs (such as bapineuzumab and lecozotan) are currently in phase 3 trials, but no clearly effective therapy appears imminent.

Contraindications: Avoid anticholinergic drugs, such as tricyclic antidepressants and antihistamines.

Precautions: Tacrine (Cognex) may cause liver toxicity. Benzodiazepines may produce paradoxical excitation. Triazolam (Halcion) can produce memory loss, confusion, or psychotic reactions. Care must be taken in the use of all drugs in these patients; they tend to tolerate them poorly and confusion may lead to dosing errors.

Alternate Therapies: Ginkgo biloba has shown some promise in clinical studies.

FOLLOW-UP

Patient Monitoring: Watch for problems with nutrition, further mental deterioration, and drug use. Provide continuing and aggressive family support. Periodically evaluate the need for nursing home placement or other assistance.

Prevention/Avoidance: None. Some data suggest that remaining intellectually active (games or puzzles), physical activity, and social interaction may reduce the risk or delay the onset.

Testing for Defects of Higher Cortical Function

A. Appearance and interpersonal behavior

Pleasant, neatly
dressed,
good
spirits

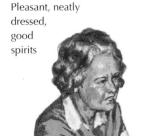

Depressed,
sloppily dressed,
careless

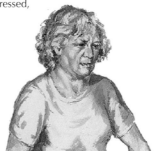

Belligerent

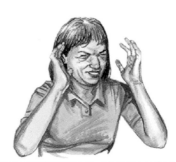

B. Language

Doctor: "Write me
a brief paragraph
about your work"

Good

Defective

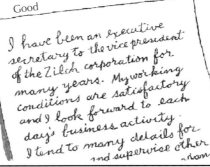

C. Memory

Doctor: "Here are three
objects: a pipe, a pen, and
a picture of Abraham Lincoln.
I want you to remember them,
and in 5 minutes I will ask
you what they were"

5 minutes later.
Patient: "I'm sorry,
I can't remember.
Did you show me
something?"

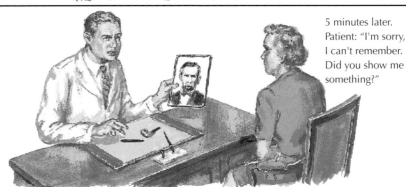

D. Constructional praxis and visual-spatial function

Doctor: "Draw me
a simple picture
of a house"

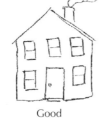

Good   Abnormal

"Draw a
clock face
for me"

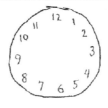

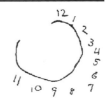

Good   Abnormal

E. Reverse counting

Doctor: "Count backward
from five to one for me"
Patient: "5...3...4...,
sorry, I can't do it"

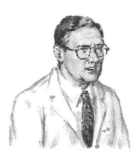

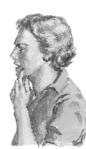

Doctor: "Spell the word "worlds"
backward for me"
Patient: "W..L..R..D..S"

Possible Complications: Progressive deterioration with metabolic changes, dehydration, drug overdose, falls, depression, and suicide.

Expected Outcome: Poor—progressive deterioration with 8- to 10-year average survival.

MISCELLANEOUS

ICD-9-CM Codes: 331.0, 290.0 (Senile dementia, uncomplicated), 290.10 (Presenile dementia, uncomplicated).

REFERENCES

Level III

Agency for Health and Research: Recognition and initial assessment of Alzheimer's disease and related dementias: Clinical Practice Guidelines 19. Rockville, Md, US Dept of Health and Human Services, 1996. AHCPR publication 97–0702.

Birks J, Grimley E, Van Dongen M: Ginkgo biloba for cognitive impairment and dementia. Cochrane Database Syst Rev 2002;4: CD003120.

Geldmacher DS, Whitehouse PJ: Evaluation of dementia. N Engl J Med 1996;335:330.

Hebert L, Scherr P, Bienias J, et al: Alzheimer disease in the US population: prevalence estimates using the 2000 census. Arch Neurol 2003;60:1119.

Lott I, Head E: Alzheimer disease and Down syndrome: factors in pathogenesis. Neurobiol Aging 2005;26:383.

Pendlebury W, Solomon PR: Alzheimer's disease. Ciba Clin Symp 1996;48:1.

Progress Report on Alzheimer's Disease 1996. Washington, DC, National Institute on Aging, US Dept of Health and Human Services, 1996. NIH publication 96–4137.

Wenk GL: Neuropathologic changes in Alzheimer's disease. J Clin Psychiatr 2003;64(Suppl 9):7.

Zamrini E: Emerging drug therapies for dementia. Geriatr Aging 2006;9:107,110.

INTRODUCTION

Description: Anemia is a reduction below normal in the oxygen-carrying capacity of the blood as reflected by the hemoglobin or hematocrit values. Women are at higher risk because of menstrual blood loss.
Prevalence: More than 20% of women, 50% to 60% of pregnant women.
Predominant Age: Reproductive most common for women.
Genetics: Hemoglobinopathies such as sickle cell disease, thalassemia, and others are associated with anemia.

ETIOLOGY AND PATHOGENESIS

Causes: Abnormalities of production (e.g., iron deficiency, chronic disease, chemotherapy, radiation). Abnormalities of destruction or loss (e.g., hemorrhage, hemolysis, sickle cell disease).
Risk Factors: Excessive blood loss (menorrhagia), poor diet, pica, malabsorption, chronic disease, endocrinopathy (thyroid). Smokers have slightly higher hemoglobin values (0.5 to 1.0 g/dL).

CLINICAL CHARACTERISTICS

Signs and Symptoms

* Asymptomatic
* Fatigue, palpitations, dyspnea, exhaustion (late signs)
* Ice craving, spooning or ridging of fingernails (iron-deficiency anemia)
* Sore mouth or dysphagia (B_{12} or iron-deficiency anemia)
* Joint and bone pain (sickle cell anemia)

DIAGNOSTIC APPROACH

* **Differential Diagnosis:** See illustration.
* **Associated Conditions:** Stomatitis, ridging and spooning of fingernails, hypersegmented polymorphonuclear neutrophils (megaloblastic anemia).

Workup and Evaluation

Laboratory: Mean corpuscular volume, reticulocyte count, blood smear, iron studies, hemoglobin electrophoresis; others based on individual patient—serum iron, total iron binding capacity, serum ferritin.
Imaging: No imaging indicated.
Special Tests: Bone marrow analysis (not necessary for the majority of patients).
Diagnostic Procedures: Laboratory evaluation.

Pathologic Findings

Based on underlying cause.

MANAGEMENT AND THERAPY

Nonpharmacologic

General Measures: Evaluation, diet counseling, control of menstrual abnormalities.
Specific Measures: Based on cause.
Diet: Adequate iron (7 to 12 mg/day) and folate (1 to 5 mg/day).
Activity: No restriction.
Patient Education: Diet counseling; American College of Obstetricians and Gynecologists Patient Education Pamphlet AP001 (Nutrition During Pregnancy).

Drug(s) of Choice

Iron supplements (ferrous sulfate 300 to 350 mg PO three times daily) for 6 to 12 months or longer. (Parenteral iron may be given to patients with severe anemia or to those who do not comply with oral therapy.)
For pernicious anemia—vitamin B_{12} 100 mg intramuscularly (IM) monthly. (Treatment of megaloblastic anemia resulting from B_{12} deficiency with folate will reverse anemia, but progressive and irreversible neurologic damage may result. B_{12} levels should always be checked if this is suspected.)
Precautions: Anaphylaxis may occur with parenteral iron.
Interactions: Ascorbic acid increases absorption of iron.

FOLLOW-UP

Patient Monitoring: Normal health maintenance, periodic evaluation of blood count.
Prevention/Avoidance: Good diet, control of excessive menstrual blood loss.
Possible Complications: Progressive and irreversible neurologic damage may result with untreated vitamin B_{12} deficiency.
Expected Outcome: Generally good response to iron therapy (iron-deficiency type).

MISCELLANEOUS

Pregnancy Considerations: Anemia more common in pregnancy.
ICD-9-CM Codes: 285.9 (others based on cause).

REFERENCES

Level III
Hillman RS, Rinder HM, Ault KA: Hematology in Clinical Practice. New York, McGraw-Hill, 2005.
De Gruchy GC: Clinical Hematology in Medical Practice. London, Blackwell Publishing, 1989.

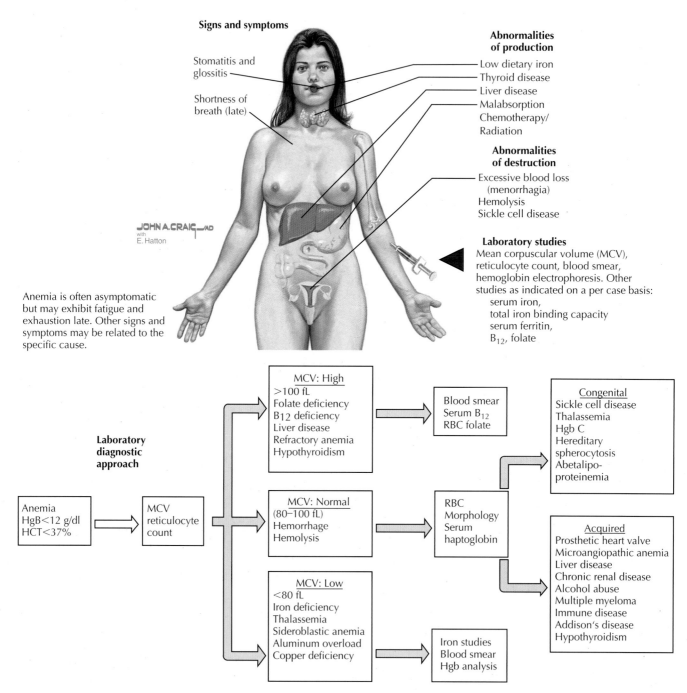

Signs and symptoms

Stomatitis and glossitis

Shortness of breath (late)

JOHN A.CRAIG—AD
with
E. Hatton

Anemia is often asymptomatic but may exhibit fatigue and exhaustion late. Other signs and symptoms may be related to the specific cause.

Abnormalities of production

Low dietary iron
Thyroid disease
Liver disease
Malabsorption
Chemotherapy/
Radiation

Abnormalities of destruction

Excessive blood loss
(menorrhagia)
Hemolysis
Sickle cell disease

Laboratory studies

Mean corpuscular volume (MCV), reticulocyte count, blood smear, hemoglobin electrophoresis. Other studies as indicated on a per case basis:
serum iron,
total iron binding capacity
serum ferritin,
B_{12}, folate

Laboratory diagnostic approach

Anemia
HgB<12 g/dl
HCT<37%

→ MCV reticulocyte count →

MCV: High
>100 fL
Folate deficiency
B_{12} deficiency
Liver disease
Refractory anemia
Hypothyroidism

→ Blood smear
Serum B_{12}
RBC folate

Congenital
Sickle cell disease
Thalassemia
Hgb C
Hereditary spherocytosis
Abetalipo-proteinemia

MCV: Normal
(80–100 fL)
Hemorrhage
Hemolysis

→ RBC Morphology
Serum haptoglobin

Acquired
Prosthetic heart valve
Microangiopathic anemia
Liver disease
Chronic renal disease
Alcohol abuse
Multiple myeloma
Immune disease
Addison's disease
Hypothyroidism

MCV: Low
<80 fL
Iron deficiency
Thalassemia
Sideroblastic anemia
Aluminum overload
Copper deficiency

→ Iron studies
Blood smear
Hgb analysis

HCT, hematocrit value; HgB hemoglobin; RBC, red blood cell.

Anorectal Fistula

INTRODUCTION

Description: An anorectal fistula involves communication between the anal or rectal canal and the perineum.
Prevalence: Common. For women, 5.6/100,000 population. The male-to-female ratio is 1.8:1.
Predominant Age: Any, average late 30s.
Genetics: No genetic pattern.

ETIOLOGY AND PATHOGENESIS

Causes: Anorectal fistulae may arise spontaneously or result from the drainage of a perirectal abscess. Patients with anal fistulae should be evaluated for the possibility of inflammatory bowel disease.
Risk Factors: Although Crohn's disease and tuberculosis are recognized risk factors, in most patients a predisposing cause is not apparent. Other risk factors include tears, puncture wounds, and internal hemorrhoids; less commonly carcinoma, radiation therapy, actinomycoses, tuberculosis, and chlamydial infections increase risk.

CLINICAL CHARACTERISTICS

Signs and Symptoms

- Intermittent perineal drainage or discharge
- Perianal lump or mass
- Pain (external sphincter) with defecation
- Anal bleeding
- Skin excoriation
- Most fistulae have involvement of the posterior midline and origin in the anorectal crypts

DIAGNOSTIC APPROACH

Differential Diagnosis

- Inflammatory bowel disease (Crohn's disease)
- Pilonidal sinus
- Perianal or other abscess
- Rectal carcinoma
- Acne inversa
- Bartholin gland abscess

Associated Conditions: Crohn's disease.

Workup and Evaluation

Laboratory: No evaluation indicated.
Imaging: If inflammatory bowel disease is suspected, lower gastrointestinal series. Fistulography (accuracy rate 16% to 48%) or magnetic resonance imaging (MRI; becoming the study of choice when evaluating complex fistulae; shown to reduce recurrence rates by identifying unknown extensions).
Special Tests: None indicated.
Diagnostic Procedures: History, physical examination, probe of fistulous tract. Anoscopy, proctoscopy, or sigmoidoscopy may be helpful.

Pathologic Findings

Inflammation and granulation change from chronic infection. Tract may be single or multiple. Internal opening is generally within an anal crypt.

MANAGEMENT AND THERAPY

Nonpharmacologic

General Measures: Evaluation, stool softening, and sitz baths.
Specific Measures: The only effective treatment is surgical, often carried out under general or spinal anesthesia in an ambulatory surgery unit. Fistulectomy or fistulotomy should not be performed in the presence of diarrhea or active inflammatory bowel disease.
Diet: High-fiber diet advisable.
Activity: No restriction.
Patient Education: Perianal care, sitz baths.

Drug(s) of Choice

Although the only effective treatment is surgery, the use of stool softeners is often beneficial.

FOLLOW-UP

Patient Monitoring: Close follow-up during postoperative period, routine health care thereafter.
Prevention/Avoidance: None.
Possible Complications: Constipation, rectovaginal fistula, recurrence.
Expected Outcome: Healing is generally good after surgical excision, although recurrence resulting from underlying disease is common.

MISCELLANEOUS

Other Notes: Goodsall-Salmon law states that fistulae with an external opening anterior to a plane passing transversely through the center of the anus will follow a straight radial course to the dentate line. Fistulae with their openings posterior to this line will follow a curved course to the posterior midline. Exceptions to this rule are external openings more than 3 cm from the anal verge, which almost always originate as a primary or secondary tract from the posterior midline, consistent with a previous horseshoe abscess.
Pregnancy Considerations: No effect on pregnancy, although may affect the choice of an episiotomy site.
ICD-9-CM Codes: 565.1.

REFERENCES

Level I
Pescatori M, Ayabaca SM, Cafaro D, et al: Marsupialization of fistulotomy and fistulectomy wounds improves healing and decreases bleeding: a randomized controlled trial. Colorectal Dis 2006;8:11.

Level II
Buchanan GN, Halligan S, Williams AB: Magnetic resonance imaging for primary fistula in ano. Br J Surg 2003;90:877.
Quah HM, Tang CL, Eu KW, et al: Meta-analysis of randomized clinical trials comparing drainage alone vs primary sphincter-cutting procedures for anorectal abscess-fistula. Int J Colorectal Dis 2006;21:602. Epub 2005 Nov 30.

Level III
Bassford T: Treatment of common anorectal disorders. Am Fam Physician 1992;45:1787.

Halligan S, Stoker J: Imaging of fistula in ano. Radiology 2006;239:18.

Hancock BD: ABC of colorectal diseases. Anal fissures and fistulas. BMJ 1992;304:904.

Jones J, Tremaine W: Evaluation of perianal fistulas in patients with Crohn's disease. Med Gen Med 2005;7:16.

Lentz GM: Anatomic defects of the abdominal wall and pelvic wall. In Katz VL, Lentz GM, Lobo RA, Gershenson DM: Comprehensive Gynecology, 5th ed. Philadelphia, Mosby/Elsevier, 2007: p 530.

Smith RP, Ling FW: Procedures in Women's Health Care. Baltimore, Williams & Wilkins, 1997: pp 153, 163, 175, 201.

Appearance and Management of Anorectal Crohn's Disease

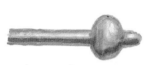

Mushroom catheter

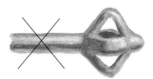

Malecot catheter (allows ingrowth of fibrous tissue, making removal difficult)

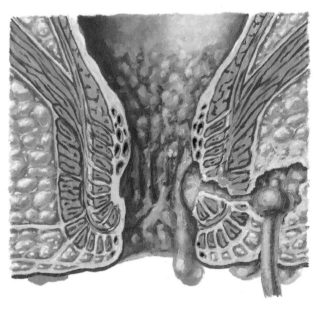

Abscess drained by placing small mushroom catheter as close to anus as possible to avoid subsequent long fistula tract

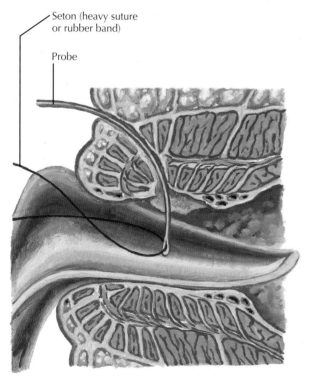

Seton (heavy suture or rubber band)

Probe

JOHN A. CRAIG—AD

Sepsis of fistula tract controlled by placing seton (avoids fistulotomy wounds, which heal poorly)

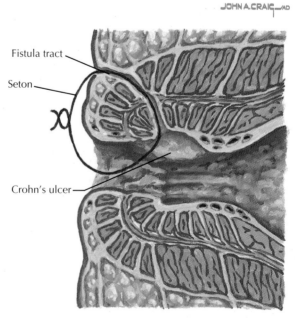

Fistula tract

Seton

Crohn's ulcer

Seton left in place between internal and external openings to prevent abscess formation and further destruction of sphincter mechanism

Types of anal fistulae

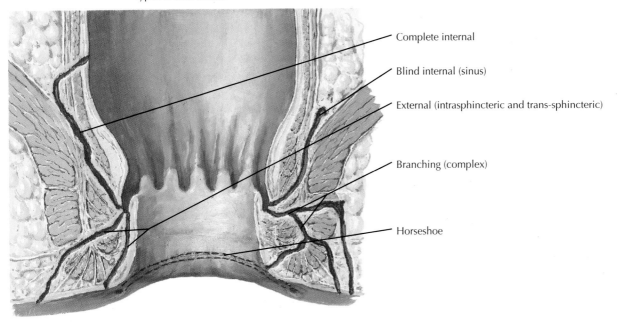

Complete internal

Blind internal (sinus)

External (intrasphincteric and trans-sphincteric)

Branching (complex)

Horseshoe

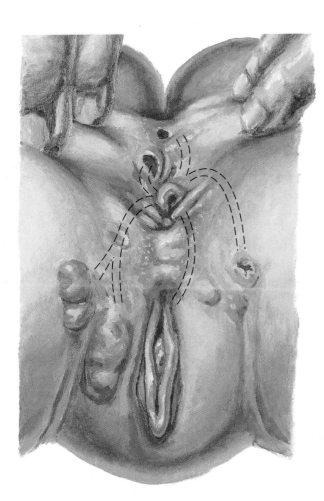

Unusually located (often multiple) anal
fistulae, abscesses, ulcers, and edematous
hemorrhoidal skin tags

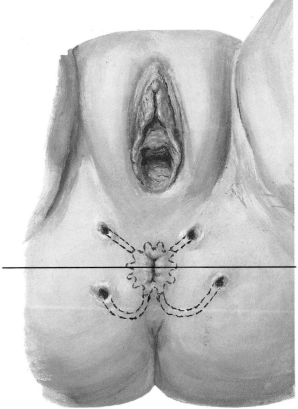

Goodsall-Salmon Law

Anxiety

INTRODUCTION

Description: Anxiety is a common acute or chronic emotion associated with physical symptoms, and it is two to three times more common in women. Subtypes include situational anxiety, adjustment disorders, panic disorders, phobias, and post-traumatic stress disorder. Obsessive-compulsive disorders are often classified in this group as well.

Prevalence: Eighteen percent of women, 40 million Americans.

Predominant Age: 20 to 45.

Genetics: Increased risk of panic disorders within monozygotic twins. Panic disorder, social phobia, and obsessive-compulsive disorders have a genetic base.

ETIOLOGY AND PATHOGENESIS

Causes: Psychosocial stressors, abnormality of the neurotransmitter system (serotonin, norepinephrine, γ-aminobutyric acid) involving the amygdala and hippocampus.

Risk Factors: Social, family or financial stress, medical illness, family history, and a lack of social support network.

CLINICAL CHARACTERISTICS

Signs and Symptoms (Vary with Subtype)

- Unrealistic or excessive worry
- Sense of impending doom
- Nervousness or instability
- Palpitations or tachycardia
- Hyperventilation or sense of suffocation
- Systemic systems (nausea, abdominal pain, paresthesias, diaphoresis, chest tightness, dizziness, muscle tension, headaches, and backaches)

DIAGNOSTIC APPROACH

Differential Diagnosis

- Cardiovascular (ischemic heart disease, valvular disease, cardiomyopathies, arrhythmias, mitral valve prolapse)
- Respiratory (asthma, emphysema, pulmonary embolism)
- Central nervous system (transient ischemia, psychomotor epilepsy, essential tremor)
- Metabolic (hyperthyroidism, adrenal insufficiency, pheochromocytoma, Cushing's syndrome, hypoglycemia, hypokalemia, hyperparathyroidism, myasthenia gravis)
- Nutritional (thiamine, pyridoxine, or folate deficiency)
- Medication/drugs (caffeinism, alcohol, cocaine, sympathomimetics, amphetamine)

Associated Conditions: Mitral valve prolapse, irritable bowel syndrome (IBS), depression, agoraphobia, substance abuse, and somatoform disorders.

Workup and Evaluation

Laboratory: No specific evaluation indicated. Tests should be based on the diagnoses being considered (e.g., thyroid function studies).

Imaging: No imaging indicated.

Special Tests: None indicated.

Diagnostic Procedures: History and psychological testing.

Pathologic Findings

None.

MANAGEMENT AND THERAPY

Nonpharmacologic

General Measures: Evaluation and assessment of cause and subtype, screening for substance abuse, counseling, establishing ties to support systems, beginning exercise program, and maintaining frequent follow-up.

Specific Measures: Psychotherapy (cognitive–behavioral therapy), medications.

Diet: No specific dietary changes indicated.

Activity: No restriction.

Patient Education: American College of Obstetricians and Gynecologists Patient Education Pamphlet AP068 (Alcohol and Women), AP083 (The Abused Woman).

Drug(s) of Choice

Acute anxiety or adjustment disorders—short-term benzodiazepines (alprazolam, 0.25 mg two to three times daily, increase in 0.25-mg increments if needed).

Generalized anxiety—azaperones (buspirone [BuSpar] 5 mg PO two to three times daily, increased every 2 to 3 days to a maximum of 60 mg/day).

Panic disorders and phobias—selective serotonin reuptake inhibitors (SSRIs; fluoxetine [Prozac] 4 mg PO, increased by 4 mg every 5 days to maximum of 40 mg, sertraline [Zoloft] 25 mg PO, increased by 25 mg every 5 days, paroxetine [Paxil]) 10 mg PO increased by 10 mg every 5 days).

Obsessive-compulsive disorders—selective serotonin reuptake inhibitors or clomipramine (Anafranil) 25 mg PO two times daily, increased to 250 mg/day.

Contraindications: Benzodiazepines are contraindicated in the first trimester of pregnancy, in patients with acute alcohol intoxication, and in patients with sleep apnea or open-angle glaucoma.

Precautions: Agents with short half-lives (e.g., alprazolam) have a high potential for dependency and withdrawal symptoms; acute withdrawal may precipitate panic attacks or seizures. Hepatic and renal function should be monitored in patients using benzodiazepines or buspirone. Breastfeeding should be discouraged in women taking chronic or high-dose benzodiazepines.

Interactions: Buspirone should not be used with monomine oxidase inhibitors (MAOIs).

Alternative Drugs

Panic disorders and phobias—imipramine (Tofranil) 10 to 25 mg PO every night, increased by 10 to 25 mg/day every 2 weeks to a maximum of 300 mg/day in adults and 100 mg/day in adolescents and elderly patients.

Anxiety

Five major types of anxiety disorders are:
·Generalized anxiety disorder
·Obsessive-compulsive disorder (OCD)
·Panic disorder
·Post-traumatic stress disorder (PTSD)
·Social phobia (or social anxiety disorder)

Clinical features

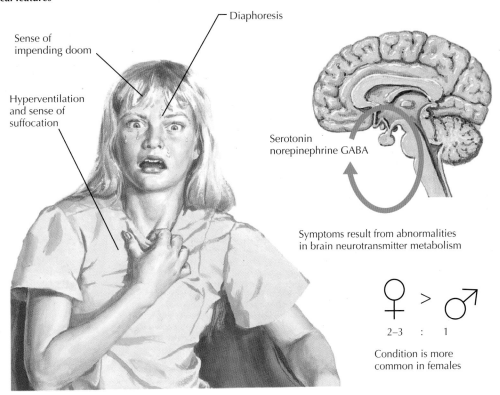

Diaphoresis

Sense of
impending doom

Hyperventilation
and sense of
suffocation

Serotonin
norepinephrine GABA

Symptoms result from abnormalities
in brain neurotransmitter metabolism

♀ > ♂

2–3 : 1

Condition is more
common in females

Anxiety may be acute or chronic and the scope of the condition includes situation
anxiety, panic disorders, phobias and adjustment, and post-traumatic disorders

Systemic somatic symptoms

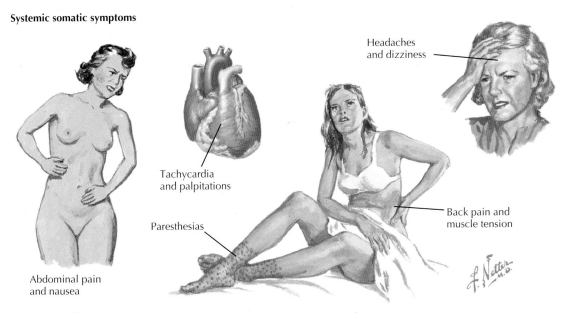

Headaches
and dizziness

Tachycardia
and palpitations

Paresthesias

Back pain and
muscle tension

Abdominal pain
and nausea

"Somatization" of anxiety results in symptoms in various systemic organ systems

FOLLOW-UP

Patient Monitoring: Frequent follow-up, identification and treatment of associated depression, periodic assessment of renal and hepatic function (based on medical therapy chosen).

Prevention/Avoidance: Stress management, relaxation training.

Possible Complications: Social withdrawal or isolation, drug dependence or side effects.

Expected Outcome: Generally good outcome. (Obsessive-compulsive disorders and post-traumatic stress disorders are more difficult to treat.)

MISCELLANEOUS

Pregnancy Considerations: Medical therapy must be adjusted based on risk and need.

ICD-9-CM Codes: 300.00 (others based on cause).

REFERENCES

Level II

Hirai M, Clum GA: A meta-analytic study of self-help interventions for anxiety problems. Behav Ther 2006;37:99. Epub 2006 Mar 24.

Spitzer R, Williams JBW, Kroenke K, et al: The PRIME-MD study: description, validation and clinical utility of a new procedure for diagnosing mental disorders in primary care. JAMA 1994; 272:1749.

Level III

Brookman RR, Sood AA: Disorders of mood and anxiety in adolescents. Adolesc Med Clin 2006;17:79.

McIntyre RS, Soczynska JK, Bottas A, et al: Anxiety disorders and bipolar disorder: a review. Bipolar Disord 2006;8:665.

Parry BL: Reproductive factors affecting the course of affective illness in women. Psychiatr Clin North Am 1989;12:207.

Ross LE, McLean LM: Anxiety disorders during pregnancy and the postpartum period: a systematic review. J Clin Psychiatry 2006;67:1285.

Roy-Byme PP: Integrated treatment of panic disorder. Am J Med 1992;suppl 1A:495.

Schneier FR: Clinical practice. Social anxiety disorder. N Engl J Med 2006;355:1029.

Tyrer P, Baldwin D: Generalised anxiety disorder. Lancet 2006;368:2156.

Asthma

INTRODUCTION

Description: Asthma is an intermittent or chronic obstructive tracheobronchial condition characterized by wheezing or cough. Adult-onset asthma is more common in women and poses potential problems during pregnancy.

Prevalence: Ten percent of the population.

Predominant Age: Adult ages 16 to 40 years (50% of patients are younger than age 10).

Genetics: Familial association with reactive airway disease, ectopic dermatitis, and allergic rhinitis.

ETIOLOGY AND PATHOGENESIS

Causes: Allergic factors (airborne pollens, molds, house dust, animal dander, feather pillows; a 2004 study showed that 71% had more than one allergy and 42% had more than three allergies), smoke or pollutants, viral upper-respiratory infections, aspirin or nonsteroidal anti-inflammatory agents, exercise, gastrointestinal reflux.

Risk Factors: Family history, viral pneumonitis in infancy.

CLINICAL CHARACTERISTICS

Signs and Symptoms

- Shortness of breath
- Wheezing and coughing (one or both)
- Prolonged exhalation
- Decreased breath sounds, hyperresonant chest
- Periodic (especially nocturnal) attacks
- Cyanosis and tachycardia
- Pulsus paradoxus, accessory muscle use for breathing, flattened diaphragm on chest radiograph or physical examination

DIAGNOSTIC APPROACH

Differential Diagnosis

- Recurrent pneumonia
- Chronic bronchitis
- Viral or fungal infection
- Aspiration (foreign body)
- Cystic fibrosis
- Tuberculosis
- Mitral valve prolapse
- Congestive heart failure
- Chronic obstructive pulmonary disease

Associated Conditions: Reflux esophagitis, sinusitis.

Workup and Evaluation

Laboratory: Complete blood count, arterial blood gases (severe cases).

Imaging: No imaging indicated. (Chest radiograph shows hyperinflation, atelectasis, or air leak, but it is nonspecific.)

Special Tests: Sweat chloride test (childhood), nasal eosinophils, pulmonary function testing (peak expiratory flow rate), allergy testing (selected patients).

Diagnostic Procedures: History, physical examination, pulmonary function testing (forced expiratory volume in 1 second, or FEV1). An excellent office screening test is to ask the patient to blow out a lit match held at arm's length. Patients with reduced FEV1 are unable to accomplish this task.

Pathologic Findings

Narrowing of large and small airways because of bronchial smooth muscle spasm, edema, and inflammation of the bronchial mucosa with increased mucus production characterize acute attacks. Chronic inflammatory changes are seen histologically. Biochemical factors related to inflammation mediators include chemical, eosinophil, and neutrophil chemotactic factors, bradykinins, and others.

MANAGEMENT AND THERAPY

Nonpharmacologic

General Measures: Evaluation, eliminate irritants, education, caffeine for mild symptoms.

Specific Measures: Mild—intermittent β-agonists via inhaler or cromolyn sodium four times daily plus low-dose inhaled steroids (beclomethasone dipropionate 400 mg/day) may add slow-release xanthines, leukotriene modifiers (montelukast, zafirlukast, pranlukast, and zileuton). Methylxanthines (theophylline and aminophylline), if sufficient control cannot be achieved with inhaled glucocorticoids and long-acting β-agonists alone. Severe—cromolyn sodium plus high-dose inhaled steroids plus theophylline (therapeutic level 10 to 20 mg/mL), inhaled β-agonist to reverse airflow obstruction. During asthma attacks patients should avoid fluid loading, intermittent positive pressure breathing, or airway mist or humidification; these worsen symptoms.

Diet: No specific dietary changes indicated. Avoid known allergens (if any).

Activity: No restriction or restriction based on pulmonary function except for those with exercise-induced asthma (e.g., cold weather, excessive activity).

Patient Education: Understanding of disease and use of inhalers, education about triggering factors and allergens.

Drug(s) of Choice

Cromoglycate and nedocromil
Steroids (beclomethasone, prednisone)
β-agonists (albuterol, bitolterol, salmeterol, terbutaline)
Methylxanthines (theophylline)
Anticholinergics (atropine, ipratropium bromide)
Leukotriene antagonists

Contraindications: Sedatives, mucolytics.

Precautions: β-agonists should only be used intermittently.

Interactions: Erythromycin and ciprofloxacin slow theophylline clearance and can increase levels by 15% to 20%.

Alternative Drugs

Histamine H_1-antagonists, methotrexate.

Postulated Mechanisms of Airway Hyperreactivity Causing Asthma

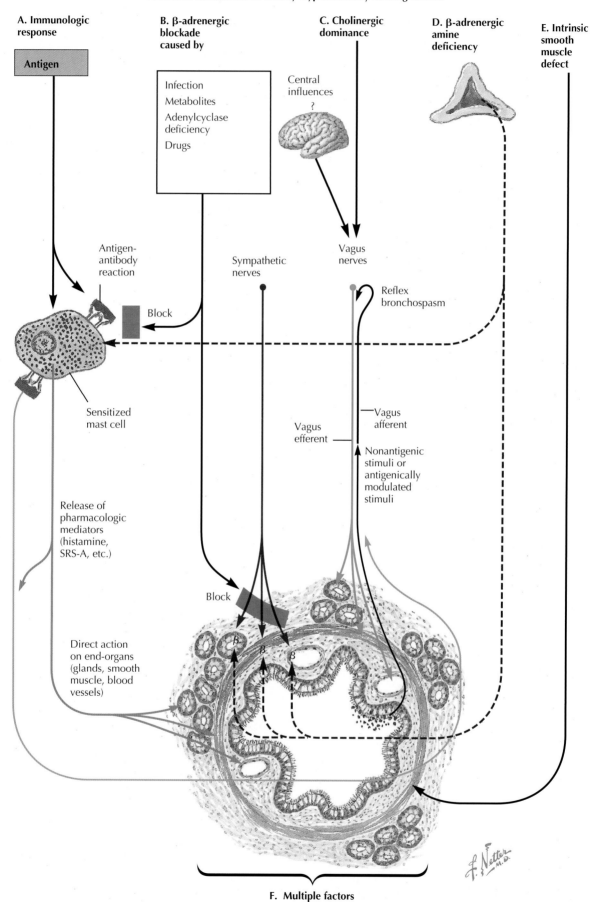

A. Immunologic response

Antigen

Antigen-antibody reaction

Block

Sensitized mast cell

Release of pharmacologic mediators (histamine, SRS-A, etc.)

Direct action on end-organs (glands, smooth muscle, blood vessels)

B. β-adrenergic blockade caused by

Infection
Metabolites
Adenylcyclase deficiency
Drugs

Sympathetic nerves

Block

β β β

C. Cholinergic dominance

Central influences
?

Vagus nerves

Vagus efferent

Vagus afferent

Reflex bronchospasm

Nonantigenic stimuli or antigenically modulated stimuli

D. β-adrenergic amine deficiency

E. Intrinsic smooth muscle defect

F. Multiple factors

FOLLOW-UP

Patient Monitoring: Normal health maintenance.

Prevention/Avoidance: Avoid known allergens, aspirin, nonsteroidal antiinflammatory and β-adrenergic blocking drugs. Have a prearranged action plan for acute attacks. Obtain annual influenza immunization. Avoid food additives known to precipitate attacks (sulfites and tartrazine).

Possible Complications: Respiratory failure, atelectasis, and pneumothorax; death. (Mortality increases with more than three emergency visits or more than two hospital admissions per year, nocturnal symptoms, history of intensive care unit admission or mechanical ventilation, steroid dependence, and history of syncope with attacks.)

Expected Outcome: Excellent with careful management.

MISCELLANEOUS

Other Notes: For those with exercise-induced asthma, activities in which the patient breathes large amounts of cold air (e.g., skiing or running) are more likely to provoke an attack, whereas swimming in an indoor, heated pool, with warm, humid air, is less likely to cause problems.

Pregnancy Considerations: Roughly 50% of patients have no change in symptoms, 25% improve, and 25% worsen. Asthma is found in 1% of pregnant patients, 15% of whom have one or more significant attacks during the gestation: the effects are highly variable but may include chronic hypoxia, intrauterine growth restriction, and (rarely) fetal death.

ICD-9-CM Codes: 493.9 (others based on type and cause).

REFERENCES

Level II
Vargas PA, Simpson PM, Gary Wheeler J, et al: Characteristics of children with asthma who are enrolled in a Head Start program. J Allergy Clin Immunol 2004;114:499.

Level III
Bank DE, Rug SE: New approaches to upper airway disease. Emerg Med Clin North Am 1995;13:473.

Barsky HE: Asthma and pregnancy: a challenge for everyone concerned. Postgrad Med 1991;89:125.

British Thoracic Society, Scottish Intercollegiate Guidelines Network (SIGN): British Guideline on the Management of Asthma. Guideline No. 63. Edinburgh, SIGN, 2004

Clark SL: Management of asthma during pregnancy. National Asthma Education Program Working Group in Asthma and Pregnancy. National Institutes of Health, National Heart, Lung and Blood Institute. Obstet Gynecol 1993;82:1036.

Greenberger PA: Asthma in pregnancy. Clin Chest Med 1992; 13:597.

Moore GJ: Asthma in pregnancy. Br J Obstet Gynecol 1994; 101:658.

National Asthma Education and Prevention Program: Expert Panel Report: Guidelines for the Diagnosis and Management of Asthma. Bethesda, Md, 1997. National Institutes of Health pub no 97–4051.

Nolan TE: Upper respiratory and pulmonary problems. Clin Obstet Gynecol 1995;38:147.

Pinnock H, Shah R: Asthma. Br Med J 2007;334:847.

Rodrigo GJ, Rodrigo C, Hall JB: Acute asthma in adults: a review. Chest 2004;125:1081.

Schatz M: Asthma during pregnancy: interrelationships and management. Ann Allergy 1992;68:23.

INTRODUCTION

Description: Cholelithiasis is the formation of stones in the gallbladder or biliary collecting system. Most stones (80%) are the result of precipitation of supersaturated cholesterol. Women are three times more likely than men to form gallstones.

Prevalence: Ten percent of the population, 1 million cases per year.

Predominant Age: Seventy percent of patients older than 40.

Genetics: Ratio of women to men is 3:1; some races at greater risk (e.g., Pima Indians). (Pigment gallstones affect men and women equally.)

ETIOLOGY AND PATHOGENESIS

Causes: The metabolic alteration leading to cholesterol stones is thought to be a disruption in the balance between hydroxymethylglutaryl coenzyme A (HMG-CoA) reductase and cholesterol 7α-hydroxylase. HMG-CoA controls cholesterol synthesis, whereas cholesterol 7α-hydroxylase controls the rate of bile acid formation. Patients who form cholesterol stones have elevated levels of HMG-CoA and depressed levels of cholesterol 7α-hydroxylase. This change in ratio increases the risk of precipitation of cholesterol as stones.

Risk Factors: Age, female gender, parity (75% of affected patients have had one or more pregnancies), obesity (15 to 20 pounds overweight 2-fold increase in risk, 50 to 75 pounds excess weight 6-fold increase in risk), estrogen use (oral), cirrhosis, diabetes, and Crohn's disease. A family history of cholelithiasis in siblings or children results in a 2-fold increase in risk.

CLINICAL CHARACTERISTICS

Signs and Symptoms

* Asymptomatic (60% to 70%; 50% become symptomatic, 20% develop complications)
* Fatty food intolerance
* Variable right upper quadrant pain with radiation to the back or scapula
* Nausea or vomiting (often mistaken for "indigestion")
* Fever usually associated with cholangitis

DIAGNOSTIC APPROACH

Differential Diagnosis

* Gastroenteritis
* Esophageal reflux
* Malabsorption
* Irritable bowel syndrome (IBS)
* Peptic ulcer disease
* Coronary artery disease
* Pneumonia
* Appendicitis

Associated Conditions: Cirrhosis, pancreatitis, and ileus.

Workup and Evaluation

Laboratory: Supportive, but often not diagnostic—complete blood count, serum bilirubin, amylase, alkaline phosphatase, and aminotransferase measurements.

Imaging: Ultrasonography of the gallbladder (96% accuracy for diagnosing sludge or a stone in the gallbladder).

Special Tests: None indicated.

Diagnostic Procedures: History, physical examination, ultrasonography, and laboratory investigation.

Pathologic Findings

Supersaturated bile, inflammation when accompanied by infection or obstruction.

MANAGEMENT AND THERAPY

Nonpharmacologic

General Measures: Watchful waiting and dietary modifications.

Specific Measures: Oral therapy, surgical extirpation, lithotripsy.

Diet: Reduced fatty food and cholesterol intake.

Activity: No restriction.

Patient Education: American College of Obstetricians and Gynecologists Patient Education Pamphlet AP064 (Weight Control: Eating Right and Keeping Fit).

Drug(s) of Choice

Ursodeoxycholic acid (Actigall) 8 to 10 mg/kg/day as two to three doses.

Contraindications: Known allergy, acute cholecystitis, abnormal liver function, calcified stones (not cholesterol based).

Precautions: The rate of stone dissolution (approximately 1 mm/mo) limits applicability for stones greater than 1.5 to 2 cm in size.

Interactions: None.

FOLLOW-UP

Patient Monitoring: Normal health maintenance

Prevention/Avoidance: Low-fat and low-cholesterol diet may delay symptoms. Oral prophylaxis during rapid weight loss has been advocated for those otherwise at risk.

Possible Complications: Acute cholecystitis, pancreatitis, ascending cholangitis, peritonitis, internal fistulization. Stones re-form in approximately 50% of patients treated with oral therapy, although the majority (85%) remain asymptomatic. Those who have recurrent symptoms respond to additional courses of oral therapy.

Expected Outcome: Generally good with either oral or surgical therapy. Oral therapy results in resolution of symptoms in 2 to 3 months. Despite this, gallstone disease is responsible for about 10,000 deaths per year in the United States.

Pathogenesis of gallstones

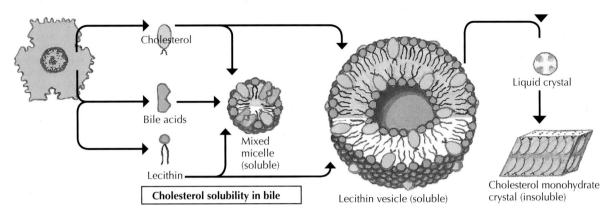

Cholesterol solubility in bile

Lecithin vesicle (soluble)

Cholesterol monohydrate crystal (insoluble)

Solubility of cholesterol in bile depends on incorporation of cholesterol in bile acid–lecithin micelles and lecithin vesicles. When bile becomes saturated with cholesterol, vesicles fuse to form liposomes, or liquid crystals, from which crystals of cholesterol monohydrate nucleate

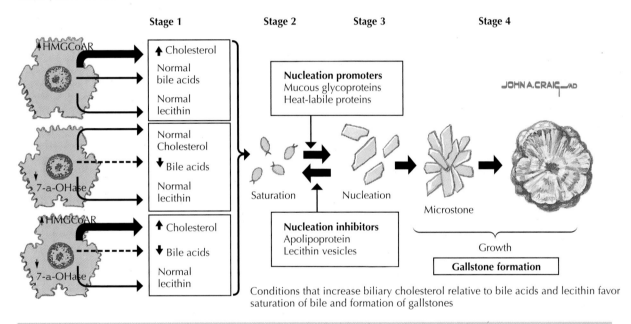

Conditions that increase biliary cholesterol relative to bile acids and lecithin favor saturation of bile and formation of gallstones

Predisposing factors

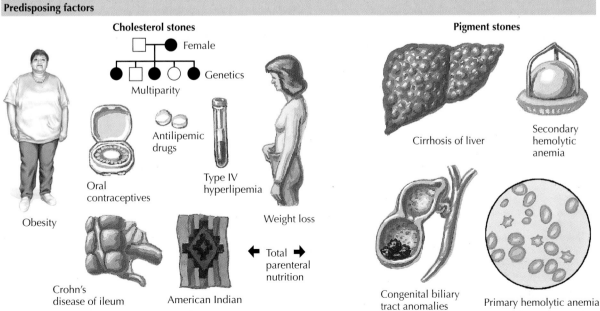

Cholesterol stones

Female
Genetics
Multiparity

Obesity

Oral contraceptives

Antilipemic drugs

Type IV hyperlipemia

Weight loss

Crohn's disease of ileum

American Indian

Total parenteral nutrition

Pigment stones

Cirrhosis of liver

Secondary hemolytic anemia

Congenital biliary tract anomalies

Primary hemolytic anemia

MISCELLANEOUS

Pregnancy Considerations: Of pregnant patients, 3% to 4% experience gallstone symptoms. Women with increased parity and multifetal pregnancies are at greatest risk.

ICD-9-CM Codes: 574.2 (others based on obstruction or inflammation).

REFERENCES

Level II

Ikard RW: Gallstones, cholecystitis and diabetes. Surg Gynecol Obstet 1990;171:528.

Maclure KM, Hayes KC, Colditz GA, et al: Dietary predictors of symptom-associated gallstones in middle-aged women. Am J Clin Nutr 1990;52:916.

Level III

Bennett GL, Balthazar EJ: Ultrasound and CT evaluation of emergent gallbladder pathology. Radiol Clin North Am 2003;41:1203.

Bhattacharya D, Ammori BJ: Contemporary minimally invasive approaches to the management of acute cholecystitis: a review and appraisal. Surg Laparosc Endosc Percutan Tech 2005;15:1.

Ko CW, Beresford SA, Schulte SJ: Incidence, natural history, and risk factors for biliary sludge and stones during pregnancy. Hepatology 2005;41:359.

Martin DJ, Vernon DR, Toouli J: Surgical versus endoscopic treatment of bile duct stones. Cochrane Database Syst Rev 2006;2:CD003327.

Ostrom NK: Women with asthma: a review of potential variables and preferred medical management. Ann Allergy Asthma Immunol 2006;96:655.

Portincasa P, Moschetta A, Palasciano G: Cholesterol gallstone disease. Lancet 2006;368:230–239.

Rees J: ABC of asthma. Prevalence. BMJ 2005;331:443.

Shaffer EA: Epidemiology and risk factors for gallstone disease: has the paradigm changed in the 21st century? Curr Gastroenterol Rep 2005;7:132.

Shaffer EA: Gallstone disease: epidemiology of gallbladder stone disease. Best Pract Res Clin Gastroenterol 2006;20:981.

Tazuma S: Gallstone disease: epidemiology, pathogenesis, and classification of biliary stones (common bile duct and intrahepatic). Best Pract Res Clin Gastroenterol 2006;20:1075.

van Erpecum KJ: Gallstone disease. Complications of bile-duct stones: acute cholangitis and pancreatitis. Best Pract Res Clin Gastroenterol 2006;20:1139.

Venneman NG, van Erpecum KJ: Gallstone disease: primary and secondary prevention. Best Pract Res Clin Gastroenterol 2006;20:1063.

Yusoff IF, Barkun JS, Barkun AN: Diagnosis and management of cholecystitis and cholangitis. Gastroenterol Clin North Am 2003;32:1145.

INTRODUCTION

Description: Constipation is the infrequent passage of hard stools, often associated with mechanical or other means to stimulate bowel movements. It often also is related to changes in the size, consistency, and ease of bowel movement in the subjective definition of constipation.

Prevalence: Very common as a sporadic problem, 8% to 10% of women.

Predominant Age: Any, more common in youth and old age.

Genetics: No genetic pattern.

ETIOLOGY AND PATHOGENESIS

Causes: Inadequate dietary fiber and fluid intake, altered gastrointestinal motility (drugs, illness, injury, laxative abuse), metabolic (hypothyroidism, diabetes), mechanical (obstruction, impaction).

Risk Factors: Poor diet and fluid intake, inactivity, medications (narcotics, iron therapy), and sedentary lifestyle.

CLINICAL CHARACTERISTICS

Signs and Symptoms

- Bowel movements fewer than three times per week
- Hard stools
- Straining to have a bowel movement
- Inability to have bowel movements without medical or mechanical interventions (enemas, manual evacuation)

DIAGNOSTIC APPROACH

Differential Diagnosis

- Hypothyroidism
- Rectocele
- Laxative abuse
- Dehydration
- Inappropriate expectation

Associated Conditions: Diverticulitis, abdominal pain.

Workup and Evaluation

Laboratory: No evaluation indicated.

Imaging: Radiography (abdominal plain film [kidneys, ureter, bladder], barium enema, defecography) may help to identify the source of the problem, but it is not required for diagnosis.

Special Tests: Rectal examination, flexible sigmoidoscopy, or colonoscopy should be considered for older patients.

Diagnostic Procedures: History and physical examination.

Pathologic Findings

None.

MANAGEMENT AND THERAPY

Nonpharmacologic

General Measures: Fluids, dietary fiber, fiber supplements, and physical activity.

Specific Measures: Mechanical assistance (enemas), mechanical disimpaction.

Diet: Increased dietary fiber and adequate fluids, fiber supplements as needed.

Activity: No restriction, activity encouraged.

Patient Education: Reassurance, diet counseling.

Drug(s) of Choice

Fiber supplements, stool softeners (docusate sodium 100 mg PO two times daily), laxatives (use with caution).

Contraindications: Bowel obstruction, peritonitis.

Precautions: Laxative abuse and dependence are common. Patients should be warned about their appropriate use.

FOLLOW-UP

Patient Monitoring: Normal health maintenance.

Prevention/Avoidance: Adequate fiber and fluid, physical activity.

Possible Complications: Impaction, fluid or electrolyte imbalance with laxative abuse, possible increase in the risk of colon cancer (proposed, but unproved).

Expected Outcome: Good with adequate diet, fluid, and activity.

MISCELLANEOUS

Pregnancy Considerations: No effect on pregnancy, although pregnancy (and associated iron supplementation) may make constipation worse.

ICD-9-CM Codes: 564.0, 306.4 (Psychogenic).

REFERENCES

Level III

Bleser SD: Chronic constipation: let symptom type and severity direct treatment. J Fam Pract 2006;55:587.

Frizelle F, Barclay M: Constipation in adults. Clin Evid 2005;14:557.

Johnson DA: Treating chronic constipation: how should we interpret the recommendations? Clin Drug Investig 2006;26:547.

Lacy BE, Weiser K: Gastrointestinal motility disorders: an update. Dig Dis 2006;24:228.

Leung FW: Etiologic factors of chronic constipation: review of the scientific evidence. Dig Dis Sci 2007;52:313. Epub 2007 Jan 12.

Longstreth GF, Thompson WG, Chey WD, et al: Functional bowel disorders. Gastroenterology 2006;130:1480.

Rapkin AJ, Mayer EA: Gastroenterologic causes of chronic pelvic pain. Obstet Gynecol Clin North Am 1993;20:663.

Thoua N, Emmanuel A: Treating functional lower gastrointestinal symptoms. Clin Med 2006;6:449.

Wald A: Constipation in the primary care setting: current concepts and misconceptions. Am J Med 2006;119:736.

Wald A: Chronic constipation: advances in management. Neurogastroenterol Motil 2007;19:4.

Functional

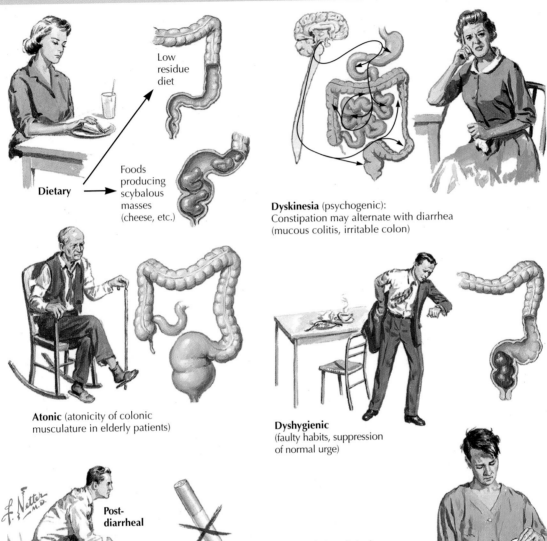

Dietary → Foods producing scybalous masses (cheese, etc.)

Low residue diet

Dyskinesia (psychogenic): Constipation may alternate with diarrhea (mucous colitis, irritable colon)

Atonic (atonicity of colonic musculature in elderly patients)

Dyshygienic (faulty habits, suppression of normal urge)

Post-diarrheal

Post-Smoking (lack of habitual reflex on cessation of smoking)

Iatrogenic (medicinal)

Hardening agents { Barium
Aluminum hydroxide
Calcium carbonate

Inspissating agents (mucilages)
Inhibitory agents (opium, anticholinergics)

Organic

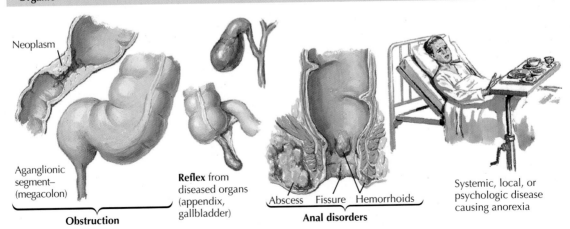

Neoplasm

Aganglionic segment– (megacolon)

Obstruction

Reflex from diseased organs (appendix, gallbladder)

Abscess   Fissure   Hemorrhoids

Anal disorders

Systemic, local, or psychologic disease causing anorexia

INTRODUCTION

Description: An idiopathic inflammatory bowel disease characterized by transmural involvement resulting in severe gastrointestinal symptoms and significant morbidity.
Prevalence: Two to 10 of 10,000.
Predominant Age: 15 to 30.
Genetics: First-degree relative for 20% of patients, more common in whites and Jews.

ETIOLOGY AND PATHOGENESIS

Causes: The inflammatory process in Crohn's disease is transmural and involves both the large and small bowel in 50% of patients.
Risk Factors: Cigarette smoking (postulated but unproved).

CLINICAL CHARACTERISTICS
Signs and Symptoms

- Abdominal pain (80% to 85%, often lasting for days or weeks; the pain described is frequently located in the mid-abdomen or right lower quadrant, although generalized pain is often present)
- Diarrhea (voluminous, watery, with occasional blood [20%])
- Fever
- Dyspareunia
- Vulvar or perineal fissures or fistulae or occasionally vulvar granulomas
- Arthritis, sclerosing cholangitis (5% to 10%)

DIAGNOSTIC APPROACH
Differential Diagnosis

- Irritable bowel syndrome (IBS)
- Ulcerative colitis
- Enteric pathogens
- Lymphoma
- Pelvic inflammatory disease (PID; acute episodes)
- Endometriosis

Associated Conditions: Arthritis, dyspareunia, vulvar or perineal fissures or fistulae, vulvar granulomas, erythema nodosum, and sclerosing cholangitis.

Workup and Evaluation

Laboratory: Complete blood count, sedimentation rate.
Imaging: Barium enema, upper gastrointestinal radiograph with small bowel follow-through.
Special Tests: Sigmoidoscopy, colonoscopy, or rectal biopsy.
Diagnostic Procedures: History, sigmoidoscopy, or colonoscopy; radiologic studies; or rectal biopsy.

Pathologic Findings

Transmural inflammation with ulceration and distortion. Areas of normal bowel (skip areas). Granulomas may be found in 15% of patients.

MANAGEMENT AND THERAPY
Nonpharmacologic

General Measures: Maintenance of weight and nutrition, perineal care.
Specific Measures: Surgical therapy (resection) often required (two thirds to three fourths of patients).
Diet: No specific dietary changes indicated; increased dietary fiber sometimes recommended.
Activity: No restriction.

Drug(s) of Choice

Mesalamine (5-aminosalicylic acid), methotrexate, or azathioprine (Imuran) for maintenance and suppression.
Prednisone (20 to 40 mg PO daily, tapered after 4 to 6 weeks) or sulfasalazine or mesalamine at increased doses for acute exacerbations. Other immunosuppressives (6-mercaptopurine, azathioprine, infliximab [Remicade]) may also be used.
For acute management, antibiotics, antidiarrheals and fluid replacements may be needed.
Precautions: Folic acid supplements should be used with mesalamine.

FOLLOW-UP

Patient Monitoring: Weight and symptoms, periodic blood count, and sedimentation rate. Endoscopy to monitor disease (as needed).
Prevention/Avoidance: None.
Possible Complications: Bowel thickening, stenosis, and internal fistula formation are common. Short bowel syndromes and malabsorption are common after repeated surgery. One study found a 2.5-fold increase in the risk of colon cancer in patients with Crohn's disease.
Expected Outcome: Need for eventual or repeated surgery very likely.

MISCELLANEOUS

Pregnancy Considerations: No effect on pregnancy.
ICD-9-CM Codes: 555.9.

REFERENCES

Level II
Ekbom A, Helmick C, Zack M: Increased risk of large-bowel cancer in Crohn's disease with colonic involvement. Lancet 1990; 336:357.

Level III
Hanauer SB, Sandborn W; Practice Parameters Committee of the American College of Gastroenterology: Management of Crohn's disease in adults. Am J Gastroenterol 2001;96:635.
Kornbluth A, Sachar DB; Practice Parameters Committee of the American College of Gastroenterology: Ulcerative colitis practice guidelines in adults (update): American College of Gastroenterology, Practice Parameters Committee. Am J Gastroenterol 2004;99:1371.
Podolsky DK: Inflammatory bowel disease. N Engl J Med 2002; 347:417.

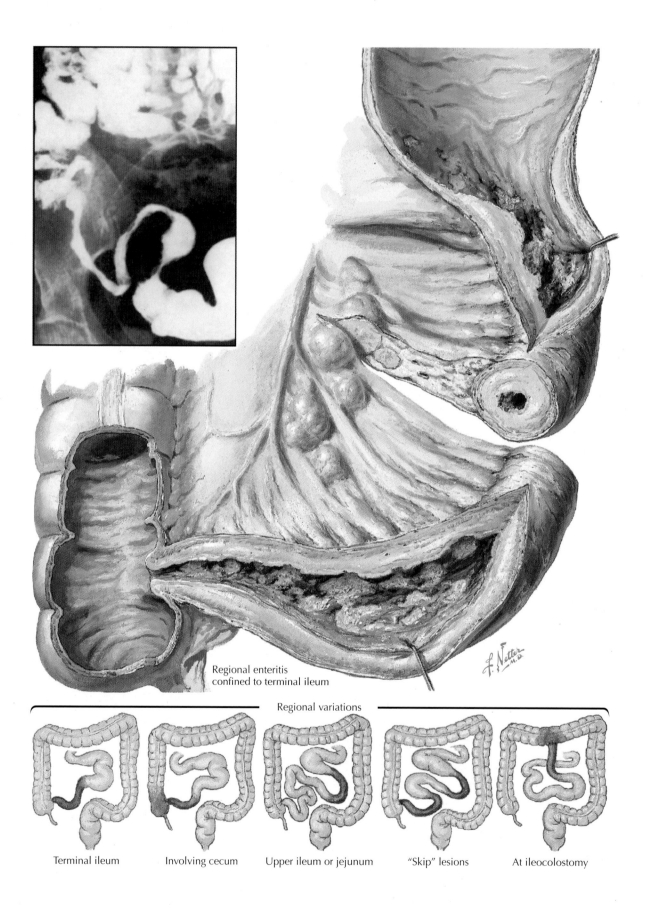

Regional enteritis
confined to terminal ileum

Regional variations

Terminal ileum   Involving cecum   Upper ileum or jejunum   "Skip" lesions   At ileocolostomy

INTRODUCTION

Description: Depression is a biochemically mediated state in which anger, frustration, loss of pleasure, and withdrawal predominate. This must be separated from normal stress reactions and grief.

Prevalence: Twenty million American adults per year, one in six to eight lifetime risk, 6% to 14% of primary care visits, 2:1 female to male ratio (1:1 after age 55). Depression is the fourth most common reason to seek medical care.

Predominant Age: Rare before puberty, commonly begins in 20s to 30s, average 40.

Genetics: Possible defect on chromosome 11 or X.

ETIOLOGY AND PATHOGENESIS

Causes: Proposed—alteration in norepinephrine or serotonin through impaired synthesis of neurotransmitters, increased breakdown or metabolism of neurotransmitters, increased uptake of neurotransmitters.

Risk Factors: Strong family history (depression, suicide, alcoholism, substance abuse). Women are at greatest risk during adolescence (up to 60% meet criteria), the premenstrual period, pregnancy, the postpartum period, perimenopause, after pregnancy loss (three times risk) and with infertility (two times risk). Women are especially vulnerable to depression after giving birth.

CLINICAL CHARACTERISTICS

Signs and Symptoms

- Depressed mood or anhedonia plus five or more other symptoms over a 2-week period:
  - Weight loss
  - Sleep changes
  - Psychomotor changes
  - Fatigue
  - Feeling of worthlessness or guilt
  - Inability to concentrate
  - Thoughts of death

  (Hallucinations and delusions may appear in profound cases.)

DIAGNOSTIC APPROACH

Differential Diagnosis

- Endocrine disorders (diabetes, pituitary, adrenal, thyroid)
- Malignancies
- Infections
- Neurologic disorders (organic brain disease)
- Autoimmune disease
- Cardiovascular, hepatic, or renal disease
- Vitamin or mineral deficiency or excess
- Medication side effect (cardiovascular drugs, hormones, anticancer agents, anti-inflammatory or anti-infective agents, amphetamines [withdrawal], L-dopa, cimetidine, ranitidine)

Associated Conditions: Chronic pain, sexual dysfunction, weight changes (up or down), bipolar disorders (manic depression), schizophrenia, and substance abuse.

Workup and Evaluation

Laboratory: No evaluation indicated (clinical diagnosis only).

Imaging: No imaging indicated unless organic brain syndrome is being considered.

Special Tests: Zung's Self-Rating Depression Scale, Beck's Depression Inventory, Criteria for Epidemiologic Studies Depression Scale, Children's Depression Inventory, or similar tests.

Diagnostic Procedures: Complete evaluation to rule out organic cause. Depression scales are helpful but are not required.

Pathologic Findings

None.

MANAGEMENT AND THERAPY

Nonpharmacologic

General Measures: Evaluation, support, and evaluation of support systems available to the patient.

Specific Measures: Psychotherapy (patients with mild depression without psychosis), medical therapy (choose agent to optimize benefit, decrease risk, and avoid drug interactions), electroshock therapy in patients with refractory conditions (controversial).

Diet: No specific dietary changes indicated.

Activity: No restriction.

Patient Education: Reassurance, careful instruction on medication use; American College of Obstetricians and Gynecologists Patient Education Pamphlet AP057 (Premenstrual Syndrome), AP091 (Postpartum Depression), AP106 (Depression).

Drug(s) of Choice

Tricyclic agents—amitriptyline (50 to 300 mg/day), doxepin (75 to 300 mg/day), imipramine (50 to 300 mg/day), nortriptyline (50 to 200 mg/day).

Monoamine oxidase inhibitors (MAOIs).

Selective serotonin reuptake inhibitors (SSRIs)—fluoxetine (10 to 80 mg/day), fluvoxamine (100 to 300 mg/day), paroxetine (10 to 50 mg/day), sertraline (50 to 200 mg/day).

Serotonin norepinephrine reuptake inhibitors (SNRIs)—venlafaxine (75 to 375 mg/day).

Noradrenergic and specific serotonergic agents—mirtazapine (15 to 45 mg/day).

Miscellaneous agents—nefazodone (200 to 600 mg/day), trazodone (150 to 400 mg/day), bupropion (300 to 400 mg/day).

Contraindications: See individual agents. Most agents are pregnancy category B. Many are contraindicated in patients with seizure disorders or cardiac arrhythmias (tricyclic agents).

Depression (Unipolar)

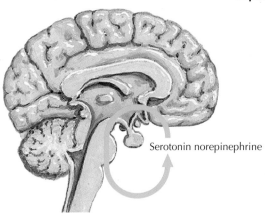

Serotonin norepinephrine

Depression is a biochemically mediated state most likely based on abnormalities in metabolism of serotonin and norepinephrine

♀ > ♂
2 : 1

Female gender predominates

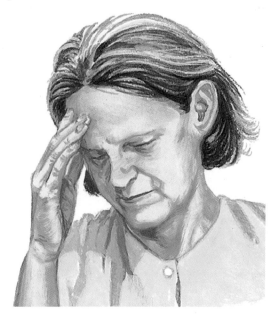

Clinical syndrome characterized by withdrawal, anger, frustration, and loss of pleasure

Associated symptoms and comorbidities

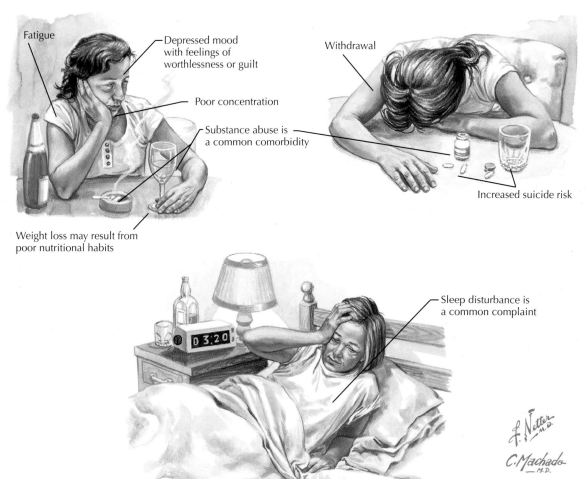

Fatigue

Depressed mood with feelings of worthlessness or guilt

Poor concentration

Substance abuse is a common comorbidity

Weight loss may result from poor nutritional habits

Withdrawal

Increased suicide risk

Sleep disturbance is a common complaint

Precautions: Monoamine oxidase inhibitors are associated with both treatment and adverse reactions that appear as emergencies. Overdoses may be lethal. Selective serotonin reuptake inhibitors are associated with nausea (20% to 35%) and sexual dysfunction (10% to 30%). Some agents can alter the dose or effectiveness of other drugs such as antihypertensive agents, digoxin, and antiseizure medications. Fluoxetine, sertraline, and paroxetine are best given in the morning. In September 2004 the U.S. Food and Drug Administration began considering a warning that some antidepressants may increase the risk of suicidal tendencies in children.

Interactions: Monoamine oxidase inhibitors and selective serotonin reuptake inhibitors or serotonin norepinephrine reuptake inhibitors may have lethal interactions and must not be used together. (Allow at least 2 weeks to elapse between therapies.) Avoid use of nonprescription drugs with pseudoephedrine, phenylephrine, or phenylpropanolamine.

Alternative Drugs

Additional tricyclic agents include clomipramine (100 to 250 mg/day), desipramine (50 to 300 mg/day), protriptyline (14 to 60 mg/day), and trimipramine (75 to 300 mg/day).

A large study conducted by the National Center for Complementary and Alternative Medicine has found that St. John's wort is not effective for treating major depression.

FOLLOW-UP

Patient Monitoring: Normal health maintenance. Monitor for recurrence, substance abuse, or suicide. Patients must be monitored every 1 to 2 weeks after they start medication and reassessed at 6 weeks. Follow-up of treatment should continue every 3 months while therapy is maintained (6 months to 2 years).

Prevention/Avoidance: None.

Possible Complications: Increased risk of general medical disorders and worsened prognosis, disability, impaired function (family, work, social, sexual), chronic pain, mortality (30,000 suicides per year in United States; adolescent girls at greatest risk).

Expected Outcome: Medical therapy is associated with 85% to 90% success rates.

MISCELLANEOUS

Pregnancy Considerations: Up to 70% of patients have depressive symptoms and 10% to 15% meet the diagnostic criteria during pregnancy. Symptoms often mimic those of pregnancy itself. Depression may result in poor nutrition, increased substance abuse, and poor fetal outcome. Drug therapy should be avoided or used sparingly in pregnancy. Postpartum depression is seen by many as a special form of depression.

ICD-9-CM Codes: 311 (Depressive disorder, not elsewhere classified), 296.2 (Major depressive disorder, single episode), 296.3 (Recurrent), 625.4 (Premenstrual syndrome).

REFERENCES

Level II

Fava GA, Ruini C, Belaise C: The concept of recovery in major depression. Psychol Med 2007;37:307.

Geddes J, Butler R, Hatcher S, et al: Depression in adults. Clin Evid 2006;15:1366.

Thachil AF, Mohan R, Bhugra D: The evidence base of complementary and alternative therapies in depression. J Affect Disord 2007;97:23. Epub 2006 Aug 22.

Level III

American College of Obstetricians and Gynecologists: Treatment with selective serotonin reuptake inhibitors during pregnancy. ACOG Committee Opinion 354. Washington, DC, ACOG, 2006.

Association of Professors of Gynecology and Obstetrics: Depressive disorders in women: diagnosis, treatment, and monitoring. Washington, DC, APGO, 1997.

Beck A: Depression Inventory. Philadelphia, Center for Cognitive Therapy, 1991.

Fancher T, Kravitz R: In the clinic. Depression. Ann Intern Med 2007;146:ITC5–1.

Klein DF, Wender PH: Understanding depression: a complete guide to its diagnosis and treatment. New York, Oxford University Press, 1993.

Maurer D, Colt R: An evidence-based approach to the management of depression. Prim Care 2006;33:923, vii.

McGrath E, Ketia GP, Strickland BR, Russo NF: Women and depression: risk factors and treatment issues. Washington, DC, American Psychological Association, 1990.

Norman TR, Burrows GD: Emerging treatments for major depression. Expert Rev Neurother 2007;7:203.

INTRODUCTION

Description: Diverticular disease involves herniation of the colon mucosa through the muscular wall. These herniations are most common in the sigmoid and distal colon, increase in prevalence with age, and can lead to significant morbidity when rupture or abscess formation occurs. Diverticulosis is the presence of these herniations, whereas diverticulitis is the symptomatic state.

Prevalence: Twenty percent of patients, increasing with age to 40% to 50% by age 60 to 80.

Predominant Age: Rare younger than age 40, most common in patients older than 50.

Genetics: No genetic pattern.

ETIOLOGY AND PATHOGENESIS

Causes: Speculative, not clearly established. Proposed—defect in colon motility with increased intraluminal pressure, exacerbated by a low-fiber diet or an intrinsic defect in the colon wall.

Risk Factors: Low-fiber diet, age older than 40, and previous diverticulitis.

CLINICAL CHARACTERISTICS

Signs and Symptoms

- Asymptomatic (75% to 90%) (diverticulosis)
- Left lower quadrant abdominal pain (worse after eating, better after bowel movement or flatus)
- Diarrhea or constipation
- Fever or chills
- Anorexia, nausea, vomiting
- Abdominal distention
- Peritonitis (rebound tenderness, guarding, rigidity, depressed bowel sounds)
- Rectal tenderness or mass on rectal examination

DIAGNOSTIC APPROACH

Differential Diagnosis

- Irritable bowel syndrome (IBS)
- Lactose intolerance
- Inflammatory bowel disease (ulcerative colitis, Crohn's disease)
- Carcinoma of the colon
- Infectious colitis
- Appendicitis
- Ectopic pregnancy (in reproductive-age women)
- Tubo-ovarian abscess

Associated Conditions: Irritable bowel syndrome.

Workup and Evaluation

Laboratory: Complete blood count, sedimentation rate, urinalysis with culture.

Imaging: Barium enema generally demonstrates diverticulosis. Supine and upright abdominal radiograph may demonstrate free air in the peritoneal cavity if rupture has occurred.

Special Tests: Colonoscopy or flexible sigmoidoscopy.

Diagnostic Procedures: History and physical examination, imaging or endoscopy.

Pathologic Findings

Herniation of colon mucosa through the muscularis, usually at the site of a perforating artery lying between two layers of serosa in the mesentery. Increased thickness of the muscular wall and narrowing of the gut lumen. With inflammation, necrosis and perforation occur.

MANAGEMENT AND THERAPY

Nonpharmacologic

General Measures: For diverticulosis—increased dietary fiber, stool softeners. Fiber supplements may be considered. For diverticulitis—evaluation, possible hospitalization (2% to 5% of patients).

Specific Measures: Patients with diverticulitis may become acutely ill with sepsis, toxicity, and peritonitis. These patients require hospitalization, fluid support, and aggressive antibiotic treatment. Surgical resection may be considered in patients with multiple attacks, fistulae, or abscesses that do not respond to medical therapy.

Diet: Increased dietary fiber is desirable both as prevention and to decrease the risk of complications in established disease. Patients who are acutely ill should receive nothing by mouth.

Activity: No restriction. Activity is encouraged to foster normal bowel function.

Patient Education: Reassurance, counseling regarding diet and the need for periodic flexible sigmoidoscopy or colonoscopy screening; American College of Obstetricians and Gynecologists Patient Education Pamphlet AP151 (A Healthy Diet, For Women 65 and Older), AP120 (Problems of the Digestive System).

Drug(s) of Choice

Antispasmodics and adjuncts—hyoscyamine (Levsin) 0.125 mg PO one to two every 4 hours for 12/24 hours), buspirone (BuSpar) 15 to 30 mg PO daily.

Antibiotics (ambulatory)—metronidazole (Flagyl) 250 to 500 mg PO every 8 hours plus amoxicillin 500 mg PO every 8 hours or ciprofloxacin (Cipro) 500 mg PO two times daily.

Symptomatic control of diarrhea or constipation as needed.

Contraindications: See individual agents. Contraindications to flexible sigmoidoscopy: absolute—active diverticulitis, acute abdomen, blood dyscrasia, or coagulopathy, cardiopulmonary disease (acute or severe), inadequate bowel preparation, subacute bacterial endocarditis or prosthetic heart valve without adequate antibiotic prophylaxis, suspected bowel perforation; relative—active infection, peritonitis, pregnancy, recent abdominal surgery.

Precautions: If narcotic pain relievers are needed, meperidine (Demerol) is preferred; others should be avoided

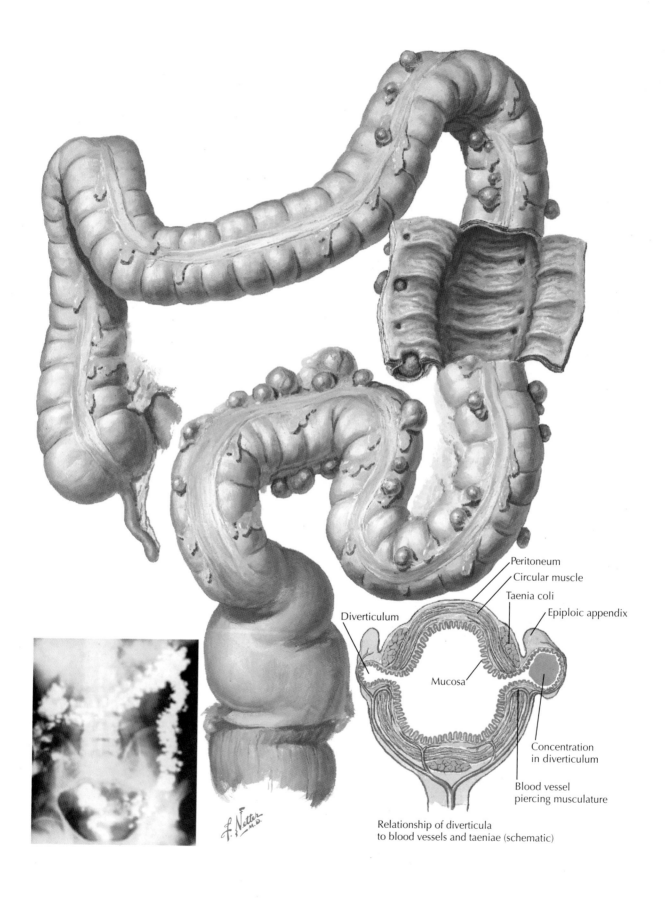

Peritoneum

Circular muscle

Taenia coli

Epiploic appendix

Diverticulum

Mucosa

Concentration
in diverticulum

Blood vessel
piercing musculature

Relationship of diverticula
to blood vessels and taeniae (schematic)

because they cause changes in bowel motility. Amino-glycosides may be associated with renal toxicity.

Interactions: See individual agents.

Alternative Drugs

Tobramycin may be used in combination with metronidazole.

FOLLOW-UP

Patient Monitoring: Normal health maintenance. Monitor for development of symptoms; perform routine flexible sigmoidoscopy and fecal occult blood screening.

Prevention/Avoidance: High-fiber diet and good bowel habits.

Possible Complications: Diverticulitis develops in 5% of patients with diverticulosis each year; lifetime risk is 50%. Enterocutaneous, enterovaginal, and perirectal fistulae may occur. Acutely, hemorrhage, perforation, abscess formation, peritonitis (with toxicity and collapse), and bowel obstruction may all occur.

Expected Outcome: With early detection and dietary change, the prognosis is good. With aggressive management of the first episode of diverticulitis, two thirds of patients do not have a recurrence. Up to 20% of those with rectal bleeding caused by diverticular disease have a recurrence of bleeding.

MISCELLANEOUS

Pregnancy Considerations: No direct effect on pregnancy, uncommon in reproductive-age women.

ICD-9-CM Codes: 562.10 (Diverticulosis of colon), 562.11 (Diverticulitis of colon).

REFERENCES

Level II

Purkayastha S, Constantinides VA, Tekkis PP, et al: Laparoscopic vs. open surgery for diverticular disease: a meta-analysis of nonrandomized studies. Dis Colon Rectum 2006;49:446.

Zarling EJ, Bernsen MB: The effect of gender on the rates of hospitalization for gastrointestinal illnesses. Am J Gastroenterol 1997;92:621.

Level III

Bogardus ST Jr: What do we know about diverticular disease? A brief overview. J Clin Gastroenterol 2006;40(7 Suppl 3):S108.

Di Mario F, Comparato G, Fanigliulo L, et al: Use of mesalazine in diverticular disease. J Clin Gastroenterol 2006;40(7 Suppl 3):S155.

D'Souza AL: Ageing and the gut. Postgrad Med J 2007;83:44.

Eglash A, Lane CH, Schneider DM: Clinical inquiries. What is the most beneficial diet for patients with diverticulosis? J Fam Pract 2006;55:813.

Floch MH, White JA: Management of diverticular disease is changing. World J Gastroenterol 2006;12:3225.

Frattini J, Longo WE: Diagnosis and treatment of chronic and recurrent diverticulitis. J Clin Gastroenterol 2006;40(7 Suppl 3):S145.

Frieri G, Pimpo MT, Scarpignato C: Management of colonic diverticular disease. Digestion 2006;73(Suppl 1):58. Epub 2006 Feb 8.

Korzenik JR: Case closed? Diverticulitis: epidemiology and fiber. J Clin Gastroenterol 2006;40(7 Suppl 3):S112.

Lundy JB, Edwards KD, Parker DM, Rivera DE: Recurrent rectal diverticulitis. Am Surg 2006;72:633.

Naliboff JA, Longmire-Cook SJ: Diverticulitis mimicking a tuboovarian abscess. Report of a case in a young woman. J Reprod Med 1996;41:921.

Salzman H, Lillie D: Diverticular disease: diagnosis and treatment. Am Fam Physician 2005;72:1229.

Simpson J, Spiller R: Colonic diverticular disease. Clin Evid 2005;14:543.

Tancer ML, Veridiano NP: Genital fistulas caused by diverticular disease of the sigmoid colon. Am J Obstet Gynecol 1996;174:1547.

Wong SK, Ho YH, Leong AP, Seow-Choen F: Clinical behavior of complicated right-sided and left-sided diverticulosis. Dis Colon Rectum 1997;40:344.

Dysmenorrhea: Primary and Secondary

INTRODUCTION

Description: Primary dysmenorrhea is painful menstruation without a clinically identifiable cause. Secondary dysmenorrhea is recurrent menstrual pain resulting from a clinically identifiable cause or abnormality.

Prevalence: Of all women, 10% to 15% are unable to function because of pain; 90% have discomfort with at least one cycle.

Predominant Age: Late teens to early 30s (primary), prevalence follows the occurrence of underlying conditions for secondary dysmenorrhea. Dysmenorrhea that begins after the age of 25 is most often secondary.

Genetics: No genetic pattern, although some suggest a familial pattern.

ETIOLOGY AND PATHOGENESIS

Causes: Primary—increased production of prostaglandin $F_2\alpha$ ($PGF_2\alpha$) resulting in increased uterine contractions (dysrhythmic) and markedly elevated intrauterine pressures (up to 400 mm Hg); possible increased sensitivity to $PGF_2\alpha$ as well. Secondary—uterine (adenomyosis, cervical stenosis and cervical lesions), congenital abnormalities (outflow obstructions, uterine anomalies), infection (chronic endometritis), intrauterine contraceptive devices, myomas (generally intracavitary or intramural), polyps; extrauterine (endometriosis, inflammation, and scarring [adhesions]); nongynecologic causes (musculoskeletal, gastrointestinal, urinary); "pelvic congestive syndrome" (debated); psychogenic (rare); tumors (myomas, benign or malignant tumors of ovary, bowel, or bladder).

Risk Factors: None known.

CLINICAL CHARACTERISTICS

Signs and Symptoms

- Primary—crampy, midline, lower abdominal pain (often demonstrated by a fist opening and closing)
  - Nausea, vomiting, and diarrhea common
  - Syncope
  - Headache
- Secondary—midline lower abdominal or low back pain accompanying menstruation
  - Pelvic heaviness or pressure
  - Symptoms specifically associated with the underlying condition

DIAGNOSTIC APPROACH

Differential Diagnosis

- Endometriosis
- Irritable bowel syndrome
- Inflammatory bowel disease
- Somatization (rare)

Abrupt onset of painful menstruation should suggest the possibility of a complication of pregnancy (abortion or ectopic pregnancy).

Associated Conditions: Menorrhagia is commonly associated.

Workup and Evaluation

Laboratory: Infrequently required, based on suspected or confirmed cause.

Imaging: For selected patients with secondary dysmenorrhea, ultrasonography of the pelvic organs may be indicated.

Special Tests: None indicated. Sigmoidoscopy may be helpful in selected patients with secondary dysmenorrhea.

Diagnostic Procedures: The absence of abnormality on pelvic examination, combined with historical characteristics, is diagnostic of primary dysmenorrhea. A pelvic examination that reveals a possible cause defines secondary dysmenorrhea.

Pathologic Findings

Based on the causative condition.

MANAGEMENT AND THERAPY

Nonpharmacologic

General Measures: Rest, analgesics (nonsteroidal antiinflammatory agents or pain relievers), heat (heating pad, hot water bottle, self-heating pads [ThermaCare]).

Specific Measures: Primary—medical management most effective, heat (heating pad, hot water bottle, or self-heating pads [ThermaCare]) appears comparable to medical management for many, transcutaneous electrical nerve stimulation (TENS) effective for selected patients, biofeedback suggested, but success poor or variable. Secondary—measures directed toward the underlying pathologic condition, modification of periods (oral contraceptives, menstrual suppression [depot medroxyprogesterone acetate, gonadotropic-releasing hormone (GnRH) agonists]), transcutaneous electrical nerve stimulation effective for selected patients, surgery for specific pathologic conditions.

Diet: No specific dietary changes indicated.

Activity: No restriction; based on patient comfort.

Patient Education: Reassurance; American College of Obstetricians and Gynecologists Patient Education Pamphlet AP046 (Dysmenorrhea), AP049 (Menstruation [Especially for Teens]), others related to underlying causes: AP013 (Important Facts About Endometriosis), AP074 (Uterine Fibroids), AP077 (Pelvic Inflammatory Disease), AP099 (Pelvic Pain).

Drug(s) of Choice

Primary—nonsteroidal antiinflammatory drugs (NSAIDs): ibuprofen 800 mg, two at onset of flow and one every 4 to 6 hours prn pain; naproxen sodium 275 mg, two at onset of flow and one every 6 to 8 hours prn pain; meclofenamate 100 mg, one at onset of flow and one every 4 to 6 hours prn pain, mefenamic acid 250 mg, two at onset of flow and one every 4 to 6 hours prn pain.

Secondary—based on pathophysiologic condition. NSAIDs or analgesics may be used.

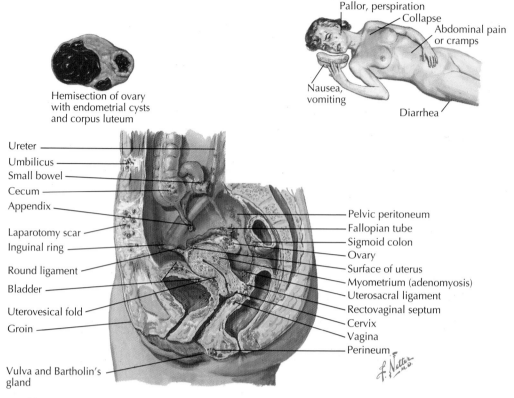

Hemisection of ovary
with endometrial cysts
and corpus luteum

Pallor, perspiration
Collapse
Abdominal pain
or cramps
Nausea, vomiting
Diarrhea

Ureter
Umbilicus
Small bowel
Cecum
Appendix
Laparotomy scar
Inguinal ring
Round ligament
Bladder
Uterovesical fold
Groin
Vulva and Bartholin's gland

Pelvic peritoneum
Fallopian tube
Sigmoid colon
Ovary
Surface of uterus
Myometrium (adenomyosis)
Uterosacral ligament
Rectovaginal septum
Cervix
Vagina
Perineum

Possible sites of endometriosis as a cause for secondary dysmenorrhea.

Contraindications: Aspirin-sensitive asthma, ulcers, inflammatory bowel disease.

Precautions: Some patients experience increased stomach upset with NSAIDs; this may be reduced by taking them with food.

Interactions: Other over-the-counter pain relievers containing NSAID compounds.

Alternative Drugs

Other rapidly acting NSAIDs may be used. Combination oral contraceptives generally provide milder periods (and contraception if necessary). Centrally acting analgesics may be added with care to avoid interaction with NSAIDs. Suppression of menstruation (depot medroxy-progesterone acetate, gonadotropic-releasing hormone agonists) may be indicated for patients with severe pain.

FOLLOW-UP

Patient Monitoring: Normal health maintenance.
Prevention/Avoidance: None.
Possible Complications: Most commonly side effects of medication. Anemia (if menorrhagia is present), others based on underlying cause.
Expected Outcome: Primary dysmenorrhea—significant relief of symptoms with medical therapy. If medical therapy does not produce pronounced improvement, the diagnosis should be reevaluated. The prevalence of primary dysmenorrhea declines with time. Secondary dysmenorrhea—based on cause and mode of therapy, resolution of symptoms is generally possible with NSAIDs, analgesics, or period modification.

MISCELLANEOUS

Pregnancy Considerations: No effect on pregnancy.
ICD-9-CM Codes: 625.3, 302.76 (Psychogenic) (others based on underlying cause).

REFERENCES

Level I
Akin MD, Weingand KW, Hengehold DA, et al: Use of continuous low-level topical heat in the treatment of dysmenorrhea. Obstet Gynecol 2001;97:343.

Level III
American College of Obstetricians and Gynecologists: Dysmenorrhea. Technical Bulletin 68. Washington, DC, ACOG, 1983.
Dawood MY: Dysmenorrhea. Clin Obstet Gynecol 1990;33:168.
Dawood MY: Primary dysmenorrhea: advances in pathogenesis and management. Obstet Gynecol 2006;108:428.
Deligeoroglou E, Tsimaris P, Deliveliotou A, et al: Menstrual disorders during adolescence. Pediatr Endocrinol Rev 2006;3(Suppl 1):150.
Doty E, Attaran M: Managing primary dysmenorrhea. J Pediatr Adolesc Gynecol 2006;19:341.
Harel Z. Dysmenorrhea in adolescents and young adults: etiology and management. J Pediatr Adolesc Gynecol 2006;19:363.
Latthe PM, Proctor ML, Farquhar CM, et al: Surgical interruption of pelvic nerve pathways in dysmenorrhea: a systematic review of effectiveness. Acta Obstet Gynecol Scand 2007;86:4. Review.
Lentz GM: Primary and secondary dysmenorrhea, premenstrual syndrome, and premenstrual dysphoric disorder. In Katz VL, Lentz GM, Lobo RA, Gershenson DM: Comprehensive Gynecology, 5th ed. Philadelphia, Mosby/Elsevier, 2007, p 901.
Proctor M, Farquhar C: Diagnosis and management of dysmenorrhoea. BMJ 2006;332:1134.
Proctor ML, Farquhar CM: Dysmenorrhoea. Clin Evid 2006;15:2429.

INTRODUCTION

Description: Abdominal, pelvic, or vaginal pain that arises during sexual thrusting, especially with deep penetration.

Prevalence: Roughly 15% of women each year (severe—less than 2% of women).

Predominant Age: Reproductive age and beyond.

Genetics: No genetic pattern.

ETIOLOGY AND PATHOGENESIS

Causes

Gynecologic—extrauterine (adhesions, chronic pelvic infection, cysts, endometriosis, pelvic relaxation [cystocele, urethrocele, rectocele, enterocele], prolapsed adnexa or adnexa adherent to vaginal apex, retained ovary syndrome, shortening of the vagina after surgery or radiation); uterine (adenomyosis, fibroids, malposition [retroversion]). Urologic—chronic urinary tract infection, detrusor dyssynergia, interstitial cystitis, urethral syndrome.

Gastrointestinal—chronic constipation, diverticular disease, inflammatory bowel disease, Crohn's disease, ulcerative colitis, irritable bowel syndrome (IBS).

Musculoskeletal—fibromyositis, hernias (abdominal, femoral), herniated disk.

Other—inadequate arousal (failure of vaginal apex expansion), pelvic tumors (benign or malignant). Care must be taken to avoid labeling any dyspareunia as purely physical or purely emotional in origin. Most often a mixture of factors causes or contributes to the problem.

Risk Factors: Positions or practices that result in particularly deep or forceful penetration, such as male superior or rear entry positions.

CLINICAL CHARACTERISTICS

Signs and Symptoms

Ache-like pain, crampy visceral pain, burning, a sense of fullness, or a feeling as if something is being bumped during deep sexual thrusting. Occasionally the pain is sharp and abrupt in character. Pain often depends on the type of sexual activity involved or the positions used.

DIAGNOSTIC APPROACH

Differential Diagnosis

* Vulvitis
* Vestibulitis
* Vaginitis
* Bartholin's gland infection, abscess, cyst
* Atrophic change
* Anxiety, depression, phobia
* Sexual or other abuse
* Pelvic mass (uterine leiomyomata, ovarian cyst)
* Shortening of the vagina after surgery or radiation

Associated Conditions: Vaginismus, orgasmic dysfunction.

WORKUP AND EVALUATION

Laboratory: No evaluation indicated.

Imaging: No imaging indicated, pelvic (abdominal or transvaginal) ultrasonography for specific indications.

Special Tests: None indicated.

Diagnostic Procedures: History (general and sexual) and careful pelvic examination. (If discomfort is produced, it is important to be sure that the sensation matches that experienced during intercourse.)

Pathologic Findings

None.

MANAGEMENT AND THERAPY

Nonpharmacologic

General Measures: Evaluation, reassurance, relaxation measures.

Specific Measures: Because dyspareunia is ultimately a symptom, the specific therapy for any form of sexual pain is focused on the underlying cause. Vaginal lubricants (water-soluble or long-acting agents such as Astroglide, Replens, Lubrin, K-Y Jelly, and others), local anesthetics (for vulvar lesions), or pelvic relaxation exercises may be appropriate while more specific therapy is under way.

Diet: No specific dietary changes indicated.

Activity: No restriction.

Patient Education: Reassurance, relaxation training, alternate sexual positions and forms of expression; American College of Obstetricians and Gynecologists Patient Education Pamphlet AP020 (Pain During Intercourse), AP042 (You and Your Sexuality [Especially for Teens]).

Drug(s) of Choice

The judicious use of anxiolytics or antidepressant medications for selected patients may be appropriate but for short periods of time only.

ALTERNATIVE THERAPIES

Modifying sexual techniques used by the couple may reduce pain with intercourse. Delaying penetration until maximal arousal has been achieved improves vaginal lubrication, ensures vaginal apex expansion, and provides an element of control for the female partner. Sexual positions that allow the women to control the direction and depth of penetration (such as woman astride) may also be of help.

FOLLOW-UP

Patient Monitoring: Normal health maintenance. Watch for signs of abuse, anxiety, or depression.

Prevention/Avoidance: None.

Possible Complications: Marital discord, orgasmic or libidinal dysfunction.

Expected Outcome: With diagnosis and treatment of the underlying cause, response should be good.

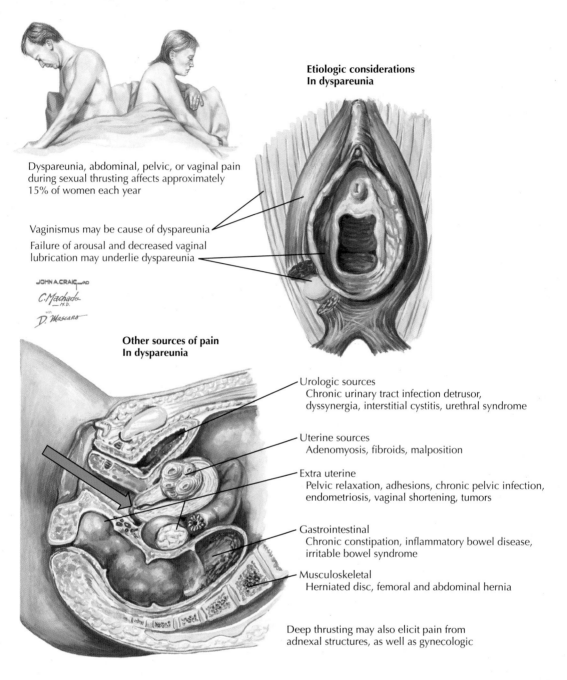

Dyspareunia, abdominal, pelvic, or vaginal pain during sexual thrusting affects approximately 15% of women each year

Vaginismus may be cause of dyspareunia

Failure of arousal and decreased vaginal lubrication may underlie dyspareunia

Etiologic considerations In dyspareunia

Other sources of pain In dyspareunia

Urologic sources
Chronic urinary tract infection detrusor, dyssynergia, interstitial cystitis, urethral syndrome

Uterine sources
Adenomyosis, fibroids, malposition

Extra uterine
Pelvic relaxation, adhesions, chronic pelvic infection, endometriosis, vaginal shortening, tumors

Gastrointestinal
Chronic constipation, inflammatory bowel disease, irritable bowel syndrome

Musculoskeletal
Herniated disc, femoral and abdominal hernia

Deep thrusting may also elicit pain from adnexal structures, as well as gynecologic

MISCELLANEOUS

Pregnancy Considerations: No effect on pregnancy. Occasionally, the coital changes necessitated by the growing uterus may result in new-onset dyspareunia. Positional changes (as noted earlier) are generally sufficient to relieve these cases.
ICD-9-CM Codes: 625.0.

REFERENCES

Level III
American College of Obstetricians and Gynecologists: Vulvodynia. ACOG Committee Opinion 345. Washington, DC, ACOG, 2006.

Fauconnier A, Chapron C: Endometriosis and pelvic pain: epidemiological evidence of the relationship and implications. Hum Reprod Update 2005;11:595. Epub 2005 Sep 19.
Fink P: Dyspareunia: current concepts. Med Aspects Hum Sex 1972;6:28.
Fordney DS: Dyspareunia and vaginismus. Clin Obstet Gynecol 1978;21:205.
Fullerton W: Dyspareunia. BMJ 1971;2:31.
Lamont JA: Female dyspareunia. Am J Obstet Gynecol 1980;136:282.
Lentz GM: Emotional aspects of gynecology: sexual dysfunction, eating disorders, substance abuse, depression, grief, loss. In Katz VL, Lentz GM, Lobo RA, Gershenson DM: Comprehensive Gynecology, 5th ed. Philadelphia, Mosby/Elsevier, 2007: p 218.
Steege JF: Dyspareunia and vaginismus. Clin Obstet Gynecol 1984;27:750.
Steege JF, Ling FW: Dyspareunia. A special type of chronic pelvic pain. Obstet Gynecol Clin North Am 1993;20:779.

INTRODUCTION

Description: Dysuria is the painful passage of urine (symptom, not diagnosis).

Prevalence: Common in women, 10% to 20% per year. One third of women during their lifetime.

Predominant Age: Any.

Genetics: No genetic pattern.

ETIOLOGY AND PATHOGENESIS

Causes: Infection and inflammation in the urethra and suburethral tissues. Most urinary tract infections in women ascend from contamination of the vulva and meatus acquired via instrumentation, trauma, or sexual intercourse. (A history of intercourse within the proceeding 24 to 48 hours is present in up to 75% of patients with acute urinary tract infection.) Coliform organisms, especially *Escherichia coli*, are the most common organisms responsible for asymptomatic bacteriuria, cystitis, and pyelonephritis. Ninety percent of first infections and 80% of recurrent infections are caused by *E. coli*, with between 10% and 20% resulting from *Staphylococcus saprophyticus*. Infection with other pathogens such as *Klebsiella* species (5%) and *Proteus* species (2%) account for most of the remaining infections. Infection with *Neisseria gonorrhoeae*, *Chlamydia trachomatis*, *Mycoplasma*, and *Ureaplasma* should all be considered when urethritis is suspected. Chemical irritation, allergic reactions, or vulvitis may all produce symptoms of dysuria.

Risk Factors: Sexual activity, instrumentation, more virulent pathogens, altered host defenses, infrequent or incomplete voiding, foreign body or stone, obstruction, or biochemical changes in the urine (diabetes, hemoglobinopathies, pregnancy) estrogen deficiency, diaphragm use, spermicides.

CLINICAL CHARACTERISTICS

Signs and Symptoms

- Painful urination
- Frequency, urgency, nocturia (commonly associated, indicate irritation of the bladder wall)
- Pelvic pressure (if cystitis is present)
- Pyuria (more than five white blood cells per high-power field in a centrifuged specimen, most prominent in first one third of voided specimen)

DIAGNOSTIC APPROACH

Differential Diagnosis

- Cystitis
- Traumatic trigonitis
- Urethral syndrome
- Interstitial cystitis
- Bladder tumors or stones
- Vulvitis and vaginitis (may give rise to external dysuria as in herpetic vulvitis)
- Urethral diverticulum
- Infection in the Skene's glands
- Detrusor instability

Associated Conditions: Dyspareunia, cystitis.

Workup and Evaluation

Laboratory: Nonpregnant women with a first episode of dysuria suggestive of urinary tract infection do not need laboratory confirmation of the diagnosis; they may be treated empirically. (Recent data suggest that this may be an acceptable strategy for women with fewer than three episodes per year, who lack fever or flank pain, and have not been treated recently for the same symptoms.) For others, urinalysis and culture should be performed. For uncentrifuged urine samples, the presence of more than one white blood cell per high-power field is 90% accurate for detecting infection. Gram stain of urine samples or sediments may help to establish the diagnosis or suggest a possible pathogen.

Imaging: No imaging indicated.

Special Tests: A sterile swab inserted into the urethra may be used to obtain material for culture and Gram stain to establish the diagnosis.

Diagnostic Procedures: History and physical examination, urinalysis. (Gentle pressure beneath the urethra or bladder trigone will often reproduce the patient's symptoms when significant urethritis is present.)

Pathologic Findings

Pyuria (hematuria may be present as well).

MANAGEMENT AND THERAPY

Nonpharmacologic

General Measures: Fluids, frequent voiding, and antipyretics. Urinary acidification (with ascorbic acid, ammonium chloride, or acidic fruit juices) and urinary analgesics (phenazopyridine [Pyridium]) may also be added based on the needs of the individual patient.

Specific Measures: Antibiotic therapy when infection is suspected.

Diet: Increased fluids and reduction of caffeine.

Activity: No restriction.

Patient Education: Reassurance; American College of Obstetricians and Gynecologists Patient Education Pamphlet AP050 (Urinary Tract Infections).

Drug(s) of Choice
(Nonpregnant Patients)

Single-dose therapy: amoxicillin 3 g, ampicillin 3.5 g, a first-generation cephalosporin 2 g, nitrofurantoin 200 mg, sulfisoxazole 2 g, trimethoprim 400 mg, trimethoprim/sulfamethoxazole (320/1600 mg).

Three- to seven-day therapy: amoxicillin 500 mg every 8 hours, a first-generation cephalosporin 500 mg every 8 hours, ciprofloxacin 250 mg every 12 hours, nitrofurantoin 100 mg every 12 hours, norfloxacin 400 mg every 12 hours, ofloxacin 200 mg every 12 hours, sulfisoxazole 500 mg every 6 hours, tetracycline 500 mg every 6 hours,

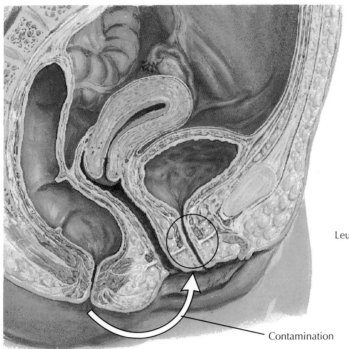

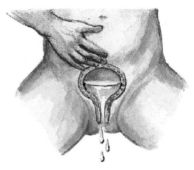

Painful urination, frequency, and urgency
are common symptoms of dysuria

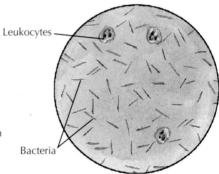

Inflammation of urethra and suburethral tissue resulting from
ascending infection caused by contamination of vulva and meatus
are often responsible for symptoms of dysuria. Coliform bacteria
are most often the responsible organism.

Bacteriuria and pyuria are common
findings on urine examinations

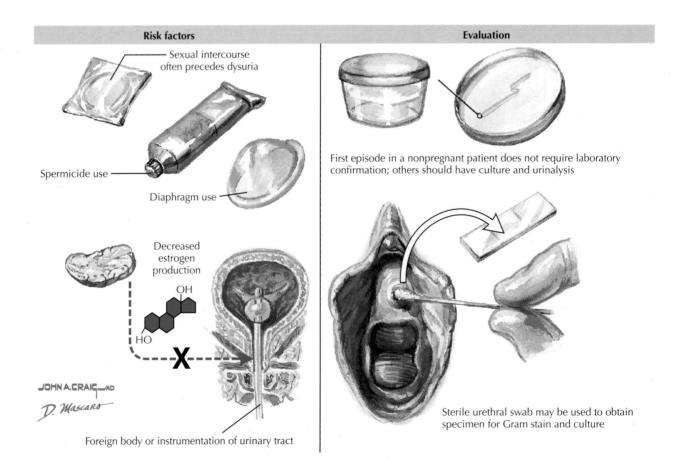

| Risk factors | Evaluation |

Sexual intercourse
often precedes dysuria

Spermicide use

Diaphragm use

First episode in a nonpregnant patient does not require laboratory
confirmation; others should have culture and urinalysis

Decreased
estrogen
production

Foreign body or instrumentation of urinary tract

Sterile urethral swab may be used to obtain
specimen for Gram stain and culture

JOHN A. CRAIG_AD
D. Mascaro

trimethoprim/sulfamethoxazole 160/800 mg every 12 hours, trimethoprim 100 (200) mg every 12 hours.

Contraindications: Known or suspected hypersensitivity.

Precautions: Urinary analgesics (phenazopyridine [Pyridium]) should be used for no longer than 48 hours and may stain some types of contact lenses.

Interactions: See individual medications.

Alternative Drugs (Pregnant Patients)

Seven-day therapy: amoxicillin 500 mg every 8 hours, a first-generation cephalosporin 500 mg every 6 hours, nitrofurantoin 100 mg every 12 hours.

FOLLOW-UP

Patient Monitoring: No follow-up is necessary after single-dose treatment or after multiday treatment for nonpregnant women who experience resolution of their symptoms. Cure for all other patients should be confirmed by urinalysis and culture. Recurrent lower tract infections require prompt evaluation. Possible causes include incorrect or incomplete (e.g., noncompliant) therapy, mechanical factors (such as obstruction or stone), or compromised host defenses.

Prevention/Avoidance: Frequent voiding, adequate fluid intake, voiding after intercourse.

Possible Complications: Urethral syndrome and interstitial cystitis. Bacteremia, septic shock, adult respiratory distress syndrome, and other serious sequelae are associated with pyelonephritis.

Expected Outcome: For most patients, symptoms (when resulting from infection) should resolve within 2 to 3 days after the initiation of therapy.

MISCELLANEOUS

Pregnancy Considerations: Those at high risk (e.g., patients with diabetes) should be monitored carefully to avoid urethritis, cystitis, and ascending infection.

ICD-9-CM Codes: 788.1 (Urinary tract infection).

REFERENCES

Level I

Greenberg RN, Reilly PM, Luppen KL, et al: Randomized study of single-dose, three-day, and seven-day treatment of cystitis in women. J Infect Dis 1986;153:277.

Level III

Car J: Urinary tract infections in women: diagnosis and management in primary care. BMJ 2006;332(7533):94.

Franco AV: Recurrent urinary tract infections. Best Pract Res Clin Obstet Gynaecol 2005;19:861. Epub 2005 Nov 17.

Mittal P, Wing DA: Urinary tract infections in pregnancy. Clin Perinatol 2005;32:749.

Nicolle L, Anderson PA, Conly J, et al: Uncomplicated urinary tract infection in women. Current practice and the effect of antibiotic resistance on empiric treatment. Can Fam Physician 2006;52:612.

Pappas P: Laboratory in the diagnosis and management of urinary tract infections. Med Clin North Am 1991;75:313.

Sheffield JS, Cunningham FG: Urinary tract infection in women. Obstet Gynecol 2005;106:1085.

Stamm W: Criteria for the diagnosis of urinary tract infection and for the assessment of therapeutic effectiveness. Infection 1992;20(Suppl 3):S151, S160.

Stamm W: Controversies in single dose therapy of acute uncomplicated urinary tract infections in women. Infection 1992;20:S272.

Stamm W, Hooton T: Management of urinary tract infections in adults. N Engl J Med 1993;329:1328.

Whelan P: Manage urinary tract infections. Practitioner 2006;250:38, 41, 43 passim.

INTRODUCTION

Description: Anorexia nervosa is a syndrome characterized by an altered body image, significant weight loss, and amenorrhea that are not caused by physical disease. Bulimia is an eating disorder characterized by an altered body image and recurrent binge eating, with or without purging through self-induced vomiting, laxative abuse, or diuretics. Exercise excess is often a part of after-binge behavior. Both affect more women than men.

Prevalence: Females, 1% to 3%. Subclinical eating disorders are common in university populations.

Predominant Age: Teens to early 20s.

Genetics: No genetic pattern.

ETIOLOGY AND PATHOGENESIS

Causes: Unknown (emotional).

Risk Factors: Anorexia nervosa—perfectionistic personality (high expectations, personal or external). Bulimia—impulsive character, low self-esteem, stress (e.g., multiple responsibilities, tight schedules), early puberty. At high risk for both: dancers, models, cheerleaders, athletes.

CLINICAL CHARACTERISTICS

Signs and Symptoms

- Insidious onset (occasionally stress related)
- Significant weight loss (15% below expected weight)
- Denial of problem
- Preoccupation with weight or body image
- Anorexia nervosa—impression of obesity rather than objective view of weight
  - Reduced food intake or refusal (often associated with elaborate eating rituals)
  - Excessive exercise (marathon running)
- Bulimia—high-calorie binges followed by severe restriction
  - Food collections or hoarding
  - Medication abuse (laxatives, diuretics, ipecac, thyroid medication)
  - Dental erosion and scarred knuckles (secondary to finger-induced vomiting)

DIAGNOSTIC APPROACH

Differential Diagnosis

- Wasting disease (tumors)
- Depression
- Hypothalamic tumor
- Food phobia
- Gastrointestinal disease
- Other emotional disorders (conversion disorder, schizophrenia, body dysmorphic disorder)

Associated Conditions: Major depression (50% to 75% of patients), obsessive-compulsive disorders (10% to 13% of patients), bipolar disorders, sexual disinterest, depression, growth arrest, hypotension and bradycardia, hypothermia, peripheral edema. Prolonged amenorrhea is associated with an increased risk of osteoporosis, which may not be reversible. Bulimia—social phobia and anxiety disorders, substance abuse, shoplifting common.

Workup and Evaluation

Laboratory: No evaluation specific for anorexia. For patients with bulimia there may be laboratory changes consistent with repeated vomiting (hypokalemia, hypomagnesemia, or hypochloremia).

Imaging: No imaging indicated.

Special Tests: Assessment of body fat.

Diagnostic Procedures: History and physical examination, Eating Attitudes Test.

Pathologic Findings

Anorexia nervosa—dry, cracked skin; sparse scalp hair; fine lanugo hair on extremities, face, and trunk; arrested maturation; pathologic fractures; cognitive defects. Bulimia—eroded dental enamel, esophagitis, Mallory-Weiss tears, parotid enlargement, gastric dilation.

MANAGEMENT AND THERAPY

Nonpharmacologic

General Measures: Psychological evaluation and support, supervised eating and exercise program, progressive increase in calories and activity as weight is regained (anorexia), limit access to bathroom for 2 hours after eating (bulimia).

Specific Measures: Hospitalization may be required, including intensive psychological assessment and therapy. Tube feedings and intravenous fluids may be required for patients with anorexia.

Diet: Supervised program of reeducation and behavior modification. For patients with anorexia, a gradual increase in caloric intake as part of a supervised program of reeducation and behavior modification.

Activity: Stepwise increase based on weight change, avoidance of goal-oriented activities.

Patient Education: Nutritional instruction, assistance with a food log; American College of Obstetricians and Gynecologists Patient Education Pamphlet AP144 (Eating Disorders), AP064 (Weight Control: Eating Right and Keeping Fit), AP045 (Exercise and Fitness: A Guide for Women).

Drug(s) of Choice

Fluoxetine (Prozac) 10 to 60 mg PO daily.

Oxazepam 15 mg or alprazolam 0.25 mg PO before meals to reduce anxiety about weight gain.

Contraindications: See specific agents.

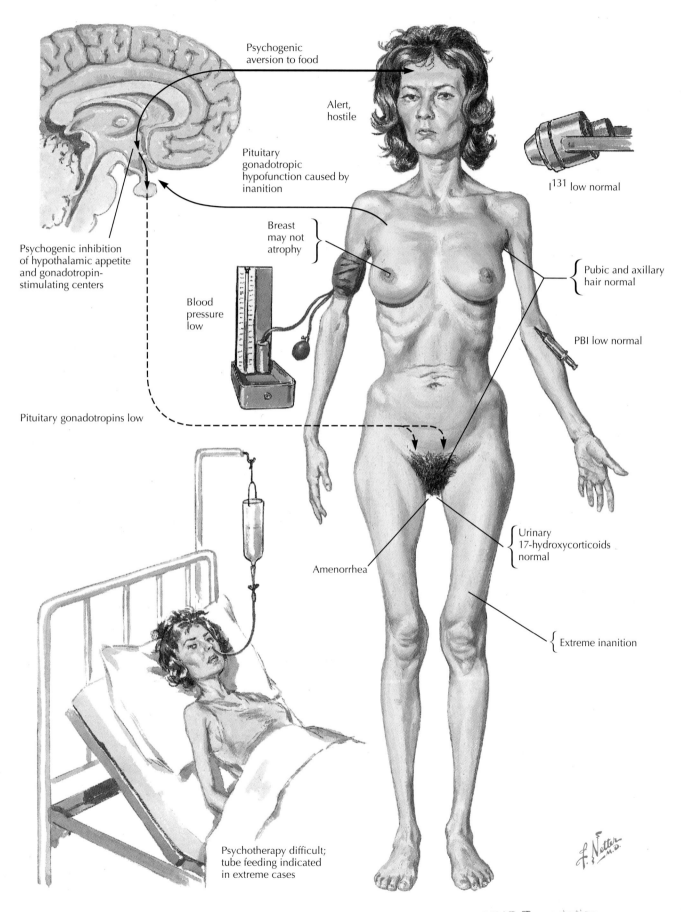

Psychogenic aversion to food

Alert, hostile

Pituitary gonadotropic hypofunction caused by inanition

Psychogenic inhibition of hypothalamic appetite and gonadotropin-stimulating centers

I^{131} low normal

Breast may not atrophy

Blood pressure low

Pubic and axillary hair normal

PBI low normal

Pituitary gonadotropins low

Urinary 17-hydroxycorticoids normal

Amenorrhea

Extreme inanition

Psychotherapy difficult; tube feeding indicated in extreme cases

BMR, basal metabolic rate; PBI, plasma protein-bound iodine.

Precautions: Starved patients tend to be more sensitive to medications or to have compromised renal, cardiac, or liver function.

Alternative Drugs

Imipramine (Tofranil) 10 mg gradually increased to 200 mg or desipramine (Norpramin) 25 mg increased gradually to 150 mg PO daily.

Lithium (Eskalith) 300 mg PO bid increased gradually until blood level of 0.6 to 1.2 mEq/L if bipolar disorder is present.

Cisapride (Propulsid) 10 to 20 mg before meals to increase gastric emptying.

Psyllium (Metamucil) 1 tablespoon every night to prevent constipation.

FOLLOW-UP

Patient Monitoring: Periodic weight measurements (weekly until stable, then monthly). Monitor for depression or suicidal ideation.

Prevention/Avoidance: Encourage healthy attitudes about weight, eating, and exercise; enhance self-esteem; and reduce stress.

Possible Complications: Drug and alcohol use/abuse, suicide, cardiac arrhythmia or arrest (potassium depletion), cardiomyopathy, suicide, necrotizing colitis, osteoporosis and osteoporotic fractures. Depression is common.

Expected Outcome: Highly variable with relapses common, better outcome with inpatient care. Bulimia may spontaneously remit.

MISCELLANEOUS

Pregnancy Considerations: Amenorrhea and infertility common in women with anorexia. For women with bulimia, the binge–purge cycle may affect fetal nutrition and growth when the behavior persists during pregnancy.

ICD-9-CM Codes: 307.1 (Anorexia), 783.6 (Bulimia).

REFERENCES

Level II

Centers for Disease Control and Prevention: Results from the National Adolescent Student Health Survey. MMWR Morb Mortal Wkly Rep 1989;38:147.

Kurtzman FD, Yager J, Landvesk J, et al: Eating disorders among selected female student populations at UCLA. J Am Diet Assoc 1989;89:45.

Legroux-Gerot I, Vignau J, Collier F, Cortet B: Bone loss associated with anorexia nervosa. Joint Bone Spine 2005;72:489.

Signorini A, De Filippo E, Panico S, et al: Long-term mortality in anorexia nervosa: a report after an 8-year follow-up and a review of the most recent literature. Eur J Clin Nutr 2007;61:119. Epub 2006 Aug 2.

Level III

Abrams SA, Silber TJ, Esteban NV, et al: Mineral balance and bone turnover in adolescents with anorexia nervosa. J Pediatr 1993;123:326.

Brunet M 2nd: Female athlete triad. Clin Sports Med 2005;24:623, ix.

Bruni V, Filicetti MF, Pontello V: Open issues in anorexia nervosa: prevention and therapy of bone loss. Ann N Y Acad Sci 2006;1092:91.

Chamay-Weber C, Narring F, Michaud PA: Partial eating disorders among adolescents: a review. J Adolesc Health 2005;37:417.

Crow SJ, Mitchell JE: Rational therapy in eating disorders. Drugs 1994;48:372.

ESHRE Capri Workshop Group: Nutrition and reproduction in women. Hum Reprod Update 2006;12:193. Epub 2006 Jan 31.

Franko DL, Keel PK: Suicidality in eating disorders: occurrence, correlates, and clinical implications. Clin Psychol Rev 2006;26:769. Epub 2006 Jul 27.

Hay PJ, Bacaltchuk J: Bulimia nervosa. Clin Evid 2005;(14):1170.

Hay PJ, Bacaltchuk J: Bulimia nervosa. Clin Evid 2006;(15):1315.

Lentz GM: Emotional aspects of gynecology: sexual dysfunction, eating disorders, substance abuse, depression, grief, loss. In Katz VL, Lentz GM, Lobo RA, Gershenson DM: Comprehensive Gynecology, 5th ed. Philadelphia, Mosby/Elsevier, 2007:, p 179.

Morris J, Twaddle S: Anorexia nervosa. BMJ 2007;334(7599):894.

Nattiv A, Agostini R, Drinkwater B, Yeager KK: The female athlete triad. The inter-relatedness of disordered eating, amenorrhea, and osteoporosis. Clin Sports Med 1994;13:405.

Warren MP, Vande Wiele RL: Clinical and metabolic features of anorexia nervosa. Am J Obstet Gynecol 1973;117:435.

Yager J, Andersen AE: Clinical practice. Anorexia nervosa. N Engl J Med 2005;353:1481.

Gastritis

INTRODUCTION

Description: Gastritis is an inflammatory condition affecting the stomach lining that results in acute or chronic indigestion, bloating, "gas," and heartburn.

Prevalence: Common.

Predominant Age: Any.

Genetics: No genetic pattern.

ETIOLOGY AND PATHOGENESIS

Causes: Generalized inflammation of the stomach lining, which, in some cases, may be infectious (*Helicobacter pylori*).

Risk Factors: Cigarette smoking, alcohol abuse, some medications (nonsteroidal anti-inflammatory drugs [NSAIDs]), bile reflux, radiation.

CLINICAL CHARACTERISTICS

Signs and Symptoms

* Nausea, vomiting, dyspepsia, heartburn, and "gas" (symptoms are most common after eating large meals, consuming certain foods)
* Upper abdominal pain or tenderness
* Hiccups

DIAGNOSTIC APPROACH

Differential Diagnosis

* Gastrointestinal reflux
* Ulcer disease (gastric or duodenal)
* Esophageal cancer
* Linitis plastica

Associated Conditions: Bleeding, dysphagia, and gastric or duodenal ulcer.

Workup and Evaluation

Laboratory: No evaluation indicated.

Imaging: No imaging indicated.

Special Tests: Gastroscopy (with or without biopsy) establishes the diagnosis but most often is not necessary.

Diagnostic Procedures: History and physical examination (suspicious), gastroscopy (diagnostic).

Pathologic Findings

Patchy erythema of the gastric mucosa (seldom full thickness) most common in the pyloric antrum.

MANAGEMENT AND THERAPY

Nonpharmacologic

General Measures: Dietary changes, elevation of the head of the bed, smoking cessation, alcohol in moderation only, antacids. (Antacids that coat [liquids] and those that tend to float on the surface of the stomach contents, such as Gaviscon, give better heartburn relief than other agents.)

Specific Measures: Eliminate medications that contribute to reduced esophageal pressure, such as diazepam and calcium channel blockers, or that may damage the esophagus (nonsteroidal anti-inflammatory drugs). Use acid-blocking therapy.

Diet: No specific dietary changes indicated.

Activity: No restriction.

Patient Education: Reassurance, diet counseling, behavior modification.

Drug(s) of Choice

Antacids.

Histamine H_2 antagonists (cimetidine 800 mg two times daily, ranitidine 400 mg four times daily, famotidine 20 mg two times daily, or nizatidine 150 mg two times daily).

Hydrogen potassium pump blocker (omeprazole 20 to 40 mg daily for 4 to 8 weeks, esomeprazole 20 to 40 mg daily for 4 to 8 weeks, or pantoprazole 40 mg daily for 8 weeks). Misoprostol (Cytotec, 100 to 200 microg PO four times daily) if mucosal injury is documented or suspected.

Contraindications: Known or suspected hypersensitivity. Misoprostol is contraindicated during pregnancy and lactation.

Precautions: If bismuth is prescribed, warn the patient about black stools. Because of a lack of long-term follow-up, hydrogen pump inhibitors may be taken for only 8 to 12 weeks.

Interactions: Multiple drug interactions are possible with agents such as cimetidine; check full prescribing information.

Alternative Drugs

In patients with *H. pylori* infection, a combination of bismuth (Pepto-Bismol) and an antibiotic (metronidazole 250 mg every 6 hours, tetracycline 500 every 6 hours, or amoxicillin 500 mg every 8 hours) has been recommended for 2 weeks. A 4-week treatment with clarithromycin (Bixin) and either omeprazole (Prilosec) or ranitidine bismuth citrate (Tritec) may also be used.

FOLLOW-UP

* **Patient Monitoring:** Normal health maintenance. If significant gastric erosion is documented, repeat gastroscopy after 6 weeks is often recommended.
* **Prevention/Avoidance:** Reduction of modifiable risk factors (e.g., smoking).
* **Possible Complications:** Chronic pain, ulcer formation, and perforation.
* **Expected Outcome:** Generally good symptomatic relief, but long-term therapy is often required.

MISCELLANEOUS

* **Pregnancy Considerations:** No direct effect on pregnancy, although severe gastritis may interfere with maternal nutrition.
* **ICD-9-CM Codes:** 535.5 (others based on cause).

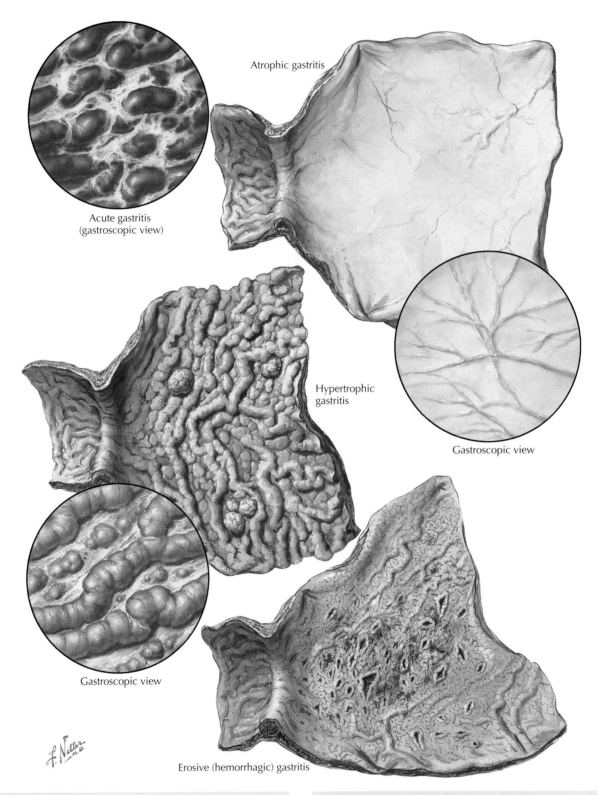

Acute gastritis
(gastroscopic view)

Atrophic gastritis

Hypertrophic
gastritis

Gastroscopic view

Gastroscopic view

Erosive (hemorrhagic) gastritis

REFERENCES

Level II

de Martel C, Parsonnet J: *Helicobacter pylori* infection and gender: a meta-analysis of population-based prevalence surveys. Dig Dis Sci 2006;51:2292. Epub 2006 Nov 7.

Graham DY, Malaty HM, Evans DG, et al: Epidemiology of *Helicobacter pylori* in an asymptomatic population in the US. Gastroenterology 1991;100:1495.

Israel DA, Peek RM Jr: The role of persistence in *Helicobacter pylori* pathogenesis. Curr Opin Gastroenterol 2006;22:3.

Level III

Feldman M, Burton ME: Drug therapy: histamine2-receptor antagonists—Standard therapy for acid-peptic disease. N Engl J Med 1990;323:1672, 1749.

Moayyedi P, Talley NJ: Gastro-oesophageal reflux disease. Lancet 2006;367(9528):2086.

Panteris V, Karamanolis DG: Different aspects in functional dyspepsia. Hepatogastroenterology 2005;52:1782.

Rapkin AJ, Mayer EA: Gastroenterologic causes of chronic pelvic pain. Obstet Gynecol Clin North Am 1993;20:663.

INTRODUCTION

Description: The reflux of gastric acid to the sensitive esophagus causes heartburn, the cardinal manifestation of gastroesophageal reflux disease (GERD).

Prevalence: Common.

Predominant Age: Generally reproductive and beyond.

Genetics: No genetic pattern.

ETIOLOGY AND PATHOGENESIS

Causes: The most common cause is decreased tone of the lower esophageal sphincter (LES). This is complicated in pregnant patients by the reduced gastric emptying and reduced esophageal sphincter tone that occur during pregnancy.

Risk Factors: Cigarette smoking, alcohol abuse, some medications or foods, pregnancy, scleroderma, sliding hiatal hernia.

CLINICAL CHARACTERISTICS

Signs and Symptoms

- Upper abdominal pain, nausea, vomiting, dyspepsia, heartburn, chest pain, and "gas" (70% to 85%; symptoms most common after large meals, consuming certain foods, and on assuming the recumbent position)
- Dysphagia (15% to 20%, suggests stricture)
- Bronchospasm/asthma (15% to 20%)

DIAGNOSTIC APPROACH

Differential Diagnosis

- Ulcer disease (gastric or duodenal)
- Chemical or infectious esophagitis
- Crohn's disease of the esophagus
- Angina pectoris
- Achalasia
- Esophageal cancer

Associated Conditions: Dysphagia. Nocturnal aspiration may occur and be mistaken for asthma.

Workup and Evaluation

Laboratory: No evaluation indicated.

Imaging: Barium swallow may demonstrate hiatal hernia or esophageal narrowing. For patients who are pregnant, this should be reserved for after completion of the pregnancy.

Special Tests: Upper gastrointestinal endoscopy eliminates other potential causes of gastroesophageal reflux disease that include esophageal motility disorders, erosive esophagitis, and peptic ulcer disease (gastric or duodenal).

Diagnostic Procedures: History (>80% accurate), physical examination, endoscopy, barium swallow.

Pathologic Findings

Acute inflammatory changes and hyperplasia of the basal layers of epithelium (85%). Squamous metaplasia of the lower esophagus may occur with chronic exposure to reflux acid (Barrett's syndrome), which may undergo dysplasia or malignant change.

MANAGEMENT AND THERAPY

Nonpharmacologic

General Measures: Dietary changes, elevation of the head of the bed, smoking cessation, alcohol in moderation only, weight loss, antacids. (Antacids that coat [liquids], and those that tend to float on the surface of the stomach contents, such as Gaviscon, give better heartburn relief than other agents.).

Specific Measures: Eliminate medications that contribute to reduced esophageal pressure, such as diazepam and calcium channel blockers, or that may damage the esophagus (nonsteroidal anti-inflammatory drugs [NSAIDs]). Use acid-blocking therapy.

Diet: Avoid eating spicy or acidic meals, chocolate, onions, garlic, peppermint, and large meals before bedtime.

Activity: No restriction.

Patient Education: Reassurance, diet counseling, behavior modification.

Drug(s) of Choice

Antacids.

Histamine H_2-antagonists (cimetidine 800 mg two times daily, ranitidine 400 mg four times daily, famotidine 20 mg two times daily, or nizatidine 150 mg two times daily).

Hydrogen potassium pump blocker (omeprazole 20 to 40 mg daily for 4 to 8 weeks, esomeprazole 20 to 40 mg daily for 4 to 8 weeks, or pantoprazole 40 mg daily for 8 weeks).

Cisapride (10 to 20 mg four times daily, before meals, and every night).

Misoprostol (Cytotec, 100 to 200 micrograms PO four times daily) if mucosal injury is documented or suspected.

Contraindications: Known or suspected hypersensitivity. Misoprostol is contraindicated during pregnancy and lactation.

Precautions: Because of a lack of long-term follow-up, hydrogen pump inhibitors may be taken only for 8 to 12 weeks.

Interactions: Multiple drug interactions are possible with agents such as cimetidine; check full prescribing information.

Alternative Drugs

Bethanechol, antiemetics, phenobarbital if necessary.

FOLLOW-UP

Patient Monitoring: Normal health maintenance

Prevention/Avoidance: Reduction of modifiable risk factors (e.g., smoking, weight loss, diet).

Possible Complications: Esophageal stricture, bleeding. Prolonged exposure of acid to the esophagus may lead to stricture formation and dysphagia. Epithelial changes

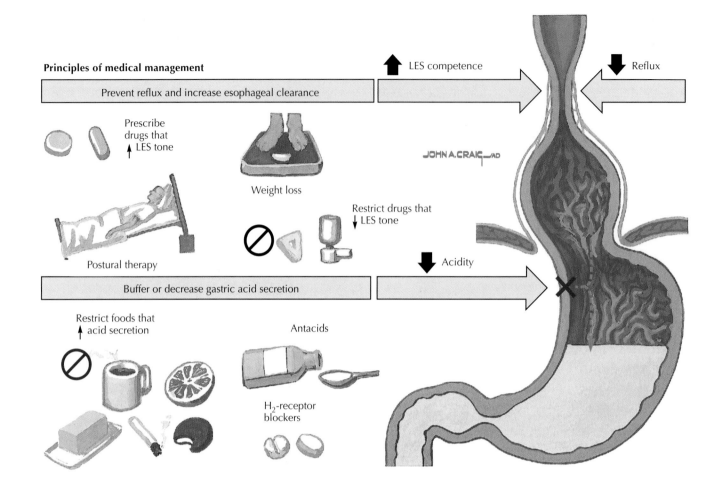

Principles of medical management

LES competence

Reflux

Prevent reflux and increase esophageal clearance

Prescribe drugs that ↑ LES tone

Weight loss

Restrict drugs that ↓ LES tone

Postural therapy

Acidity

Buffer or decrease gastric acid secretion

Restrict foods that ↑ acid secretion

Antacids

H₂-receptor blockers

JOHN A. CRAIG—AD

---

induced in the lower esophagus are also associated with an increased risk of esophageal cancer.

Expected Outcome: Generally good symptomatic relief, but long-term therapy is often required.

MISCELLANEOUS

Pregnancy Considerations: No effect on pregnancy, although may worsen during pregnancy because of reduced esophageal tone and increased intra-abdominal pressure caused by the expanding uterus.

ICD-9-CM Codes: 530.11.

REFERENCES

Level II
Chang AB, Lasserson TJ, Kiljander TO, et al: Systematic review and meta-analysis of randomised controlled trials of gastro-oesophageal reflux interventions for chronic cough associated with gastro-oesophageal reflux. BMJ 2006;332(7532):11. Epub 2005 Dec 5.

Qadeer MA, Phillips CO, Lopez AR, et al: Proton pump inhibitor therapy for suspected GERD-related chronic laryngitis: a meta-analysis of randomized controlled trials. Am J Gastroenterol 2006;101:2646. Epub 2006 Oct 13.

Ulualp SO, Roland PS, Toohill RJ, Shaker R: Prevalence of gastro-esophagopharyngeal acid reflux events: an evidence-based systematic review. Am J Otolaryngol 2005;26:239.

Level III
DeVault KR, Castell DO: Guidelines for the diagnosis and treatment of gastroesophageal reflux disease. Arch Intern Med 1995; 155:2165.

Feldman M, Burton ME: Drug therapy: histamine2-receptor antagonists-standard therapy for acid-peptic disease. N Engl J Med 1990;323:1672, 1749.

Fennerty MB, Sampliner RE, Garewall HS: Barrett's oesophagus—cancer risk, biology and therapeutic management. Aliment Pharmacol Ther 1993;7:339.

Kahrilas PJ: Gastroesophageal reflux disease. JAMA 1996;276:983.

Kahrilas PJ, Lee TJ: Pathophysiology of gastroesophageal reflux disease. Thorac Surg Clin 2005;15:323.

Locke GR 3rd: Current medical management of gastroesophageal reflux disease. Thorac Surg Clin 2005;15:369.

Moayyedi P, Talley NJ: Gastro-oesophageal reflux disease. Lancet 2006;367(9528):2086.

Nava-Ocampo AA, Velazquez-Armenta EY, Han JY, Koren G: Use of proton pump inhibitors during pregnancy and breastfeeding. Can Fam Physician 2006;52:853.

Rapkin AJ, Mayer EA: Gastroenterologic causes of chronic pelvic pain. Obstet Gynecol Clin North Am 1993;20:663.

Turcotte S, Duranceau A: Gastroesophageal reflux and cancer. Thorac Surg Clin 2005;15:341.

Hair Loss

INTRODUCTION

Description: Patients often experience hair loss in the early stages of pregnancy, in the immediate postpartum period, or in the postmenopausal years. For some this may be of sufficient volume to cause concern or cosmetic problems.

Prevalence: Of postmenopausal women, 37% have some hair loss. Loss of hair 1 to 2 months after delivery (telogen effluvium) is common.

Predominant Age: Older than 50 years.

Genetics: Androgenic alopecia follows autosomal dominance with incomplete penetrance.

ETIOLOGY AND PATHOGENESIS

Causes: Accelerated hair loss may come about any time there is an abrupt change in hormonal patterns and is the result of a higher number of hair follicles entering into the resting, or telogen, phase of hair growth. Hair follicles have cycles of growth (anagen), followed by a resting phase (telogen) of 3 to 9 months, and then resumption of normal growth. Alterations in hormones may induce an increased number of follicles to enter telogen. If this is the situation, the lost hair will be regained in time. Stress and some medications (anticoagulants, retinoids, beta blockers, chemotherapeutic agents) may also cause similar hair loss. The relative androgen dominance found in postmenopausal women not receiving hormone replacement therapy might also cause male pattern hair loss (temporal balding, androgenic alopecia).

Risk Factors: Pregnancy, delivery, hormonal contraception, scalp disease, family history of baldness, nutritional deprivation, drug or toxin exposure.

CLINICAL CHARACTERISTICS

Signs and Symptoms

- Hair loss
- Pruritus, scaling, and broken hairs (tinea)
- Tapered, easily removed hair near the edge of patches (alopecia areata)

DIAGNOSTIC APPROACH

Differential Diagnosis

- Telogen effluvium (as seen after pregnancy)
- Anagen effluvium (loss that includes growing hairs and may progress to complete baldness)
- Cicatricial alopecia (resulting from scarring)
- Androgenic alopecia
- Traction alopecia (trauma)
- Tinea capitis
- Drug, poison, or chemotherapy exposure
- Local infection or dermatitis
- Endocrinopathy (polycystic ovaries, adrenal hyperplasia, pituitary hyperplasia)

Associated Conditions: Alopecia areata, Down syndrome, vitiligo, and diabetes; traction alopecia; behavior aberrations.

Workup and Evaluation

Laboratory: No evaluation indicated except as dictated by specific differential diagnoses being considered.

Imaging: No imaging indicated.

Special Tests: Inspection of hair shafts, skin scraping for fungi.

Diagnostic Procedures: History, physical examination, inspection of hair shafts.

Pathologic Findings

If the base of the hair shaft is smooth, it came from natural (telogen) loss; if the base has the follicular bulb still attached (a white swelling at the end), the loss may be due to dermatologic or other disease conditions, and consultation is suggested.

MANAGEMENT AND THERAPY

Nonpharmacologic

General Measures: Evaluation, reassurance often is all that is required (telogen effluvium is self-limited).

Specific Measures: Based on cause, most are self-limited or reverse with correction of the underlying problem. For postmenopausal women, hormone replacement therapy often arrests or reverses hair loss.

Diet: No specific dietary changes indicated.

Activity: No restriction.

Patient Education: Reassurance and information about hair growth.

Drug(s) of Choice

For androgenic effluvium: topical minoxidil (Rogaine) 2% (approximately 40% response rate in 1 year).

For alopecia areata: high-potency topical steroids.

For tinea capitis: 6- to 8-week therapy with either griseofulvin (ultramicrosize) 250 to 375 mg PO daily or ketoconazole 200 mg PO daily and careful hand washing.

Contraindications: Griseofulvin is contraindicated in pregnant patients and in those with porphyria and hepatocellular failure. Ketoconazole and itraconazole should not be used concomitantly with cisapride (Propulsid).

Precautions: Topical minoxidil can cause eye irritation. Griseofulvin use is associated with the possibility of photosensitivity, lupus-like syndromes, oral thrush, and granulocytopenia. Ketoconazole and itraconazole may be associated with hepatotoxicity.

Interactions: Minoxidil may potentiate the actions of other antihypertensive agents. Griseofulvin can interact with both barbiturates and warfarin. Ketoconazole and itraconazole may interact with warfarin, histamine H_2 blockers, digoxin, isoniazid, rifampin, and phenytoin.

Alternative Drugs

Finasteride (Propecia) has been used for male pattern baldness in men, but it is ineffective for postmenopausal hair loss for women and is contraindicated during pregnancy.

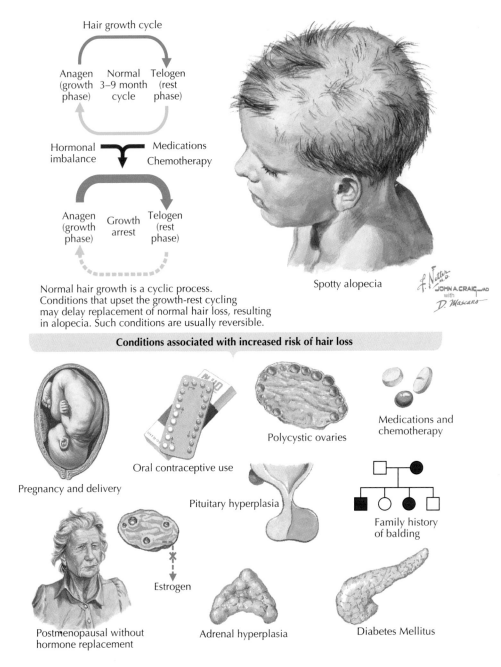

Hair growth cycle

Anagen (growth phase) — Normal 3–9 month cycle — Telogen (rest phase)

Hormonal imbalance   Medications Chemotherapy

Anagen (growth phase) — Growth arrest — Telogen (rest phase)

Normal hair growth is a cyclic process. Conditions that upset the growth-rest cycling may delay replacement of normal hair loss, resulting in alopecia. Such conditions are usually reversible.

Spotty alopecia

Conditions associated with increased risk of hair loss

Pregnancy and delivery

Oral contraceptive use

Polycystic ovaries

Medications and chemotherapy

Pituitary hyperplasia

Family history of balding

Postmenopausal without hormone replacement

Estrogen

Adrenal hyperplasia

Diabetes Mellitus

FOLLOW-UP

Patient Monitoring: Normal health maintenance. With ketoconazole and itraconazole periodic assessment of liver function is prudent.
Prevention/Avoidance: None.
Possible Complications: Social withdrawal.
Expected Outcome: Most hair loss is not permanent; a gradual return may be expected in 3 to 6 months after any causes have been eliminated. Only cicatricial alopecia is associated with permanent damage to the hair follicles.

MISCELLANEOUS

Pregnancy Considerations: No effect on pregnancy, although delivery is often the trigger for increased hair loss.

ICD-9-CM Codes: 704.02 (Telogen effluvium), 704.00 (Alopecia, unspecified), 704.01 (Alopecia areata), 704.09 (Other alopecias).

REFERENCES

Level III
Burke KE: Hair loss. What causes it and what can be done about it. Postgrad Med 1989;85:52.
Elewski BE: Clinical diagnosis of common scalp disorders. J Investig Dermatol Symp Proc 2005;10:190.
Hordinsky MK: Medical treatment of noncicatricial alopecia. Semin Cutan Med Surg 2006;25:51.
Hunt N, McHale S: The psychological impact of alopecia. BMJ 2005;331(7522):951.
Powell J, Stone N, Dawber RPR: An Atlas of Hair and Scalp Diseases (The Encyclopedia of Visual Medicine Series). Boston, Blackwell Scientific Publications, 2001.
Roberts WE: Dermatologic problems of older women. Dermatol Clin 2006;24:271, viii.

INTRODUCTION

Description: The tension headache is the most common form of headache. Tension headaches are caused by abnormal neuronal sensitivity and pain facilitation and/or contracted muscles of the neck and scalp. Cluster headaches are a type of recurrent headache characterized as unilateral and "stabbing" that are associated with symptoms of histamine release such as nasal stuffiness. These occur in episodic waves of frequent headaches separated by days, weeks, or years of remission. Migraine headaches are recurrent severe headaches that last 4 to 72 hours and are accompanied by neurologic, gastrointestinal, and autonomic changes. These may or may not be preceded by a characteristic aura.

Prevalence: Ninety percent of women experience tension headaches. Cluster headaches occur in 4 of 100,000 women per year. Migraine headaches affect 15% to 20% of women. Approximately 10% of tension headache sufferers also have migraine headaches.

Predominant Age: Tensions headaches—any age, 60% begin after age 20, rarely do they start after age 50. Cluster headaches—ages 20 to 30. Migraine headaches—ages 25 to 55 (peak 30 to 49), first attack generally between adolescence and 20.

Genetics: Women are more often affected by tension headaches than men (88% versus 69%); 40% have a family history of headache. Cluster headaches are four times more common in women than in men; migraines are three times more common in women. Of migraine sufferers, 89% have a family history of headache.

ETIOLOGY AND PATHOGENESIS

Causes: Tension headache—abnormal neuronal sensitivity and pain facilitation; no correlation to muscle contraction. They generally build in intensity in relation to stress. Cluster headache—unknown; postulated: disorders of histamine release or sensitivity, serotonin metabolism or transmission, hypothalamic circadian rhythm, or cerebral artery autoregulation. Migraine headache—unknown; postulated: genetically linked vascular disruption secondary to neurochemical change, serotonin or norepinephrine metabolism, or tachykinin abnormality. These alterations may result in distention of and inflammation of cranial blood vessels. A strong relationship with female sex hormones is suspected.

Risk Factors: Tension headache—physical or emotional stress, poor posture, depression, obstructive sleep apnea, excess caffeine. Cluster headache—allergies, alcohol, tobacco, nitroglycerine, high altitudes, sleep-cycle disruption, stress. Migraine headache—more common in upper-income patients (1.6 times), 60% to 70% of women note a link with menstruation (14% of women have migraine headaches only during menses). Precipitating factors: some foods, stress or stress relief (let down), missed meals, excessive sleep.

CLINICAL CHARACTERISTICS
Signs and Symptoms

Tension headache—dull, aching, and constant pain of mild to moderate intensity lasting from 30 minutes to 7 days, often located in the temples, around the head in a band, or up the back of the neck. It is rare, but some patients experience chronic tension-type headaches characterized by occurring 15 days/month for 6 months or longer.
- Pressing or tightening quality (nonpulsating)
- Bilateral symmetry
- Not aggravated by physical activity
- No nausea or vomiting, photophobia or phonophobia (may have one but not both)
- Teeth grinding common

Cluster headache—unilateral or orbital distribution (90% of headaches recur on the same side)
- Sharp, stabbing, or "ice pick" in character
- Symptoms of histamine release (nasal stuffiness and rhinorrhea, facial flushing, lacrimation, edema of eyelids)
- Symptoms are relieved when the patient is moving around
- Strong association with sleep
- Duration of less than 1 hour
- No aura or prodrome
- Annual recurrence common

Migraine headache—May be preceded by aura (20%)
- May begin with dull ache
- Unilateral pain (30% to 40%, may switch sides from attack to attack)
- Pulsating quality (60%), rapid onset
- Moderate to severe intensity
- Made worse by activity
- Frequently accompanied by nausea (90%), vomiting (60%), photophobia (80%), blurred vision, scalp tenderness and neck stiffness, restlessness, irritability, nasal congestion, facial edema
- Menstrual migraine is characterized by onset between 1 day before and 4 days after menstruation. (First day is most common.) This pattern is found in 15% of patients.

DIAGNOSTIC APPROACH
Differential Diagnosis

- Depression
- Cervical spondylosis
- Temporomandibular joint syndrome
- Analgesic dependency
- Anemia
- Medication or toxin exposure
- Dental disease
- Chronic sinusitis (cluster, migraine)
- Temporal arteritis
- Trigeminal neuralgia
- Pheochromocytoma

Associated Conditions: Tension headache has been associated with an increased risk of epilepsy (4-fold). Cluster headaches are associated with seasonal allergy. Migraine headache are associated with increased risk of peptic ulcer and coronary heart disease. Epilepsy, depression, anxiety, Raynaud's phenomenon, mitral valve prolapse, stroke (debated), motion sickness, and panic disorders are more common in patients with migraine headaches.

Workup and Evaluation

Laboratory: No evaluation indicated.
Imaging: No imaging indicated. (Computed tomography, electroencephalogram, and other evaluations are not indicated unless there is the new onset of headaches after age 50.)
Special Tests: None indicated.
Diagnostic Procedures: History.

Pathologic Findings

None.

MANAGEMENT AND THERAPY

Nonpharmacologic

General Measures: Tension headache—over-the-counter analgesics, rest, fluids, massage of shoulders, neck, or temples. Cluster headache—over-the-counter analgesics; rest; fluids; avoidance of alcohol, bright lights, and noise. Migraine headache—rest; fluids; analgesics; avoidance of alcohol, bright lights, and noise. Compression over the temporal artery may help. Biofeedback has been suggested but results vary.

Specific Measures: Nonsteroidal antiinflammatory drugs, stress reduction techniques, and biofeedback are indicated for tension headache. Prophylaxis is most effective for cluster headaches. Migraine headaches should be treated with medical therapy for acute attacks and prophylaxis against recurrent headaches.

Diet: No specific dietary changes indicated. (Caffeine restriction has been suggested.) Patients should avoid alcohol or food known to hasten attacks.

Activity: No restriction, avoidance of known precipitating activities. Improved general fitness and strengthening may reduce incidence. Bed rest for severe migraine attacks.

Patient Education: American College of Obstetricians and Gynecologists Patient Education Pamphlet AP124 (Headache).

Drug(s) of Choice

Tension headache—over-the-counter analgesics, nonsteroidal antiinflammatory drugs, antidepressants (when appropriate).

Cluster headache—prophylaxis: ergotamine (1 to 2 mg PO 2 hours before likely attack, e.g., sleep), verapamil (80 mg PO four times daily), lithium carbonate (Eskalith, 300 mg PO two to four times daily), methysergide (Sansert, 2 mg three or four times daily); acute attacks: oxygen (100%, 7 to 10 L/min via mask for 10 to 15

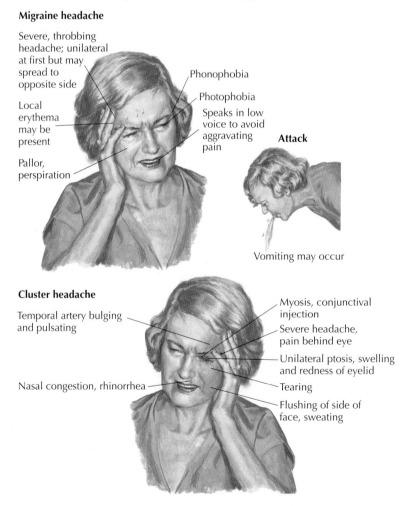

Migraine headache

Severe, throbbing headache; unilateral at first but may spread to opposite side

Local erythema may be present

Pallor, perspiration

Phonophobia

Photophobia

Speaks in low voice to avoid aggravating pain

Attack

Vomiting may occur

Cluster headache

Temporal artery bulging and pulsating

Nasal congestion, rhinorrhea

Myosis, conjunctival injection

Severe headache, pain behind eye

Unilateral ptosis, swelling and redness of eyelid

Tearing

Flushing of side of face, sweating

Muscle contraction headache

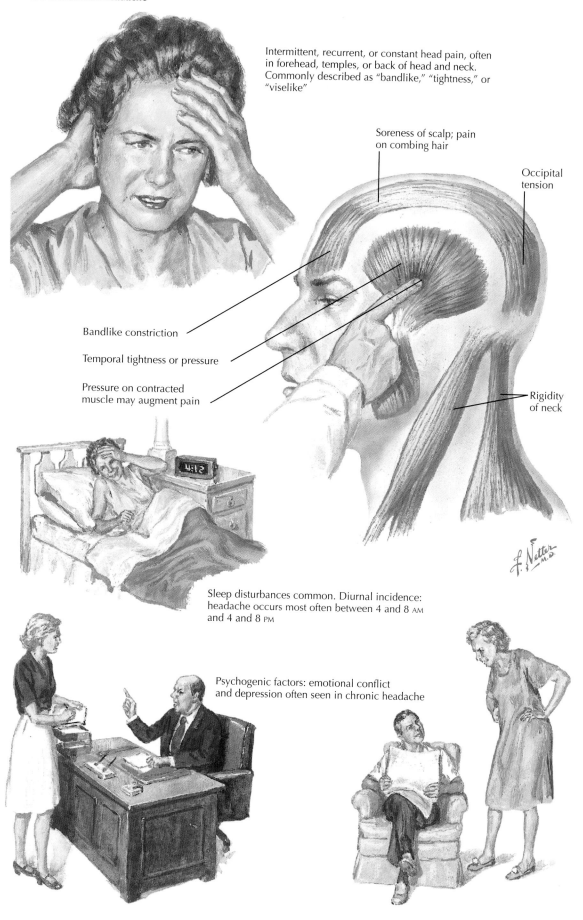

Intermittent, recurrent, or constant head pain, often in forehead, temples, or back of head and neck. Commonly described as "bandlike," "tightness," or "viselike"

Soreness of scalp; pain on combing hair

Occipital tension

Bandlike constriction

Temporal tightness or pressure

Pressure on contracted muscle may augment pain

Rigidity of neck

Sleep disturbances common. Diurnal incidence: headache occurs most often between 4 and 8 AM and 4 and 8 PM

Psychogenic factors: emotional conflict and depression often seen in chronic headache

Triggers of Migraine

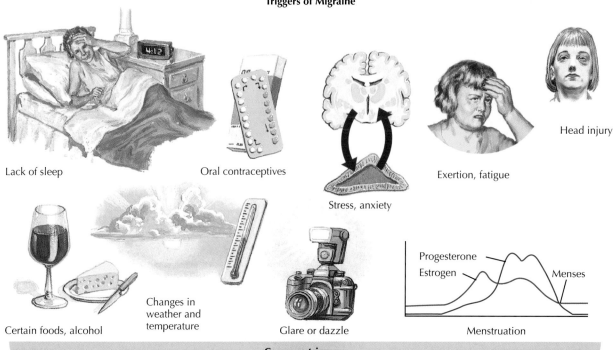

Lack of sleep

Oral contraceptives

Stress, anxiety

Exertion, fatigue

Head injury

Certain foods, alcohol

Changes in weather and temperature

Glare or dazzle

Progesterone
Estrogen
Menses
Menstruation

Common triggers

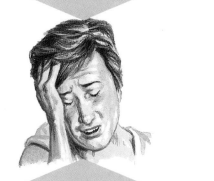

JOHN A. CRAIG—MD

C. Machado—M.D.

Common triggers

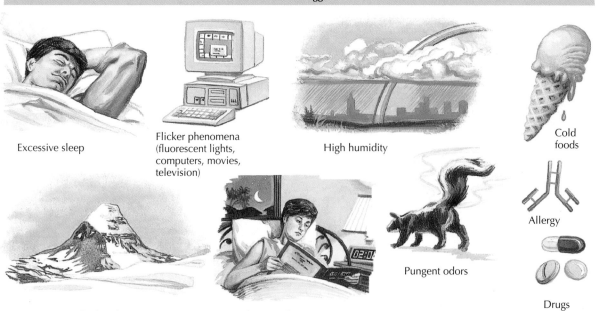

Excessive sleep

Flicker phenomena (fluorescent lights, computers, movies, television)

High humidity

Cold foods

Allergy

Drugs

High altitude

Reading or refractive errors

Pungent odors

minutes), sumatriptan (Imitrex, 6 mg SC or 100 mg PO, may repeat dose once in 24 hours when separated by at least 1 hour), dihydroergotamine mesylate (DHE 45, 1 mg IM or IV). Although the symptoms of cluster headaches are consistent with histamine release, treatment with antihistamines is ineffective.

Migraine headache: nonsteroidal antiinflammatory drugs (may provide relieve for some or may abort the headache if taken early in the attack), ergotamine preparations (ergotamine tartrate rectally at onset, may repeat in 1 hour or ergotamine tartrate 1 mg with caffeine 100 mg [Cafergot], 2 PO at onset, repeat every 30 min up to six per day, dihydroergotamine mesylate 1 mg IM or 2 to 3 mg intranasally at onset, 3 mg in 24 hours maximum), serotonin agonists (sumatriptan 6 mg SC or 100 mg PO or 5 to 20 mg intranasally at onset may repeat once in 24 hours with a minimum of 1 hour separation, naratriptan 1 to 2.5 mg PO, may repeat in 4 hours, 5 mg in 24 hours maximum, zolmitriptan 2.5 mg PO, may repeat in 2 hours, 10 mg in 24 hours maximum).

Contraindications: Aspirin-sensitive asthma, known or suspected sensitivity. See individual medications for others.

Precautions: Overuse of analgesics may lead to habituation and "analgesic rebound headaches" perpetuating the cycle of headache and analgesic use. Avoid the use of narcotic analgesics, especially oral agents in patients with cluster headaches; may convert attack to chronic form. Significant side effects are possible with most migraine therapy—see individual agents. Use vasoactive agents with care in patients with cardiovascular disease.

Alternative Drugs

Cluster headache—indomethacin 25 mg PO four times daily, nifedipine 40 to 120 mg/day.

Migraine headache—antiemetics and phenothiazines may abort migraine headaches or help to relieve associated symptoms. Metoclopramide may be used to reduce nausea. Narcotic analgesics may be used for patients who do not achieve relief with other measures or cannot take other agents.

FOLLOW-UP

Patient Monitoring: Normal health maintenance. Anticipate episodic recurrences for cluster and migraine headaches.

Prevention/Avoidance: Stress reduction, muscle strengthening and training, and biofeedback. For cluster headaches the prophylactic use of antihistamines should be considered during the times of year when the patient is most likely to have a recurrence. During the same period, alcoholic beverages and tobacco should be avoided because they may trigger an attack. These patients should also avoid sleep-cycle disruption. Patients who suffer from migraine headache should have adequate rest and fluids and avoid known triggers. Prophylactic medical therapy may be warranted for patients with two or more attacks per month. Prophylaxis may be attempted using beta blockers, divalproex, calcium antagonists, antidepressants, or serotonin antagonists.

Possible Complications: Headaches that are of sudden onset; begin after age 50; are dramatically different from past experience; have an accelerating pattern; are brought on by exertion, sexual activity, coughing, or sneezing; or are accompanied by focal neurologic signs are ominous and demand aggressive evaluation for possible intracranial or other pathologic cause. Patients with cluster or migraine headaches have an increased risk for peptic ulcers and gastrointestinal injury (from medications), caffeine dependence, coronary heart disease, and suicide.

Expected Outcome: Tension headaches generally resolve with rest and analgesics, although intermittent recurrence is common without lifestyle changes. Cluster headaches commonly have seasonal or annual recurrence patterns. Prolonged remission also is common. Migraines can generally be controlled, but recurrence is common. Severity and frequency tend to decline with age.

MISCELLANEOUS

Pregnancy Considerations: No effect on pregnancy. Pregnancy does not appear to affect the frequency of tension headaches. Cluster headaches are very rare in pregnancy. Migraine headaches may worsen in the first trimester of pregnancy and generally become less severe in the second and third trimesters. Pregnancy may alter medical therapy because of adverse effects of medications on the pregnant patient or fetus.

ICD-9-CM Codes: 307.81 (Tension headache), 346.2 (Cluster headache), 346.9 (Migraine), 346.0 (Classical migraine).

REFERENCES

Level I
Sulak P, Willis S, Kuehl T, et al: Headaches and oral contraceptives: impact of eliminating the standard 7-day placebo interval. Headache 2007;47:27.

Level II
Granella F, Sances G, Zanferrari C, et al: Migraine without aura and reproductive life events. A clinical epidemiologic study in 1300 women. Headache 1993;33:385.
Kudrow L: The relationship of headache frequency to hormone use in migraine. Headache 1975;15:36.
Loder E, Rizzoli P, Golub J: Hormonal management of migraine associated with menses and the menopause: a clinical review. Headache 2007;47:329.

Level III
American College of Obstetricians and Gynecologists: Use of hormonal contraception in women with coexisting medical conditions. ACOG Practice Bulletin 73. Washington, DC, ACOG, 2006.
APGO Educational Series on Women's Health Issues. Strategies for the Management of Headache. Washington, DC, APGO, 1998.
Brandes JL: The influence of estrogen on migraine: a systematic review. JAMA 2006;295:1824.
Cairns BE: The influence of gender and sex steroids on craniofacial nociception. Headache 2007;47:319.
Edelson RN: Menstrual migraine and other hormonal aspects of migraine. Headache 1985;25:376.
Headache Classification Committee of the International Headache Society: Classification and diagnostic criteria for headache disorders, cranial neuralgia, and facial pain. Cephalagia 1988;8:1.
Laube DW: Headache. In Ling FW, Laube DW, Nolan TE, et al., eds: Primary Care in Gynecology. Baltimore, Williams & Wilkins, 1996;87.
Loder EW: Menstrual migraine: pathophysiology, diagnosis, and impact. Headache 2006;46(Suppl 2):S55.
Silberstein SD: The role of sex hormones in headache. Neurology 1992;42:37.

INTRODUCTION

Description: Hematuria is the presence of blood, either microscopically or macroscopically, in the urine. Hematuria is a symptom only and requires further evaluation to establish a cause. Hematuria should be considered an indication of malignancy until proven otherwise.
Prevalence: Common in women.
Predominant Age: Any age, most common in reproductive years in association with urinary tract infections.
Genetics: No genetic pattern.

ETIOLOGY AND PATHOGENESIS

Causes: Disruption of the uroepithelium by infection, neoplasia (benign or malignant), or mechanical trauma (trauma, stone).
Risk Factors: Sexual activity, instrumentation, urinary tract infection, foreign body, or stone.

CLINICAL CHARACTERISTICS
Signs and Symptoms

* Painless (or otherwise) passage of blood in the urine

DIAGNOSTIC APPROACH
Differential Diagnosis

* Renal or bladder cancer
* Lower urinary tract infection (urethritis, cystitis)
* Pyelonephritis
* Urolithiasis
* Endometriosis involving the urinary tract
* Traumatic trigonitis
* Interstitial cystitis
* Coagulopathy (iatrogenic or natural)
* Contamination of the urine from another source (vaginal, rectal, anal, factitious)

Associated Conditions: Dysuria, urinary frequency, and urinary tract infections.

Workup and Evaluation

Laboratory: Urinalysis, urine culture and sensitivity (based on other symptoms present).
Imaging: Intravenous or retrograde pyelography. Renal ultrasonography may reveal dilation of the collecting system.
Special Tests: Cystoscopy may be necessary for selected patients. Urine should be collected and passed through a fine screen or mesh if a stone is suspected.
Diagnostic Procedures: History and physical examination, urinalysis.

Pathologic Findings

Based on cause.

MANAGEMENT AND THERAPY
Nonpharmacologic

General Measures: Evaluation, hydration.
Specific Measures: Based on the underlying cause; infection should be treated with appropriate antibiotics; stones and tumors require more extensive diagnosis and eventual removal (or passage).
Diet: Adequate fluid intake.
Activity: No restriction except those imposed by the causative process.
Patient Education: Reassurance; American College of Obstetricians and Gynecologists Patient Education Pamphlet AP050 (Urinary Tract Infections).

Drug(s) of Choice

Drug choice is based on cause.

FOLLOW-UP

Patient Monitoring: Normal health maintenance.
Prevention/Avoidance: None.
Possible Complications: Failure to diagnose a malignancy in a timely manner. With large-volume bleeding, clotting with urethral obstruction is theoretically possible.
Expected Outcome: For most patients, complete resolution of their symptoms occurs with appropriate treatment of the base problem.

MISCELLANEOUS

Pregnancy Considerations: No effect on pregnancy except that caused by the underlying condition.
ICD-9-CM Codes: 599.7.

REFERENCES

Level III
Ahmed Z, Lee J: Asymptomatic urinary abnormalities. Hematuria and proteinuria. Med Clin North Am 1977;81:641.
Ahn JH, Morey AF, McAninch JW: Workup and management of traumatic hematuria. Emerg Med Clin North Am 1988;16:145.
Cohen RA, Brown RS: Clinical practice. Microscopic hematuria. N Engl J Med 2003;348:2330.
Feld LG, Waz WR, Perez LM, Joseph DB: Hematuria. An integrated medical and surgical approach. Pediatr Clin N Am 1997;44:119.
Foresman WH, Messing EM: Bladder cancer: natural history, tumor markers, and early detection strategies. Semin Surg Oncol 1977;13:299.
Mahan JD, Turman MA, Mentser MI: Evaluation of hematuria, proteinuria, and hypertension in adolescents. Pediatr Clin North Am 1997;44:1573.
McCarthy JJ: Outpatient evaluation of hematuria: locating the source of bleeding. Postgrad Med 1997;101:125.
Pashos CL, Botteman MF, Laskin BL, Redaelli A: Bladder cancer: epidemiology, diagnosis, and management. Cancer Pract 2002;10:311.

Hematuria

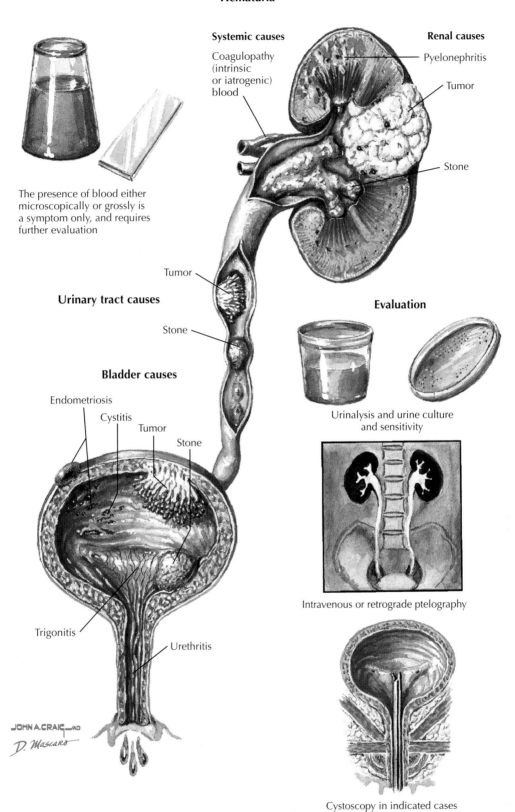

Systemic causes

Coagulopathy (intrinsic or iatrogenic) blood

Renal causes

Pyelonephritis

Tumor

Stone

The presence of blood either microscopically or grossly is a symptom only, and requires further evaluation

Tumor

Stone

Urinary tract causes

Bladder causes

Endometriosis

Cystitis

Tumor

Stone

Trigonitis

Urethritis

Evaluation

Urinalysis and urine culture and sensitivity

Intravenous or retrograde ptelography

Cystoscopy in indicated cases

Rodgers MA, Hempel S, Aho T, et al: Diagnostic tests used in the investigation of adult haematuria: a systematic review. BJU Int 2006;98:1154. Epub 2006 Jul 28.

Rosenstein D, McAninch JW: Urologic emergencies. Med Clin North Am 2004;88:495.

Tomson C, Porter T: Asymptomatic microscopic or dipstick haematuria in adults: which investigations or which patients? A review of the evidence. BJU Int 2002;90:185.

Wai CY, Miller DS: Urinary bladder cancer. Clin Obstet Gynecol 2002;45:844.

INTRODUCTION

Description: A hemorrhoid is a symptomatic dilation of the hemorrhoidal venous plexus resulting in perianal swelling, itching, pain, hematochezia, and fecal soiling.

Prevalence: Fifty percent to 80 percent of all Americans.

Predominant Age: Adult, more common after pregnancy.

Genetics: No genetic pattern.

ETIOLOGY AND PATHOGENESIS

Causes: Dilated rectal venous plexus with varying degrees of inflammation.

Risk Factors: Pregnancy, obesity, chronic cough, constipation, heavy lifting, sedentary work or lifestyle, hepatic disease, colon malignancy, portal hypertension, loss of muscle tone resulting from age, surgery, episiotomy, anal intercourse, or neurologic disease (multiple sclerosis).

CLINICAL CHARACTERISTICS

Signs and Symptoms

- Rectal bleeding
- Anal protrusion
- Anal itching and pain (especially with thrombosis or ulceration)
- Constipation and straining for bowel movement
- Rectal incontinence and soiling
- Hematochezia and stool mucus
- Anal fissure, infection, or ulceration
- Hemorrhoidal thrombosis

DIAGNOSTIC APPROACH

Differential Diagnosis

- Colon cancer
- Colon polyps
- Soiling caused by loss of anal tone (anal intercourse, multiple sclerosis, episiotomy)
- Pinworms
- Rectocele
- Fecal impaction
- Anal fissure or fistula

Associated Conditions: Liver disease, pregnancy, portal hypertension, and constipation.

Workup and Evaluation

Laboratory: No evaluation indicated.

Imaging: No imaging indicated.

Special Tests: None indicated.

Diagnostic Procedures: History and physical examination.

Pathologic Findings

Enlarged hemorrhoidal veins with stasis and inflammation are common.

MANAGEMENT AND THERAPY

Nonpharmacologic

General Measures: Stool softeners, bowel movement regulation, and topical medications.

Specific Measures: Surgical therapy is appropriate for those patients with debilitating symptoms or for whom medical therapy has failed (15% to 20% of patients). Banding of internal hemorrhoids is better accepted by patients than traditional surgical therapy. Hemorrhoidal banding requires a minimum of equipment and is well suited to the office or outpatient surgical setting. Some aching is generally experienced for several days after hemorrhoid banding procedures. Sitz baths and topical analgesics such as witch hazel are generally sufficient.

Diet: Increased dietary fiber.

Activity: Avoid prolonged sitting, straining, or heavy lifting. Encourage physical fitness.

Patient Education: Reassurance, diet instruction.

Drug(s) of Choice

Dietary fiber supplements.

Stool softeners—docusate sodium (Colace, Dialose, Sof-Lax) 50 to 300 mg PO daily (larger doses are generally divided over the day).

Topical analgesic sprays or ointments—benzocaine (Americaine, Hurricaine) 20% spray or gel, dibucaine (Nupercainal) 1% ointment.

Antipruritics and antiinflammatory agents—hydrocortisone (Anusol-HC, Analpram-HC, Cortenema, Cortifoam, Epifoam, Proctofoam-HC), pramoxine 1% (Fleet rectal pads, Analpram-HC), witch hazel 50% (Tucks pads or gel).

Astringents—Preparation H.

Contraindications to Surgical Therapy: Acquired immunodeficiency syndrome (AIDS) or immunocompromise, anorectal fissures, bleeding diathesis or blood dyscrasia, inflammatory bowel disease, portal hypertension, rectal prolapse, undiagnosed anorectal tumor, undiagnosed rectal bleeding.

Precautions: See individual agents.

Interactions: Docusate sodium may potentiate the hepatotoxicity of other drugs; see individual agents.

Alternative Drugs

Flavanoids have been advocated but a recent meta-analysis was unable to document efficacy.

FOLLOW-UP

Patient Monitoring: Normal health maintenance.

Prevention/Avoidance: Avoidance of constipation (bowel regularity); weight loss (if appropriate); physical fitness; avoidance of prolonged sitting, straining, or heavy lifting.

Possible Complications: Thrombosis, bleeding, secondary infection, ulceration, anemia, and rectal incontinence.

Expected Outcome: Resolution (spontaneous resolution or with medication), recurrence common.

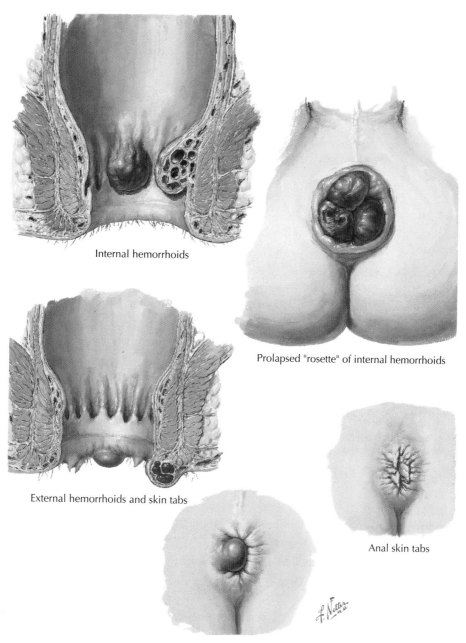

Internal hemorrhoids

Prolapsed "rosette" of internal hemorrhoids

External hemorrhoids and skin tabs

Anal skin tabs

Thrombosed external hemorrhoid

MISCELLANEOUS

Pregnancy Considerations: No effect on pregnancy. Hemorrhoids are extremely common as pregnancy progresses. Dietary prophylaxis and symptomatic therapy early reduce the severity of symptoms. At least partial resolution after delivery is expected.

ICD-9-CM Codes: 455.6, 455.3 (External), 455.0 (Internal), 455.7 (Thrombosed).

REFERENCES

Level II
Alonso-Coello P, Mills E, Heels-Ansdell D, et al: Fiber for the treatment of hemorrhoids complications: a systematic review and meta-analysis. Am J Gastroenterol 2006;101:181.

Alonso-Coello P, Zhou Q, Martinez-Zapata MJ, et al: Meta-analysis of flavonoids for the treatment of haemorrhoids. Br J Surg 2006;93:909.

Quijano CE, Abalos E: Conservative management of symptomatic and/or complicated haemorrhoids in pregnancy and the puerperium. Cochrane Database Syst Rev 2005;20(3):CD004077.

Level III
Bleday R, Pena JP, Rothenberger DA, et al: Symptomatic hemorrhoids: current incidence and complications of operative therapy. Dis Colon Rectum 1992;35:477.

Gearhart SL: Symptomatic hemorrhoids. Adv Surg 2004;38:167.

Mazier WP: Hemorrhoids, fissures, and pruritus ani. Surg Clin North Am 1994;74:1277.

Medich DS, Fazio VW: Hemorrhoids, anal fissure, and carcinoma of the colon, rectum, and anus during pregnancy. Surg Clin North Am 1995;75:77.

Nisar PJ, Scholefield JH: Managing haemorrhoids. BMJ 2003; 327(7419):847.

Parangi S, Levine D, Henry A, et al: Surgical gastrointestinal disorders during pregnancy. Am J Surg 2007;193:223.

Wald A: Constipation, diarrhea, and symptomatic hemorrhoids during pregnancy. Gastroenterol Clin North Am 2003;32:309, vii.

INTRODUCTION

Description: Hyperthyroidism is excess production of thyroid hormone. Hyperthyroidism is three times more common in women and may result in menstrual irregularity or fertility disturbances, or it may complicate pregnancy. It may occur because of Graves' autoimmune disease (most common) or toxic single or multinodular goiters. Rarely, trophoblastic tumors or dermoid cysts may be the cause.

Prevalence: One of 1000 women.

Predominant Age: 20 to 40 years.

Genetics: Graves' disease may follow a familial pattern.

ETIOLOGY AND PATHOGENESIS

Causes: Graves' disease—an autoimmune disease in which thyroid-stimulating immunoglobulins bind to thyroid-stimulating hormone (TSH) receptors mimicking the action of thyroid-stimulating hormone and causing excess secretion of triiodothyronine (T_3) and thyroxine (T_4). Goiter and exophthalmos are common. Toxic single or multinodular goiter—one or more autonomous benign nodules that slowly grow. Exophthalmos and myxedema are generally absent.

Risk Factors: Family history, other autoimmune disorders, and iodine deprivation followed by replacement.

CLINICAL CHARACTERISTICS

Signs and Symptoms

- Nervousness (85%)
- Palpitations, tachycardia (>100 beats/min) and dyspnea (75%)
- Heat intolerance (70%)
- Fatigue and weakness (60%)
- Weight loss (50%), increased appetite (40%)
- Palpable goiter (90%)
- Tremor (65%)
- Exophthalmos (35%)

DIAGNOSTIC APPROACH

Differential Diagnosis

- Physiologic changes of pregnancy
- Anxiety
- Malignancy
- Diabetes
- Pregnancy
- Menopause
- Pheochromocytoma
- Substance abuse (caffeine, diet preparations, cocaine)
- Struma ovarii

Associated Conditions: Other autoimmune diseases (Graves' disease).

Workup and Evaluation

Laboratory: Sensitive thyroid-stimulating hormone (below normal), T_3 radioimmunoassay (RIA) (>200 ng/

mL), T_4 radioimmunoassay (>160 nmol/L), free thyroxine index (>12).

Imaging: Radioiodine thyroid scan (diffuse uptake in Graves' disease; focal uptake in nodular goiter).

Special Tests: None indicated.

Diagnostic Procedures: History, physical examination, and laboratory studies.

Pathologic Findings

Graves' disease—diffuse hyperplasia; toxic nodules—discrete nodule formation.

MANAGEMENT AND THERAPY

Nonpharmacologic

General Measures: Evaluation, education about the need for continuing therapy, beta blockers for symptoms of tachycardia or tremor.

Specific Measures: Antithyroid medication, therapeutic radioiodine, surgical reduction of thyroid or excision of nodules.

Diet: No specific dietary changes indicated. Maintain adequate calories to avoid weight loss.

Activity: No restriction, as tolerated.

Patient Education: Education regarding need for compliance with medication and follow-up; American College of Obstetricians and Gynecologists Patient Education Pamphlet AP128 (Thyroid Disease).

Drug(s) of Choice

For thyrotoxic crisis—propylthiouracil (PTU) 15 to 20 mg PO every 4 hours during the first day in addition to other therapies.

Initial treatment: PTU 30 to 300 mg PO three times daily (no more than 300 mg/day during pregnancy), maintain at 25 to 300 mg PO two times daily, methimazole (Tapazole, MMI) 15 to 60 mg PO daily, maintain at 5 to 30 mg PO daily; radioiodine therapy: sodium iodine (I^{131}); adjunctive therapy: propranolol (Inderal) 40 to 240 mg PO daily.

Contraindications: Radioiodine therapy is contraindicated in pregnancy (may cause fetal hypothyroidism or malformation). Propranolol is contraindicated in the presence of congestive heart failure, asthma, chronic bronchitis, and hypoglycemia and during pregnancy.

Precautions: Both PTU and methimazole may cause agranulocytosis, dermatitis, or hepatotoxicity.

Interactions: PTU may potentiate the actions of anticoagulants.

Alternative Drugs

Ipodate sodium (Oragrafin) 0.5 g PO four times daily.

FOLLOW-UP

Patient Monitoring: Normal health maintenance, follow thyroid function test twice yearly. After radioiodine therapy, thyroid function should be checked at 6 and 12 weeks, 6 months, and then yearly.

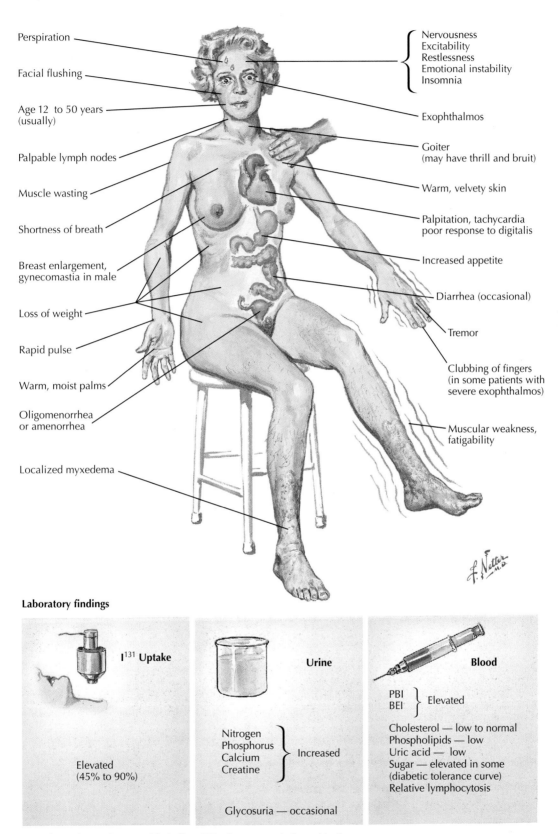

Perspiration

Facial flushing

Age 12 to 50 years
(usually)

Palpable lymph nodes

Muscle wasting

Shortness of breath

Breast enlargement,
gynecomastia in male

Loss of weight

Rapid pulse

Warm, moist palms

Oligomenorrhea
or amenorrhea

Localized myxedema

Nervousness
Excitability
Restlessness
Emotional instability
Insomnia

Exophthalmos

Goiter
(may have thrill and bruit)

Warm, velvety skin

Palpitation, tachycardia
poor response to digitalis

Increased appetite

Diarrhea (occasional)

Tremor

Clubbing of fingers
(in some patients with
severe exophthalmos)

Muscular weakness,
fatigability

Laboratory findings

I^{131} **Uptake**

Elevated
(45% to 90%)

Urine

Nitrogen
Phosphorus
Calcium
Creatine
Increased

Glycosuria — occasional

Blood

PBI
BEI
Elevated

Cholesterol — low to normal
Phospholipids — low
Uric acid — low
Sugar — elevated in some
(diabetic tolerance curve)
Relative lymphocytosis

BEI, plasma butanol-extractable iodine; PBI, plasma protein-bound iodine.

Prevention/Avoidance: None.

Possible Complications: Hypothyroidism after medical therapy, vision change or loss caused by ophthalmopathy, pretibial myxedema or cardiac failure, muscle wasting and proximal muscle weakness. Surgical therapy—hypoparathyroidism, recurrent laryngeal nerve damage, hypothyroidism.

Expected Outcome: With early diagnosis and adequate treatment, a good outcome is expected.

MISCELLANEOUS

Pregnancy Considerations: Difficult to diagnose in pregnancy. Increased risk of spontaneous abortion. Thyrotoxicosis often improves during pregnancy only to relapse postpartum—must be alert for this possibility. Any goiter is abnormal. Doses of PTU and methimazole must be reduced. Radioiodine therapy is contraindicated.

ICD-9-CM Codes: Based on cause.

REFERENCES

Level III

American College of Obstetricians and Gynecologists: Thyroid Disease in Pregnancy. ACOG Practice Bulletin 37. Washington, DC, ACOG, 2002.

Azizi F: The safety and efficacy of antithyroid drugs. Expert Opin Drug Saf 2006;5:107.

Casey BM, Leveno KJ: Thyroid disease in pregnancy. Obstet Gynecol 2006;108:1283.

Cooper DS: Hyperthyroidism. Lancet 2003;362(9382):459.

Cooper DS: Antithyroid drugs. N Engl J Med 2005;352:905.

Lao TT: Thyroid disorders in pregnancy. Curr Opin Obstet Gynecol 2005;17:123.

Lazarus JH: Thyroid dysfunction: reproduction and postpartum thyroiditis. Semin Reprod Med 2002;20:381.

Lazarus JH: Thyroid disorders associated with pregnancy: etiology, diagnosis, and management. Treat Endocrinol 2005;4:31.

McKeown NJ, Tews MC, Gossain VV, Shah SM: Hyperthyroidism. Emerg Med Clin North Am 2005;23:669, viii.

Mestman JH: Hyperthyroidism in pregnancy. Best Pract Res Clin Endocrinol Metab 2004;18:267.

Nayak B, Burman K: Thyrotoxicosis and thyroid storm. Endocrinol Metab Clin North Am 2006;35:663, vii.

Pearce EN, Farwell AP, Braverman LE: Thyroiditis. N Engl J Med 2003 Jun 26;348(26):2646. Erratum in: N Engl J Med 2003 Aug 7;349(6):620.

Redmond GP: Thyroid dysfunction and women's reproductive health. Thyroid 2004;14(Suppl 1):S5.

Schindler AE: Thyroid function and postmenopause. Gynecol Endocrinol 2003;17:79.

Soldin OP: Thyroid function testing in pregnancy and thyroid disease: trimester-specific reference intervals. Ther Drug Monit 2006; 28:8.

Stagnaro-Green A: Postpartum thyroiditis. Best Pract Res Clin Endocrinol Metab 2004;18:303.

INTRODUCTION

Description: Reduced or inadequate circulating levels of thyroid hormone. Women are 5 to 10 times more likely than men to suffer from hypothyroidism. Menstrual disturbances may be the first indication of this abnormality. Some women develop a transient (3 to 4 months) hypothyroid state (painless subacute thyroiditis) after giving birth.

Prevalence: Five to 10 of 1000 general population, 6% to 10% of women older than age 65.

Predominant Age: Older than age 40.

Genetics: No genetic pattern for idiopathic type, may be associated with type II autoimmune polyglandular syndrome (*HLA-DR3, HLA-DR4*).

ETIOLOGY AND PATHOGENESIS

Causes: Idiopathic or autoimmune (most common when goiter is present)—after ablative medical or surgical therapy. Postpartum thyroiditis (silent)—abnormalities of thyroid-stimulating hormone (TSH) or thyrotropin-releasing hormone (TRH) production or release.

Risk Factors: Age, other autoimmune disease, ablative therapy, pituitary failure.

CLINICAL CHARACTERISTICS

Signs and Symptoms

- Weakness, lethargy, fatigue
- Cold intolerance, hypothermia
- Menstrual disturbances (dysfunctional bleeding, amenorrhea, menorrhagia)
- Decreased memory, hearing loss
- Constipation
- Dry, coarse skin, brittle hair
- Periorbital puffiness, swelling of hands and feet
- Bradycardia, narrowed pulse pressure
- Anemia
- Cardiomegaly, pericardial effusion

DIAGNOSTIC APPROACH

Differential Diagnosis

- Depression
- Congestive heart failure
- Dementia
- Amyloidosis
- Nephrotic syndrome
- Chronic nephritis

Associated Conditions: Anemia, bipolar disorder, depression, diabetes mellitus, hypercholesterolemia, hyponatremia, idiopathic adrenocorticoid deficiency, mitral valve prolapse, myasthenia gravis, vitiligo.

Workup and Evaluation

Laboratory: Sensitive TSH (>4 micro IU/mL), triiodothyronine (T_3) resin uptake (increased), thyroxine (T_4) radioimmunoassay (decreased), free thyroxine index (low).

Imaging: No imaging indicated.

Special Tests: None indicated.

Diagnostic Procedures: History, physical examination, and laboratory studies.

Pathologic Findings

The thyroid may be small and atrophic, normal, or enlarged.

MANAGEMENT AND THERAPY

Nonpharmacologic

General Measures: Evaluation, education about need for continuing therapy.

Specific Measures: Thyroid replacement mediation.

Diet: High-bulk diet to avoid constipation.

Activity: No restriction.

Patient Education: Education regarding need for compliance with medication and follow-up; American College of Obstetricians and Gynecologists Patient Education Pamphlet AP128 (Thyroid Disease).

Drug(s) of Choice

Levothyroxine (Synthroid, Levothroid) 50 to 100 microgram PO daily, increase by 25 microgram/day every 4 to 6 weeks until TSH is in normal range.

Contraindications: Adrenocorticoid insufficiency (uncorrected), thyrotoxic heart disease.

Precautions: The initial dose should be reduced in elderly patients.

Interactions: The dose of insulin, oral hypoglycemics, and anticoagulants may need to be adjusted after thyroid therapy is initiated. Other possible interactions may be seen with oral contraceptives, estrogen and cholestyramine. Ferrous sulfate may decrease the absorption of thyroid replacement medications.

FOLLOW-UP

Patient Monitoring: Thyroid status should be checked every 6 weeks until stable, then every 6 months. Because of the prevalence of hypothyroidism in older women, a baseline assessment should be obtained at age 45 and periodic screening (biannually) is recommended in patients older than age 60.

Prevention/Avoidance: None.

Possible Complications: Life threatening—coma (myxedema coma) and hypothermia. (Treatment is with intravenous thyroid hormone replacement and steroid therapy. Supportive therapy [oxygen, assisted ventilation, fluid replacement] and intensive-care nursing may be indicated.) Others—treatment-induced congestive heart failure, increased susceptibility to infection, megacolon, organic psychosis with paranoia, infertility and amenorrhea, or osteoporosis resulting from overtreatment.

Expected Outcome: With treatment, return to normal function. Relapse will occur if therapy is discontinued.

Primary myxedema

Pituitary myxedema (differential features)

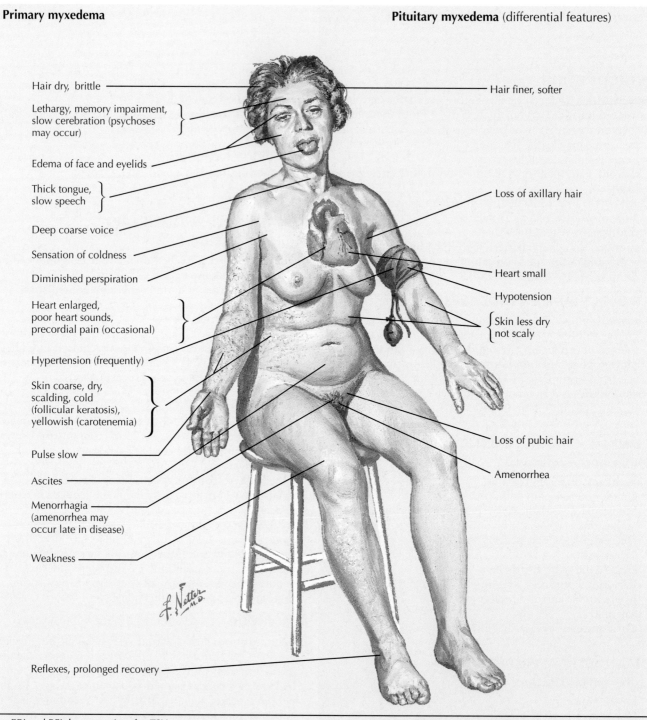

Hair dry, brittle

Lethargy, memory impairment, slow cerebration (psychoses may occur)

Edema of face and eyelids

Thick tongue, slow speech

Deep coarse voice

Sensation of coldness

Diminished perspiration

Heart enlarged, poor heart sounds, precordial pain (occasional)

Hypertension (frequently)

Skin coarse, dry, scalding, cold (follicular keratosis), yellowish (carotenemia)

Pulse slow

Ascites

Menorrhagia (amenorrhea may occur late in disease)

Weakness

Reflexes, prolonged recovery

Hair finer, softer

Loss of axillary hair

Heart small

Hypotension

Skin less dry not scaly

Loss of pubic hair

Amenorrhea

PBI and BEI; low – no rise after TSH	Low, but rise after TSH
I^{131}; 24-hour uptake low – no rise after TSH	Low, but rise after TSH
Cholesterol; elevated (usually)	Normal (usually)
Uric acid; elevated in males and postmenopausal females	Same
Urinary gonadotropins; positive	Absent
17-Ketosteroids; low	Lower

BEI, plasma butanol-extractable iodine; PBI, plasma protein-bound iodine. TSH, thyroid-stimulating hormone.

MISCELLANEOUS

Pregnancy Considerations: Medication may need to be adjusted. TSH levels should be checked monthly during the first trimester. TSH levels should be checked at 6 weeks postpartum. Women who develop postpartum thyroiditis have a 30% chance of developing hypothyroidism in the future. Any goiter during pregnancy is abnormal.

ICD-9-CM Codes: Based on cause.

REFERENCES

Level II

Grozinsky-Glasberg S, Fraser A, Nahshoni E, et al: Thyroxine-triiodothyronine combination therapy versus thyroxine monotherapy for clinical hypothyroidism: meta-analysis of randomized controlled trials. J Clin Endocrinol Metab 2006;91:2592.

Level III

American College of Obstetricians and Gynecologists: Thyroid Disease in Pregnancy. ACOG Practice Bulletin 37. Washington, DC, ACOG, 2002.

Bach-Huynh TG, Jonklaas J: Thyroid medications during pregnancy. Ther Drug Monit 2006;28:431.

Barzel US: Hypothyroidism: diagnosis and management. Clin Geriatr Med 1995;11:239.

Boelaert K, Franklyn JA: Thyroid hormone in health and disease. J Endocrinol 2005;187:1.

Casey BM: Subclinical hypothyroidism and pregnancy. Obstet Gynecol Surv 2006;61:415; quiz 423.

Casey BM, Leveno KJ: Thyroid disease in pregnancy. Obstet Gynecol 2006;108:1283.

Davis LE, Leveno KJ, Cunningham FG: Hypothyroidism complicating pregnancy. Obstet Gynecol 1988;72:108.

Hypothyroidism in the pregnant woman. Drug Ther Bull 2006;44:53.

Lao TT: Thyroid disorders in pregnancy. Curr Opin Obstet Gynecol 2005;17:123.

Lazarus JH: Thyroid disorders associated with pregnancy: etiology, diagnosis, and management. Treat Endocrinol 2005;4:31.

Lazarus JH, Premawardhana LD: Screening for thyroid disease in pregnancy. J Clin Pathol 2005;58:449.

Mandel SJ, Larsen PR, Seely EW, Brent GA: Increased need for thyroxine during pregnancy in women with primary hypothyroidism. N Engl J Med 1990;323:91.

Pearce EN, Farwell AP, Braverman LE. Thyroiditis. N Engl J Med 2003;348:2646. Erratum in: N Engl J Med. 2003;349:620.

Redmond GP: Thyroid dysfunction and women's reproductive health. Thyroid 2004;14(Suppl 1):S5.

Schindler AE: Thyroid function and postmenopause. Gynecol Endocrinol 2003;17:79.

Soldin OP: Thyroid function testing in pregnancy and thyroid disease: trimester-specific reference intervals. Ther Drug Monit 2006;28:8.

Wartofsky L, Van Nostrand D, Burman KD: Overt and "subclinical" hypothyroidism in women. Obstet Gynecol Surv 2006;61:535.

THE CHALLENGE

To assist couples who experience difficulty conceiving through normal means.

Scope of the Problem: The inability to conceive and bear children affects 8% to 18% of the American population. Under ordinary circumstances, 80% to 90% of normal couples conceive during 1 year of attempting pregnancy. Infertility is generally defined as failure to conceive after 1 year of regular, unprotected intercourse. Infertility may be further subdivided into primary and secondary types based on the patient's past reproductive history; patients with infertility who are nulligravid are in the primary infertility group; those who have achieved a pregnancy more than 1 year previously, regardless of the outcome of that pregnancy, are grouped in the secondary infertility group. Slightly more than one half of infertility patients fall into the primary group.

Objectives of Management: To establish the relevant cause or causes and develop strategies that result in conception and delivery. With improved understanding of the physiology of conception and a wide range of technologies that may be brought to bear to assist with procreation, 85% of "infertile" couples may be helped.

TACTICS

Relevant Pathophysiology: The male partner brings to the union sperm-laden semen, which is deposited in the vagina during intercourse. The average ejaculate has a volume of between 1 and 15 mL and contains more than 20 million spermatozoa. The survival of sperm in the female genital tract is thought to be at least 96 hours and may be as long as 8 days. However, it is probable that sperm are capable of fertilizing an egg for only the first 24 to 48 hours after ejaculation. The woman's gametic contribution, the oocyte, is released from the ovary during the mid-cycle process of ovulation, 14 days before the onset of menstruation, regardless of the total cycle length. Progesterone is produced by the luteinized follicle, producing a characteristic increase of between 0.5°F and 1°F in basal body temperature. The oocyte may be fertilized during the first 24 hours after ovulation only. Generally, fertilization takes place in the distal portion of the fallopian tube. Pregnancy does not result unless the zygote passes into the uterine cavity at the correct time (3 to 5 days after fertilization), encounters a receptive endometrium, and can successfully implant and grow.

Strategies: To achieve pregnancy, three critical elements must be in place: (1) a sperm must be available, (2) an egg must be available, and (3) the sperm and egg must meet at a time and place conducive to fertilization. It is the investigation of these three elements that constitutes the evaluation of the infertile couple.

Patient Education: Reassurance; American College of Obstetricians and Gynecologists Patient Education Booklet AP136 (Evaluating Infertility), AP137 (Treating Infertility).

IMPLEMENTATION

Special Considerations: While the evaluation of infertility proceeds, couples should be instructed to continue to attempt pregnancy through intercourse timed to the most fertile days of the cycle. Between one third and one half of all infertility problems may be diagnosed in the first phase of evaluation. The medical definition of infertility differs from that of fecundity, which refers to the physical ability of a woman to have children. Women with impaired fecundity include those who find it physically difficult or medically inadvisable to conceive and those who fail to conceive after 36 months of regular, unprotected intercourse. In short, fecundity deals with childbearing ability and fertility deals with childbearing performance. When dealing with the question of infertility, establishing the diagnosis is not the problem; the problem is identifying the underlying pathophysiologic causes. Unlike most areas of medicine, the provider must deal with two patients at the same time because it is the couple that is infertile, not the man or woman. When the relative frequency of causes is considered, it is apparent that male and female factors are present in roughly equal proportion, with a small remainder that are idiopathic. This is important to keep in mind during counseling. The distribution of causes is also helpful in designing a logical and efficient strategy for the evaluation of the infertile couple.

REFERENCES

Level III

Aitken RJ: Sperm function tests and fertility. Int J Androl 2006;29:69; discussion 105.

Al-Inany H: Female infertility. Clin Evid 2006;(15):2465.

American College of Obstetricians and Gynecologists: Management of Infertility Caused by Ovulatory Dysfunction. ACOG Practice Bulletin 34. Washington, DC, ACOG, 2002.

American College of Obstetricians and Gynecologists: Polycystic Ovary Syndrome. ACOG Practice Bulletin 41. Washington, DC, ACOG, 2002.

American College of Obstetricians and Gynecologists: Selective Estrogen Receptor Modulators. ACOG Practice Bulletin 39. Washington, DC, ACOG, 2002.

American College of Obstetricians and Gynecologists: Perinatal Risks Associated with Assisted Reproductive Technology. ACOG Committee Opinion 324. Washington, DC, ACOG, 2005.

Cheung AP: Assisted reproductive technology: both sides now. J Reprod Med 2006;51:283.

Grainger DA, Frazier LM, Rowland CA: Preconception care and treatment with assisted reproductive technologies. Matern Child Health J 2006;10(5 Suppl):S161.

Harrison EC, Taylor JS: IVF therapy for unexplained infertility. Am Fam Physician 2006;73:63.

Holzer H, Casper R, Tulandi T: A new era in ovulation induction. Fertil Steril 2006;85:277.

Homburg R: Clomiphene citrate—End of an era? A mini-review. Hum Reprod 2005;20:2043. Epub 2005 May 5.

Keefe DL, Parry JP: New approaches to assisted reproductive technologies. Semin Reprod Med 2005;23:301.

Lobo RA: Infertility. In Katz VL, Lentz GM, Lobo RA, Gershenson DM. Comprehensive Gynecology, 5th ed. Philadelphia, Mosby/Elsevier, 2007:p 1001.

Infertility

Ovulatory phase

Basal body temperature (BBT) detects signs of ovulation

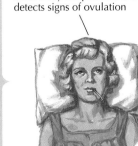

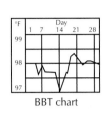

BBT chart

Preovulatory follicle

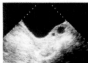

Ruptured follicle

Serial follicular ultrasound monitors follicular rupture

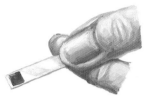

Ovulation detection kit detects urinary metabolites of luteinizing hormone (LH)

Luteal phase

Progesterone

Corpus luteum

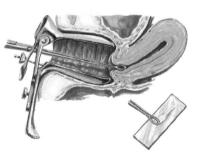

Spot urine test. Detects urinary metabolites of progesterone (measure of corpus luteum function)

Positive

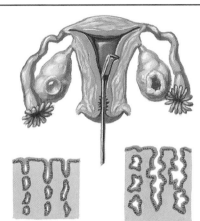

Endometrial biopsy and dating provides evidence of functioning corpus luteum and end organ response

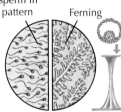

Proliferative phase

Secretory phase

Postcoital analysis

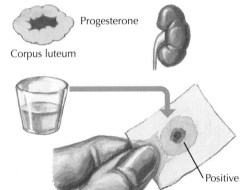

Postcoital mucus specimen from endocervical canal placed on slide for testing

Motile sperm in orderly pattern   Ferning

Optimal postcoital test. Adequate motile sperm and cervical mucus with high water content. Increased ferning and spinnbarkeit

Sluggish sperm in low numbers   Nonferning mucus

Suboptimal postcoital test. Few sluggish sperm in thick, cellular mucus. Decreased ferning and spinnbarkeit

Semen analysis

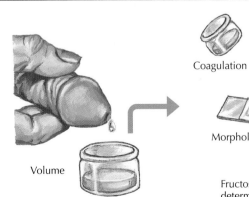

Volume

Coagulation   25–30 min   Liquefaction

Morphology/motility

JOHN A. CRAIG—AD

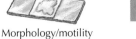

Fructose determination (if azospermic)

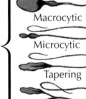

Normal

Macrocytic

Microcytic

Tapering

Bicephalic

Morphology

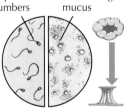

Maroulis GB, Koutlaki N: Preimplantation genetic diagnosis. Ann N Y Acad Sci 2006;1092:1001.

Messinis IE: Ovulation induction: a mini review. Hum Reprod 2005;20:2688. Epub 2005 Jul 8.

Mosher WD, Pratt WF: Fecundity and infertility in the United States, 1965–1988. Advance Data 1990;192:1.

Office of Technology Assessment: Infertility: Medical and Social Choices. Washington, DC, Congress of the United States, 1988:25.

Practice Committee of the American Society for Reproductive Medicine: Endometriosis and infertility. Fertil Steril 2006;86(5 Suppl):S156.

Practice Committee of the American Society for Reproductive Medicine: Smoking and infertility. Fertil Steril 2006;86(5 Suppl):S172.

Practice Committee of the American Society for Reproductive Medicine: Use of clomiphene citrate in women. Fertil Steril 2006;86(5 Suppl):S187.

Practice Committee of the American Society for Reproductive Medicine: Aging and infertility in women. Fertil Steril 2006;86(5 Suppl):S248.

Practice Committee of the American Society for Reproductive Medicine: Optimal evaluation of the infertile female. Fertil Steril 2006;86(5 Suppl):S264.

Reddy UM, Wapner RJ, Rebar RW, Tasca RJ: Infertility, assisted reproductive technology, and adverse pregnancy outcomes: executive summary of a National Institute of Child Health and Human Development workshop. Obstet Gynecol 2007;109:967.

Rowe T: Fertility and a woman's age. J Reprod Med 2006;51:157.

Setji TL, Brown AJ: Polycystic ovary syndrome: diagnosis and treatment. Am J Med 2007;120:128.

Trokoudes KM, Skordis N, Picolos MK: Infertility and thyroid disorders. Curr Opin Obstet Gynecol 2006;18:446.

Urman B, Yakin K: Ovulatory disorders and infertility. J Reprod Med 2006;51:267.

Van Voorhis BJ: Outcomes from assisted reproductive technology. Obstet Gynecol 2006;107:183.

Van Voorhis BJ: Clinical practice. In vitro fertilization. N Engl J Med 2007;356:379.

Wilson EE: Assisted reproductive technologies and multiple gestations. Clin Perinatol 2005;32:315, v.

INTRODUCTION

Description: A syndrome of intermittent abdominal pain, constipation, and diarrhea related to hypermotility of the gut.

Prevalence: First described in 1818 and accounts for 50% of all visits to gastroenterologists; 2.4 to 3.5 million physician visits per year and an estimated 2.2 million prescriptions. Despite the prevalence of irritable bowel syndrome (IBS), only approximately 25% of those with IBS seek care, and only 1% of those with IBS are referred to specialists or become chronic health care users.

Predominant Age: Young to middle age.

Genetics: No genetic pattern, 2 : 1 female : male ratio.

ETIOLOGY AND PATHOGENESIS

Causes: Colonic wall motility is altered in these patients, with evidence suggesting altered colonic wall sensitivity. Patients with IBS have altered motor reactivity to various stimuli, including meals, psychological stress, and balloon distention of the rectosigmoid, resulting in altered transit time, which in turn results in pain, constipation, and diarrhea. Studies of patients with and without IBS have shown that there are significantly higher levels of 5-hydroxytryptamine (5-HT) in those patients with IBS, supporting a possible causal role.

Risk Factors: None known; prior infectious gastroenteritis has been postulated as a risk factor.

CLINICAL CHARACTERISTICS

Signs and Symptoms

- Intermittent abdominal pain (often worse before menses)
- Bloating and nausea
- Alternating constipation and diarrhea

Symptoms are generally worse 1 to 1½ hours after meals, with 50% of patients experiencing pain that lasts for hours or days; pain may last for weeks in up to 20% of patients. Pain is generally worse with high-fat meals, stress, depression, or menstruation and is better after bowel movements. There are three common clinical variants: (1) "spastic colitis" characterized by chronic abdominal pain and constipation; (2) intermittent diarrhea, which is usually painless; and (3) a combination of both with alternating diarrhea and constipation (see box).

DIAGNOSTIC APPROACH

Differential Diagnosis

- Bacterial or parasitic infections
- Somatization
- Laxative abuse
- Iatrogenic diarrhea (dietary—e.g., tea, coffee, food poisoning)
- Ulcerative colitis or Crohn's disease
- Lactose intolerance
- Diverticular disease

Associated Conditions: High prevalence of psychopathologic conditions among IBS sufferers; a greater likelihood of somatization disorders, stress, anxiety disorders, depression, hysteria, and hypochondriases.

Workup and Evaluation

Laboratory: No evaluation indicated.

Imaging: No imaging indicated.

Special Tests: Flexible sigmoidoscopy or colonoscopy may be considered for selected patients.

Diagnostic Procedures: History and exclusion of other pathologic conditions.

Pathologic Findings

None.

MANAGEMENT AND THERAPY

Nonpharmacologic

General Measures: Because many of these patients have hysterical, depressive, and bipolar personality disorders, psychological support is important. In some studies, placebo response rates are as high as 80%.

Specific Measures: Mild sedation with phenobarbital and tranquilizers may offer some relief, although long-term success is generally poor.

Diet: Bulk agents and increased dietary fiber; reduction in alcohol, fat, caffeine, and sorbitol. Both fasting and probiotic diets have been suggested with variable results.

Activity: No restriction.

Patient Education: Diet (increased fiber) and stress management. Biofeedback and relaxation techniques may be of some help.

Drug(s) of Choice

Bulk-forming agents including Guar gum.

Emerging 5-HT$_3$ receptor-blocking agents, although two recently introduced agents (alosetron and tegaserod) have been withdrawn because of side effects. Melatonin has shown promise in some trials.

Contraindications: Bowel obstruction or fecal impaction, known or suspected allergy to agent or any component.

Precautions: Empiric therapy may be started during the process of evaluation but should not be continued indefinitely without the establishment of a diagnosis. Bulk-forming agents must be taken with adequate fluid intake to prevent obstruction and provide optimal effects.

FOLLOW-UP

Patient Monitoring: Normal health maintenance.

Prevention/Avoidance: High-fiber diet, stress reduction.

Possible Complications: Continued dependency on others; adverse effects of work, school, or home functions. Relapses are common.

Expected Outcome: Transient response is often good with most therapies. Long-term relapse is common.

MISCELLANEOUS

Pregnancy Considerations: No effect on pregnancy.

ICD-9-CM Codes: 564.1.

INTRODUCTION

Description: Pain located in the lower portion of the back (generally between the level of the iliac spines and the lower ribs) with radiation to the abdomen, pelvis, legs, or trunk. In women, gynecologic processes are often implicated (correctly or incorrectly) in this complaint. Low back pain is especially common during pregnancy.

Prevalence: Common (80% suffer some form of low back pain during their lifetime).

Predominant Age: 25 to 45 years.

Genetics: No genetic pattern.

ETIOLOGY AND PATHOGENESIS

Causes: Normal aging aggravated by trauma, injury, or pregnancy.

Risk Factors: Obesity, poor posture, improper lifting, age, sedentary lifestyle, osteoporosis, psychosocial factors (secondary gain), and trauma.

CLINICAL CHARACTERISTICS

Signs and Symptoms

- Pain and discomfort between the level of the iliac spines and the lower ribs, generally sudden in onset after an injury or gradually over the subsequent 24 hours
- Radiation of pain to buttocks or posterior thighs (stopping at the knees); referred pain, not radicular; back pain greater than leg pain
- Pain aggravated by back motion, lifting, coughing, straining, bending, or twisting; relieved by rest
- Normal sensory, motor, and reflex findings;, decreased range of motion

DIAGNOSTIC APPROACH

Differential Diagnosis

- Gynecologic disease (pregnancy, endometriosis, pelvic inflammatory disease)
- Gastrointestinal disease (duodenal ulcer, pancreatitis, irritable bowel syndrome, diverticulitis)
- Urinary tract disease (pyelonephritis, nephrolithiasis)
- Disc herniation or degenerative disease
- Osteoporotic fracture
- Fibromyalgia
- Spinal stenosis
- Spondylolisthesis
- Ankylosing spondylitis
- Arthritis (hip or back)
- Neoplasia (primary or metastatic)
- Fictitious complaint (somatization, secondary gain)

Associated Conditions: Chronic pain states (pelvic pain, headaches), radiculopathy, obesity, and psychosocial disease. Secondary gain often complicates both the diagnosis and treatment of low back pain. Warning signs of significant secondary gain include pending litigation or compensation, depression, hostility, and prolonged use of potent analgesics.

Workup and Evaluation

Laboratory: No evaluation indicated unless suggested by nonmechanical symptoms or atypical patterns of pain.

Imaging: Generally not required. When indicated (persistent pain, atypical symptoms)—anteroposterior, lateral, and spot films of L_5–S_1 area. Bone scan if tumor, trauma, or infection is suspected.

Special Tests: Computed tomography, magnetic resonance imaging, or myelography only for specific cause.

Diagnostic Procedures: History and physical examination (with special attention to the back and hips).

Pathologic Findings

Based on cause.

MANAGEMENT AND THERAPY

Nonpharmacologic

General Measures: Bed rest, short-term analgesics or anti-inflammatory agents, massage, or manipulation.

Specific Measures: Muscle relaxants, Williams' flexion exercises, physical therapy, topical low-level continuous heat therapy, transcutaneous electrical nerve stimulation (TENS).

Diet: No specific dietary changes indicated. Weight reduction, if appropriate.

Activity: Restricted activity for 3 to 6 weeks, then a gradual return to normal activity as tolerated. Patients should begin Williams' flexion exercises as prevention for future injuries.

Patient Education: Posture and activity counseling, home back exercises; American College of Obstetricians and Gynecologists Patient Education Pamphlet AP115 (Easing Back Pain During Pregnancy).

Drug(s) of Choice

Nonsteroidal anti-inflammatory drugs, muscle relaxants—cyclobenzaprine (Flexeril) 10 mg PO three times daily, diazepam (Valium) 5 to 10 mg PO two times daily.

Contraindications: See individual agents. Aspirin-sensitive asthma for most agents.

Precautions: See individual agents. Ulcer or renal disease for most agents.

Interactions: See individual agents.

FOLLOW-UP

Patient Monitoring: Normal health maintenance.

Prevention/Avoidance: Muscle-strengthening exercises, care in lifting, maintenance of reasonable weight. Avoid tasks that aggravate (heavy lifting, bending, twisting, sudden movements). Weight reduction, if appropriate.

Possible Complications: Chronic low back pain, pain medication dependence, and dependency state resulting from secondary gain.

Expected Outcome: Gradual improvement with analgesics, muscle relaxants, massage, and exercise (1 to 6 weeks).

Effects of lumbar hyperlordosis on spinal nerve roots

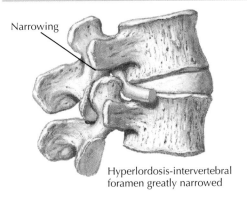
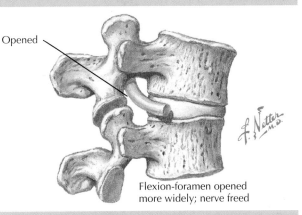

Narrowing

Opened

Hyperlordosis-intervertebral foramen greatly narrowed

Flexion-foramen opened more widely; nerve freed

Treatment of lumbar strain

Acute	**Chronic and prophylactic**
Absolute bed rest	Reduction of weight
Warm tub baths, heat pad, hydrocollator	Correction of posture
Sedation	Firm mattress, bed board
Firm mattress, bed board	Daily low back exercises
Diathermy, massage	Regular sports activity compatible
Local anesthetic infiltration to trigger zones	with age and physique
Occasionally corset, brace, or strapping	

Exercises for chronic lumbar strain (starting positions in outline)

1. Lie on back, arms on chest, knees bent. Press small of back firmly down to floor, tightening muscles of abdomen and buttocks, thus tilting pubis forward, exhale simultaneously. Hold for count of 10, relax and repeat

2. Lie on back, arms at sides, knees bent. Draw knees up and pull them firmly to chest with clasped hands several times. Relax and repeat. Also, repeat exercise using one leg at a time

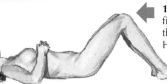

3. Lie on back, knees bent, arms folded on chest or at sides. Sit up using abdominal muscles and reach forward. Return slowly to starting position

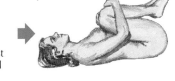

4. Begin in a runner's starting position (one leg extended, the other forward as shown, hands on floor). Press downward and forward several times, flexing front knee and bringing abdomen to thigh. Repeat with legs reversed

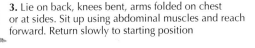

6. Sit on chair, hands folded in lap. Bend forward, bringing chin between knees. Return slowly to starting position while tensing abdominal muscles. Relax and repeat

5. Stand with hands on back of chair. Squat, straightening hollow of back. Return to starting position and repeat

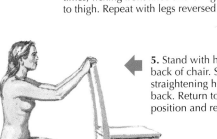
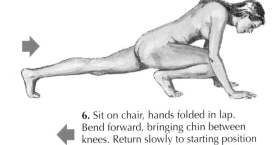

Exercises are best done on hard, padded surface like carpeted floor. Start slowly. Do each only once or twice a day, then progressively to 10 or more times within limits of comfort. Pain, but not mild discomfort, is indication to stop

MISCELLANEOUS

Pregnancy Considerations: No effect on pregnancy, although pregnancy (and the postural changes brought about by it) may worsen existing low back pain. Some relief is gained when the fetus descends into the pelvis in the last days of the gestation, but the sudden return to upright and the constant bending to care for a newborn make this improvement short-lived.

ICD-9-CM Codes: Based on cause.

REFERENCES

Level I

Donzelli S, Di Domenica E, Cova AM, et al: Two different techniques in the rehabilitation treatment of low back pain: a randomized controlled trial. Eura Medicophys 2006;42:205.

Gale GD, Rothbart PJ, Li Y: Infrared therapy for chronic low back pain: a randomized, controlled trial. Pain Res Manag 2006;11:193.

Goins ML, Wimberley DW, Yuan PS, et al: Nucleus pulposus replacement: an emerging technology. Spine J 2005;5(6 Suppl):317S-.

Katz J, Pennella-Vaughan J, Hetzel RD, et al: A randomized, placebo-controlled trial of bupropion sustained release in chronic low back pain. J Pain 2005;6:656.

Kovacs F, Abraira V, Santos S, et al; Spanish Back Pain Research Network: A comparison of two short education programs for improving low back pain-related disability in the elderly: a cluster randomized controlled trial. Spine 2007;32:1053.

Linde K, Witt CM, Streng A, et al: The impact of patient expectations on outcomes in four randomized controlled trials of acupuncture in patients with chronic pain. Pain 2007;128:264. Epub 2007 Jan 25.

Mayer JM, Mooney V, Matheson LN, et al: Continuous low-level heat wrap therapy for the prevention and early phase treatment of delayed-onset muscle soreness of the low back: a randomized controlled trial. Arch Phys Med Rehabil 2006;87:1310.

Mayer JM, Ralph L, Look M, et al: Treating acute low back pain with continuous low-level heat wrap therapy and/or exercise: a randomized controlled trial. Spine J 2005;5:395.

Tavafian SS, Jamshidi A, Mohammad K, Montazeri A: Low back pain education and short term quality of life: a randomized trial. BMC Musculoskelet Disord 2007 Feb 28;8:21.

Warke K, Al-Smadi J, Baxter D, et al: Efficacy of transcutaneous electrical nerve stimulation (TENS) for chronic low-back pain in a multiple sclerosis population: a randomized, placebo-controlled clinical trial. Clin J Pain 2006;22:812.

Ximenes A, Robles M, Sands G, Vinueza R: Valdecoxib is as efficacious as diclofenac in the treatment of acute low back pain. Clin J Pain 2007;23:244.

Level II

Allan L, Richarz U, Simpson K, Slappendel R: Transdermal fentanyl versus sustained release oral morphine in strong-opioid naive patients with chronic low back pain. Spine 2005;30:2484.

Demoulin C, Crielaard JM, Vanderthommen M: Spinal muscle evaluation in healthy individuals and low-back-pain patients: a literature review. Joint Bone Spine 2007;74:9–13. Epub 2006 Nov 13.

Farasyn A, Meeusen R: Validity of the new Backache Index (BAI) in patients with low back pain. Spine J 2006;6:565.

Katz JN: Lumbar disc disorders and low-back pain: socioeconomic factors and consequences. J Bone Joint Surg Am 2006;88(Suppl 2):21.

Rivero-Arias O, Gray A, Frost H, et al: Cost-utility analysis of physiotherapy treatment compared with physiotherapy advice in low back pain. Spine 2006;31:1381.

Level III

American Academy of Orthopedic Surgeons: Clinical Policy; Low Back Musculoligamentous Injury (Sprain/Strain). AAOS Bulletin 3638. Rosemont, Ill, AAOS, 1991.

American College of Obstetricians and Gynecologists: Chronic Pelvic Pain. ACOG Practice Bulletin 51. Washington, DC, ACOG, 2004.

International Association for the Study of Pain: Classification of chronic pain, descriptions of chronic pain syndromes and definitions of pain terms. Pain 1986;3(suppl):S1.

Shelerud RA: Epidemiology of occupational low back pain. Clin Occup Environ Med 2006;5:501, v.

Smith RP, Ling FW: Back examination. In Procedures in Women's Health Care. Baltimore, Williams & Wilkins, 1997:367.

Yelland MJ, Schluter PJ: Defining worthwhile and desired responses to treatment of chronic low back pain. Pain Med 2006;7:38.

INTRODUCTION

Description: Melanoma is the malignant degeneration of cells from the melanocytic (pigment) system. Although generally a skin lesion, melanomas may arise in any pigmented tissue (such as the eye). The vulva accounts for 5% to 10% of all malignant melanomas in women, despite containing only 1% of the skin surface.

Prevalence: Found in 4.5 of 100,000, 2007: 59,940 cases, 8110 deaths.

Predominant Age: 20 to 40 years (50% of patients).

Genetics: Familial dysplastic nevus syndrome (if history includes a family member with melanoma, lifetime risk is 100%).

ETIOLOGY AND PATHOGENESIS

Causes: Unknown, may be related to ultraviolet (A and B) light exposure.

Risk Factors: Previous dysplastic nevi, multiple pigmented lesions, fair complexion, freckling, blue eyes and blond hair, adolescent blistering sunburn (twofold increase in risk), family history of melanoma.

CLINICAL CHARACTERISTICS

Signs and Symptoms

- Asymptomatic
- Pigmented lesion with irregular border and variegation in color
- Bleeding, scaling, size, or texture change in any pigmented lesion (ABCDE mnemonic—**a**symmetry, **b**order irregularity, **c**olor variegation, **d**iameter 0.6 mm on back or lower leg [in whites] or hand, feet, and nails [in African Americans], **e**levation above the skin surface)

DIAGNOSTIC APPROACH

Differential Diagnosis

- Junctional nevus
- Dysplastic nevus
- Malignant melanoma (the risk of malignancy is greatest in nevi that are more than 5 mm in diameter, have irregular borders, are asymmetrical, or have variegated coloration)
- Pigmented basal or squamous cell carcinoma
- Seborrheic keratoses

Associated Conditions: Junctional nevus, dysplastic nevus.

Workup and Evaluation

Laboratory: No evaluation indicated.

Imaging: No imaging indicated, used only to evaluate metastases (brain, bone, lymph nodes).

Special Tests: Excisional biopsy for all vulvar nevi or suspicious nevi anywhere on the body. All lesions should be submitted for histologic examination; they never should be removed destructively.

Diagnostic Procedures: Physical examination and excisional biopsy.

Pathologic Findings

Superficial spreading melanoma (70% of cases), nodular (vertical growth, 15%), acral lentiginous (2% to 8%), lentigo maligna (4% to 10%).

MANAGEMENT AND THERAPY

Nonpharmacologic

General Measures: Evaluation, biopsy of suspicious lesions, instruction on prevention (use of sunscreen, avoidance of excessive exposure).

Specific Measures: Surgical excision with 1-cm margin for lesions, <2 mm thick, 3 cm for thicker lesions.

Diet: No specific dietary changes indicated.

Activity: Sun exposure reduction and protection.

Patient Education: Risks of sun exposure, use of sunscreen products, characteristics of suspicious lesions.

Drug(s) of Choice

Adjuvant therapy with bacillus Calmette-Guérin and levamisole plus dacarbazine.

Contraindications: See individual agents.

Precautions: See individual agents.

Interactions: See individual agents.

FOLLOW-UP

Patient Monitoring: Frequent (every 3 to 6 months) total body inspection for abnormal or changing nevi. Annual chest radiograph (6% of recurrences diagnosed this way). Weekly self-examination.

Prevention/Avoidance: Avoidance of excessive sun exposure, especially blistering sunburn. Sunscreen use.

Possible Complications: Disease progression or spread, cosmetic damage by excision.

Expected Outcome: Prognosis is based on staging—5-year survival if no local or distant spread, 70%; <0.85-mm thick, 95% to 100%; lymphatic involvement, 5%.

MISCELLANEOUS

Pregnancy Considerations: Although rarely seen in pregnancy, melanoma is exacerbated by this condition. Although any malignant metastasis to the fetus is rare, melanomas represent up to one third of all malignancies found. Melanoma is one of the few malignancies that spreads to the placenta, and metastatic melanoma is a threat to both the fetus and mother. If a woman has had melanoma, it is recommended that she wait 2 or more years before planning a pregnancy.

ICD-9-CM Codes: Based on location and severity of disease.

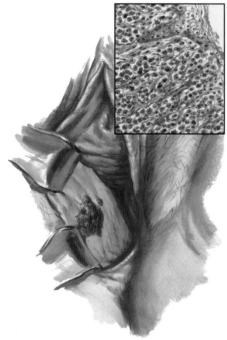

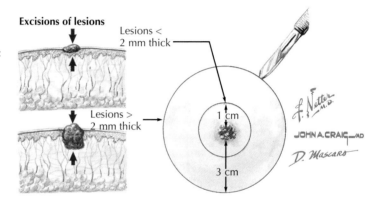

Risk factors
UVA and UVB
radiation

Family history of
melanoma or
dysplastic nevi

Blue eyes

Freckles

Blonde hair
and fair skin

Blistering
sunburn in
adolescence

Clinical considerations

Typical clinical appearance of melanoma
exhibiting features of "ABCDE" mnemonic
A) Asymmetry
B) Border irregularity
C) Color variegation
D) Diameter >6 mm
E) Elevation above skin surface

Wide excision of dysplastic nevi and suspected
melanomas is based on thickness of lesion—1 cm
border recommended for lesions less than 2 mm
thick, and 3 cm border for lesions greater than
2 mm thick

UV, ultraviolet.

Excisions of lesions

Lesions <
2 mm thick

Lesions >
2 mm thick

1 cm

3 cm

REFERENCES

Level II
Beyeler M, Dummer R: Cutaneous melanoma: uncommon presentations. Clin Dermatol 2005;23:587.

Chiu V, Won E, Malik M, Weinstock MA: The use of mole-mapping diagrams to increase skin self-examination accuracy. J Am Acad Dermatol 2006;55:245. Epub 2006 May 15.

Giblin AV, Thomas JM: Incidence, mortality and survival in cutaneous melanoma. J Plast Reconstr Aesthet Surg 2007;60:32. Epub 2006 Jul 7.

Gokaslan H, Sismanoglu A, Pekin T, et al: Primary malignant melanoma of the vagina: a case report and review of the current treatment options. Eur J Obstet Gynecol Reprod Biol 2005;121:243.

Lens M: Cutaneous melanoma: interferon alpha adjuvant therapy for patients at high risk for recurrent disease. Dermatol Ther 2006;19:9.

Level III
Berwick M, Wiggins C: The current epidemiology of cutaneous malignant melanoma. Front Biosci 2006;11:1244.

Bishop JN, Harland M, Bishop DT: The genetics of melanoma. Br J Hosp Med (Lond) 2006;67:299.

Bishop JN, Harland M, Randerson-Moor J, Bishop DT: Management of familial melanoma. Lancet Oncol 2007;8:46.

Driscoll MS, Grant-Kels JM: Nevi and melanoma in pregnancy. Dermatol Clin 2006;24:199, vi.

Dunton CJ, Kautzky M, Hanau C: Malignant melanoma of the vulva: a review. Obstet Gynecol Surv 1995;57:739.

Fecher LA, Cummings SD, Keefe MJ, Alani RM: Toward a molecular classification of melanoma. J Clin Oncol 2007;25:1606.

King DM: Imaging of metastatic melanoma. Cancer Imaging 2006;6:204.

Menzies SW: Cutaneous melanoma: making a clinical diagnosis, present and future. Dermatol Ther 2006;19:32.

Niendorf KB, Tsao H: Cutaneous melanoma: family screening and genetic testing. Dermatol Ther 2006;19:1.

NIH Consensus Development Panel on Early Melanoma: Diagnosis and treatment of early melanoma. JAMA 1992;268:1314.

Patrick RJ, Fenske NA, Messina JL: Primary mucosal melanoma. J Am Acad Dermatol 2007;56:828. Epub 2007 Mar 8.

Rager EL, Bridgeford EP, Ollila DW: Cutaneous melanoma: update on prevention, screening, diagnosis, and treatment. Am Fam Physician 2005;72:269.

Rouzier R, Haddad B, Atallah D, et al: Surgery for vulvar cancer. Clin Obstet Gynecol 2005;48:869.

Tarhini AA, Agarwala SS: Cutaneous melanoma: available therapy for metastatic disease. Dermatol Ther 2006;19:19.

Wiggins CL, Berwick M, Bishop JA: Malignant melanoma in pregnancy. Obstet Gynecol Clin North Am 2005;32:559.

Myofascial Syndromes

INTRODUCTION

Description: Myofascial syndrome is characterized by muscular and fascial pain associated with localized tenderness and pain referred to sites that are often remote. Myofascial pain syndromes and fibromyalgia frequently demonstrate trigger-point involvement. These syndromes may present as chronic lower abdominal or pelvic pain that is easily confused with gynecologic causes.

Prevalence: Three percent of the population.

Predominant Age: Sedentary middle-aged women.

Genetics: No genetic pattern. More common in women (80% to 90%). Several studies indicate that women who have a family member with fibromyalgia are more likely to have fibromyalgia themselves.

ETIOLOGY AND PATHOGENESIS

Causes: Abnormal spasm of a small portion of a muscle resulting in an extremely taut, tender band of muscle (trigger point). Compression of this site elicits local tenderness and often reproduces the referred pain. Most trigger points are located at or near areas of moving or sliding muscle surfaces, although they are not limited to these locations. Genetics and physical and emotional stressors are possible contributory factors to the development of the illness.

Risk Factors: Stress, sleep deprivation, trauma, depression, and weather changes.

CLINICAL CHARACTERISTICS

Signs and Symptoms

- Chronic pain referred to remote sites.
- "Trigger points" (hypersensitive areas overlying muscles that induce spasm and pain) that induce or reproduce the patient's symptoms. (Trigger points may be found throughout the body but are most common in the abdominal wall, back, and pelvic floor when pelvic pain is the symptom.) Most patients have 11 or more trigger points.
- Pain is worse in the morning, with stress or weather change, after nonrestorative sleep. Pain is better with activity, stress reduction, and rest.
- Two criteria established by the American College of Rheumatology: a history of widespread pain lasting more than 3 months and the presence of tender points.

DIAGNOSTIC APPROACH

Differential Diagnosis

- Somatization
- Sympathetic dystrophy
- Muscle strain or sprain
- Polymyalgia rheumatica
- Temporal arteritis
- Irritable bowel syndrome (IBS)
- Low back strain or sprain

Associated Conditions: Chronic pain syndromes, irritable bowel syndrome, depression, reduced physical endurance, and social withdrawal.

Workup and Evaluation

Laboratory: No evaluation indicated. Screening with an erythrocyte sedimentation rate (normal) may be helpful. Others based on diagnosis being considered.

Imaging: No imaging indicated.

Special Tests: None indicated.

Diagnostic Procedures: History and physical examination generally sufficient.

Pathologic Findings

A trigger point is often felt as an extremely taut band of muscle. (Normal muscle should not be tender to firm compression and does not contain taut bands.)

MANAGEMENT AND THERAPY

Nonpharmacologic

General Measures: Evaluation, analgesics, heat (low-level continuous topical heat [ThermaCare], hot packs, ultrasound therapy), and general conditioning exercises.

Specific Measures: Transcutaneous electrical nerve stimulation (TENS), trigger-point injections. A 22-gauge needle is selected for trigger-point injection because of the amount of movement within tissue often required to probe for and block a taut muscle bundle. Thinner needles may bend or break under these circumstances. The length of the needle should be sufficient to allow the entire trigger point to be reached without indenting the skin or having the hub at the skin surface. Superficial trigger points may also be treated with a "spray-and-stretch" technique. (The area overlying the trigger point is sprayed with a coolant or freezing spray [e.g., ethyl chloride] for several seconds, and the muscle is forcibly stretched by passive extension.) Hypnosis may also be used.

Diet: No specific dietary changes indicated.

Activity: No restriction except that caused by pain.

Patient Education: American College of Obstetricians and Gynecologists Patient Education Pamphlet AP099 (Pelvic Pain).

Drug(s) of Choice

Nonsteroidal anti-inflammatory drugs (NSAIDs).

Sleep aids—flurazepam (Dalmane) 15 mg PO every night, triazolam (Halcion) 0.125 mg PO every night, amitriptyline (Elavil) 20 to 25 mg PO every night.

Muscle relaxants—cyclobenzaprine (Flexeril) 10 mg PO three times a day.

Local anesthetic for injection (generally 1% lidocaine without epinephrine, limit injection to approximately 10 mL/site).

Emerging: Adjuvant therapy with gabapentin and 5-HT$_3$ receptor-blocking agents has been advocated in some studies.

Myofascial Syndromes

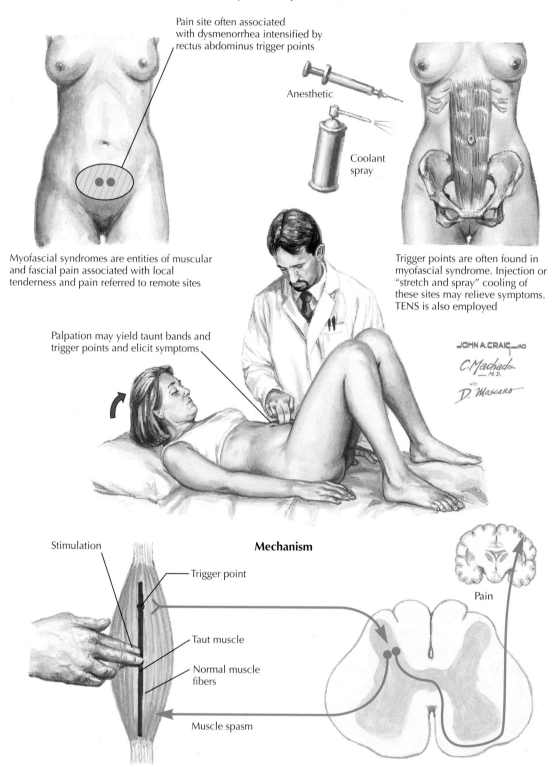

Pain site often associated with dysmenorrhea intensified by rectus abdominus trigger points

Anesthetic

Coolant spray

Myofascial syndromes are entities of muscular and fascial pain associated with local tenderness and pain referred to remote sites

Trigger points are often found in myofascial syndrome. Injection or "stretch and spray" cooling of these sites may relieve symptoms. TENS is also employed

Palpation may yield taut bands and trigger points and elicit symptoms

JOHN A. CRAIG—AD
C. Machado—M.D.
with
D. Mascaro

Mechanism

Stimulation

Trigger point

Taut muscle

Normal muscle fibers

Muscle spasm

Pain

Symptoms cause abnormal spasm of small portion of muscle, resulting in extremely taut, tender band of muscle (trigger point). Compression of this site elicits local tenderness and often produces referred pain

Contraindications: See individual agents. Trigger-point injections should not be attempted when infection is present near the planned site.

Precautions: Watch for side effects or dependence.

Alternative Drugs

Trazodone (Desyrel) 50 mg PO every night.

FOLLOW-UP

Patient Monitoring: Normal health maintenance, monitor for medication side effects.

Prevention/Avoidance: Adequate restorative sleep, stress reduction, physical fitness, and activity.

Possible Complications: Depression, reduced physical endurance, social withdrawal, chronic pain, work compromise or absence. The most common complications of trigger-point injection are local ecchymoses and anesthetic agent toxicity. The latter is best avoided by strictly limiting the total dose given. Infection is rare if the skin is first disinfected and areas of frank infection are avoided.

Expected Outcome: Improvement with medical therapy generally is seen in 2 to 4 weeks. With the identification of a specific trigger point and the use of trigger point injection, results should be good. (Response to trigger point injection routinely persists longer than the duration of action of the anesthetic agent used. This frequently extends to permanent relief after only one or two injections.)

MISCELLANEOUS

Pregnancy Considerations: No effect on pregnancy. Pregnancy may limit some therapies. Pregnancy is generally not a contraindication to trigger-point injections.

ICD-9-CM Codes: Based on type and location.

REFERENCES

Level I

Garvey TA, Marks MR, Wiesel SW: A prospective, randomized, double-blind evaluation of trigger-point injection therapy for low-back pain. Spine 1989;14:962.

Gobel H, Heinze A, Reichel G, et al; Dysport Myofascial Pain Study Group: Efficacy and safety of a single botulinum type A toxin complex treatment (Dysport) for the relief of upper back myofascial pain syndrome: results from a randomized double-blind placebo-controlled multicentre study. Pain 2006;125:82. Epub 2006 Jun 5.

Graboski CL, Gray DS, Burnham RS: Botulinum toxin A versus bupivacaine trigger point injections for the treatment of myofascial pain syndrome: a randomised double blind crossover study. Pain 2005;118:170. Epub 2005 Oct 3.

Kamanli A, Kaya A, Ardicoglu O, et al: Comparison of lidocaine injection, botulinum toxin injection, and dry needling to trigger points in myofascial pain syndrome. Rheumatol Int 2005;25:604. Epub 2004 Sep 15.

Level III

American College of Obstetricians and Gynecologists: Chronic pelvic pain. ACOG Practice Bulletin 51. Washington, DC, ACOG, 2004.

Borg-Stein J: Treatment of fibromyalgia, myofascial pain, and related disorders. Phys Med Rehabil Clin N Am 2006;17:491, viii.

Campbell SM: Regional myofascial pain syndromes. Rheum Dis Clin North Am 1989;15:31.

Ling FW, Slocumb JC: Use of trigger point injections in chronic pelvic pain. Obstet Gynecol Clin North Am 1993;20:809.

McClaflin RR: Myofascial pain syndrome. Primary care strategies for early intervention. Postgrad Med 1994;96:56.

Rothschild B: Diagnosing and treating fibrositis and fibromyalgia. Geriatr Consultant 1990;9:26.

Slocumb JC: Neurologic factors in chronic pelvic pain: trigger points and the abdominal pelvic pain syndrome. Am J Obstet Gynecol 1984;149:536.

Wolfe F, Smythe HA, Yunus MB, et al: The American College of Rheumatology criteria for the classification of fibromyalgia. Arthritis Rheum 1990;33:160.

INTRODUCTION

Description: Obesity is a state of increased fat and lean body mass (>20% higher ideal weight, body mass index [BMI] >28) associated with increased health risks. Obesity affects more women than men and is of special concern to adolescents and older women. Weight gained during pregnancy (in excess of that related to the pregnancy) is often not lost.

Prevalence: Varies with age: 30% to 40% of women.

Predominant Age: Any.

Genetics: Of the variance in body mass, 20% to 30% may be genetically determined. Rare genetic syndromes have been described.

ETIOLOGY AND PATHOGENESIS

Causes: Calorie consumption in excess of expenditure, insulinoma, hypothalamic disorders, Cushing' syndrome, corticosteroid drugs.

Risk Factors: Parental obesity, pregnancy, sedentary lifestyle, high-fat diet (higher calorie density), low socioeconomic status.

CLINICAL CHARACTERISTICS

Signs and Symptoms

- Increased body mass and fat (male pattern obesity [abdominal] is associated with the greatest health risk)

DIAGNOSTIC APPROACH

Differential Diagnosis

- Pathologic process other than excess dietary consumption

Associated Conditions: Increased morbidity and mortality (see Complications), cholelithiasis. Recent studies indicate an increase in the risks of ovarian and breast cancers.

Workup and Evaluation

Laboratory: No evaluation indicated. Consider thyroid testing in selected patients. Determine serum cholesterol, triglycerides, or glucose levels to assess risk factors for complications.

Imaging: No imaging indicated.

Special Tests: Body mass index = weight (kg)/height (m^2), waist to hip circumference ratio (normal female gynecoid pattern is greater than 0.85).

Diagnostic Procedures: Physical examination, body mass index.

Pathologic Findings

Hypertrophy and/or hyperplasia of adipocytes. Cardiomegaly or hepatomegaly is common.

MANAGEMENT AND THERAPY

Nonpharmacologic

General Measures: Risk assessment, diet and exercise counseling. Assistance with diet planning or selection of a commercial program.

Specific Measures: Behavior modification and hypnosis have been applied with variable success. In select patients (body mass index >40) surgical intervention (stapling or bypass) may be indicated. Surgery is the most effective long-term therapy for morbid obesity.

Diet: Restriction to 500 kcal below maintenance generally provides the best sustainable loss (1 lb/week). Very-low-calorie diets are associated with increased risk and occasional deaths.

Activity: A program of physical activity should accompany any calorie-restriction diet. Activity by itself is generally ineffective.

Patient Education: Diet and exercise instruction, behavior modification; American College of Obstetricians and Gynecologists Patient Education Pamphlet AP045 (Exercise and Health: A Guide for Women), AP064 (Weight Control: Eating Right and Keeping Fit), AP101 (Cholesterol and Your Health).

Drug(s) of Choice

Drug therapy is not generally recommended. However, orlistat (Xenical) 120 mg PO three times a day, taken during or up to 1 hour after meals containing fat, may be recommended. In 2007 a reduced dose version of orlistat (Alli) was introduced as an over-the-counter adjunct for weight loss. With these agents, high-fat meals should be avoided to reduce cramping and diarrhea.

Contraindications: See individual agents. Most are contraindicated in the presence of atherosclerosis or other heart disease, hypertension, hyperthyroidism, or glaucoma. Patients with chronic malabsorption syndromes or cholestasis should avoid orlistat.

Precautions: Relapse common, abuse potential is high for stimulants. Diarrhea, fatty stools, increased frequency of bowel movements, fecal incontinence, abdominal pain, and nausea may occur with orlistat therapy.

Interactions: Some agents may cause arrhythmias with general anesthetic agents. Orlistat can interact with cyclosporine, fat-soluble vitamin absorption, and warfarin.

Alternative Drugs

Phenylpropanolamine (over-the-counter preparations).

FOLLOW-UP

Patient Monitoring: Long-term follow-up, screening for complications of drug therapy or obesity itself.

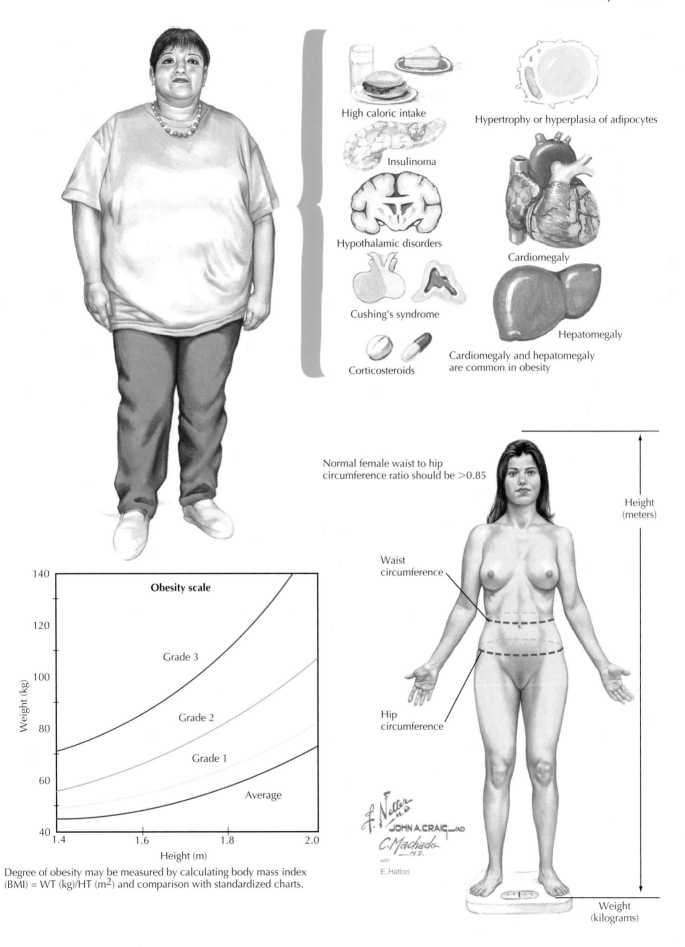

High caloric intake

Hypertrophy or hyperplasia of adipocytes

Insulinoma

Hypothalamic disorders

Cardiomegaly

Cushing's syndrome

Hepatomegaly

Corticosteroids

Cardiomegaly and hepatomegaly are common in obesity

Normal female waist to hip circumference ratio should be >0.85

Height (meters)

Waist circumference

Hip circumference

Obesity scale

Grade 3

Grade 2

Grade 1

Average

Weight (kg)

Height (m)

Degree of obesity may be measured by calculating body mass index (BMI) = WT (kg)/HT (m^2) and comparison with standardized charts.

Weight (kilograms)

Prevention/Avoidance: Diet and exercise counseling (especially important for adolescents and children).

Possible Complications: Significant increase in risk for cardiovascular disease, diabetes mellitus, hypertension, hyperlipidemia, cholelithiasis, cholecystitis, osteoarthritis, gout, thromboembolism, and sleep apnea.

Expected Outcome: Long-term maintenance is difficult and relapses are common. Individual motivation is the best predictor of success.

MISCELLANEOUS

Pregnancy Considerations: Obesity complicates pregnancy, and pregnancy is often the time of onset of obesity for many women. Weight gain should be monitored and adjusted downward for patients who are obese. Orlistat is a Category B medication.

ICD-9-CM Codes: 278.00, 278.01 (Morbid).

REFERENCES

Level I

Ebbeling CB, Leidig MM, Feldman HA, et al: Effects of a low-glycemic load vs low-fat diet in obese young adults: a randomized trial. JAMA 2007;297:2092.

Gardner CD, Kiazand A, Alhassan S, et al: Comparison of the Atkins, Zone, Ornish, and LEARN diets for change in weight and related risk factors among overweight premenopausal women: the A TO Z Weight Loss Study: a randomized trial. JAMA 2007;297:969.

Mathus-Vliegen EM, de Wit LT: Health-related quality of life after gastric banding. Br J Surg 2007;94:457.

McMillan-Price J, Petocz P, Atkinson F, et al: Comparison of 4 diets of varying glycemic load on weight loss and cardiovascular risk reduction in overweight and obese young adults: a randomized controlled trial. Arch Intern Med 2006;166:1466.

Scholze J, Grimm E, Herrmann D, et al: Optimal treatment of obesity-related hypertension: the Hypertension-Obesity-Sibutramine (HOS) study. Circulation 2007;115:1991. Epub 2007 Apr 2.

Level II

Alexander CI, Liston WA: Operating on the obese woman—A review. BJOG 2006;113:1167.

Carmichael AR: Obesity and prognosis of breast cancer. Obes Rev 2006;7:333.

Janssen I, Mark AE: Elevated body mass index and mortality risk in the elderly. Obes Rev 2007;8:41.

Olsen CM, Green AC, Whiteman DC, et al: Obesity and the risk of epithelial ovarian cancer: a systematic review and meta-analysis. Eur J Cancer 2007;43:690. Epub 2007 Jan 12.

Level III

Bray GA: Obesity. Endocrinol Metab Clin North Am 1996;25.

Catalano PM: Management of obesity in pregnancy. Obstet Gynecol 2007;109:419.

Danford D, Fletcher JW: Methods for voluntary weight loss and control. National Institutes of Health Technology Assessment Conference. Ann Intern Med 1993;119:41.

ESHRE Capri Workshop Group: Nutrition and reproduction in women. Hum Reprod Update 2006;12:193. Epub 2006 Jan 31.

Gray AD, Power ML, Zinberg S, Schulkin J: Assessment and management of obesity. Obstet Gynecol Surv 2006;61:742.

Haslam D, Sattar N, Lean M: ABC of obesity. Obesity—Time to wake up. BMJ 2006;333:640.

Kral JG: ABC of obesity. Management: Part III—Surgery. BMJ 2006;333:900.

Lawlor DA, Lean M, Sattar N: ABC of obesity: obesity and vascular disease. BMJ 2006;333:1060.

Lean M, Lara J, Hill JO: ABC of obesity. Strategies for preventing obesity. BMJ 2006;333:959.

Legato MJ: Gender-specific aspects of obesity. Int J Fertil Womens Med 1997;42:184.

Malnick SD, Knobler H: The medical complications of obesity. QJM 2006;99:565. Epub 2006 Aug 17.

Milewicz A, Jedrzejuk D: Clinical aspects of obesity in the gynecological endocrinology practice. Maturitas 2007 Feb56:113. Epub 2006 Sep 12.

Mitrakou A: Women"s health and the metabolic syndrome. Ann N Y Acad Sci 2006;1092:33.

Pasquali R: Obesity, fat distribution and infertility. Maturitas 2006;54:363. Epub 2006 May 24.

Pasquali R, Gambineri A, Pagotto U: The impact of obesity on reproduction in women with polycystic ovary syndrome. BJOG 2006;113:1148. Epub 2006 Jul 7.

Pettigrew R, Hamilton-Fairley D: Obesity and female reproductive function. Br Med Bull 1997;53:341.

Pujol P, Galtier-Dereure F, Bringer J: Obesity and breast cancer risk. Hum Reprod 1997;12:116.

Ramsay JE, Greer I, Sattar N: ABC of obesity. Obesity and reproduction. BMJ 2006;333:1159.

Regulation of body weight. Science 1998;280:1363.

Schneider JG, Tompkins C, Blumenthal RS, Mora S: The metabolic syndrome in women. Cardiol Rev 2006;14:286.

Wyatt SB, Winters KP, Dubbert PM: Overweight and obesity: prevalence, consequences, and causes of a growing public health problem. Am J Med Sci 2006;331:166.

Yu CK, Teoh TG, Robinson S: Obesity in pregnancy. BJOG 2006;113:1117. Epub 2006 Aug 10.

Osteoporosis

INTRODUCTION

Description: Osteoporosis is characterized by loss of bone mass (calcium) that puts the patient at risk for fracture with minimal trauma or during activities of daily living. This process disproportionately affects older women and results in significant morbidity and mortality. Estimates of medical costs are as high as $10 billion each year in the United States.

Prevalence: Of women older than age 75 years (not receiving estrogen replacement), 40% have spine, hip, or forearm fractures; 80% of hip fractures occur in this group.

Predominant Age: Postmenopausal.

Genetics: More common in some races (Caucasian/oriental, thought to be a function of peak bone mass).

ETIOLOGY AND PATHOGENESIS

Causes: Alcohol use/abuse, chronic illness, diabetes mellitus, estrogen loss, especially early menopause, excessive caffeine use, family history of osteoporosis, high parity, high protein intake, inactivity/sedentary lifestyle, inadequate vitamin D intake or sun exposure, low body weight, medical therapy (anticonvulsants, corticosteroids, excess thyroid hormone replacement, long-term heparin or tetracycline use, loop diuretics, chemotherapy), poor diet/inadequate calcium intake (<1000 mg/day), white race or Asian, radiation therapy, smoking.

Risk Factors: Menopause (without estrogen replacement), inactivity, presence of other causes as listed previously. (Women suffer roughly a 10-fold increase in the normal rate of bone loss for a period of about 10 years beginning with the loss of ovarian function. This results in an average lifetime loss of approximately 35% of cortical bone mass and 50% of the more metabolically active trabecular bone. By comparison, men lose only about two thirds this amount.)

CLINICAL CHARACTERISTICS

Signs and Symptoms

- Asymptomatic
- Spinal, hip, or forearm fractures (with or without pain, fractures should be suspected in idiopathic back pain in at-risk patients)
- Loss of height (up to 4 to 8 inches)
- Development of kyphoscoliosis ("dowager's hump")

DIAGNOSTIC APPROACH

Differential Diagnosis

- Metastatic tumor (breast)
- Paget disease (osteitis deformans)
- Multiple myeloma
- Unreported trauma (abuse, elder abuse)
- Cushing' syndrome

Associated Conditions: Dyspareunia, vulvodynia, atrophic vulvitis, increased risk of cardiovascular disease, hot flashes and flushes, sleep disturbances, urinary incontinence, and others associated with hypoestrogenic states.

Workup and Evaluation

Laboratory: No evaluation specifically indicated.

Imaging: Dual-energy x-ray absorptiometry (DEXA) or quantitative computed tomography. Routine radiographic studies (e.g., chest radiograph) do not detect changes until almost 30% of bone has been lost (approximately equal to fracture threshold, 1 g/cm^2).

Special Tests: Urinary tests for bone metabolites are investigational only.

Diagnostic Procedures: Radiographic assessment of bone mass.

Pathologic Findings

Loss of bone calcium, thinning of trabeculae, microfractures, macrofractures (spine, hips, forearms).

MANAGEMENT AND THERAPY

Nonpharmacologic

General Measures: Smoking cessation, alcohol and caffeine intake in moderation, weightbearing exercise, adequate dietary calcium or supplementation.

Specific Measures: Bisphosphonates, calcitonin (infrequently used, reserved for selected patients as a therapeutic agent, not as prevention), selective estrogen receptor modulators (SERMs). Estrogen replacement therapy (when indicated for other reasons) will provide protection but is no longer considered sufficient to justify risks, based on the results of the Women's Health Initiative (WHI) study, although significant concerns about the methodologies of this study exist.

Diet: Adequate dietary intake of calcium (1000 to 1500 mg/day) and vitamin D (400 to 800 IU daily). (Supplementation of vitamin D beyond this dose is generally not warranted.)

Activity: Weightbearing exercise or exercise against resistance. Low-impact activities for those with established bone loss.

Patient Education: Reassurance; American College of Obstetricians and Gynecologists Patient Education Pamphlet AP048 (Preventing Osteoporosis), AP047 (The Menopause Years), AP045 (Exercise and Fitness), AP066 (Hormone Replacement Therapy).

Drug(s) of Choice

Bisphosphonates—alendronate sodium (Fosamax) 10 mg PO daily (must be taken on arising for the day, with a full glass of water, and nothing by mouth for 30 minutes), risedronate sodium (Actonel) 30 mg PO weekly, ibandronate sodium (Boniva) 150 mg PO monthly or 3 mg IM every 3 months. Zoledronic acid has recently been approved for once yearly intravenous therapy. (New agents under development include bazedoxifene, with and without a combined estrogen.)

Selective estrogen receptor modulators (also known as tissue selective estrogens). Many of these agents have bone activity and have been shown to protect or increase bone mass. For most, no current data show a reduction in fracture rate, but this is expected to be the case when studies of longer-term use become available.

Estrogen replacement therapy (with progesterone if indicated). See "Menopause" for dosage options. (Estrogen's effect on bone protection appears to depend on obtaining a relatively normal [premenopausal] blood level [40 to 60 pg/mL] and is not affected by the route of therapy.)

Radiographic Findings in Axial Osteoporosis

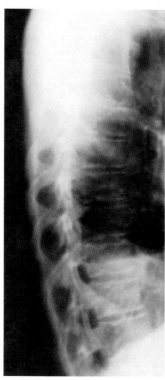

Mild osteopenia in post-menopausal women. Vertebrae appear "washed-out"; no kyphosis or vertebral collapse

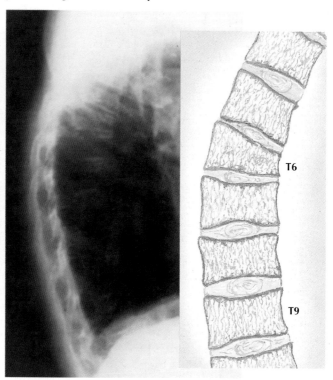

Anterior wedge compression at T6 in same patient 16 1/2 years later. Patient has lymphoma, with multiple biconcave ("codfish") vertebral bodies and kyphosis. Focal lesion at T6 suggests neoplasm

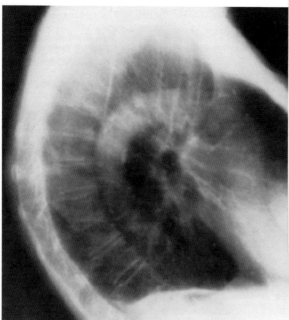

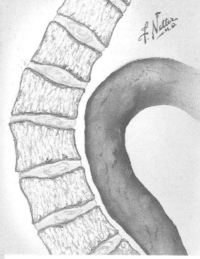

Severe kyphosis in postmenopausal woman. Mild, multiple biconcavity and wedging of vertebrae. Extensive calcification of aorta

Progression of Scoliotic Curve in Adult

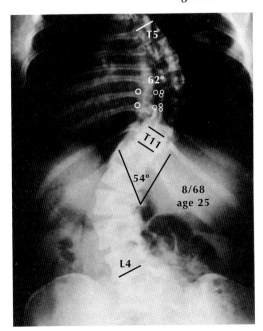
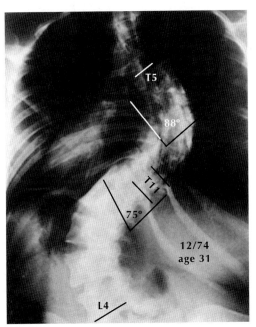

Right thoracic curve of 62° and left lumbar curve of 54° in 25-year-old woman. Curve and grade II spondylolisthesis of L5 detected but not treated during adolescence. Curve increased slowly during adulthood

Increased curves in same woman at age 31 after two closely spaced pregnancies. Thoracic curve progressed to 88° and lumbar curve to 75° Spondylolisthesis increased to grade III

Reproduced from Keim HA: The Adolescent Spine. New York, Grune & Stratton, 1976.

Progressive Spinal Deformity in Osteoporosis

Age
55 years

Age
65 years

Age
75 years

Compression fractures of thoracic vertebrae lead to loss of height and progressive thoracic kyphosis (dowager's hump). Lower ribs eventually rest on iliac crests, and downward pressure on viscera causes abdominal distention

Contraindications: See "Menopause." Alendronate is contraindicated in patients with esophageal stricture or difficulty swallowing, an inability to sit or stand for 30 to 60 minutes, and in nursing mothers.

Precautions: See "Menopause." Patients must remain upright after the ingestion of bisphosphonates to avoid esophageal irritation. Long-term use may be associated with impaired mineralization; therefore, bisphosphonates should be given cyclically. (Infrequent cases of osteonecrosis of the jaw have been reported in bisphosphonate users.) Vitamin D should be used judiciously, if at all, because doses that increase calcium absorption are close to doses that result in bone resorption. If calcitonin is used, it must be given with adequate calcium intake to avoid secondary hyperparathyroidism.

Interactions: See "Menopause." Calcium supplements and antacids may interfere with the absorption of some bisphosphonates and must be taken later in the day.

Alternative Drugs

Calcium supplements should be reserved for those with inadequate intake or a food intolerance that prevents achievement of sufficient dietary levels. Calcium carbonate provides the greatest percentage of elemental calcium, and calcium citrate is highly absorbable, making both acceptable supplements. When used, these should be taken in divided doses over the course of the day. Excessive intake of calcium supplements has been associated with an increased risk of stone formation and should be discouraged.

FOLLOW-UP

Patient Monitoring: Normal health maintenance and continued (lifelong) compliance with medical therapy must be encouraged. Periodic measurement of height may detect asymptomatic spinal fractures.

Prevention/Avoidance: Estrogen replacement therapy at menopause (when otherwise indicated), good diet (adequate calcium and vitamin D intake), and exercise (weightbearing and otherwise). Elimination or reduction of bone toxins (smoking and excess alcohol consumption).

Possible Complications: After hip fracture, half of patients require assistance walking and 15% to 30% are institutionalized, often for the rest of their lives. Roughly, one of five patients with a hip fracture dies within 6 months of the fracture. Fracture of the hip is the twelfth leading cause of death for women.

Expected Outcome: The rate of bone loss may be slowed by medical interventions, but these are most successful if instituted early. Estrogen replacement (when started early) is associated with a reduction by about 50% in the rate of hip and arm fractures in postmenopausal women. This value has been reported to increase to more than 90% when estrogen is used for more than 5 years. Vertebral fractures may be reduced by as much as 80% for these same women.

MISCELLANEOUS

Pregnancy Considerations: No effect on pregnancy (generally not a consideration). Most bisphosphonates are pregnancy category C medications.

ICD-9-CM Codes: 733.01 (Postmenopausal).

REFERENCES

Level I

Black DM, Delmas PD, Eastell R, et al; HORIZON Pivotal Fracture Trial: Once-yearly zoledronic acid for treatment of postmenopausal osteoporosis. N Engl J Med 2007;356:1809.

Goss AN: Bisphosphonate-associated osteonecrosis of the jaws. Climacteric 2007;10:5.

Reid IR, Mason B, Horne A, et al: Randomized controlled trial of calcium in healthy older women. Am J Med 2006;119:777.

Level II

Boonen S: Bisphosphonate efficacy and clinical trials for postmenopausal osteoporosis: similarities and differences. Bone 2007;40:S26.

Chesnut CH: Treating osteoporosis with bisphosphonates and addressing adherence: a review of oral ibandronate. Drugs 2006;66:1351.

Level III

American College of Obstetricians and Gynecologists: Osteoporosis. ACOG Practice Bulletin 50. Washington, DC, ACOG, 2004.

American College of Obstetricians and Gynecologists: Selective estrogen receptor modulators. ACOG Practice Bulletin 39. Washington, DC, ACOG, 2002.

Benhamou CL: Effects of osteoporosis medications on bone quality. Joint Bone Spine 2007;74:39. Epub 2006 Nov 28.

Clunie G: Update on postmenopausal osteoporosis management. Clin Med 2007;7:48.

Dennison E, Mohamed MA, Cooper C: Epidemiology of osteoporosis. Rheum Dis Clin North Am 2006;32:617.

Derk CT: Osteoporosis in premenopause. When are screening and treatment prudent? Postgrad Med 2006;119:8.

Gass M, Dawson-Hughes B: Preventing osteoporosis-related fractures: an overview. Am J Med 2006;119:S3.

Hadjidakis DJ, Androulakis II: Bone remodeling. Ann N Y Acad Sci 2006;1092:385.

Hosking D, Chilvers CED, Christiansen C, et al: Prevention of bone loss with alendronate in postmenopausal women. N Engl J Med 1998;338:485.

Kim DH, Vaccaro AR: Osteoporotic compression fractures of the spine; current options and considerations for treatment. Spine J 2006;6:479.

Lambrinoudaki I, Christodoulakos G, Botsis D: Bisphosphonates. Ann N Y Acad Sci 2006;1092:397.

Liberman UA: Long-term safety of bisphosphonate therapy for osteoporosis: a review of the evidence. Drugs Aging 2006;23:289.

Llorens R: A review of osteoporosis: diagnosis and treatment. Mo Med 2006;103:612.

Lobo RA: Menopause. In Katz VL, Lentz GM, Lobo RA, Gershenson DM: Comprehensive Gynecology, 5th ed. Philadelphia, Mosby/Elsevier, 2007:1050.

Mauck KF, Clarke BL: Diagnosis, screening, prevention, and treatment of osteoporosis. Mayo Clin Proc 2006;81:662.

McCarus DC: Fracture prevention in postmenopausal osteoporosis: a review of treatment options. Obstet Gynecol Surv 2006;61:39.

Miller RG: Osteoporosis in postmenopausal women. Therapy options across a wide range of risk for fracture. Geriatrics 2006;61:24.

Mosekilde L, Vestergaard P, Langdahl B: Fracture prevention in postmenopausal women. Clin Evid 2006;15:1543.

Poole KE, Compston JE: Osteoporosis and its management. BMJ 2006;333:1251.

Pyon EY: Once-monthly ibandronate for postmenopausal osteoporosis: review of a new dosing regimen. Clin Ther 2006;28:475.

Reid DM: Once-monthly dosing: an effective step forward. Bone 2006;38:S18. Epub 2006 Mar 13.

Raisz LG: Clinical practice. Screening for osteoporosis. N Engl J Med 2005;353:164.

Riggs BL, Melton LJ III: Medical progress: involutional osteoporosis. N Engl J Med 1986;314:1676.

Rizer MK: Osteoporosis. Prim Care 2006;33:943, vii.

Rosen CJ: Clinical practice. Postmenopausal osteoporosis. N Engl J Med 2005;353:595.

Sambrook P, Cooper C: Osteoporosis. Lancet 2006;367:2010.

THE CHALLENGE

To identify patients who may benefit from pessary therapy and to effectively select, fit, and monitor pessary use.

Scope of the Problem: As our population ages, the prevalence of pelvic relaxation disorders will increase. Pessary therapy offers an attractive, effective, nonsurgical therapy for many of these patients. Patients with symptomatic pelvic relaxation, uterine retroversion, cervical incompetence, or urinary incontinence may benefit from this form of therapy. It is estimated that 10% to 15% of women suffer from anterior vaginal wall support failure, and this increases to 30% to 40% after menopause.

Objectives of Management: To provide symptomatic relief for patients with pelvic relaxation without causing iatrogenic harm.

TACTICS

Relevant Pathophysiology: Pessaries act either by using existing pelvic support mechanisms or by diffusing the forces acting on pelvic structures over a wide area so that support and reposition are achieved. Available in a variety of types and sizes, the most commonly used forms of pessaries for pelvic relaxation are the ring (or doughnut), the ball, and the cube. To varying degrees, the pessary occludes the vagina and holds the pelvic organs in a relatively normal position. The type of pessary chosen is based on the indications of the individual patient. Pessaries are available in both latex and polyurethane types. The latex type is often less expensive but tends to deteriorate over time; polyurethane pessaries are less likely to retain odor or cause irritation.

Strategies: Pessaries are fitted and placed in the vagina in much the same way as a contraceptive diaphragm (see Chapter 249). The pessary is lubricated with a water-soluble lubricant, folded or compressed, and inserted into the vagina. The pessary is next adjusted so that it is in the proper position based on the type: ring and lever pessaries should sit behind the cervix (when present) and rest in the retropubic notch, the Gellhorn pessary should be contained entirely within the vagina with the plate resting above the levator plane, the Gehrung pessary must bridge the cervix with the limbs resting on the levator muscles on each side, and the ball or cube pessaries should occupy and occlude the upper vagina. All pessaries must allow the easy passage of an examining finger between the pessary and the vaginal wall in all areas. Examination 5 to 7 days after initial fitting is required to confirm proper placement, hygiene, and the absence of pressure-related problems (vaginal trauma or necrosis). Earlier evaluation (in 24 to 48 hours) may be advisable for patients who are debilitated or require additional assistance.

Patient Education: Reassurance; American College of Obstetricians and Gynecologists Patient Education Pamphlet AP012 (Pelvic Support Problems), AP081 (Urinary Incontinence).

IMPLEMENTATION

Special Considerations: Pessaries offer an excellent alternative to surgical repair, but the use of a pessary requires the cooperation and involvement of the patient. Patients who are unable or unwilling to manage the periodic insertion and removal of the device are poor candidates for their use. Pessaries are not well tolerated and do not provide optimal support in patients who have low estrogen levels. For this reason, many suggest a minimum of 30 days of topical estrogen therapy (for those not already receiving estrogen replacement) before a trial of pessary therapy. Patients who are going to use a pessary should be instructed on both proper insertion and removal techniques. Ring pessaries should be removed by hooking a finger into the opening of the pessary, gently compressing the device, and then withdrawing the pessary with gentle traction. Cube pessaries must also be compressed, but the suction created between the faces of the cube and the vaginal wall must be broken by gently separating the device from the vaginal sidewall. The locator string often attached to these pessaries should not be used for traction. Inflatable pessaries should be deflated before removal. Gellhorn and Gehrung pessaries are removed by a reversal of their insertion steps.

REFERENCES

Level I

Cundiff GW, Amundsen CL, Bent AE, et al: The PESSRI study: symptom relief outcomes of a randomized crossover trial of the ring and Gellhorn pessaries. Am J Obstet Gynecol 2007;196: 405.e1.

Level II

Shaikh S, Ong EK, Glavind K, et al: Mechanical devices for urinary incontinence in women. Cochrane Database Syst Rev 2006;3: CD001756.

Level III

American College of Obstetricians and Gynecologists: Urinary incontinence in women. ACOG Practice Bulletin 63. Washington, DC, ACOG, 2005.

American College of Obstetricians and Gynecologists: Pelvic organ prolapse. ACOG Practice Bulletin 79. Washington, DC, ACOG, 2007.

Anders K: Devices for continence and prolapse. BJOG 2004;111:61.

Appell RA, Davila GW: Treatment options for patients with suboptimal response to surgery for stress urinary incontinence. Curr Med Res Opin 2007;23:285.

Deger RB, Menzin AW, Mikuta JJ: The vaginal pessary: past and present. Postgrad Obstet Gynecol 1993;13:1.

Greenhill JP: The nonsurgical management of vaginal relaxation. Clin Obstet Gynecol 1972;15:1083.

Jelovsek JE, Maher C, Barber MD: Pelvic organ prolapse. Lancet 2007;369:1027.

Lentz GM: Anatomic defects of the abdominal wall and pelvic floor. In Katz VL, Lentz GM, Lobo RA, Gershenson DM: Comprehensive Gynecology, 5th ed. Philadelphia, Mosby/Elsevier, 2007:514.

Smith RP, Ling FW: Procedures in women's health care. Baltimore, Williams & Wilkins, 1997:127.

Sulak PJ, Kuehl TJ, Shull BL: Vaginal pessaries and their use in pelvic relaxation. J Reprod Med 1993;38:919.

Trowbridge ER, Fenner DE: Conservative management of pelvic organ prolapse. Clin Obstet Gynecol 2005;48:668.

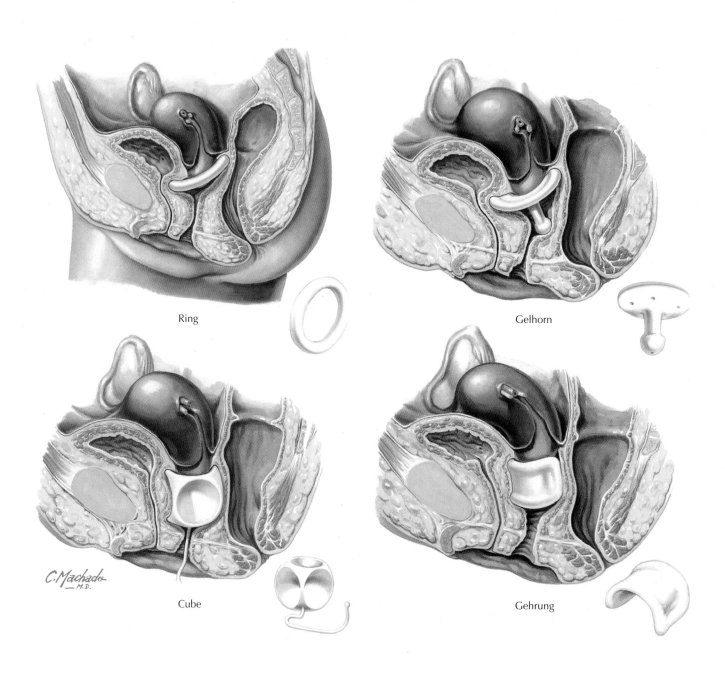

Ring

Gelhorn

Cube

Gehrung

INTRODUCTION

Description: Postcoital bleeding is vaginal bleeding that occurs following sexual intercourse.
Prevalence: Common.
Predominant Age: Reproductive age and beyond.
Genetics: No genetic pattern.

ETIOLOGY AND PATHOGENESIS

Causes: Uterine (pregnancy, endometrial polyps, endometrial hyperplasia, endometrial carcinoma, leiomyomata), cervical (polyps, cervicitis, cervical erosion, cervical dysplasia or neoplasia), vaginal (trauma, infection, atrophy), perineal (vulvar lesions, hemorrhoids).
Risk Factors: Hypoestrogenic states (menopause without estrogen replacement, vigorous intercourse, and nonconsensual intercourse [rape]).

CLINICAL CHARACTERISTICS

Signs and Symptoms

* Painless vaginal bleeding related to (after) intercourse

DIAGNOSTIC APPROACH

Differential Diagnosis

* Pregnancy (normal or abnormal)
* Cervical polyps
* Endometrial polyps
* Uterine leiomyomata
* Cervicitis or cervical lesions (including cancer)
* Endometrial cancer
* Endometriosis
* Vaginitis (including atrophic vaginitis)
* Coagulopathy (acquired or iatrogenic)
* Nongynecologic sources of bleeding (e.g., perineal or rectal)

Associated Conditions: Endometrial cancer, endometrial polyps or carcinoma, and uterine leiomyomata.

Workup and Evaluation

Laboratory: No evaluation indicated.
Imaging: No imaging indicated.
Special Tests: None indicated.
Diagnostic Procedures: History and physical examination often point to possible causes for further evaluation.

Pathologic Findings

Based on underlying pathologic condition.

MANAGEMENT AND THERAPY

Nonpharmacologic

General Measures: Evaluation.
Specific Measures: Focused on underlying cause.

Diet: No specific dietary changes indicated.
Activity: No restriction.
Patient Education: Reassurance; American College of Obstetricians and Gynecologists Patient Education Pamphlet AP095 (Abnormal Uterine Bleeding).

Drug(s) of Choice

Based on cause.

FOLLOW-UP

Patient Monitoring: Normal health maintenance.
Prevention/Avoidance: None.
Possible Complications: Sexual dysfunction (rare).
Expected Outcome: Return to normal sexual function with reassurance and correction of the causative process.

MISCELLANEOUS

Pregnancy Considerations: No effect on pregnancy. Slightly more common during pregnancy.
ICD-9-CM Codes: 626.7.

REFERENCES

Level I
Bain C, Parkin DE, Cooper KG: Is outpatient diagnostic hysteroscopy more useful than endometrial biopsy alone for the investigation of abnormal uterine bleeding in unselected premenopausal women? A randomised comparison. BJOG 2002;109:805.
Tahir MM, Bigrigg MA, Browning JJ, et al: A randomised controlled trial comparing transvaginal ultrasound, outpatient hysteroscopy and endometrial biopsy with inpatient hysteroscopy and curettage. Br J Obstet Gynaecol 1999;106:1259.

Level II
Davidson KG, Dubinsky TJ: Ultrasonographic evaluation of the endometrium in postmenopausal vaginal bleeding. Radiol Clin North Am 2003;41:769.
Shapley M, Jordan J, Croft PR: A systematic review of postcoital bleeding and risk of cervical cancer. Br J Gen Pract 2006;56:453.

Level III
American College of Obstetricians and Gynecologists: Diagnosis and treatment of cervical carcinomas. ACOG Practice Bulletin 35. Washington, DC, ACOG, 2002.
American College of Obstetricians and Gynecologists: Vaginitis. ACOG Practice Bulletin 72. Washington, DC, ACOG, 2006.
Cowan BD, Morrison JC: Management of abnormal genital bleeding in girls and women. N Engl J Med 1991;324:1710.
Field CS: Dysfunctional uterine bleeding. Primary Care 1988;15:561.
Neese RE: Managing abnormal vaginal bleeding. Postgrad Med 1991;89:205.
Smith-Bindman R, Kerlikowske K, Feldstein VA, et al: Endovaginal ultrasound to exclude endometrial cancer and other endometrial abnormalities. JAMA 1998;280:1510.
Zuber TJ: Endometrial biopsy. Am Fam Physician 2001;63:1131, 1137.

Postcoital Bleeding

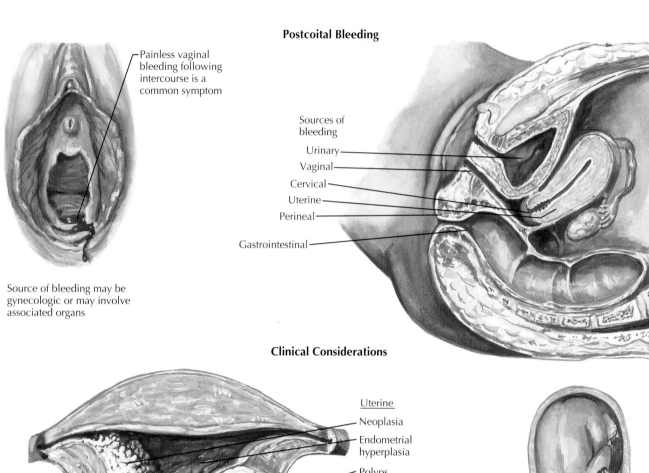

Painless vaginal bleeding following intercourse is a common symptom

Source of bleeding may be gynecologic or may involve associated organs

Sources of bleeding
Urinary
Vaginal
Cervical
Uterine
Perineal
Gastrointestinal

Clinical Considerations

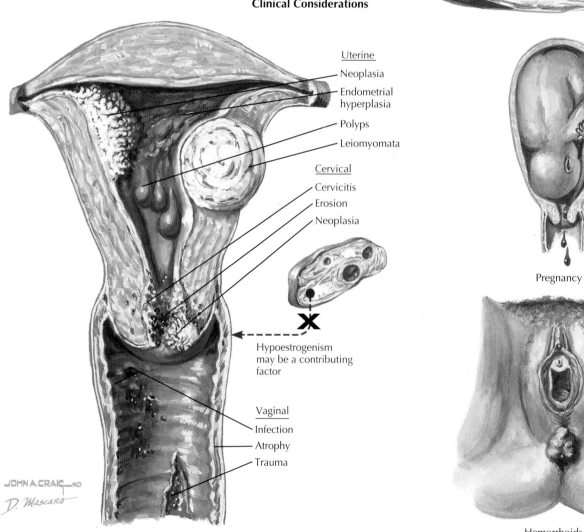

Uterine
Neoplasia
Endometrial hyperplasia
Polyps
Leiomyomata

Cervical
Cervicitis
Erosion
Neoplasia

Hypoestrogenism may be a contributing factor

Vaginal
Infection
Atrophy
Trauma

JOHN A. CRAIG—AD
D. Mascaro

Pregnancy

Hemorrhoids

Premenstrual Syndrome

INTRODUCTION

Description: Premenstrual syndrome (PMS) involves physical and emotional symptoms characterized by their relationship to menses. Symptoms are confined to a period of not more than 14 days before the onset of menstrual flow with complete resolution at, or soon after, the end of menstrual flow.

Prevalence: Reproductive (25% to 85%; 5% to 10% affect lifestyle, 2% to 5% meet strict criteria).

Predominant Age: Reproductive; most commonly 30s and 40s.

Genetics: Family tendency, but no confirmed genetic pattern.

ETIOLOGY AND PATHOGENESIS

Causes: The physiologic foundations of PMS, premenstrual dysphoric disorder (PMDD), and premenstrual magnification (PMM) have yet to be established. The most promising research into a cause of PMS has been in the areas of β-endorphins and serotonin.

Risk Factors: None known.

CLINICAL CHARACTERISTICS

Signs and Symptoms

Physical or emotional symptoms confined to a period of not more than 14 days before the onset of menstrual flow with complete resolution at, or soon after, the end of menstrual flow. More than 150 different signs and symptoms have been described under the rubric of PMS. (The character of the symptoms is not important—only the timing of their appearance. Symptoms that are present at all times but worsen before menses or those that appear at irregular intervals do not meet the criteria for PMS; they should be classified as premenstrual magnification.)

DIAGNOSTIC APPROACH

Differential Diagnosis

- Breast disorders
- Chronic fatigue states
- Drug and substance abuse
- Endocrinologic disorders
- Family, marital, and social stress
- Gastrointestinal conditions
- Gynecologic disorders
- Idiopathic edema
- Psychiatric and psychologic disorders

Associated Conditions: Bipolar disorders, sleep disorders, chronic pain states, and somatization.

Workup and Evaluation

Laboratory: Complete blood count, liver enzyme studies, endocrine studies (androgens, follicle-stimulating hormone [FSH]/luteinizing hormone [LH], glucose tolerance test, prolactin, thyroid function studies [highly sensitive thyroid-stimulating hormone, thyronine, thyrotropin-releasing hormone stimulation]), all to rule out other conditions.

Imaging: No imaging indicated.

Special Tests: Prospective menstrual calendar or other diary for a 3-month period to establish the diagnosis.

Diagnostic Procedures: History, physical examination, prospective menstrual calendar or diary. Research has shown that up to 80% of patients who present with self-diagnosed "PMS" fail to meet strict criteria for this diagnosis. Most are found to have other conditions ranging from mood disorders to irritable bowel syndrome or endometriosis. This observation makes it imperative that no therapy be instituted until the diagnosis can be firmly established.

Pathologic Findings

None.

MANAGEMENT AND THERAPY

Nonpharmacologic

General Measures: Lifestyle changes (aerobic exercise [20 to 45 minutes, three times weekly], smoking cessation, stress reduction), dietary changes and supplementation (adequate protein and complex carbohydrates; avoidance of alcohol, caffeine, and simple sugars; eating frequent small meals and plenty of fresh fruits and vegetables; reduction of dietary fat to <15%; salt restriction; increased dietary or supplemental fiber; 1000 mg calcium daily; magnesium 200 mg daily during luteal phase; vitamin B_6 50 to 200 mg daily; vitamin E 150 to 300 IU daily) all have been advocated but with few data to support the recommendations.

Specific Measures: Generally based on specific symptoms. A favorable response should be expected for 80% of patients with PMS and 50% of those with premenstrual magnification.

Diet: See previous.

Activity: Aerobic exercise (20 to 45 minutes, three times weekly).

Patient Education: Reassurance; American College of Obstetricians and Gynecologists Patient Education Pamphlets AP057 (Premenstrual Syndrome), AP106 (Depression).

Drug(s) of Choice

Hydrochlorothiazide 25 to 50 mg daily, luteal phase (for fluid retention).

Alprazolam 0.25 mg three to four times daily or atenolol 25 mg two to three times daily (for agitation and anxiety).

Buspirone 5 mg three times daily or fluoxetine 20 mg daily (in the morning) for mood swings.

Third-generation oral contraceptives (e.g., desogestrel-containing).

Danazol sodium 200 mg daily, luteal phase or continuous gonadotropin-releasing hormone (GnRH) agonists (depot leuprolide 3.75 mg IM monthly for a maximum of 6 months or nafarelin acetate nasal spray, 200 microgram twice daily for a maximum of 6 months).

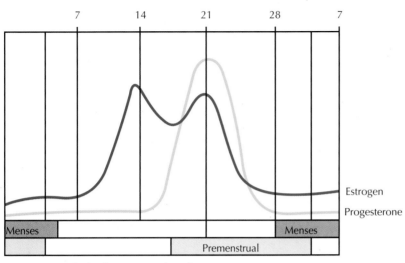

Cycle of premenstrual syndrome

Syndrome characterized by pelvic pain, fluid retention, breast discomfort, and mood changes in days preceding menses

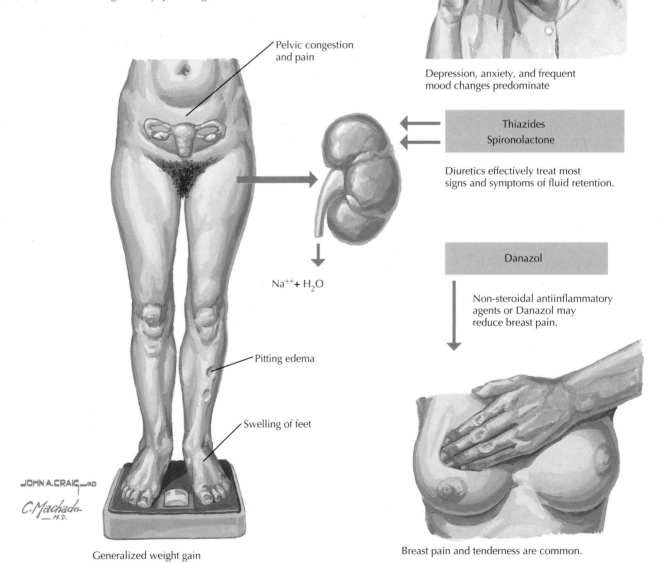

Pelvic congestion and pain

Depression, anxiety, and frequent mood changes predominate

Thiazides
Spironolactone

Diuretics effectively treat most signs and symptoms of fluid retention.

$Na^{++} + H_2O$

Danazol

Non-steroidal antiinflammatory agents or Danazol may reduce breast pain.

Pitting edema

Swelling of feet

Generalized weight gain

Breast pain and tenderness are common.

Contraindications: See individual agents.
Precautions: See individual agents.

FOLLOW-UP

Patient Monitoring: Normal health maintenance.
Prevention/Avoidance: General stress reduction appears to blunt the cyclic symptoms experienced.
Possible Complications: Social withdrawal or isolation, work or family disruption. The rate of suicide increases during the luteal phase.
Expected Outcome: Symptoms can generally be resolved through the process of diagnosis, providing insight and control to the patient, and pharmacologic intervention.

MISCELLANEOUS

Pregnancy Considerations: No effect on pregnancy. Patients with a history of PMS may have exaggerated response to the hormonal changes associated with pregnancy.
ICD-9-CM Codes: 625.4.

REFERENCES

Level I

Facchinetti F, Borella P, Sances G, et al: Oral magnesium successfully relieves premenstrual mood changes. Obstet Gynecol 1991;78:177.

Goodale IL, Domar AD, Benson H: Alleviation of premenstrual syndrome symptoms with the relaxation response. Obstet Gynecol 1990;75:649.

London RS, Murphy L, Kitlowski KE, Reynolds MA:. Efficacy of alpha-tocopherol in the treatment of the premenstrual syndrome. J Reprod Med 1987;32:400.

Schmidt PJ, Nieman LK, Danaceau MA, et al: Differential behavioral effects of gonadal steroids in women with and in those without premenstrual syndrome. N Engl J Med 1998;338:209.

Steiner M, Steinberg S, Stewart D, et al: Fluoxetine in the treatment of premenstrual dysphoria. Canadian Fluoxetine/Premenstrual Dysphoria Collaborative Study Group. N Engl J Med 1995;332:1529.

Thys-Jacobs, Starkey P, Bernstein D, Tian J: Calcium carbonate and the premenstrual syndrome: effects on premenstrual and menstrual symptoms. Premenstrual Syndrome Study Group. Am J Obstet Gynecol 1998;179:444.

Yonkers KA, Halbreich U, Freeman E, et al: Symptomatic improvement of premenstrual dysphoric disorder with sertraline treatment. A randomized controlled trial. Sertraline Premenstrual Dysphoric Collaborative Study Group. JAMA 1997;278:983

Level II

Ford O, Lethaby A, Mol B, Roberts H: Progesterone for premenstrual syndrome. Cochrane Database Syst Rev 2006;4:CD003415.

Freeman E, Rickels K, Sondheimer S, Scharlop B: Diagnostic classifications from daily symptom ratings of women who seek treatment for premenstrual symptoms. Am J Gynecol Health 1987;1:17.

Garris PD, Sokol MS, Kelly K, et al: Leuprolide acetate treatment of catamenial pneumothorax. Fertil Steril 1994;61:173.

Kornstein SG, Pearlstein TB, Fayyad R, et al: Low-dose sertraline in the treatment of moderate-to-severe premenstrual syndrome: efficacy of 3 dosing strategies. J Clin Psychiatr 2006;67:1624.

Krasnik C, Montori VM, Guyatt GH, et al: Medically Unexplained Syndromes Study Group. The effect of bright light therapy on depression associated with premenstrual dysphoric disorder. Am J Obstet Gynecol 2005;193:658.

Level III

American College of Obstetricians and Gynecologists: Premenstrual syndrome. ACOG Practice Bulletin 15. Washington, DC, ACOG, 2000.

Braverman PK: Premenstrual syndrome and premenstrual dysphoric disorder. J Pediatr Adolesc Gynecol 2007;20:3.

Claman F, Miller T: Premenstrual syndrome and premenstrual dysphoric disorder in adolescence. J Pediatr Health Care 2006; 20:329.

Futterman LA, Rapkin AJ: Diagnosis of premenstrual disorders. J Reprod Med 2006;51:349.

Kroll R, Rapkin AJ: Treatment of premenstrual disorders. J Reprod Med 2006;51:359.

Lentz GM: Primary and secondary dysmenorrhea, premenstrual syndrome, and premenstrual dysphoric disorder. In Katz VL, Lentz GM, Lobo RA, Gershenson DM: Comprehensive Gynecology, 5th ed. Philadelphia, Mosby/Elsevier, 2007:906.

Moline ML: Pharmacologic strategies for managing premenstrual syndrome. Clin Pharm 1993;12:181.

Plouffe L Jr, Trott EA: Premenstrual syndrome: new concepts and recent therapeutic breakthroughs. Postgrad Obstet Gynecol 1995;15:1.

Rubinow DR: The premenstrual syndrome: new views. JAMA 1992;268:1908.

Winer SA, Rapkin AJ: Premenstrual disorders: prevalence, etiology and impact. J Reprod Med 2006;51:339.

INTRODUCTION

Description: Pruritus ani is acute or chronic itching (generally intense) of the anal and perianal skin. Patients also may have complaints of vulvar itching or of a vaginal infection that has not responded to therapy.
Prevalence: Common.
Predominant Age: All ages.
Genetics: No genetic pattern.

ETIOLOGY AND PATHOGENESIS

Causes: Anal disease—fissures, fistulae, infection (bacterial, fungal, pinworms, scabies), neoplasia, hemorrhoids, leakage of stool. Dermatologic processes—psoriasis, eczema, fecal irritation, contact dermatitis, seborrheic dermatitis, vulvitis, chemical dermatitis (diarrheal irritation), dietary intolerance (coffee, cola, tomatoes, chocolate). Other—excessively zealous hygiene, psychologic problems.
Risk Factors: Hemorrhoids, obesity.

CLINICAL CHARACTERISTICS

Signs and Symptoms

- Anal and perianal itching
- Perianal erythema
- Anal fissures
- Excoriation
- Bleeding after bowel movement

DIAGNOSTIC APPROACH

Differential Diagnosis

- Vulvitis
- Vaginitis
- Pruritus vulvae
- Contact dermatitis
- Psoriasis
- Bacterial or fungal infection
- Parasites (pinworms, scabies)
- Diabetes mellitus
- Liver disease
- Anxiety
- Atopic dermatitis
- Menopausal perineal atrophy

Associated Conditions: Vaginitis, secondary infection, diabetes mellitus, psoriasis, and hemorrhoids.

Workup and Evaluation

Laboratory: No evaluation indicated. Selective testing based on differential diagnosis being considered (e.g., fasting and postprandial glucose levels, skin scrapings for fungi, stool for ova and parasites).
Imaging: No imaging Indicated.

Special Tests: None indicated. Anoscopy for anal diseases.
Diagnostic Procedures: History and physical examination.

Pathologic Findings

Excoriation common.

MANAGEMENT AND THERAPY

Nonpharmacologic

General Measures: Evaluation, perineal hygiene, cool sitz baths, moist soaks, or the application of soothing solutions such as Burow's solution. Patients should be advised to wear loose-fitting clothing and keep the area dry and well ventilated. Avoid soaps; water-moistened cotton balls or baby wipes provide a portable cleansing option. Nonmedicated talcum powder may be used to absorb moisture. If overnight itching and excoriation are a problem, patients should wear cotton gloves during sleep to avoid excoriation.
Specific Measures: Antihistamines, especially at night when itching is often intense, and sedation may be desirable. Crotamiton (Eurax) may be applied topically, twice daily, to suppress itching. Occasionally, the use of a topical anesthetic, such as 2% lidocaine (Xylocaine) jelly, may be required. Other therapies based on causal agent.
Diet: No specific dietary changes needed. If food allergy or irritation is suspected, diet change is indicated (reduce caffeine, spices, citrus, vitamin C, milk products, alcohol).
Activity: No restriction.
Patient Education: Reassurance, counseling about perineal hygiene, risk reduction.

Drug(s) of Choice

Burow's solution (Domeboro, aluminum acetate 5% aqueous solution, three to four times daily for 30 to 60 minutes).
Crotamiton (Eurax) may be applied topically, twice daily.
Topical analgesic sprays or ointments—benzocaine (Americaine, Hurricane) 20% spray or gel, dibucaine (Nupercainal) 1% ointment.
Antipruritics and antiinflammatory agents—hydrocortisone (Anusol-HC, Analpram-HC, Cortenema, Cortifoam, Epifoam, Proctofoam-HC), pramoxine 1% (Fleet rectal pads, Analpram-HC), witch hazel 50% (Tucks pads or gel).
Astringents—Preparation H.

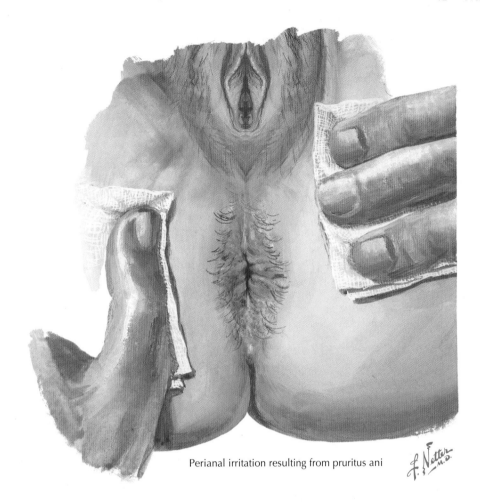

Perianal irritation resulting from pruritus ani

FOLLOW-UP

Patient Monitoring: Normal health maintenance.

Prevention/Avoidance: Perineal hygiene, hormone replacement therapy, and avoidance of local irritants and laxatives.

Possible Complications: Secondary infection caused by excoriation, lichenification.

Expected Outcome: Good, with identification of underlying causation.

MISCELLANEOUS

Pregnancy Considerations: No effect on pregnancy

ICD-9-CM Codes: 698.0.

REFERENCES

Level I

Lysy J, Sistiery-Ittah M, Israelit Y, et al: Topical capsaicin—A novel and effective treatment for idiopathic intractable pruritus ani: a randomised, placebo controlled, crossover study. Gut 2003;52:1323.

Level III

Alexander S: Dermatological aspects of anorectal disease. Clin Gastroenterol 1975;4:651.

Jones DJ: ABC of colorectal diseases. Pruritus ani. BMJ 1992;305:575.

INTRODUCTION

Description: Rape and sexual assault encompass manual, oral, and genital contact by one person without the consent of the other in a way that would be considered sexual in a consensual situation. It does not require penetration, ejaculation, force, or evidence of resistance—only the lack of consent. The legal definition varies slightly by location, but it often includes elements of fear, fraud, coercion, or threat. In some areas, the mentally incompetent, those under the influence of drugs or alcohol, or minors are deemed incapable of giving consent for any otherwise-consensual sexual activity, resulting in "statutory rape." Rape trauma syndrome is a well-recognized set of behaviors that occurs after a sexual assault. These responses are organized into three phases: the acute phase, lasting from hours to days; a middle, or readjustment, phase, lasting from days to weeks; and a final reorganization or resolution phase that involves lifelong changes.

Prevalence: Rape constitutes 5% to 10% of violent crime, 601 of 100,000 women. It is the most underreported crime in the United States. Rape trauma syndrome occurs in virtually every case.

Predominant Age: Any age.

ETIOLOGY AND PATHOGENESIS

Causes: One fourth to one half of all rapes occur at home (either the victim's or the attacker's), but only one third of these involve a male intruder. Most attackers are known to the victims. Of recurrent victims, about 25% have been raped by someone well known to them, such as an ex-lover, employer, coworker, neighbor, or relative, and two thirds are vulnerable because of mental impairment, substance abuse, or a psychiatric disorder. Weapons are used in 30% to 50% of sexual assaults (handguns are most common). Approximately 50% of campus rapes occur during dates. Estimates of sexual violence occurring in the setting of a dating relationship indicate that 10% to 25% of high school students and 20% to 50% of college students have experienced some form of sexual violence. Rape trauma syndrome can follow rape or other forms of intense physical or emotional trauma.

Risk Factors: Studies indicate that alcohol use is involved in more than one half of all rapes of college students. Rape trauma syndrome is more common in those older than 40, those assaulted in their homes by a stranger, and those with a history of previous mental illness.

CLINICAL CHARACTERISTICS

Signs and Symptoms

- Rape—history of nonconsensual sexual activity
  - Physical signs of sexual activity (not limited to vaginal intercourse)
  - Physical signs of trauma or coercion (including impairment resulting from drugs, alcohol, or mental abilities)
- Rape trauma syndrome—acute (decompensation, inability to cope, volatile emotions, fear, guilt, anger, depression, and problems concentrating are common; flashbacks are frequent; ideation is often disturbed)
  - Middle, or readjustment (resolution of many issues [may not be functional], flashbacks, nightmares, and phobias may develop)
  - Reorganization (recognizes that event was an assault over which she could have no control)

DIAGNOSTIC APPROACH

Differential Diagnosis

- Consensual intercourse
- Nonsexual trauma
- Rape trauma syndrome—depression
  - Mania
  - Psychosis

Associated Conditions: Pregnancy, sexually transmitted infections, and depression.

Workup and Evaluation

Laboratory: As outlined in Special Tests, as well as serum pregnancy test, cervical cultures for sexually transmitted infections, a screening serologic test for syphilis and human immunodeficiency virus (HIV), hepatitis antigens, urinalysis (often with culture).

Imaging: No imaging indicated unless the possibility of internal injuries is suspected.

Special Tests: Special rape evaluation kits are available in many jurisdictions and should be used if available. Wood's light (ultraviolet light) causes semen stains to fluoresce.

Diagnostic Procedures: Examination under general anesthesia is also indicated any time the patient is unable to urinate or there is hematuria, lower abdominal tenderness, or signs of occult blood loss such as hypovolemia.

Pathologic Findings

The physical examination is normal in one half of rape victims. Common sites of lacerations are the vaginal wall, the lateral fornices, and the cul-de-sac.

MANAGEMENT AND THERAPY

Nonpharmacologic

General Measures: Support with compassion, care, and sensitivity. The primary goal is to provide reassurance and a return of control. Support and assistance should be provided in moving through the stages of resolution. Because one of the pivotal aspects of sexual assault is the loss of control, every effort should be made to allow the patient control over even the most trivial aspect of the physical examination.

Specific Measures: There are three basic responsibilities in the care of someone who may have been raped or abused: the detection and treatment of serious injuries, the preservation of evidence, and protection against sequelae. All women deserve intensive follow-up and counseling. Assist in recognizing and adapting to the changes that make up the rape trauma syndrome.

Diet: No specific dietary changes indicated.

Activity: No restriction.

Patient Education: American College of Obstetricians and Gynecologists Patient Education Pamphlet AP114 (Emergency Contraception), AP009 (How to Prevent Sexually Transmitted Diseases), AP068 (Alcohol and Women), AP083 (Domestic Violence).

Drug(s) of Choice

Pregnancy interdiction—levonorgestrel 0.75 mg (Plan B) PO every 12 hours for two doses, diethylstilbestrol 25 mg PO twice a day for 5 days with prochlorperazine (Compazine) 10 mg PO every 8 hours or ethinyl estradiol 0.05 mg plus norgestrel 0.5 mg (Ovral) two tablets PO twice a day for 2 to 5 days, ethinyl estradiol 0.1 mg plus levonorgestrel 0.5 mg (Preven, no longer marketed) 2 PO every 12 hours for two doses.

Sexually transmitted infection prophylaxis—ceftriaxone 250 mg IM or spectinomycin 2 g IM, both followed by tetracycline 500 mg PO four times a day for 7 days or doxycycline 100 mg PO twice a day for 7 days.

Prophylaxis—tetanus toxoid should be given if indicated.

Contraindications: Known or suspected allergy, preexisting pregnancy.

Precautions: Nausea is common with high-dose estrogen pregnancy interdiction.

Alternative Drugs

Pregnancy interdiction—ethinyl estradiol, 5 mg PO daily for 5 days or conjugated estrogen, 10 mg PO four times a day for 5 days. An intrauterine contraceptive device may be placed as an alternative to drug therapy for pregnancy interdiction.

Sexually transmitted infection prophylaxis—amoxicillin 3 g PO or ampicillin 3.5 g PO plus probenecid 1 g PO as initial therapy, then follow as previous.

Erythromycin esterase 500 mg PO four times a day for 7 days may be substituted for tetracycline or doxycycline.

FOLLOW-UP

Patient Monitoring: Follow-up contacts by the health care provider, social service agencies, or support groups should be made early and often. Contacts at 1 to 2 weeks, a month, and periodically thereafter provide support and identify evolving problems. Physical reevaluation should be performed at 1 and 6 weeks to check for delayed symptoms or signs of pelvic infection, bleed-

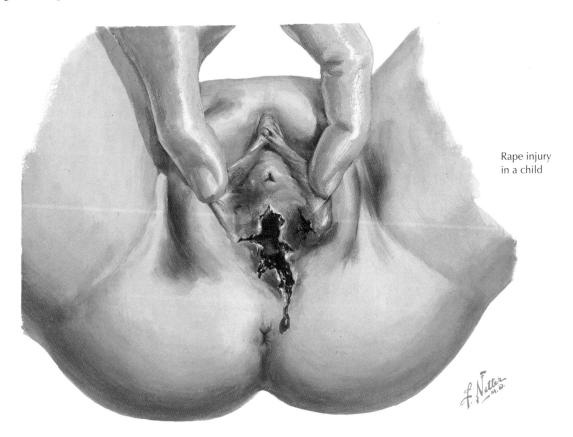

Rape injury in a child

Straddle injuries, such as falling on the crossbar of a brother's bicycle, will generally cause symmetric trauma and usually involves the anterior and posterior portions of the vulva and surrounding perineum. Trauma restricted to the 3- to 9-o'clock positions of the vulva is suggestive of abuse.

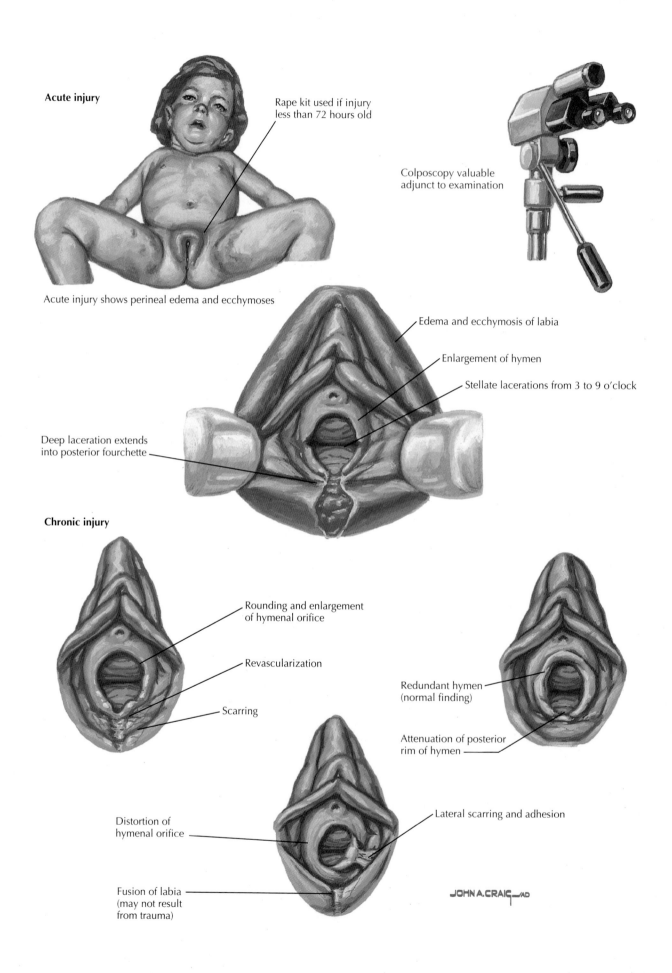

Acute injury

Rape kit used if injury less than 72 hours old

Colposcopy valuable adjunct to examination

Acute injury shows perineal edema and ecchymoses

Edema and ecchymosis of labia

Enlargement of hymen

Stellate lacerations from 3 to 9 o'clock

Deep laceration extends into posterior fourchette

Chronic injury

Rounding and enlargement of hymenal orifice

Revascularization

Scarring

Redundant hymen (normal finding)

Attenuation of posterior rim of hymen

Distortion of hymenal orifice

Lateral scarring and adhesion

Fusion of labia (may not result from trauma)

JOHN A. CRAIG—AD

ing abnormalities, delayed menses, suicidal ideation, or other possible sequelae of the attack. Retesting for human immunodeficiency virus and hepatitis B status should be done at 12 to 18 weeks. Health care providers should watch for a failure to move to resolution and the emergence of dysfunctional adaptations.

Prevention/Avoidance: Avoidance of high-risk situations, especially those involving alcohol or drugs.

Possible Complications: The risk of acquiring a sexually transmitted disease is uncertain but is estimated to be 3% to 5% or less. The risk of becoming infected with human immunodeficiency virus is unknown. When pregnancy interdiction is undertaken within 72 hours, efficacy approaches 90%. Efficacy is greater the earlier the interdiction is instituted; therapy may still be undertaken beyond 72 hours with declining results. Roughly one third of rape victims suffer long-term psychiatric problems.

Expected Outcome: If both physical and mental traumas are addressed in a proactive manner, results should be good. This must include risk avoidance to reduce the chance of recurrence. (Up to one fifth of rape victims have been victims previously.) Even with care and support, the last phase of the rape trauma syndrome is often accompanied by painful transitions, frequently involving significant changes in lifestyle, work, or friends. Insomnia, depression, somatic complaints, and poor self-esteem are common during this phase. For some, this phase can be extremely disruptive and prolonged. Roughly one third of rape victims suffer long-term psychiatric problems. The risk of this is greatest for those older than 40, those assaulted in their homes by a stranger, and those with a history of previous mental illness.

MISCELLANEOUS

Pregnancy Considerations: No effect on preexisting pregnancy. If pregnancy interdiction fails, the agents used are teratogenic and a therapeutic abortion is recommended.

ICD-9-CM Codes: V71.5 (Alleged, observation or examination), 308 (Acute reaction to stress), 308.0 (Predominant disturbance of emotions), 308.3 (Other acute reactions to stress), 308.4 (Mixed disorders as reaction to stress).

REFERENCES

Level II

Ranney ML, Gee EM, Merchant RC: Nonprescription availability of emergency contraception in the United States: current status, controversies, and impact on emergency medicine practice. Ann Emerg Med 2006;47:461. Epub 2005 Sep 13.

Rocca CH, Schwarz EB, Stewart FH, et al: Beyond access: acceptability, use and nonuse of emergency contraception among young women. Am J Obstet Gynecol 2007;196:29.e1; discussion 90.e1.

Level III

American College of Obstetricians and Gynecologists: Sexually transmitted diseases in adolescents. ACOG Committee Opinion 301. Washington, DC, ACOG, 2004.

American College of Obstetricians and Gynecologists: Emergency contraception. ACOG Practice Bulletin 69. Washington, DC, ACOG, 2005.

Burgess WA, Holmstrom LL: Rape trauma syndrome. Am J Psychiatry 1974;131:981.

Burgess WA, Holmstrom LL: Adaptive strategies and recovery from rape. Am J Psychiatry 1979;136:1278.

Cantu M, Coppola M, Lindner AJ: Evaluation and management of the sexually assaulted woman. Emerg Med Clin North Am 2003;21:737.

Chrisler JC, Ferguson S: Violence against women as a public health issue. Ann N Y Acad Sci 2006;1087:235.

Danielson CK, Holmes MM: Adolescent sexual assault: an update of the literature. Curr Opin Obstet Gynecol 2004;16:383.

Gerber GL, Cherneski L: Sexual aggression toward women: reducing the prevalence. Ann N Y Acad Sci 2006;1087:35.

Hampton HL: Care of the woman who has been raped. N Engl J Med 1995;332:234.

Hicks DJ: Rape: Sexual assault. Am J Obstet Gynecol 1980;137:931.

Lentz GM: Rape, incest, and domestic violence. In Katz VL, Lentz GM, Lobo RA, Gershenson DM: Comprehensive Gynecology, 5th ed. Philadelphia, Mosby/Elsevier, 2007:203.

INTRODUCTION

Description: Sexual dysfunction/anorgasmia is a lack of interest in sexual expression or sexual contact or the inability to achieve orgasm. Most studies indicate that only 30% to 40% of women are able to experience orgasm during intercourse and up to 15% of sexually active women have never experienced sexual release.

Genetics: No genetic pattern.

Prevalence: Most experience libidinal dysfunction episodically. Of sexually active women, 10% to 15% experience orgasmic failure; most experience it episodically. In "happy" or "very happy" marriages, sexual dysfunction occurs in almost two thirds of women, with three fourths reporting sexual difficulties that fall short of true dysfunction (such as lack of interest or inability to relax). In one survey, almost one half the women reported trouble becoming sexually excited, one third had trouble maintaining excitement, and one third were completely disinterested in sex. Almost half of the women reported difficulties in achieving orgasm, and 15% had never been able to have an orgasm at all.

Predominant age: Reproductive and beyond.

Genetics: No genetic pattern.

CLINICAL CHARACTERISTICS

Signs and Symptoms

- Libidinal dysfunction:
  - Disinterest in or avoidance of sexual expression
  - Lack of pleasure from sexual encounters
- Orgasmic dysfunction:
  - Failure to obtain sexual release through any means.

Causes: The most common causes of sexual dysfunction are relationship problems, intrapsychic factors, and medical factors. Relationship problems are an obvious source for sexual problems, but both the patient and her doctor often overlook them. Marital or relationship stresses may be acted out by sexual distancing, orgasmic failure, or exploitation. Anger, hidden agendas, lack of trust, or infidelity may be expressed through the withdrawal of intimacy. Libidinal mismatches are common, but when combined with poor communication, they lead to dysfunction. Dual-income families may not realize the impact fatigue and a fast-paced lifestyle may be having on their ability to express warmth and be sexually expressive. Medical factors that influence sexual performance include drug and alcohol use, depression, anxiety, chronic illness, pregnancy, untreated menopause, and the effects of surgical therapies.

Once proximation (the process of courting, flirting, and desire that begins progress toward physical sexual expression) and arousal have occurred, orgasmic success requires effective stimulation, of a sufficient quality over a sufficient time, provided in a supportive environment. Failures in any of these areas may present as orgasmic problems. Medical factors that influence sexual performance include drug and alcohol use, depression, anxiety, chronic illness, pregnancy, untreated menopause, and the effects of surgical therapies.

Risk factors: Abuse, restrictive rearing, depression, fatigue, sleep disorders

DIAGNOSTIC APPROACH

Differential Diagnosis

- Depression and affective disorders
- Relational stress
- Physical or sexual abuse (current or past)
- Alcohol or drug use or abuse
- Conditioning (repeated orgasmic failure, restrictive rearing)
- Inappropriate expectations (inaccurate perception of "normal," "correct," or "expected")
- Multiple sclerosis or other neurologic process
- Other sexual dysfunction (arousal, lubrication, dyspareunia, etc.) presenting as orgasmic failure

Workup and Evaluation

Laboratory: No evaluation indicated.

Imaging: No imaging indicated.

Special Tests: None indicated.

Diagnostic Procedures: History.

Pathologic Findings

None.

MANAGEMENT AND THERAPY

General Measures: Reassurance, evaluation, stress reduction, relaxation training, encourage communication, sensate focusing (pleasuring). One of the simplest models for sexual therapy is the PLISSIT model. This model is made up of four levels of intervention: **P**ermission, **L**imited **I**nformation, **S**pecific **S**uggestions, and **I**ntensive **T**herapy. These steps are applied in order. At each step a large number of dysfunctions will be resolved, leaving few patients who require referral for intensive or specialized therapy.

- **Permission:** Many patients only need permission for what they are doing or want to do.
- **Limited Information:** When permission is not enough, providing limited information often will be the solution to the problem.
- **Specific Suggestion:** These do not have to be exotic, complex, or imaginative. In most cases, they will be obvious and suggested by the situation.
- **Intensive Therapy:** When the problem is more complex, or deep seated, the intensive, specialized therapy of a trained sexual therapist, psychiatrist, psychologist, or other specialist should be considered.

Specific Measures: Specific suggestions for scheduled time together (including nonsexual time), sexual counseling as needed. Many patients who do not achieve orgasm during intercourse are fully orgasmic with additional manual stimulation, oral–genital stimulation, a vibrator, or masturbation. (About 30% to 40% of women require concurrent clitoral stimulation to achieve orgasm.) This is common enough that it should be viewed as a problem only if it is a source of concern for the patient or her partner.

Diet: No specific dietary changes indicated. (There are no true aphrodisiacs, but if the patient believes a food will enhance sexuality, it should not be denied.)

Activity: No restriction.

Patient Education: American College of Obstetricians and Gynecologists Patient Education Booklet AP042 (Your and Your Sexuality), AP072 (Sexuality and Sexual Problems)

Bacos CS: The sex bible: The complete guide to sexual love. Beverly, MA, Quiver, 2006.

Comfort A: The new joy of sex. New York, Crown Publishers, Inc, 2002.

Keeling B: Sexual healing: The complete guide to overcoming common sexual problems. Alameda, CA, Hunter House Publishing, 2006.

Drug(s) of Choice

None. (Hormone replacement therapy for postmenopausal women may improve sexual function, especially if vaginal

Goals of sexual counseling or therapy

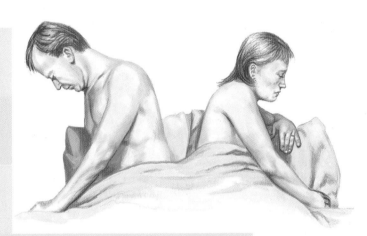

Sex is more than intercourse
  Look at larger picture of sensuality

Leave each encounter feeling good
  Feel good—don't ask for orgasm

Give and receive pleasure
  Enjoy giving and accepting pleasure

Open good communications
  Listen without feeling criticized, provide cooperative communications

Learn to say "yes" instead of "no" (or at least "maybe")
  Learn to suggest alternatives, break rejection cycle

Improve the quality, not necessarily the quantity
  Better sex is better than more sex

Have fun, not work
  Sex shouldn't be work—requires interesting and interested partners

Allow "space" for each other
  Allow distance without abandonment

Go slowly, provide reassurance
  Take your time

From: Smith RP: Gynecology in Primary Care. Baltimore, Williams & Wilkins, 1997, p 527.

dryness or atrophy play a role in the dysfunction. Testosterone treatment improves libido but does not result in improved sexual functioning and is generally not indicated as a treatment for sexual dysfunction except in women who are surgically menopausal.)

Alternative Therapies

Biofeedback, relaxation therapy, marital or psychological counseling as needed.

Patient Monitoring: Normal health maintenance.

Prevention/Avoidance: Communication, maintenance of general health, adequate rest and exercise. Many patients who do not achieve orgasm during intercourse are fully orgasmic with additional manual stimulation, oral–genital stimulation, a vibrator, or masturbation. (About 30% to 40% of women require concurrent clitoral stimulation to achieve orgasm.) This is common enough that it should be viewed as a problem only if it is a source of concern for the patient or her partner.

Possible complications: Social withdrawal, depression, marital discord.

Expected outcome: Generally good with a mixture of reassurance, sexual counseling, stress reduction, and graded exercises as appropriate.

Associated conditions: Orgasmic dysfunction, dyspareunia, depression.

Pregnancy considerations: No effect on pregnancy.

Synonyms: Inhibited desire.

ICD-9-CM Codes: 302.71 (Libidinal dysfunction), 302.73 (Orgasmic dysfunction)

REFERENCES

Level III

Alexander B: Disorders of sexual desire: diagnosis and treatment of decreased libido. Am Fam Physician 1993;47:832.

Amato P: Categories of female sexual dysfunction. Obstet Gynecol Clin North Am 2006;33:527.

Carey JC: Disorders of sexual desire and arousal. Obstet Gynecol Clin North Am 2006;33:549.

Duddle M, Brown ADG: The clinical management of sexual dysfunction. Clin Obstet Gynecol 1980;7:293.

Goldstein I, Meston CM, Davis S, Trais A: Women's sexual function and dysfunction: study, diagnosis and treatment. London, Informa Healthcare, 2005

Gracia CR, Freeman EW, Sammel MD, et al: Hormones and sexuality during transition to menopause. Obstet Gynecol 2007; 109:831.

Hatzimouratidis K, Hatzichristou D: Sexual dysfunctions: classifications and definitions. J Sex Med 2007;4:241.

Kingsberg S: Testosterone treatment for hypoactive sexual desire disorder in postmenopausal women. J Sex Med 2007;4:227.

Lentz GM: Emotional aspects of gynecology: sexual dysfunction, eating disorders, substance abuse, depression, grief, loss. In Katz VL, Lentz GM, Lobo RA, Gershenson DM: Comprehensive Gynecology, 5th ed. Philadelphia, Mosby/Elsevier, 2007:184.

McGloin L, Carey JC: Orgasmic dysfunction. Obstet Gynecol Clin North Am 2006;33:579.

Redelman M: A general look at female orgasm and anorgasmia. Sex Health 2006;3:143.

Shen WW, Sata LS: Inhibited female orgasm resulting from psychotropic drugs. J Reprod Med 1983;28:497.

Smith RP: Gynecology in primary care. Baltimore, Williams & Wilkins, 1997:193, 517.

Stimmel GL, Gutierrez MA: Counseling patients about sexual issues. Pharmacotherapy 2006;26:1608.

Zeiss AM, Rosen GM, Zeiss RA: Orgasm during intercourse: a treatment strategy for women. J Consult Clin Psychol 1977;45:89.

INTRODUCTION

Description: Infection by *Haemophilus ducreyi* results in chancroid, one of a group of infrequently encountered sexually transmitted diseases (STDs). Chancroid is more common than syphilis in some areas of Africa and Southeast Asia, but it is uncommon in the United States.

Prevalence: In the United States, 1500 cases per year, generally in small, sporadic outbreaks.

Predominant Age: Younger reproductive.

Genetics: No genetic pattern.

ETIOLOGY AND PATHOGENESIS

Causes: *H. ducreyi* is not capable of infecting intact skin; thus, the lesions of chancroid tend to be found in areas traumatized by sexual activity. Material from the vulvar ulcers is virulent and can infect other body sites.

Risk Factors: Sexual trauma and exposure to the infective agent, prostitution, and human immunodeficiency virus (HIV) infection.

CLINICAL CHARACTERISTICS

Signs and Symptoms

- One to three painful "soft chancres" 3 to 10 days after exposure (these break down over about 2 weeks to form shallow, progressive ulcers with red, ragged, undermined edges, with little surrounding inflammation; autoinoculation is common, resulting in lesions at various stages of evolution)
- Unilateral adenopathy progressing to massive enlargement and inflammation ("buboes," 50%)

  (The combination of a painful ulcer and tender inguinal adenopathy, symptoms occurring in one third of patients, suggests chancroid; when accompanied by suppurative inguinal adenopathy, they are almost pathognomonic. A definitive diagnosis of chancroid requires identification of *H. ducreyi* on special culture media that is not widely available from commercial sources; even using these media, sensitivity is ≤80%.)

DIAGNOSTIC APPROACH

Differential Diagnosis

- Herpes simplex
- Syphilis
- Granuloma inguinale
- Lymphogranuloma venereum

Associated Conditions: Other sexually transmitted infections, HIV. (About 10% of persons who have chancroid acquired in the United States are coinfected with *Treponema pallidum* or herpes simplex virus (HSV); this percentage is higher in persons acquiring chancroid outside the United States.)

Workup and Evaluation

Laboratory: Gram stain and culture of material from open ulcers. Because of the growing association with HIV, serum testing for HIV infections is highly recommended.

Imaging: No imaging indicated.

Special Tests: None indicated.

Diagnostic Procedures: The diagnosis is established based on clinical findings, finding the gram-negative coccobacillus on smears from the primary lesion, or (rarely) on culture of aspirates of the bubo. Biopsy is also diagnostic, although not often performed.

Pathologic Findings

The *H. ducreyi* bacillus is a gram-positive, nonmotile, facultative anaerobe that can be seen in chains on Gram stain or in culture. Superficial and deep ulcers with granulomatous inflammation are found on biopsy.

MANAGEMENT AND THERAPY

Nonpharmacologic

General Measures: Evaluation, culture or Gram stain, topical cleansing, and care.

Specific Measures: Antibiotic treatment for patient and her sexual partner(s). Fluctuant nodes may be drained by aspiration through adjacent normal tissue, but incision and drainage delay healing and should not be attempted.

Diet: No specific dietary changes indicated.

Activity: No sexual activity until lesions have healed.

Patient Education: American College of Obstetricians and Gynecologists Patient Education Pamphlet AP009 (How to Prevent Sexually Transmitted Diseases). Patients should be advised to have all sexual partners seen for diagnosis and treatment.

Drug(s) of Choice

Azithromycin 1 g PO single dose or ceftriaxone 250 mg IM single dose or ciprofloxacin 500 mg PO twice a day for 3 days or erythromycin 500 mg PO four times a day. Treatment must continue for no less than 10 days or until the lesions heal, whichever is longer.

Contraindications: Erythromycin estolate and ciprofloxacin are contraindicated in pregnancy and should not be used. Ciprofloxacin is contraindicated in patients younger than 18 years of age.

Precautions: See individual agents. The safety of azithromycin in pregnancy has not been established.

Interactions: See individual agents.

Alternative Drugs

Trimethoprim 160 mg plus sulfamethoxazole 800 mg PO twice a day. Treatment must continue for no less than 10 days or until the lesions heal, whichever is longer.

Amoxicillin 500 mg plus clavulanic acid 125 mg (Augmentin) PO every 8 hours for 7 days.

FOLLOW-UP

Patient Monitoring: Follow-up evaluation for cure (improvement in 3 to 7 days), culture or other tests

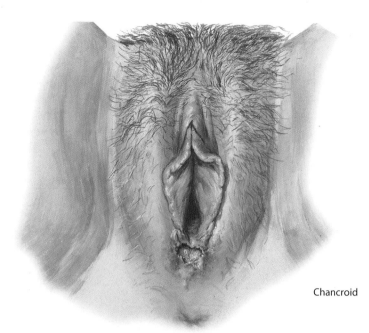

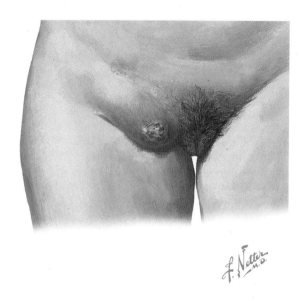

Chancroid

should be carried out, as well as screening for other sexually transmitted diseases. (As with all sexually transmitted diseases, all sexual partners who have had sexual contact with the patient within the preceding 10 days should be screened and treated for probable infections.)

Prevention/Avoidance: Use of barrier contraception (condoms, diaphragm), limitation or elimination of risky behavior (sexual promiscuity).

Possible Complications: Buboes may rupture and drain, causing extensive soft-tissue and skin damage. Chronic draining sinus tracts and abscesses may occur. Scarring is common.

Expected Outcome: If detected early, successful treatment with minimal sequelae may be expected. Buboes, if present, may take several weeks to resolve. Up to 10% of patients have a recurrence at the site of old ulcers.

MISCELLANEOUS

Pregnancy Considerations: No effect on pregnancy, although the possibility of vertical transmission of other associated conditions (such as HIV infection) should be considered.

ICD-9-CM Codes: 099.0.

REFERENCES

Level I

Al-Tawfiq JA, Palmer KL, Chen CY, et al: Experimental infection of human volunteers with *Haemophilus ducreyi* does not confer protection against subsequent challenge. J Infect Dis 1999;179:1283.

Kaul R, Kimani J, Nagelkerke NJ, et al; Kibera HIV Study Group: Monthly antibiotic chemoprophylaxis and incidence of sexually transmitted infections and HIV-1 infection in Kenyan sex workers: a randomized controlled trial. JAMA 2004;291:2555.

Malonza IM, Tyndall MW, Ndinya-Achola JO, et al: A randomized, double-blind, placebo-controlled trial of single-dose ciprofloxacin versus erythromycin for the treatment of chancroid in Nairobi, Kenya. J Infect Dis 1999;180:1886.

Palmer KL, Thornton AC, Fortney KR, et al: Evaluation of an isogenic hemolysin-deficient mutant in the human model of *Haemophilus ducreyi* infection. J Infect Dis 1998;178:191.

Thornton AC, O'Mara EM Jr, Sorensen SJ, et al: Prevention of experimental *Haemophilus ducreyi* infection: a randomized, controlled clinical trial. J Infect Dis 1998;177:1608.

Level II

American College of Obstetricians and Gynecologists: Sexually transmitted diseases in adolescents. ACOG Committee Opinion 301. Washington, DC, ACOG, 2004.

Chen CY, Mertz KJ, Spinola SM, Morse SA: Comparison of enzyme immunoassays for antibodies to *Haemophilus ducreyi* in a community outbreak of chancroid in the United States. J Infect Dis 1997;175:1390.

Dillon SM, Cummings M, Rajagopalan S, McCormack WC: Prospective analysis of genital ulcer disease in Brooklyn, New York. Clin Infect Dis 1997;24:945.

Level III

Abeck D, Freinkel AL, Korting HC, et al: Immunohistochemical investigations of genital ulcers caused by *Haemophilus ducreyi*. Int J STD AIDS 1997;8:585.

Centers for Disease Control and Prevention: Sexually transmitted diseases treatment guidelines, 2006. MMWR 2006;55:15.

Eckert LO, Lentz GM: Infections of the lower genital tract. In Katz VL, Lentz GM, Lobo RA, Gershenson DM: Comprehensive Gynecology, 5th ed. Philadelphia, Mosby/Elsevier, 2007:582.

Eichmann A: Chancroid. Curr Probl Dermatol 1996;4:20.

Wilkinson EJ, Stone IK: Atlas of vulvar disease. Baltimore, Williams & Wilkins, 1995:137.

Sexually Transmitted Infections: Chlamydia Trachomatis

46

INTRODUCTION

Description: The second most common sexually transmitted disease (STD) and most common bacterial STD is infection caused by *Chlamydia trachomatis*. More common than *Neisseria gonorrhoeae* by 3-fold, infections with *C. trachomatis* can be the source of significant complications and infertility.

Prevalence: Twenty percent of pregnant patients, 30% of sexually active adolescent women. Up to 40% of all sexually active women have antibodies suggesting prior infection. In 2005, 976,445 chlamydia infections were reported to the Centers for Disease Control and Prevention (CDC) from 50 states and the District of Columbia (496.5 cases per 100,000 females), up 5.1% from 2004.

Predominant Age: 15 to 30 years (85%), peak age 15 to 19 years. The Centers for Disease Control and Prevention recommend screening all sexually active women younger than age 26 years.

Genetics: No genetic pattern.

ETIOLOGY AND PATHOGENESIS

Causes: Infection by the obligate intracellular organism *C. trachomatis*. Chlamydia has a long incubation period (average, 10 days) and may persist in the cervix as a carrier state for many years.

Risk Factors: The risk of contracting chlamydial infection is five times greater with three or more sexual partners and four times higher for patients using no contraception or nonbarrier methods of birth control. Other factors are age younger than 26 years, new partner within the preceding 3 months, other sexually transmitted diseases, vaginal douching.

CLINICAL CHARACTERISTICS

Signs and Symptoms

- Frequently asymptomatic
- Cervicitis; pelvic inflammatory disease (PID); or, much less common, lymphogranuloma venereum
- Less common: nongonococcal urethritis and inclusion conjunctivitis
- Eversion of the cervix with mucopurulent cervicitis supports the diagnosis but not pathognomic

DIAGNOSTIC APPROACH

Differential Diagnosis

- Gonorrhea
- PID
- Septic abortion
- Appendicitis
- Gastroenteritis
- **Associated Conditions:** Infertility, ectopic pregnancy, mucopurulent cervicitis, PID, chronic pelvic pain, and endometritis.

Workup and Evaluation

Laboratory: Cultures on cycloheximide-treated McCoy cells are specific and may be used to confirm the diagnosis, but these cultures are expensive, difficult to perform, and often not available. Two clinical screening tests are an enzyme-linked immunoassay (enzyme-linked immunosorbent assay) performed on cervical secretions and a monoclonal antibody test carried out on dried smears. When trying to obtain cervical cultures for chlamydia, plastic- or metal-shafted rayon- or cotton-tipped swabs are preferred. Wood-shafted or calcium alginate swabs reduce the yield of material when transport media are used because of leeching of toxic products into the media. Newer screening techniques using patient-collected vaginal swabs or urine specimens may be used but are not widely available.

Imaging: No imaging indicated. Ultrasonography may demonstrate free fluid in the cul-de-sac when pelvic inflammation is present.

Special Tests: None indicated.

Diagnostic Procedures: Physical examination, suspicion, and cervical culture.

Pathologic Findings

This infection tends to involve the mucosal layers and not the entire structure. As a result, extensive damage may occur without dramatic symptoms if the fallopian tubes become infected.

MANAGEMENT AND THERAPY

Nonpharmacologic

General Measures: Evaluation and diagnosis.

Specific Measures: Aggressive antibiotic therapy should be instituted in those suspected of infection. Approximately 45% of patients with chlamydial infection have coexisting gonorrhea; the therapy chosen should consider this.

Diet: No specific dietary changes indicated.

Activity: No restriction. (Sexual continence required until infection is resolved.)

Patient Education: American College of Obstetricians and Gynecologists Patient Education Pamphlet AP009 (How to Prevent Sexually Transmitted Diseases). Patients should be advised to have all sexual partners seen for diagnosis and treatment.

Drug(s) of Choice

Azithromycin (1 g PO, single dose) compares favorably with the standard 7-day course of doxycycline, while providing better compliance and fewer side effects. A meta-analysis of 12 randomized clinical trials of azithromycin versus doxycycline for the treatment of genital chlamydial infection demonstrated that the treatments were equally efficacious, with microbial cure rates of 97% and 98%, respectively.

127

Doxycycline (100 mg PO twice a day for 7 days) may also be used.

Contraindications: Quinolones (Ofloxacin), tetracyclines (including doxycycline), and erythromycin estolate are contraindicated in pregnancy and should not be used.

Precautions: Pregnant patients with chlamydial infections should be treated with azithromycin, amoxicillin (500 mg PO three times a day for 7 days), erythromycin base, or erythromycin ethylsuccinate.

Alternative Drugs

Erythromycin (erythromycin base 500 mg PO four times a day for 7 days or erythromycin ethylsuccinate 800 mg PO four times a day for 7 days) may be substituted for tetracycline in patients who are tetracycline-sensitive or pregnant. For patients who cannot tolerate erythromycin, amoxicillin (500 mg PO three times a day for 7 to 10 days) may be substituted.

Ofloxacin (300 mg PO twice a day for 7 days).

Levofloxacin (500 mg orally once daily for 7 days).

FOLLOW-UP

Patient Monitoring: Follow-up evaluation for cure with culture or other tests (3 to 4 weeks after therapy) and screening for other sexually transmitted diseases should be performed. (As with all sexually transmitted diseases, all sexual partners within the preceding 30 days should be screened and treated for probable infections.)

Prevention/Avoidance: Use of barrier contraception (condoms, diaphragm), limitation or elimination of risky behavior (sexual promiscuity).

Possible Complications: Infertility, chronic pelvic pain. If PID occurs, the risk of infertility roughly doubles with each subsequent episode resulting in a 40% rate of infertility after only three episodes. Women with documented salpingitis have a 4-fold increase in their rate of ectopic pregnancy and 5% to 15% of women require surgery because of damage caused by PID.

Expected Outcome: If detected early, successful treatment with minimal sequelae may be expected. Significant permanent damage is common despite treatment because of the indolent course of most infections and thus the late institution of therapy.

MISCELLANEOUS

Pregnancy Considerations: No effect on pregnancy. Neonatal conjunctivitis and ophthalmia neonatorum may result if an infant does not receive adequate prophylaxis. Even with standard protection (1% $AgNO_3$ or 0.5% erythromycin ointment), complete protection is not assured.

ICD-9-CM Codes: 099.5.

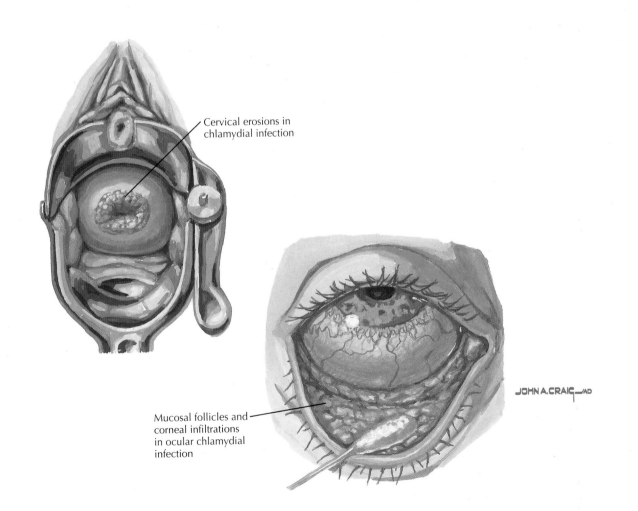

Cervical erosions in chlamydial infection

Mucosal follicles and corneal infiltrations in ocular chlamydial infection

JOHN A. CRAIG—AD

REFERENCES

Level I

Adair CD, Gunter M, Stovall TG, et al: Chlamydia in pregnancy: a randomized trial of azithromycin and erythromycin. Obstet Gynecol 1998;91:165.

Jacobson GF, Autry AM, Kirby RS, et al: A randomized controlled trial comparing amoxicillin and azithromycin for the treatment of *Chlamydia trachomatis* in pregnancy. Am J Obstet Gynecol 2001;184:1352.

Silverman NS, Sullivan M, Hochman M, et al: A randomized, prospective trial comparing amoxicillin and erythromycin for the treatment of *Chlamydia trachomatis* in pregnancy. Am J Obstet Gynecol 1994;170:829.

Level II

Cook RL, Hutchison SL, Ostergaard L, et al: Systematic review: noninvasive testing for *Chlamydia trachomatis* and *Neisseria gonorrhoeae*. Ann Intern Med 2005;142:914.

Lau C-Y, Qureshi AK: Azithromycin versus doxycycline for genital chlamydial infections: a meta-analysis of randomized clinical trials. Sex Transmit Dis 2002;29:497.

Lyss SB, Kamb ML, Peterman TA, et al: *Chlamydia trachomatis* among patients infected with and treated for *Neisseria gonorrhoeae* in sexually transmitted disease clinics in the United States. Ann Intern Med 2003;139:178.

Martin DH, Mroczkowski TF, Dalu ZA, et al: A controlled trial of a single dose of azithromycin for the treatment of chlamydial urethritis and cervicitis: the azithromycin for Chlamydial Infections Study Group. N Engl J Med 1992;327:921.

Ness RB, Trautmann G, Richter HE, et al: Effectiveness of treatment strategies of some women with pelvic inflammatory disease: a randomized trial. Obstet Gynecol 2005;106:573.

Ostergaard L, Andersen B, Olesen F, Moller JK: Efficacy of home sampling for screening of *Chlamydia trachomatis*: randomized study. BMJ 1998;317:26.

Peterman TA, Tian LH, Metcalf CA, et al; RESPECT-2 Study Group: High incidence of new sexually transmitted infections in the year following a sexually transmitted infection: a case for rescreening. Ann Intern Med 2006;145:564–72. Summary for patients in: Ann Intern Med 2006;145:I44.

Tanaka M, Nakayama H, Sagiyama K, et al: Evaluation of a new amplified enzyme immunoassay (EIA) for the detection of *Chlamydia trachomatis* in male urine, female endocervical swab, and patient-obtained vaginal swab specimens. J Clin Pathol 2000;53:350.

Level III

American College of Obstetricians and Gynecologists: Sexually transmitted diseases in adolescents. ACOG Committee Opinion 301. Washington, DC, ACOG, 2004.

Centers for Disease Control and Prevention: Recommendations for the prevention and management of *Chlamydia trachomatis* infections, 1993. MMWR 1993;42:1.

Centers for Disease Control and Prevention: Sexually transmitted diseases treatment guidelines, 2006. MMWR 2006;55:21, 38.

Crossman SH: The challenge of pelvic inflammatory disease. Am Fam Physician 2006;73:859.

Eckert LO, Lentz GM: Infections of the lower genital tract. In Katz VL, Lentz GM, Lobo RA, Gershenson DM: Comprehensive Gynecology, 5th ed. Philadelphia, Mosby/Elsevier, 2007:600.

Faro S: Chlamydia trachomatis: female pelvic infection. Am J Obstet Gynecol 1991;164:1767.

Jones RB: New treatments for *Chlamydia trachomatis*. Am J Obstet Gynecol 1991;164:1789.

Lee HH, Chernesky MA, Schachter J, et al: Diagnosis of *Chlamydia trachomatis* genitourinary infection in women by ligase chain reaction assay of urine. Lancet 1995;345:213.

Low N: Screening programmes for chlamydial infection: when will we ever learn? BMJ 2007;334:725.

Mangione-Smith R, McGlynn EA, Hiatt L: Screening for chlamydia in adolescents and young women. Arch Pediatr Adolesc Med 2000;154:1108.

Miller KE: Diagnosis and treatment of *Chlamydia trachomatis* infection. Am Fam Physician 2006;73:1411.

Morrison RP. New insights into a persistent problem—Chlamydial infections. J Clin Invest 2003;111:1647.

Osser S, Persson K: Chlamydial antibodies in women who suffer miscarriage. Br J Obstet Gynaecol 1996;103:137.

Peipert JF: Clinical practice. Genital chlamydial infections. N Engl J Med 2003;349:2424.

Skolnik NS: Screening for *Chlamydia trachomatis* infection. Am Fam Physician 1995;51:821.

Stamm WE: *Chlamydia trachomatis* infections: progress and problems. J Infect Dis 1999;179:S380.

INTRODUCTION

Description: Condyloma acuminata are raised, warty lesions caused by infection by the human papillomavirus (HPV).

Prevalence: Most common sexually transmitted disease: 500,000 cases per year.

Predominant Age: 16 to 25 years.

Genetics: No genetic pattern.

ETIOLOGY AND PATHOGENESIS

Causes: Caused by infection by HPV (most frequently serotypes 6 and 11; 90%). This DNA virus is found in 2% to 4% of all women, and up to 60% of patients have evidence of the virus when polymerase chain reaction techniques are used. The virus is hardy and may resist even drying, making transmission and autoinoculation common. Some evidence suggests that fomite transmission rarely could occur. The virus is most commonly spread by skin-to-skin (generally sexual) contact and has an incubation period of 3 weeks to 8 months, with an average of 3 months. Roughly 65% of patients acquire the infection after intercourse with an infected partner.

Risk Factors: Multiple sexual partners; the presence of other vaginal infections such as candidiasis, trichomoniasis, or bacterial vaginosis; smoking; and oral contraceptive use.

CLINICAL CHARACTERISTICS

Signs and Symptoms

- Asymptomatic (<2% have condyloma)
- Painless, raised, soft, fleshy growths on the vulva, vagina, cervix, urethral meatus, perineum, and anus (mild irritation or discharge may accompany secondary infections). Symmetrical lesions across the midline of the genital area common (condyloma may also be found on the tongue or within the oral cavity, the urethra, bladder, or rectum). (Roughly one third of women with vulvar lesions also have vaginal warts or intraepithelial neoplasia [VAIN], and approximately 40% have cervical involvement. Cervical condyloma are generally flatter and may be identified through colposcopic examination; by Pap test; or through the application of 3% to 5% acetic acid to make apparent the raised, white, shiny plaques.)
- Abnormal cervical cytologic changes common

DIAGNOSTIC APPROACH

Differential Diagnosis

- Condyloma lata (syphilis)
- Papilloma

Associated Conditions: Other sexually transmitted infections (*Trichomonas* infection or bacterial vaginosis), abnormal cervical cytologic changes, vulvar and vaginal neoplasia.

Workup and Evaluation

Laboratory: No evaluation indicated. (Tests for syphilis when indicated.)

Imaging: No imaging indicated.

Special Tests: Colposcopic examination; Pap test; or the application of 3% to 5% acetic acid to make apparent the raised, white, shiny plaques. Serotyping is not currently indicated. Biopsy is indicated if the warts are pigmented, indurated, fixed, bleeding, or ulcerated.

Diagnostic Procedures: Physical examination, colposcopy, and biopsy.

Pathologic Findings

Sessile (keratotic) lesions.

MANAGEMENT AND THERAPY

Nonpharmacologic

General Measures: Local hygiene.

Specific Measures: The treatment of small, uncomplicated venereal warts is generally by cytolytic topical agents, such as podophyllin (Podophyllum resin); bichloracetic or trichloroacetic acid (TCA); or physical ablative methods such as laser, cryotherapy, or electrodesiccation. In rare selected patients, surgical excision or tangential shaving may be used.

Diet: No specific dietary changes indicated.

Activity: Sexual continence until partner(s) are examined and treated.

Patient Education: American College of Obstetricians and Gynecologists Patient Education Pamphlet AP009 (How to Prevent Sexually Transmitted Diseases). Patients should be advised to have all sexual partners seen for diagnosis and treatment.

Drug(s) of Choice

Podophyllin (20% to 50% in tincture of benzoin, 25% ointment), podophyllotoxin (0.5% solution, Condylox), bichloracetic or trichloroacetic acid (80% to 100% solution), carefully applied to the warts, protecting the adjacent skin, and allowed to remain for between 30 minutes and 4 hours before being washed off the lesions. With most topical therapy, slough of the treated lesions happens in 2 to 4 days. Treatment may be repeated every 7 to 14 days as needed. Patients may self-apply podofilox (0.5% solution or gel, twice a day for 3 days) or Imiquimod (5% cream, Aldara, every night three times per week for up to 16 weeks).

Contraindications: Podophyllin may not be used during pregnancy because of absorption, potentially resulting in neural or myelotoxicity.

Precautions: To limit toxicity with podophyllin, treatments should be limited to less than 0.5 mL total volume and less than 10 cm^2 in area. Imiquimod should be washed from the vulva in the morning (after 6 to 10 hours).

Alternative Drugs

Treatment with 5-fluorouracil 1% or 5% cream is often used as primary therapy or as an adjunct for cervical or vaginal lesions (applied daily until edema, erythema, or vesiculation occurs). Therapy with autologous vaccine, dinitrochlorobenzene, and interferon has been advocated but has yet to gain a significant place in clinical practice.

FOLLOW-UP

Patient Monitoring: The patient should be seen weekly until no further lesions are found. Because these patients are at higher risk for cervical neoplasia, close follow-up with Pap tests, colposcopy, or both, at 6- to 12-month intervals is recommended. Follow-up serologic testing for syphilis and human immunodeficiency virus (HIV) infection as indicated. The sexual partners of patients with HPV should also be screened for genital warts.

Prevention/Avoidance: Limitation or elimination of risky behavior (sexual promiscuity). The use of condoms has not been shown to reduce the spread of HPV but should still be encouraged to reduce the spread of other sexually transmitted diseases. Qvadravalent HPV vaccine (types 6, 11, 16, and 18; Guardasil) should provide some measure of protection though its primary indication is to reduce the risk of cervical cancer.

Possible Complications: Those who are immunocompromised, such as patients who have received a transplant, patients with acquired immune deficiency syndrome (AIDS), or pregnant patients, may experience rapid and exuberant growth of condyloma. External factors that suppress the immune system (steroids, cigarette smoking, metabolic deficiencies, and infections with other viruses such as herpes) may have similar effects. Several subtypes (16, 18, 31, 33, 35, and others) are associated with the development of cervical neoplasia. Roughly 90% of patients with cervical squamous cell carcinoma have evidence of HPV DNA present in their cervical tissues. It is currently thought that a cocarcinogen, such as smoking, other viruses, or nutritional factors are required before malignant transformation may take place.

Expected Outcome: The success rate for resolution of overt warts is approximately 75%, with a recurrence rate of 65% to 80%. If lesions persist or continually recur, cryosurgery, electrodesiccation, surgical excision, or laser vaporization may be required. If cryotherapy is chosen, three to six treatments are often required, but cure rates are higher than those for podophyllin and comparable with those for laser ablation (60% to 80%). Even with laser ablation, recurrence rates are reported to vary from 25% to 100%. Scarring is rare. HPV types 16, 18, 31, 33, and 35 are found occasionally in visible

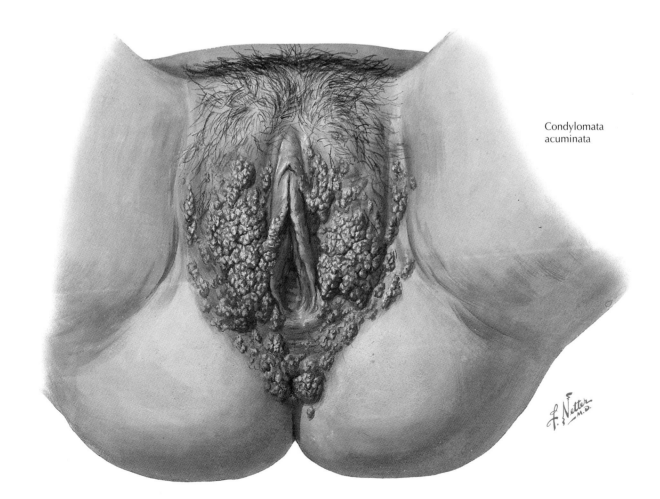

Condylomata
acuminata

genital warts and have been associated with external genital (i.e., vulvar, penile, and anal) squamous intraepithelial neoplasia (i.e., squamous cell carcinoma in situ, bowenoid papulosis, erythroplasia of Queyrat, or Bowen's disease of the genitalia). For this reason, recurrent lesions or those that do not respond as expected should be further investigated.

MISCELLANEOUS

Pregnancy Considerations: Pregnant patients may experience rapid and exuberant growth of condyloma, and lesions are more resistant to therapy. Extensive vaginal or vulvar lesions may require cesarean delivery to avoid extensive lacerations and suturing problems.
ICD-9-CM Codes: 078.11.

REFERENCES

Level I
Georgala S, Katoulis AC, Befon A, et al: Oral inosiplex in the treatment of cervical condylomata acuminata: a randomized placebo-controlled trial. BJOG 2006;113:1088.
Vandepapeliere P, Barrasso R, Meijer CJ, et al: Randomized controlled trial of an adjuvanted human papillomavirus (HPV) type 6 L2E7 vaccine: infection of external anogenital warts with multiple HPV types and failure of therapeutic vaccination. J Infect Dis 2005;192:2099. Epub 2005 Nov 11.

Level II
Bonnez W, Elswick RK Jr, Bailey-Farchione A, et al: Efficacy and safety of 0.5% podofilox solution in the treatment and suppression of anogenital warts. Am J Med 1994;96:420.
Conley LJ, Ellenbrock TV, Bush TJ, et al: HIV-1 infection and risk of vulvovaginal and perianal condylomata acuminata and intraepithelial neoplasia: a prospective cohort study. Lancet 2002; 359:108.
Jha PK, Beral V, Peto J, et al: Antibodies to human papillomavirus and to other genital infectious agents and invasive cervical cancer risk. Lancet 1993;341:1116.

Level III
American College of Obstetricians and Gynecologists: Human papillomavirus. ACOG Practice Bulletin 61. Washington, DC, ACOG, 2005.
American College of Obstetricians and Gynecologists: Human papillomavirus vaccination. ACOG Committee Opinion 344. Washington, DC, ACOG, 2006.
Brotzman GL: Evaluating the impact of HPV-related diseases: cervical cancer and genital warts. J Fam Pract 2005;Suppl HPV Prevention:S3.
Eckert LO, Lentz GM: Infections of the lower genital tract. In Katz VL, Lentz GM, Lobo RA, Gershenson DM: Comprehensive Gynecology, 5th ed. Philadelphia, Mosby/Elsevier, 2007:576.
Hagensee ME, Cameron JE, Leigh JE, Clark RA: Human papillomavirus infection and disease in HIV-infected individuals. Am J Med Sci 2004;328:57.
Horowitz BJ: Interferon therapy for condylomatous vulvitis. Obstet Gynecol 1989;73:446.
Kodner CM, Nasraty S: Management of genital warts. Am Fam Physician 2004;70:2335.

INTRODUCTION

Description: Infection with gonorrhea, a gram-negative intracellular diplococcus, remains common, accounting for 358,366 new cases of gonorrhea in the United States in 2006.

Prevalence: Roughly 3 of 1000 sexually active women and as many as 7% of pregnant patients; 120.9 per 100,000 women.

Predominant Age: 15 to 30 (85%), highest age 15 to 19 years.

Genetics: No genetic pattern.

ETIOLOGY AND PATHOGENESIS

Causes: Infection by the gram-negative intracellular diplococcus, *Neisseria gonorrhoeae.*

Risk Factors: It is estimated that the rate of infection with one act of intercourse with an infected partner is 20% for men but 60% to 80% for women. (For this reason, any patient exposed to gonorrhea within the preceding month should be cultured and treated presumptively.) This rate increases to 60% to 80% for both sexes with four or more exposures. The groups with the highest risk are adolescents, drug users, and sex workers.

CLINICAL CHARACTERISTICS
Signs and Symptoms

- Asymptomatic (50%)
- Malodorous, purulent discharge from the urethra, Skene duct, cervix, vagina, or anus (even without rectal intercourse) 3 to 5 days after exposure (40% to 60%)
- Simultaneous urethral infection (70% to 90%)
- Infection of the pharynx (10% to 20%)
- Gonococcal conjunctivitis (can rapidly lead to blindness)
- Polyarthritis
- Septic abortion or postabortal sepsis

DIAGNOSTIC APPROACH
Differential Diagnosis

- Chlamydial infection
- Pelvic inflammatory disease (PID)
- Septic abortion
- Appendicitis
- Gastroenteritis

Associated Conditions: Infertility, ectopic pregnancy, mucopurulent cervicitis, pelvic inflammatory disease (10% to 40% of untreated cases), chronic pelvic pain, and endometritis.

Workup and Evaluation

Laboratory: Culture on Thayer-Martin agar plates kept in a CO_2-rich environment. Cervical cultures provide 80% to 95% diagnostic sensitivity. Cultures should also be obtained from the urethra and anus, although these additional cultures do not significantly increase the sensitivity of testing. A Gram stain of any cervical discharge for the presence of gram-negative intracellular diplococcus supports the presumptive diagnosis but does not establish it (sensitivity 50% to 70%, specificity 97%). A solid-phase enzyme immunoassay may also be used. Even when the diagnosis is established by other methods, all cases of gonorrhea should have cultures obtained to assess antibiotic susceptibility, although therapy should not be delayed pending the results.

Imaging: No imaging indicated. Ultrasonography may demonstrate free fluid in the cul-de-sac when pelvic inflammation is present.

Special Tests: None indicated.

Diagnostic Procedures: Physical examination, suspicion, and cervical culture.

Pathologic Findings

Gram-negative intracellular diplococcus associated with diffuse inflammatory reaction (transluminal in the fallopian tube).

MANAGEMENT AND THERAPY
Nonpharmacologic

General Measures: Evaluation and diagnosis.

Specific Measures: Aggressive antibiotic therapy should be instituted in patients suspected of having an infection.

Diet: No specific dietary changes indicated.

Activity: No restriction. (Sexual continence is required until the infection has resolved.)

Patient Education: American College of Obstetricians and Gynecologists Patient Education Pamphlet AP009 (How to Prevent Sexually Transmitted Diseases). Patients should be advised to have all sexual partners seen for diagnosis and treatment.

Drug(s) of Choice

Ceftriaxone 125 mg IM or cefixime 400 mg PO single dose or

Ciprofloxacin 500 mg PO single dose or

Ofloxacin 400 mg orally in a single dose* or

Levofloxacin 250 mg orally in a single dose*

Contraindications: Quinolones (Ofloxacin), tetracyclines (including doxycycline), and erythromycin estolate are contraindicated in pregnancy and should not be used.

Precautions: See individual agents.

Interactions: See individual agents.

---

*Quinolones should not be used for infections in men who have sex with men or in patients with a history of recent foreign travel or partners' travel, infections acquired in California or Hawaii, or infections acquired in other areas with increased quinolone-resistant *N. gonorrhoeae* (QRNG) prevalence.

Gonorrhea in the Female

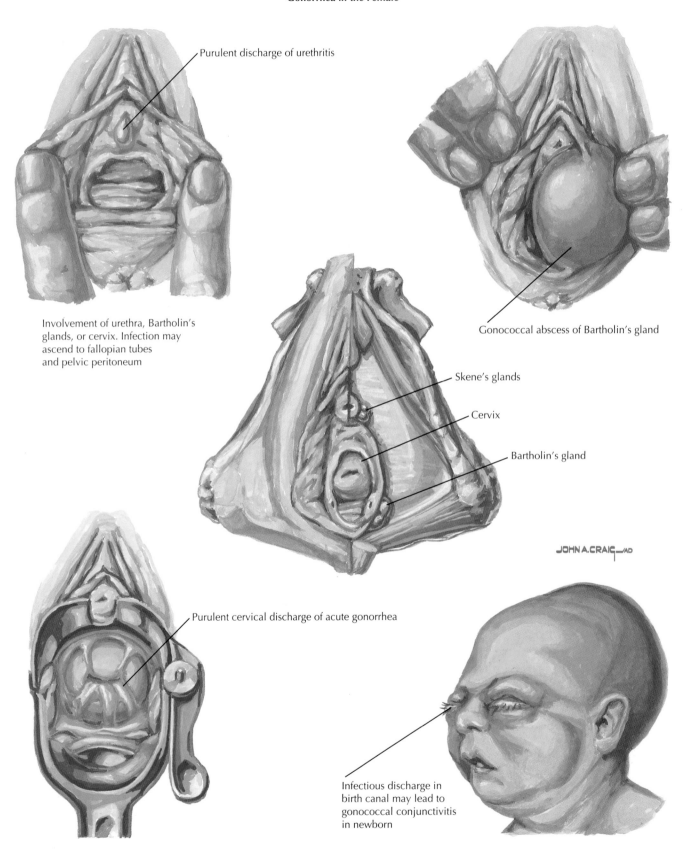

Purulent discharge of urethritis

Involvement of urethra, Bartholin's glands, or cervix. Infection may ascend to fallopian tubes and pelvic peritoneum

Gonococcal abscess of Bartholin's gland

Skene's glands

Cervix

Bartholin's gland

JOHN A. CRAIG—AD

Purulent cervical discharge of acute gonorrhea

Infectious discharge in birth canal may lead to gonococcal conjunctivitis in newborn

Alternative Drugs

Spectinomycin 2 g IM as single dose.

Ceftriaxone 125 mg IM and cefixime 400 mg PO as single dose.

Ceftizoxime 500 mg IM, cefotaxime 500 mg IM, or cefotetan 1 g IM, all as single dose.

Cefoxitin 2 g IM plus probenecid 1 g PO.

Cefuroxime axetil 1 g PO or cefpodoxime proxetil 200 mg PO, both as single dose.

Enoxacin 400 mg PO, lomefloxacin 400 mg PO, or norfloxacin 800 mg PO, all as single dose.

FOLLOW-UP

Patient Monitoring: When patients are treated with the currently recommended ceftriaxone–doxycycline, therapy failure is rare and a follow-up culture is not necessary. Reexamination of the patient in 1 to 2 months for the possibility of reinfection may be warranted in patients at high risk. (As with all sexually transmitted diseases, all sexual partners within the preceding 30 days should be screened and treated for probable infections.)

Prevention/Avoidance: Use of barrier contraception (condoms, diaphragm), limitation or elimination of risky behavior (sexual promiscuity).

Possible Complications: Damage caused by *N. gonorrhoeae* infection causes an increased risk of recurrent pelvic infection, chronic pelvic pain, or infertility resulting from tubal damage or hydrosalpinx formation. The impact of a gonorrheal infection is much greater for women than it is for men. For every three men infected, two women are hospitalized for 1 or more days. For every 18 men infected, 1 woman undergoes surgery. It is estimated that one episode of gonorrhea is associated with a 15% infertility rate; this increases to 75% for three or more infections. The risk of an ectopic pregnancy is increased 7 to 10 times in women with a history of salpingitis. Neonatal infections acquired from a mother with gonorrhea may result in conjunctivitis or pneumonia. Pregnant patients are more likely to experience disseminated gonococcal infection. They account for 7% to 40% of all cases.

Expected Outcome: If detected early, successful treatment with minimal sequelae may be expected. Significant permanent damage is common despite treatment because of the indolent course of many infections and the late institution of therapy.

MISCELLANEOUS

Pregnancy Considerations: Pregnant patients should be treated with ceftriaxone 250 mg IM as a single dose. Erythromycin (erythromycin base, 500 mg PO four times a day for 7 days) may be added if there is a possibility of a coexisting chlamydial infection. Neonatal conjunctivitis and ophthalmia neonatorum may result if the infant does not receive adequate prophylaxis.

ICD-9-CM Codes: 098.0 (Acute, lower genital tract), 098.1 (Acute, upper genital tract) (others based on chronicity and organ involved).

REFERENCES

Level II

Centers for Disease Control and Surveillance: Decreased susceptibility of *Neisseria gonorrhoeae* to fluoroquinolones—Ohio and Hawaii, 1992–1994. MMWR 1994;43:325.

Golden MR, Whittington WL, Handsfield HH, et al: Effect of expedited treatment of sex partners on recurrent or persistent gonorrhea or chlamydial infection. N Engl J Med 2005;352:676.

Lyss SB, Kamb ML, Peterman TA, et al: Chlamydia trachomatis among patients infected with and treated for *Neisseria gonorrhoeae* in sexually transmitted disease clinics in the United States. Ann Intern Med 2003;139:178.

Phillips RS, Hanff PA, Wertheimer A, Aronson MD: Gonorrhea in women seen for routine gynecologic care: criteria for testing. Am J Med 1988;85:177.

Ramus R, Mayfield J, Wendel G: Evaluation of the current CDC recommended treatment guidelines for gonorrhea in pregnancy. Am J Obstet Gynecol 1996;174:409.

Level III

Centers for Disease Control and Prevention: Sexually transmitted disease surveillance, 2004. Atlanta, GA, U.S. Department of Health and Human Services, CDC, National Center for HIV, STD, and TB Prevention, 2005.

Centers for Disease Control and Prevention: Sexually transmitted diseases treatment guidelines, 2006. MMWR 2006;55:21, 38.

Centers for Disease Control and Prevention: Updated recommended treatment regimens for gonococcal infections and associated conditions—United States, April 2007. MMWR 2007;56;332.

Eckert LO, Lentz GM: Infections of the lower genital tract. In Katz VL, Lentz GM, Lobo RA, Gershenson DM: Comprehensive Gynecology, 5th ed. Philadelphia, Mosby/Elsevier, 2007:599.

Sexually Transmitted Infections: Granuloma Inguinale (Donovanosis)

INTRODUCTION

Description: Granuloma inguinale (also called donovanosis) is relatively common in the tropics, New Guinea, and Caribbean areas but accounts for less than 100 cases per year in the United States. This infection is caused by the intracellular gram-negative bacterium *Klebsiella granulomatis* (formerly known as *Calymmatobacterium granulomatis)*.

Prevalence: Uncommon, 100 cases per year in United States, up to 25% of the population in some subtropical areas.

Predominant Age: Younger reproductive.

Genetics: No genetic pattern.

ETIOLOGY AND PATHOGENESIS

Causes: Infection is caused by the bipolar, gram-negative bacterium *K. granulomatis.*

Risk Factors: Sexual trauma and exposure to the infective agent.

CLINICAL CHARACTERISTICS

Signs and Symptoms

- Single or multiple painless subcutaneous papules that evolve to raised, beefy-red, granulomatous lesions that bleed on contact, undergo ulceration and necrosis, and heal slowly (lesions are confined to the genitalia in 80% of patients; lesions generally appear within 2 weeks of exposure)
- Painless papules with rolled borders and friable base
- Marked adenopathy not present
- Hypertrophic, necrotic, or sclerotic variants exist

DIAGNOSTIC APPROACH

Differential Diagnosis

- Chancroid
- Lymphogranuloma venereum
- Herpes simplex
- Syphilis

Associated Conditions: Brawny edema of the external genitalia.

Workup and Evaluation

Laboratory: Gram stain and culture of material from open ulcers. Culture for other sexually transmitted infections should also be considered.

Imaging: No imaging indicated.

Special Tests: Samples for biopsy may be taken from the edge of the ulcer to confirm the diagnosis. A crushed tissue smear may be examined for Donovan bodies.

Diagnostic Procedures: Diagnosis is established clinically or through the identification of intracytoplasmic bacteria (Donovan bodies) in mononuclear cells.

Pathologic Findings

Granulation tissue associated with an extensive chronic inflammatory cell infiltrate and endarteritis. The ulcer is filled with fibrinous exudate and necrosis; plasma cells and mononuclear cells predominate. Donovan bodies (large vacuolated histiocytes with encapsulated bacilli) are diagnostic. Granuloma inguinale extends by local infiltration and by lymphatic permeation in later stages.

MANAGEMENT AND THERAPY

Nonpharmacologic

General Measures: Evaluation, culture or Gram stain, topical cleansing and care.

Specific Measures: Antibiotic therapy.

Diet: No specific dietary changes indicated.

Activity: No restriction. (Sexual continence required until infection is resolved.)

Patient Education: American College of Obstetricians and Gynecologists Patient Education Pamphlet AP009 (How to Prevent Sexually Transmitted Diseases). Patients should be advised to have all sexual partners seen for diagnosis and treatment.

Drug(s) of Choice

Doxycycline 100 mg PO twice a day for a minimum of 3 weeks or

Azithromycin 1 g PO once per week for at least 3 weeks and until all lesions have completely healed or

Ciprofloxacin 750 mg PO twice a day for at least 3 weeks and until all lesions have completely healed or

Erythromycin base 500 mg PO four times a day for at least 3 weeks and until all lesions have completely healed or

Trimethoprim-sulfamethoxazole, one double-strength tablet PO twice a day for a minimum of 3 weeks.

Contraindications: Known or suspected allergy.

Precautions: Tetracyclines should not be used during pregnancy if at all possible because staining of teeth and inhibition of bone growth are both possible. Sulfonamides should not be used during pregnancy.

Interactions: See individual agents.

Alternative Drugs

Ciprofloxacin 750 mg PO twice a day for a minimum of 3 weeks.

Erythromycin 500 mg PO four times a day for a minimum of 3 weeks.

If lesions fail to show improvement after the first week of treatment, chloramphenicol (500 mg PO three times a day) or gentamicin (1 mg/kg twice a day) should be considered.

FOLLOW-UP

Patient Monitoring: Because of relapse and late scarring, these patients should be followed carefully for several weeks. Follow-up evaluation for cure with culture or

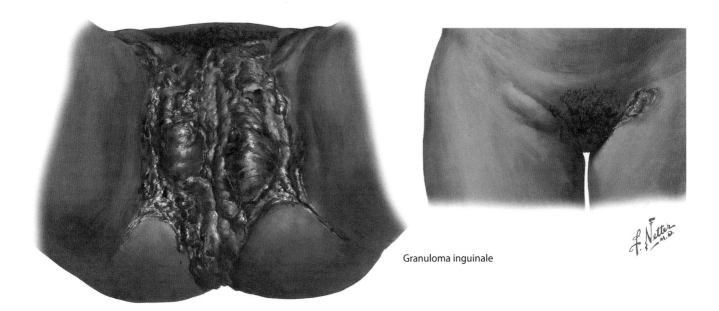

Granuloma inguinale

other tests should be carried out, as should screening for other sexually transmitted diseases. (As with all sexually transmitted diseases, all sexual partners within the preceding 30 days should be screened and treated for probable infections as well.)

Prevention/Avoidance: None.

Possible Complications: Secondary infection or significant scarring may occur in patients with untreated disease.

Expected Outcome: Gradual healing with antibiotic treatment, but scarring and vulvar stenosis are common and may require surgical treatment.

MISCELLANEOUS

Pregnancy Considerations: No direct effect on pregnancy. Women who are pregnant or lactating should be treated with erythromycin plus parenteral aminoglycoside (e.g., gentamicin).

ICD-9-CM Codes: 099.2.

REFERENCES

Level III

Centers for Disease Control and Prevention: Sexually transmitted diseases treatment guidelines, 2006. MMWR 2006;55:20–1.

Eckert LO, Lentz GM: Infections of the lower genital tract. In Katz VL, Lentz GM, Lobo RA, Gershenson DM: Comprehensive Gynecology, 5th ed. Philadelphia, Mosby/Elsevier, 2007:580–2.

Goens JL, Schwartz RA, De Wolf K: Mucocutaneous manifestations of chancroid, lymphogranuloma venereum and granuloma inguinale. Am Fam Physician 1994;49:415–8, 423–5.

Keck JW: Ulcerative lesions. Clin Fam Pract 2005;7:13–30.

Krieger JN: Biology of sexually transmitted diseases. Urol Clin North Am 1984;11:15–25.

Kuberski T: Granuloma inguinale (donovanosis). Sex Transm Dis 1980;7:29.

Lynch PJ: Therapy of sexually transmitted diseases. Med Clin North Am 1982;66:915–25.

Rackel RE, Bope ET: Granuloma inguinale. In Conn's Current therapy 2005, 57th ed. St. Louis, Saunders, 2005:859.

INTRODUCTION

Description: Infection by the herpes simplex virus (HSV) results in recurrent symptoms that range from uncomfortable to disabling, and there is a special risk to the neonate when herpes infection occurs during pregnancy.

Prevalence: Forty-five to 50 million recurrent cases; 1 million new cases per year; one in four women have been infected.

Predominant Age: 15 to 30 years (85%).

Genetics: No genetic pattern.

ETIOLOGY AND PATHOGENESIS

Causes: Roughly 80% of genital herpes infections are caused by HSV type 2, with the remaining 20% caused by the HSV type 1 virus. (Up to 50% of first-episode cases of genital herpes are caused by HSV-1.) Exposure to type 1 virus often happens in childhood and causes oral "cold sores." Previous infection with type 1 virus appears to provide some immunity to type 2 infections. The incubation period from infection to symptoms is generally approximately 6 days (range 3 to 9), with first episodes lasting from 10 to 12 days. The majority of patients with symptomatic, first-episode genital HSV-2 infection subsequently have recurrent episodes; recurrences are less frequent after initial genital HSV-1 infection.

Risk Factors: Roughly 75% of sexual partners of infected individuals contract the disease if intercourse occurs during viral shedding. Patients are infectious during the period from first prodrome through crusting of the lesions. Viral shedding may also occur asymptomatically. (Persons unaware that they have the infection or who are asymptomatic when transmission occurs transmit the majority of genital herpes infections.) Nonsexual transmission has not been documented.

CLINICAL CHARACTERISTICS

Signs and Symptoms

- Prodromal phase—mild paresthesia and burning (beginning approximately 2 to 5 days after infection)
- Progresses to very painful vesicular and ulcerated lesions, 3 to 7 days after exposure (may prompt hospitalization in up to 10% of patients)
- Dysuria caused by vulvar lesions, urethral and bladder involvement, or autonomic dysfunction (may lead to urinary retention)
- Malaise, low-grade fever, and inguinal adenopathy (40%)
- Systemic symptoms, including aseptic meningitis, fever, headache, and meningismus, can be found in 70% of patients 5 to 7 days after the appearance of the genital lesions in primary infections

DIAGNOSTIC APPROACH

Differential Diagnosis

- Chancroid
- Syphilis
- Granuloma inguinale
- Folliculitis

Associated Conditions: Other sexually transmitted diseases, cervicitis.

Workup and Evaluation

Laboratory: Viral cultures (including type-specific serologic tests) of material taken by swab from the lesions (95% sensitivity). Smears of vesicular material may also be stained with Wright's stain to visualize giant multinucleated cells with characteristic eosinophilic intranuclear inclusions.

Imaging: No imaging indicated.

Special Tests: Scrapings from the base of vesicles may be stained using immunofluorescence techniques to detect the presence of viral particles.

Diagnostic Procedures: History, physical examination, viral culture, and serologic testing.

Pathologic Findings

The virus replicates in the parabasal and intermediate cells of the skin. It passes from cell to cell until it encounters nerve cell endings, providing access to local ganglia. Typical lesions consist of clear vesicles that lyse, progressing to shallow, painful ulcers with a red border. These may coalesce, becoming secondarily infected and necrotic.

MANAGEMENT AND THERAPY

Nonpharmacologic

General Measures: Topical cleansing, sitz baths followed by drying with a heat lamp or hair dryer, analgesics.

Specific Measures: Topical analgesics (lidocaine [Xylocaine] 2% jelly, nonprescription throat spray with phenol), antiviral agents. If secondary infections occur, therapy with a local antibacterial cream, such as Neosporin, is appropriate.

Diet: No specific dietary changes indicated.

Activity: Pelvic rest until lesions have healed.

Patient Education: American College of Obstetricians and Gynecologists Patient Education Pamphlet AP009 (How to Prevent Sexually Transmitted Diseases). Patients should be advised to have all sexual partners seen for diagnosis and treatment. (Counseling regarding the natural history of genital herpes, sexual and perinatal transmission, and methods to reduce transmission is integral to clinical management.)

Drug(s) of Choice

Acute (begun within 48 hours of onset)—acyclovir ointment (Zovirax or generic 5% applied locally every 3 hours) or acyclovir (400 mg PO three times a day or 200 mg PO five times a day while lesions are present) or famciclovir (Famvir 250 mg PO three times a day for 7 to 10 days) or valacyclovir (Valtrex, 1 g PO twice a day for 5 days) will decrease the duration of symptoms and viral shedding. However, these later therapies have not been shown to decrease the likelihood of recurrence and the shortening of symptom duration is often minimal.

For frequent recurrences or suppression—acyclovir (200 mg PO three times a day or 400 mg PO twice a day, increased to five times per day with lesions) or famciclovir (Famvir, 125 mg PO twice a day for 5 days during outbreaks) or valacyclovir (Valtrex 500 mg to 1 gm PO daily) is effective in decreasing frequency and severity of flare-ups, but use is limited to less than 6 months.

Contraindications: Known or suspected hypersensitivity. Acyclovir is pregnancy category C; famciclovir and valacyclovir are pregnancy category B. Suppressive therapy should not be used for pregnant patients.

Precautions: Thrombotic thrombocytopenic purpura/hemolytic uremic syndrome has been reported in some patients with human immunodeficiency virus (HIV) taking valacyclovir. It has not been encountered in

Lesions of Herpes Simplex

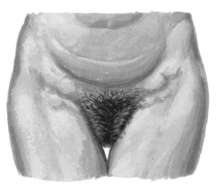

Regional lymphadenopathy, common in genital herpes

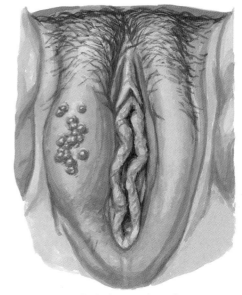

Marked edema and vesicle formation in primary herpes

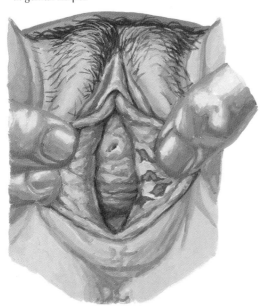

Ulcerative lesions of genitalia

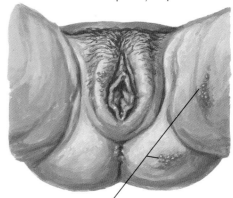

Autoinoculation lesions

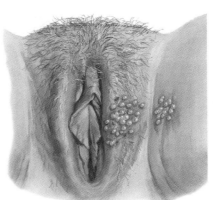

Herpes genitalis

patients who are immunocompetent. Antiviral agents should be used with caution in patients with compromised renal function.

Interactions: Antiviral agents may interact with or enhance the effects of nephrotoxic agents.

Alternative Drugs

In severe infections, acyclovir 5 to 10 mg/kg IV every 8 hours for 5 to 7 days may be required.

FOLLOW-UP

Patient Monitoring: Normal health maintenance. Watch for possible recurrence.

Prevention/Avoidance: Sexual continence during prodrome to full healing, use of condoms to reduce risk, sexual monogamy.

Possible Complications: Between 60% and 90% of patients have recurrences of the herpetic lesions in the first 6 months after initial infection. Although generally shorter and milder, these recurrent attacks are no less virulent.

Expected Outcome: Healing of the lesions is generally complete. Inguinal adenopathy may persist for several weeks after the resolution of the vulvar lesions. Suppuration is uncommon. Complete resolution of all symptoms occurs in 2 to 4 weeks.

MISCELLANEOUS

Pregnancy Considerations: Significant risk to neonate if acute infection or viral shedding is occurring at the time of delivery or rupture of the membranes. Infection is also associated with an increased risk of early fetal loss. The risk for transmission to the neonate from an infected mother is high (30% to 50%) among women who acquire genital herpes near the time of delivery and is low (<1%) among women with histories of recurrent herpes at term or who acquire genital HSV during the first half of pregnancy. Women with recurrent genital herpetic lesions at the onset of labor should give birth by cesarean delivery to prevent neonatal herpes; however, this does not completely eliminate the risk. Acyclovir may be administered orally to pregnant women with first-episode genital herpes or severe recurrent herpes and should be administered IV to pregnant women with severe HSV infection. Acyclovir treatment late in pregnancy reduces the frequency of cesarean deliveries among women who have recurrent genital herpes by diminishing the frequency of recurrences at term.

ICD-9-CM Codes: 054.11 (Vulvovaginal).

REFERENCES

Level I

Aoki FY, Tyring S, Diaz-Mitoma F, et al: Single-day patient initiated famciclovir therapy for recurrent genital herpes: a randomized, double-blind, placebo-controlled trial. Clin Infect Dis 2006;42:8.

Sheffield JS, Hill JB, Hollier LM, et al: Valacyclovir prophylaxis to prevent recurrent herpes at delivery: a randomized clinical trial. Obstet Gynecol 2006;108:141.

Watts DH, Brown ZA, Money D, et al: A double-blind, randomized, placebo-controlled trial of acyclovir in late pregnancy for the reduction of herpes simplex virus shedding and cesarean delivery. Am J Obstet Gynecol 2003;188:836.

Level II

Andrews WW, Kimberlin DF, Whitley R, et al: Valacyclovir therapy to reduce recurrent genital herpes in pregnant women. Am J Obstet Gynecol 2006;194:774.

Benedetti JK, Corey L, Ashley R: Recurrence rates in genital herpes after symptomatic first-episode infection. Ann Intern Med 1994;121:847.

Bryson Y, Dillon M, Bernstein DI, et al: Risk of acquisition of genital herpes simplex virus type 2 in sex partners of persons with genital herpes: a prospective couple study. J Infect Dis 1993;167:942.

Cone RW, Swenson PD, Hobson AC, et al: Herpes simplex virus detection from genital lesions: a comparative study using antigen detection (HerpChek) and culture. J Clin Microbiol 1993;31:1774.

Corey L, Wald A, Patel R, et al: Once-daily valacyclovir to reduce the risk of transmission of genital herpes. N Engl J Med 2004;350:11.

Eckert LO, Lentz GM: Infections of the lower genital tract. In Katz VL, Lentz GM, Lobo RA, Gershenson DM: Comprehensive Gynecology, 5th ed. Philadelphia, Mosby/Elsevier, 2007:578.

Gottlieb SL, Douglas JM Jr, Foster M, et al: Incidence of herpes simplex virus type 2 infection in 5 sexually transmitted disease (STD) clinics and the effect of HIV/STD risk-reduction counseling. J Infect Dis 2004;190:1059.

Gupta R, Wald A, Krantz E, et al: Valacyclovir and acyclovir for suppression of shedding of herpes simplex virus in the genital tract. J Infect Dis 2004;190:1374. Epub 2004 Sep 20.

Nagot N, Ouedraogo A, Foulongne V, et al; ANRS 1285 Study Group: Reduction of HIV-1 RNA levels with therapy to suppress herpes simplex virus. N Engl J Med 2007;356:790.

Oxman MN, Levin MJ, Johnson GR, et al; Shingles Prevention Study Group: A vaccine to prevent herpes zoster and postherpetic neuralgia in older adults. N Engl J Med 2005;352:2271.

Roberts CM, Pfister JR, Spear SJ: Increasing proportion of herpes simplex virus type 1 as a cause of genital herpes infection in college students. Sex Transmit Dis 2003;30:801.

Scott LL, Hollier LM, McIntire D, et al: Acyclovir suppression to prevent recurrent genital herpes at delivery. Infect Dis Obstet Gynecol 2002;10:71.

Sheffield JS, Hollier LM, Hill JB, et al: Acyclovir prophylaxis to prevent herpes simplex virus recurrence at delivery: a systematic review. Obstet Gynecol 2003;102:1396.

Stone KM, Reiff-Eldridge R, White AD, et al: Pregnancy outcomes following systemic prenatal acyclovir exposure: conclusions from the International Acyclovir Pregnancy Registry, 1984–1999. Birth Defects Research (Part A) 2004;70:201.

Level III

American College of Obstetricians and Gynecologists: Gynecologic herpes simplex virus infections. ACOG Practice Bulletin 57. Washington, DC, ACOG, 2004.

American College of Obstetricians and Gynecologists: Sexually transmitted diseases in adolescents. ACOG Committee Opinion 301. Washington, DC, ACOG, 2004.

Centers for Disease Control and Prevention: Sexually transmitted diseases treatment guidelines, 2006. MMWR 2006;55:16.

Engelberg R, Carrell D, Krantz E, et al: Natural history of genital herpes simplex virus type 1 infection. Sex Transmit Dis 2003;30:174.

Sen P, Barton SE: Genital herpes and its management. BMJ 2007;334:1048.

Tita AT, Grobman WA, Rouse DJ: Antenatal herpes serologic screening: an appraisal of the evidence. Obstet Gynecol 2006;108:1247.

Sexually Transmitted Infections: Human Immunodeficiency Virus

INTRODUCTION

Description: Infection by the human immunodeficiency virus (HIV) preferentially involves the immune system and leads to progressive deterioration in immune function. Infection produces a spectrum of disease that progresses from a clinically latent, asymptomatic state to acquired immune deficiency syndrome (AIDS) as a late manifestation. The speed of this progression varies. In untreated patients, the time between infection and the development of AIDS ranges from a few months to 17 years (median: 10 years). Women make up the fastest-growing group of individuals with HIV. Many states have specific laws governing HIV screening, reporting, disclosure, and breach of confidence. All care providers should become familiar with the requirements imposed in their area.

Prevalence: Two million Americans, or 0.7% of the entire population.

Predominant Age: Median age 35 years; 84% of cases occur at ages 15 to 44. In the United States in 2004, HIV/AIDS was the leading cause of death among African American women ages 25 to 34 years.

Genetics: No genetic pattern.

ETIOLOGY AND PATHOGENESIS

Causes: Infection with HIV, a retrovirus that preferentially infects helper lymphocytes but may infect macrophages, cells of the central nervous system, and possibly the placenta. Incubation from infection to clinical symptoms ranges from 5 days to 3 months, with an average of 2 to 4 weeks.

Risk Factors: Sexual activity (multiple partners or infected partner—37% of all infections), parenteral exposure to blood (sharing needles, inadvertent needle stick), perinatal exposure of infants. There is no evidence that HIV infection may be transmitted by casual contact, immune globulin preparations, hepatitis B vaccine, or contact with biting insects. HIV infection following donor insemination has been reported.

CLINICAL CHARACTERISTICS

Signs and Symptoms

- Nonspecific symptoms, often mimicking mononucleosis with aseptic meningitis (90%) (Febrile pharyngitis is the most common, with fever, sweats, lethargy, arthralgia, myalgia, headache, photophobia, and lymphadenopathy lasting up to 2 weeks.)
- Signs of loss of immune function: fever, weight loss, malaise, lymphadenopathy, central nervous system dysfunction, abnormal Pap test result, recurrent cervical intraepithelial neoplasia (CIN), oral or vaginal candidiasis
Patients are often diagnosed late in the progress of the disease (up to 40% within 1 year of developing full-blown AIDS).

DIAGNOSTIC APPROACH

Differential Diagnosis

- Mononucleosis

Associated Conditions: Gynecologic—abnormal Pap test results, cervical intraepithelial neoplasia and cervical cancer, condyloma acuminata, increased risk of pregnancy loss.

Workup and Evaluation

Laboratory: Enzyme-linked immunosorbent assay (ELISA) with positive results confirmed by Western blot analysis (sensitivity and specificity >99%). (Informed consent is recommended before testing. False-positive Western blot test results are uncommon and are found on the order of less than 1 in 130,000.) Antibodies may not be detectable until 6 to 12 weeks after infection. Other tests include complete blood count, with differential white count, electrolytes, glucose 6-phosphate dehydrogenase, hepatitis B screen, liver and renal function tests, platelet count, Venereal Disease Research Laboratory (VDRL), or rapid plasma reagent (RPR) test.

Imaging: No imaging indicated.

Special Tests: Tests for tuberculosis (tuberculin skin test with control [Candida, mumps, tetanus]) and other infections should be considered in individuals with HIV, Pap test.

Diagnostic Procedures: Enzyme-linked immunosorbent assay and Western blot analysis.

Pathologic Findings

Reduced CD4 counts and diffuse evidence of immunocompromise.

MANAGEMENT AND THERAPY

Nonpharmacologic

General Measures: Health maintenance, avoidance of stress and infection.

Specific Measures: Management is focused on stabilization of HIV disease, prevention of opportunistic infections, and prevention of perinatal transmission. When CD4 counts are less than 200, antibiotic prophylaxis should be started.

Diet: No specific dietary changes indicated.

Activity: No restriction.

Patient Education: American College of Obstetricians and Gynecologists Patient Education Pamphlet AP009 (How to Prevent Sexually Transmitted Diseases). Patient counseling should include the risk of infections associated with sexual behavior, intravenous drug use, the risk of transmission to an infant, the availability of treatment to reduce that risk, and the risk and benefits of treatment for the patient.

Clinical course and features

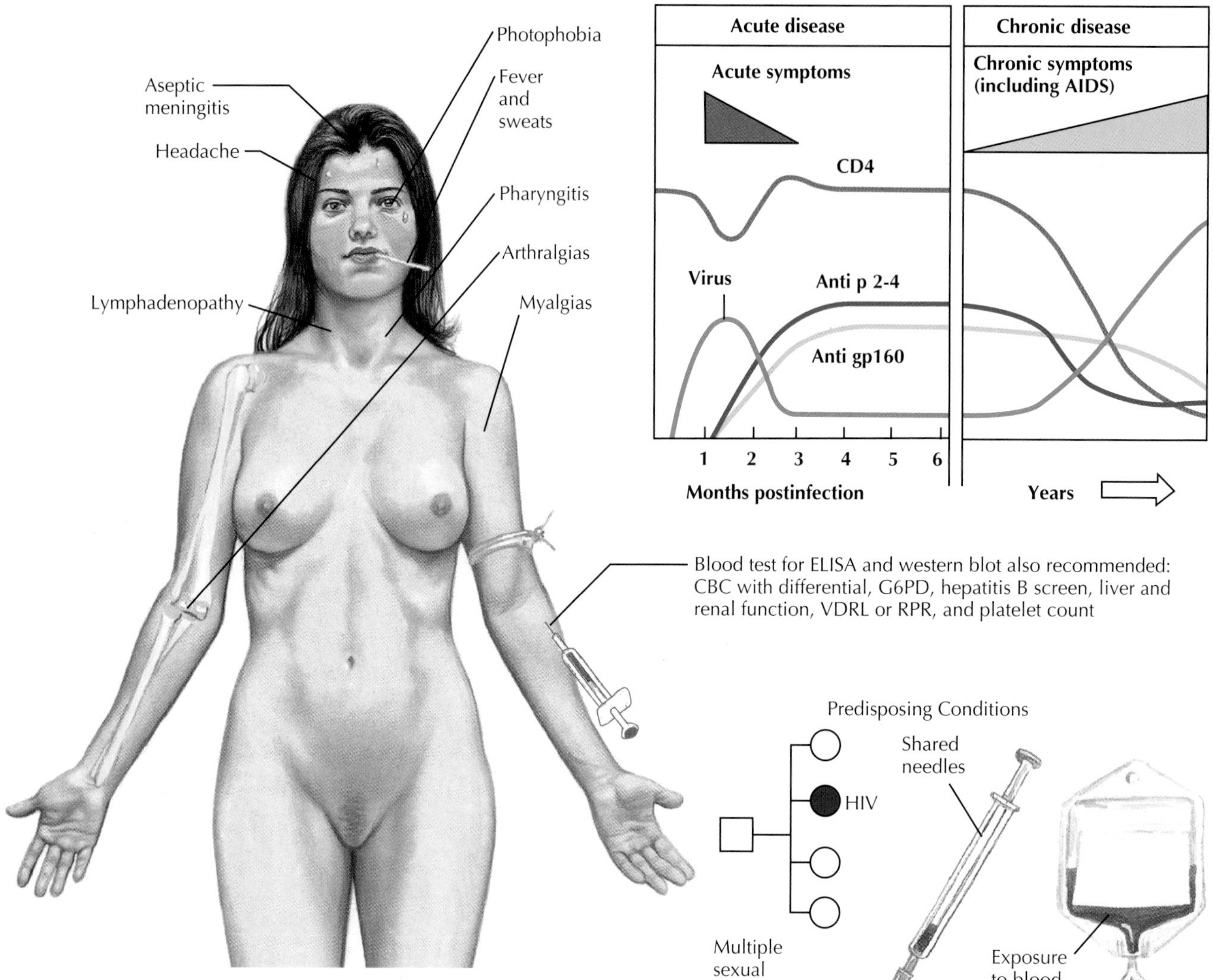

Aseptic meningitis
Headache
Lymphadenopathy
Photophobia
Fever and sweats
Pharyngitis
Arthralgias
Myalgias

Acute symptoms are often nonspecific, mimicking mononucleosis with weight loss and malaise

Acute disease	Chronic disease
Acute symptoms	Chronic symptoms (including AIDS)

CD4
Virus
Anti p 2-4
Anti gp160

1 2 3 4 5 6
Months postinfection

Years

Blood test for ELISA and western blot also recommended: CBC with differential, G6PD, hepatitis B screen, liver and renal function, VDRL or RPR, and platelet count

Predisposing Conditions

HIV
Shared needles
Multiple sexual partners
Exposure to blood products

Signs of loss of immune function

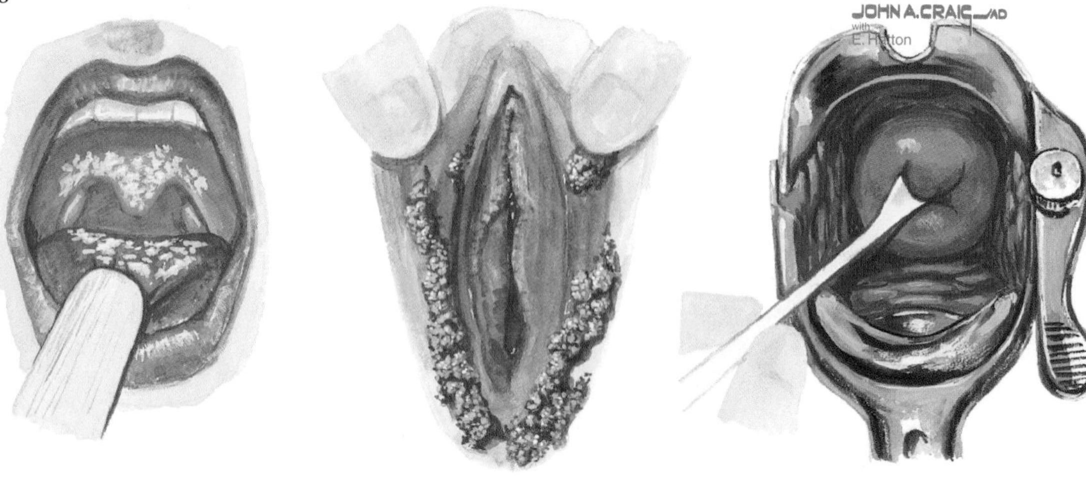

Oral or vaginal candidiasis

Condyloma acuminata

Abnormal Pap smear

AIDS, acquired immunodeficiency syndrome; CBC, complete blood count; ELISA, enzyme-linked immunosorbent assay; G6PD, glucose 6-phosphate dehydrogenase, RPR, rapid plasma reagent; VDRL, Venereal Disease Research Laboratory.

Drug(s) of Choice

Zidovudine (ZVD, 100 mg PO five times daily) is used to reduce vertical transmission during pregnancy. Multiple drug therapy is common for individuals with HIV, but the best combination has yet to be determined, and guidelines are rapidly changing. Referral to a specialist is recommended.

Prophylactic drugs—trimethoprim (160 mg) sulfamethoxazole (800 mg) daily as prophylaxis for those at risk (CD4 <200). (Significant infections must be treated specifically and aggressively.)

FOLLOW-UP

Patient Monitoring: Increased frequency of monitoring, including periodic assessment of blood and CD4 counts.

Prevention/Avoidance: Avoidance of risky behaviors such as intravenous drug use or multiple sexual partners, universal precautions for health care workers, consistent use of condoms, substance abuse prevention and treatment programs, and counseling programs. Prophylaxis after acute exposure (e.g., needle stick) with zidovudine singly or in combination with other agents has been shown to reduce the risk of infection.

Possible Complications: Opportunistic infections (bacterial, mycotic, and viral), increased risk of malignancy (cervical, Kaposi sarcoma, lymphoma), central nervous system dysfunction.

Expected Outcome: After recovery from the initial infection, the patient enters a carrier state during which symptoms are absent, but viral shedding occurs. Immune dysfunction generally becomes apparent roughly 10 years after the initial infection. The development of immunocompromise is rare before 3 years after infection, and less than 35% develop symptoms of AIDS before 5 years. Despite continuing progress in treatment of HIV infection and AIDS, the outcome is generally poor.

MISCELLANEOUS

Pregnancy Considerations: Significant risk of vertical transmission and worsening of maternal disease. Prenatal screening and suppressive strategies have reduced the risk of vertical transmission to approximately 2%.

ICD-9-CM Codes: V08, 042 (With symptoms).

REFERENCES

Level I

Catanzaro AT, Koup RA, Roederer M, et al; Vaccine Research Center 006 Study Team: Phase 1 safety and immunogenicity evaluation of a multiclade HIV-1 candidate vaccine delivered by a replication-defective recombinant adenovirus vector. J Infect Dis 2006;194:1638. Epub 2006 Nov 8.

Gallant JE, DeJesus E, Arribas JR, et al; Study 934 Group: Tenofovir DF, emtricitabine, and efavirenz vs. zidovudine, lamivudine, and efavirenz for HIV. N Engl J Med 2006;354:251.

Gulick RM, Ribaudo HJ, Shikuma CM, et al; AIDS Clinical Trials Group (ACTG) A5095 Study Team: Three- vs four-drug antiretroviral regimens for the initial treatment of HIV-1 infection: a randomized controlled trial. JAMA 2006;296:769.

Hurwitz BE, Klaus JR, Llabre MM, et al: Suppression of human immunodeficiency virus type 1 viral load with selenium supplementation: a randomized controlled trial. Arch Intern Med 2007;167:148.

Lockman S, Shapiro RL, Smeaton LM, et al: Response to antiretroviral therapy after a single, peripartum dose of nevirapine. N Engl J Med 2007;356:135.

Pitisuttithum P, Gilbert P, Gurwith M, et al; Bangkok Vaccine Evaluation Group: Randomized, double-blind, placebo-controlled efficacy trial of a bivalent recombinant glycoprotein 120 HIV-1 vaccine among injection drug users in Bangkok, Thailand. J Infect Dis 2006;194:1661. Epub 2006 Nov 3.

Level II

Nagot N, Ouedraogo A, Foulongne V, et al; ANRS 1285 Study Group: Reduction of HIV-1 RNA levels with therapy to suppress herpes simplex virus. N Engl J Med 2007;356:790.

Pilcher CD, Eron JJ Jr, Vemazza PL, et al: Sexual transmission during the incubation period of primary HIV infection. JAMA 2001;286:1713.

Strategies for Management of Antiretroviral Therapy (SMART) Study Group; El-Sadr WM, Lundgren JD, Neaton JD, et al: CD4+ count-guided interruption of antiretroviral treatment. N Engl J Med 2006;355:2283.

Waller SC: A meta-analysis of condom effectiveness in reducing sexually transmitted HIV. Soc Sci Med 1993;36:1635.

Wawer MJ, Gray RH, Sewankambo NK, et al: Rates of HIV-1 transmission per coital act, by stage of HIV-1 infection, in Rakai, Uganda. J Infect Dis 2005;191:1403.

Level III

Bardequez AD: Management of HIV infection for the childbearing age woman. Clin Obstet Gynecol 1996;39:344.

Centers for Disease Control and Prevention: Sexually transmitted diseases treatment guidelines, 2006. MMWR 2006;55:10.

Letvin NL: Progress in the development of an HIV-1 vaccine. Science 1998;280:1875.

Panel on Antiretroviral Guidelines for Adult and Adolescents: Guidelines for the use of antiretroviral agents in HIV-infected adults and adolescents. Department of Health and Human Services. 2006;1. Available at http://www.aidsinfo.nih.gov/ContentFiles/AdultandAdolescentsGL.pdf. Accessed June 1, 2007.

Piot P: AIDS: from crisis management to sustained strategic response. Lancet 2006;368:526.

Simon V, Ho DD, Abdool Karim Q: HIV/AIDS epidemiology, pathogenesis, prevention, and treatment. Lancet 2006;368:489.

U.S. Department of Health and Human Services: Treatment of opportunistic infections. Washington, DC, U.S. Department of Health and Human Services, National Institutes of Health, CDC, 2006. Available at http://www.aidsinfo.nih.gov. Accessed June 1, 2007.

Sexually Transmitted Infections: Human Papillomavirus

INTRODUCTION

Description: Infection by one or more subtypes (of the more than 100 known) of human papillomaviruses (HPV) causes epithelial proliferations at cutaneous and mucosal surfaces. Some serotypes are associated with warty growths on the hands, feet, and other locations (including genital warts). Some high-risk serotypes are found in more than 99% of cervical cancers.

Prevalence: Thought to be the most common sexually transmitted disease in the world. About 20 million people are currently infected with HPV. At least 50% of sexually active people acquire genital HPV infection at some point in their lives. One study estimated that 64% to 82% of adolescent girls were infected with at least one strain of HPV. By age 50, at least 80% of women will have acquired genital HPV infection. About 6.2 million Americans acquire a new genital HPV infection yearly.

Predominant Age: Reproductive and beyond.

Genetics: No genetic pattern to infection. The genetic characterization of the virus has led to the identification of those serotypes that are oncogenic.

ETIOLOGY AND PATHOGENESIS

Causes: Exposure to the DNA human papillomavirus. More than 40 serotypes are know to be sexually transmissible. Vertical transmission from mother to child during childbirth can occur and rarely results in laryngeal polyps (approximately 2/100,000 births). Papillomaviruses initiate infection in the basal layer of the epithelium, and viral genome amplification occurs in differentiating cells. After infection, differentiating epithelial cells that are normally nondividing remain in an active cell cycle. This can result in a thickened, sometimes exophytic, epithelial lesion. The virus is released as cells exfoliate from the epithelium. Research indicates that HPVs produce proteins (designated E5, E6, E7) that interfere with tumor suppressor p53 proteins that arrest the cell cycle when there is DNA damage.

Risk Factors: Direct contact with an infected individual; therefore, having multiple sexual partners or contact with a person with multiple sexual partners increases the risk. Viral persistence is more likely in those with reduced immunity and tobacco smokers. Other epidemiologic factors associated with risk of cervical cancer include long-term use of oral contraceptives, coinfections such as chlamydia, parity, and nutritional factors.

CLINICAL CHARACTERISTICS

Signs and Symptoms

- Most are asymptomatic and are cleared spontaneously (70% by 1 year and more than 90% within 2 years; median infection: 8 months)
- Persistent infections may be associated with warty growths at the site of infection (condyloma acuminata)

and cellular changes associated with dysplasia or cancer (including cancers of the anus, vulva, vagina, cervix, and some cancers of the oropharynx).

The incubation period required before symptoms appear is highly variable and varies from several weeks to years.

DIAGNOSTIC APPROACH

Differential Diagnosis

- Secondary syphilis (Condyloma lata), other viral) infections.

Associated Conditions: Other sexually transmitted diseases.

Workup and Evaluation

Laboratory: No evaluation indicated (see special tests).

Imaging: No imaging indicated.

Special Tests: HPV serotyping for those with abnormal cervical cytology (Pap tests), colposcopy for those with persistently abnormal cytology or for surveillance of those with high-risk serotypes.

Diagnostic Procedures: Serotyping of HPV obtained from cervical cells can be performed but is not indicated on a routine or screening basis. Generally, this testing is reserved for those with abnormal cervical cytology (ASCUS [atypical squamous cells of undetermined significance] or above Pap tests). These tests will identify 13 high-risk serotypes. (Because most younger patients will clear even high-risk serotypes with no sequela, recommendations for serotyping and aggressive follow-up of abnormal Pap test results are changing to more conservative management schemes.)

Pathologic Findings

Cellular atypia (koilocytotic changes) may be found in infected cells. Recent research suggests the degree of atypia may be a function of the serotype involved.

MANAGEMENT AND THERAPY

Nonpharmacologic

General Measures: There is no specific therapy available or indicated for HPV infection—most (>90%) infections are cleared by the body with little or no symptoms or sequela.

Specific Measures: Only those directed at the specific symptoms generated by persistent infection; condyloma or cervical epithelial change.

Diet: No specific dietary changes indicated.

Activity: No restriction.

Patient education: Reassurance; American College of Obstetricians and Gynecologists Patient Education Booklet AP073 (Human Papillomavirus [HPV] Infection), AP163 (Cancer of the Cervix), AP161 (Abnormal

Pap Test Results), AP149 (Cancer of the Vulva and Vagina)

Drug(s) of Choice

None.

Contraindications: The HPV vaccine is currently contraindicated in those with known allergies to any of its components and those who are currently pregnant.

Precautions: None.

Interactions: Quadrivalent HPV vaccine can be administered at the same visit as other age-appropriate vaccines, such as the tetanus, diphtheria, and pertussis (Tdap) and quadrivalent meningococcal conjugate (MCV4) vaccines.

HPV Serotypes and Common Clinical Conditions

Disease	HPV Strain
Anogenital warts	6 and 11(90% of cases), 42, 43, 44, 55, and others
Cervical cancer, vulvar squamous cancer	16 and 18 (70% of cases), 31, 33, 35, 39, 45, 51
Common warts	2, 7
Epidermodysplasia verruciformis	More than 15 strains
Flat cutaneous warts	3, 10
Focal epithelial hyperplasia	12, 32
Oral papillomas	6, 7, 11, 16, 32
Oropharyngeal squamous cell carcinoma	16 and others
Plantar warts	1, 2, 4
Respiratory papillomatosis	6 and 11

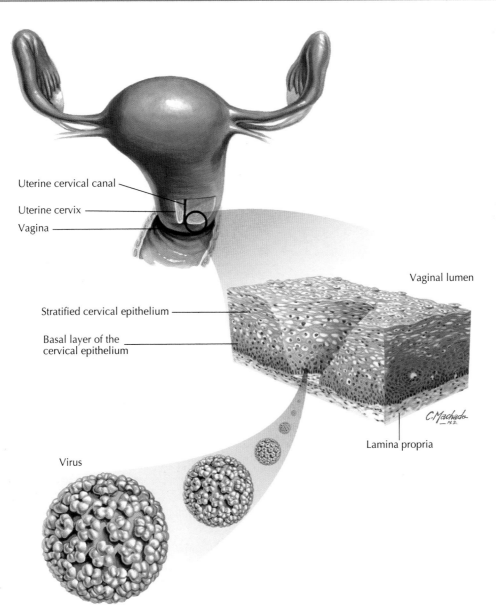

Uterine cervical canal
Uterine cervix
Vagina
Vaginal lumen
Stratified cervical epithelium
Basal layer of the cervical epithelium
Lamina propria
Virus

FOLLOW-UP

Patient Monitoring: Normal health maintenance. Frequent cervical monitoring (cytology and/or colposcopy) for those found to have persistent high-risk serotypes.

Prevention/Avoidance: Abstinence. Condom use is thought to reduce the risk of transmission. (A study among newly sexually active college women demonstrated a 70% reduction in HPV infection when their partners used condoms consistently and correctly.) A vaccine that provides immunity against high-risk types 16 and 18 (thought to account for 70% of cervical cancers) and low-risk types 6 and 11 (associated with condyloma accuminata). The vaccine is made up of a noninfectious virus-like particle formed from a single protein (L1) from the virus. Other vaccines against other high-risk serotypes will be introduced soon. The currently available vaccine is given as a series of three injections over 6 months (0, 2, and 6 months) and may be associated with local pain, swelling, itching and redness, fever, nausea, or dizziness. The vaccine is currently indicated for women ages 9 to 26.

Possible complications: Both high- and low-risk types of HPV can cause the growth of abnormal cells, but generally only the high-risk types (16, 18, 31, 33, 35, 39, 45, 51, 52, 56, 58, 59, 68, 69, and possibly a few others) are associated with cervical cancer. These high-risk types may cause flat condyloma that are often difficult to see compared with the more exuberant warts caused by low-risk types such as types 6 and 11. HPV 16 is the most common high-risk type, found in almost half of all cervical cancers (HPV 18 accounts for 10% to 12% of cervical cancers). HPV 16 is also one of the most common types found in women without cancer. High-risk types can be detected in 99% of cervical cancers. It is important to note that most infections by both high- and low-risk types are cleared spontaneously and do not cause clinical problems.

Expected outcome: Most infections clear spontaneously. For those with persistent infections, warty growths, dysplastic cellular changes, and epithelial cancers may emerge over time.

MISCELLANEOUS

Pregnancy Considerations: No direct effect on pregnancy. Vertical transmission to the infant during delivery may occur. Although vaccination during pregnancy is contraindicated, lactating women may receive the vaccine.

Other Notes: All warts are caused by papillomaviruses, but each type of HPV grows only in specific areas of the body. Those types associated with common warts found on the hands and feet are not transmitted sexually.

Patients with low-grade squamous intraepithelial lesions (LSIL) or high-grade squamous intraepithelial lesions (HSIL) on Pap test results almost always have high-risk HPV on serotyping; thus, typing for these patients does not add anything to their management and is usually not indicated for these individuals. Between 5% and 30% of individuals infected with HPV are infected with multiple serotypes.

ICD-9-CM Codes: 079.4 (Human papillomavirus), 795.05 (cervical high-risk human papillomavirus [HPV] DNA test positive), 078.1 (viral warts), 078.11 (condyloma accuminata).

REFERENCES

Level I

Koutsky LA, Ault KA, Wheeler CM, et al: A controlled trial of a human papillomavirus type 16 vaccine. New Engl J Med 2002;347:1645.

Level II

Dunne EF: Prevalence of HPV infection among females in the United States. JAMA 2007;297:813.

Munoz N, Bosch FX, de Sanjosé S, et al: Epidemiologic classification of human papillomavirus types associated with cervical cancer. New Engl J Med 2003;348:518.

Srodon M, Stoler MH, Baber GB, Kurman RJ: The distribution of low and high-risk HPV types in vulvar and vaginal intraepithelial neoplasia (VIN and VaIN). Am J Surg Pathol 2006;30:1513.

Villa LL, Costa RL, Petta CA, et al: High sustained efficacy of a prophylactic quadrivalent human papillomavirus types 6/11/16/18 L1 virus-like particle vaccine through 5 years of follow-up. Br J Cancer 20064;95:1459. Epub 2006 Nov 21.

Winer RL, Hughes JP, Feng Q, et al: Condom use and the risk of genital human papillomavirus infection in young women. N Engl J Med 2006;354:2645.

Zuna RE, Allen RA, Moore WE, et al: Distribution of HPV genotypes in 282 women with cervical lesions: evidence for three categories of intraepithelial lesions based on morphology and HPV type. Mod Pathol 2007;20:167. Epub 2006 Dec 22.

Level III

American College of Obstetricians and Gynecologists: Sexually transmitted diseases in adolescents. ACOG Committee Opinion 301. Washington, DC, ACOG, 2004.

American College of Obstetricians and Gynecologists: Human papillomavirus. ACOG Practice Bulletin 61. Washington, DC, ACOG, 2005.

American College of Obstetricians and Gynecologists: Human papillomavirus vaccination. ACOG Committee Opinion 344. Washington, DC, ACOG, 2006.

Clifford GM, Goncalves MA, Franceschi S; HPV and HIV Study Group: Human papillomavirus types among women infected with HIV: a meta-analysis. AIDS 2006;20:2337.

Cox JT: Epidemiology and natural history of HPV. J Fam Pract 2006;Suppl:3.

Dunne EF, Markowitz LE: Genital human papillomavirus infection. Clin Infect Dis 20061;43:624. Epub 2006 Jul 26.

Eckert LO, Lentz GM: Infections of the lower genital tract. In Katz VL, Lentz GM, Lobo RA, Gershenson DM: Comprehensive Gynecology, 5th ed. Philadelphia, Mosby/Elsevier, 2007:576.

Lowy DR, Schiller JT: Prophylactic human papillomavirus vaccines. J Clin Invest 2006;116:1167.

Markowitz LE, Dunne EF, Saraiya M, et al: Quadrivalent human papillomavirus vaccine. MMWR 2007;56:1. Available at: http://www.cdc.gov/mmwr/preview/mmwrhtml/ rr5602a1.htm. Accessed May 13, 2007.

Scheurer ME, Tortolero-Luna G, Adler-Storthz K: Human papillomavirus infection: biology, epidemiology, and prevention. Int J Gynecol Cancer 2005;15:727.

Trottier H, Franco EL: The epidemiology of genital human papillomavirus infection. Vaccine 2006;24:S1.

Walboomers JM, Jacobs MV, Manos MM, et al: Human papillomavirus is a necessary cause of invasive cervical cancer worldwide. J Pathol 1999;189:12.

Weaver BA: Epidemiology and natural history of genital human papillomavirus infection. J Am Osteopath Assoc 2006;106:S2.

Wiley D, Masongsong E: Human papillomavirus: the burden of infection. Obstet Gynecol Surv 2006;61:S3.

Sexually Transmitted Infections: Lymphogranuloma Venereum

INTRODUCTION

Description: Lymphogranuloma venereum (LVG) is a potentially destructive infection caused by one of a number of serotypes (L-1, L-2, L-3) of *Chlamydia trachomatis*. Although uncommon in the United States, this infection causes significant morbidity.

Prevalence: Uncommon (600 cases per year in the United States).

Predominant Age: Younger reproductive.

Genetics: LVG is 20 times more common in men than in women.

ETIOLOGY AND PATHOGENESIS

Causes: LGV is caused by several serotypes of *Chlamydia trachomatis*.

Risk Factors: Sexual trauma and exposure to the infective agent.

CLINICAL CHARACTERISTICS

Signs and Symptoms

* Painless vesicle that heals quickly leaving no scar, generally located on posterior aspect of vulva or vestibule
* Proctitis, tenesmus, or bloody rectal discharge in ano-rectal infections (anal intercourse)
* Progressive adenopathy with bubo formation (groove sign—the "groove sign" is not specific to LGV; it may also be seen in other inflammatory processes such as acne inversa)
* Severe fibrosis and scarring (elephantiasis, "esthiomene"; rectal stenosis may occur)

DIAGNOSTIC APPROACH

Differential Diagnosis

* Granuloma inguinale
* Chancroid
* Herpes simplex
* Syphilis
* Cancer (vulvar or colon)

Associated Conditions: Other sexually transmitted infections, human immunodeficiency virus (HIV), dyspareunia, rectal stricture or stenosis.

Workup and Evaluation

Laboratory: Complement fixation test (a titer of greater than 1:64 is highly suspicious for LGV). Approximately 20% of patients with LGV will have false-positive Venereal Disease Research Laboratory (VDRL) test results.

Imaging: No imaging indicated.

Special Tests: None indicated. (Biopsy of the lesions is not diagnostic because of the nonspecific damage present. Enlarged lymph nodes should not be biopsied or opened: chronic sinuses will result.)

Diagnostic Procedures: Complement fixation testing—80% of patients have a titer of 1:16 or greater. Genital and lymph node specimens (i.e., lesion swab or bubo aspirate) may be tested for *C. trachomatis* by culture, direct immunofluorescence, or nucleic acid detection.

Pathologic Findings

None (nonspecific inflammatory changes).

MANAGEMENT AND THERAPY

Nonpharmacologic

General Measures: Evaluation, culture or Gram stain, topical cleansing and care.

Specific Measures: Antibiotic therapy. Treatment should be started even before results of confirmatory tests are received.

Diet: No specific dietary changes indicated.

Activity: No restriction. (Sexual continence required until infection is resolved.)

Patient Education: American College of Obstetricians and Gynecologists Patient Education Pamphlet AP009 (How to Prevent Sexually Transmitted Diseases). Patients should be advised to have all sexual partners seen for diagnosis and treatment.

Drug(s) of Choice

Doxycycline 100 PO twice a day for 3 weeks or tetracycline, 500 mg PO four times a day, for 3 weeks.

Contraindications: Erythromycin estolate and tetracyclines are contraindicated in pregnancy and should not be used.

Precautions: Doxycycline is contraindicated in pregnant women.

Interactions: See individual agents.

Alternative Drugs

Erythromycin (500 mg PO four times a day for 3 weeks) or sulfadiazine (2 g PO loading dose, 1 g PO four times a day for 14 to 21 days) may be substituted. Azithromycin (1.0 g PO once weekly for 3 weeks) has been suggested but clinical data are lacking.

FOLLOW-UP

Patient Monitoring: Follow-up evaluation for cure with culture or other tests should be carried out, as should screening for other sexually transmitted diseases. (As with all sexually transmitted diseases, all sexual partners within the preceding 30 days should be screened and treated for probable infections as well.)

Prevention/Avoidance: Use of barrier contraception (condoms, diaphragm), limitation or elimination of risky behavior (sexual promiscuity).

Possible Complications: In one third of patients, abscess formation, rupture, and fistula formation occur. Chronic progressive lymphangitis with chronic edema and sclerosing fibrosis may occur, causing extensive destruction of the vulva. Rectal stenosis also may occur and may be life threatening.

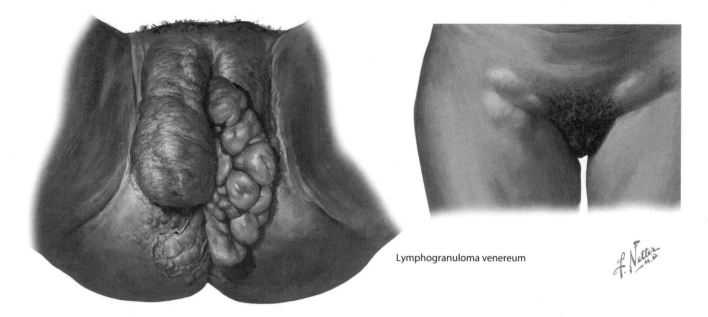

Lymphogranuloma venereum

Expected Outcome: If detected early, successful treatment with minimal sequelae may be expected. Long-term scarring and disfigurement are common.

MISCELLANEOUS

Pregnancy Considerations: No effect on pregnancy, although the possibility of vertical transmission of other associated conditions (such as human immunodeficiency virus infection) should be considered. Doxycycline use is contraindicated in pregnant women.

ICD-9-CM Codes: 099.1.

REFERENCES

Level I
Martin DH, Mroczkowski TF, Dalu ZA, et al: A controlled trial of a single dose of azithromycin for the treatment of chlamydial urethritis and cervicitis. The Azithromycin for Chlamydial Infections Study Group. N Engl J Med 1992;327:921.

Level II
Daling JR, Weiss NS, Hislop et al: Sexual practices, sexually transmitted diseases, and the incidence of anal cancer. N Engl J Med 1987;317:973.

Golden N, Hammerschlag M, Neuhoff S, Gleyzer A: Prevalence of Chlamydia trachomatis cervical infection in female adolescents. Am J Dis Child 1984;138:562.

McLelland BA, Anderson PC: Lymphogranuloma venereum. Outbreak in a university community. JAMA 1976;235:56.

Osewe PL, Peterman TA, Ransom RL, et al: Trends in the acquisition of sexually transmitted diseases among HIV-positive patients at STD clinics, Miami 1988–1992. Sex Transm Dis 1996;23:230.

Pearlman MD, McNeeley SG: A review of the microbiology, immunology and clinical implications of Chlamydia trachomatis infections. Obstet Gynecol Surv 1992;47:448.

Level III
Abrams AJ: Lymphogranuloma venereum. JAMA 1968;205:199.

Anonymous: Treatment for Neisseria gonorrhoeae and Chlamydia trachomatis. N Engl J Med 1984;311:124–6.

Anonymous: Screening and treatment of chlamydial infections. N Engl J Med 1989;321:1046.

Ballard RC, Ye H, Matta A, et al: Treatment of chancroid with azithromycin. Int J STD AIDS 1996;7:9.

Bell TA, Grayston JT: Centers for Disease Control guidelines for prevention and control of Chlamydia trachomatis infections. Summary and commentary. Ann Intern Med 1986;104:524.

Campbell WF, Dodson MG: Clindamycin therapy for Chlamydia trachomatis in women. Am J Obstet Gynecol 1990;162:343.

Centers for Disease Control and Prevention: Sexually transmitted diseases treatment guidelines, 2006. MMWR 2006;55:21.

Eckert LO, Lentz GM: Infections of the lower genital tract. In Katz VL, Lentz GM, Lobo RA, Gershenson DM: Comprehensive Gynecology, 5th ed. Philadelphia, Mosby/Elsevier, 2007:582.

Goens JL, Schwartz RA, De Wolf K: Mucocutaneous manifestations of chancroid, lymphogranuloma venereum and granuloma inguinale. Am Fam Physician 1994;49:415, 423.

Pruessner HT, Hansel NK, Griffiths M: Diagnosis and treatment of chlamydial infections. Am Fam Physician 1986;34:81.

Sevinsky LD, Lambierto A, Casco R, Woscoff A: Lymphogranuloma venereum: tertiary stage. Int J Dermatol 1997;36:47.

INTRODUCTION

Description: Molluscum contagiosum is a papillary lesion caused by viral infection (pox virus) that is spread by skin to skin contact, first described in 1817.

Prevalence: Two of 100,000, 1 of 40 to 60 patients with gonorrhea, about 1% of all skin disorders in the United States.

Predominant Age: Early reproductive.

Genetics: No genetic pattern.

ETIOLOGY AND PATHOGENESIS

Causes: Molluscum contagiosum is caused by the largest member of the pox virus group. This mildly contagious DNA virus infects epithelial tissues, and autoinoculation to other sites is common. The appearance of lesions ranges from 1 week to 6 months, with an average incubation period of 6 weeks. (The virus can also infect other primates and kangaroos.)

Risk Factors: Sexual activity and direct exposure to the infective agent.

CLINICAL CHARACTERISTICS

Signs and Symptoms

- Asymptomatic
- After several weeks of incubation, a round, umbilicated papule, 1 to 5 mm in size, with a yellow, waxy core of cheesy material (these lesions may grow slowly for months; they may be solitary or occur in clusters) may occur
- Eczema (10%)

The lesions of molluscum are highly contagious, and appropriate precautions should be used when examining the lesions or material from the lesions to avoid infection or spread.

DIAGNOSTIC APPROACH

Differential Diagnosis

- Sebaceous cysts
- Folliculitis
- Herpes simplex
- Dermal papilloma
- Nevus

Associated Conditions: Other sexually transmitted infections.

Workup and Evaluation

Laboratory: No evaluation indicated. Because patients who are immunosuppressed are at higher risk for molluscum, testing for human immunodeficiency virus infection should be considered.

Imaging: No imaging indicated.

Special Tests: Material from the lesions is examined microscopically; inclusion bodies are seen in material from the core of the lesion.

Diagnostic Procedures: Clinical picture and examination of material from lesion.

Pathologic Findings

Eosinophilic inclusion bodies (intracytoplasmic) in material from the core of the lesion.

MANAGEMENT AND THERAPY

Nonpharmacologic

General Measures: Local care.

Specific Measures: Molluscum lesions may go away on their own in 6 to 9 months but can persist, via autoinoculation, for up to 4 years. Treatment is based on obliterating the lesion. This is done by desiccation, cryotherapy, curettage, laser ablation, or chemical cautery (AgNO$_3$; may cause hyperpigmentation and scarring). Curettage of the base of the lesion (with the tip of an 18-gauge needle or curette) is also curative. Bleeding may be controlled with Monsel's solution (ferric subsulfate solution 20%).

Diet: No specific dietary changes indicated.

Activity: No restriction. (Sexual continence required until infection is resolved.)

Patient Education: American College of Obstetricians and Gynecologists Patient Education Pamphlet AP009 (How to Prevent Sexually Transmitted Diseases). Patients should be advised to have all sexual partners seen for diagnosis and treatment.

Drug(s) of Choice

None.

FOLLOW-UP

Patient Monitoring: Follow-up should occur in 1 month to look for new lesions.

Prevention/Avoidance: Limitation or elimination of risky behavior (sexual promiscuity).

Possible Complications: Local secondary infection.

Expected Outcome: Good response to lesion destruction—generally heals with little or no scarring.

MISCELLANEOUS

Pregnancy Considerations: No effect on pregnancy.

ICD-9-CM Codes: 078.0.

REFERENCES

Level I

Hanna D, Hatami A, Powell J, et al: A prospective randomized trial comparing the efficacy and adverse effects of four recognized treatments of molluscum contagiosum in children. Pediatr Dermatol 2006;23:574.

Level II

Hughes P: Treatment of molluscum contagiosum with the 585-nm pulsed dye laser. Dermatol Surg 1998;24:229.

Clinical findings

Magnified view showing typical umbilicated lesion

Keratin plug

Inclusion bodies

Scattered distribution of molluscum lesions over perineum, buttocks, and thighs. Lesions spread by physical contact and autoinoculation

Histologic section of molluscum lesions showing pox virus inclusion bodies and central core of keratin

Evaluation and management

Application of liquid nitrogen to lesion using cotton swab

JOHN A. CRAIG _AD
with
E. Hatton

Local eradication of lesions can be obtained with desiccation, cryotherapy, laser ablation, chemical cautery, or curettage

Human immunodeficiency virus (HIV) testing may be warranted because molluscum is a common complication in immunosuppressed patients

Papa C, Berger R: Venereal herpes-like molluscum contagiosum: treatment with tretinoin. Cutis 1976;18:537.

Smith MA, Singer C: Sexually transmitted viruses other than HIV and papillomavirus. Urol Clin North Am 1992;19:47.

Tyring SK: Molluscum contagiosum: the importance of early diagnosis and treatment. Am J Obstet Gynecol 2003;189:S12.

Weller R, O'Callaghan CJ, MacSween RM, White MI: Scarring in Molluscum contagiosum: comparison of physical expression and phenol ablation. BMJ 1999;319:1540.

Level III

Blattner RJ: Molluscum contagiosum: eruptive infection in atopic dermatitis. J Pediatr 1967;70:997.

Brown ST, Nalley JF, Kraus SJ: Molluscum contagiosum. Sex Transm Dis 1981;8:227.

de la Maza LM, Peterson EM: Genital infections. Med Clin North Am 1983;67:1059.

Cohen J, Powderly WG: Infectious diseases, 2nd ed. New York, Elsevier, 2004:2053.

Eckert LO, Lentz GM: Infections of the lower genital tract. In Katz VL, Lentz GM, Lobo RA, Gershenson DM: Comprehensive Gynecology, 5th ed. Philadelphia, Mosby/Elsevier, 2007:575.

Gottlieb SL, Myskowski PL: Molluscum contagiosum. Int J Dermatol 1994;33:453.

Margolis S: Genital warts and molluscum contagiosum. Urol Clin North Am 1984;11:163.

Reed RJ, Parkinson RP: The histogenesis of molluscum contagiosum. Am J Surg Pathol 1977;1:161.

INTRODUCTION

Description: *Phthirus humanus* (pubic or crab lice) and *Sarcoptes scabiei* (scabies or itch mite) are parasitic insects that may be transferred through sexual activity or through contact with contaminated clothing or bedding.

Prevalence: Three million cases per year in the United States.

Predominant Age: Reproductive.

ETIOLOGY AND PATHOGENESIS

Causes: Parasitic insects (*P. humanus* [pubic or crab lice] and *S. scabiei* [scabies or itch mite]).

Risk Factors: Contact with infected person or fomites.

Genetics: No genetic pattern.

CLINICAL CHARACTERISTICS

Signs and Symptoms

- Intense itching (greatest at night), most frequently in the area of the pubic hair
- Infestations occur most frequently in the area of the pubic hair. Spread to other hairy areas can and does take place. Scabies infections are not confined to hairy area but may be found in any area of the body.

DIAGNOSTIC APPROACH

Differential Diagnosis

- Dermatoses
- Contact dermatitis
- Norwegian (crusted) scabies

Associated Conditions: Other sexually transmitted diseases.

Workup and Evaluation

Laboratory: No evaluation indicated.

Imaging: No imaging indicated.

Special Tests: Close inspection of the affected area generally reveals nits, feces, burrows, or the insects themselves.

Diagnostic Procedures: History and physical examination, microscopic examination of nits.

Pathologic Findings

Inflammatory reaction to the bite, burrow, and feces of the insect.

MANAGEMENT AND THERAPY

Nonpharmacologic

General Measures: Local cleansing, soothing creams, or lotions may be used.

Specific Measures: Topical applications of insecticide. Other family members should be treated and the home disinfected at the same time. Scabies—bedding and clothing should be decontaminated (i.e., either machine washed, machine dried using the hot cycle, or dry cleaned) or removed from body contact for at least 72 hours. Fumigation of living areas is unnecessary.

Diet: No specific dietary changes indicated.

Activity: No restriction.

Patient Education: American College of Obstetricians and Gynecologists Patient Education Pamphlet AP009 (How to Prevent Sexually Transmitted Diseases). Patients should be advised to have all sexual partners seen for diagnosis and treatment.

Drug(s) of Choice

Permethrin cream (5%) applied to all areas of the body from the neck down and washed off 8 to 14 hours later. Topical applications of lindane 1% (Kwell) lotion and shampoo applied for 4 minutes, then washed off. Malathion 0.5% lotion applied for 8 to 12 hours and washed off or Ivermectin 250 μg/kg repeated in 2 weeks

Contraindications: Lindane is contraindicated in premature neonates, pregnant or lactating patients, children younger than 2 years of age, or patients with Norwegian (crusted) scabies. Patients with seizure disorders or known or suspected hypersensitivity should not use the product.

Precautions: Care must be taken to avoid the eyes. The dose of lindane should be reduced in elderly patients because of increased skin absorption. Lindane should not be used immediately after a bath or shower, and it should not be used by persons who have extensive dermatitis. (Seizures have occurred when lindane was applied after a bath or used by patients who had extensive dermatitis. Aplastic anemia after lindane use also has been reported.) Lindane is not recommended as first-line therapy because of toxicity. It should only be used as an alternative if the patient cannot tolerate other therapies or if other therapies have failed.

Interactions: Oils and ointments may increase the rate of absorption and should not be used.

Alternative Drugs

Crotamiton (Eurax) (10%) applied to all areas of the body from the neck down for two nights; on the third night, wash off the medication. Repeat the cycle beginning the fourth night.

FOLLOW-UP

Patient Monitoring: Normal health maintenance. Patients should be warned that the rash and pruritus of scabies might persist for up to 2 weeks after treatment.

Prevention/Avoidance: Sexual monogamy.

Possible Complications: Secondary skin infection from scratching.

Expected Outcome: Generally good response to insecticide therapy. Reinfection is possible if each partner, family members, and fomites are not all treated simultaneously.

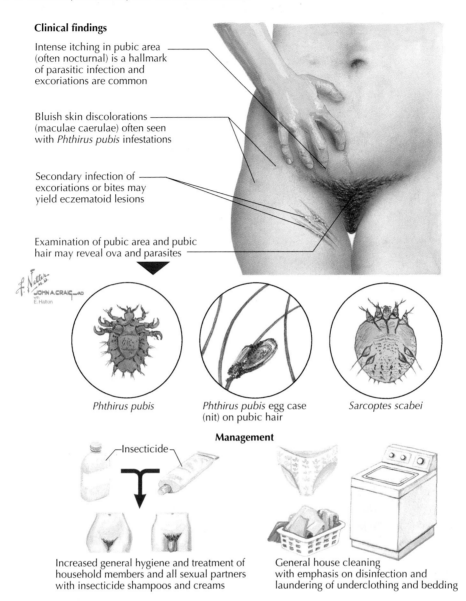

Clinical findings

Intense itching in pubic area (often nocturnal) is a hallmark of parasitic infection and excoriations are common

Bluish skin discolorations (maculae caerulae) often seen with *Phthirus pubis* infestations

Secondary infection of excoriations or bites may yield eczematoid lesions

Examination of pubic area and pubic hair may reveal ova and parasites

Phthirus pubis

Phthirus pubis egg case (nit) on pubic hair

Sarcoptes scabei

Management

Insecticide

Increased general hygiene and treatment of household members and all sexual partners with insecticide shampoos and creams

General house cleaning with emphasis on disinfection and laundering of underclothing and bedding

MISCELLANEOUS

Pregnancy Considerations: No direct effect on pregnancy. Lindane is contraindicated during pregnancy.
ICD-9-CM Codes: 132.2 (*Phthirus pubis*), 131.0 (Scabies).

REFERENCES

Level II
Burkhart CG: Relationship of treatment-resistant head lice to the safety and efficacy of pediculicides. Mayo Clin Proc 2004;79:661.
Dawes M, Hicks NR, Fleminger M, et al: Evidence based case report: treatment for head lice. BMJ 1999;318:385.
Fischer TF: Lindane toxicity in a 24-year-old woman. Ann Emerg Med 1994;24:972.
Meinking TL, Taplin D, Hermida JL, et al: The treatment of scabies with ivermectin. N Engl J Med 1995;333:26.
Pearlman DL: A simple treatment for head lice: dry-on, suffocation-based pediculicide. Pediatrics 2004;114:e275.

Level III
Centers for Disease Control and Prevention: Sexually transmitted diseases treatment guidelines, 2006. MMWR 2006;55:79.
Chosidow O: Clinical practices. Scabies. N Engl J Med 2006;354:1718.

Crissey JT: Scabies and pediculosis pubis. Urol Clin North Am 1984;11:1716.
Eckert LO, Lentz GM: Infections of the lower genital tract. In Katz VL, Lentz GM, Lobo RA, Gershenson DM: Comprehensive Gynecology, 5th ed. Philadelphia, Mosby/Elsevier, 2007:573.
Faber BM: The diagnosis and treatment of scabies and pubic lice. Primary Care Update Ob/Gyn 1996;3:20.
Flinders DC, De Schweinitz P: Pediculosis and scabies. Am Fam Physician 2004;69:341.
Gurevitch AW: Scabies and lice. Pediatr Clin North Am 1985;32:987.
Heukelbach J, Feldmeier H: Ectoparasites—The underestimated realm. Lancet 2004;363:889.
Heukelbach J, Feldmeier H: Scabies. Lancet 2006;367:1767.
Hook EW 3rd, Stamm WE: Sexually transmitted diseases in men. Med Clin North Am 1983;67:235.
Hosidow O: Scabies and pediculosis. Lancet 2000;355:819.
Johnston G, Sladden M: Scabies: diagnosis and treatment. BMJ 2005;331:619.
Nash B: Treating head lice. BMJ 2003;326:1256.
Roberts RJ: Clinical practice. Head lice. N Engl J Med 2002; 346:1645.
Rosen T, Brown TJ: Cutaneous manifestations of sexually transmitted diseases. Med Clin North Am 1998;82:1081, vi.
Smith RP: Gynecology in primary care. Baltimore, Williams & Wilkins, 1997:549.

INTRODUCTION

Description: Since antiquity, syphilis has been the prototypic venereal disease. This disease presents with an easily overlooked first stage and, if left untreated, can slowly progress to a disabling disease noted for central nervous system, cardiac, and musculoskeletal involvement.

Prevalence: Increasing; 9,756 new cases (1,458 women) were reported in 2006.

Predominant Age: 15 to 30 years (85%).

Genetics: No genetic pattern.

ETIOLOGY AND PATHOGENESIS

Causes: *Treponema pallidum* is one of a very small group of spirochetes that are virulent for humans. This motile anaerobic spirochete can rapidly invade even intact moist mucosa (epithelium).

Risk Factors: It is estimated that roughly one third of patients exposed to early syphilis acquire the disease.

CLINICAL CHARACTERISTICS

Signs and Symptoms (Based on Stage)

- Painless chancres (shallow, firm, punched out, with a smooth base and rolled edges; on the vulva, anus, rectum, pharynx, tongue, lips, fingers, or the skin of almost any part of the body) 10 to 60 days (average, 21 days) after inoculation
- Low-grade fever; headache; malaise; sore throat; anorexia; generalized lymphadenopathy; a diffuse, symmetrical, asymptomatic maculopapular rash over the palm and soles ("money palms"); mucous patches; condyloma lata (second stage)
- Cardiac or ophthalmic manifestations, auditory abnormalities, or gummatous lesions (tertiary stage)

DIAGNOSTIC APPROACH

Differential Diagnosis

- Herpes vulvitis
- Condyloma acuminata
- Lymphogranuloma venereum
- Chancroid

Associated Conditions: Tabes dorsalis, aortic aneurysm, and gummas.

Workup and Evaluation

Laboratory: The Venereal Disease Research Laboratory (VDRL) and rapid plasma reagin (RPR) tests are nonspecific and good screening tests because they are rapid and inexpensive. The fluorescent treponemal antibody absorption or microhemagglutination *T. pallidum* tests are specific treponemal antibody tests that are confirmatory or diagnostic; they are not used for routine screening but are useful to rule out a false-positive screening test result. If neurosyphilis is suspected, a lumbar puncture with a Venereal Disease Research Laboratory performed on the spinal fluid is required. (Unless clinical signs or symptoms of neurologic or ophthalmic involvement are present, cerebrospinal fluid analysis is not recommended for routine evaluation of patients who have primary or secondary syphilis.) Screening for human immunodeficiency virus (HIV) infection should also be strongly considered. False-positive screening results may occur in patients with lupus, hepatitis, sarcoidosis, recent immunization, or drug abuse or during pregnancy. These test results may be falsely negative in the second stage of the disease as a result of high levels of anticardiolipin antibody that interfere with the test (prozone phenomenon). Up to 30% of patients with a primary lesion have negative test results. (Approximately 15% to 25% of patients treated during the primary stage revert to being serologically nonreactive after 2 to 3 years.)

Imaging: No imaging indicated.

Special Tests: The diagnosis may be made by identifying motile spirochetes on darkfield microscopic examination of material from primary or secondary lesions or lymph node aspirates or through direct fluorescent antibody (DFA) testing.

Diagnostic Procedures: Physical examination, suspicion, serologic testing.

Pathologic Findings

Based on stage of disease.

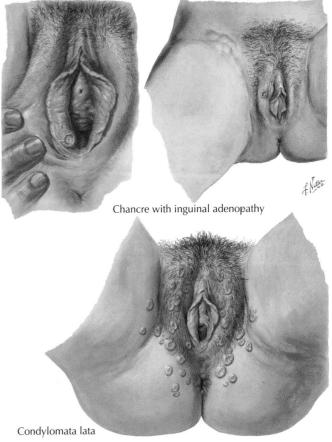

Chancre with inguinal adenopathy

Condylomata lata

Superficial Syphilitic Lesions

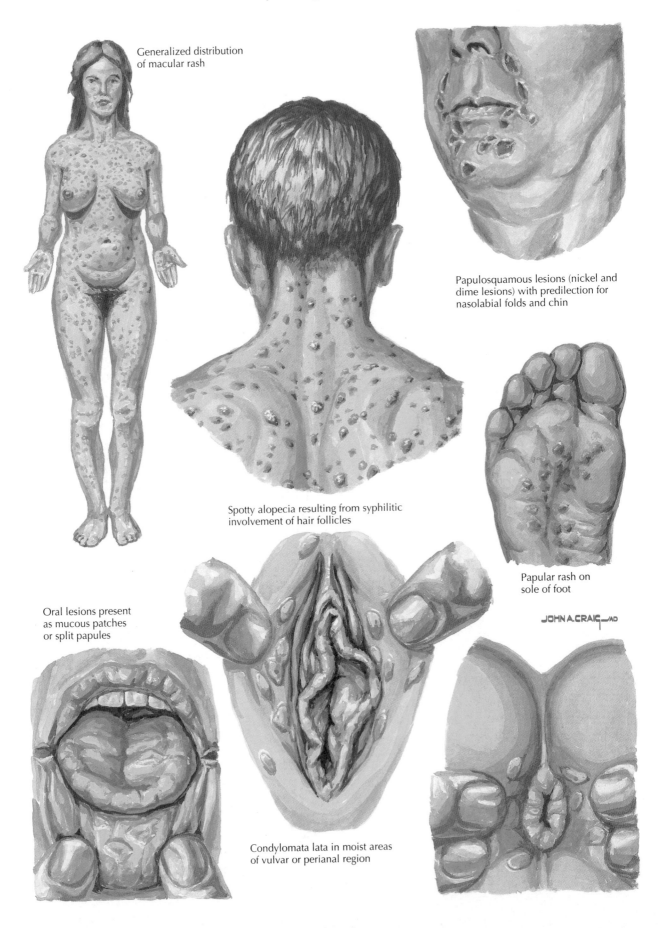

Generalized distribution of macular rash

Papulosquamous lesions (nickel and dime lesions) with predilection for nasolabial folds and chin

Spotty alopecia resulting from syphilitic involvement of hair follicles

Papular rash on sole of foot

Oral lesions present as mucous patches or split papules

JOHN A. CRAIG—AD

Condylomata lata in moist areas of vulvar or perianal region

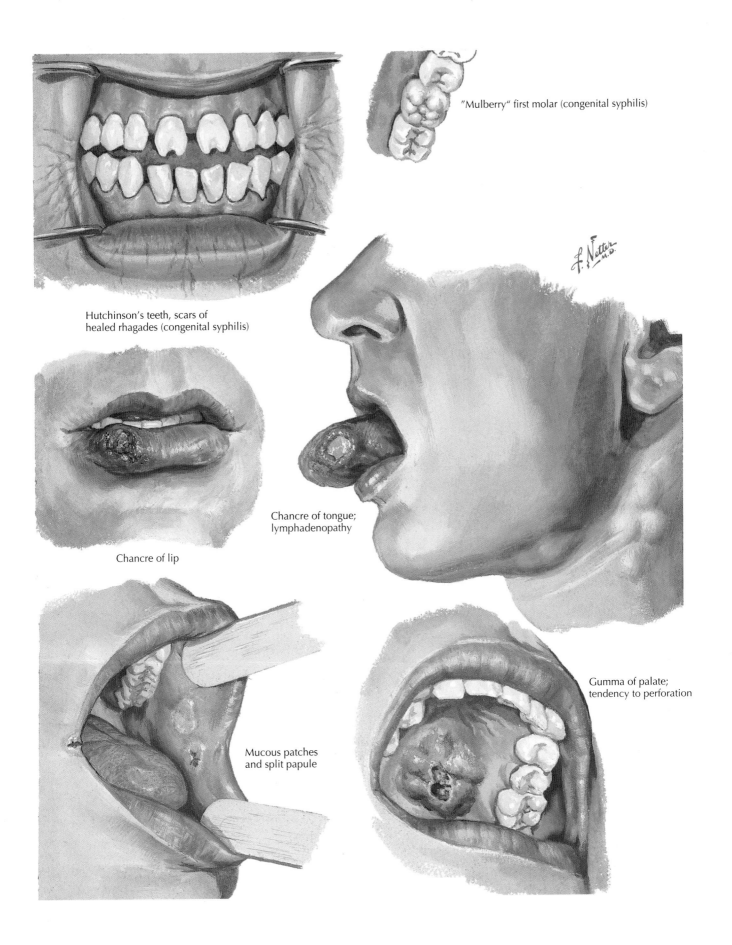

"Mulberry" first molar (congenital syphilis)

Hutchinson's teeth, scars of
healed rhagades (congenital syphilis)

Chancre of lip

Chancre of tongue;
lymphadenopathy

Mucous patches
and split papule

Gumma of palate;
tendency to perforation

MANAGEMENT AND THERAPY
Nonpharmacologic

General Measures: Evaluation and diagnosis.
Specific Measures: Antibiotic therapy based on stage of disease.
Diet: No specific dietary changes indicated.
Activity: No restriction. (Sexual continence required until infection is resolved.)
Patient Education: American College of Obstetricians and Gynecologists Patient Education Pamphlet AP009 (How to Prevent Sexually Transmitted Diseases). Patients should be advised to have all sexual partners (within 90 days of diagnosis) seen for diagnosis and treatment.

Drug(s) of Choice

Benzathine penicillin G 2.4 million units IM in a single dose. (Tertiary: benzathine penicillin G 7.2 million units total, administered as three doses of 2.4 million units IM each at 1-week intervals.) Penicillin G, administered parenterally, is the preferred drug for treatment of all stages of syphilis. Dosage is based on stage of disease.
Contraindications: Known or suspected allergy.

Alternative Drugs

Doxycycline (100 mg PO twice a day) or tetracycline (500 mg PO four times a day), both for 14 to 28 days. Pregnant patients who are allergic to penicillin should be desensitized and then treated with penicillin.

FOLLOW-UP

Patient Monitoring: Screening for other sexually transmitted diseases. (As with all sexually transmitted diseases, all sexual partners within the preceding 90 days should be screened and treated for probable infections as well.)
Prevention/Avoidance: Limitation or elimination of risky behavior (sexual promiscuity).
Possible Complications: If untreated, crippling damage to the central nervous or skeletal systems, heart, or great vessels often ensues in the form of destructive, necrotic, granulomatous lesions (gummas), which develop from 1 to 10 years after the initial infection. Serious cardiovascular or neurologic complications occur in 5% to 20% of patients.
Expected Outcome: Early treatment is associated with resolution; permanent damage may occur if disease is treated at a later stage. The Jarisch-Herxheimer reaction is an acute febrile reaction frequently accompanied by headache, myalgia, and other symptoms that usually occurs within the first 24 hours after any therapy for syphilis.

MISCELLANEOUS

Pregnancy Considerations: Parenteral penicillin G is the only therapy with documented efficacy for syphilis during pregnancy. Transplacental spread of syphilis occurs at any time during pregnancy and can result in congenital syphilis. Transplacental infection occurs in roughly 50% of patients with untreated primary or secondary disease. Half of these patients have premature deliveries or stillbirths. Pregnant women with syphilis in any stage who report penicillin allergy should be desensitized and treated with penicillin.
ICD-9-CM Codes: 091.0 (Primary, genital chancre), 091.3 (Secondary) (others based on organ system and extent of disease).

REFERENCES

Level I
Hook EW III, Martin DH, Stephens J, et al: A randomized, comparative pilot study of azithromycin versus benzathine penicillin G for treatment of early syphilis. Sex Transmit Dis 2002;29:486.

Riedner G, Rusizoka M, Todd J, et al: Single-dose azithromycin versus penicillin G benzathine for the treatment of early syphilis. N Engl J Med 2005;353:1236.

Rolfs RT, Joesoef MR, Hendershot EF, et al: A randomized trial of enhanced therapy for early syphilis in patients with and without human immunodeficiency virus infection: the Syphilis and HIV Study Group. N Engl J Med 1997;337:307.

Level II
Alexander JM, Sheffield JS, Sanchez PJ, et al: Efficacy of treatment for syphilis in pregnancy. Obstet Gynecol 1999;93:5.

Berry MC, Dajani AS: Resurgence of congenital syphilis. Infect Dis Clin North Am 1992;6:19.

El-Zaatari MM, Martens MG, Anderson GD: Incidence of the prozone phenomenon in syphilis serology. Obstet Gynecol 1994;84:609.

Fonck K, Claeys P, Bashir F, et al: Syphilis control during pregnancy: effectiveness and sustainability of a decentralized program. Am J Public Health 2001;91:705.

Hollier LM, Harstad TW, Sanchez PJ, et al: Fetal syphilis: clinical and laboratory characteristics. Obstet Gynecol 2001;97:947.

Romanowski B, Sutherland R, Fick GH, et al: Serologic response to treatment of infectious syphilis. Ann Intern Med 1991;114:1005.

St Louis ME, Wasserheit JN: Elimination of syphilis in the United States. Science 1998;281:353.

Walker GJ: Antibiotics for syphilis diagnosed during pregnancy. Cochrane Database Syst Rev 2001;3:CD001143.

Level III
Birnbaum NR, Goldschmidt RH, Buffett WO: Resolving the common clinical dilemmas of syphilis. Am Fam Physician 1999;59:2233, 2245.

Centers for Disease Control and Prevention: Sexually transmitted diseases treatment guidelines, 2006. MMWR 2006;55:22.

Clay JC: Antenatal screening for syphilis. BMJ 1989;299:409.

Doherty L, Fenton KA, Jones J, et al: Syphilis: old problem, new strategy. BMJ 2002;325:153.

Drusin LM: Syphilis: clinical manifestations, diagnosis, and treatment. Urol Clin North Am 1984;11:121.

Eckert LO, Lentz GM: Infections of the lower genital tract. In Katz VL, Lentz GM, Lobo RA, Gershenson DM: Comprehensive Gynecology, 5th ed. Philadelphia, Mosby/Elsevier, 2007:583.

Emmert DH, Kirchner JT: Sexually transmitted diseases in women. Gonorrhea and syphilis. Postgrad Med 2000;107:181, 189, 193.

Pope V: Use of treponemal tests to screen for syphilis. Infect Med 2004;21:399.

Riedner G, Rusizoka M, Todd J, et al: Single-dose azithromycin versus penicillin G benzathine for the treatment of early syphilis. N Engl J Med 2005;353:1236.

Rolfs RT: Treatment of syphilis, 1993. Clin Infect Dis 1995;20:S23.

Wong TY, Mihm MC Jr: Primary syphilis. N Engl J Med 1994;331:1492.

Sexually Transmitted Infections: Trichomonas Vaginalis

INTRODUCTION

Description: Infection by the anaerobic flagellate protozoan, *Trichomonas vaginalis* is most often acquired by sexual contact with an infected person.

Prevalence: Roughly 3 million cases per year, 25% of "vaginal infections."

Predominant Age: 15 to 50 (may occur at any age).

Genetics: No genetic pattern.

ETIOLOGY AND PATHOGENESIS

Causes: *T. vaginalis*, an anaerobic flagellate protozoan.

Risk Factors: Multiple sexual partners, vaginal pH that is less acidic. (Blood, semen, or bacterial pathogens increase the risk.) Of asymptomatic partners of women with *Trichomonas* infections, 30% to 80% have a positive culture. The incubation period for *Trichomonas* infections is thought to be between 4 and 28 days. *Trichomonas* has been reported (rarely) in virginal patients, supporting the possibility of nonsexual transmission.

CLINICAL CHARACTERISTICS

Signs and Symptoms

- Forty percent may be asymptomatic; a carrier state may exist for many years
- Vulvar itching or burning
- Copious discharge with a rancid odor (generally thin, runny, and yellow–green to gray in color, "frothy" in 25%)
- "Strawberry" punctation of the cervix and upper vagina (15%)
- Dysuria
- Dyspareunia
- Edema or erythema of the vulva

DIAGNOSTIC APPROACH

Differential Diagnosis

- Bacterial vaginitis
- Bacterial vaginosis
- Chlamydial cervicitis
- Gonococcal cervicitis

Associated Conditions: Other sexually transmitted infections (specifically, gonorrhea and chlamydial infection).

Workup and Evaluation

Laboratory: Culture or monoclonal antibody staining may be obtained but are seldom necessary. Evaluation for concomitant sexually transmitted infections should be strongly considered. Detection of *Trichomonas* by Pap test results in an error rate of 50%. (Alternative tests include OSOM Trichomonas Rapid Test [Genzyme Diagnostics, Cambridge, Massachusetts], an immunochromatographic capillary flow dipstick technology, and the Affirm VP III [Becton Dickinson, San Jose, California], a nucleic acid probe test that evaluates for *T. vaginalis*, *Gardnerella vaginalis*, and *Candida albicans*. These tests have a sensitivity of >83% and a specificity of >97%, although false-positive results are common when prevalence is low.)

Imaging: No imaging indicated.

Special Tests: Vaginal pH 6 to 6.5 or higher.

Diagnostic Procedures: Physical examination, microscopic examination of vaginal secretions in normal saline (sensitivity of only approximately 60% to 70%).

Pathologic Findings

T. vaginalis is a fusiform protozoan, slightly larger than a white blood cell, with three to five flagella extending from the narrow end that provide active movement.

MANAGEMENT AND THERAPY

Nonpharmacologic

General Measures: Perineal hygiene, education regarding sexually transmitted infections.

Specific Measures: Medical therapy, vaginal acidification.

Diet: No specific dietary changes indicated. Avoid alcohol during metronidazole or tinidazole treatment.

Activity: Sexual continence until partner(s) are examined and treated.

Patient Education: American College of Obstetricians and Gynecologists Patient Education Pamphlet AP009 (How to Prevent Sexually Transmitted Diseases), AP028 (Vaginitis: Causes and Treatments). Patients should be advised to have all sexual partners seen for diagnosis and treatment.

Drug(s) of Choice

Metronidazole 2 g PO as a single dose or metronidazole 250 mg twice a day for 7 days. For recurrences where reinfection is excluded, metronidazole 500 mg PO twice a day for 7 days or tinidazole 2 g PO single dose.

Contraindications: Metronidazole is relatively contraindicated in the first trimester of pregnancy (pregnancy category B). Multiple studies and meta-analyses have not demonstrated a consistent association between metronidazole and teratogenic or mutagenic effects. Tinidazole is pregnancy category C.

Precautions: Metronidazole or tinidazole may produce a disulfiram-like reaction resulting in nausea, vomiting, headaches or other symptoms if the patient ingests alcohol. Patients should not use these agents if they have taken disulfiram in the preceding 2 weeks. Metronidazole must be used with care or the dose should be reduced in patients with hepatic disease.

Interactions: Metronidazole may potentiate the effects of warfarin or coumarin and alcohol (as noted earlier).

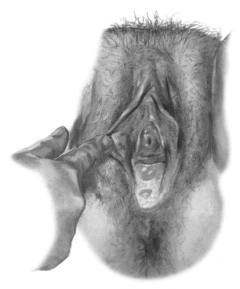

Trichomoniasis

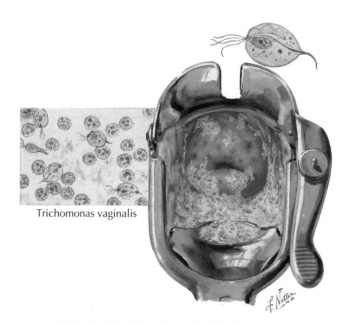

Trichomonas vaginalis

Alternative Drugs

Tinidazole 2 g PO in a single dose. Topical clotrimazole, povidone iodine (topical), hypertonic (20%) saline douches. (Metronidazole gel is considerably less efficacious for the treatment of trichomoniasis (<50%) than oral preparations of metronidazole and should not be used.)

FOLLOW-UP

Patient Monitoring: Follow-up serologic testing for syphilis and human immunodeficiency virus (HIV) infection as indicated.

Prevention/Avoidance: Sexual monogamy, condom use for intercourse.

Possible Complications: Cystitis, infections of the Skene's or Bartholin's glands, increased risk of pelvic inflammatory disease (PID), pelvic pain, infertility, and other sequelae of sexually transmitted infections.

Expected Outcome: Resistance to metronidazole is uncommon (<5% with low-dose therapy, high-level resistance is rare). Most treatment failures are actually caused by reinfection or failure to comply with treatment.

MISCELLANEOUS

Pregnancy Considerations: Vaginal infections are associated with an increased risk of premature rupture of membranes, preterm delivery, and low birthweight. Data do not suggest that metronidazole treatment results in a reduction in perinatal morbidity. Discontinue breastfeeding during metronidazole treatment and for 12 to 24 hours after the last dose. While using tinidazole, discontinue breastfeeding during treatment and for 3 days after the last dose.

ICD-9-CM Codes: 131.0, 131.01 (Vaginal).

REFERENCES

Level I

Lossick JG: Single-dose metronidazole treatment for vaginal trichomoniasis. Obstet Gynecol 1980;56:508.

Tidwell BH, Lushbaugh WB, Laughlin MD, et al: A double-blind placebo-controlled trial of single-dose intravaginal versus single-dose oral metronidazole in the treatment of trichomonal vaginitis. J Infect Dis 1994;170:242.

Level II

Burtin P, Taddio A, Ariburnu O, et al: Safety of metronidazole in pregnancy: a meta-analysis. Obstet Gynecol 1995;172:525.

Caro-Paton T, Carvajal A, Martin de Diego I, et al: Is metronidazole teratogenic? A meta-analysis. Br J Clin Pharmacol 1997;44:179.

Forna F, Gulmezoglu AM: Interventions for treating trichomoniasis in women. Cochrane Database Syst Rev 2003;2:CD000218.

Klebanoff MA, Carey JC, Hauth JC, et al; National Institute of Child Health and Human Development Network of Maternal-Fetal Medicine Units: Failure of metronidazole to prevent preterm delivery among pregnant women with asymptomatic *Trichomonas vaginalis* infection. N Engl J Med 2001;345:487.

Okun N, Gronau KA, Hannah ME: Antibiotics for bacterial vaginosis or *Trichomonas vaginalis* in pregnancy: a systematic review. Obstet Gynecol 2005;105:857.

Piper JM, Mitchel EF, Ray WA: Prenatal use of metronidazole and birth defects: no association. Obstet Gynecol 1993;82:348.

Wiese W, Patel SR, Patel SC, et al: A meta-analysis of the Papanicolaou smear and wet mount for the diagnosis of vaginal trichomoniasis. Am J Med 2000;108:301.

Level III

American College of Obstetricians and Gynecologists: Sexually transmitted diseases in adolescents. ACOG Committee Opinion 301. Washington, DC, ACOG, 2004.

American College of Obstetricians and Gynecologists: Vaginitis. ACOG Practice Bulletin 72. Washington, DC, ACOG, 2006.

Anderson MR, Klink K, Cohrssen A: Evaluation of vaginal complaints. JAMA 2004;291:1368.

Centers for Disease Control and Prevention: Sexually transmitted diseases treatment guidelines, 2006. MMWR 2006;55:52.

Eckert LO: Clinical practice. Acute vulvovaginitis. N Engl J Med 2006;355:1244.

Eckert LO, Lentz GM: Infections of the lower genital tract. In Katz VL, Lentz GM, Lobo RA, Gershenson DM: Comprehensive Gynecology, 5th ed. Philadelphia, Mosby/Elsevier, 2007:591.

Lossick JG: Sexually transmitted vaginitis. Urol Clin North Am 1984;11:141.

McLellan R, Spence MR, Brockman M, et al: The clinical diagnosis of trichomoniasis. Obstet Gynecol 1982;60:30.

Moldwin RM: Sexually transmitted protozoal infections. *Trichomonas vaginalis, Entamoeba histolytica,* and *Giardia lamblia.* Urol Clin North Am 1992;19:93.

Sobel JD: Vaginitis. N Engl J Med 1997;337:1896.

Thomason JL, Gelbart SM: *Trichomonas vaginalis.* Obstet Gynecol 1989;74:536.

Thrombophlebitis

INTRODUCTION

Description: Thrombophlebitis is an inflammatory condition of the veins with secondary thrombosis. This may occur in two forms: aseptic or suppurative (septic). The vessels may be either superficial or deep. Risk factors may be present, or the onset may be idiopathic. Risk varies with location and cause.

Prevalence: Two million cases per year in the United States, 10% of nosocomial infections, intravascular (venous or arterial) catheter-related—88 of 100,000.

Predominant Age: Septic—childhood; aseptic—age 20 to 30 years; superficial—older than 40 years.

Genetics: Uncommon—antithrombin III, proteins C and S, and factor XII deficiencies (autosomal dominant with variable penetrance), factor V Leiden or prothrombin C-20210-a genes.

ETIOLOGY AND PATHOGENESIS

Causes: Sepsis (*Staphylococcus aureus* [65% to 75%], multiple organisms [14%]), hypercoagulable states (congenital deficiencies, malignancy, pregnancy, high-dose oral contraceptives, Behçets syndrome, Buerger's disease, factor V Leiden deficiency), venous stasis (varicose veins), injury to vessel wall. Septic thrombophlebitis may be caused by *Candida albicans* in unusual cases. (Virchow triad: intimal damage [trauma, infection, or inflammation], stasis, or changes in the blood constituents [changes in coagulability].)

Risk Factors: Trauma (general or vascular), prolonged immobility (hospitalization, prolonged air travel), advanced age, obesity, pregnancy or puerperium, recent surgery, intravascular catheters, steroid or high-dose estrogen therapy (high-dose oral contraceptives), high altitude, hemoglobinopathies, malignancy, nephrotic syndrome, homocystinuria, congenital abnormality.

CLINICAL CHARACTERISTICS

Signs and Symptoms

- Asymptomatic
- Generalized limb pain or swelling
- Swelling, tenderness, redness along the course of the vein
- Fever (70% of patients)
- Warmth, erythema, tenderness, or lymphangitis (32%)
- Systemic sepsis (84% in suppurative cases)
- Red, tender cord
- Swelling of collateral veins

DIAGNOSTIC APPROACH

Differential Diagnosis

- Cellulitis
- Erythema nodosa
- Cutaneous polyarteritis nodosa
- Sarcoid
- Kaposi's sarcoma
- Ruptured synovial cyst (Baker's cyst)
- Lymphedema
- Muscle tear, sprain, strain
- Venous obstruction (secondary to tumor, lymph node enlargement)

Associated Conditions: Budd-Chiari syndrome (hepatic vein thrombosis), renal vein thrombosis, homocystinuria, hypercoagulability states (antiphospholipid antibody syndrome), Behçets syndrome, and varicose veins.

Workup and Evaluation

Laboratory: Complete blood count, blood culture (positive in 80% to 90% of superficial cases), D-dimer assay, coagulation profiles (antithrombin III levels are suppressed during the acute event—evaluations for abnormal levels should await completion of therapy), activated partial thromboplastin time (APTT) and prothrombin time (PT) to monitor anticoagulant therapy. For patients with septic thrombosis—periodic white blood cell counts.

Imaging: Contrast venography is the "gold standard" for diagnosis. Doppler studies of vascular flow may be effective for some deep vessels. Chest radiography or spiral computed tomography if embolism is suspected.

Special Tests: Impedance plethysmography, I^{125}-fibrinogen scans (not widely available and requires 41 hours), bone or gallium scans for associated periosteal sepsis, ventilation/perfusion scans of the lungs if an embolism is suspected. Duplex ultrasound evaluation is becoming the diagnostic study of choice to search for venous thrombosis.

Diagnostic Procedures: History, physical examination, imaging or other diagnostic study (impedance plethysmography, ^{125}I-fibrinogen scans).

Pathologic Findings

Clot is attached to vessel wall with variable degrees of inflammation present in the vessel wall. Enlargement of the vessel with thickening is common. Perivascular suppuration or hemorrhage may be seen.

MANAGEMENT AND THERAPY

Nonpharmacologic

General Measures: For superficial aseptic conditions—heat, elevation, observation. For deep or septic thrombophlebitis—hospitalization, anticoagulation, bed rest for 1 to 5 days with progressive return to normal activity. Patients with deep vein thrombosis confined to the calf (distal to the popliteal system) may be managed as outpatients.

Specific Measures: Heparin anticoagulation initially followed by oral maintenance therapy (warfarin) for 3 to 6 months for first episodes or 12 months for recurrent episodes. Filtering devices ("umbrellas") should be considered for those who cannot receive anticoagulation

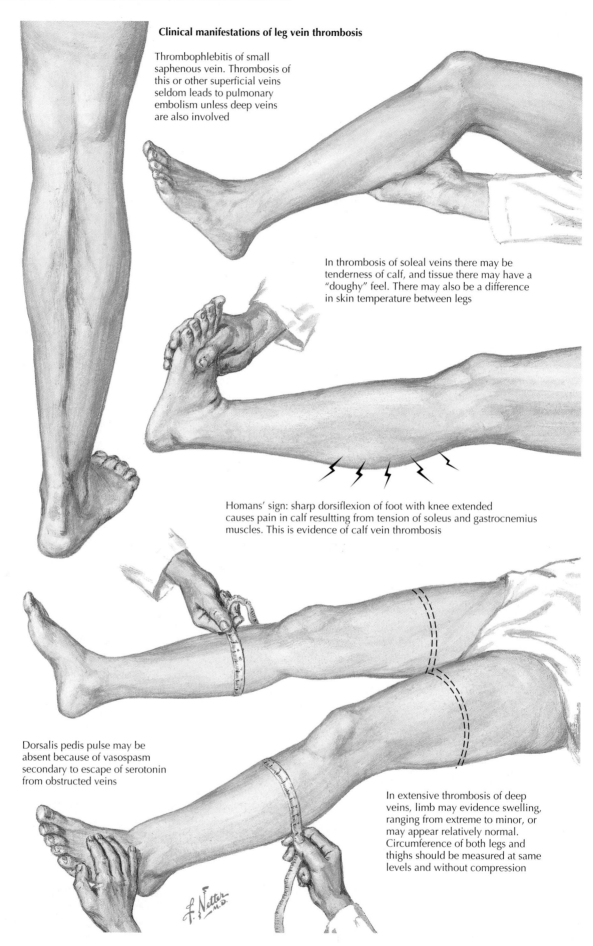

Clinical manifestations of leg vein thrombosis

Thrombophlebitis of small saphenous vein. Thrombosis of this or other superficial veins seldom leads to pulmonary embolism unless deep veins are also involved

In thrombosis of soleal veins there may be tenderness of calf, and tissue there may have a "doughy" feel. There may also be a difference in skin temperature between legs

Homans' sign: sharp dorsiflexion of foot with knee extended causes pain in calf resultting from tension of soleus and gastrocnemius muscles. This is evidence of calf vein thrombosis

Dorsalis pedis pulse may be absent because of vasospasm secondary to escape of serotonin from obstructed veins

In extensive thrombosis of deep veins, limb may evidence swelling, ranging from extreme to minor, or may appear relatively normal. Circumference of both legs and thighs should be measured at same levels and without compression

therapy or those with evidence of emboli. Surgical excision of involved superficial veins (and tributaries) may be required.

Diet: No specific dietary changes indicated.

Activity: Initially, bed rest for deep or extensive thrombosis with gradual return to activity in 1 to 5 days. No restriction once acute episode is resolved.

Patient Education: Patients who have had an episode of thrombosis should be instructed in risk reduction and warning signs that require reevaluation.

Drug(s) of Choice

Heparin 5000 to 10,000 U IV bolus followed by 1000 U per hour IV (may also use bolus of 80 U/kg, followed by 18 U/kg/hour). Dosage must be titrated based on APTT: target >2 times control. Low molecular weight heparin (LMWH) may also be used.

Maintenance with warfarin (Coumadin) starting at 1 to 5 days. Initial dose 5 to 10 mg PO daily, adjusted based on PT: target >1.3 to 1.5 times control (international normalized ratio [INR] of 2.0 to 3.0). (Intermittent subcutaneous heparin therapy with 15,000 U twice a day may also be used.)

Antibiotic therapy should be added for any patient suspected of sepsis (nafcillin 2 g IV every 6 hours, gentamicin 1 to 1.7 mg/kg IV).

Contraindications: Acute bleeding, recent neurosurgical procedure, known adverse reaction. Warfarin is contraindicated in pregnancy—these patients must continue heparin therapy. Relative contraindications—recent hemorrhage or surgery, peptic ulcer disease (severe), recent nonembolic stroke.

Precautions: Patients should continue to receive heparin until the target PT level is reached. Heparin therapy may cause thrombocytopenia. Intramuscular injections should be avoided while patients are receiving anticoagulant therapy. Warfarin therapy may be associated with necrotic skin lesions in a small number of patients (warfarin necrosis). Desogestrel-containing oral contraceptives are associated with a higher incidence of thromboembolism than other oral contraceptive formulations. This difference is small (20 to 30 of 100,000 versus 10 to 15 of 100,000 for levonorgestrel and 4 of 100,000 for nonpregnant women).

Interactions: Agents that prolong or intensify the action of anticoagulants—alcohol, allopurinol, amiodarone, steroids, androgens, many antimicrobials, cimetidine, chloral hydrate, disulfiram, all nonsteroidal antiinflammatory agents, sulfinpyrazone, tamoxifen, thyroid hormone, vitamin E, ranitidine, salicylates. Agents such as aminoglutethimide, antacids, barbiturates, carbamazepine, cholestyramine, diuretics, griseofulvin, rifampin, and oral contraceptives reduce the efficacy of oral anticoagulants.

Alternative Drugs

Thrombolytic agents (urokinase, streptokinase, tissue plasminogen activator) are effective in dissolving clots but remain investigational for the treatment of thrombosis. For mild superficial clots, nonsteroidal antiinflammatory agents may be used.

FOLLOW-UP

Patient Monitoring: Patients must be carefully monitored for embolization or further thrombosis. At the start of heparin therapy, the APTT must be monitored several times daily until the dose has been stabilized. The dose of warfarin must be monitored with periodic evaluation of the PT. Monitoring should be done daily until the target has been achieved, weekly for several weeks, and then monthly during maintenance therapy. Periodic checks should be made for hematuria and fecal occult blood.

Prevention/Avoidance: Avoid prolonged immobilization. Active prophylaxis (e.g., for patients after surgery) using low-dose subcutaneous heparin, low molecular weight heparin (enoxaparin), mechanical leg compression, and early ambulation. Changing intravenous sites every 48 hours reduces the risk of infection and inflammation.

Possible Complications: Pulmonary embolism (fatal in up to 20% of patients), phlegmasia cerulens dolens (rare). Hematuria or gastrointestinal bleeding may occur while patients are receiving anticoagulants. Any bleeding must be investigated and not presumed to be related to therapy; therapy may unmask an underlying condition such as cancer or ulcer disease. After thrombophlebitis, persistent pain and swelling of the limb may occur. Septic thrombophlebitis is associated with bacteremia (85%), septic emboli (45%), or abscess formation or pneumonia (45%).

Expected Outcome: Superficial thrombophlebitis and distal deep disease generally respond to prompt therapy with eventual resolution of symptoms. Up to 20% of proximal thrombosis may lead to embolization.

MISCELLANEOUS

Pregnancy Considerations: The use of warfarin is contraindicated. Patients who must receive anticoagulant therapy should be given heparin or low molecular weight heparin (intermittent subcutaneous therapy). Pregnancy causes a 49-fold increase in the incidence of phlebitis. Risk is increased with increased maternal age, multiparity, multiple pregnancy, hypertension, and preeclampsia.

ICD-9-CM Codes: Based on location and type.

REFERENCES

Level I

Agnelli G, Piovella F, Buoncristiani P, et al: Enoxaparin plus compression stockings compared with compression stockings alone in the prevention of venous thromboembolism after elective neurosurgery. N Engl J Med 1998;339:80.

Pinede L, Ninet J, Duhaut P, et al; Investigators of the "Duree Optimale du Traitement AntiVitamines K" (DOTAVK) Study: Comparison of 3 and 6 months of oral anticoagulant therapy after a first episode of proximal deep vein thrombosis or pulmonary embolism and comparison of 6 and 12 weeks of therapy after isolated calf deep vein thrombosis. Circulation 2001;103:2453.

Prandoni P, Tormene D, Pesavento R, Vesalio Investigators Group: High vs. low doses of low-molecular-weight heparin for the treatment of superficial vein thrombosis of the legs: a double-blind, randomized trial. J Thromb Haemost 2005;3:1152.

Scurr JH, Machin SJ, Bailey-King S, et al: Frequency and prevention of symptomless deep-vein thrombosis in long-haul flights: a randomised trial. Lancet 2001;357:1485.

Superficial Thrombophlebitis Treated by Enoxaparin Study Group: A pilot randomized double-blind comparison of a low-molecular-weight heparin, a nonsteroidal anti-inflammatory agent, and placebo in the treatment of superficial vein thrombosis. Arch Intern Med 2003;163:1657.

Level II

Anonymous: Low-molecular-weight heparin in the treatment of patients with venous thromboembolism. The Columbus Investigators. N Engl J Med 1997;337:657.

Anonymous: Prevention of pulmonary embolism and deep vein thrombosis with low dose aspirin: Pulmonary Embolism Prevention (PEP) trial. Lancet 2000;355:1295.

Daniel KR, Jackson RE, Kline JA: Utility of lower extremity venous ultrasound scanning in the diagnosis and exclusion of pulmonary embolism in outpatients. Ann Emerg Med 2000;35:547.

Grady D, Sawaya G: Postmenopausal hormone therapy increases risk of deep vein thrombosis and pulmonary embolism. Am J Med 1998;105:41.

Joffe HV, Kucher N, Tapson VF, Goldhaber SZ; Deep Vein Thrombosis (DVT) FREE Steering Committee: Upper-extremity deep vein thrombosis: a prospective registry of 592 patients. Circulation 2004;110:1605. Epub 2004 Sep 7.

Kamran SI, Downey D, Ruff RL: Pneumatic sequential compression reduces the risk of deep vein thrombosis in stroke patients. Neurology 1998;50:1683–8.

Lepercq J, Conard J, Borel-Derlon A, et al: Venous thromboembolism during pregnancy: a retrospective study of enoxaparin safety in 624 pregnancies. BJOG 2001;108:1134

Lutter KS, Kerr TM, Roedersheimer LR: Superficial thrombophlebitis diagnosed by duplex scanning. Surgery 1991;110:42.

Tagalakis V, Kahn SR, Libman M, Blostein M: The epidemiology of peripheral vein infusion thrombophlebitis: a critical review. Am J Med 2002;113:146.

Level III

American College of Obstetricians and Gynecologists: Thromboembolism in pregnancy. ACOG Practice Bulletin 19. Washington, DC, ACOG, 2000.

American College of Obstetricians and Gynecologists: Prevention of deep vein thrombosis and pulmonary embolism. ACOG Practice Bulletin 20. Washington, DC, ACOG, 2000.

American College of Obstetricians and Gynecologists: Air travel during pregnancy. ACOG Committee Opinion 261. Washington, DC, ACOG, 2001.

American College of Obstetricians and Gynecologists: Safety of Lovenox in pregnancy. ACOG Committee Opinion 276. Washington, DC, ACOG, 2002.

Katz VL: Postoperative counseling and management. In Katz VL, Lentz GM, Lobo RA, Gershenson DM: Comprehensive Gynecology, 5th ed. Philadelphia, Mosby/Elsevier, 2007:672.

Samlaskie CP, James WD: Superficial thrombophlebitis. I. Primary hypercoagulable states. J Am Acad Dermatol 1990;22:975.

Samlaskie CP, James WD: Superficial thrombophlebitis. II. Secondary hypercoagulable states. J Am Acad Dermatol 1990;23:1.

Vandenbroucke JP, Helmerhorst FM, Bloemenkamp KW, Rosendaal FR: Third-generation oral contraceptive and deep venous thrombosis: from epidemiologic controversy to new insight in coagulation. Am J Obstet Gynecol 1997;177:887.

Weinman EE, Salzman EW: Deep-vein thrombosis. N Engl J Med 1994;331:1630.

INTRODUCTION

Description: Toxic shock syndrome (TSS) is caused by toxins produced by an often asymptomatic infection with *Staphylococcus aureus*. Although most commonly associated with prolonged tampon use, about 10% of TSS cases are associated with other conditions.

Prevalence: Seen in 1 to 2 per 100,000 women 15 to 44 years of age (last active surveillance done in 1987).

Predominant Age: 30 to 60 years.

Genetics: No genetic pattern.

ETIOLOGY AND PATHOGENESIS

Causes: *S. aureus* exotoxins (TSS toxin-1, enterotoxins A, B, and C). For toxic shock to develop, three conditions must be met: there must be colonization by the bacteria, it must produce toxin, and there must be a portal of entry for the toxin. The presence of foreign bodies, such as a tampon, is thought to reduce magnesium levels, which promotes the formation of toxin by the bacteria.

Risk Factors: Infection by *S. aureus*, use of super-absorbency tampons, prolonged use of regular tampons, use of barrier contraceptive devices, nasal surgery, and postoperative staphylococcal wound infections.

CLINICAL CHARACTERISTICS

Signs and Symptoms

* Most common—rapid onset of fever greater than 38.9°C (102°F), hypotension, diffuse rash (the rash caused by TSS is commonly absent in places where clothing presses tightly against the skin). Hypotension may progress to severe and intractable hypotension and multisystem dysfunction.
* Other typical findings—agitation; arthralgias; confusion; diarrhea; erythema of pharynx, vulva, or vagina; conjunctiva; headache; myalgias; nausea; vomiting
* Desquamation, particularly on the palms and soles, can occur 1 to 2 weeks after onset of the illness

DIAGNOSTIC APPROACH

Differential Diagnosis

* Other exanthems (acute rheumatic fever, bullous impetigo, drug reaction, erythema multiforme, Kawasaki disease, leptospirosis, meningococcemia, Rocky Mountain spotted fever, rubella, rubeola, scarlet fever, viral disease)
* Gastrointestinal illness (appendicitis, dysentery, gastroenteritis, pancreatitis, staphylococcal food poisoning)
* Acute pyelonephritis
* Hemolytic uremic syndrome
* Legionnaires' disease
* Pelvic inflammatory disease (PID)
* Reye's syndrome
* Rhabdomyolysis
* Septic shock
* Stevens-Johnson syndrome
* Systemic lupus erythematosus
* Tick typhus

Associated Conditions: Other sources—surgical wounds (including dilation and curettage), nonsurgical focal infections, cellulitis, subcutaneous abscesses, mastitis, infected insect bites, postpartum (including transmission to the neonate), nonmenstrual vaginal conditions, vaginal infection, pelvic inflammatory disease, steroid cream use. Even the use of laminaria to dilate the cervix has been reported to be associated with rare cases.

Workup and Evaluation

Laboratory: Cultures for *S. aureus*, complete blood count, liver and renal function studies.

Imaging: No imaging indicated.

Special Tests: None indicated.

Diagnostic Procedures: History and physical findings.

Pathologic Findings

Lymphocyte depletion, subepidermic cleavage planes, cervical or vaginal ulcers.

Characteristics That Define Toxic Shock Syndrome

* Fever >38.9°C (102°F)
* Diffuse, macular, erythematous rash
* Desquamation of palms and soles 1 to 2 weeks after onset
* Hypotension (<90 torr systolic or orthostatic change)
* Negative blood, pharyngeal, and cerebrospinal fluid culture
* Negative serologic tests for measles, leptospirosis, Rocky Mountain spotted fever
* Three or more of the following organ systems:
  Cardiopulmonary (respiratory distress, pulmonary edema, heart block, myocarditis)
  Central nervous (disorientation or altered sensorium)
  Gastrointestinal (vomiting, diarrhea)
  Hematologic (thrombocytopenia of ≤100,000/mm³)
  Hepatic (> 2-fold elevation of total bilirubin or liver enzymes, serum albumin >2 g/dL)
* Mucous membrane inflammation (vaginal, oropharyngeal, conjunctival)
* Musculoskeletal (myalgia, >2-fold elevation of creatine phosphokinase)
* Renal (pyuria, >2-fold elevation of blood urea nitrogen or creatinine)

MANAGEMENT AND THERAPY

Nonpharmacologic

General Measures: Rapid evaluation and supportive intervention. Aggressive support and treatment of the attendant shock is paramount. (Frank shock is common by the time the patient is first seen for care.)

Specific Measures: The site of infection must be identified and drained, most commonly by removing the contaminated tampon. Antibiotic therapy with a β-

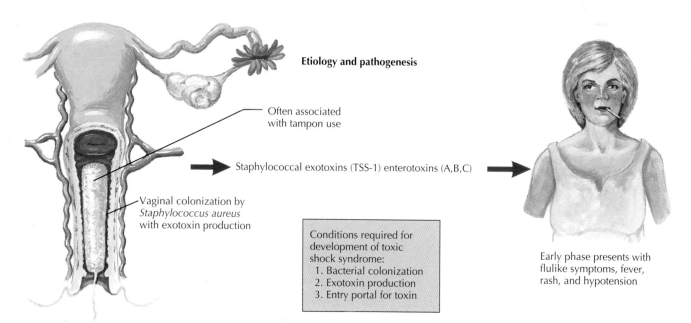

Etiology and pathogenesis

Often associated with tampon use

Staphylococcal exotoxins (TSS-1) enterotoxins (A,B,C)

Vaginal colonization by *Staphylococcus aureus* with exotoxin production

Conditions required for development of toxic shock syndrome:
1. Bacterial colonization
2. Exotoxin production
3. Entry portal for toxin

Early phase presents with flulike symptoms, fever, rash, and hypotension

Clinical features of toxic shock syndrome

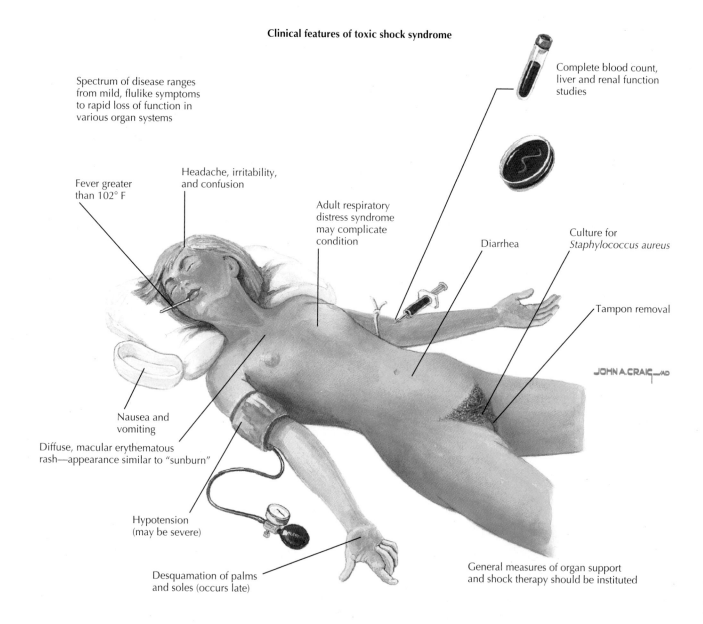

Spectrum of disease ranges from mild, flulike symptoms to rapid loss of function in various organ systems

Fever greater than 102° F

Headache, irritability, and confusion

Adult respiratory distress syndrome may complicate condition

Complete blood count, liver and renal function studies

Diarrhea

Culture for *Staphylococcus aureus*

Tampon removal

Nausea and vomiting

Diffuse, macular erythematous rash—appearance similar to "sunburn"

Hypotension (may be severe)

Desquamation of palms and soles (occurs late)

General measures of organ support and shock therapy should be instituted

JOHN A.CRAIG—AD

lactamase-resistant antistaphylococcal agent should be started but does not alter the initial course of the illness. Other support (e.g., mechanical ventilation, pressor agents) as needed.

Diet: As tolerated and dictated by the patient's clinical status during acute phase.

Activity: Bed rest during initial diagnosis and therapy.

Patient Education: American College of Obstetricians and Gynecologists Patient Education Pamphlet AP049 (Menstruation [Especially for Teens]), AP041 (Growing Up [Especially for Teens]).

Drug(s) of Choice

Oxacillin or nafcillin 100 mg/kg/day given in divided doses every 6 hours.

Contraindications: Known or suspected allergy.

Precautions: The dose of oxacillin must be reduced if renal failure is present.

Interactions: See individual agents.

Alternative Drugs

Clindamycin 25 mg/kg/day given in divided doses every 8 hours. Vancomycin 30 mg/kg/day given in divided doses every 6 hours.

FOLLOW-UP

Patient Monitoring: Intense monitoring is required during the initial phase of treatment. After resolution, normal health maintenance.

Prevention/Avoidance: Frequent changes of tampons. Use of sanitary pads at night. Although the risk of recurrence is low (10% to 15%), patients who have had TSS should refrain from the use of tampons in the future.

Possible Complications: Adult respiratory distress syndrome is a common sequela of TSS and patients must be monitored for the development of this complication. Acute renal failure, alopecia, and nail loss also may occur.

Expected Outcome: Although the prognosis for patients with TSS is generally good, mortality rates of 5% to 10% are common.

MISCELLANEOUS

Pregnancy Considerations: Uncommon during pregnancy. May occur postpartum as a complication of operative delivery, endometritis, episiotomy infection, or nursing.

ICD-9-CM Codes: 040.89.

REFERENCES

Level II

Broome CV: Epidemiology of toxic shock syndrome in the United States. Rev Infect Dis 1989;11:S14.

Chesney PJ, Davis JP, Purdy WK, et al: Clinical manifestations of toxic shock syndrome. JAMA 1981;246:741.

Davis JP, Vergernot JM, Amsterdam LE, et al: Long-term effects of toxic shock syndrome in women: sequelae, subsequent pregnancy, menstrual history, and long-term trends in catamenial product use. Rev Infect Dis 1989;11:S50.

Gavanta S. Reingold AL, Hightower AW et al: Active surveillance for toxic shock syndrome in the United States. 1986. Rev Infect Dis 1989:2:S28.

Hajjeh RA, Reingold A, Weil A, et al: Toxic shock syndrome in the United States: surveillance update, 1979–1996. Emerg Infect Dis J 1999;5:6.

Kain KC, Schulzer M, Chow AW: Clinical spectrum of nonmenstrual toxic shock syndrome (TSS): comparison with menstrual TSS by multivariate discriminant analyses. Clin Infect Dis 1993;16:100.

Martin SR, Foley MR: Intensive care in obstetrics: an evidence-based review. Am J Obstet Gynecol 2006;195:673.

Reingold AL, Shards KN, Dan BB, Broome CV: Toxic-shock not associated with menstruation. A review of 54 cases. Lancet 1982;1:1.

Sutkin G, Capelle SD, Schlievert PM, Creinin MD: Toxic shock syndrome after laminaria insertion. Obstet Gynecol 2001;98:959.

Level III

Centers for Disease Control and Prevention: Toxic-shock syndrome—United States. MMWR 1990;39:421.

Centers for Disease Control and Prevention: Toxic-shock syndrome—United States. 1980. MMWR 1997;46:492.

Eckert LO, Lentz GM: Infections of the lower genital tract. In Katz VL, Lentz GM, Lobo RA, Gershenson DM: Comprehensive Gynecology, 5th ed. Philadelphia, Mosby/Elsevier, 2007:596.

Reingold AL: Toxic shock syndrome: an update. Am J Obstet Gynecol 1991;165:1236.

Schuchat A, Broome CV: Toxic shock syndrome and tampons. Epidemiologic Reviews 1991;13:99.

Ulcerative Colitis

INTRODUCTION

Description: Ulcerative colitis is an inflammatory bowel disease characterized by an inflammation limited to the mucosa of the large bowel and found primarily in the descending colon and rectum (although the entire colon may be involved). The disease is characterized by intermittent bouts of symptoms interspersed by periods of quiescence.

Prevalence: Seventy to 150 in 100,000.

Predominant Age: 20 to 50 years, 20% of patients are younger than 21. (Usually starts between the ages of 15 and 30, and less frequently between 50 and 70 years of age).

Genetics: Family history present in up to 20% (ulcerative colitis or Crohn disease). More common in some ethnic groups (e.g., Jews).

ETIOLOGY AND PATHOGENESIS

Causes: An inflammatory process limited to the mucosa of the large bowel and found primarily in the descending colon and rectum, although the entire colon may be involved. Genetic, infectious, immunologic, and psychologic factors have been postulated to underlie the process.

Risk Factors: Family history. Negatively related to smoking.

CLINICAL CHARACTERISTICS

Signs and Symptoms

- Abdominal pain (generally mild to moderate; the pain is frequently relieved by a bowel movement, but many report the sensation of incomplete evacuation)
- Diarrhea (voluminous, watery, with occasional blood)
- Fever and weight loss
- Arthralgias and arthritis (15% to 20%)
- Aphthous ulcers of the mouth (5% to 10%)

DIAGNOSTIC APPROACH

Differential Diagnosis

- Irritable bowel syndrome (IBS; ulcerative colitis may be differentiated from irritable bowel syndrome by the frequent presence of fever or bloody stools in ulcerative colitis)
- Crohn disease
- Hemorrhoids
- Colon carcinoma
- Diverticulitis
- Infectious diarrhea (*Escherichia coli*, *Salmonella*, *Shigella*, *Entamoeba histolytica*)
- Iatrogenic (antibiotic associated)
- Radiation proctitis/colitis

Associated Conditions: Ocular complications (uveitis, cataracts, keratopathy, corneal ulceration, retinopathy; 4% to 10% of patients), liver and biliary complications (cirrhosis, 1% to 5%; sclerosing cholangitis, 1% to 4%; bile-duct carcinoma), ankylosing spondylitis, and osteoporosis.

Workup and Evaluation

Laboratory: No specific evaluation indicated. Complete blood count to evaluate blood loss or inflammation. Albumen and potassium levels may be reduced or liver functions test results may be elevated.

Imaging: Barium enema (air contrast).

Special Tests: Sigmoidoscopy, colonoscopy, or rectal biopsy.

Diagnostic Procedures: History, sigmoidoscopy, barium enema, or rectal biopsy.

Pathologic Findings

Superficial inflammation with ulceration is common. Hyperemia and hemorrhage also are common. The rectum is involved in 95% of cases, but the inflammation extends proximally in a continuous manner, at times even involving the terminal ileum.

MANAGEMENT AND THERAPY

Nonpharmacologic

General Measures: Evaluation and control of inflammation, prevention of complications, maintenance of nutrition (including adequate iron intake).

Specific Measures: Severe exacerbations may require hospitalization. Patients whose disease is refractory to antibiotic therapy may require surgical resection. (Between 25% and 40% of patients with ulcerative colitis eventually undergo colectomy because of massive bleeding, severe illness, rupture of the colon, or risk of cancer.)

Diet: No specific dietary changes indicated except for those based on other indications (such as lactose intolerance).

Activity: No restriction.

Drug(s) of Choice

Sulfasalazine 1 to 4 g PO daily (useful for both mild flare-ups and chronic suppression; approximately 10% of patients require chronic suppressive therapy).

Steroid enemas or mesalamine (5-aminosalicylic acid [5-ASA]) enemas or suppositories.

Prednisone 40 to 60 mg PO daily for flare-ups (tapered off over 2 months).

Contraindications: Known or suspected allergy or intolerance.

Precautions: Antidiarrheal agents may precipitate toxic megacolon.

Interactions: See individual agents.

Alternative Drugs

Azathioprine and 6-mercapto-purine (6-MP) may be used for patients who have not responded to 5-ASAs or corticosteroids or who are dependent on corticosteroids. Other oral 5-ASA derivatives are being studied. Antidiarrheal agents (diphenoxylate-atropine and loperamide) may be used but may precipitate toxic megacolon. Preliminary studies with Tetomilast (OPC-6535), a novel

Intestinal complications

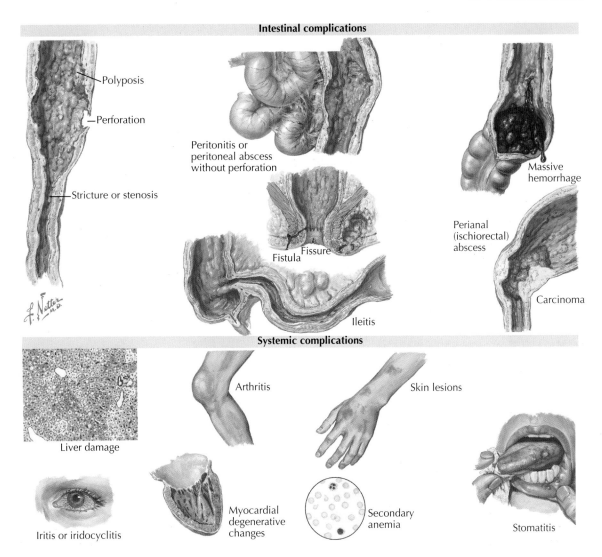

Polyposis

Perforation

Stricture or stenosis

Peritonitis or peritoneal abscess without perforation

Massive hemorrhage

Perianal (ischiorectal) abscess

Fistula
Fissure

Ileitis

Carcinoma

Systemic complications

Liver damage

Arthritis

Skin lesions

Iritis or iridocyclitis

Myocardial degenerative changes

Secondary anemia

Stomatitis

thiazole compound, failed to achieve statistically significant effects, but trends suggest possible utility.

FOLLOW-UP

Patient Monitoring: Normal health maintenance, periodic follow-up to monitor status of disease and possible complications. Colonoscopy to watch for the possible development of cancer should be performed every 1 to 2 years beginning 7 to 8 years after the onset of disease. Annual testing of liver function is desirable.

Prevention/Avoidance: None (prevention of complications as previously mentioned).

Possible Complications: Perforation, toxic megacolon, hepatic disease, bowel stricture and obstruction, colon cancer (30% after 25 years, less for left-sided disease). Mortality for initial attack is approximately 5%.

Expected Outcome: Highly variable; 75% to 85% of patients experience relapses, 20% require colectomy. Colon cancer risk is the greatest factor affecting long-term prognosis and management.

MISCELLANEOUS

Pregnancy Considerations: No effect on pregnancy. Of patients with inactive disease, 30% have relapses during pregnancy, 15% in the first trimester. Treatment with sulfasalazine does not affect the outcome of the pregnancy. It is recommended that pregnancy be delayed until the disease is in remission.

ICD-9-CM Codes: 556.9.

REFERENCES

Level I
Ardizzone S, Maconi G, Russo A, et al: Randomised controlled trial of azathioprine and 5-aminosalicylic acid for treatment of steroid dependent ulcerative colitis. Gut 2006;55:47. Epub 2005 Jun 21.

Level II
Rutgeerts P, Sandborn WJ, Feagan BG, et al: Infliximab for induction and maintenance therapy for ulcerative colitis. N Engl J Med 2005;353:2462.
van Staa TP, Card T, Logan RF, Leufkens HG: 5-Aminosalicylate use and colorectal cancer risk in inflammatory bowel disease: a large epidemiological study. Gut 2005;54:1573. Epub 2005 Jun 30.

Level III
Cima RR, Pemberton JH: Medical and surgical management of chronic ulcerative colitis. Arch Surg 2005;140:300.
Hannauer SB: Inflammatory bowel disease. N Engl J Med 1996;334:841.
Rapkin AJ, Mayer EA: Gastroenterologic causes of chronic pelvic pain. Obstet Gynecol Clin North Am 1993;20:663.

INTRODUCTION

Description: Urinary incontinence is a sign, a symptom, and a disease all at the same time. Bypass incontinence is continuous incontinence occurring when the normal continence mechanism is bypassed, as with fistulae. Symptoms may be intermittent or continuous, making the establishment of a diagnosis difficult in some patients. Overflow incontinence is continuous or intermittent insensible loss of small volumes of urine resulting from an overfilled or atonic bladder.

Prevalence: Of all women who have hysterectomies, 0.05% develop a fistula and subsequent bypass incontinence. Overflow incontinence is uncommon and generally follows trauma, instrumentation, surgery, or anesthesia.

Predominant Age: Mid-reproductive age and onward. Overflow incontinence is more common in later years.

Genetics: No genetic pattern.

ETIOLOGY AND PATHOGENESIS

Causes: Bypass incontinence—fistulae may result from surgical or obstetric trauma, irradiation, or malignancy, although the most common cause by far (in developed countries) is unrecognized surgical trauma (obstructed labor in other parts of the world). Roughly 75% of fistulae occur after abdominal hysterectomy. Signs of a urinary fistula (watery discharge) usually occur from 5 to 30 days after surgery, although they may be present in the immediate postoperative period.

Overflow incontinence—trauma (vulvar, perineal, radical pelvic surgery), irritation/infection (chronic cystitis, herpetic vulvitis, herpes zoster), anesthesia (spinal, epidural, caudal), pressure (uterine leiomyomata, pregnancy), anatomic defect (cystocele, retroversion, or prolapse of the uterus), neurologic disorder (multiple sclerosis, diabetes, spinal cord tumors, herniated disc, stroke, amyloid disease, pernicious anemia, Guillain-Barré syndrome, neurosyphilis), systemic disease (hypothyroidism, uremia), medications (antihistamines, appetite suppressants, β-adrenergic agents, parasympathetic blockers, vincristine, carbamazepine), radiation therapy, behavioral problems (psychogenic, infrequent voiding).

Risk Factors: Bypass incontinence—surgery or radiation treatment. Most common after uncomplicated hysterectomy, although pelvic adhesive disease, endometriosis, or pelvic tumors increase the individual risk. **Overflow incontinence**—none known other than causes listed previously.

CLINICAL CHARACTERISTICS

Signs and Symptoms

Bypass Incontinence

- Continuous loss of urine (often from the vagina or rectum)
- Fistulae from the vagina to the bladder (vesicovaginal), urethra (urethrovaginal), or ureter (ureterovaginal).

(Rarely, communication between the bladder and the uterus [vesicouterine] may also occur through the same mechanisms. Multiple fistulae are present in up to 15% of patients.)

Overflow Incontinence

- Frequent loss of small volumes of urine (may or may not be related to increases in intraabdominal pressure)
- Midline lower abdominal mass (with or without tenderness) that disappears with catheterization
- Ability for spontaneous voiding may or may not be compromised

DIAGNOSTIC APPROACH

Differential Diagnosis

Bypass Incontinence

- Overflow incontinence
- Urge incontinence
- Ectopic ureter

Overflow Incontinence

- Other forms of incontinence (stress, bypass/fistula)
- Chronic urinary tract infections
- Urinary tract obstruction
- Neurologic conditions presenting as an adynamic bladder

Associated Conditions: Vulvitis, vaginitis.

Workup and Evaluation

Laboratory: No evaluation indicated. Urinalysis is generally recommended, although results are nonspecific. Abrupt-onset incontinence in older patients should suggest infection, which may be confirmed through urinalysis or culture.

Imaging: Ureterovaginal fistulae should be evaluated by excretory urography to evaluate possible ureteral dilation or obstruction. Retrograde urography, with the passage of ureteral stents, may also be required. Ultrasonography demonstrates a distended bladder in patients with overflow incontinence.

Special Tests: If a vesicovaginal fistula is found, cystoscopy is required to evaluate the location of the fistula in relation to the ureteral opening and bladder trigone. For those with overflow incontinence that is either recurrent or unrelated to an obvious cause, urodynamics testing (including a cystometrogram) should be considered.

Diagnostic Procedures: When a fistula is suspected, the installation of a dilute solution of methylene blue (or sterile milk) into the bladder while a tampon is in place in the vagina documents a vesicovaginal fistula. A ureterovaginal fistula may be documented in a similar fashion using intravenous indigo carmine. For patients with overflow incontinence, physical examination and catheter drainage of the bladder are diagnostic. Urodynamics testing (cystometrogram) generally confirms the diagnosis.

Pathologic Findings

Based on cause. A distended, often hypotonic bladder is typical of patients with overflow incontinence.

MANAGEMENT AND THERAPY

Nonpharmacologic

General Measures: Bypass incontinence—urinary diversion, protection of the vulva from continuous moisture (zinc oxide, diaper rash preparations). **Overflow incontinence**—treatment of urinary tract infection (if present).

Specific Measures: Bypass incontinence—vesicovaginal fistulae that occur in the immediate postoperative period should be treated by large-caliber transurethral catheter drainage. Spontaneous healing is evident within 2 to 4 weeks. Similarly, in patients with a ureterovaginal fistula, prompt placement of a ureteral stent, left in place for 2 weeks, allows spontaneous healing for roughly 25% of patients. Surgical repair of genitourinary fistulae is generally delayed 2 to 4 months to allow complete healing of the original insult. In all cases, successful surgical repair consists of meticulous dissection of the fistulous tract and careful reapproximation of tissues. **Overflow incontinenc**e—prompt and continuous drainage if

retention is present, timed voiding to reduce bladder volume, suprapubic pressure or Crede maneuver to reduce residual volume.

Diet: No specific dietary changes indicated.

Activity: No restriction.

Patient Education: Reassurance; American College of Obstetricians and Gynecologists Patient Education Pamphlet AP081 (Urinary Incontinence).

Drug(s) of Choice

Bypass incontinence—none.

Overflow incontinence—pharmacologic therapy for these patients is often unsatisfactory and many require long-term catheter drainage or intermittent self-catheterization to manage their problem.

Urinary tract antibiotics if infection is present.

Acetylcholine-like drugs (bethanechol chloride [Urecholine] 10 to 50 mg three to four times per day; may also be given as 2.5 to 5 mg SC).

Contraindications: Overflow incontinence—Hyperthyroidism, peptic ulcer, latent or active bronchial asthma, pronounced bradycardia or hypotension, vasomotor instability, coronary artery disease, epilepsy, or Parkinsonism.

Precautions: Overflow incontinence—it is preferred that bethanechol be given when the stomach is empty

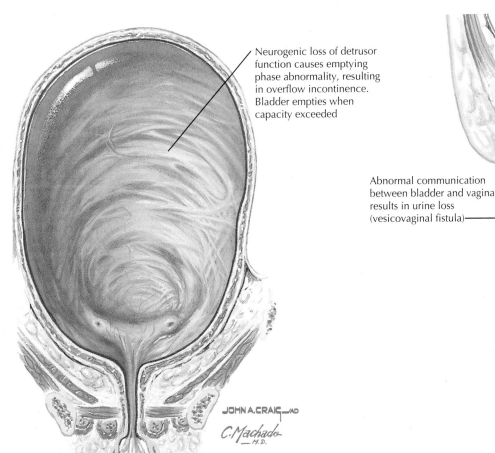

Neurogenic loss of detrusor function causes emptying phase abnormality, resulting in overflow incontinence. Bladder empties when capacity exceeded

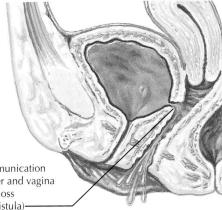

Abnormal communication between bladder and vagina results in urine loss (vesicovaginal fistula)

JOHN A. CRAIG—AD
C. Machado—M.D.

(1 hour before or 2 hours after meals). The sterile solution must not be given IM or IV. Bethanechol should not be given if the integrity of either the bladder wall or the gastrointestinal tract is in question or may be mechanically obstructed.

Interactions: Overflow incontinence—bethanechol should be used with extreme care in patients receiving ganglion-blocking compounds.

Alternate Therapies: Overflow incontinence—intermittent self-catheterization, electrical stimulation, reduction cystoplasty, urinary diversion.

FOLLOW-UP

Patient Monitoring: Normal health maintenance. Patients are at increased risk for urinary tract infections, vaginitis, and vulvitis. Patients who have experienced overflow incontinence have an increased risk of recurrence.

Prevention/Avoidance: Careful surgical technique should be used to reduce the risk of fistula formation. Surveillance in situations that predispose to retention (e.g., after regional anesthesia, childbirth).

Possible Complications: Social isolation and vulvar and perineal irritation are common complications of any type of urinary incontinence. Ascending urinary tract infection (including pyelonephritis) may occur if a fistula or bladder distention is present.

Expected Outcome: Recurrence after surgical repair of a fistula is common, especially in patients who have undergone radiation therapy for malignancies. For patients with time-limited causes for overflow incontinence, a complete resolution with drainage should be expected. For patients with idiopathic retention or retention caused by chronic causation, frequent recurrence, possible dependence on self-catheterization, urinary diversion, and electrical stimulation are possible.

MISCELLANEOUS

Pregnancy Considerations: No effect on pregnancy, although pregnancy (and vaginal delivery) increases the risk of urinary retention and overflow incontinence. Obstructed labor is a major cause of vesicovaginal fistula in developing countries.

ICD-9-CM Codes: Bypass incontinence—788.30, 788.37 (Continuous leakage); **overflow incontinence**—788.39, 788.21 (Incomplete bladder emptying), 788.37 (Continuous leakage of urine), 788.34 (Without sensory awareness).

REFERENCES

Level II

Freeman RM: The role of pelvic floor muscle training in urinary incontinence. BJOG 2004;111:37.

Level III

Abrams P, Blaivas JG, Stanton SL, Andersen JT: The standardization of terminology of lower urinary tract function produced by the International Continence Society Committee on Standardization of Terminology. Scand J Urol Nephrol 1988;114:5.

American College of Obstetricians and Gynecologists: Genitourinary tract changes. Obstet Gynecol 2004;104:56S.

American College of Obstetricians and Gynecologists: Urinary incontinence in women. Obstet Gynecol 2005;105:1533.

Consensus Conference: Urinary incontinence in adults. JAMA 1989;261:2685.

Diaz-Ball FL, Moore CA: A diagnostic aid for vesicovaginal fistula. J Urol 1969;102:424.

Dubeau CE: The aging lower urinary tract. J Urol 2006;175:S11.

Katz VL: Postoperative counseling and management. In Katz VL, Lentz GM, Lobo RA, Gershenson DM: Comprehensive Gynecology, 5th ed. Philadelphia, Mosby/Elsevier, 2007:681.

Lentz GM: Urogynecology. In Katz VL, Lentz GM, Lobo RA, Gershenson DM: Comprehensive Gynecology, 5th ed. Philadelphia, Mosby/Elsevier, 2007:561.

Norton P, Brubaker L: Urinary incontinence in women. Lancet 2006;367:57.

Norton PA: Urinary incontinence. Clin Obstet Gynecol 1990;33:293.

Sims JM: On the treatment of vesico-vaginal fistula. Am J Med Sci 1852;23:59.

Smith PP, McCrery RJ, Appell RA: Current trends in the evaluation and management of female urinary incontinence. CMAJ 2006;175:1233.

Sutherland SE, Goldman HB: Treatment options for female urinary incontinence. Med Clin North Am 2004;88:345.

Symmonds RE: Incontinence: Vesical and urethral fistulas. Clin Obstet Gynecol 1984;27:499.

Urinary Incontinence Guideline Panel: Urinary incontinence in adults: Clinical Practice Guidelines. Rockville, MD: Agency for Health Care Policy and Research, U.S. Dept of Health and Human Services, 1992. AHCPR publication 92–0038.

Wall LL: Obstetric vesicovaginal fistula as an international public-health problem. Lancet 2006;368:1201.

INTRODUCTION

Description: Urinary incontinence is a sign, a symptom, and a disease all at the same time. Stress incontinence is limited almost exclusively to women. Stress incontinence is the passive loss of urine in response to increased intraabdominal pressure, such as that caused by coughing, laughing, or sneezing.

Prevalence: Stress incontinence affects 10% to 15% of all women and 30% to 60% of women after menopause.

Predominant Age: Mid-reproductive age and onward. Stress incontinence becomes more common during the 40s and beyond and is most common after menopause.

Genetics: No genetic pattern.

ETIOLOGY AND PATHOGENESIS

Causes: Unequal transmission of intraabdominal pressure to the bladder and urethra. Generally associated with an anatomic defect such as a cystocele, urethrocele, or cystourethrocele. The degree of incontinence is often not correlated with the scale of pelvic relaxation.

Risk Factors: Multiparity, obesity, chronic cough, heavy lifting, intrinsic tissue weakness or atrophic changes resulting from estrogen loss.

CLINICAL CHARACTERISTICS

Signs and Symptoms

- Loss of small spurts of urine in association with transient increases in intraabdominal pressure
- Associated cystocele, urethrocele, or cystourethrocele

DIAGNOSTIC APPROACH

Differential Diagnosis

- Mixed incontinence (stress and urge)
- Urge incontinence (detrusor instability)
- Intrinsic sphincter defect (ISD)
- Low pressure urethra
- Urinary tract fistula
- Urinary tract infection
- Urethral diverticulum
- Overflow incontinence

Associated Conditions: Vulvitis, vaginitis, pelvic relaxation, uterine prolapse, other hernias, recurrent urinary tract infection.

Workup and Evaluation

Laboratory: No evaluation indicated. Urinalysis is generally recommended, although results are nonspecific. Abrupt-onset incontinence in older patients should suggest infection, which may be confirmed through urinalysis or culture.

Imaging: Radiographic studies are sometimes performed as a part of complex urodynamics studies but are generally of limited utility.

Special Tests: A "Q-tip test" is generally recommended, although it as a poor predictive value. (A cotton-tipped applicator dipped in 2% lidocaine [Xylocaine] is placed in the urethra and rotation anteriorly with straining is measured. Greater than 30 degrees is abnormal.) An evaluation of urinary function is advisable, especially if surgical therapy is being considered. In the past, the functional significance of a cystourethrocele was gauged by elevating the bladder neck (using fingers or an instrument) and asking the patient to strain (referred to as a Bonney or Marshall-Marchetti test). This test has fallen out of favor as nonspecific and unreliable.

Diagnostic Procedures: The best way to confirm stress incontinence is by pelvic examination—loss is best demonstrated by having the patient strain or cough while the vaginal opening is observed (preferably while the patient is standing). Urodynamics testing (simple or complex) may be used to evaluate other possible causes of incontinence.

Pathologic Findings

Based on cause. Evidence of a loss of support for the urethra and/or bladder is generally apparent on physical examination in patients with stress urinary incontinence.

MANAGEMENT AND THERAPY

Nonpharmacologic

General Measures: Weight reduction, treatment of chronic cough (if present), timed voiding, topical or systemic estrogen replacement or therapy as indicated (rendered controversial by the Women's Health Initiative [WHI] study).

Specific Measures: Pessary therapy, pelvic muscle exercises (Kegel exercises), collagen injections (for intrinsic sphincter defect), surgical repair; limited role for medical therapy.

Diet: No specific dietary changes indicated.

Activity: No restriction, although some reduction in heavy lifting may be prudent.

Patient Education: Reassurance; American College of Obstetricians and Gynecologists Patient Education Pamphlet AP081 (Urinary Incontinence), AP166 (Surgery for Urinary Incontinence).

Drug(s) of Choice

Phenylpropanolamine (75 to 150 mg PO daily) may improve mild stress incontinence.

Phenylpropanolamine plus chlorpheniramine (75 mg/ 12 mg PO every 6 hours) is better tolerated than phenylpropanolamine alone.

Imipramine hydrochloride (Tofranil) 50 to 150 mg PO daily is good for mixed incontinence and enuresis. Use with care in elderly patients.

Duloxetine, a potent and relatively balanced serotonin and noradrenaline reuptake inhibitor, has been evaluated in phase II and phase III clinical trials and was found to be efficacious and safe in the treatment of women with moderate to severe stress urinary incontinence symptoms. Approval for use in the United States has been delayed.

Stress Incontinence

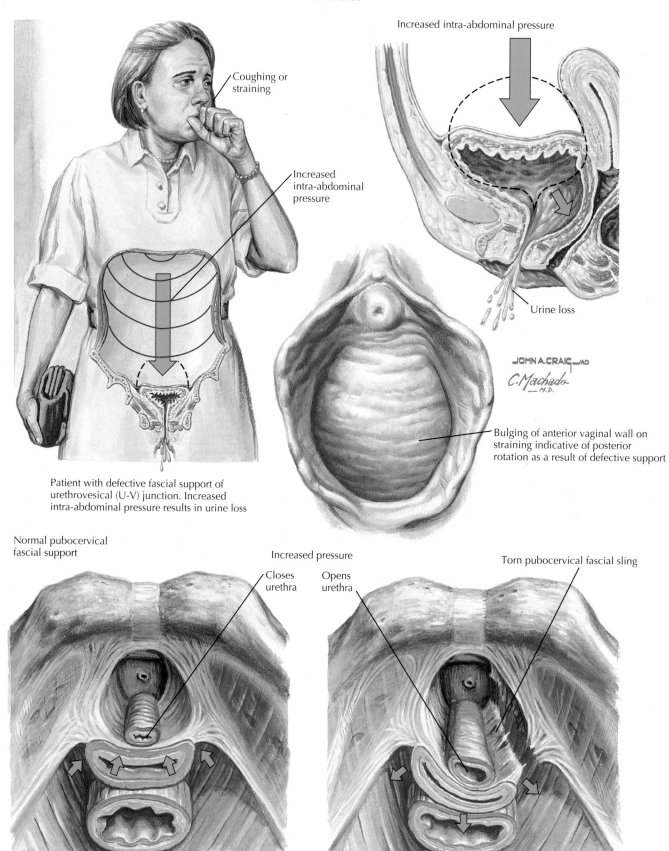

Coughing or straining

Increased intra-abdominal pressure

Patient with defective fascial support of urethrovesical (U-V) junction. Increased intra-abdominal pressure results in urine loss

Increased intra-abdominal pressure

Urine loss

Bulging of anterior vaginal wall on straining indicative of posterior rotation as a result of defective support

JOHN A. CRAIG—AD
C. Machado—M.D.

Normal pubocervical fascial support

Increased pressure

Closes urethra

Increased intra-abdominal pressure forces urethra against intact pubocervical fascia, closing urethra and maintaining continence

Opens urethra

Torn pubocervical fascial sling

Defective fascial support allows posterior rotation of U-V junction because of increased pressure, opening urethra and causing urine loss

Estrogen, either topically or systemically, is often prescribed to improve tissue tone, reduce irritation, and prepare tissues for surgical or pessary therapy.

Contraindications: Known or suspected sensitivity to medication, undiagnosed vaginal bleeding, breast cancer.

Precautions: Alpha-blocking agents used to treat hypertension may reduce urethral tone sufficiently to result in stress incontinence in patients with reduced pelvic support. Patients treated with angiotensin-converting enzyme inhibitors may develop a cough as a side effect of medication, worsening incontinence symptoms and accelerating the appearance or worsening of a cystourethrocele.

Interactions: See individual agents.

Alternate Therapies: None at this time.

FOLLOW-UP

Patient Monitoring: Normal health maintenance. Patients are at increased risk for urinary tract infections, vaginitis, and vulvitis.

Prevention/Avoidance: The role of elective cesarean delivery in reducing pelvic floor trauma has been debated, but there are data to suggest that nerve damage in the pelvic floor may occur late in pregnancy without the trauma of vaginal delivery, resulting in an increased risk of eventual stress incontinence even with cesarean delivery.

Possible Complications: Social isolation and vulvar and perineal irritation are common complications of any type of urinary incontinence.

Expected Outcome: Generally favorable results may be obtained for patients with symptoms of stress incontinence through the use of a carefully chosen and fitted pessary. Surgical therapy is associated with 40% to 95% success in long-term correction of the anatomic defect and the associated symptoms. (Success rates vary based on the type of procedure performed and duration of follow-up.)

MISCELLANEOUS

Pregnancy Considerations: No effect on pregnancy, although pregnancy (and vaginal delivery) may contribute to a worsening of pelvic support problems.

ICD-9-CM Codes: 625.6.

REFERENCES

Level I

Carey MP, Goh JT, Rosamilia A, et al: Laparoscopic versus open Burch colposuspension: a randomised controlled trial. BJOG 2006;113:999.

Kinn AC, Lindskog M: Estrogens and phenylpropanolamine in combination for stress urinary incontinence in postmenopausal women. Urology 1988;32:273.

Kitchener HC, Dunn G, Lawton V, et al; COLPO Study Group: Laparoscopic versus open colposuspension—Results of a prospective randomized controlled trial. BJOG 2006;113:1007.

Laurikainen E, Valpas A, Kivela A, et al: Retropubic compared with transobturator tape placement in treatment of urinary incontinence: a randomized controlled trial. Obstet Gynecol 2007;109:4.

Meschia M, Pifarotti P, Bernasconi F, et al: Tension-free vaginal tape (TVT) and intravaginal slingplasty (IVS) for stress urinary incontinence: a multicenter randomized trial. Am J Obstet Gynecol 2006;195:1338. Epub 2006 Jun 12.

Oelke M, Roovers JP, Michel MC: Safety and tolerability of duloxetine in women with stress urinary incontinence. BJOG 2006;113:22.

Level II

Albo ME, Richter HE, Brubaker L, et al; Urinary Incontinence Treatment Network: Burch colposuspension versus fascial sling to reduce urinary stress incontinence. N Engl J Med 2007;356:2143. Epub 2007 May 21.

Atherton MJ, Stanton SL: The tension-free vaginal tape reviewed: an evidence-based review from inception to current status. BJOG 2005;112:534.

Brubaker L, Cundiff GW, Fine P, et al; Pelvic Floor Disorders Network: Abdominal sacrocolpopexy with Burch colposuspension to reduce urinary stress incontinence. N Engl J Med 2006;354:1557.

Dean N, Herbison P, Ellis G, Wilson D: Laparoscopic colposuspension and tension-free vaginal tape: a systematic review. BJOG 2006;113:1345.

Federkiw DM, Sand PK, Retzky SS, Johnson DC: The cotton swab test. Receiver-operating characteristic curves. J Reprod Med 1995;40:42.

Freeman RM: The role of pelvic floor muscle training in urinary incontinence. BJOG 2004;111:37.

Stanton SL: Mid-urethral tapes: which? Review of available commercial mid-urethral tapes for the correction of stress incontinence. BJOG 2004;111:41.

Level III

Abrams P, Blaivas JG, Stanton SL, Andersen JT: The standardization of terminology of lower urinary tract function produced by the International Continence Society Committee on Standardization of Terminology. Scand J Urol Nephrol 1988;114:5.

American College of Obstetricians and Gynecologists: Genitourinary tract changes. Obstet Gynecol 2004;104:56S.

American College of Obstetricians and Gynecologists: Urinary incontinence in women. Obstet Gynecol 2005;105:15335.

American College of Obstetricians and Gynecologists: Pelvic organ prolapse. ACOG Practice Bulletin 79. Obstet Gynecol 2007;109:461.

Anders K: Devices for continence and prolapse. BJOG 2004;111:61.

Bombieri L: Is there a role for colposuspension? BJOG 2004;111:46.

Consensus Conference: Urinary incontinence in adults. JAMA 1989;261:2685.

Drutz H: Duloxetine in women awaiting surgery. BJOG 2006;113:17.

Freeman RM: Initial management of stress urinary incontinence: pelvic floor muscle training and duloxetine. BJOG 2006;113:10.

Lentz GM: Urogynecology. In Katz VL, Lentz GM, Lobo RA, Gershenson DM: Comprehensive Gynecology, 5th ed. Philadelphia, Mosby/Elsevier, 2007:551.

Mariappan P, Ballantyne Z, N'Dow JM, Alhasso AA: Serotonin and noradrenaline reuptake inhibitors (SNRI) for stress urinary incontinence in adults. Cochrane Database Syst Rev 2005:CD004742.

Norton P, Brubaker L: Urinary incontinence in women. Lancet 2006;367:57.

Norton PA: Urinary incontinence. Clin Obstet Gynecol 1990;33:293.

Nygaard IE, Heit M: Stress urinary incontinence. Obstet Gynecol 2004;104:607.

Ramsay IN: The treatment of stress incontinence—Is there a role for laparoscopy? BJOG 2004;111:49.

Smith PP, McCrery RJ, Appell RA: Current trends in the evaluation and management of female urinary incontinence. CMAJ 2006;175:1233.

Sutherland SE, Goldman HB: Treatment options for female urinary incontinence. Med Clin North Am 2004;88:345.

Urinary Incontinence Guideline Panel: Urinary incontinence in adults: Clinical Practice Guidelines. Rockville, MD: Agency for Health Care Policy and Research, U.S. Dept of Health and Human Services, 1992. AHCPR publication 92–0038.

Videla FLG, Wall LL. Diagnosing stress incontinence without multichannel urodynamic studies. Obstet Gynecol 1998;91:965.

Wagg A. Urinary incontinence—Older people: where are we now? BJOG 2004;111:15.

INTRODUCTION

Description: Urinary incontinence is a sign, a symptom, and a disease all at the same time. Urge incontinence is the involuntary loss of urine accompanied by a sense of urgency or impending loss and is associated with increased bladder activity.

Prevalence: Urge incontinence accounts for 35% of patients with incontinence.

Predominant Age: Mid-reproductive age and onward. Urge incontinence becomes more common during the 40s and beyond and is most common after menopause.

Genetics: No genetic pattern.

ETIOLOGY AND PATHOGENESIS

Causes: Allergy, bladder stone, bladder tumor, caffeinism, central nervous system tumors, detrusor muscle instability, interstitial cystitis, multiple sclerosis, Parkinson's disease, radiation cystitis, radical pelvic surgery, spinal cord injury, urinary tract infections (Urinary tract infections [UTI]; acute or chronic).

Risk Factors: Frequent UTIs.

CLINICAL CHARACTERISTICS

Signs and Symptoms

- Reduced bladder capacity and early, intense sensations of bladder fullness
- Spontaneous and uninhibitable contractions of the bladder muscles, resulting in large-volume, uncontrolled urine loss
- Loss possibly provoked by activities such as hand washing or a change in position or posture or after (not during) changes in intra-abdominal pressure such as a cough or sneeze

DIAGNOSTIC APPROACH

Differential Diagnosis

- Mixed incontinence (stress and urge)
- Stress incontinence
- UTI
- Urinary tract fistula
- Interstitial cystitis
- Urethritis

Associated Conditions: Vulvitis, vaginitis, nocturia, enuresis (bed-wetting).

Workup and Evaluation

Laboratory: No evaluation indicated. Urinalysis is generally recommended, although results are nonspecific. Abrupt-onset incontinence in older patients should suggest infection, which may be confirmed through urinalysis or culture.

Imaging: Radiographic studies are sometimes performed as a part of complex urodynamics studies but are generally of limited utility.

Special Tests: Measurement of postvoid urinary residual volume.

Diagnostic Procedures: History and physical examination, urodynamics testing (simple or complex), and evaluation of sphincter tone and function (as an indication of neurologic function) are the best ways to establish the diagnosis of urge incontinence.

Pathologic Findings

Based on cause. Patients with urge incontinence have a reduced bladder capacity, early first sensation, and uninhibited bladder contractions.

Other Causes of Incontinence

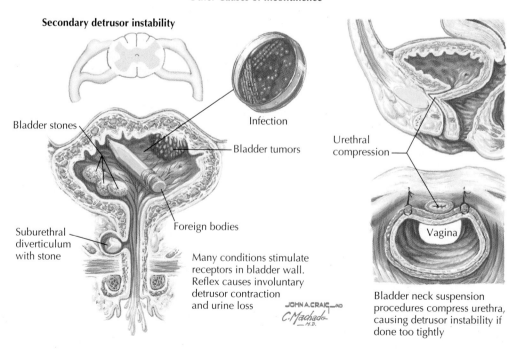

Secondary detrusor instability

Bladder stones

Infection

Bladder tumors

Suburethral diverticulum with stone

Foreign bodies

Many conditions stimulate receptors in bladder wall. Reflex causes involuntary detrusor contraction and urine loss

JOHN A. CRAIG —MD
C. Machado
M.D.

Urethral compression

Vagina

Bladder neck suspension procedures compress urethra, causing detrusor instability if done too tightly

Detrusor Instability and Hyperreflexia

Detrusor instability

Detrusor hyperreflexia

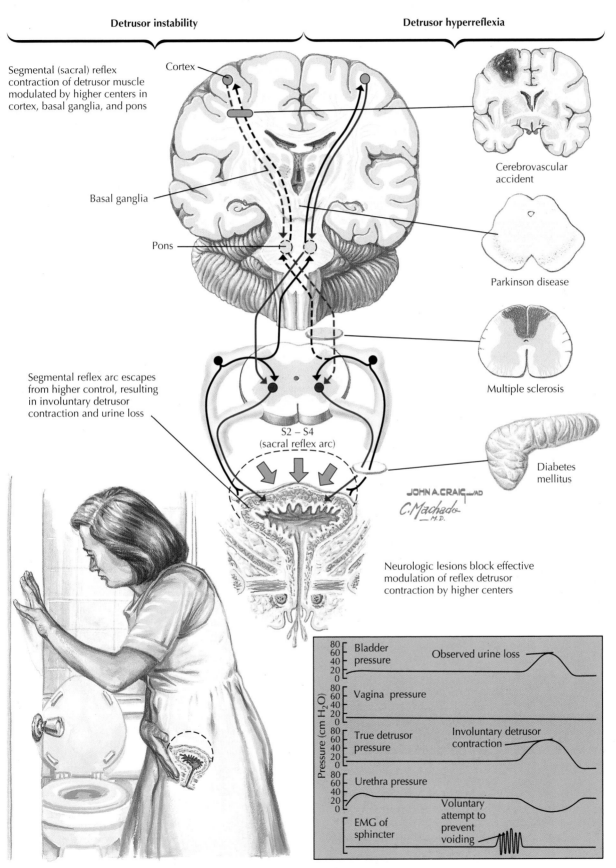

Segmental (sacral) reflex contraction of detrusor muscle modulated by higher centers in cortex, basal ganglia, and pons

Cortex

Basal ganglia

Pons

Cerebrovascular accident

Parkinson disease

Segmental reflex arc escapes from higher control, resulting in involuntary detrusor contraction and urine loss

Multiple sclerosis

S2 – S4 (sacral reflex arc)

Diabetes mellitus

JOHN A. CRAIG—AD
C. Machado —M.D.

Neurologic lesions block effective modulation of reflex detrusor contraction by higher centers

Urgency and urge incontinence typical of detrusor instability or hyperreflexia

Cystometry documents involuntary detrusor contraction in bladder filling phase

Bladder pressure — Observed urine loss

Vagina pressure

True detrusor pressure — Involuntary detrusor contraction

Urethra pressure

EMG of sphincter — Voluntary attempt to prevent voiding

Pressure (cm H$_2$O)

MANAGEMENT AND THERAPY

Nonpharmacologic

General Measures: Treatment of any UTI present, timed voiding.

Specific Measures: Medical therapy; limited role for surgical repair.

Diet: No specific dietary changes indicated. Reduction in caffeine use and other bladder irritants may help some patients with symptoms of urgency incontinence.

Activity: No restriction.

Patient Education: Reassurance; American College of Obstetricians and Gynecologists Patient Education Pamphlet AP081 (Urinary Incontinence).

Drug(s) of Choice

Flavoxate hydrochloride (Urispas) 100 to 200 mg PO three times a day to four times a day (fewer side effects, more expensive than some).

Imipramine hydrochloride (Tofranil) 25 to 50 mg PO twice a day to three times a day (good for mixed incontinence and enuresis, 60% to 75% effective).

Oxybutynin hydrochloride (Ditropan) 5 to 10 mg PO three times a day to four times a day (side effects common [75%], 60% to 80% effective).

Phenylpropanolamine hydrochloride (Propadrine) 50 mg PO twice a day (α-adrenergic sympathomimetic).

Propantheline bromide (Pro-Banthine) 15 to 30 mg PO three times a day to four times a day (few side effects, variable absorption, 60% to 80% effective).

Darifenacin (Enablex) 7.5 mg PO daily (works by blocking the M3 muscarinic acetylcholine receptor, which is primarily responsible for bladder muscle contractions).

Solifenacin (Vesicare) 5 mg PO daily (urinary antispasmodic of the anticholinergic class).

Contraindications: Most agents are contraindicated in patients with urinary retention, narrow-angle glaucoma, or known or suspected hypersensitivity.

Precautions: Anticholinergic drugs must be used with caution in patients with obstructive gastrointestinal disease or tachycardia. Dry mouth is experienced by 40% to 50% of patients. Darifenacin and solifenacin are contraindicated in urinary retention, gastric retention, or uncontrolled narrow-angle glaucoma and are pregnancy category C.

Interactions: Patients taking cytochrome P450 3A4 inhibitors (macrolide antibiotics or antifungal agents) must reduce their doses of tolterodine tartrate.

Alternate Therapies: Tolterodine tartrate (Detrol) 1 to 2 mg PO twice a day, dicyclomine hydrochloride (Bentyl) 20 mg IM four times a day (requires parenteral use), terodiline hydrochloride (Micturin) 12.5 to 25 mg PO twice a day (available outside of United States, carries some risk of esophageal and gastric erosions).

FOLLOW-UP

Patient Monitoring: Normal health maintenance. Patients are at increased risk for UTIs, vaginitis, and vulvitis.

Prevention/Avoidance: Avoidance of and prompt treatment for UTIs are thought to reduce the risk of developing urgency incontinence in the future.

Possible Complications: Social isolation and vulvar and perineal irritation are common complications of any type of urinary incontinence.

Expected Outcome: Patients with urge incontinence can expect generally good results with medical therapy and timed voiding.

MISCELLANEOUS

Pregnancy Considerations: No effect on pregnancy. Pregnancy often induces frequency and urgency because of bladder compression by the fetal presenting part near term. Bethanechol, darifenacin, and solifenacin are pregnancy category C drugs.

ICD-9-CM Codes: 788.31.

REFERENCES

Level I

Green SA, Alon A, Ianus J, et al: Efficacy and safety of a neurokinin-1 receptor antagonist in postmenopausal women with overactive bladder with urge urinary incontinence. J Urol 2006;176:2535; discussion 2540.

Level II

Freeman RM: The role of pelvic floor muscle training in urinary incontinence. BJOG 2004;111:37.

Level III

Abrams P, Blaivas JG, Stanton SL, Andersen JT: The standardization of terminology of lower urinary tract function produced by the International Continence Society Committee on Standardization of Terminology. Scand J Urol Nephrol 1988;114:5.

American College of Obstetricians and Gynecologists: Genitourinary tract changes. Obstet Gynecol 2004;104:56S-61S.

American College of Obstetricians and Gynecologists: Urinary incontinence in women. Obstet Gynecol 2005;105:1533.

American College of Obstetricians and Gynecologists: Pelvic organ prolapse. ACOG Practice Bulletin 79. Obstet Gynecol 2007; 109:461.

Consensus Conference: Urinary incontinence in adults. JAMA 1989;261:2685.

Dubeau CE: The aging lower urinary tract. J Urol 2006;175:S11.

Gibbs CF, Johnson TM 2nd, Ouslander JG: Office management of geriatric urinary incontinence. Am J Med 2007;120:211.

Lentz GM: Urogynecology. In Katz VL, Lentz GM, Lobo RA, Gershenson DM: Comprehensive Gynecology, 5th ed. Philadelphia, Mosby/Elsevier, 2007:559.

Norton P, Brubaker L: Urinary incontinence in women. Lancet 2006;367:57.

Norton PA: Urinary incontinence. Clin Obstet Gynecol 1990; 33:293.

Smith PP, McCrery RJ, Appell RA: Current trends in the evaluation and management of female urinary incontinence. CMAJ 2006;175:1233.

Sutherland SE, Goldman HB: Treatment options for female urinary incontinence. Med Clin North Am 2004;88:345.

Urinary Incontinence Guideline Panel: Urinary incontinence in adults: Clinical Practice Guidelines. Rockville, MD: Agency for Health Care Policy and Research, U.S. Dept of Health and Human Services, 1992. AHCPR publication 92–0038.

Wagg A: Urinary incontinence—Older people: where are we now? BJOG 2004;111:15.

Wall LL: Diagnosis and management of urinary incontinence due to detrusor instability. Obstet Gynecol Surv 1990;45:1s.

Wein AJ, Rackley RR: Overactive bladder: a better understanding of pathophysiology, diagnosis and management. J Urol 2006;175: S5.

INTRODUCTION

Description: An infection of the urinary tract causes urethritis, cystitis (including trigonitis), or pyelonephritis. Urinary tract infections (UTIs) are much more common in women because of their shortened urethral length and exposure of the urinary tract to trauma and pathogens during sexual activity.

Prevalence: Seen in 3% to 8% of patients (second most common type of infection in the body, 8.3 million visits per year), with roughly 45% of women aged 15 to 60 experiencing at least one UTI.

Predominant Age: Any, increases with older age.

Genetics: No genetic pattern.

ETIOLOGY AND PATHOGENESIS

Causes: Most UTIs in women ascend from contamination of the urethra, acquired via instrumentation, trauma, or sexual intercourse. (A history of intercourse within the preceding 24 to 48 hours is present in up to 75% of patients with acute UTI.) Coliform organisms, especially *Escherichia coli*, are the most common organisms responsible for asymptomatic bacteriuria, cystitis, and pyelonephritis. Ninety percent of first infections and 80% of recurrent infections are caused by *E. coli*, with between 10% and 20% resulting from *Staphylococcus saprophyticus*. Infection with other pathogens such as *Klebsiella* species (5%) and *Proteus* species (2%) account for most of the remaining infections. Anaerobic bacteria, *Trichomonas*, and yeasts are rare sources of infections except in patients with diabetes, patients who are immunosuppressed, or those requiring chronic catheterization. Infection with *Neisseria gonorrhoeae*, *Chlamydia trachomatis*, *Mycoplasma*, and *Ureaplasma* should all be considered when urethritis is suspected.

Risk Factors: Sexual activity, instrumentation, more virulent pathogens, altered host defenses, infrequent or incomplete voiding, foreign body or stone, obstruction, or biochemical changes in the urine (diabetes, hemoglobinopathies, pregnancy), estrogen deficiency, diaphragm use, and spermicides.

CLINICAL CHARACTERISTICS

Signs and Symptoms

- Asymptomatic (5%)
- Frequency, urgency, nocturia, or dysuria
- Pelvic pressure (cystitis)
- Fever and chills (pyelonephritis)
- Pyuria (more than five white cells per high power field in a centrifuged specimen)
- Hematuria (infrequent)
- Costovertebral angle tenderness (pyelonephritis)
- Suprapubic tenderness (cystitis)

DIAGNOSTIC APPROACH

Differential Diagnosis

- Traumatic trigonitis
- Urethral syndrome
- Interstitial cystitis
- Bladder tumors or stones
- Vulvitis and vaginitis (may give rise to external dysuria)
- Urethral diverticulum
- Infection in the Skene's glands
- Detrusor instability

Associated Conditions: Dyspareunia.

Workup and Evaluation

Laboratory: Nonpregnant women with a first episode of classic symptoms suggestive of UTI do not need laboratory confirmation of the diagnosis; they may be treated empirically. (Recent data suggest that this may be an acceptable strategy for women with fewer than three episodes per year, those who lack fever or flank pain, and those who have not been treated recently for the same symptoms.) Others should have a urinalysis and culture performed. For uncentrifuged urine samples, the presence of more than one white blood cell per high power field gives 90% accuracy in detecting infection. Gram stain of urine samples or sediments may help establish the diagnosis or suggest a possible pathogen.

Imaging: No imaging indicated.

Special Tests: When urethritis is suspected, a swab inserted into the urethra may be used to obtain material for culture and Gram stain to establish the diagnosis.

Diagnostic Procedures: History and physical examination, urinalysis.

Pathologic Findings

Pyuria with white blood cell casts common.

MANAGEMENT AND THERAPY

Nonpharmacologic

General Measures: Fluids, frequent voiding, and antipyretics. Urinary acidification (with ascorbic acid, ammonium chloride, or acidic fruit juices) and urinary analgesics (phenazopyridine [Pyridium]) may also be added based on the needs of the individual patient.

Specific Measures: Antibiotic therapy.

Diet: Increased fluids and reduction of caffeine.

Activity: No restriction.

Patient Education: Reassurance; American College of Obstetricians and Gynecologists Patient Education Pamphlet AP050 (Urinary Tract Infections).

Drug(s) of Choice

Nonpregnant patients: single-dose therapy—amoxicillin 3 g, ampicillin 3.5 g, cephalosporin (first generation) 2 g, nitrofurantoin 200 mg, sulfisoxazole 2 g, trimethoprim (TMP) 400 mg, TMP/sulfamethoxazole 320/1600 mg, fosfomycin tromethamine (Monurol) 3 gm PO.

Three- to 7-day therapy—amoxicillin 500 mg every 8 hours, cephalosporin (first generation) 500 mg every 8 hours, ciprofloxacin 250 mg every 12 hours, nitrofurantoin 100 mg every 12 hours, norfloxacin 400 mg every

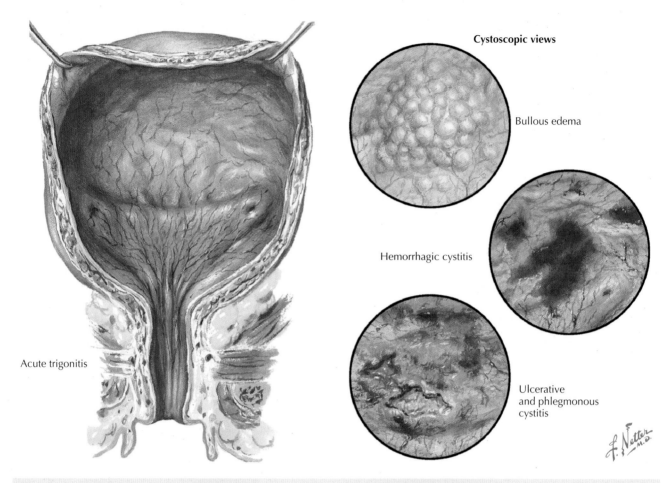

Cystoscopic views

Bullous edema

Hemorrhagic cystitis

Ulcerative
and phlegmonous
cystitis

Acute trigonitis

Common Clinical And Laboratory Features Of Acute Pyelonephritis

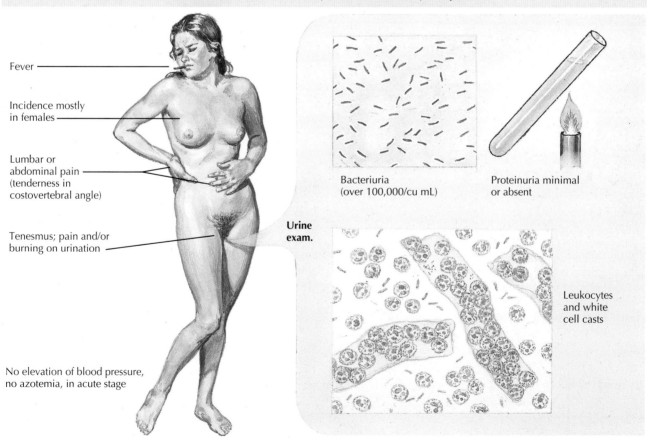

Fever

Incidence mostly
in females

Lumbar or
abdominal pain
(tenderness in
costovertebral angle)

Tenesmus; pain and/or
burning on urination

Urine
exam.

No elevation of blood pressure,
no azotemia, in acute stage

Bacteriuria
(over 100,000/cu mL)

Proteinuria minimal
or absent

Leukocytes
and white
cell casts

12 hours, ofloxacin 200 mg every 12 hours, sulfisoxazole 500 mg every 6 hours, tetracycline 500 mg every 6 hours, TMP/sulfamethoxazole 160/800 mg every 12 hours, TMP 200 mg every 12 hours.

Contraindications: Known or suspected hypersensitivity.

Precautions: Urinary analgesics (phenazopyridine [Pyridium]) should be used for no longer than 48 hours and may stain some types of contact lenses.

Interactions: See individual medications.

Alternative Drugs

Pregnant patients: 7-day therapy—amoxicillin 500 mg every 8 hours, cephalosporin (first generation) 500 mg every 6 hours, nitrofurantoin 100 mg every 12 hours.

FOLLOW-UP

Patient Monitoring: No follow-up is necessary after single-dose treatment or multiday treatment for non-pregnant women who experience resolution of their symptoms. Confirmation of cure for all other patients should be carried out with urinalysis and culture. Those with recurrent infections should be evaluated for possible causes, and a program of patient-initiated single-dose therapy should be begun as needed for prophylaxis (after intercourse, daily, or three times weekly based on patient need). Possible causes of recurrent infection include incorrect or incomplete (e.g., noncompliant) therapy, mechanical factors (such as obstruction or stone), or compromised host defenses.

Prevention/Avoidance: Frequent voiding, adequate fluid intake, and voiding after intercourse.

Possible Complications: Urethral syndrome and interstitial cystitis. Bacteremia, septic shock, adult respiratory distress syndrome, and other serious sequelae are associated with pyelonephritis. Recurrence rates may be as high as 20% (90% represent reinfection). Up to one third of patients may develop pyelonephritis.

Expected Outcome: For most patients, symptoms should resolve within 2 to 3 days of the initiation of therapy. Some authors estimate that up to 50% of infections resolve without intervention.

MISCELLANEOUS

Pregnancy Considerations: Asymptomatic bacteriuria is more common during pregnancy (5%). Those at high risk (e.g., patients with diabetes) should be monitored carefully.

ICD-9-CM Codes: 599.0, 646.6 (Complicating pregnancy).

REFERENCES

Level I
Greenberg RN, Reilly PM, Luppen KL, et al: Randomized study of single-dose, three-day, and seven-day treatment of cystitis in women. J Infect Dis 1986;153:277.

Level II
Ambulatory Care Visits to Physician Offices, Hospital Outpatient Departments, and Emergency Departments: United States, 1999–2000. Vital and Health Statistics. Series 13, No. 157. Hyattsville, MD, National Center for Health Statistics, Centers for Disease Control and Prevention, U.S. Dept. of Health and Human Services, 2004.

Level III
American College of Obstetricians and Gynecologists: Urinary incontinence in women. ACOG Practice Bulletin 63. Obstet Gynecol 2005;105:1533.

Car J: Urinary tract infections in women: diagnosis and management in primary care. BMJ 2006;332:94.

Colgan R, Nicolle LE, McGlone A, Hooton TM: Asymptomatic bacteriuria in adults. Am Fam Physician 2006;74:985.

Franco AV: Recurrent urinary tract infections. Best Pract Res Clin Obstet Gynaecol 2005;19:861. Epub 2005 Nov 17.

Kunin CM: Urinary tract infections in females. Clin Infect Dis 1994;18:1.

Lentz GM: Urogynecology. In Katz VL, Lentz GM, Lobo RA, Gershenson DM: Comprehensive Gynecology, 5th ed. Philadelphia, Mosby/Elsevier, 2007:545.

Macejko AM, Schaeffer AJ: Asymptomatic bacteriuria and symptomatic urinary tract infections during pregnancy. Urol Clin North Am 2007;34:35.

Mittal P, Wing DA: Urinary tract infections in pregnancy. Clin Perinatol 2005;32:749.

Nicolle L, Anderson PA, Conly J, et al: Uncomplicated urinary tract infection in women. Current practice and the effect of antibiotic resistance on empiric treatment. Can Fam Physician 2006;52:612.

Pappas P: Laboratory in the diagnosis and management of urinary tract infections. Med Clin North Am 1991;75:313.

Sheffield JS, Cunningham FG: Urinary tract infection in women. Obstet Gynecol 2005;106:1085.

Stamm W: Criteria for the diagnosis of urinary tract infection and for the assessment of therapeutic effectiveness. Infection 1992;20:S151, S160.

Stamm W: Controversies in single dose therapy of acute uncomplicated urinary tract infections in women. Infection 1992;20:S272.

Stamm W, Hooton T: Management of urinary tract infections in adults. N Engl J Med 1993;329:1328.

Whelan P: Manage urinary tract infections. Practitioner 2006;250:38, 41, 43 passim.

THE CHALLENGE

An important part of the evaluation of urinary symptoms or incontinence of any type is urodynamic testing of bladder function. This may be performed in the office setting using readily available equipment or may require complex equipment and expertise.

Scope of the Problem: Almost one half of all women have involuntary loss of a few drops of urine at some time in their lifetime, with 10% to 15% of women suffering significant, recurrent loss. It has been estimated that more than one fourth of women of reproductive age experience some degree of urinary incontinence. This number increases to 30% to 40% of women after the age of menopause.

Objectives of Test: To evaluate bladder function and aid in the diagnosis of bladder symptoms such as urgency and incontinence.

TACTICS

Relevant Pathophysiology: The bladder is designed to gradually distend as urine is delivered by the ureters. This distention proceeds with little or no change in bladder pressure (normal compliance). When bladder volume reaches a certain point (generally 150 to 200 mL) the first sensation of bladder fullness occurs. Additional increases in volume can be accomplished with an increasing sense of urgency but without uninhibited bladder contraction or incontinence. When bladder emptying is allowed, it should happen in an expeditious and efficient manner. Although the specific content of urodynamics testing varies, at a minimum it includes cystometrics and provocative tests (such as coughing or straining while the bladder is full). Most centers include sophisticated evaluation of bladder compliance and contractility, cystoscopy, and evaluations of the voiding process itself. Pressure profiles of the bladder and urethra, electromyography, and fluoroscopic examinations may also be included.

Strategies: Simple office cystometrics—the patient should be in a relaxed, supine position with her bladder emptied. The patient is catheterized with sterile technique using a straight catheter. Any residual urine is caught, measured for volume, and sent for culture to detect occult infection. The bladder is slowly filled (with sterile, warmed saline) by gravity at a rate of less than 3 mL per second. The patient is asked to report her first sensation of bladder fullness, and the volume infused at that point is noted. Filling continues in 25-mL aliquots until the patient is unable to tolerate more, and this volume is recorded as the maximal bladder capacity. Any upward movement of the fluid column, intense sensation of urgency, or leakage around the catheter is abnormal, suggests detrusor instability, and should be noted. (More exact measurements of bladder function may be made by assembling intravenous tubing, a spinal manometer [or limb of extra tubing], and a three-way connector. The pressure inside the fluid column may be monitored, and the presence of bladder contractions can be more easily detected and documented. When this greater degree of accuracy is required, many prefer to proceed to formal urodynamics testing.) The catheter is removed, and the patient is asked to cough several times; leakage should be noted. Leakage that occurs immediately after removal, is prolonged, or is of large volume suggests detrusor instability. These maneuvers may be repeated in the standing position.

Complex urodynamic testing—the procedures used in multichannel urodynamic test vary somewhat with the specifics of the equipment being used and local custom. Instead of the use of a simple straight catheter (as previous), bladder filling is accomplished by a catheter system equipped with sensors that can monitor bladder and urethral pressure. (Referenced pressures from the rectum or vagina may also be recorded.) Following filling of the bladder, the catheter may be slowly pulled through the length of the urethra to measure both pressure and functional urethral length. After provocative tests are performed, the patient is asked to empty her bladder on a special commode that can measure flow rate and volume. Some centers augment these studies with radiographic evaluations of the bladder and urethra.

Patient Education: American College of Obstetricians and Gynecologists Patient Education Pamphlet AP081 (Urinary Incontinence), AP050 (Urinary Tract Infections), AP012 (Pelvic Support Problems), AP166 (Surgery for Urinary Incontinence).

IMPLEMENTATION

Special Considerations: "Urinary incontinence" may be a sign, a symptom, or a condition. It is defined as a condition in which involuntary loss of urine may be objectively demonstrated, and the loss presents a social or hygienic problem. The volume of the loss is not as important as the impact it has on the patient and her life.

An assessment of voiding may be carried out by filling the bladder with 200 mL of fluid and listening to the patient's voiding from outside a bathroom door or while the patient voids behind a screen. The volume of flow (rate) may be estimated by the sound; the duration of flow may be timed with a stopwatch. Sophisticated measures of voiding parameters are typically included in formal urodynamics testing.

Residual bladder volume may also be measured by specialized ultrasonographic techniques.

REFERENCES

Level I
Chin-Peuckert L, Rennick JE, Jednak R, et al: Should warm infusion solution be used for urodynamic studies in children? A prospective randomized study. J Urol 2004;172:1657.

Level II
Jarvis GJ, Hall S, Stamp S, et al: An assessment of urodynamic examination in incontinent women. Br J Obstet Gynaecol 1980;87:893.
Robinson D, Anders K, Cardozo L, et al: Can ultrasound replace ambulatory urodynamics when investigating women with irritative urinary symptoms? BJOG 2002;109:145.

Yalcin I, Versi E, Benson JT, et al: Validation of a clinical algorithm to diagnose stress urinary incontinence for large studies. J Urol 2004;171:2321.

Level III

American College of Obstetricians and Gynecologists: Urinary incontinence in women. ACOG Practice Bulletin 63. Obstet Gynecol 2005;105:1533.

Bradley WE, Timm GW: Cystometry VI. Interpretation. Urology 1976;7:231.

Lentz GM: Urogynecology. In Katz VL, Lentz GM, Lobo RA, Gershenson DM: Comprehensive Gynecology, 5th ed. Philadelphia, Mosby/Elsevier, 2007:543.

Massey A, Abrams P: Urodynamics of the female lower urinary tract. Urol Clin North Am 1985;12:231.

Nygaard IE, Heit M: Stress urinary incontinence. Obstet Gynecol 2004;104:607.

Smith RP, Ling FW: Procedures in women's health care. Baltimore, Williams & Wilkins, 1997:411, 415.

Sutherst JR, Brown MC: Comparison of single and multichannel cystometry in diagnosing bladder instability. BMJ 1984;288:1720.

Walters MD, Realini JP: The evaluation and treatment of urinary incontinence in women: a primary care approach. J Am Board Fam Pract 1992;5:289.

Office Testing Procedures

Standing stress test

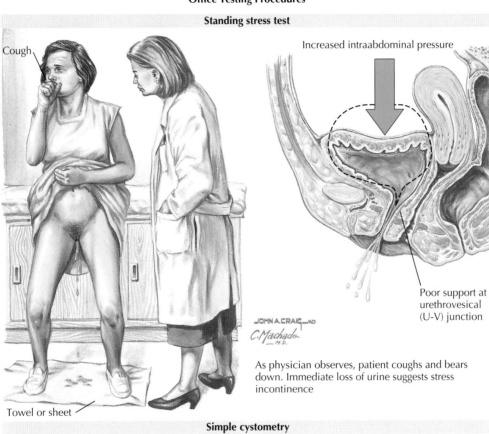

Cough

Increased intraabdominal pressure

Poor support at urethrovesical (U-V) junction

As physician observes, patient coughs and bears down. Immediate loss of urine suggests stress incontinence

Towel or sheet

Simple cystometry

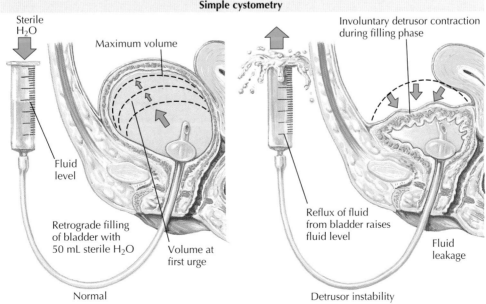

Sterile H$_2$O

Maximum volume

Involuntary detrusor contraction during filling phase

Fluid level

Retrograde filling of bladder with 50 mL sterile H$_2$O

Volume at first urge

Reflux of fluid from bladder raises fluid level

Fluid leakage

Normal

Detrusor instability

Complex Cystometry

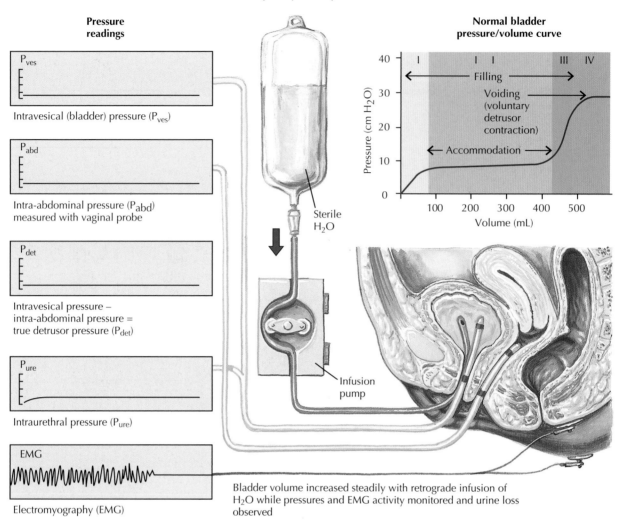

Pressure readings

P_{ves}

Intravesical (bladder) pressure (P_{ves})

P_{abd}

Intra-abdominal pressure (P_{abd}) measured with vaginal probe

P_{det}

Intravesical pressure – intra-abdominal pressure = true detrusor pressure (P_{det})

P_{ure}

Intraurethral pressure (P_{ure})

EMG

Electromyography (EMG)

Sterile H_2O

Infusion pump

Normal bladder pressure/volume curve

Filling

Voiding (voluntary detrusor contraction)

Accommodation

Bladder volume increased steadily with retrograde infusion of H_2O while pressures and EMG activity monitored and urine loss observed

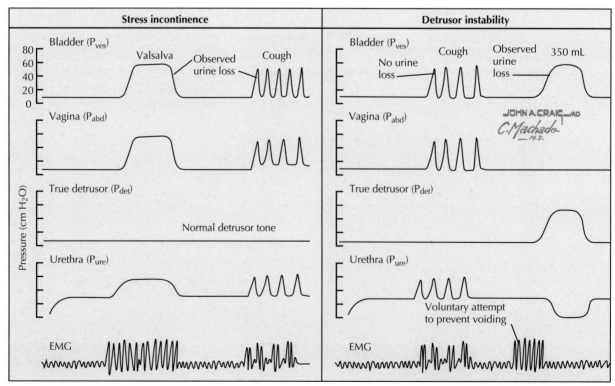

Stress incontinence

Bladder (P_{ves})

Valsalva — Observed urine loss — Cough

Vagina (P_{abd})

True detrusor (P_{det})

Normal detrusor tone

Urethra (P_{ure})

Pressure (cm H_2O)

EMG

Detrusor instability

Bladder (P_{ves})

No urine loss — Cough — Observed urine loss — 350 mL

Vagina (P_{abd})

True detrusor (P_{det})

Urethra (P_{ure})

Voluntary attempt to prevent voiding

EMG

JOHN A. CRAIG—MD
C. Machado —M.D.

Varicose Veins

INTRODUCTION

Description: Varicose veins are dilated, elongated, and tortuous superficial veins with incompetent or congenitally absent valves. Although these may occur anywhere in the body, they are most common in the legs, where gravity produces reverse flow. Varicose veins are five times more common in women than in men.

Prevalence: Twenty percent of adults, one out of two people older than age 50.

Predominant Age: Middle age and beyond.

Genetics: Familial as an X-linked dominant condition.

ETIOLOGY AND PATHOGENESIS

Causes: Faulty or absent valves in one or more perforating veins that may result in secondary incompetence at the saphenofemoral junction. Other causes—deep vein thrombophlebitis, increased venous pressure from any source (e.g., obstruction by tumor, pregnancy, pelvic mass).

Risk Factors: Pregnancy, family history, prolonged standing.

CLINICAL CHARACTERISTICS

Signs and Symptoms

- Asymptomatic
- Leg pain or cramps (worse during menstruation)
- Dilated, tortuous superficial veins
- Spider veins (idiopathic telangiectases)
- Limb edema
- Superficial ulceration

DIAGNOSTIC APPROACH

Differential Diagnosis

- Radiculopathy (nerve root compression)
- Arthritis
- Peripheral neuritis

Associated Conditions: Stasis ulcers and dermatitis.

Workup and Evaluation

Laboratory: No evaluation indicated.

Imaging: Doppler studies may be used to evaluate the possibility of deep vein thrombosis but are generally not required for the diagnosis of varicose veins.

Special Tests: Trendelenburg-Brodie test (elevate leg, compress greater saphenous vein at mid-thigh, have patient stand: rapid refilling of vein indicates incompetent communicating veins).

Diagnostic Procedures: History and physical examination.

Pathologic Findings

Elongated, tortuous veins with medial fibrosis and absent or atrophic valves.

MANAGEMENT AND THERAPY

Nonpharmacologic

General Measures: Frequent rest, elevation of affected limb, lightweight compression (hosiery), avoidance of proximal compression (girdles).

Specific Measures: Superficial veins may be eliminated with intracapillary injection of hypertonic saline (20% to 25%) or 1% to 3% solution of sodium tetradecyl sulfate (must be followed by compression for up to 3 weeks). Ligation or stripping of the saphenous veins should be considered in patients with pain, ulcers, recurrent phlebitis, or significant cosmetic problems.

Diet: No specific dietary changes indicated. Weight loss when appropriate.

Activity: Active exercise routines including walking, use of elastic stockings (applied before arising), avoidance of prolonged standing or inactivity.

Patient Education: Education about risk factors and avoidance; American College of Obstetricians and Gynecologists Patient Education Pamphlet AP119 (Exercise During Pregnancy), AP045 (Exercise and Fitness: A Guide for Women).

Drug(s) of Choice

None.

Precautions: Some authors suggest that oral contraceptives not be used within 6 weeks of sclerotherapy.

Alternative Drugs

Antibiotic therapy for infected ulcers.

FOLLOW-UP

Patient Monitoring: Normal health maintenance, evaluation for progression of disease or emergence of complications (skin ulcers).

Prevention/Avoidance: Avoidance of prolonged standing or inactivity, use of compression stockings, exercise, weight loss, leg elevation when at rest.

Possible Complications: Petechial hemorrhages, chronic edema, superficial ulceration and infection, chronic pigment change, eczema.

Expected Outcome: Generally a chronic condition with control possible through treatment.

MISCELLANEOUS

Pregnancy Considerations: No effect on pregnancy. Pregnancy often worsens existing disease and increases the risk of future occurrence. Use of compression stockings should be encouraged for those at increased risk.

ICD-9-CM Codes: 454.1.

Clinical Features

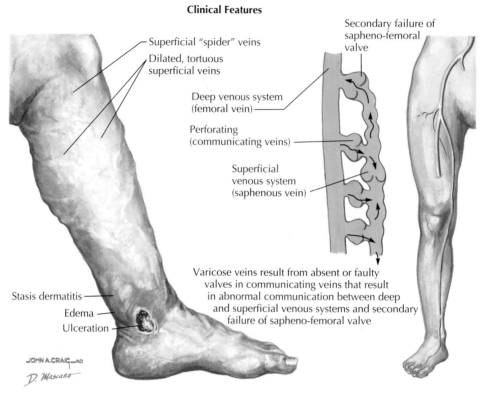

- Superficial "spider" veins
- Dilated, tortuous superficial veins
- Deep venous system (femoral vein)
- Perforating (communicating veins)
- Superficial venous system (saphenous vein)
- Secondary failure of sapheno-femoral valve
- Stasis dermatitis
- Edema
- Ulceration

Varicose veins result from absent or faulty valves in communicating veins that result in abnormal communication between deep and superficial venous systems and secondary failure of sapheno-femoral valve

JOHN A. CRAIG—MD
D. Mascaro

Trendelenburg-Brodie Test of Venous Valve Competence

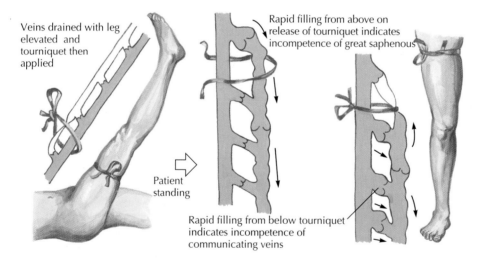

Veins drained with leg elevated and tourniquet then applied

Patient standing

Rapid filling from above on release of tourniquet indicates incompetence of great saphenous

Rapid filling from below tourniquet indicates incompetence of communicating veins

REFERENCES

Level I

Lorenz D, Gabel W, Redtenbacher M, et al: Randomized clinical trial comparing bipolar coagulating and standard great saphenous stripping for symptomatic varicose veins. Br J Surg 2007;94:434.

Michaels JA, Brazier JE, Campbell WB, et al: Randomized clinical trial comparing surgery with conservative treatment for uncomplicated varicose veins. Br J Surg 2006;93:175.

Level III

American College of Obstetricians and Gynecologists: Prevention of deep vein thrombosis and pulmonary embolism. ACOG Practice Bulletin 21. Washington, DC, ACOG, 2000.

Baccaglini U, Spreafico G, Castoro C, Sorrentino P: Sclerotherapy of varicose veins of the lower limbs. Consensus paper. North American Society of Phlebology. Dermatol Surg 1996;22:883.

Green D: Sclerotherapy for the permanent eradication of varicose veins: theoretical and practical considerations. J Am Acad Dermatol 1998;38:461.

Eberhardt RT, Raffetto JD: Chronic venous insufficiency. Circulation 2005;111:2398.

Helmerhorst FM, Bloemenkamp KW, Rosendaal FR, Vandenbroucke JP: Oral contraceptives and thrombotic disease: risk of venous thromboembolism. Thromb Haemost 1997;78:327.

Hobson J. Venous insufficiency at work. Angiology 1997;48:577.

Houghton AD, Panayiotopoulos Y, Taylor PR: Practical management of primary varicose veins. Br J Clin Pract 1996;50:103.

Rajendran S, Rigby AJ, Anand SC: Venous leg ulcer treatment and practice—Part 4: Surgery and pharmaceutical therapies. J Wound Care 2007;16:155.

Ramelet AA: Complications of ambulatory phlebectomy. Dermatol Surg 1997;23:947.

Sapira JD: The art and science of bedside diagnosis. Baltimore, Williams & Wilkins, 1990:368.

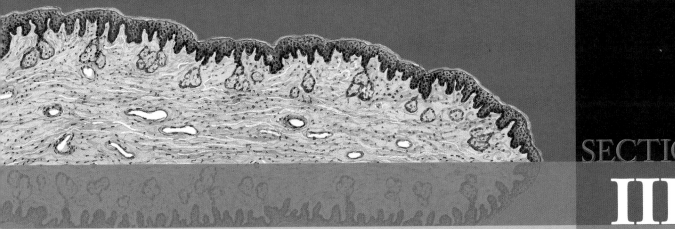

Vulvar Disease

INTRODUCTION

Description: An infection may occur in one or both Bartholin's glands, resulting in swelling and/or abscess formation. Usually the process is unilateral and marked by pain and swelling. Systemic symptoms are minimal except in advanced cases.

Prevalence: Two percent of adult women develop infection or enlargement of one or both Bartholin's glands.

Predominant Age: Of Bartholin's gland infections, 85% occur during the reproductive years (peak: 20 to 29 years).

Genetics: No genetic pattern.

ETIOLOGY AND PATHOGENESIS

Causes: Infection by *Neisseria gonorrhoeae* (80%), secondary infection by other organisms (e.g., *Escherichia coli*).

Risk Factors: Exposure to sexually transmitted disease, trauma.

CLINICAL CHARACTERISTICS

Signs and Symptoms

- Cystic, painful swelling of the labia in the area of the Bartholin's gland (at 5 and 7 o'clock positions on the vulva) developing rapidly over 2 to 4 days; cysts can range in size to 8 cm or greater
- Fever and malaise (uncommon)

DIAGNOSTIC APPROACH

Differential Diagnosis

- Cellulitis
- Necrotizing fasciitis
- Mesonephric cysts of the vagina
- Lipomas
- Fibromas
- Hernias
- Hydrocele
- Epidermal inclusion or sebaceous cyst
- Bartholin's gland malignancy (rare)
- Neurofibroma
- Kaposi sarcoma (generally associated with immunocompromise)

Associated Conditions: Dyspareunia.

Workup and Evaluation

Laboratory: Because bartholinitis or Bartholin's gland abscess may be gonococcal in origin, further evaluation for other sexually transmitted disease is prudent. Most often, culture-positive cysts are secondarily infected by coliform organisms or are polymicrobial, limiting the value of routine culture from the cyst.

Imaging: No imaging indicated.

Special Tests: None indicated.

Diagnostic Procedures: Inspection.

Pathologic Findings

Inflammation, dilation of the Bartholin gland duct, abscess formation.

MANAGEMENT AND THERAPY

Nonpharmacologic

General Measures: Evaluation, perineal hygiene.

Specific Measures: Mild infections may respond to antibiotic or topical therapies. Warm to hot sitz baths provide relief and promote drainage. Spontaneous drainage typically occurs in 1 to 4 days. Simple drainage is associated with recurrence; therefore, placement of a Word catheter, packing with iodoform gauze, or surgical marsupialization of the gland is desirable.

Diet: No specific dietary changes indicated.

Activity: No restriction.

Patient Education: Reassurance; American College of Obstetricians and Gynecologists Patient Education Pamphlet AP088 (Disorders of the Vulva), AP009 (How to Prevent Sexually Transmitted Diseases).

Drug(s) of Choice

Ampicillin (500 mg PO four times a day) or other broad-spectrum antibiotic if cellulitis is present.

Ceftriaxone 125 mg IM or cefixime 400 mg PO single dose or ciprofloxacin 500 mg PO single dose for gonorrhea.

Contraindications: Known hypersensitivity or allergy to agent.

Alternative Therapies

Excision of the gland is often difficult and is associated with significant risk of morbidity, including intraoperative hemorrhage, hematoma formation, secondary infection, scar formation, and dyspareunia. For these reasons, excision is not generally recommended.

FOLLOW-UP

Patient Monitoring: Follow up to monitor for spontaneous drainage or the need for surgical intervention.

Prevention/Avoidance: Reduced exposure to sexually transmitted disease and vulvar trauma.

Possible Complications: Chronic cyst formation.

Expected Outcome: Recurrences occur in 5% to 10% of patients after marsupialization.

MISCELLANEOUS

Pregnancy Considerations: No effect on pregnancy.

ICD-9-CM Codes: 616.3.

REFERENCES

Level II

Aghajanian A, Bernstein L, Grimes DA: Bartholin's duct abscess and cyst: a case-control study. South Med J 1994;87:26.

Bartholin's Gland: Abscess/Infection

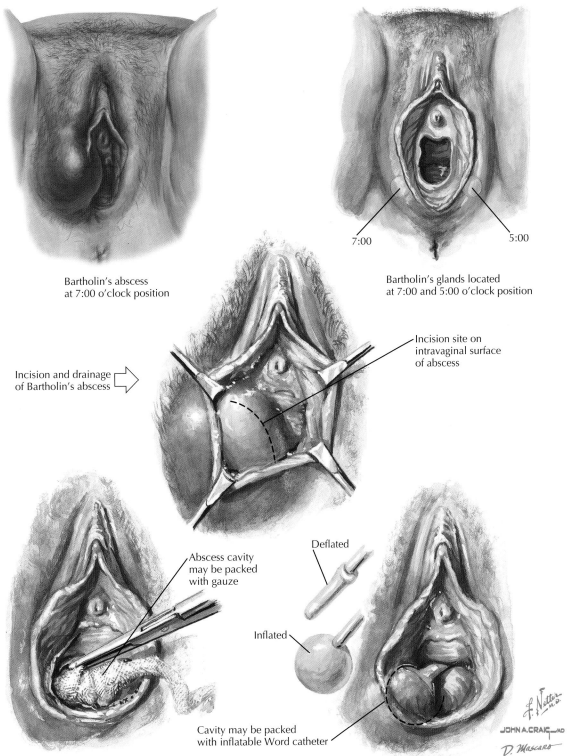

Bartholin's abscess
at 7:00 o'clock position

Bartholin's glands located
at 7:00 and 5:00 o'clock position

7:00   5:00

Incision site on
intravaginal surface
of abscess

Incision and drainage
of Bartholin's abscess

Abscess cavity
may be packed
with gauze

Deflated

Inflated

Cavity may be packed
with inflatable Word catheter

Eilber KS, Raz S: Benign cystic lesions of the vagina: a literature review. J Urol 2003;170:717.

Laartz BW, Cooper C, Degryse A, Sinnott JT: Wolf in sheep's clothing: advanced Kaposi sarcoma mimicking vulvar abscess. South Med J 2005;98:475. Review.

Level III

Cheetham DR: Bartholin's cyst: marsupialization or aspiration? Am J Obstet Gynecol 1985;152:569.

Eckert LO, Lentz GM: Infections of the lower genital tract. In Katz VL, Lentz GM, Lobo RA, Gershenson DM: Comprehensive Gynecology, 5th ed. Philadelphia, Mosby/Elsevier, 2007:571.

Hill DA, Lense JJ: Office management of Bartholin gland cysts and abscesses. Am Fam Physician 1998;57:1611, 1619.

Omole F, Simmons BJ, Hacker Y: Management of Bartholin's duct cyst and gland abscess. Am Fam Physician 2003;68:135.

Smith RP: Gynecology in primary care. Baltimore, Williams & Wilkins, 1997:606, 622.

INTRODUCTION

Description: A chronic cystic dilation of Bartholin's gland and duct, generally secondary to past infection.

Prevalence: Two percent of adult women develop infection or enlargement of one or both Bartholin's glands.

Predominant Age: Of Bartholin's gland cysts, 85% occur during the reproductive years (peak: 20 to 29 years). Occurrence after age 40 years is rare and should raise concerns about malignancy.

Genetics: No genetic pattern.

ETIOLOGY AND PATHOGENESIS

Causes: Bartholin's gland infection or abscess leading to obstruction of the duct.

Risk Factors: Exposure to sexually transmitted disease, trauma, prior Bartholin's gland abscesses.

CLINICAL CHARACTERISTICS

Signs and Symptoms

Smaller, more chronic cysts, caused by obstruction of the Bartholin duct, may be identified by gentle palpation at the base of the labia majora. These cysts are smooth, firm, and tender with varying degrees of induration and overlying erythema. The cysts may be clear, yellow, or bluish in color.

DIAGNOSTIC APPROACH

Differential Diagnosis

- Epidermal inclusion or sebaceous cyst
- Mesonephric cysts of the vagina
- Lipomas
- Fibromas
- Hernias
- Hydrocele
- Bartholin's gland malignancy (rare)
- Neurofibroma
- Kaposi sarcoma (generally associated with immuno-compromise)

Associated Conditions: Dyspareunia.

Workup and Evaluation

Laboratory: No evaluation indicated. (More than 80% of cultures of material from Bartholin's gland cysts are sterile.)

Imaging: No imaging indicated.

Special Tests: None indicated.

Diagnostic Procedures: Inspection.

Pathologic Findings

Cystic dilation of the duct and/or gland, often with chronic induration or inflammation.

MANAGEMENT AND THERAPY

Nonpharmacologic

General Measures: Evaluation, perineal hygiene.

Specific Measures: Asymptomatic small Bartholin's cysts require no therapy. Larger or symptomatic cysts require surgical marsupialization. If surgery is undertaken, it should be reserved for a time when any infection is quiescent.

Diet: No specific dietary changes indicated.

Activity: No restriction.

Patient Education: Reassurance; American College of Obstetricians and Gynecologists Patient Education Pamphlet AP088 (Disorders of the Vulva).

Drug(s) of Choice

None indicated.

Alternative Therapies

Excision of the gland is often difficult and is associated with significant risk of morbidity, including intraoperative hemorrhage, hematoma formation, secondary infection, scar formation, and dyspareunia. For these reasons, excision is not generally recommended.

FOLLOW-UP

Patient Monitoring: Normal health maintenance.

Prevention/Avoidance: Reduced exposure to sexually transmitted disease and vulvar trauma.

Possible Complications: Dyspareunia, recurrent inflammation.

Expected Outcome: Recurrences occur in 5% to 10% of patients following marsupialization.

MISCELLANEOUS

Pregnancy Considerations: No effect on pregnancy.

ICD-9-CM Codes: 616.2.

REFERENCES

Level II

Aghajanian A, Bernstein L, Grimes DA: Bartholin's duct abscess and cyst: a case-control study. South Med J 1994;87:26.

Eilber KS, Raz S: Benign cystic lesions of the vagina: a literature review. J Urol 2003;170:717.

Laartz BW, Cooper C, Degryse A, Sinnott JT: Wolf in sheep's clothing: advanced Kaposi sarcoma mimicking vulvar abscess. South Med J 2005;98:475. Review.

Level III

Cheetham DR: Bartholin's cyst: Marsupialization or aspiration? Am J Obstet Gynecol 1985;152:569.

Bartholin's Gland: Cysts

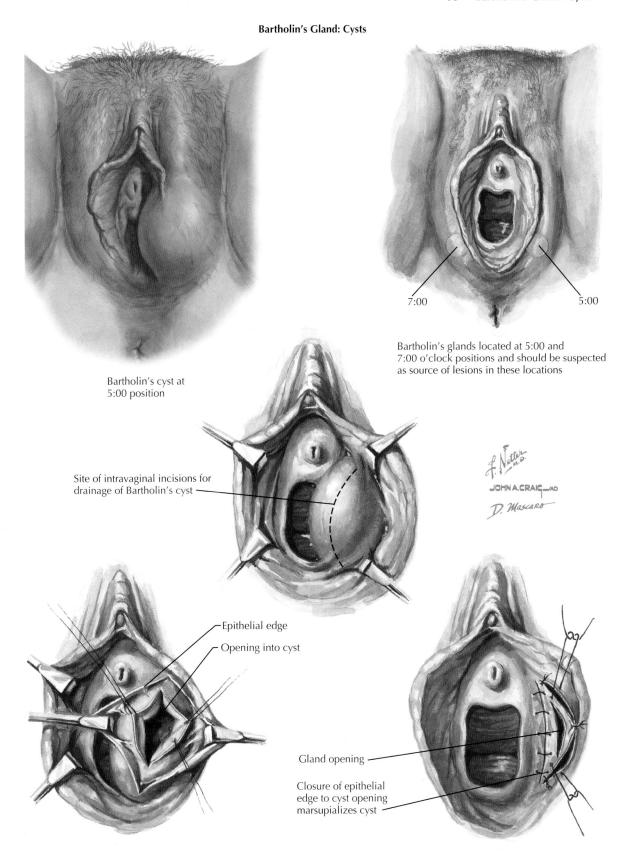

Bartholin's cyst at
5:00 position

7:00   5:00

Bartholin's glands located at 5:00 and
7:00 o'clock positions and should be suspected
as source of lesions in these locations

Site of intravaginal incisions for
drainage of Bartholin's cyst

Epithelial edge

Opening into cyst

Gland opening

Closure of epithelial
edge to cyst opening
marsupializes cyst

Hill DA, Lense JJ: Office management of Bartholin gland cysts and abscesses. Am Fam Physician 1998;57:1611, 1619.
Katz VL: Benign gynecologic lesions. In Katz VL, Lentz GM, Lobo RA, Gershenson DM: Comprehensive Gynecology, 5th ed. Philadelphia, Mosby/Elsevier, 2007:421.

Omole F, Simmons BJ, Hacker Y: Management of Bartholin's duct cyst and gland abscess. Am Fam Physician 2003;68:135.
Smith RP: Gynecology in primary care. Baltimore, Williams & Wilkins, 1997:603.

INTRODUCTION

Description: Contact vulvitis is characterized by vulvar irritation caused by contact with an irritant or allergen.

Prevalence: Relatively common.

Predominant Age: Any, but most common in reproductive and menopausal years.

Genetics: No genetic pattern.

ETIOLOGY AND PATHOGENESIS

Causes: Irritants may be primary or immunologic in character. The list of potential irritants can be extensive, including "feminine hygiene" sprays, deodorants and deodorant soaps, tampons or pads (especially those with deodorants or perfumes), tight-fitting undergarments or those made of synthetic fabric, colored or scented toilet paper, and laundry soap or fabric softener residues. Even topical contraceptives, latex condoms, lubricants, "sexual aids," or semen may be the source of irritation. Soiling of the vulva by urine or feces can also create significant symptoms. Severe dermatitis of the vulva resulting from contact with poison ivy or poison oak is found occasionally.

Risk Factors: Exposure to allergen (most often cosmetic or local therapeutic agents), immunosuppression, or diabetes.

CLINICAL CHARACTERISTICS

Signs and Symptoms

- Diffuse reddening of the vulvar skin accompanied by itching or burning
- Symmetric, red, edematous change in the tissues
- Ulceration with weeping sores and secondary infection possible

DIAGNOSTIC APPROACH

Differential Diagnosis

- Vaginal infection
- Local *Candida* infection
- Vulvar dermatoses
- Atrophic vulvitis
- Vulvar dystrophy
- Pinworms
- Psoriasis
- Seborrheic dermatitis
- Neurodermatitis
- Impetigo
- Acne inversa

Associated Conditions: Dyspareunia, dysuria.

Workup and Evaluation

Laboratory: Examination of vaginal secretions under saline and 10% KOH (potassium hydroxide) to rule out possible vaginal infection.

Imaging: No imaging indicated.

Special Tests: Vulvar biopsy rarely required, although it may be diagnostic.

Diagnostic Procedures: A careful history, combined with the withdrawal of the suspected cause, usually both confirms the diagnosis and constitutes the needed therapy.

Pathologic Findings

Vulvar biopsy shows chronic inflammatory change and infiltration by histiocytes.

MANAGEMENT AND THERAPY

Nonpharmacologic

General Measures: Perineal hygiene (keep the perineal area clean and dry; avoid tight undergarments or those made of synthetic fabric); education regarding prevention; encourage completion of the prescribed course of therapy.

Specific Measures: Removal of identified (or possible) allergens, topical therapy.

Diet: No specific dietary changes indicated.

Activity: No restriction.

Patient Education: Reassurance, education about avoidance or risk reduction; American College of Obstetricians and Gynecologists Patient Education Pamphlet AP088 (Disorders of the Vulva).

Drug(s) of Choice

Wet compresses or soaks using Burow's solution (aluminum acetate 2.5% to 5% solution, three to four times daily for 30 to 60 minutes), followed by air drying or drying with a hair dryer (on cool setting). (Loose-fitting clothing and the sparing use of a nonmedicated baby powder may facilitate the drying process.)

Steroid creams (hydrocortisone 0.5% to 1%) or fluorinated corticosteroids (Valisone 0.1%, Synalar 0.01%) applied two to three times a day if needed.

Precautions: Further evaluation is warranted (including biopsy) if initial therapy does not produce significant improvement.

Alternative Drugs

Eucerin cream may be used to rehydrate the skin and reduce itching.

FOLLOW-UP

Patient Monitoring: Normal health maintenance.

Prevention/Avoidance: Avoidance of possible allergens.

Possible Complications: Excoriation, chronic vulvar change (thickening).

Expected Outcome: With removal of causative agent, complete resolution should be expected.

MISCELLANEOUS

Pregnancy Considerations: No effect on pregnancy.

ICD-9-CM Codes: 616.10.

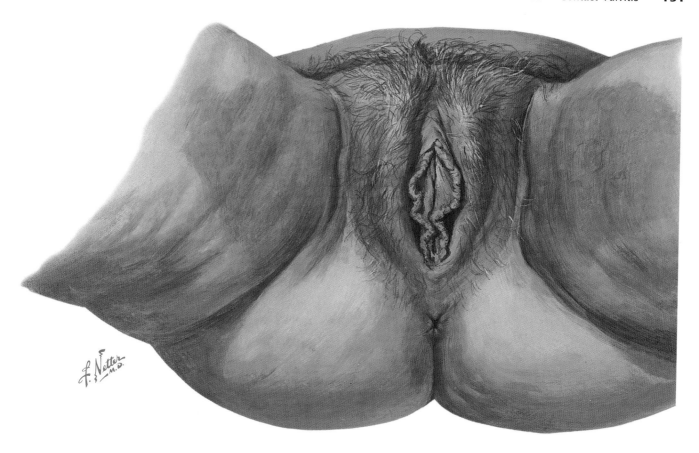

REFERENCES

Level II

Chang TW: Familial allergic seminal vulvovaginitis. Am J Obstet Gynecol 1976;126:442.

Fisher AA: Allergic reaction to feminine hygiene sprays. Arch Dermatol 1973;108:801.

Moraes PS: Allergic vulvovaginitis induced by house dust mites: a case report. J Allergy Clin Immunol 1998;101:557.

Nyirjesy P, Peyton C, Weitz MV, et al: Causes of chronic vaginitis: analysis of a prospective database of affected women. Obstet Gynecol 2006;108:1185.

Rigg D, Miller MM, Metzger WJ: Recurrent allergic vulvovaginitis: treatment with *Candida albicans* allergen immunotherapy. Am J Obstet Gynecol 1990;162:332.

Witkin SS, Jeremias J, Ledger WJ: A localized vaginal allergic response in women with recurrent vaginitis. J Allergy Clin Immunol 1988;81:412.

Level III

American College of Obstetricians and Gynecologists: Vaginitis. ACOG Practice Bulletin 72. Obstet Gynecol 2006;107:1195.

McKay M: Vulvar dermatoses. Clin Obstet Gynecol 1991;34:614.

McKay M: Vulvitis and vulvovaginitis: cutaneous considerations. Am J Obstet Gynecol 1991;165:1176.

Nanda VS: Common dermatoses. Am J Obstet Gynecol 1995;173:488.

Smith RP: Gynecology in primary care. Baltimore, Williams & Wilkins, 1997:603.

Summers P: Vaginitis in 1993. Clin Obstet Gynecol 1993;36:105.

INTRODUCTION

Description: Pain that occurs with sexual penetration is considered to be insertional dyspareunia. This may be in the form of mild discomfort that may be tolerated, pain that completely prevents intromission, or any level of pain in between. In severe cases, pain may lead to severe vaginal spasms that interfere with penetration (vaginismus).

Prevalence: Roughly 15% of women each year (severe—less than 2% of women).

Predominant Age: Reproductive and beyond.

Genetics: No genetic pattern.

ETIOLOGY AND PATHOGENESIS

Causes: Congenital factors (duplication of the vagina, hymenal stenosis, vaginal agenesis, vaginal septum), cystitis (acute or chronic), hemorrhoids, inadequate lubrication (abuse [current or past], arousal disorders, insufficient foreplay, medication, phobias), pelvic (levator) muscle spasm, pelvic scarring (episiotomy, surgical repairs [colporrhaphy]), proctitis, trauma (acute or chronic sequelae), urethral diverticula, urethral syndrome, urethritis (bacterial or chlamydial), vaginismus, vulvar (atrophic vulvitis, chancroid, chemical irritation [deodorants, adjuncts, lubricants]), herpes vulvitis, hypertrophic vulvar dystrophy, lichen sclerosus, lymphogranuloma venereum, vestibulitis, vulvitis (infectious), vulvodynia.

Risk Factors: Those associated with causal pathologic conditions.

CLINICAL CHARACTERISTICS

Signs and Symptoms

Sharp, burning, or pinching discomfort felt externally (vulva and perineum) during attempts at vaginal penetration (not limited to the penis). The discomfort is generally localized to the vulva, perineum, or outer portion of the vagina. The symptoms may help to localize the cause but are often generalized and nonspecific.

DIAGNOSTIC APPROACH

Differential Diagnosis

- Vulvitis (including condyloma)
- Vestibulitis
- Vaginitis
- Bartholin's gland infection, abscess, cyst
- Atrophic change
- Anxiety, depression, phobia
- Sexual or other abuse
- Postherpetic neuralgia
- Hymenal stenosis
- Hymenal caruncle

Associated Conditions: Vaginismus, orgasmic dysfunction.

Workup and Evaluation

Laboratory: No evaluation indicated. Urinalysis, microscopic examination of vaginal secretions, and cultures (cervical and urethral) only for the evaluation of specific processes and clinical suspicion.

Imaging: No imaging indicated.

Special Tests: Colposcopic examination of the vulva and introitus if vestibulitis is suspected.

Diagnostic Procedures: History and pelvic examination.

Pathologic Findings

None.

MANAGEMENT AND THERAPY

Nonpharmacologic

General Measures: Evaluation, reassurance, and relaxation measures. Vaginal lubricants (water-soluble or long-acting agents such as Astroglide, Replens, Lubrin, K-Y Jelly, and others), local anesthetics (for vulvar lesions), or pelvic relaxation exercises may be appropriate while more specific therapy is under way. These may be especially useful during the early phase of therapy when arousal may be compromised by the experience of pain.

Specific Measures: Because dyspareunia is ultimately a symptom, the specific therapy for any form of sexual pain is focused on the underlying cause.

Diet: No specific dietary changes indicated.

Activity: No restriction.

Patient Education: Reassurance, relaxation training, progressive desensitization; American College of Obstetricians and Gynecologists Patient Education Pamphlet AP020 (Pain During Intercourse), AP042 (You and Your Sexuality [Especially for Teens]).

Drug(s) of Choice

The judicious use of anxiolytics or antidepressant medications for selected patients may be appropriate but for short periods of time only.

Alternative Therapies

Modifying the sexual techniques used by the couple may reduce pain with intercourse. Delaying penetration until maximal arousal has been achieved improves vaginal lubrication, ensures vaginal apex expansion, and provides an element of control for the female partner. Sexual positions that allow the women to control the direction and depth of penetration (such as woman astride) may also be of help.

FOLLOW-UP

Patient Monitoring: Normal health maintenance. Watch for signs of abuse, anxiety, or depression.

Prevention/Avoidance: None.

Self-perpetuating sexual pain

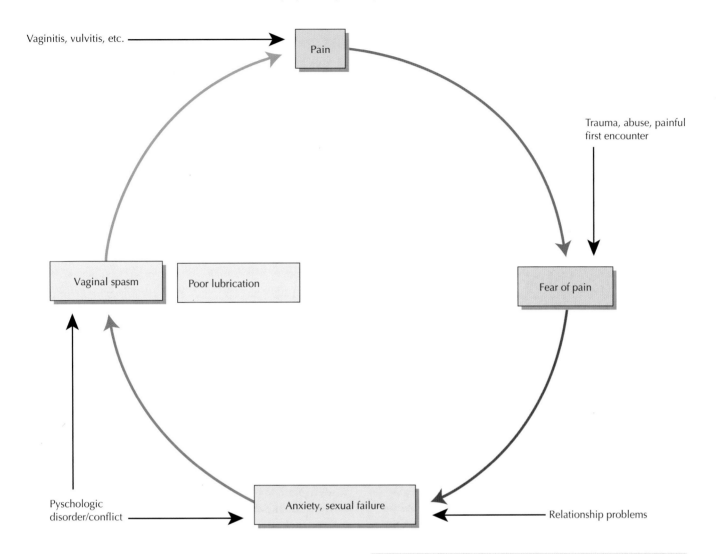

Possible Complications: Marital discord, orgasmic or libidinal dysfunction.

Expected Outcome: With diagnosis and treatment of the underlying cause, response should be good.

MISCELLANEOUS

Pregnancy Considerations: No effect on pregnancy.
ICD-9-CM Codes: 625.0.

REFERENCES

Level I
Abbott JA, Jarvis SK, Lyons SD, et al: Botulinum toxin type A for chronic pain and pelvic floor spasm in women: a randomized controlled trial. Obstet Gynecol 2006;108:915.

Level II
Munday P, Green J, Randall C, et al: Vulval vestibulitis: a common cause of dyspareunia? BJOG 2005;112:500.
Zolnoun DA, Hartmann KE, Steege JF: Overnight 5% lidocaine ointment for treatment of vulvar vestibulitis. Obstet Gynecol 2003;102:84.

Level III
American College of Obstetricians and Gynecologists: Vulvodynia. ACOG Committee Opinion 345. Obstet Gynecol 2006;108:1049.

Basson R, Schultz WW: Sexual sequelae of general medical disorders. Lancet 2007;369:409.
Edwards L: New concepts in vulvodynia. Am J Obstet Gynecol 2003;189:S24.
Fink P: Dyspareunia: current concepts. Med Aspects Hum Sex 1972;6:28.
Fordney DS: Dyspareunia and vaginismus. Clin Obstet Gynecol 1978;21:205.
Fullerton W: Dyspareunia. BMJ 1971;2:31.
Lentz GM: Emotional aspects of gynecology: sexual dysfunction, eating disorders, substance abuse, depression, grief, loss. In Katz VL, Lentz GM, Lobo RA, Gershenson DM: Comprehensive Gynecology, 5th ed. Philadelphia, Mosby/Elsevier, 2007:218.
National Institutes of Health: National Institutes of Health State-of-the-Science Conference statement: Management of menopause-related symptoms. Ann Intern Med 2005;142:1003. Epub 2005 May 27.
Peckham EM, Maki DG, Patterson JJ, Hafez GR: Focal vulvitis: a characteristic syndrome and cause of dyspareunia. Features, natural history, and management. Am J Obstet Gynecol 1986;154:855.
Ryan L, Hawton K: Female dyspareunia. BMJ 2004;328:1357.
Steege JF: Dyspareunia and vaginismus. Clin Obstet Gynecol 1984;27:750.
Steege JF, Ling FW: Dyspareunia. A special type of chronic pelvic pain. Obstet Gynecol Clin North Am 1993;20:779.

INTRODUCTION

Description: Female circumcision is removal of part or all of the external genitalia including the labia majora, labia minora, the clitoris, or all three. Female circumcision (female genital mutilation, infibulation) is generally performed as a ritual process, often without benefit of anesthesia and frequently under unsterile conditions. The resulting scarring may preclude intromission. The amount and location of tissue removed determine the type of infibulation:

- **Type I**—excision of the prepuce, with or without excision of part or the entire clitoris
- **Type II**—excision of the clitoris with partial or total excision of the labia minora (most common form)
- **Type III**—excision of part or all of the external genitalia and stitching/narrowing of the vaginal opening (infibulation)
- **Type IV**—pricking, piercing, or incising of the clitoris, labia, or both; stretching of the clitoris, labia, or both; cauterization by burning of the clitoris and surrounding tissue

Other forms of female genital mutilation include the following:

- Scraping of the tissue surrounding the vaginal orifice (angurya cuts) or cutting of the vagina (gishiri cuts)
- Introduction of corrosive substances or herbs into the vagina to cause bleeding or for the purpose of tightening or narrowing it
- Any other procedure that falls under the definition given previously

Prevalence: Approximately 168,000 women in the United States, approximately 96% of women in some African countries (e.g., Somalia). (Amnesty International estimates that it is performed on more than 130 million women worldwide.)

Predominant Age: Majority performed during early teens.

Genetics: No genetic pattern.

ETIOLOGY AND PATHOGENESIS

Causes: Performed as part of ritual or religious beliefs, generally without the permission and often without the cooperation of the young girl herself.

Risk Factors: Most common in some African and Southeast Asian cultures.

CLINICAL CHARACTERISTICS

Signs and Symptoms

- Significant scarring and deformity of the external genital structures, often to the point of complete obliteration of vaginal introitus (varies with the type and extent of the procedure performed)
- Obstruction may be sufficient to result in amenorrhea or dysmenorrhea
- Dyspareunia
- Orgasmic dysfunction
- Libidinal dysfunction
- Obstruction or hindrance to vaginal delivery

DIAGNOSTIC APPROACH

Differential Diagnosis

- Childhood burn injuries
- Intersex condition
- Imperforate hymen

Associated Conditions: Dyspareunia, libidinal dysfunction, and orgasmic dysfunction.

Workup and Evaluation

Laboratory: No evaluation indicated.
Imaging: No imaging indicated.
Special Tests: None indicated.
Diagnostic Procedures: History and physical examination.

Pathologic Findings

Absent or grossly scarred and deformed external genital tissues.

MANAGEMENT AND THERAPY

Nonpharmacologic

General Measures: Evaluation, support, and culturally sensitive education.

Specific Measures: Surgical opening of fused or scarred genital tissue may be necessary to allow for menstrual hygiene and sexual function. An anterior episiotomy, with or without subsequent repair, may be required at the time of childbirth (see the following).

Diet: No specific dietary changes indicated.
Activity: No restriction.
Patient Education: Culturally sensitive discussion of female anatomy, sexuality, and menstrual hygiene.

Drug(s) of Choice

None.

FOLLOW-UP

Patient Monitoring: Normal health maintenance. (Cervical samples for cytologic examination may be difficult to obtain in patients with extensive scarring until or unless surgical revision is performed.)

Prevention/Avoidance: Education of parents of young girls in cultures at risk for the procedure.

Possible Complications: Acutely (at the time of the procedure)—bleeding and infection (including tetanus), urinary retention, pain. Long term—sexual dysfunction, difficulty with menstrual hygiene, recurrent vaginal or urinary tract infections, retrograde menstruation, hematocolpos, chronic pelvic inflammatory disease.

Expected Outcome: Sexual sequelae are often lifelong despite surgical revision (especially when clitoridectomy has been performed).

MISCELLANEOUS

Pregnancy Considerations: No effect on pregnancy, but presence may complicate conception and delivery. Delivery may require an anterior episiotomy with atten-

Female Circumcision

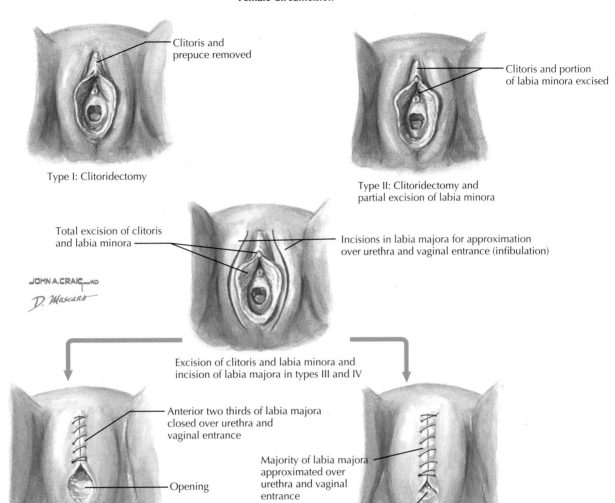

Type I: Clitoridectomy

Clitoris and prepuce removed

Clitoris and portion of labia minora excised

Type II: Clitoridectomy and partial excision of labia minora

Total excision of clitoris and labia minora

Incisions in labia majora for approximation over urethra and vaginal entrance (infibulation)

JOHN A. CRAIG—AD
D. Mascaro

Excision of clitoris and labia minora and incision of labia majora in types III and IV

Anterior two thirds of labia majora closed over urethra and vaginal entrance

Opening

Majority of labia majora approximated over urethra and vaginal entrance

Opening

Type III: Modified (intermediate infibulation)—allows moderate posterior opening

Type IV: Total infibulation— allows only small posterior opening for urine and menstrual flow

dant increased risk of bleeding. (Subsequent repair of the episiotomy is illegal in some locations such as the United Kingdom and others because this amounts to reinfibulation.)

ICD-9-CM Codes: 624.4 (Old laceration or scarring of the vulva).

REFERENCES

Level II

Elmusharaf S, Elhadi N, Almroth L: Reliability of self reported form of female genital mutilation and WHO classification: cross sectional study. BMJ 2006;333:124. Epub 2006 Jun 27.
WHO study group on female genital mutilation and obstetric outcome; Banks E, Meirik O, Farley T, et al: Female genital mutilation and obstetric outcome: WHO collaborative prospective study in six African countries. Lancet 2006;367:1835.

Level III

Adams KM, Gardiner LD, Assefi N: Healthcare challenges from the developing world: post-immigration refugee medicine. BMJ 2004;328:1548.

Aziz FA: Gynecologic and obstetric complications of female circumcision. J Gynaecol Obstet 1980;17:560.
Baker CA, Gilson GJ, Vill MD, Curet LB: Female circumcision: obstetric issues. Am J Obstet Gynecol 1993;169:1616.
Council on Scientific Affairs, American Medical Association: Female genital mutilation. JAMA 1995;274:1714.
Cuntner LP: Female genital mutilation. Obstet Gynecol Surv 1985;40:437.
Khaled K, Vause S: Genital mutilation: a continued abuse. Br J Obstet Gynaecol 1996;103:86.
Lentz GM: Rape, incest, and domestic violence. In Katz VL, Lentz GM, Lobo RA, Gershenson DM: Comprehensive Gynecology, 5th ed. Philadelphia, Mosby/Elsevier, 2007:207.
Toubia N: Female circumcision as a public health issue. N Engl J Med 1994;331:712.
World Health Organization: Female genital mutilation. Fact sheet 241, 2000. Available at: http://www.who.int/mediacentre/factsheets/fs241/en/l. Accessed June 7, 2007.

INTRODUCTION

Description: Acne inversa (formerly hidradenitis suppurativa) is a chronic, unrelenting, refractory infection of the skin and subcutaneous tissue initiated by obstruction and subsequent inflammation of follicles and apocrine glands, with resultant sinus and abscess formation. This process may involve the axilla, vulva, and perineum.

Prevalence: Uncommon. Four to five times more common in females; reported to occur in as many as 4% of women in some studies.

Predominant Age: Reproductive (not found before puberty).

Genetics: Suggestions of family pattern, but genetic link remains unproved. (In some studies, as many as 38% of patients have a similarly affected relative.)

ETIOLOGY AND PATHOGENESIS

Causes: Recurrent infections that arise in subcutaneous nodules. Proposed—hypersensitivity to androgens.

Risk Factors: None known. Proposed—excessive heat, perspiration, tight clothing, and obesity.

CLINICAL CHARACTERISTICS

Signs and Symptoms

- Recurrent and chronic inflammatory and ulcerated portions of labia associated with pain and foul-smelling discharge
- Multiple draining sinuses and abscesses

DIAGNOSTIC APPROACH

Differential Diagnosis

- Sexually transmitted disease (granuloma inguinale, lymphogranuloma venereum)
- Crohn disease
- Fox-Fordyce disease
- Bacterial folliculitis and furunculosis

Associated Conditions: Dyspareunia, vulvodynia.

Workup and Evaluation

Laboratory: No evaluation indicated.

Imaging: No imaging indicated.

Special Tests: Biopsy of the affected area may be necessary to establish the diagnosis.

Diagnostic Procedures: History, physical, and biopsy of affected area.

Pathologic Findings

Inflammation of the apocrine glands with occlusion of ducts, cystic dilation, and inspissation of keratin material. Multiple draining sinuses and abscesses are common.

MANAGEMENT AND THERAPY

Nonpharmacologic

General Measures: Perineal hygiene, sitz baths, loose-fitting clothing.

Specific Measures: Most effective therapy is based on early, aggressive, wide excision of affected area. Topical therapy with antibiotics, topical steroids, oral contraceptives, antiandrogens, and isotretinoin may be used in early or mild cases.

Diet: No specific dietary changes indicated.

Activity: No restriction. Patients frequently abandon intercourse because of pain, discharge, odor, or embarrassment.

Patient Education: Reassurance; American College of Obstetricians and Gynecologists Patient Education Pamphlet AP088 (Disorders of the Vulva).

Drug(s) of Choice

Antibiotics (tetracycline 2 g PO daily, clindamycin topical daily), topical steroids, oral contraceptives, antiandrogens (finasteride: Proscar, Propecia, etc.), and isotretinoin (Accutane) 0.5 to 2.0 mg/kg in two divided doses for 15 to 20 weeks. A second course may be considered after a 2-month hiatus.

Contraindications: Isotretinoin must not be taken during pregnancy. Therefore, isotretinoin should not be given to women who are or may become pregnant.

Precautions: Isotretinoin should be given with food. Isotretinoin has been associated with the development of pseudotumor cerebri. Periodic assessment of liver function, cholesterol and triglyceride levels, and white blood counts should be carried out on patients receiving isotretinoin therapy.

Interactions: See individual agents.

Alternative Drugs

Dexamethasone or gonadotropin-releasing hormone agonists have been proposed, but costs and side effects limit their use.

Infliximab (Remicade) and other immunosuppressant agents have shown promise but are second-line therapies reserved for resistant cases.

FOLLOW-UP

Patient Monitoring: Normal health maintenance, watch for periodic worsening or secondary infection.

Prevention/Avoidance: Meticulous perineal hygiene; keep the affected area dry.

Possible Complications: Secondary infection, abscess formation, scarring, sexual dysfunction.

Expected Outcome: Relapses and chronic infections are common. With surgical excision, results are generally good, but scarring and dyspareunia may persist or result.

MISCELLANEOUS

Pregnancy Considerations: No effect on pregnancy. Isotretinoin should not be given to women who are or may become pregnant.

ICD-9-CM Codes: 705.83.

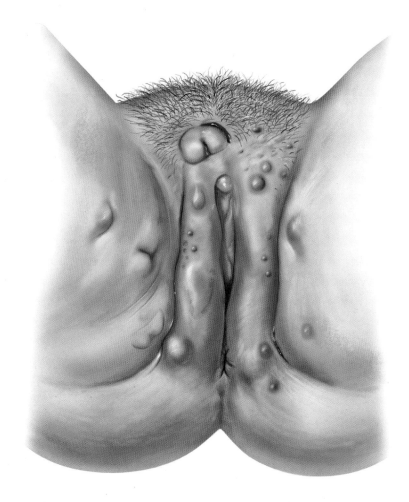

REFERENCES

Level I
Sullivan TP, Welsh E, Kerdel FA, et al: Infliximab for acne inversa. Br J Dermatol 2003;149:1046.

Level II
Brocard A, Knol AC, Khammari A, Dreno B: Acne inversa and zinc: a new therapeutic approach. A pilot study. Dermatology 2007;214:325.

Fardet L, Dupuy A, Kerob D, et al: Infliximab for severe acne inversa: transient clinical efficacy in 7 consecutive patients. J Am Acad Dermatol 2007;56:624. Epub 2007 Jan 22.

Greenbaum AR: Modified abdominoplasty as a functional reconstruction for recurrent hidradenitis suppurativa of the lower abdomen and groin. Plast Reconstr Surg 2007;119:764.

Joseph MA, Jayaseelan E, Ganapathi B, Stephen J: Acne inversa treated with finasteride. J Dermatolog Treat 2005;16:75.

Kagan RJ, Yakuboff KP, Warner P, Warden GD: Surgical treatment of acne inversa: a 10-year experience. Surgery 2005; 138:734; discussion 740.

Mendonca CO, Griffiths CE: Clindamycin and rifampicin combination therapy for acne inversa. Br J Dermatol 2006;154:977.

Moul DK, Korman NJ: The cutting edge. Severe acne inversa treated with adalimumab. Arch Dermatol 2006;142:1110.

Sherman AL, Reid R: CO_2 laser for suppurative hidradenitis of the vulva. J Reprod Med 1991;36:113.

Thielen AM, Barde C, Saurat JH: Long-term infliximab for severe acne inversa. Br J Dermatol 2006;155:1105.

Thomas R, Barnhill D, Bibro M, Hoskins W: Acne inversa: a case presentation and review of the literature. Obstet Gynecol 1985;66:592.

Level III
Ather S, Chan DS, Leaper DJ, Harding KG: Surgical treatment of acne inversa: case series and review of the literature. Int Wound J 2006;3:159.

Attanoos RL, Appleton MA, Douglas-Jones AG: The pathogenesis of acne inversa: a closer look at apocrine and apoeccrine glands. Br J Dermatol 1995;133:254.

Basta A, Madej JG Jr: Hidradenoma of the vulva. Incidence and clinical observations. Eur J Gynecol Oncol 1990;11:185.

Brown TJ, Rosen T, Orengo IF: Acne inversa. South Med J 1998; 91:1107.

Katz VL: Benign gynecologic lesions. In Katz VL, Lentz GM, Lobo RA, Gershenson DM: Comprehensive Gynecology, 5th ed. Philadelphia, Mosby/Elsevier, 2007:431.

Kelly AM, Cronin P: MRI features of acne inversa and review of the literature. AJR Am J Roentgenol 2005;185:1201.

Mitchell KM, Beck DE: Acne inversa. Surg Clin North Am 2002;82:1187

Sellheyer K, Krahl D: "Acne inversa" is acne inversa! An appeal to (finally) abandon a misnomer. Int J Dermatol 2005; 44:535.

Shah N: Acne inversa: a treatment challenge. Am Fam Physician 2005;72:1547.

Slade DE, Powell BW, Mortimer PS: Acne inversa: pathogenesis and management. Br J Plast Surg 2003;56:451.

Hymenal Stenosis

INTRODUCTION

Description: Hymenal stenosis is thickening or narrowing of the hymenal opening resulting in difficulty in tampon use and intercourse.
Prevalence: Uncommon.
Predominant Age: Congenital, although generally diagnosed in the early reproductive years.
Genetics: No genetic pattern.

ETIOLOGY AND PATHOGENESIS

Causes: Congenital narrowing of the hymen or scarring after trauma or surgery (e.g., previous excision, trauma).
Risk Factors: Introital surgery (for iatrogenic cases).

CLINICAL CHARACTERISTICS

Signs and Symptoms

- Insertional dyspareunia
- Difficulty with tampon use
- Narrowing of the vaginal introitus

DIAGNOSTIC APPROACH

Differential Diagnosis

- Vulvar vestibulitis
- Vaginismus
- Other vulvitis
- Cribriform hymen

Associated Conditions: Dyspareunia, orgasmic or libidinal dysfunction.

Workup and Evaluation

Laboratory: No evaluation indicated.
Imaging: No imaging indicated.
Special Tests: None indicated.
Diagnostic Procedures: History and physical examination.

Pathologic Findings

None.

MANAGEMENT AND THERAPY

Nonpharmacologic

General Measures: Evaluation, reassurance.
Specific Measures: Gentle digital dilation, surgical excision.
Diet: No specific dietary changes indicated.
Activity: No restriction.

Drug(s) of Choice

None.

FOLLOW-UP

Patient Monitoring: Normal health maintenance.
Prevention/Avoidance: None.
Possible Complications: Sexual dysfunction.

Expected Outcome: Generally good, but secondary problems (such as sexual dysfunction) often may persist.

MISCELLANEOUS

Pregnancy Considerations: No effect on pregnancy once achieved. Generally no effect on the route of delivery. Delivery (with or without an episiotomy) often results in improvement or resolution of symptoms.
ICD-9-CM Codes: 623.3.

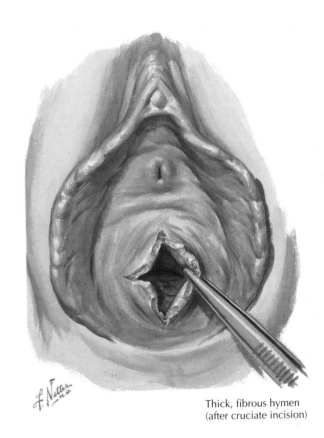

Thick, fibrous hymen
(after cruciate incision)

REFERENCES

Level II

Berenson AB, Chacko MR, Wiemann CM, et al: A case-control study of anatomic changes resulting from sexual abuse. Am J Obstet Gynecol 2000;182:820.
Berenson AB, Grady JJ: A longitudinal study of hymenal development from 3 to 9 years of age. J Pediatr 2002;140:600.
McCann J, Miyamoto S, Boyle C, Rogers K: Healing of hymenal injuries in prepubertal and adolescent girls: a descriptive study. Pediatrics 2007;119:e1094. Epub 2007 Apr 9.

Level III

Posner JC, Spandorfer PR: Early detection of imperforate hymen prevents morbidity from delays in diagnosis. Pediatrics 2005;115:1008.
Smith RP: Gynecology in primary care. Baltimore, Williams & Wilkins, 1997:517.

Hyperplastic Vulvar Dystrophy (Squamous Cell Hyperplasia)

INTRODUCTION

Description: Hypertrophic vulvar dystrophy causes a thickening of the vulvar skin over the labia majora, outer aspects of the labia minora, and clitoral areas. Eczematous inflammation or hyperkeratosis may be present.

Prevalence: Common, 40% to 45% of non-neoplastic epithelial disorders.

Predominant Age: Middle to late reproductive and beyond.

Genetics: No genetic pattern.

ETIOLOGY AND PATHOGENESIS

Causes: Unknown. Dermal reaction to chronic itch-scratch cycle. Often associated with or worsened by stress.

Risk Factors: Genital atrophy (postmenopausal), recurrent vulvitis.

CLINICAL CHARACTERISTICS

Signs and Symptoms

- Vulvar itching (almost always present)
- Dusky-red to thickened-white appearance of the vulva
- Fissuring and excoriations (common)

DIAGNOSTIC APPROACH

Differential Diagnosis

- Vulvar cancer (premalignant or malignant changes)
- Chronic mycotic vulvitis
- Contact vulvitis
- Psoriasis
- Lichen sclerosus

Associated Conditions: Vulvodynia, vulvar pruritus, and dyspareunia.

Workup and Evaluation

Laboratory: No evaluation indicated.

Imaging: No imaging indicated.

Special Tests: Biopsy may be required to confirm the diagnosis. Cultures for *Candida* or other dermatophytes should be considered.

Diagnostic Procedures: History, physical examination, colposcopy, or biopsy of lesions.

Pathologic Findings

Thickening of the epithelium with acanthosis, elongation of the epithelial folds, and chronic inflammatory changes (lymphocytes and plasma cells) occur. Hyperkeratosis may be present.

MANAGEMENT AND THERAPY

Nonpharmacologic

General Measures: Perineal hygiene, sitz baths, stress reduction. Reduce or eliminate sources of irritation such as candidiasis or contact allergy. Wearing white cotton gloves (especially at night) reduces the tissue damage caused by scratching.

Specific Measures: Treatment is focused on interrupting the itch-scratch-rash-itch cycle. Topical steroids, perineal soothing agents, and agents to reduce itching are most effective. If significant improvement is not achieved in 3 months, biopsy is indicated.

Diet: No specific dietary changes indicated.

Activity: No restriction.

Patient Education: Reassurance; American College of Obstetricians and Gynecologists Patient Education Pamphlet AP088 (Disorders of the Vulva).

Drug(s) of Choice

Fluocinolone acetonide (0.025% or 0.01%), triamcinolone acetonide (0.01%) or betamethasone valerate (Valisone 0.1%), or a similar corticosteroid applied two to three times daily may give relief. Once relief is achieved, treatment should switch to hydrocortisone 2.5% cream or ointment.

For itching: diphenhydramine hydrochloride (Benadryl) or hydroxyzine hydrochloride (Atrax) used at night.

Contraindications: See individual agents.

Precautions: Fluorinated steroids should be used for short periods only and replaced with hydrocortisone or nonsteroidal therapies when possible.

Interactions: See individual agents.

Alternative Drugs

Topical clobetasol propionate (0.05%) may be used if relief of pruritus is not achieved with less potent agents.

Subcutaneous injections of triamcinolone (5-mg suspension mixed with 2 mL of saline) or alcohol (0.1 to 0.2 mL of absolute alcohol) have been reported but should be reserved for the most intractable disease.

Topical progestins and androgens have been advocated as alternative therapies.

FOLLOW-UP

Patient Monitoring: Constant vigilance is required to watch for possible premalignant or malignant changes that can often mimic these lesions and those of lichen sclerosus.

Prevention/Avoidance: Avoidance of local irritants.

Possible Complications: Vulvar cancer may be overlooked; excoriation is common with secondary infection possible.

Expected Outcome: Generally good if itch-scratch cycle is broken.

MISCELLANEOUS

Pregnancy Considerations: No effect on pregnancy.

ICD-9-CM Codes: 624.3.

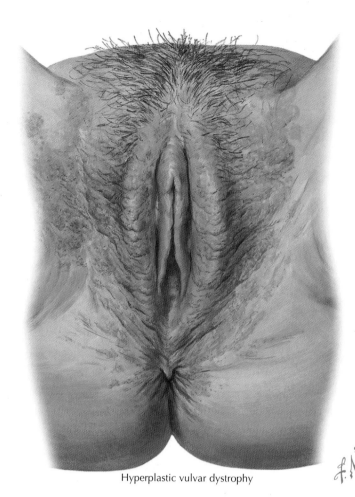

Hyperplastic vulvar dystrophy

REFERENCES

Level I

Bousema MT, Romppanen U, Geiger JM, et al: Acitretin in the treatment of severe lichen sclerosus et atrophicus of the vulva: a double-blind, placebo-controlled study. J Am Acad Dermatol 1994; 30:225.

Li C, Bian D, Chen W, et al: Focused ultrasound therapy of vulvar dystrophies: a feasibility study. Obstet Gynecol 2004;104:915.

Level II

Cario GM, House MJ, Paradinas FJ: Squamous cell carcinoma of the vulva in association with mixed vulvar dystrophy in an 18-year-old girl. Case report. Br J Obstet Gynaecol 1984;91:87.

Cattaneo A, Bracco GL, Maestrini G, et al: Lichen sclerosis and squamous hyperplasia of the vulva. A clinical study of medical treatment. J Reprod Med 1991;36:301.

Friedrich EG Jr: Topical testosterone for benign vulvar dystrophy. Obstet Gynecol 1971;37:677.

Japaze H, Garcia-Bunuel R, Woodruff JD: Primary vulvar neoplasia: a review of in situ and invasive carcinoma, 1935–1972. Obstet Gynecol 1977;49:404.

Jasionowski EA, Jasionowski P: Topical progesterone in treatment of vulvar dystrophy: preliminary report of five cases. Am J Obstet Gynecol 1977;127:667.

Level III

American College of Obstetricians and Gynecologists: Vulvodynia. ACOG Committee Opinion 345. Obstet Gynecol 2006;108:1049.

Friedrich EG Jr: Vulvar dystrophy. Clin Obstet Gynecol 1985; 28:178.

Frumovitz M, Bodurka DC: Neoplastic disease of the vulva. In Katz VL, Lentz GM, Lobo RA, Gershenson DM: Comprehensive Gynecology, 5th ed. Philadelphia, Mosby/Elsevier, 2007:783.

Jasionowski EA, Jasionowski PA: Further observations on the effect of topical progesterone on vulvar disease. Am J Obstet Gynecol 1979;134:565.

Maloney ME: Exploring the common vulvar dermatoses. Contemp Obstet/Gynecol 1988;29:91.

McKay M: Vulvar dermatoses. Clin Obstet Gynecol 1991;34:614.

Murphy FR, Lipa M, Haberman HF: Familial vulvar dystrophy of lichen sclerosus type. Arch Dermatol 1982;118:329.

Nanda VS: Common dermatoses. Am J Obstet Gynecol 1995; 173:488.

Imperforate Hymen

75

INTRODUCTION

Description: An imperforate hymen is the most commonly encountered anomaly resulting from abnormalities in the development or canalization of the Müllerian ducts.

Prevalence: Uncommon.

Predominant Age: Generally not diagnosed until puberty.

Genetics: No genetic pattern.

ETIOLOGY AND PATHOGENESIS

Causes: Failure of the endoderm of the urogenital sinus and the epithelium of the vaginal vestibule to fuse and perforate during embryonic development.

Risk Factors: None known.

CLINICAL CHARACTERISTICS

Signs and Symptoms

- Vaginal obstruction
- Primary amenorrhea
- Cyclic abdominal pain
- Hematocolpos

DIAGNOSTIC APPROACH

Differential Diagnosis

- Vaginal agenesis
- Hermaphroditism

Associated Conditions: Endometriosis, vaginal adenosis, infertility, chronic pelvic pain, sexual dysfunction, and hematocolpos.

Workup and Evaluation

Laboratory: No evaluation indicated.

Imaging: Ultrasonography to evaluate the upper genital tract.

Special Tests: None indicated.

Diagnostic Procedures: History and physical examination.

Pathologic Findings

None.

MANAGEMENT AND THERAPY

Nonpharmacologic

General Measures: Evaluation, reassurance.

Specific Measures: Incision of hymenal membrane and drainage of vaginal canal.

Diet: No specific dietary changes indicated.

Activity: No restriction.

Drug(s) of Choice

None.

FOLLOW-UP

Patient Monitoring: Normal health maintenance.

Prevention/Avoidance: None.

Possible Complications: Hematocolpos, endometriosis, hymenal scarring and narrowing after surgical excision.

Expected Outcome: Generally good with early resection. Delayed diagnosis is associated with reduced fertility caused by secondary damage (endometriosis).

MISCELLANEOUS

Pregnancy Considerations: No effect on pregnancy, although often associated with conditions that do affect fertility, such as endometriosis. Reproductive outlook is best when diagnosis and treatment occur early.

ICD-9-CM Codes: 752.42.

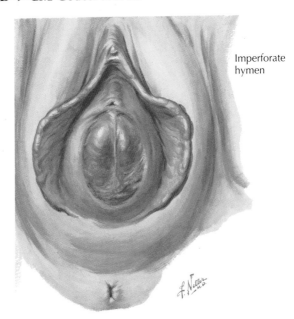

Imperforate hymen

REFERENCES

Level II

Dickson CA, Saad S, Tesar JD: Imperforate hymen with hematocolpos. Ann Emerg Med 1985;14:467.

Friedman M, Gal D, Peretz BA: Management of imperforate hymen with the carbon dioxide laser. Obstet Gynecol 1989;74:270.

Greiss FC, Mauzy CH: Congenital anomalies in women: an evaluation of diagnosis, incidence, and obstetric performance. Am J Obstet Gynecol 1961;82:330.

Posner JC, Spandorfer PR: Early detection of imperforate hymen prevents morbidity from delays in diagnosis. Pediatrics 2005; 115:1008.

Usta IM, Awwad JT, Usta JA, et al: Imperforate hymen: report of an unusual familial occurrence. Obstet Gynecol 1993;82:655.

Level III

American College of Obstetricians and Gynecologists: Vaginal agenesis: diagnosis, management, and routine care. ACOG Committee Opinion 355. Obstet Gynecol 2006;108:1605.

Baramki TA: The treatment of congenital anomalies in girls and women. J Reprod Med 1984;29:376.

Katz VL, Lentz GM: Congenital abnormalities of the female reproductive tract. In Katz VL, Lentz GM, Lobo RA, Gershenson DM: Comprehensive Gynecology, 5th ed. Philadelphia, Mosby/Elsevier, 2007;245.

Winderl LM, Silverman RK: Prenatal diagnosis of congenital imperforate hymen. Obstet Gynecol 1995;85:857.

INTRODUCTION

Description: Labial adhesions are agglutination of the labial folds resulting in fusion in the midline.

Prevalence: One percent to 2% of female children.

Predominant Age: Peak 2 to 6 years; may be found at any age up to puberty. May also occur in postmenopausal women with significant vulvar atrophy.

Genetics: No genetic pattern.

ETIOLOGY AND PATHOGENESIS

Causes: Local inflammation and the hypoestrogenic environment of preadolescence.

Risk Factors: Labial infections or irritation.

CLINICAL CHARACTERISTICS

Signs and Symptoms

- Fusion of the labia majora in the midline (extends from just below the clitoris to the posterior fourchette)
- Retention of urine in the vestibule or vagina resulting in irritation, discharge, and odor

DIAGNOSTIC APPROACH

Differential Diagnosis

- Intersex
- Female circumcision
- Sexual abuse

Associated Conditions: Urinary tract infection.

Workup and Evaluation

Laboratory: No evaluation indicated.

Imaging: No imaging indicated.

Special Tests: None indicated.

Diagnostic Procedures: History and physical examination.

Pathologic Findings

None.

MANAGEMENT AND THERAPY

Nonpharmacologic

General Measures: Evaluation, reassurance, perineal hygiene, and sitz baths.

Specific Measures: Topical estrogen cream, gentle traction to separate the labia (only after estrogen pretreatment; generally not necessary and strongly discouraged). Surgical treatment is almost never required.

Diet: No specific dietary changes indicated.

Activity: No restriction.

Patient Education: Reassurance; American College of Obstetricians and Gynecologists Patient Education Pamphlet AP041 (Growing Up [Especially for Teens]).

Drug(s) of Choice

Topical estrogen cream (Premarin vaginal cream, Dienestrol cream)—small portion applied to the vulva twice a day for 7 to 10 days. May be continued one to three times a week if desired, although generally not necessary.

Contraindications: Undiagnosed vaginal bleeding.

FOLLOW-UP

Patient Monitoring: Normal health maintenance.

Prevention/Avoidance: Good perineal hygiene.

Possible Complications: Vaginitis, urinary tract infection, urinary retention, or vaginal cyst formation.

Expected Outcome: Excellent.

MISCELLANEOUS

ICD-9-CM Codes: 624.9.

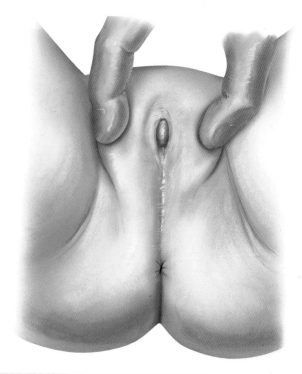

REFERENCES

Level II

Aribarg A: Topical oestrogen therapy for labial adhesions in children. Br J Obstet Gynaecol 1975;82:424.

Bacon JL: Prepubertal labial adhesions: evaluation of a referral population. Am J Obstet Gynecol 2002;187:327.

Johnson N, Lilford RJ, Sharpe D: A new surgical technique to treat refractory labial fusion in the elderly. Am J Obstet Gynecol 1989;161:289.

Stovall TG, Murman D: Urinary retention secondary to labial adhesions. Adolesc Pediatr Gynecol 1988;1:203.

Yano K, Hosokawa K, Takagi S, et al: Y-V advancement flaps for labial adhesions in postmenopausal women. Plast Reconstr Surg 2002;109:2614.

Level III

Davis AJ, Katz VL: Pediatric and adolescent gynecology. In Katz VL, Lentz GM, Lobo RA, Gershenson DM: Comprehensive Gynecology, 5th ed. Philadelphia, Mosby/Elsevier, 2007:263.

Muram D: Labial adhesions in sexually abused children. JAMA 1988;259:352.

Smith RP: Gynecology in primary care. Baltimore, Williams & Wilkins, 1997:177.

INTRODUCTION

Description: Lichen planus is a non-neoplastic epithelial disorder that affects glabrous skin, hair-bearing skin and scalp, nails, mucous membranes, or the oral cavity and the vulva.
Prevalence: Unknown, but relatively common.
Predominant Age: 30 to 60 years.
Genetics: No genetic pattern.

ETIOLOGY AND PATHOGENESIS

Causes: Unknown. Proposed—autoimmune disorder, possibly initiated by certain drugs such as beta blockers, angiotensin-converting enzyme (ACE) inhibitors.
Risk Factors: None known.

CLINICAL CHARACTERISTICS

Signs and Symptoms

- Red erosion and ulceration of the vulva and inner aspects of the labia minora (may precede oral lesions by years; 33% of patients)
- Loss of the labia minora with scarring, adhesions, and narrowing common (complete obliteration of the vagina possible); dyspareunia and postcoital bleeding common
- Oral lesions—reticulated gray, lacy pattern (Wickham's striae) with gingivitis (vulvar involvement in 50% of patients with oral lesions)

DIAGNOSTIC APPROACH

Differential Diagnosis:

- Amebiasis
- Behçet's syndrome
- Candidiasis
- Dermatophyte infection
- Lichen sclerosus
- Neurodermatitis
- Pemphigus and pemphigoid (cicatricial or bullous type)
- Plasma cell vulvitis
- Psoriasis
- Squamous cell hyperplasia
- Systemic lupus erythematosus
- Vulvar intraepithelial neoplasia (VIN III)

Associated Conditions: Hair loss and a history of papular lesions on the skin (ankle, dorsal surface of the hands, and flexor surfaces of the wrists and forearms).

Workup and Evaluation

Laboratory: No evaluation indicated.
Imaging: No imaging indicated.
Special Tests: Skin biopsy (taken from the nearby intact skin or mucous membranes rather than the ulcer). Direct immunofluorescence testing on fresh tissue.
Diagnostic Procedures: History, physical examination, and biopsy.

Pathologic Findings

Chronic inflammatory cell infiltrate (lymphocytes and plasma cells) involving the superficial dermis and the basal and parabasal epithelium. Liquefaction necrosis with colloid bodies may be present. Prominent acanthosis with a prominent granular layer and hyperkeratosis. Ulceration and bullae may be present. Hyperkeratosis is absent in the vulvar tissues.

MANAGEMENT AND THERAPY

Nonpharmacologic

General Measures: Evaluation, local cleansing, antipruritics.
Specific Measures: Therapy is often difficult, chronic, and prone to failure or relapse. Therapies include steroids, retinoids, griseofulvin, dapsone, cyclosporine, and surgery. Vaginal dilators may be necessary to maintain vaginal caliber.
Diet: No specific dietary changes indicated.
Activity: No restriction.
Patient Education: Reassurance; American College of Obstetricians and Gynecologists Patient Education Pamphlet AP088 (Disorders of the Vulva).

Drug(s) of Choice

Topical steroids (betamethasone valerate 0.1% ointment or hydrocortisone 25 mg vaginal suppository daily) or
Griseofulvin (250 mg PO twice a day) or
Dapsone (50 to 100 mg PO daily; after negative results of screening for glucose-6-phosphate dehydrogenase) or
Isotretinoin (Accutane) 0.5 to 1 mg/kg/day in divided doses (or etretinate [Tegison] 0.75 to 1 mg/kg/day in two doses) or
Cyclosporine (1 mg/kg/day, increased weekly by 0.5 mg/kg/day up to 3 to 5 mg/kg/day).
Contraindications: Vulvar cancer. Isotretinoin and etretinate are teratogenic and must not be given during pregnancy or if there is a potential for pregnancy.
Precautions: Continued or prolonged use of topical steroids may result in thinning of the skin outside the area of lichen sclerosus with subsequent atrophy and traumatic injury (splitting and cracking). The use of dapsone, isotretinoin, etretinate, or cyclosporine requires careful monitoring of complete blood counts, liver function tests, cholesterol, triglycerides, electrolytes, urea nitrogen, creatinine, and creatinine clearance. Reliable contraception must be maintained if isotretinoin or etretinate is used.
Interactions: See individual agents.

FOLLOW-UP

Patient Monitoring: Because malignant change is possible, long-term follow-up is required.
Prevention/Avoidance: None.

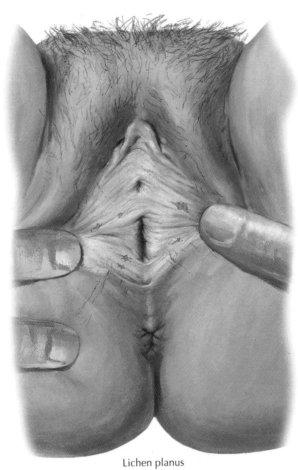

Lichen planus

Possible Complications: Vulvar lesions are often chronic and may undergo malignant change.

Expected Outcome: Chronic therapy required with relapses common.

MISCELLANEOUS

Pregnancy Considerations: No effect on pregnancy.
ICD-9-CM Codes: 697.0.

REFERENCES

Level II

Anderson M, Kutzner S, Kaufman RH: Treatment of vulvovaginal lichen planus with vaginal hydrocortisone suppositories. Obstet Gynecol 2002;100:359.

Cooper SM, Wojnarowska F: Influence of treatment of erosive lichen planus of the vulva on its prognosis. Arch Dermatol 2006;142:289.

Eisen D: The vulvovaginal-gingival syndrome of lichen planus. The clinical characteristics of 22 patients. Arch Dermatol 1994;130:1379.

Franck JM, Young AW Jr: Squamous cell carcinoma in situ arising within lichen planus of the vulva. Dermatol Surg 1995;21:890.

Jensen JT, Bird M, Leclair CM: Patient satisfaction after the treatment of vulvovaginal erosive lichen planus with topical clobetasol and tacrolimus: a survey study. Am J Obstet Gynecol 2004;190:1759.

Lewis FM, Shah M, Harrington CI: Vulvar involvement in lichen planus: a study of 37 women. Br J Dermatol 1996;135:89.

Level III

Edwards L, Friedrich EG Jr: Desquamative vaginitis: lichen planus in disguise. Obstet Gynecol 1988;71:832.

Katz VL: Benign gynecologic lesions. In Katz VL, Lentz GM, Lobo RA, Gershenson DM: Comprehensive Gynecology, 5th ed. Philadelphia, Mosby/Elsevier, 2007:431.

Lotery HE, Galask RP: Erosive lichen planus of the vulva and vagina. Obstet Gynecol 2003;101:1121.

Mann MS, Kaufman RH: Erosive lichen planus of the vulva. Clin Obstet Gynecol 1991;34:605.

Pelisse M: Erosive vulvar lichen planus and desquamative vaginitis. Semin Dermatol 1996;15:47.

Valdatta L, Tuinder S, Thione A, et al: Lichen planus cutis and squamous cell carcinoma. Plast Reconstr Surg 2004;113:1085.

INTRODUCTION

Description: Lichen sclerosus is a chronic condition of the vulvar skin characterized by thinning, distinctive skin changes and inflammation. It is non-neoplastic and involves glabrous skin and the vulva. The term *lichen sclerosus et atrophicus* has been dropped because the epithelium is metabolically active, not atrophic. (At one time, the condition was referred to as *kraurosis vulvae*.)

Prevalence: Common.

Predominant Age: Late reproductive to early menopausal (however, may be seen as early as 6 months).

Genetics: No genetic pattern.

ETIOLOGY AND PATHOGENESIS

Causes: Unknown. Proposed—immunologic (autoimmune), genetic, inactive or deficient androgen receptors, epidermal growth factor deficiency.

Risk Factors: None known.

CLINICAL CHARACTERISTICS

Signs and Symptoms

- Intense itching common (99%)
- Thinned, atrophic-appearing skin, with linear scratch marks or fissures (the skin often has a "cigarette-paper" or parchment-like appearance); these changes frequently extend around the anus in a figure-eight configuration
- Atrophic changes result in thinning, or even loss, of the labia minora and significant narrowing of the introitus
- Fissures, scarring, and synechiae cause marked pain for some patients

DIAGNOSTIC APPROACH

Differential Diagnosis

- Lichen simplex (hyperplastic vulvar dystrophy)
- Scleroderma
- Vitiligo
- Paget's disease
- Vulvar candidiasis
- Squamous cell hyperplasia or carcinoma (when thickening is present)

Associated Conditions: Dyspareunia, vulvodynia, vulvar pruritus, hypothyroidism, vulvar squamous cancer (5% lifetime risk).

Workup and Evaluation

Laboratory: Thyroid function studies should be considered because up to one third of patients have coexisting hypothyroidism.

Imaging: No imaging indicated.

Special Tests: Culture or KOH (potassium hydroxide) wet preparations of skin scrapings may help to evaluate the possibility of candidiasis. Punch biopsy of the skin will establish the diagnosis.

Diagnostic Procedures: History, physical examination, and biopsy of affected clerea.

Pathologic Findings

Loss of normal vulvar architecture with loss of rete pegs; a homogeneous dermis with edema, fibrin, and loss of vascularity; elastic fibers; and dermal collagen. Chronic inflammation is common, and spongiosis of the basilar epithelial cells is often present. Ulceration or hypertrophy may be present as a result of rubbing or scratching.

MANAGEMENT AND THERAPY

Nonpharmacologic

General Measures: Evaluation, perineal hygiene, cool sitz baths, moist soaks, or the application of soothing solutions such as Burow's solution. Patients should be advised to wear loose-fitting clothing and keep the area dry and well ventilated. Emollients such as petroleum jelly may help to reduce local drying.

Specific Measures: Topical steroid therapy is preferred over the traditional testosterone cream. Surgical excision is occasionally required if medical therapy fails. This is associated with a high rate of recurrence and the risk of postsurgical scarring.

Diet: No specific dietary changes indicated.

Activity: No restriction.

Patient Education: Reassurance; American College of Obstetricians and Gynecologists Patient Education Pamphlet AP088 (Disorders of the Vulva), AP028 (Vaginitis: Causes and Treatments), AP020 (Pain During Intercourse).

Drug(s) of Choice

Burow's solution (Domeboro, aluminum acetate 5% aqueous solution, three to four times daily for 30 to 60 minutes).

Crotamiton 10% (Eurax) may be applied topically, twice daily. High-potency prednisolone analogs (clobetasol propionate, Cormax, Temovate) 0.05% twice a day for 30 days, every night for 30 days, then daily.

Fluorinated corticosteroids (Valisone 0.1%, Synalar 0.01%) applied two to three times a day for 2 weeks. Lower-potency steroids (hydrocortisone) may be used after initial therapy or in children.

Testosterone propionate in petrolatum (2%) applied two to three times daily for up to 6 months.

Contraindications: Vulvar cancer.

Precautions: Continued or prolonged use of topical steroids may result in thinning of the skin outside the area of lichen sclerosus with subsequent atrophy and traumatic injury (splitting and cracking). Prolonged testosterone propionate therapy may be associated with clitoral enlargement or pain, local burning, or erythema. Rarely, hirsutism may result.

Alternative Drugs

In selected patients, intralesional steroids (Kenalog-10) may be used.

Topical progesterone (400 mg in oil with 4 oz of Aquaphor, applied twice a day) may be substituted for testosterone cream in children.

Topical tacrolimus has been studied in a limited number of patients, but it does not work as fast or as effectively as potent topical corticosteroids.

FOLLOW-UP

Patient Monitoring: Frequent follow-up (3 to 6 months) is required to watch for recurrence or worsening of symptoms.

Prevention/Avoidance: None.

Possible Complications: Scarring and narrowing of the introitus may be sufficient to preclude intercourse. Excoriation with secondary infections may occur. Areas that become hyperplastic as a result of scratching are thought to be at increased risk for premalignant or malignant changes (squamous cell carcinoma—lifetime risk of 3% to 5%).

Expected Outcome: Initial response is generally good, but recurrence is common, often necessitating lifelong therapy.

MISCELLANEOUS

Pregnancy Considerations: No effect on pregnancy (generally not a consideration).

ICD-9-CM Codes: Based on location and severity of disease.

REFERENCES

Level II

Bohm M, Frieling U, Luger TA, Bonsmann G: Successful treatment of anogenital lichen sclerosus with topical tacrolimus. Arch Dermatol 2003;139:922.

Bornstein J, Heifetz S, Kellner Y, et al: Clobetasol dipropionate 0.05% versus testosterone propionate 2% topical application for severe vulvar lichen sclerosus. Am J Obstet Gynecol 1998;178:80.

Bracco GL, Carli P, Sonni L, et al: Clinical and histologic effects of topical treatments of vulvar lichen sclerosus: a critical evaluation. J Reprod Med 1993;38:37.

Cattaneo A, Bracco GL, Maestrini G, et al: Lichen sclerosis and squamous hyperplasia of the vulva. A clinical study of medical treatment. J Reprod Med 1991;36:301.

Kunstfeld R, Kirnbauer R, Stingl G, Karlhofer FM: Successful treatment of vulvar lichen sclerosus with topical tacrolimus. Arch Dermatol 2003;139:850.

Luesley DM, Downey GP: Topical tacrolimus in the management of lichen sclerosus. BJOG 2006;113:832.

Paslin D: Treatment of lichen sclerosus with topical dihydrotestosterone. Obstet Gynecol 1991;78:1046.

Renaud-Vilmer C, Cavelier-Balloy B, Porcher R, Dubertret L: Vulvar lichen sclerosus: effect of long-term topical application of a potent steroid on the course of the disease. Arch Dermatol 2004;140:709.

Level III

Elchalal U, Gilead L, Bardy D, et al: Treatment of vulvar lichen sclerosus in the elderly: an update. Obstet Gynecol Surv 1995;50:155.

Flynt J, Gallup DG: Childhood lichen sclerosus. Obstet Gynecol 1979;53:79S.

Goldstein AT, Burrows LJ: Surgical treatment of clitoral phimosis caused by lichen sclerosus. Am J Obstet Gynecol 2007;196:126.

Hewitt J: Lichen sclerosus. J Reprod Med 1986;31:781.

Katz VL: Benign gynecologic lesions. In Katz VL, Lentz GM, Lobo RA, Gershenson DM: Comprehensive Gynecology, 5th ed. Philadelphia, Mosby/Elsevier, 2007:431.

Maloney ME: Exploring the common vulvar dermatoses. Contemp Ob/Gyn 1988;29:91.

Mann MS, Kaufman RH: Erosive lichen planus of the vulva. Clin Obstet Gynecol 1991;34:605.

Neill S: Treatment for lichen sclerosus. BMJ 1990;301:555.

Powell JJ, Wojnarowska F: Lichen sclerosus. Lancet 1999;353:1777.

Scrimin F, Rustja S, Radillo O, et al: Vulvar lichen sclerosus: an immunologic study. Obstet Gynecol 2000;95:147.

Soper DE, Patterson JW, Hurt WG, et al: Lichen planus of the vulva. Obstet Gynecol 1988;72:74.

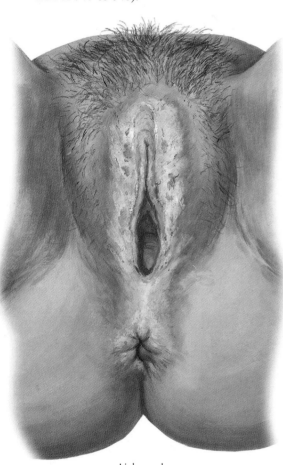

Lichen sclerosus

INTRODUCTION

Description: Squamous cell cancer of the vulva generally presents as an exophytic ulcer or hyperkeratotic plaque. It may arise as a solitary lesion or develop hidden within hypertrophic or other vulvar skin changes, making diagnosis difficult and often delayed.

Prevalence: Fewer than 5000 cases per year, 4% of gynecologic malignancies. (The incidence of vulvar cancer increased by approximately 20% between 1973 and 2000, likely related to increased exposure to human papillomavirus [HPV].)

Predominant Age: In situ 40 to 49, invasive 65 to 70.

Genetics: No genetic pattern.

ETIOLOGY AND PATHOGENESIS

Causes: Unknown. Thought to be associated with human papillomavirus.

Risk Factors: Infection with human papillomavirus (molecular analysis had detected human papillomavirus DNA in 40% of vulvar cancers), smoking, immunosuppression, lichen sclerosus.

CLINICAL CHARACTERISTICS

Signs and Symptoms

- Itching, irritation, cracking, or bleeding of the vulva, most common on the posterior two thirds of the labia majus
- Ulcerated exophytic lesion or hyperkeratotic plaque (late in disease)

DIAGNOSTIC APPROACH

Differential Diagnosis

- Hypertrophic vulvar dystrophy
- Lichen sclerosus

Associated Conditions: Hyperplastic vulvar dystrophy.

Workup and Evaluation

Laboratory: No evaluation indicated.

Imaging: No imaging indicated.

Special Tests: Biopsy of any suspicious lesion.

Diagnostic Procedures: History, physical examination, and vulvar biopsy.

Pathologic Findings

Histologic types include squamous cell (90%), melanoma (5%), basaloid, warty, verrucous, giant cell, spindle cell, acantholytic squamous cell (adenoid squamous), lymphoepithelioma-like, basal cell, and Merkel cell. Sarcoma accounts for approximately 2% of vulvar cancers. Metastatic tumors from other sources are rare, but they do occur.

MANAGEMENT AND THERAPY

Nonpharmacologic

General Measures: Early evaluation (generally by biopsy). (The majority of women have had symptoms for more than 6 months before a diagnosis is made.)

Specific Measures: Initial treatment consists of wide local excision (1-cm margins). Subsequent therapy, including node dissections and adjunctive therapy (radiation), is determined by the stage of disease, cell type, and surgical margins.

Diet: No specific dietary changes indicated.

Activity: No restriction, except as dictated by surgical therapy.

Patient Education: American College of Obstetricians and Gynecologists Patient Education Pamphlet AP088 (Disorders of the Vulva).

Drug(s) of Choice

None.

FOLLOW-UP

Patient Monitoring: Careful follow-up for recurrence or additional new lesions. Any patient who has had human papillomavirus–related dysplasia should avoid the vulvar use of topical steroids because this may increase the risk of recurrence.

Prevention/Avoidance: None.

Possible Complications: Distant spread and disease progression, secondary infection. Wound breakdown after surgical excision is common.

Expected Outcome: If tumor invasion is less than 1 mm, the risk of lymph node involvement is essentially 0 and high success rates may be expected. Five-year survival rates decline with advancing stage: 20% with deep node involvement. Overall 5-year survival is 70%.

MISCELLANEOUS

Pregnancy Considerations: No effect on pregnancy, although the presence of a pregnancy may affect surgical therapeutic options.

ICD-9-CM Codes: Specific to cell type and location.

REFERENCES

Level II

Ansink AC, Sie-Go DM, van der Velden J, et al: Identification of sentinel lymph nodes in vulvar carcinoma patients with the aid of a patent blue V injection: a multicenter study. Cancer 1999; 86:652.

Maggino T, Landoni F, Sartori E, et al: Patterns of recurrence in patients with squamous cell carcinoma of the vulva. A multicenter CTF Study. Cancer 2000;89:116.

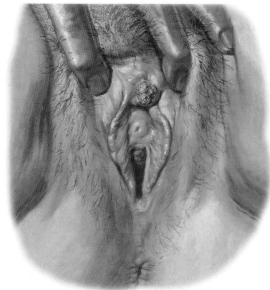

Carcinoma of the clitoris

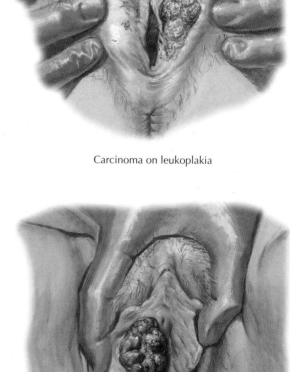

Carcinoma on leukoplakia

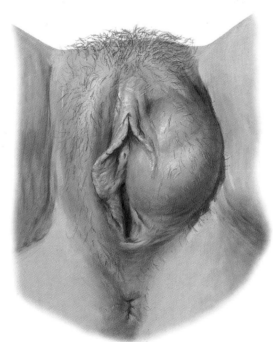

Sarcoma of the labium

Metastatic
hypernephroma

Rhodes CA, Cummins C, Shafi MI: The management of squamous cell vulval cancer: a population based retrospective study of 411 cases. Br J Obstet Gynaecol 1998;105:200.

Level III

Canavan TP, Cohen D: Vulvar cancer. Am Fam Physician 2002;66:1269.

DiSaia PJ. Management of superficially invasive vulvar carcinoma. Clin Obstet Gynecol 1985;28:196.

Frumovitz M, Bodurka DC: Neoplastic disease of the vulva. In Katz VL, Lentz GM, Lobo RA, Gershenson DM: Comprehensive Gynecology, 5th ed. Philadelphia, Mosby/Elsevier, 2007:790.

Hacker NF, Van der Velden J: Conservative management of early vulvar cancer. Cancer 1993;71:1673.

Kurman RJ, Norris HJ, Wilkinson EJ: In Rosai J, ed. Atlas of tumor pathology: tumors of the cervix, vagina and vulva, Vol 4. Washington, DC, AFIP, 1992.

Tyring SK: Vulvar squamous cell carcinoma: guidelines for early diagnosis and treatment. Am J Obstet Gynecol 2003;189:S17.

INTRODUCTION

Description: Vulvar hematoma is swelling of one or both labia because of interstitial bleeding, most often after blunt trauma.

Predominant Age: Most common in childhood and teen years but may occur at any age.

Genetics: No genetic pattern.

ETIOLOGY AND PATHOGENESIS

Causes: Blunt trauma (straddle injury, sexual abuse, rape, water skiing), vaginal surgery or delivery, varicose veins of vulva.

Risk Factors: Sports activities; uncommonly, consensual intercourse.

CLINICAL CHARACTERISTICS

Signs and Symptoms

- Painful swelling of one or both labia
- Dark blue or black discoloration
- Bleeding from vulva if laceration is present

DIAGNOSTIC APPROACH

Differential Diagnosis

- Bartholin's gland cyst or abscess
- Varicose veins of vulva
- Lymphogranuloma venereum
- Acne inversa

Associated Conditions: The presence of vaginal lacerations must always be considered.

Workup and Evaluation

Laboratory: No evaluation indicated.
Imaging: No imaging indicated.
Special Tests: None indicated.
Diagnostic Procedures: History and gentle visualization, speculum examination if vaginal trauma also suspected or possible.

Pathologic Findings

None.

MANAGEMENT AND THERAPY

Nonpharmacologic

General Measures: Analgesics (avoid aspirin), pressure, ice packs.
Specific Measures: Surgical drainage for rapidly expanding hematomas or those more than 10 cm in diameter.

Children with vulvar trauma should have a tetanus toxoid booster if none has been given in the preceding 5 years.

Diet: No specific dietary changes indicated.
Activity: Bed rest until condition is stable; return to activity as tolerated.

Drug(s) of Choice

Nonaspirin analgesics.

FOLLOW-UP

Patient Monitoring: Observation for expanding hematoma, hemodynamic monitoring if blood loss severe.
Prevention/Avoidance: Proper footwear during sports.
Possible Complications: Chronic expanding hematoma with fibrosis and pain.
Expected Outcome: Most hematomas gradually resolve with conservative management only.

MISCELLANEOUS

Pregnancy Considerations: No effect on pregnancy; rarely may complicate delivery if present before or during labor. More often, delivery precedes hematoma formation.
ICD-9-CM Codes: 624.5, 664.5 (Vulvar hematoma following delivery).

REFERENCES

Level II

Benrubi G, Neuman C, Nuss RC, Thompson RJ: Vulvar and vaginal hematomas: a retrospective study of conservative versus operative management. South Med J 1987;80:991.

Naumann RO, Droegemueller W: Unusual etiology of vulvar hematomas. Am J Obstet Gynecol 1982;142:357.

Niv J, Lessing JB, Hartuv J, Peyser MR: Vaginal injury resulting from sliding down a water chute. Am J Obstet Gynecol 1992;166:930.

Level III

Gianini GD, Method MW, Christman JE: Traumatic vulvar hematomas. Assessing and treating nonobstetric patients. Postgrad Med 1991;89:115.

Huddock JJ, Dupayne N, McGeary JA: Traumatic vulvar hematomas. Am J Obstet Gynecol 1955;70:1064.

Katz VL: Benign gynecologic lesions. In Katz VL, Lentz GM, Lobo RA, Gershenson DM: Comprehensive Gynecology, 5th ed. Philadelphia, Mosby/Elsevier, 2007:426.

Propst AM, Thorp JM Jr: Traumatic vulvar hematomas: conservative versus surgical management. South Med J 1998;91:144.

Ridgeway LE: Puerperal emergency: vaginal and vulvar hematomas. Obstet Gynecol Clin North Am 1995;22:275.

Smith RP: Gynecology in primary care. Baltimore, Williams & Wilkins, 1997:603.

Vulvar Hematoma

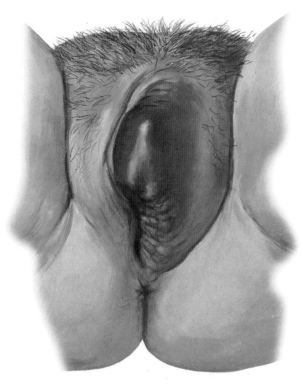

Typical appearance of vulvar hematoma,
a hematoma involving one or both labia

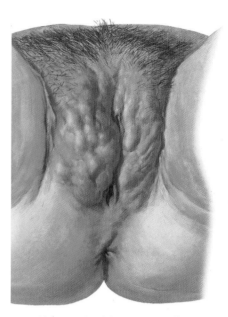

Vulvar varicosities, trauma and
childbirth may all contribute to
vulvar hematoma formation

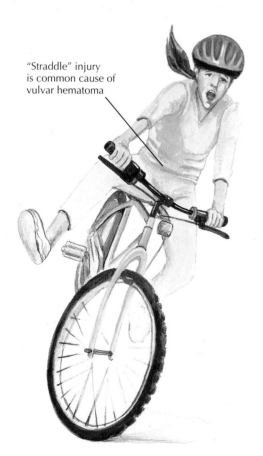

"Straddle" injury
is common cause of
vulvar hematoma

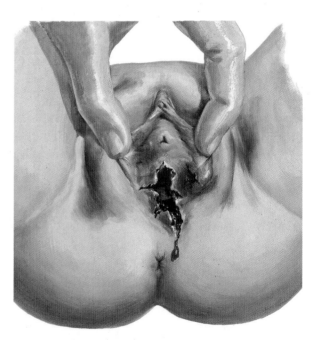

Presence of vulvar hematoma in children most
often due to "straddle" injury, but should raise
concern of sexual abuse, especially if lacerations
are present

Vulvar Lesions

THE CHALLENGE

The skin of the vulva is subject to all the changes that affect skin elsewhere in the body. In addition, the tissues of the vulva represent a rich ecosystem, with interactions between tissues, fluids, hormones, and microbes.

Scope of the Problem: In gynecologic practices, two or more patients a day with these concerns is the norm.

Objectives of Management: To establish a timely diagnosis and management plan for those patients with vulvar lesions.

TACTICS

Relevant Pathophysiology: The skin of the vulva is like that of other areas of the body with stratified squamous epithelium; hair follicles; and sebaceous, sweat, and apocrine glands. Just as in other areas of the body, the vulva is susceptible to inflammatory and dermatologic diseases. Intertrigo, acne inversa, psoriasis, seborrheic dermatitis, Fox-Fordyce disease, fifth disease, changes caused by Behçet's or Crohn's diseases, viral infections, and parasites may all affect the skin of the vulva. The skin of the vulva is also vulnerable to irritation from vaginal secretions, recurrent urinary loss, or contact with external irritants (such as soap residue, perfumes, fabric softeners, or infestation by pinworms). Changes may occur because of the effects of diabetes or hormonal alterations and dermatoses such as hypertrophic dystrophy, lichen sclerosus, psoriasis, and others.

Strategies: The character of the lesion or vulvar findings may be used to establish a working diagnosis for the patient with a vulvar lesion. Processes that result in lesions that occupy a superficial location are different from those that cause processes deep within the tissues of the vulva. It is important to keep in mind that many conditions that cause vulvar lesions may present in several forms. Consequently, in any decision tree based on lesion morphology, some diagnoses may be represented at the end of more than one branch (e.g., seborrheic keratosis or nevus).

Patient Education: American College of Obstetricians and Gynecologists Patient Education Pamphlet AP088 (Disorders of the Vulva).

IMPLEMENTATION

Special Considerations: In addition to the diagnoses discussed in the preceding, several other significant possibilities must always be considered when diffuse symptoms and findings are present: atopic dermatitis, contact dermatitis, fixed drug reaction, and factitial vulvitis. When cystic structures are encountered, the possibility of congenital remnants such as mesothelial cysts (cysts of the canal of Nuck), Wolffian duct remnants, and periurethral cysts must be considered. Lipomas, neurofibromas, rhabdomyomas, schwannomas, and leiomyomas may present as fleshy tumors of the vulva. Of special importance are lesions that involve significant necrosis: necrotizing fasciitis and pyoderma gangrenosum. Both of these processes represent a significant threat to the life and health of the patient and require prompt and aggressive treatment.

REFERENCES

Level III

Katz VL: Benign gynecologic lesions. In Katz VL, Lentz GM, Lobo RA, Gershenson DM: Comprehensive Gynecology, 5th ed. Philadelphia, Mosby/Elsevier, 2007:419.

McKay M: Vulvar dermatoses. Clin Obstet Gynecol 1991;34:614.

Nanda VS: Common dermatoses. Am J Obstet Gynecol 1995; 173:488.

Peckham EM, Maki DG, Patterson JJ, Hafez GR: Focal vulvitis: a characteristic syndrome and cause of dyspareunia. Features, natural history, and management. Am J Obstet Gynecol 1986;154:855.

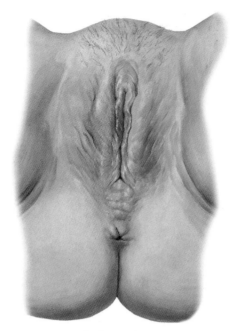

Senile atrophy

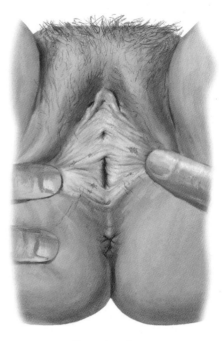

Kraurosis vulvae

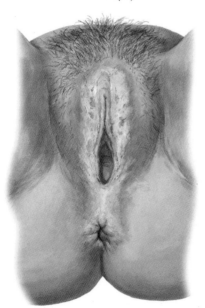

Leukoplakia

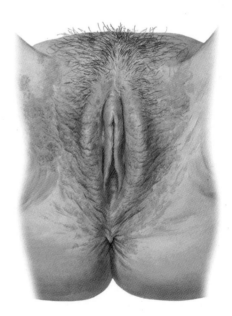

Lichenification

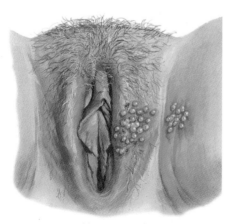

Herpes genitalis

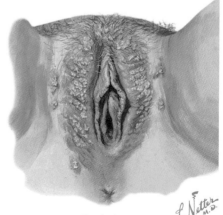

Psoriasis

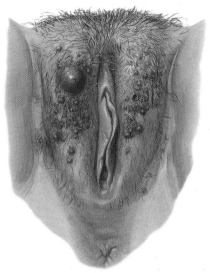

Folliculitis and furunculosis

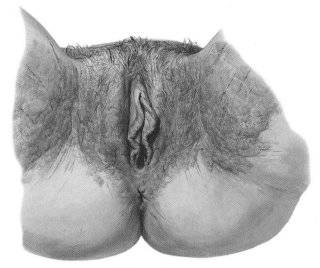

Tinea cruris

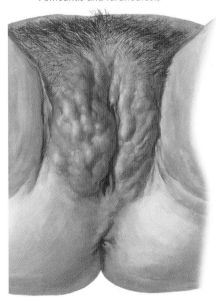

Varicose veins

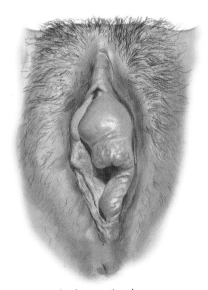

Angioneurotic edema

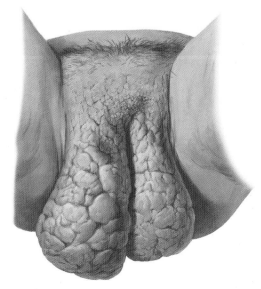

Elephantiasis

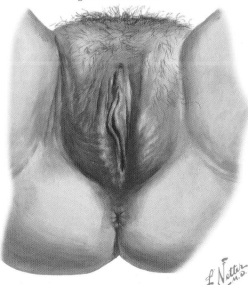

Diabetic vulvitis

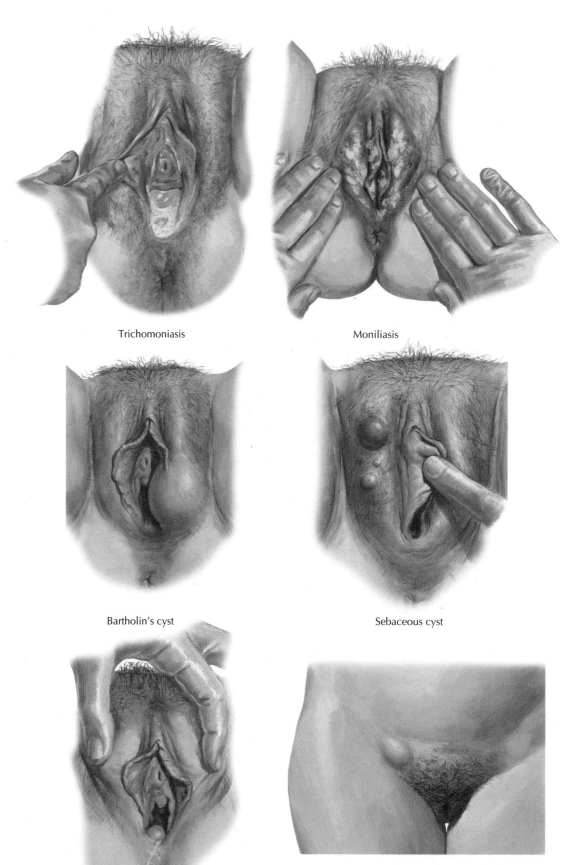

Trichomoniasis

Moniliasis

Bartholin's cyst

Sebaceous cyst

Inclusion cyst

Cyst of Canal of Nuck

INTRODUCTION

Description: Vulvar vestibulitis is an uncommon syndrome of intense sensitivity of the skin of the posterior vaginal introitus and vulvar vestibule, with progressive worsening, which leads to loss of function.

Prevalence: Some estimates place it at 15% of all women, but significant, disabling symptoms are much less common.

Predominant Age: 19 to 81 years, median age 36.

Genetics: No genetic pattern.

ETIOLOGY AND PATHOGENESIS

Causes: Unknown. High degree of association with human papillomavirus but no causal link established. Despite the implication of the term, true inflammation is not a characteristic of this process.

Risk Factors: None known. It has been postulated that the use of oral contraceptives may increase the risk or severity of vulvar vestibulitis and that users who experience symptoms should switch to other methods of contraception. Strong evidence for either causation or significant improvement is lacking.

CLINICAL CHARACTERISTICS

Signs and Symptoms

- Intense pain and tenderness at the posterior introitus and vestibule, most often present for 2 to 5 years. (Some authors suggest that symptoms must be present for more than 6 months before the diagnosis is made.)
- Unable to use tampons (33%) or have intercourse (entry dyspareunia, 100%)
- Focal inflammation, punctation, and ulceration of the perineal and vaginal epithelium
- Punctate areas (1 to 10) of inflammation 3 to 10 mm in size may be seen between the Bartholin's glands (75%), hymenal ring, and middle perineum

DIAGNOSTIC APPROACH

Differential Diagnosis

- Vaginismus
- Chronic vulvitis
- Atrophic vaginitis
- Hypertrophic vulvar dystrophy
- Recurrent vaginal infections
- Herpes vulvitis
- Vulvar dermatoses
- Contact (allergic) vulvitis

Associated Conditions: Sexual dysfunction, dyspareunia, and vulvodynia.

Workup and Evaluation

Laboratory: No evaluation indicated.

Imaging: No imaging indicated.

Special Tests: Colposcopy of the vulva (using 3% acetic acid) may reveal the characteristic punctate and aceto-white areas.

Diagnostic Procedures: History, physical examination, mapping of sensitive areas, and colposcopy.

Pathologic Findings

Small inflammatory punctate lesions varying in size from 3 to 10 mm, often with superficial ulceration. The Bartholin gland openings may be inflamed as well. The area involved may be demarcated by light touching with a cotton-tipped applicator, although the level of discomfort is often out of proportion to the physical findings. Microscopic inflammation of minor vestibular glands may be seen.

MANAGEMENT AND THERAPY

Nonpharmacologic

General Measures: Evaluation, perineal hygiene, cool sitz baths, moist soaks, or the application of soothing solutions such as Burow's solution. Patients should be advised to wear loose-fitting clothing and keep the area dry and well ventilated.

Specific Measures: Topical anesthetics and antidepressants (amitriptyline hydrochloride) may reduce pain and itch. Interferon injections may provide relief in up to 60% of patients. Refractory disease may require surgical resection or laser ablation.

Diet: No specific dietary changes indicated. (Reducing urinary oxylate through dietary means has been suggested but remains unproved.)

Activity: No restriction (pelvic rest often recommended when symptoms are maximal).

Patient Education: Reassurance: American College of Obstetricians and Gynecologists Patient Education Pamphlet AP088 (Disorders of the Vulva), AP020 (Pain During Intercourse).

Drug(s) of Choice

Lidocaine (Xylocaine) 2% jelly (or 5% cream) topically as needed.

Antidepressants (amitriptyline hydrochloride [Elavil] 25 mg PO every night or 10 mg PO three times a day).

Interferon injections three times weekly for 4 weeks, introducing 1 million units at each of 12 areas (clock face) by the completion of the course.

Contraindications: Interferon injections cannot be given during pregnancy.

Precautions: Patients should be warned that interferon injections are associated with flulike symptoms and that a clinical response may not be seen for up to 3 months. Patients should abstain from intercourse during the series of injections.

FOLLOW-UP

Patient Monitoring: Frequent follow-up and monitoring are required. Frustration for both the patient and provider is common.

Prevention/Avoidance: None.

Vulvar Vestibulitis

Vulvar vestibulitis is syndrome of intense sensitivity of skin of posterior vaginal introitus and vulvar vestibule resulting in dyspareunia and pain on attempted use of tampons.

Area most commonly involved is posterior to Bartholin's glands.

Opening of minor vestibular glands

Orifice of Bartholin's gland

Bartholin's gland

Level of discomfort is usually out of proportion to degree of physical findings, which include 1 to 10 small (3–10 mm) areas of punctate inflammation, some with ulceration in perineal and vaginal epithelium

Involved area may be demarcated by light touch with cotton-tipped applicator

JOHN A.CRAIG—AD
D. MASCARO

Hymenal ring

Bartholin's gland opening may be inflamed

Punctate erosions on erythematous base found in vestibule and introitus

Magnified view of vestibule

Possible Complications: Secondary infection, sexual dysfunction.

Expected Outcome: Spontaneous remission in one third of patients over the course of 6 months. Chronic, continuing pain most common. Surgical therapy is associated with 50% to 60% success.

MISCELLANEOUS

Pregnancy Considerations: No effect on pregnancy.
ICD-9-CM Codes: 616.10.

REFERENCES

Level II

David GD: The management of vulvar vestibulitis syndrome with the carbon dioxide laser. J Gynecol Surg 1989;5:87.

Goetsch MF: Vulvar vestibulitis: prevalence and histologic features in a general gynecologic practice population. Am J Obstet Gynecol 1991;164:1609.

Zolnoun DA, Hartmann KE, Steege JF: Overnight 5% lidocaine ointment for treatment of vulvar vestibulitis. Obstet Gynecol 2003;102:84.

Level III

American College of Obstetricians and Gynecologists: Vulvodynia. ACOG Committee Opinion 345. Obstet Gynecol 2006;108:1049.

Baggish MS, Miklos JR: Vulvar pain syndrome: a review. Obstet Gynecol Surv 1995;50:618.

Bornstein J, Zarfati D, Goldik Z, Abramovici H: Vulvar vestibulitis: physical or psychosexual problem? Obstet Gynecol 1999;93:876.

Danielsson I, Eisemann M, Sjoberg I, Wikman M: Vulvar vestibulitis: a multi-factorial condition. BJOG 2001;108:456.

Edwards L: New concepts in vulvodynia. Am J Obstet Gynecol 2003;189:S24.

Fischer G, Spurrett B, Fischer A: The chronically symptomatic vulva: aetiology and management. Br J Obstet Gynaecol 1995;102:773.

Katz VL: Benign gynecologic lesions. In Katz VL, Lentz GM, Lobo RA, Gershenson DM: Comprehensive Gynecology, 5th ed. Philadelphia, Mosby/Elsevier, 2007:427.

Marinoff SC, Turner ML: Vulvar vestibulitis syndrome: an overview. Am J Obstet Gynecol 1991;165:1228.

Metts JF: Vulvodynia and vulvar vestibulitis: challenges in diagnosis and management. Am Fam Physician 1999;59:1547, 1561.

Peckham EM, Maki DG, Patterson JJ, Hafez GR: Focal vulvitis: a characteristic syndrome and cause of dyspareunia. Features, natural history, and management. Am J Obstet Gynecol 1986;154:855.

Stewart DE, Reicher AE, Gerulath AH, Boydel KM: Vulvodynia and psychological distress. Obstet Gynecol 1994;84:587.

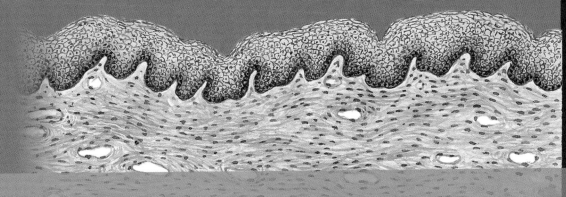

Vaginal Disease

INTRODUCTION

Description: Loss of support for the anterior vagina, through rupture or attenuation of the pubovesicocervical fascia, is manifested by descent or prolapse of the urethra (urethrocele) or bladder (cystocele).

Prevalence: Ten percent to 15% of women, 30% to 40% after menopause.

Predominant Age: 40 and older, increasing with age.

Genetics: No genetic pattern.

ETIOLOGY AND PATHOGENESIS

Causes: Loss of normal tissue integrity or tissue disruption as a result of trauma (childbirth, obstetric injury, surgery).

Risk Factors: Multiparity, obesity, chronic cough, heavy lifting, intrinsic tissue weakness or atrophic changes caused by estrogen loss. Some authors include smoking as a risk factor.

CLINICAL CHARACTERISTICS

Signs and Symptoms

- Asymptomatic
- Pelvic pressure or "heaviness"
- Stress incontinence, frequency, hesitancy, incomplete voiding, or recurrent infections
- Bulging of tissue at the vaginal opening
- Descent of the anterior vaginal wall during straining
- Positive results on "Q-tip test"

DIAGNOSTIC APPROACH

Differential Diagnosis

- Urethral diverticulum
- Skene's gland cyst, tumor, or abscess
- Anterior enterocele
- Gartner's duct cyst
- Urgency incontinence

Associated Conditions: Stress urinary incontinence, pelvic relaxation, uterine prolapse, and other hernias.

Workup and Evaluation

Laboratory: No evaluation indicated; perform urinalysis if urinary tract infection is suspected.

Imaging: No imaging indicated.

Special Tests: A "Q-tip test" is generally recommended, although it has a poor predictive value. (A cotton-tipped applicator dipped in 2% lidocaine [Xylocaine] is placed in the urethra, and rotation anteriorly with straining is measured. Greater than 30 degrees is abnormal.) An evaluation of urinary function is advisable, especially if surgical therapy is being considered. In the past, the functional significance of a cystourethrocele was gauged by elevating the bladder neck (using fingers or an instrument) and asking the patient to strain (referred to as a Bonney or Marshall-Marchetti test). This test has fallen out of favor as nonspecific and unreliable.

Diagnostic Procedures: Pelvic examination—best demonstrated by having the patient strain or cough and observing the vaginal opening through the separated labia. When a urethrocele or cystocele is present, a downward movement and forward rotation of the vaginal wall toward the introitus are demonstrated. A Sims speculum or the lower half of a Graves, Peterson, or other vaginal speculum may be used to retract the posterior vaginal wall, facilitating the identification of the support defect. The bladder should be partially filled (100 to 250 mL) during this examination.

Pathologic Findings

No characteristic histologic change. Chronic irritation or keratinization secondary to mechanical trauma may be found with complete prolapse.

MANAGEMENT AND THERAPY

Nonpharmacologic

General Measures: Weight reduction, treatment of chronic cough (if present), topical or systemic estrogen replacement or therapy as indicated.

Specific Measures: Pessary therapy (the intermittent use of a large [super] tampon may suffice for some patients), pelvic muscle exercises, surgical repair; limited role for medical therapy.

Diet: No specific dietary changes indicated.

Activity: Avoidance of heavy lifting and straining may slow the rate of progression or risk of recurrence.

Patient Education: Reassurance; American College of Obstetricians and Gynecologists Patient Education Pamphlet AP0012 (Pelvic Support Problems), AP081 (Urinary Incontinence).

Drug(s) of Choice

None. (Estrogen, either topically or systemically, is often prescribed to improve tissue tone, reduce irritation, and prepare tissues for surgical or pessary therapy.)

Contraindications: Undiagnosed vaginal bleeding, breast cancer.

Precautions: Alpha-adrenergic blocking agents used to treat hypertension may reduce urethral tone sufficiently to result in stress urinary incontinence in patients with reduced pelvic support. Patients treated with angiotensin-converting enzyme (ACE) inhibitors may develop a cough as a side effect of medication, worsening incontinence symptoms and accelerating the appearance or worsening of a cystourethrocele.

FOLLOW-UP

Patient Monitoring: Normal health maintenance.

Prevention/Avoidance: None.

Possible Complications: Compromise of ureteral drainage may be found in patients with significant downward displacement of the trigone. Recurrent urinary tract infections may occur if the support defect leads to significant residual urine. Vaginal ulceration, bleeding, infection, or pain frequently accompanies complete prolapse.

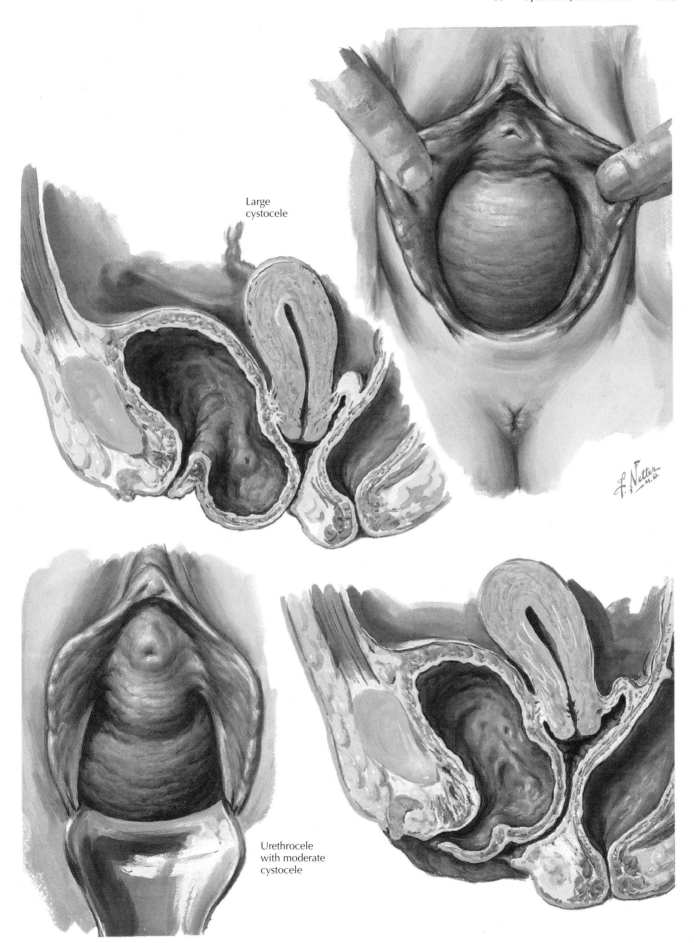

Large
cystocele

Urethrocele
with moderate
cystocele

Expected Outcome: Generally favorable reduction in symptoms may be obtained with a carefully chosen and fitted pessary. Surgical therapy is associated with 95% success in long-term correction of the anatomic defect and the associated symptoms.

MISCELLANEOUS

Pregnancy Considerations: No effect on pregnancy, although pregnancy (and vaginal delivery) may cause or contribute to a worsening of pelvic support problems.

ICD-9-CM Codes: 618.0, (618.4 [With uterine prolapse], 618.3 [Complete], 618.2 [Incomplete]).

REFERENCES

Level I
Sand PK, Koduri S, Lobel RW, et al: Prospective randomized trial of polyglactin 910 mesh to prevent recurrence of cystoceles and rectoceles. Am J Obstet Gynecol 2001;184:1357; discussion 1362.

Level II
Colombo M, Vitobello D, Proietti F, Milani R: Randomised comparison of Burch colposuspension versus anterior colporrhaphy in women with stress urinary incontinence and anterior vaginal wall prolapse. BJOG 2000;107:544.

Cross CA, Cespedes RD, McGuire EJ: Treatment results using pubovaginal slings in patients with large cystoceles and stress incontinence. J Urol 1997;158:431.

Federkiw DM, Sand PK, Retzky SS, Johnson DC: The cotton swab test. Receiver-operating characteristic curves. J Reprod Med 1995; 40:42.

Fielding JR: MR imaging of pelvic floor relaxation. Radiol Clin North Am 2003;41:747.

Kinn AC, Lindskog M: Estrogens and phenylpropanolamine in combination for stress urinary incontinence in postmenopausal women. Urology 1988;32:273.

Level III
American College of Obstetricians and Gynecologists: Urinary incontinence in women. ACOG Practice Bulletin 63. Obstet Gynecol 2005;105:1533.

American College of Obstetricians and Gynecologists: Pelvic organ prolapse. ACOG Practice Bulletin 79. Obstet Gynecol 2007; 109:461.

Lentz GM: Anatomic defects of the abdominal wall and pelvic wall. In Katz VL, Lentz GM, Lobo RA, Gershenson DM: Comprehensive Gynecology, 5th ed. Philadelphia, Mosby/Elsevier, 2007: 506.

Marinkovic SP, Stanton SL: Incontinence and voiding difficulties associated with prolapse. J Urol 2004;171:1021.

Smith RP: Gynecology in primary care. Baltimore, Williams & Wilkins, 1997:577.

INTRODUCTION

Description: Enterocele is loss of support for the apex of the vagina, through rupture or attenuation of the pubovesicocervical fascia, manifested by descent or prolapse of the vaginal wall and underlying peritoneum, most commonly after abdominal or vaginal hysterectomy. An enterocele may occur when the uterus is present and tissue damage or weakness allows herniation behind the cervix and between the uterosacral ligaments.

Prevalence: Ten percent to 15% of women, 30% to 40% after menopause.

Predominant Age: 40 and older, increasing with age.

Genetics: No genetic pattern.

ETIOLOGY AND PATHOGENESIS

Causes: Loss or rupture of the normal support mechanisms in the pouch of Douglas. There is true herniation of the peritoneal cavity between the uterosacral ligaments and into the rectovaginal septum. Unlike a cystocele, urethrocele, or rectocele, the herniated tissue contains a true sac lined by parietal peritoneum.

Risk Factors: Multiparity, obesity, chronic cough, heavy lifting, intrinsic tissue weakness, or atrophic changes resulting from estrogen loss. Some authors include smoking as a risk factor.

CLINICAL CHARACTERISTICS

Signs and Symptoms

- Asymptomatic
- Pelvic pressure or "heaviness"
- Bulging of tissue at the vaginal opening
- Descent of the apical vaginal wall during straining

DIAGNOSTIC APPROACH

Differential Diagnosis

- Urethral diverticulum
- Cystocele
- Rectocele
- Vaginal prolapse (generally includes an enterocele)
- Gartner's duct cyst

Associated Conditions: Pelvic relaxation, vaginal prolapse, other hernias, and bowel obstruction (rare).

Workup and Evaluation

Laboratory: No evaluation indicated.

Imaging: No imaging indicated.

Special Tests: When the enterocele prolapses to beyond the introitus, transillumination may reveal loops of small bowel or omentum within the sac.

Diagnostic Procedures: Pelvic examination—best demonstrated by having the patient strain or cough and observing the vaginal opening through the separated labia. Rectovaginal examination differentiates this condition from a rectocele.

Pathologic Findings

No characteristic histologic change. Chronic irritation or keratinization secondary to mechanical trauma may be found when the enterocele descends to the level of the vulva or beyond.

MANAGEMENT AND THERAPY

Nonpharmacologic

General Measures: Weight reduction, treatment of chronic cough (if present), topical or systemic estrogen replacement or therapy as indicated.

Specific Measures: Pessary therapy (generally when the uterus is absent), surgical repair (abdominal or vaginal approach—McCall or Halban repair).

Diet: No specific dietary changes indicated.

Activity: No restriction.

Patient Education: Reassurance; American College of Obstetricians and Gynecologists Patient Education Pamphlet AP0012 (Pelvic Support Problems).

Drug(s) of Choice

None. (Estrogen, either topically or systemically, is often prescribed to improve tissue tone, reduce irritation, and prepare tissues for surgical or pessary therapy.)

Contraindications: Undiagnosed vaginal bleeding, breast cancer.

FOLLOW-UP

Patient Monitoring: Normal health maintenance.

Prevention/Avoidance: Maintenance of normal weight, use of surgical techniques at the time of hysterectomy that minimize the risk of enterocele formation (most commonly, this is plication of the uterosacral and cardinal ligaments).

Possible Complications: Bowel obstruction (rare).

Expected Outcome: Generally, favorable reduction of symptoms may be obtained with a carefully chosen and fitted pessary. Surgical therapy is associated with 95% success in long-term correction of the anatomic defect and the associated symptoms.

MISCELLANEOUS

Pregnancy Considerations: Generally not a consideration.

ICD-9-CM Codes: 618.6.

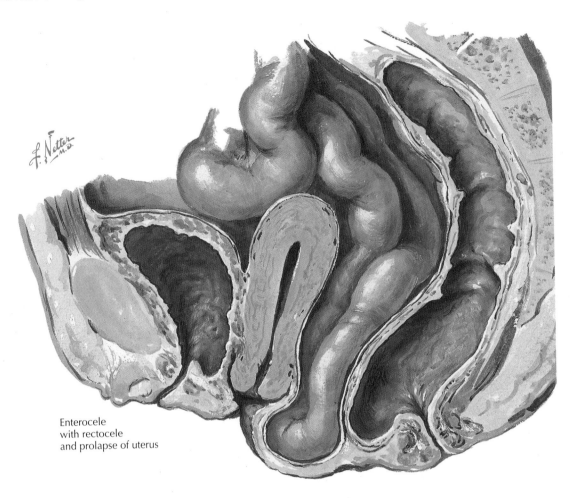

Enterocele
with rectocele
and prolapse of uterus

REFERENCES

Level II
Kelvin FM, Maglinte DD: Dynamic evaluation of female pelvic organ prolapse by extended proctography. Radiol Clin North Am 2003;41:395.

Nasr AO, Tormey S, Aziz MA, Lane B: Vaginal herniation: case report and review of the literature. Am J Obstet Gynecol 2005;193:95.

Level III
American College of Obstetricians and Gynecologists: Pelvic organ prolapse. ACOG Practice Bulletin 79. Obstet Gynecol 2007;109:461.

Chou Q, Weber AM, Piedmonte MR: Clinical presentation of enterocele. Obstet Gynecol 2000;96:599.

Kobashi KC, Leach GE: Pelvic prolapse. J Urol 2000;164:1879.

Lentz GM: Anatomic defects of the abdominal wall and pelvic wall. In Katz VL, Lentz GM, Lobo RA, Gershenson DM: Comprehensive Gynecology, 5th ed. Philadelphia, Mosby/Elsevier, 2007:511.

Smith RP: Gynecology in primary care. Baltimore, Williams & Wilkins, 1997:577.

Fistulae: Gastrointestinal and Urinary Tract

INTRODUCTION

Description: A fistula is an abnormal communication between two cavities or organs. In gynecology, this usually refers to a communication between the gastrointestinal or urinary tract and genital tract. (Connections directly to the skin are not discussed here.)

Prevalence: Gastrointestinal fistulae are uncommon; urinary tract fistulae are estimated to occur after 1 of 200 abdominal hysterectomies.

Predominant Age: Reproductive and beyond.

Genetics: No genetic pattern.

ETIOLOGY AND PATHOGENESIS

Causes: Urinary tract fistulae may result from surgical or obstetric trauma, irradiation, or malignancy, although the most common cause by far is unrecognized surgical trauma. Roughly 75% of urinary tract fistulae occur after abdominal hysterectomy. Signs of a urinary fistula (watery discharge) usually occur from 5 to 30 days after surgery (average 8 to 12), although they may be present in the immediate postoperative period. Fistulae between the gastrointestinal tract and vagina may be precipitated by the same injuries that cause genitourinary fistulae; most common are obstetric injuries and complications of episiotomies (lower one third of vagina). Fistulae may also follow hysterectomy or enterocele repair (upper one third of vagina). Inflammatory bowel disease or pelvic radiation therapy may hasten or precipitate fistula formation.

Risk Factors: Gastrointestinal—obstetric tears, puncture wounds, inflammatory bowel disease, intra-abdominal surgery, carcinoma, radiation therapy, perirectal abscess. Although Crohn's disease, lymphogranuloma venereum, or tuberculosis are recognized risk factors, these are uncommon. **Urinary tract**—surgery or radiation treatment. Urinary tract fistulae are most common after uncomplicated hysterectomy, although pelvic adhesive disease, endometriosis, or pelvic tumors increase the individual risk.

CLINICAL CHARACTERISTICS

Signs and Symptoms

Gastrointestinal Fistulae

- Foul vaginal discharge
- Marked vaginal and vulvar irritation
- Fecal incontinence and soiling and the passage of fecal matter or gas from the vagina, pathognomonic
- Dyspareunia common
- Dark-red rectal mucosa or granulation tissue apparent in vaginal canal at the site of the fistula

Urinary Tract Fistulae

- Continuous incontinence (occasionally made worse by position change or an increase in intra-abdominal pressure as with a cough or laugh)
- Vaginal and perineal wetness and irritation
- Granulation tissue at site of fistula

DIAGNOSTIC APPROACH

Differential Diagnosis

Gastrointestinal Fistulae

- Inflammatory bowel disease (Crohn's disease)
- Pilonidal sinus
- Perianal or other abscess
- Rectal carcinoma

Urinary Tract Fistulae

- Overflow incontinence
- Urge incontinence

Associated Conditions: Inflammatory bowel disease, bacterial vaginitis, dyspareunia, vaginitis, vulvitis, and urinary tract infection.

Workup and Evaluation

Laboratory: No evaluation indicated. (Evaluation of renal function [serum creatinine] is prudent but not diagnostic.)

Imaging: If inflammatory bowel disease is suspected, lower gastrointestinal series. Intravenous or retrograde pyelography may be useful.

Special Tests: Gastrointestinal fistulae—methylene blue may be instilled in the rectum with a tampon in place; staining indicates a communication. Sigmoidoscopy should be considered. **Urinary tract fistulae**—a tampon placed in the vagina with dye instilled into the bladder or dye given, usually intravenously, to be excreted by the kidney may be used to help find a fistula. Cystoscopy may help identify vesicovaginal fistulae.

Diagnostic Procedures: History, physical examination, probe of fistulous tract. Anoscopy, proctoscopy, sigmoidoscopy, or intravenous or retrograde pyelography may be helpful. Cystoscopy may be required to evaluate the location of a urinary tract fistula in relation to the ureteral opening and bladder trigone and to exclude the possibility of multiple fistulae.

Pathologic Findings

Inflammation and granulation changes from chronic infection. Tract may be single or multiple. Chronic bacterial vaginitis is generally present. Fistulae may be from the vagina to the bladder (vesicovaginal), to the urethra (urethrovaginal), or to the ureter (ureterovaginal). Rarely, communication between the bladder and the uterus (vesicouterine) may also occur.

MANAGEMENT AND THERAPY

Nonpharmacologic

General Measures: Gastrointestinal fistulae—evaluation, stool softening, treatment of vaginitis. **Urinary**

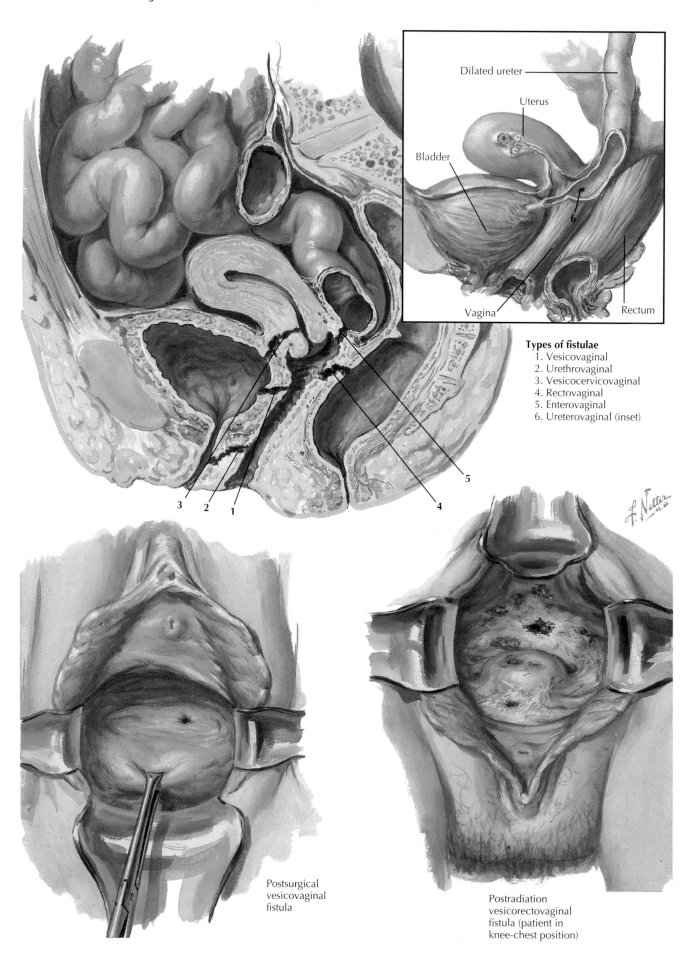

Dilated ureter

Uterus

Bladder

6

Vagina

Rectum

Types of fistulae
1. Vesicovaginal
2. Urethrovaginal
3. Vesicocervicovaginal
4. Rectovaginal
5. Enterovaginal
6. Ureterovaginal (inset)

3 2 1

5

4

Postsurgical
vesicovaginal
fistula

Postradiation
vesicorectovaginal
fistula (patient in
knee-chest position)

tract fistulae—urinary diversion (see the following text), protection of the vulva from continuous moisture (zinc oxide cream or diaper rash preparations).

Specific Measures: Gastrointestinal fistulae—for those that do not heal spontaneously (three fourths of fistulae), the only effective treatment is surgical. When the fistula is small, this is often carried out with the patient under general or spinal anesthesia in an ambulatory surgery unit. Fistulectomy or fistulotomy should not be performed in the presence of tissue edema or inflammation, diarrhea, or active inflammatory bowel disease. **Urinary tract fistulae**—vesicovaginal fistulae that occur in the immediate postoperative period should be treated by large-caliber transurethral catheter drainage. Spontaneous healing is evident within 2 to 4 weeks (20% of patients). Similarly, in patients with a ureterovaginal fistula, prompt placement of a ureteral stent, left in place for 2 weeks, allows spontaneous healing for roughly 30% of patients. When these conservative therapies fail, full surgical correction is required.

Diet: Low-residue diet advisable for patients with a gastrointestinal fistula.

Activity: No restriction. (Pelvic rest after surgical repair, until healing is completed.)

Patient Education: Perianal care, sitz baths; American College of Obstetricians and Gynecologists Patient Education Pamphlet AP081 (Urinary Incontinence).

Drug(s) of Choice

Although the only effective treatment is surgical, the use of stool softeners is often beneficial. If diarrhea is present, diphenoxylate hydrochloride (Lomotil) or a similar drug should be used to control symptoms. Treatment of coexisting vaginitis should be instituted.

Urinary antisepsis should be considered when necessary.

FOLLOW-UP

Patient Monitoring: Patients with a gastrointestinal fistula should be closely followed during the postoperative period (hospital discharge is generally delayed until after the first bowel movement). Maintain routine health care. When a ureteral fistula has been repaired, follow-up intravenous pyelography should be planned for 3, 6, and 12 months to check for delayed stricture.

Prevention/Avoidance: Careful surgical and obstetric techniques including preoperative and perioperative bladder drainage, good visualization, careful dissection, and care in placement of hemostatic sutures.

Possible Complications: Upper genital tract infection, recurrence, ascending urinary tract infection (including pyelonephritis).

Expected Outcome: Healing is generally good after surgical excision, although recurrence, when the original fistulae were caused by underlying disease or radiation therapy, is common.

MISCELLANEOUS

Pregnancy Considerations: No direct effect on pregnancy, although some causal processes may result in lower fertility or other effects on reproduction.

ICD-9-CM Codes: 619.1 (Gastrointestinal), 619.0 (Urinary tract).

REFERENCES

Level II

Alexander AA, Liu JB, Merton DA, Nagle DA: Fecal incontinence: transvaginal US evaluation of anatomic causes. Radiology 1996; 199:529.

Meeks GR, Sams JO 4th, Field KW, et al: Formation of vesicovaginal fistula: the role of suture placement into the bladder during closure of the vaginal cuff after transabdominal hysterectomy. Am J Obstet Gynecol 1997;177:1298.

Level III

Alvarez RD: Gastrointestinal complications in gynecologic surgery: a review for the general gynecologist. Obstet Gynecol 1988; 72:533.

American College of Obstetricians and Gynecologists: Urinary incontinence in women. ACOG Practice Bulletin 63. Obstet Gynecol 2005;105:1533.

Bassford T: Treatment of common anorectal disorders. Am Fam Physician 1992;45:1787.

Gerber GS, Schoenberg HW: Female urinary tract fistulas. J Urol 1993;149:229.

Katz VL: Postoperative counseling and management. In Katz VL, Lentz GM, Lobo RA, Gershenson DM: Comprehensive Gynecology, 5th ed. Philadelphia, Mosby/Elsevier, 2007:681.

Lentz GM: Anatomic defects of the abdominal wall and pelvic wall. In Katz VL, Lentz GM, Lobo RA, Gershenson DM: Comprehensive Gynecology, 5th ed. Philadelphia, Mosby/Elsevier, 2007:530.

Michelassi F, Melis M, Rubin M, Hurst RD: Surgical treatment of anorectal complications in Crohn's disease. Surgery 2000;128: 597.

Saclarides TJ: Rectovaginal fistula. Surg Clin North Am 2002; 82:1261.

Smith RP: Gynecology in primary care. Baltimore, Williams & Wilkins, 1997:577.

Smith RP, Ling FW: Procedures in women's health care. Baltimore, Williams & Wilkins, 1997:153, 163, 175, 201.

Symmonds RE: Incontinence: vesical and urethral fistulas. Clin Obstet Gynecol 1984;27:499.

INTRODUCTION

Description: Failure of the normal support mechanisms between the rectum and the vagina results in rectocele—herniation of the posterior vaginal wall and underlying rectum into the vaginal canal and eventually to, and through, the introitus.

Prevalence: Ten percent to 15% of women, 30% to 40% after menopause.

Predominant Age: Postmenopausal.

Genetics: No genetic pattern.

ETIOLOGY AND PATHOGENESIS

Causes: Loss of normal tissue integrity or tissue disruption as a result of trauma (childbirth, obstetric injury, surgery).

Risk Factors: Multiparity, obesity, chronic cough, heavy lifting, intrinsic tissue weakness, or atrophic changes resulting from estrogen loss. Some authors include smoking as a risk factor.

CLINICAL CHARACTERISTICS

Signs and Symptoms

- Bulging of the posterior vaginal wall
- Difficulty passing stool (may require manual splinting of the posterior vaginal wall to have a bowel movement)
- Dyspareunia uncommon but may occur

DIAGNOSTIC APPROACH

Differential Diagnosis

- Enterocele
- Rectovaginal hematoma
- Rectal cancer
- Vaginal inclusion cyst (after obstetric trauma or episiotomy)

Associated Conditions: Stress urinary incontinence, pelvic relaxation, uterine prolapse, other hernias, and vaginal outlet relaxation.

Workup and Evaluation

Laboratory: No evaluation indicated.

Imaging: Transvaginal ultrasonography may be used to assess the presence of an enterocele if not clinically apparent. Defecography has been used in some research settings but has not gained a major role in routine clinical practice.

Special Tests: None indicated.

Diagnostic Procedures: Pelvic examination—best demonstrated by having the patient strain or cough and observing the vaginal opening through the separated labia. A Sims speculum or the lower half of a Graves, Peterson, or other vaginal speculum (inserted upside down) may be inserted to retract the anterior vaginal wall, facilitating the identification of the support defect.

Pathologic Findings

No characteristic histologic change. Chronic irritation or keratinization secondary to mechanical trauma may be found with complete prolapse.

MANAGEMENT AND THERAPY

Nonpharmacologic

General Measures: Weight reduction, treatment of chronic cough (if present), topical or systemic estrogen replacement or therapy as indicated. Bowel regularity, facilitated by fiber or stool softeners, may reduce symptoms.

Specific Measures: Pessary therapy, pelvic muscle exercises, surgical repair; limited role for medical therapy.

Diet: No specific dietary changes indicated.

Activity: Avoidance of heavy lifting and straining may slow the rate of progression or risk of recurrence.

Patient Education: Reassurance; American College of Obstetricians and Gynecologists Patient Education Pamphlet AP012 (Pelvic Support Problems).

Drug(s) of Choice

None. (Estrogen, either topically or systemically, is often prescribed to improve tissue tone, reduce irritation, and prepare tissues for surgical or pessary therapy.)

Contraindications: Undiagnosed vaginal bleeding, breast cancer.

FOLLOW-UP

Patient Monitoring: Normal health maintenance.

Prevention/Avoidance: None.

Possible Complications: Laxative abuse/dependence. Vaginal ulceration, bleeding, infection, or pain frequently accompanies complete prolapse.

Expected Outcome: Generally favorable reduction of symptoms may be obtained with a carefully chosen and fitted pessary. Surgical therapy is associated with 95% success in long-term correction of the anatomic defect and the associated symptoms.

MISCELLANEOUS

Pregnancy Considerations: No effect on pregnancy, although pregnancy (and vaginal delivery) may cause or contribute to a worsening of pelvic support problems.

ICD-9-CM Codes: 618.0 (Without uterine prolapse), 618.4 (With uterine prolapse).

REFERENCES

Level I

Paraiso MF, Barber MD, Muir TW, Walters MD: Rectocele repair: a randomized trial of three surgical techniques including graft augmentation. Am J Obstet Gynecol 2006;195:1762.

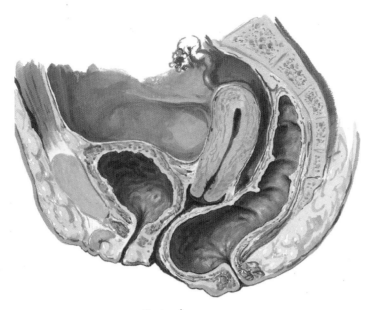

Rectocele

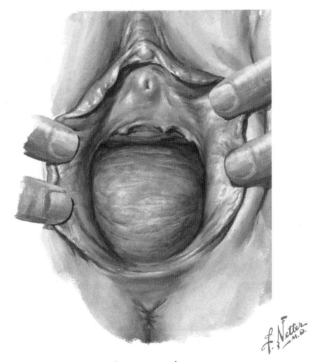

Large rectocele

Sand PK, Koduri S, Lobel RW, et al: Prospective randomized trial of polyglactin 910 mesh to prevent recurrence of cystoceles and rectoceles. Am J Obstet Gynecol 2001;184:1357.

Level II

Cundiff GW, Fenner D: Evaluation and treatment of women with rectocele: focus on associated defecatory and sexual dysfunction. Obstet Gynecol 2004;104:1403.

Level III

American College of Obstetricians and Gynecologists: Pelvic organ prolapse. ACOG Practice Bulletin 79. Obstet Gynecol 2007;109:461.

Bump RC, Mattiasson A, Bø K, et al: The standardization of terminology of female pelvic organ prolapse and pelvic floor dysfunction. Am J Obstet Gynecol 1996;175:10.

Kobashi KC, Leach GE: Pelvic prolapse. J Urol 2000;164:1879.

Lentz GM: Anatomic defects of the abdominal wall and pelvic wall. In Katz VL, Lentz GM, Lobo RA, Gershenson DM: Comprehensive Gynecology, 5th ed. Philadelphia, Mosby/Elsevier, 2007:510.

Monga A: Management of the posterior compartment. BJOG 2004;111:73.

Smith RP: Gynecology in primary care. Baltimore, Williams & Wilkins, 1997:577.

INTRODUCTION

Description: Sarcoma botryoides is a rare form of sarcoma (embryonal rhabdomyosarcoma) generally found in the vagina of young girls. Rarely, these tumors may arise from the cervix. Although the cervical form of sarcoma is histologically similar to the vaginal form, the prognosis for the cervical form is better.

Prevalence: Rare.

Predominant Age: Generally younger than 8 years, two thirds younger than 2, most common neoplasm of the lower genital tract in premenarchal girls.

Genetics: No genetic pattern.

ETIOLOGY AND PATHOGENESIS

Causes: Unknown. Arises in the subepithelial layers of the vagina, often multicentric.

Risk Factors: None known.

CLINICAL CHARACTERISTICS

Signs and Symptoms

- Vaginal bleeding
- Vaginal mass (resembles a cluster of grapes, may be hemorrhagic, myxoid, or both)

DIAGNOSTIC APPROACH

Differential Diagnosis

- Urethral prolapse
- Vaginal polyp (pseudosarcoma botryoides)
- Endodermal sinus tumor (yolk sac tumor)
- Precocious puberty

Associated Conditions: None.

Workup and Evaluation

Laboratory: No specific evaluation indicated.

Imaging: No specific imaging indicated, only that necessary to evaluate tumor location and spread.

Special Tests: Biopsy of the mass.

Diagnostic Procedures: Physical examination, histologic tests.

Pathologic Findings

Tumor is often multicentric with loose myxomatous stroma containing malignant pleomorphic cells and eosinophilic rhabdomyoblasts that have characteristic cross striations (strap cells).

MANAGEMENT AND THERAPY

Nonpharmacologic

General Measures: Evaluation.

Specific Measures: Surgical excision combined with multiagent chemotherapy. Adjunctive radiation therapy has also been advocated but is generally reserved for those with residual disease. (Some recent studies have suggested that surgery can be delayed until after chemotherapy has been given, although long-term data are lacking.)

Diet: No specific dietary changes indicated.

Activity: No restriction.

Drug(s) of Choice

Adjunctive multiagent chemotherapy only.

FOLLOW-UP

Patient Monitoring: Once surgery and chemotherapy have been completed, monitoring for recurrence and general health maintenance.

Prevention/Avoidance: None.

Possible Complications: These are aggressive tumors; dissemination and recurrence are common. Spread is through direct invasion and metastasis to lymph nodes and distant sites (by hematogenous routes). The cause of death is generally by direct local extension.

Expected Outcome: Overall the prognosis is poor. Small series suggest that with the combination of surgical resection and combination chemotherapy, survival in more than 80% may be expected. Among those who survive, normal (eventual) pubertal changes and pregnancy have been reported.

MISCELLANEOUS

Pregnancy Considerations: No effect on pregnancy for those who survive and achieve conception.

ICD-9-CM Codes: M8910/3.

REFERENCES

Level II

Behtash N, Mousavi A, Tehranian A, et al: Embryonal rhabdomyosarcoma of the uterine cervix: case report and review of the literature. Gynecol Oncol 2003;91:452.

Hilgers RD: Pelvic exenteration for vaginal embryonal rhabdomyosarcoma: a review. Obstet Gynecol 1975;45:175.

Mitchell M, Talerman A, Sholl JS, et al: Pseudosarcoma botryoides in pregnancy: report of a case with ultrastructural observations. Obstet Gynecol 1987;70:522.

Level III

Copeland LJ, Gershenson DM, Saul PB, et al: Sarcoma botryoides of the female genital tract. Obstet Gynecol 1985;66:262.

Davos I, Abell MR: Sarcomas of the vagina. Obstet Gynecol 1976;47:342.

Dotters DJ, Katz VL: Malignant diseases of the vagina. In Katz VL, Lentz GM, Lobo RA, Gershenson DM: Comprehensive Gynecology, 5th ed. Philadelphia, Mosby/Elsevier, 2007:808.

Golbang P, Khan A, Scurry J, et al: Cervical sarcoma botryoides and ovarian Sertoli-Leydig cell tumor. Gynecol Oncol 1997;67:102.

Gruessner SE, Omwandho CO, Dreyer T, et al: Management of stage I cervical sarcoma botryoides in childhood and adolescence. Eur J Pediatr 2004;163:452. Epub 2004 Jun 2.

Hilgers RD, Malkasian GD, Soule EH: Embryonal rhabdomyosarcoma (botryoid type) of the vagina. Am J Obstet Gynecol 1970;107:484.

Rutledge F, Sullivan MP: Sarcoma botryoides. Ann N Y Acad Sci 1967;124:694.

Tscherne G: Female genital tract malignancies during puberty. Uterine and cervical malignancies. Ann N Y Acad Sci 1997;816:331.

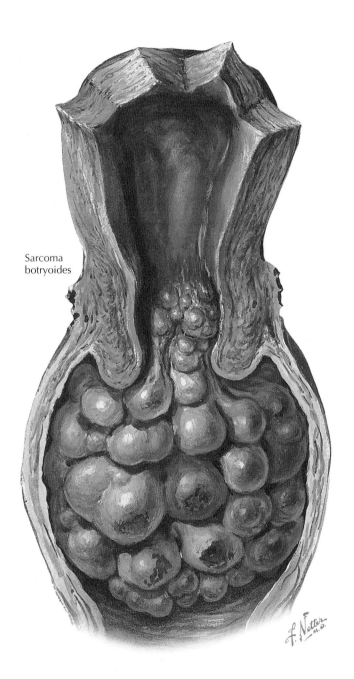

Sarcoma
botryoides

INTRODUCTION

Description: A transverse vaginal septum is a partial or complete obstruction of the vagina generally found at the junction of the upper third and lower two thirds of the vaginal canal. The septum is generally less than 1 cm in thickness and may or may not have a small opening to the upper genital tract. (The location and thickness are highly variable.)

Prevalence: One of 72,000 to 75,000 females.

Predominant Age: Present at birth but generally not diagnosed until puberty.

Genetics: No genetic pattern.

ETIOLOGY AND PATHOGENESIS

Causes: Incomplete canalization of the Müllerian tubercle and sinovaginal bulb.

Risk Factors: Partial septa have been reported in women exposed in utero to diethylstilbestrol (DES).

CLINICAL CHARACTERISTICS

Signs and Symptoms

- Blind, shortened vaginal pouch
- Primary amenorrhea
- Mucocolpos
- Hematocolpos
- Hematometra
- Foul vaginal discharge (with incomplete septum)
- Vaginal/abdominal mass without bulging of the vaginal outlet (hematocolpos and mucocolpos may be associated with urinary tract obstruction if very large)

DIAGNOSTIC APPROACH

Differential Diagnosis

- Vaginal agenesis
- Imperforate hymen

Associated Conditions: Endometriosis, infertility, amenorrhea, hematocolpos, and dyspareunia.

Workup and Evaluation

Laboratory: No evaluation indicated.

Imaging: Ultrasonography may be used to evaluate the presence and condition of the upper genital tract.

Special Tests: None indicated.

Diagnostic Procedures: Pelvic examination.

Pathologic Findings

None.

MANAGEMENT AND THERAPY

Nonpharmacologic

General Measures: Evaluation, reassurance.

Specific Measures: Transverse vaginal septa must be excised surgically. When the septum is thick, recon-struction with skin grafts or flaps may be required. In extreme cases, a neovagina must be surgically created. (Once drainage of the upper tract is obtained, vaginal reconstruction may be delayed to a later date.)

Diet: No specific dietary changes indicated.

Activity: No restriction.

Patient Education: Reassurance, education about possible effects on fertility and sexual function (for most patients there will be little or no effect).

Drug(s) of Choice

None.

FOLLOW-UP

Patient Monitoring: Once a normal vaginal canal has been restored, normal health maintenance. Patients must be monitored for narrowing of the vagina at the level of the removed septum or vaginal reanastomosis.

Prevention/Avoidance: None.

Possible Complications: It is rare, but a mucocolpos can cause serious and life-threatening compression of surrounding organs, leading to hydroureter, hydronephrosis, rectal compression and obstruction, restricted diaphragmatic excursion, compression of the vena cava, and cardiorespiratory failure. Fistulae to the urinary tract may occur. Prolonged obstruction of menstrual outflow is associated with the development of endometriosis and pelvic scarring (often extensive); chronic pelvic pain, dyspareunia, and infertility may result. Pregnancy rates for patients with corrected transverse septa range from 25% to 50% based on location of the septum and series report.

Expected Outcome: With timely diagnosis and treatment, the prognosis is good.

MISCELLANEOUS

Pregnancy Considerations: No effect on pregnancy once pregnancy is achieved. Pregnancy success is greatest with septa that are lower in the vagina and repaired early. Based on the extent of vaginal reconstruction performed and the degree of subsequent scarring, cesarean delivery may be elected.

ICD-9-CM Codes: 752.49.

REFERENCES

Level II

McKusick VA, Weiboecher RG, Gragg GW: Recessive inheritance of a congenital malformation syndrome. JAMA 1968; 204:113.

Rock JA, Zacur HA, Dlugi AM, et al: Pregnancy success following surgical correction of imperforate hymen and complete transverse vaginal septum. Obstet Gynecol 1982;59:448.

Level III

American College of Obstetricians and Gynecologists: Vaginal agenesis: diagnosis, management, and routine care. ACOG Committee Opinion 355. Obstet Gynecol 2006;108:1605.

Transverse Vaginal Septum

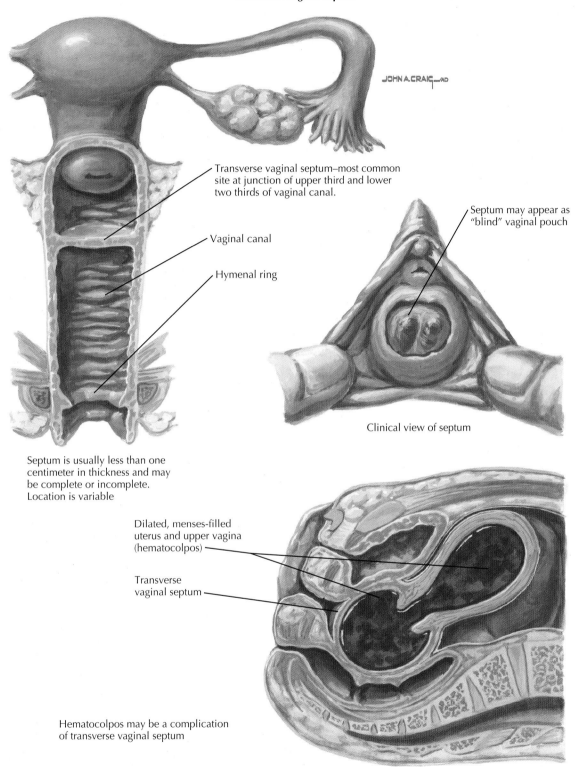

Transverse vaginal septum–most common site at junction of upper third and lower two thirds of vaginal canal.

Vaginal canal

Hymenal ring

Septum may appear as "blind" vaginal pouch

Clinical view of septum

Septum is usually less than one centimeter in thickness and may be complete or incomplete. Location is variable

Dilated, menses-filled uterus and upper vagina (hematocolpos)

Transverse vaginal septum

Hematocolpos may be a complication of transverse vaginal septum

JOHN A. CRAIG—AD

Brenner P, Sedlis A, Cooperman H: Complete imperforate transverse vaginal septum. Obstet Gynecol 1965;25:135.

Katz VL, Lentz GM: Congenital abnormalities of the female reproductive tract. In Katz VL, Lentz GM, Lobo RA, Gershenson DM: Comprehensive Gynecology, 5th ed. Philadelphia, Mosby/Elsevier, 2007:248.

Lilford RJ, Morton K, Dewhurst J: The diagnosis and management of the imperforate vaginal membrane in the pre-pubertal child. Pediatr Adolesc Gynecol 1983;1:115.

Lopez C, Balogun M, Ganesan R, Olliff JF: MRI of vaginal conditions. Clin Radiol 2005;60:648.

McKusick VA: Transverse vaginal septum (hydrometrocolpos). Birth Defects 1971;7:326.

INTRODUCTION

Description: Cystic masses in the vaginal wall are uncommon and may arise from either congenital (Gartner's duct cysts) or acquired (epithelial inclusion cysts) processes.

Prevalence: One of 200 women.

Predominant Age: Generally from adolescence to middle reproductive years.

Genetics: No genetic pattern.

ETIOLOGY AND PATHOGENESIS

Causes: Congenital (Gartner's duct cyst or remnant, generally found in the anterior lateral vaginal wall), structural (urethral diverticulum, loss of vaginal wall support), acquired (inclusion cyst, >50% of cysts).

Risk Factors: Episiotomy or obstetric laceration, gynecologic surgery.

CLINICAL CHARACTERISTICS

Signs and Symptoms

- Asymptomatic
- May be associated with a sense of fullness
- Dyspareunia (uncommon)
- Difficulty with tampon insertion or retention
- Cystic mass lesion (1 to 5 cm) found generally in the lateral vaginal wall (congenital) or in midline posteriorly (acquired)

DIAGNOSTIC APPROACH

Differential Diagnosis

- Urethral diverticulum
- Cystocele
- Urethrocele
- Rectocele
- Bartholin's gland cyst
- Vaginal adenosis
- Vaginal endometriosis
- Perirectal abscess
- Vaginal fibromyoma

Associated Conditions: Slightly higher rate of upper genital tract malformations when embryonic remnants persist.

Workup and Evaluation

Laboratory: No evaluation indicated.

Imaging: No imaging indicated.

Special Tests: Vaginal adenosis may be excluded by staining with Lugol's solution (adenosis will not stain).

Diagnostic Procedures: History and physical examination.

Pathologic Findings

Most embryonic cysts are lined by cuboidal epithelium. Stratified epithelium suggests an inclusion (acquired) cyst.

MANAGEMENT AND THERAPY

Nonpharmacologic

General Measures: Evaluation and reassurance.

Specific Measures: Surgical excision if the mass is symptomatic or its cause is uncertain; otherwise no therapy is required.

Diet: No specific dietary changes indicated.

Activity: No restriction.

Patient Education: Reassurance; American College of Obstetricians and Gynecologists Patient Education Pamphlet AP012 (Pelvic Support Problems).

Drug(s) of Choice

None.

FOLLOW-UP

Patient Monitoring: Normal health maintenance.

Prevention/Avoidance: None.

Possible Complications: Mechanical irritation or interference with intercourse or childbirth (rare), infection (rare).

Expected Outcome: Some care must be used in the excision of large cysts so that vaginal scarring and stenosis do not occur; otherwise, surgical therapy should be successful.

MISCELLANEOUS

Pregnancy Considerations: No effect on pregnancy.

ICD-9-CM Codes: 623.8 (Inclusion), 752.41 (Embryonal).

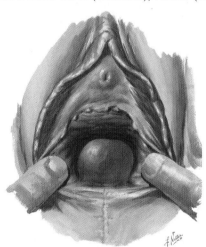

Inclusion cyst

REFERENCES

Level II

Dwyer PL, Rosamilia A: Congenital urogenital anomalies that are associated with the persistence of Gartner's duct: a review. Am J Obstet Gynecol 2006;195:354. Epub 2006 Apr 21.

Eilber KS, Raz S: Benign cystic lesions of the vagina: a literature review. J Urol 2003;170:717.

Junaid TA, Thomas SM: Cysts of the vulva and vagina: a comparative study. Int J Gynaecol Obstet 1981;19:239.

Level III

Deppisch LM: Cysts of the vagina. Obstet Gynecol 1975;45:623.

Dmochowski RR, Ganabathi K, Zimmern PE, Leach GE: Benign female periurethral masses. J Urol 1994;152:1943.

Robboy SJ, Ross JS, Prat J, et al: Urogenital sinus origin of mucinous and ciliated cysts of the vulva. Obstet Gynecol 1978;51:347.

90

Vaginal Dryness

INTRODUCTION

Description: Vaginal dryness is characterized by loss of normal vaginal moisture resulting in irritation, itching, or pain with intercourse. This loss may result from alterations in vaginal physiology caused by infection or the loss of estrogen stimulation (atrophic change). This may also occur situationally because of inadequate or inappropriate sexual stimulation, sexual phobia, or pain.

Prevalence: Common in menopausal women not receiving estrogen replacement therapy. Estimated to affect one in five women around the time of menopause and more than half of women after 5 years without normal estrogen levels.

Predominant Age: Postmenopausal.

Genetics: No genetic pattern.

ETIOLOGY AND PATHOGENESIS

Causes: Loss of estrogen stimulation (menopause), vaginitis, arousal disorders.

Risk Factors: Menopause without estrogen replacement, vaginal infection.

CLINICAL CHARACTERISTICS

Signs and Symptoms

- Sensation of vaginal dryness
- Vaginal itching or irritation
- Insertional dyspareunia
- Dry, inflamed vaginal tissues seen on pelvic examination
- Loss of normal vaginal rugae

DIAGNOSTIC APPROACH

Differential Diagnosis

- Lichen sclerosus
- Vaginitis
- Vulvar vestibulitis
- Libidinal dysfunction/arousal disorders

Associated Conditions: Dyspareunia, vaginitis, and menopause.

Workup and Evaluation

Laboratory: Microscopic examination of vaginal secretions if infection is suspected.

Imaging: No imaging indicated.

Special Tests: A vaginal maturation index may confirm atrophic change but is seldom required.

Diagnostic Procedures: History and physical examination.

Pathologic Findings

Postmenopausal: Thinned, pale vaginal epithelium with loss of rugations, low moisture content, increased pH (usually >5), inflammation and small petechiae. **Infection:** based on organism present.

MANAGEMENT AND THERAPY

Nonpharmacologic

General Measures: Evaluation, topical moisturizers or lubricants (as needed or long acting).

Specific Measures: Estrogen replacement therapy or treatment of vaginal infection (when appropriate). Counseling regarding sexuality, arousal, foreplay, and coital technique (if needed).

Diet: No specific dietary changes indicated.

Activity: No restriction.

Patient Education: Reassurance; American College of Obstetricians and Gynecologists Patient Education Pamphlet AP047 (The Menopause Years), AP066 (Hormone Replacement Therapy), AP028 (Vaginitis: Causes and Treatment), AP020 (Pain During Intercourse).

Drug(s) of Choice

Estrogen replacement therapy when appropriate (see "Menopause").

Water-soluble lubricants for intercourse.

Long-acting emollients (Replens, etc.).

Contraindications: Known or suspected allergy or intolerance to any agent.

Precautions: Petroleum-based products (e.g., Vaseline) are difficult to remove and may lead to additional irritation.

FOLLOW-UP

Patient Monitoring: Normal health maintenance.

Prevention/Avoidance: Estrogen replacement after menopause.

Possible Complications: Vaginal lacerations and secondary infection, vulvar excoriations, sexual dysfunction.

Expected Outcome: Generally good results with topical or systemic therapy for estrogen loss. Good response to therapy for vaginitis.

MISCELLANEOUS

Pregnancy Considerations: No effect on pregnancy (generally not an issue).

ICD-9-CM Codes: Based on cause.

REFERENCES

Level I

Barnabei VM, Cochrane BB, Aragaki AK, et al; Women's Health Initiative Investigators: Menopausal symptoms and treatment-related effects of estrogen and progestin in the Women's Health Initiative. Obstet Gynecol 2005;105:1063.

Loprinzi CL, Abu-Ghazaleh S, Sloan JA, et al: Phase III randomized double-blind study to evaluate the efficacy of a polycarbophil-based vaginal moisturizer in women with breast cancer. J Clin Oncol 1997;15:969.

Level II

Ayton RA, Darling GM, Murkies AL, et al: A comparative study of safety and efficacy of continuous low dose oestradiol released from

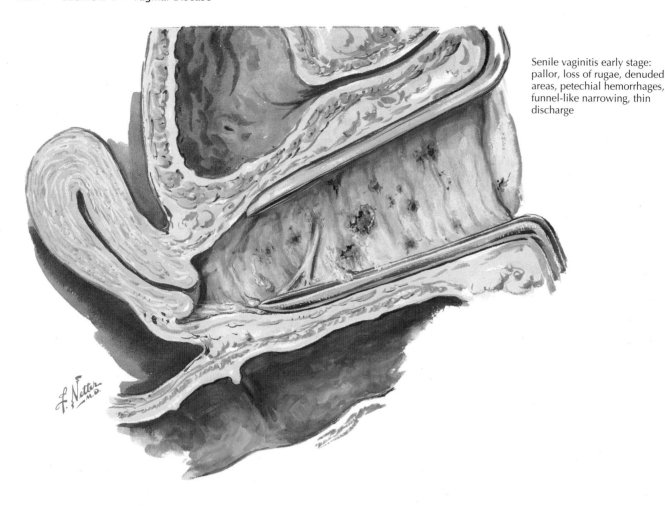

Senile vaginitis early stage: pallor, loss of rugae, denuded areas, petechial hemorrhages, funnel-like narrowing, thin discharge

a vaginal ring compared with conjugated equine oestrogen vaginal cream in the treatment of postmenopausal urogenital atrophy. Br J Obstet Gynaecol 1996;103:351.

Barnabei VM, Grady D, Stovall DW, et al: Menopausal symptoms in older women and the effects of treatment with hormone therapy. Obstet Gynecol 2002;100:1209.

Brown JS, Vittinghoff E, Kanaya AM, et al; Heart and Estrogen/Progestin Replacement Study Research Group: Urinary tract infections in postmenopausal women: effect of hormone therapy and risk factors. Obstet Gynecol 2001;98:1045.

Bygdeman M, Swahn ML: Replens versus dienoestrol cream in the symptomatic treatment of vaginal atrophy in postmenopausal women. Maturitas 1996;23:259.

Chompootaweep S, Nunthapisud P, Trivijitsilp P, et al: The use of two estrogen preparations (a combined contraceptive pill versus conjugated estrogen cream) intravaginally to treat urogenital symptoms in postmenopausal Thai women: a comparative study. Clin Pharmacol Ther 1998;64:204.

Woods NF, Mitchell ES: Symptoms during the perimenopause: prevalence, severity, trajectory, and significance in women's lives. Am J Med 2005;118:14.

Level III

American College of Obstetricians and Gynecologists: Use of botanicals for management of menopausal symptoms. ACOG Practice Bulletin 28. Washington, DC, ACOG, 2001.

American College of Obstetricians and Gynecologists: Vaginitis. ACOG Practice Bulletin 72. Obstet Gynecol 2006;107:1195.

Avis NE, Brockwell S, Colvin A: A universal menopausal syndrome? Am J Med 2005;118:37.

Coope J: Hormonal and non-hormonal interventions for menopausal symptoms. Maturitas 1996;23:159.

Hickey M, Davis SR, Sturdee DW: Treatment of menopausal symptoms: what shall we do now? Lancet 2005;366:409.

Lobo RA: Menopause. In Katz VL, Lentz GM, Lobo RA, Gershenson DM: Comprehensive Gynecology, 5th ed. Philadelphia, Mosby/Elsevier, 2007:1050.

Van Voorhis BJ: Genitourinary symptoms in the menopausal transition. Am J Med. 2005;118:47.

91

Vaginal Lacerations

INTRODUCTION

Description: Nonobstetric lacerations of the vaginal wall or introitus are most often the result of sexual trauma (80%, consensual or otherwise).

Prevalence: Uncommon, but specific prevalence is unknown.

Predominant Age: Reproductive (most common at younger than age 25).

Genetics: No genetic pattern.

ETIOLOGY AND PATHOGENESIS

Causes: Intercourse (80%), saddle or water skiing injury, sexual assault, penetration by foreign objects.

Risk Factors: Virginity, vaginismus, postpartum and postmenopausal vaginal atrophy, hysterectomy, alcohol or other drug use.

CLINICAL CHARACTERISTICS

Signs and Symptoms

- Vaginal bleeding (may be profuse and prolonged)
- Acute pain during intercourse (25%, lacerations of the distal vagina or introitus)
- Persistent pain after intercourse (the location of the pain is somewhat dependent on the location of the laceration)

DIAGNOSTIC APPROACH

Differential Diagnosis

- Cervical polyp (as source of bleeding)
- Menstrual bleeding
- Threatened abortion
- Granulation tissue in healing incision (episiotomy, other vaginal surgery)
- Sexual abuse/rape

Associated Conditions: Vaginal atrophy, sexual dysfunction, alcohol or drug use/abuse.

Workup and Evaluation

Laboratory: Complete blood count.

Imaging: No imaging indicated.

Special Tests: None indicated.

Diagnostic Procedures: History and physical examination (history is often misleading or false).

Pathologic Findings

The most common site of coital laceration is the posterior fornix, followed by the right and left fornices.

MANAGEMENT AND THERAPY

Nonpharmacologic

General Measures: Rapid assessment and hemodynamic stabilization (when appropriate).

Specific Measures: Surgical closure of the laceration, evaluation of the integrity of the urinary and gastrointestinal tract; may include exploratory laparotomy or laparoscopy in cases of evisceration or peritoneal breach.

Diet: No specific dietary changes indicated.

Activity: Pelvic rest (no tampons, douches, or intercourse) until healing has occurred.

Patient Education: Reassurance; American College of Obstetricians and Gynecologists Patient Education Pamphlet AP083 (Domestic Violence), AP020 (Pain During Intercourse).

Drug(s) of Choice

Local or general anesthesia for surgical repair.

Treatment with an antibiotic is generally not required, except if a peritoneal breach is present.

FOLLOW-UP

Patient Monitoring: Normal health maintenance after healing has been completed.

Prevention/Avoidance: Avoidance of alcohol or drug use, careful consensual intercourse, adequate vaginal lubrication.

Possible Complications: Vaginal evisceration, excessive blood loss. In rare cases, death has been reported.

Expected Outcome: Generally good healing; the risk of recurrence is based on cause.

MISCELLANEOUS

Pregnancy Considerations: No effect on pregnancy unless the health or safety of the mother is compromised.

ICD-9-CM Codes: Based on location and cause.

REFERENCES

Level I
Garcia V, Rogers RG, Kim SS, et al: Primary repair of obstetric anal sphincter laceration: a randomized trial of two surgical techniques. Am J Obstet Gynecol 2005;192:1697.

Level II
Haefner HK, Andersen F, Johnson MP: Vaginal laceration following a jet-ski accident. Obstet Gynecol 1991;78:986.
Hartmann K, Viswanathan M, Palmieri R, et al: Outcomes of routine episiotomy: a systematic review. JAMA 2005;293:2141.
McCann J, Miyamoto S, Boyle C, Rogers K: Healing of hymenal injuries in prepubertal and adolescent girls: a descriptive study. Pediatrics 2007;119:e1094. Epub 2007 Apr 9.
Niv J, Lessing JB, Hartuv J, Peyser MR: Vaginal injury resulting from sliding down a water chute. Am J Obstet Gynecol 1992; 166:930.
Smith NC, Van Coeverden de Groot HA, Gunston KD: Coital injuries of the vagina in nonvirginal patients. S Afr Med J 1983; 64:746.

Level III
Ahnaimugan S, Asuen MI: Coital laceration of the vagina. Aust N Z J Obstet Gynaecol 1980;20:180.
American College of Obstetricians and Gynecologists: Episiotomy. ACOG Practice Bulletin 71. Obstet Gynecol 2006; 107:957.

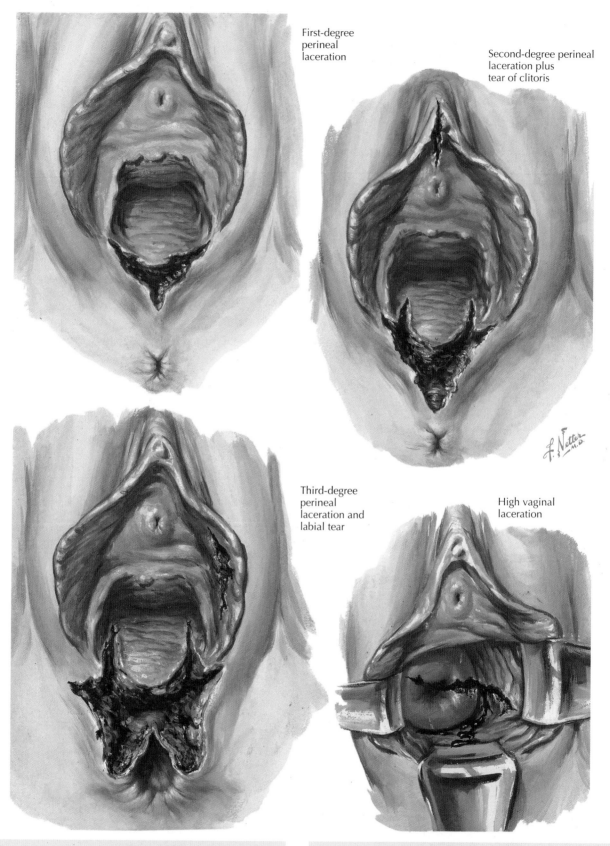

First-degree
perineal
laceration

Second-degree perineal
laceration plus
tear of clitoris

Third-degree
perineal
laceration and
labial tear

High vaginal
laceration

Barrett KF, Bledsoe S, Greer BE, Droegemueller W: Tampon-
    induced vaginal or cervical ulceration. Am J Obstet Gynecol
    1977;127:332.
Friedel W, Kaiser IH: Vaginal evisceration. Obstet Gynecol
    1975;45:315.

Katz VL: Benign gynecologic lesions. In Katz VL, Lentz GM, Lobo
    RA, Gershenson DM: Comprehensive Gynecology, 5th ed. Phila-
    delphia, Mosby/Elsevier, 2007:436.
Rafla N: Vaginismus and vaginal tears. Am J Obstet Gynecol
    1988;158:1043.

INTRODUCTION

Description: Vaginal prolapse is loss of the normal support mechanism, resulting in descent of the vaginal wall down the vaginal canal. In the extreme, this may result in the vagina becoming everted beyond the vulva to a position outside the body. Vaginal prolapse is generally found only after hysterectomy and is a special form of enterocele.

Prevalence: Depends on the severity of the original defect, type of surgery originally performed and other risk factors (estimated to be between 0.1% to 18.2% of patients who have had a hysterectomy).

Predominant Age: Late reproductive and beyond.

Genetics: No genetic pattern.

ETIOLOGY AND PATHOGENESIS

Causes: Loss of normal structural support because of trauma (childbirth), surgery, chronic intra-abdominal pressure elevation (such as obesity, chronic cough, or heavy lifting), or intrinsic weakness. A recurrence within 1 to 2 years of surgery is considered a failure of technique.

Risk Factors: Birth trauma, chronic intra-abdominal pressure elevation (such as obesity, chronic cough, or heavy lifting), intrinsic tissue weakness, or atrophic changes resulting from estrogen loss.

CLINICAL CHARACTERISTICS

Signs and Symptoms

- Pelvic pressure or heaviness, backache
- Mass or protrusion at the vaginal entrance
- New onset or paradoxical resolution of urinary incontinence

DIAGNOSTIC APPROACH

Differential Diagnosis

- Cystocele
- Urethrocele
- Rectocele
- Bartholin's cyst
- Vaginal cyst or tumor

Associated Conditions: Urinary incontinence, pelvic pain, dyspareunia, intermenstrual or postmenopausal bleeding. A cystourethrocele, rectocele, and/or enterocele is almost always present when complete prolapse has occurred.

Workup and Evaluation

Laboratory: No evaluation indicated.

Imaging: No imaging indicated.

Special Tests: Urodynamics testing may be considered if there is altered voiding or continence.

Diagnostic Procedures: History and physical examination.

Pathologic Findings

Tissue change common because of mechanical trauma and desiccation.

MANAGEMENT AND THERAPY

Nonpharmacologic

General Measures: Weight reduction, modification of activity (lifting); address factors such as chronic cough.

Specific Measures: Pessary therapy, surgical repair (culdoplasty, plication of the uterosacral ligaments, sacrospinous ligament fixation, mesh-based support, or colpocleisis). When surgical repair is undertaken, attention must also focus on correction of any anterior or posterior vaginal wall support problems.

Diet: No specific dietary changes indicated.

Activity: No restriction, although heavy lifting or strenuous activities may predispose to the development or recurrence of prolapse.

Patient Education: Reassurance; American College of Obstetricians and Gynecologists Patient Education Pamphlet AP012 (Pelvic Support Problems), AP081 (Urinary Incontinence).

Drug(s) of Choice

Estrogen replacement therapy (for postmenopausal patients) improves tissue tone and healing and is often prescribed before surgical repair or as an adjunct to pessary therapy.

Contraindications: Estrogen therapy should not be used if undiagnosed vaginal bleeding is present.

FOLLOW-UP

Patient Monitoring: Normal health maintenance. If a pessary is used, frequent follow-up (both initially and long term) is required.

Prevention/Avoidance: Maintenance of normal weight, avoidance of known (modifiable) risk factors.

Possible Complications: Thickening or ulceration of the vaginal tissues, urinary incontinence, kinking of the ureters, and obstipation. Complications of surgical repair include intraoperative hemorrhage, nerve damage (sciatic), damage to the rectum, damage to the ureters, postoperative infection, and complications of anesthesia.

Expected Outcome: Vaginal prolapse tends to worsen with time. If uncorrected, complete prolapse is associated with vaginal skin changes, ulceration, and bleeding.

MISCELLANEOUS

ICD-9-CM Codes: 618.0, 618.5 (Vaginal vault prolapse after hysterectomy).

Vaginal Prolapse

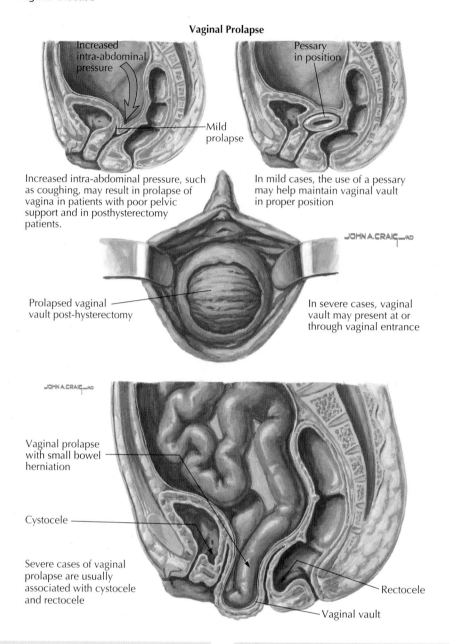

Increased intra-abdominal pressure, such as coughing, may result in prolapse of vagina in patients with poor pelvic support and in posthysterectomy patients.

In mild cases, the use of a pessary may help maintain vaginal vault in proper position

Prolapsed vaginal vault post-hysterectomy

In severe cases, vaginal vault may present at or through vaginal entrance

Vaginal prolapse with small bowel herniation

Cystocele

Severe cases of vaginal prolapse are usually associated with cystocele and rectocele

Rectocele

Vaginal vault

REFERENCES

Level I

Cundiff GW, Amundsen CL, Bent AE, et al: The PESSRI study: symptom relief outcomes of a randomized crossover trial of the ring and Gellhorn pessaries. Am J Obstet Gynecol 2007;196:405.e1.

Meschia M, Pifarotti P, Bernasconi F, et al: Porcine skin collagen implants to prevent anterior vaginal wall prolapse recurrence: a multicenter, randomized study. J Urol 2007;177:192.

Paraiso MF, Barber MD, Muir TW, Walters MD: Rectocele repair: a randomized trial of three surgical techniques including graft augmentation. Am J Obstet Gynecol 2006;195:1762.

Roovers JP, van der Vaart CH, van der Bom JG, et al: A randomised controlled trial comparing abdominal and vaginal prolapse surgery: effects on urogenital function. BJOG 2004;111:50.

Level II

Kahn MA, Breitkopf CR, Valley MT, et al: Pelvic Organ Support Study (POSST) and bowel symptoms: straining at stool is associated with perineal and anterior vaginal descent in a general gynecologic population. Am J Obstet Gynecol 2005;192:1516.

Morley GW, Delancey JOL: Sacrospinous ligament fixation for eversion of vagina. Am J Obstet Gynecol 1988;158:872.

Nichols DH: Sacrospinous fixation for massive eversion of vagina. Am J Obstet Gynecol 1982;142:901.

Swift S, Woodman P, O'Boyle A, et al: Pelvic Organ Support Study (POSST): the distribution, clinical definition, and epidemiologic condition of pelvic organ support defects. Am J Obstet Gynecol 2005;192:795.

Level III

American College of Obstetricians and Gynecologists: Pelvic organ prolapse. ACOG Practice Bulletin 79. Obstet Gynecol 2007;109:461.

Birnbaum SJ: Rational therapy for the prolapsed vagina. Am J Obstet Gynecol 1973;115:411.

Cutner AS, Elneil S: The vaginal vault. BJOG 2004;111:79.

Delancey JOL: Anatomic aspects of vaginal eversion after hysterectomy. Am J Obstet Gynecol 1992;166:1717.

Lentz GM: Anatomic defects of the abdominal wall and pelvic wall. In Katz VL, Lentz GM, Lobo RA, Gershenson DM: Comprehensive Gynecology, 5th ed. Philadelphia, Mosby/Elsevier, 2007:517.

Percy NM, Perl JI: Total colpectomy. Surg Gynecol Obstet 1961;113:174.

INTRODUCTION

Description: Atrophic vaginitis is characterized by degeneration (atrophy) of vaginal tissues caused by the loss of ovarian steroids.

Prevalence: Occurs in 100% of postmenopausal women who do not receive estrogen replacement.

Predominant Age: 50+ (or after surgical menopause).

Genetics: No genetic pattern.

ETIOLOGY AND PATHOGENESIS

Causes: Loss of estrogen stimulation as a result of surgery, chemotherapy (alkylating agents), radiation, or natural cessation of ovarian function (menopause).

Risk Factors: Loss of ovarian function because of age, chemotherapy, radiation, or surgery.

CLINICAL CHARACTERISTICS

Signs and Symptoms

- Vaginal dryness, burning, and itching
- Pain or bleeding with intercourse (may be associated with lacerations)
- Thin, shiny, red epithelium with a smooth surface (loss of rugae)

DIAGNOSTIC APPROACH

Differential Diagnosis

- Vaginal infections
- Vulvitis (including dermatologic causes)
- Chemical vaginitis
- Changes after radiation exposure
- Lichen sclerosus

Associated Conditions: Menopause, dyspareunia, vulvodynia, atrophic vulvitis, urinary frequency, urinary urgency, urgency incontinence, increased risk of other menopause-related conditions including osteoporosis, increased risk of cardiovascular disease, hot flashes and flushes, or sleep disturbances.

Workup and Evaluation

Laboratory: No evaluation indicated.

Imaging: No imaging indicated.

Special Tests: A vaginal maturation index may be performed but is generally not required.

Diagnostic Procedures: History and clinical inspection generally sufficient.

Pathologic Findings

Thinned epithelium with loss of rugae and rete pegs (on biopsy).

MANAGEMENT AND THERAPY

Nonpharmacologic

General Measures: Vaginal moisturizers.

Specific Measures: Topical or systemic estrogen (estrogen/progestin) therapy.

Diet: No specific dietary changes indicated.

Activity: No restriction, supplemental lubricants for intercourse (if necessary).

Patient Education: Reassurance; American College of Obstetricians and Gynecologists Patient Education Pamphlet AP047 (The Menopause Years), AP066 (Hormone Replacement Therapy), AP028 (Vaginitis: Causes and Treatments).

Drug(s) of Choice

(Most common drug dosages shown. Note: Because of concerns raised by the Women's Health Initiative [WHI] study, topical estrogen therapy has become preferred over oral therapy unless otherwise indicated. This does not avoid systemic absorption, which may actually be increased in the presence of significant atrophy; see below.)

Topical—17β-estradiol (transdermal) (0.05 to 0.10 μg/day), conjugated equine estrogens (0.625 mg/g), estradiol (0.1 mg/g), estropipate (1.5 mg/g).

Oral estrogens—conjugated equine estrogens (0.625 to 1.25 mg/day), diethylstilbestrol, esterified estrogens (0.625 to 1.25 mg/day), ethinyl estradiol (0.05 mg/day), micronized estradiol (0.5 to 1 mg/day), piperazine estrone sulfate, estropipate, quinestrol.

Injectable estrogens—conjugated equine estrogens, estradiol benzoate, estradiol cypionate, estradiol valerate (oil), estradiol valerate (oil), estrone (aqueous), ethinyl estradiol, polyestradiol phosphate.

Contraindications (Systemic Therapy): Active liver disease, carcinoma of the breast (current), chronic liver damage (impaired function), known sensitivity to topical vehicles, endometrial carcinoma (current), recent thrombosis (with or without emboli), unexplained vaginal bleeding.

Precautions: Up to 25% of estrogen placed in the vagina may be absorbed into the circulation. This amount may be even greater for patients with atrophic changes. Continuous estrogen exposure without periodic or concomitant progestins increases the risk of endometrial carcinoma 6-fold to 8-fold when the uterus is present.

Interactions: See individual agents.

Alternative Drugs

Topical moisturizers.

FOLLOW-UP

Patient Monitoring: Normal health maintenance. Patients may be at slightly greater risk for vaginal infections or trauma.

Prevention/Avoidance: Estrogen replacement therapy at menopause.

Possible Complications: Reduced resistance to infection, dyspareunia, and traumatic injury during intercourse.

Expected Outcome: Reversal of symptoms, reestablishment of normal physiology.

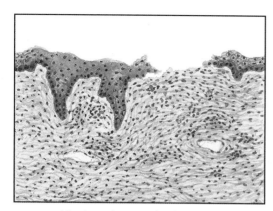

Histology of vagina after the menopause

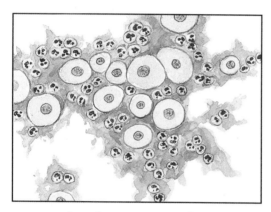

Smear from postmenopausal vagina

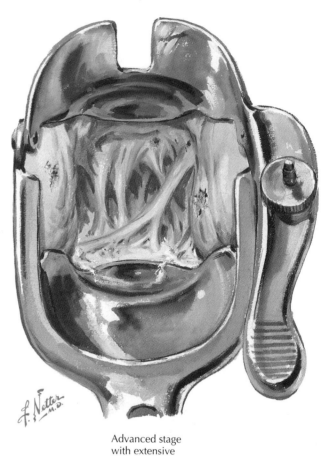

Advanced stage
with extensive
adhesions

MISCELLANEOUS

Pregnancy Considerations: Menopause is associated with the loss of fertility.

ICD-9-CM Codes: 627.3 (Postmenopausal atrophic vaginitis).

REFERENCES

Level I

Barnabei VM, Cochrane BB, Aragaki AK, et al; Women's Health Initiative Investigators: Menopausal symptoms and treatment-related effects of estrogen and progestin in the Women's Health Initiative. Obstet Gynecol 2005;105:1063.

Parsons A, Merritt D, Rosen A, et al; Study Groups on the Effects of Raloxifene HCI With Low-Dose Premarin Vaginal Cream. Effect of raloxifene on the response to conjugated estrogen vaginal cream or nonhormonal moisturizers in postmenopausal vaginal atrophy. Obstet Gynecol 2003;101:346.

Simon JA, Bouchard C, Waldbaum A, et al: Low dose of transdermal estradiol gel for treatment of symptomatic postmenopausal women: a randomized controlled trial. Obstet Gynecol 2007;109:588.

Speroff L: Efficacy and tolerability of a novel estradiol vaginal ring for relief of menopausal symptoms. Obstet Gynecol 2003;102:823.

Level II

Ayton RA, Darling GM, Murkies AL, et al: A comparative study of safety and efficacy of continuous low dose oestradiol released from a vaginal ring compared with conjugated equine oestrogen vaginal cream in the treatment of postmenopausal urogenital atrophy. Br J Obstet Gynaecol. 1996;103:351.

Barnabei VM, Grady D, Stovall DW, et al: Menopausal symptoms in older women and the effects of treatment with hormone therapy. Obstet Gynecol 2002;100:1209.

Woods NF, Mitchell ES: Symptoms during the perimenopause: prevalence, severity, trajectory, and significance in women's lives. Am J Med 2005;118:14.

Level III

American College of Obstetricians and Gynecologists: Use of botanicals for management of menopausal symptoms. ACOG Practice Bulletin 28. Washington, DC, ACOG, 2001.

American College of Obstetricians and Gynecologists: Vaginitis. ACOG Practice Bulletin 72. Obstet Gynecol 2006;107:1195.

Avis NE, Brockwell S, Colvin A: A universal menopausal syndrome? Am J Med 2005;118:37.

Butler RN, Lewis MI, Hoffman E, Whitehead ED: Love and sex after 60: how to evaluate and treat the sexually active woman. Geriatrics 1994;49:33.

Coope J: Hormonal and non-hormonal interventions for menopausal symptoms. Maturitas 1996;23:159.

Hickey M, Davis SR, Sturdee DW: Treatment of menopausal symptoms: what shall we do now? Lancet 2005;366:409.

Jones KP: Estrogen replacement therapy. Clin Obstet Gynecol 1992;35:854.

Lobo RA: Menopause. In Katz VL, Lentz GM, Lobo RA, Gershenson DM: Comprehensive Gynecology, 5th ed. Philadelphia, Mosby/Elsevier, 2007:1050.

Van Voorhis BJ: Genitourinary symptoms in the menopausal transition. Am J Med 2005;118:47.

Vaginitis: Bacterial (Nonspecific) and Bacterial Vaginosis

INTRODUCTION

Description: Bacterial vaginitis is a vaginal infection caused by an overgrowth of normal or pathogenic bacteria that results in irritation, inflammation, and clinical symptoms. Bacterial vaginosis is a change in vaginal ecology caused by an overgrowth of anaerobic bacteria, often with an absence of clinical symptoms. It should be noted that bacterial vaginosis does not engender an inflammatory response and is therefore technically not a type of vaginitis.

Prevalence: Roughly 6 million cases per year, 50% of "vaginal infections."

Predominant Age: 15 to 50 (may occur at any age).

Genetics: No genetic pattern.

ETIOLOGY AND PATHOGENESIS

Causes: Bacterial vaginitis—overgrowth of normal or pathologic bacteria with an inflammatory response (which distinguishes this from bacterial vaginosis). Bacterial vaginosis—a polymicrobial process that involves the loss of normal lactobacilli, an increase in anaerobic bacteria (especially *Gardnerella vaginalis*, *Bacteroides* sp., *Peptococcus* sp., and *Mobiluncus* sp.), and a change in the chemical composition of the vaginal secretions. There is a 1000-fold increase in the number of bacteria present and a 1000:1 anaerobic/aerobic bacteria ratio (normal 5:1), high levels of mucinases; phospholipase A_2, lipases, proteases, arachidonic acid, and prostaglandins are all present. Amines (cadaverine and putrescine) are made through bacterial decarboxylation of arginine and lysine. These amines are more volatile at an alkaline pH, such as that created by the addition of 10% KOH (potassium hydroxide) or semen (roughly a pH of 7), giving rise to the odor found with the "whiff test" or reported by these patients after intercourse.

Risk Factors: Systemic processes—diabetes, pregnancy, and debilitating disease. Anything that alters the normal vaginal flora—smoking, numbers of sexual partners, vaginal contraceptives used, some forms of sexual expression such as oral sex, antibiotic use, hygiene practices and douching, menstruation, and immunologic status.

CLINICAL CHARACTERISTICS

Signs and Symptoms

Bacterial Vaginitis

* Vulvar burning or irritation
* Increased discharge (often with odor)
* Dysuria
* Dyspareunia
* Edema or erythema of the vulva

Bacterial Vaginosis

* Asymptomatic (20% to 50% of patients)
* Increased discharge
* Vaginal odor (often more pronounced after intercourse)
* Vulvar burning or irritation

Uncommon

* Dysuria
* Dyspareunia
* Edema or erythema of the vulva

DIAGNOSTIC APPROACH

Differential Diagnosis

* Chlamydial cervicitis
* Gonococcal cervicitis
* *Trichomonas vaginalis* infection
* Vaginal candidiasis

Associated Conditions: Other vaginal or sexually transmitted infections, cervicitis, and vulvitis. Ascending infections including endometritis, pelvic inflammatory disease, postoperative vaginal cuff cellulitis, preterm rupture of the membranes and endomyometritis, increased early pregnancy loss, and decreased success with in vitro fertilization.

Workup and Evaluation

Laboratory: Culture or monoclonal antibody staining may be obtained to evaluate other causes but are seldom necessary. Evaluation for concomitant sexually transmitted infections should be considered.

Imaging: No imaging indicated.

Special Tests: Vaginal pH 5 to 5.5, "whiff" test—the addition of 10% potassium hydroxide to vaginal secretions to liberate volatile amines, causing a "fishy" odor (bacterial vaginosis).

Diagnostic Procedures: Physical examination, microscopic examination of vaginal secretions in normal saline. For bacterial vaginosis, the diagnosis requires three of the following: homogeneous discharge, pH 5 to 5.5, clue cells (>20%), positive "whiff" test. Commercial tests (such as for proline iminopeptidase activity) exist but are generally not necessary to establish the diagnosis.

Pathologic Findings

Increased white blood cells and bacteria when vaginal secretions are viewed under normal saline suggest vaginitis. Clue cells may be present but are often absent in vaginitis. For bacterial vaginosis, clue cells must represent 20% or more of epithelial cells seen.

MANAGEMENT AND THERAPY

Nonpharmacologic

General Measures: Perineal hygiene, education regarding sexually transmitted infections.

Specific Measures: Medical therapy, vaginal acidification.

Diet: No specific dietary changes indicated.

Activity: No restriction.

Patient Education: Reassurance; American College of Obstetricians and Gynecologists Patient Education Pamphlet AP028 (Vaginitis: Causes and Treatments),

AP009 (How to Prevent Sexually Transmitted Diseases).

Drug(s) of Choice

Oral—metronidazole (Flagyl, Protostat) 500 mg twice daily for 7 days (90% to 100% cure), oral ampicillin, 500 mg every 6 hours for 7 days.

Topical—clindamycin (5 g of cream, 100 mg of clindamycin) every night at bedtime for 7 days, metronidazole (5 g of cream, 37.5 mg of metronidazole) twice a day for 5 days.

Contraindications: Metronidazole is relatively contraindicated in the first trimester of pregnancy.

Precautions: Oral metronidazole is associated with the potential for systemic side effects including a metallic taste in the mouth and stomach upset. Topical metronidazole is currently available in two forms: one for dermatologic use and one for intravaginal use. The pH of these two preparations is quite different, making it important to specify the form on the prescription to avoid significant chemical irritation. Some concerns have been raised about the risk of inducing antibiotic resistance through the use of topical clindamycin, although the clinical significance is uncertain.

Interactions: Because of a disulfiram-like reaction, patients must be warned to avoid alcohol intake during metronidazole therapy.

Alternative Drugs

Oral—tetracycline, 250 to 500 mg twice a day for 7 days, clindamycin, 300 to 450 mg every 6 hours for 7 days.

Topical—topical triple sulfa (cream or suppositories) twice a day for 7 to 10 days, vaginal acidification (Aci-Jel, Amino-Cerv, boric acid), povidone iodine, as a douche or gel.

FOLLOW-UP

Patient Monitoring: Normal health maintenance.

Prevention/Avoidance: It is thought that bacterial vaginosis develops 5 to 10 days after exposure to the involved bacteria. *Gardnerella* may be found in 90% of male partners of women with bacterial vaginosis. Hence, sexual transmission is postulated, although bacterial vaginosis can occur in virginal women. The role of condoms in prevention is debated.

Possible Complications: Cystitis, cervicitis, infections of Skene's or Bartholin's glands, increased risk of pelvic inflammatory disease, pelvic pain, and infertility. Increased risk of upper genital tract infections and postoperative infections if surgery is performed while bacterial vaginosis is present. Increased risk of premature delivery, premature rupture of the membranes, and chorioamnionitis when bacterial vaginosis is present during pregnancy.

Expected Outcome: Most treatment failures are actually caused by reinfection or failure to comply with treatment.

MISCELLANEOUS

Pregnancy Considerations: Vaginal infections are associated with an increased risk of prematurity and premature rupture of the membranes.

ICD-9-CM Codes: 616.10.

REFERENCES

Level I

Sanchez S, Garcia PJ, Thomas KK, et al: Intravaginal metronidazole gel versus metronidazole plus nystatin ovules for bacterial vaginosis: a randomized controlled trial. Am J Obstet Gynecol 2004; 191:1898.

Sobel JD, Ferris D, Schwebke J, et al: Suppressive antibacterial therapy with 0.75% metronidazole vaginal gel to prevent recurrent bacterial vaginosis. Am J Obstet Gynecol 2006;194:1283. Epub 2006 Apr 21.

Level II

Beigi RH, Austin MN, Meyn LA, et al: Antimicrobial resistance associated with the treatment of bacterial vaginosis. Am J Obstet Gynecol 2004;191:1124.

Leitich H, Brunbauer M, Bodner-Adler B, et al: Antibiotic treatment of bacterial vaginosis in pregnancy: a meta-analysis. Am J Obstet Gynecol 2003;188:752.

Ness RB, Hillier SL, Kip KE, et al: Bacterial vaginosis and risk of pelvic inflammatory disease. Obstet Gynecol 2004;104:761.

Okun N, Gronau KA, Hannah ME: Antibiotics for bacterial vaginosis or *Trichomonas vaginalis* in pregnancy: a systematic review. Obstet Gynecol 2005;105:857.

Ugwumadu A, Reid F, Hay P, Manyonda I: Natural history of bacterial vaginosis and intermediate flora in pregnancy and effect of oral clindamycin. Obstet Gynecol 2004;104:114.

Level III

American College of Obstetricians and Gynecologists: Assessment of risk factors for preterm birth. ACOG Practice Bulletin 31. Obstet Gynecol 2001;98:709.

American College of Obstetricians and Gynecologists: Vaginitis. ACOG Practice Bulletin 72. Obstet Gynecol 2006;107:1195.

Anderson MR, Klink K, Cohrssen A: Evaluation of vaginal complaints. JAMA 2004;291:1368.

Centers for Disease Control and Prevention: Sexually transmitted diseases treatment guidelines, 2006. MMWR 2006;55:50.

Eckert LO, Lentz GM: Infections of the lower genital tract. In Katz VL, Lentz GM, Lobo RA, Gershenson DM: Comprehensive Gynecology, 5th ed. Philadelphia, Mosby/Elsevier, 2007:590.

Faro S: Bacterial vaginitis. Clin Obstet Gynecol 1991;34:582.

Friese K: The role of infection in preterm labour. BJOG 2003; 110:52.

Ledger WJ: Historical review of the treatment of bacterial vaginosis. Am J Obstet Gynecol 1993;169:474.

Mitchell H: Vaginal discharge—Causes, diagnosis, and treatment. BMJ 2004;328:1306.

Owen MK, Clenney TL: Management of vaginitis. Am Fam Physician 2004;70:2125.

Spiegel CA: Bacterial vaginosis. Clin Microbiol Rev 1991;4:485.

Sweet RL: New approaches for the treatment of bacterial vaginosis. Am J Obstet Gynecol 1994;169:479.

Thomason JL, Gelbart SM, Scaglione NJ: Bacterial vaginosis: current review with indications for asymptomatic therapy. Am J Obstet Gynecol 1991;165:1210.

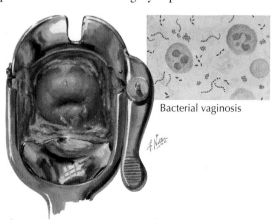

Bacterial vaginosis

INTRODUCTION

Description: Monilial vaginitis is a vaginal infection caused by ubiquitous fungi found in the air or as common inhabitants of the vagina, rectum, and mouth.

Prevalence: Twenty-five percent to 40% of "vaginal infections;" 75% of women experience one or more lifetime occurrences.

Predominant Age: 15 to 50 (rare outside this range except for those receiving estrogen replacement after menopause).

Genetics: No genetic pattern.

ETIOLOGY AND PATHOGENESIS

Causes: *Candida albicans* (80% to 95%), *Candida glabrata*, *Candida tropicalis*, or others (5% to 20%).

Risk Factors: Altered vaginal ecosystem (stress, antibiotic use, pregnancy, diabetes, depressed immunity, topical contraceptives, and warm and moist environment).

CLINICAL CHARACTERISTICS

Signs and Symptoms (15% asymptomatic carrier rate)

- Vulvar itching or burning (intense)
- External dysuria, dyspareunia
- Tissue erythema, edema, and excoriations
- Thick, adherent, plaquelike discharge with a white to yellow color (generally odorless)
- Vulvar excoriations

DIAGNOSTIC APPROACH

Differential Diagnosis

- Bacterial vaginitis
- Bacterial vaginosis
- *Trichomonas* vaginal infection
- Contact vulvitis (allergic vulvitis)
- Atrophic vulvitis
- Vulvar dermatoses
- Pinworms

Associated Conditions: Diabetes, immunosuppression or compromise (as risk factors for infection), chronic vulvitis.

Workup and Evaluation

Laboratory: Culture (Nickerson's or Sabouraud media) or monoclonal antibody staining may be obtained but are seldom necessary.

Imaging: No imaging indicated.

Special Tests: Vaginal pH 4 to 4.5.

Diagnostic Procedures: Physical examination, microscopic examination of vaginal secretions in normal saline and 10% KOH (potassium hydroxide).

Pathologic Findings

Branching and budding of vaginal monilia distinguish monilial vaginitis from lint or other foreign material. The use of 10% potassium hydroxide lyses white blood cells and renders epithelial cells "ghostlike," making identification easier.

MANAGEMENT AND THERAPY

Nonpharmacologic

General Measures: Perineal hygiene (keep the perineal area clean and dry, avoid tight undergarments or those made of synthetic fabric), education regarding prevention, encourage completion of the prescribed course of therapy.

Specific Measures: Medical therapy.

Diet: No specific dietary changes indicated.

Activity: No restriction.

Patient Education: Reassurance; American College of Obstetricians and Gynecologists Patient Education Pamphlet AP028 (Vaginitis: Causes and Treatments).

Drug(s) of Choice

Imidazoles—miconazole (Monistat, 200-mg suppositories, every night at bedtime for 3 days, 2% cream, 5 g every night at bedtime for 7 days), clotrimazole (Femcare, Gyne-Lotrimin, Mycelex, 100-mg inserts, every night at bedtime for 7 days, 1% cream, 5 g every night at bedtime for 7 days), butoconazole (Femstat, 2% cream, 5 g every night at bedtime for 3 days), tioconazole (Vagistat, 6.5% ointment, 4.6 g every night at bedtime).

Triazoles—terconazole (Terazol, 80-mg suppositories, every night at bedtime for 3 days, 0.8% cream, 5 g every night at bedtime for 3 days, 0.4% cream, 5 g every night at bedtime for 7 days), fluconazole (Diflucan, 150 mg PO single dose).

Contraindications: Known or suspected hypersensitivity or allergy. Imidazoles are contraindicated during the first trimester of pregnancy. Fluconazole is a pregnancy category C drug.

Precautions: Topical steroid preparations should be avoided. Use of oral ketoconazole requires baseline and follow-up liver function studies. Gastrointestinal side effects are common with oral therapies.

Interactions: Oral fluconazole should be used with caution in patients taking oral hypoglycemics, coumarin-type anticoagulants, phenytoin, cyclosporine, rifampin, or theophylline.

Alternative Drugs

Povidone iodine (topical), gentian violet (1%), boric acid (600-mg capsules placed high in the vagina twice daily).

FOLLOW-UP

Patient Monitoring: Normal health maintenance, frequent recurrences should suggest host compromise (e.g., diabetes, human immunodeficiency virus, anemia).

Prevention/Avoidance: Good perineal hygiene, clothing and activities that allow perineal ventilation (cotton underwear, loose clothing).

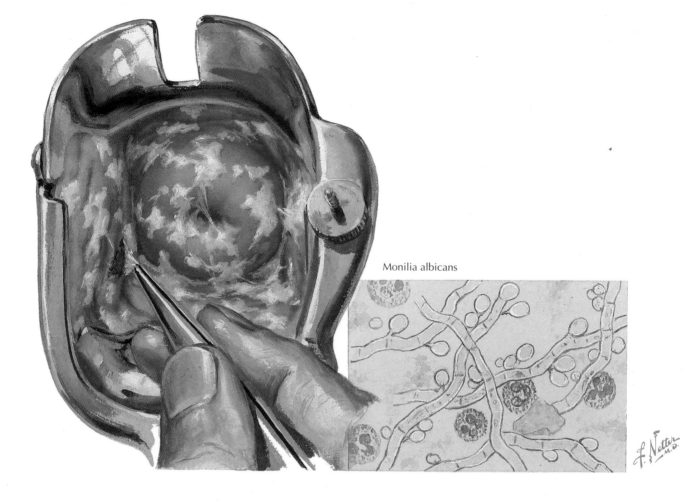

Monilia albicans

Possible Complications: Vulvar excoriation caused by scratching, chronic vulvitis, secondary vaginal or vulvar infections.

Expected Outcome: A small number (<5%) of fungal infections are resistant to imidazole therapy. Organisms causing these infections are generally susceptible to triazoles. Roughly 30% of patients experience a recurrence of symptoms within a month (related to a continuing exposure, a change in host defenses [such as altered cellular immunity], or the ability of the fungus to burrow beneath the epithelium of the vagina).

MISCELLANEOUS

Pregnancy Considerations: Vaginal infections are associated with an increased risk of premature delivery and premature rupture of the membranes.

ICD-9-CM Codes: 112.1.

REFERENCES

Level I

Phillips AJ: Treatment of non-albicans *Candida* vaginitis with amphotericin B vaginal suppositories. Am J Obstet Gynecol 2005;192:2009.

Level II

Javanovic R, Congema E, Nguyen H: Antifungal agents vs. boric acid for treating chronic mycotic vulvovaginitis. J Reprod Med 1991;36:593.

Level III

American College of Obstetricians and Gynecologists: Vaginitis. ACOG Practice Bulletin 72. Obstet Gynecol 2006;107:1195.

Anderson MR, Klink K, Cohrssen A: Evaluation of vaginal complaints. JAMA 2004;291:1368.

Centers for Disease Control and Prevention: Sexually transmitted diseases treatment guidelines, 2006. MMWR 2006;55:54.

Eckert LO: Clinical practice. Acute vulvovaginitis. N Engl J Med 2006;355:1244.

Eckert LO, Lentz GM: Infections of the lower genital tract. In Katz VL, Lentz GM, Lobo RA, Gershenson DM: Comprehensive Gynecology, 5th ed. Philadelphia, Mosby/Elsevier, 2007:594.

Forssman L, Milsom I: Treatment of recurrent vaginal candidiasis. Am J Obstet Gynecol 1985;152:959.

Horowitz BJ: Candidiasis: specification and therapy. Curr Prob Obstet Gynecol Fertil 1990;8:233.

Marrazzo J: Vulvovaginal candidiasis. BMJ 2002;325:586.

Mitchell H: Vaginal discharge—Causes, diagnosis, and treatment. BMJ 2004;328:1306.

INTRODUCTION

Description: *Trichomonas* vaginitis is a vaginal infection by an anaerobic flagellate protozoan, *Trichomonas vaginalis*.

Prevalence: Roughly 3 million cases per year, 25% of "vaginal infections."

Predominant Age: 15 to 50 (may occur at any age)

Genetics: No genetic pattern.

ETIOLOGY AND PATHOGENESIS

Causes: *Trichomonas vaginalis*, an anaerobic flagellate protozoan.

Risk Factors: Multiple sexual partners, vaginal pH that is less acid (blood, semen, or bacterial pathogens increase the risk).

CLINICAL CHARACTERISTICS

Signs and Symptoms (40% may be asymptomatic)

- Vulvar itching or burning
- Copious discharge with a rancid odor (generally thin, runny, and yellow–green to gray in color, "frothy" in 25%)
- "Strawberry" punctation of the cervix and upper vagina (15%, pathognomonic when present)
- Dysuria
- Dyspareunia
- Edema or erythema of the vulva

DIAGNOSTIC APPROACH

Differential Diagnosis

- Bacterial vaginitis
- Bacterial vaginosis
- Chlamydial cervicitis
- Gonococcal cervicitis

Associated Conditions: Other sexually transmitted infections (specifically gonorrhea and chlamydia).

Workup and Evaluation

Laboratory: Culture or monoclonal antibody testing may be obtained but is seldom necessary. Evaluation for concomitant sexually transmitted infections should be strongly considered. U.S. Food and Drug Administration–cleared tests for trichomoniasis in women include OSOM Trichomonas Rapid Test (Genzyme Diagnostics, Cambridge, Massachusetts), an immunochromatographic capillary flow dipstick technology, and a nucleic acid probe test that evaluates for *T. vaginalis*, *Gardnerella vaginalis*, and *C. albicans* (Affirm VP III, Becton Dickinson, San Jose, California). These tests have a sensitivity of more than 83% and a specificity of more than 97% but require 10 to 45 minutes to complete. (False-positive results may occur in low-prevalence populations.)

Imaging: No imaging indicated.

Special Tests: Vaginal pH 6 to 6.5 or higher.

Diagnostic Procedures: Physical examination, microscopic examination of vaginal secretions in normal saline (sensitivity of 60% to 70%).

Pathologic Findings

Trichomonas is a fusiform protozoon slightly larger than a white blood cell with three to five flagella, which provide active movement, extending from the narrow end.

MANAGEMENT AND THERAPY

Nonpharmacologic

General Measures: Perineal hygiene, education regarding sexually transmitted infections.

Specific Measures: Medical therapy, vaginal acidification.

Diet: No specific dietary changes indicated; avoid alcohol during metronidazole treatment.

Activity: Sexual abstinence until partner(s) are examined and treated.

Patient Education: Reassurance; American College of Obstetricians and Gynecologists Patient Education Pamphlet AP028 (Vaginitis: Causes and Treatments), AP009 (How to Prevent Sexually Transmitted Diseases).

Drug(s) of Choice

Metronidazole 1 g in AM and PM 1 day (may also use a single 2-g dose), tinidazole 2 g orally in a single dose, or metronidazole 500 mg twice a day for 7 days. (All sexual partners should be treated at the same time.)

Contraindications: Metronidazole and tinidazole are relatively contraindicated in the first trimester of pregnancy.

Precautions: Metronidazole and tinidazole may produce disulfiram-like reactions, resulting in nausea, vomiting, headaches, or other symptoms if the patient ingests alcohol. Patients should not use metronidazole or tinidazole if they have taken disulfiram in the preceding 2 weeks. Metronidazole and tinidazole must be used with care or the dose must be reduced in patients with hepatic disease.

Interactions: Metronidazole and tinidazole may potentiate the effects of warfarin or coumarin or alcohol (as noted previously).

Alternative Drugs

Topical clotrimazole, povidone iodine (topical), hypertonic (20%) saline douches. (Metronidazole gel is considerably less efficacious [<50%] than oral preparations and is unlikely to achieve therapeutic levels in the urethra or perivaginal glands; therefore, use of the gel is not recommended.)

FOLLOW-UP

Patient Monitoring: Follow-up serologic testing for syphilis and human immunodeficiency virus infection as indicated.

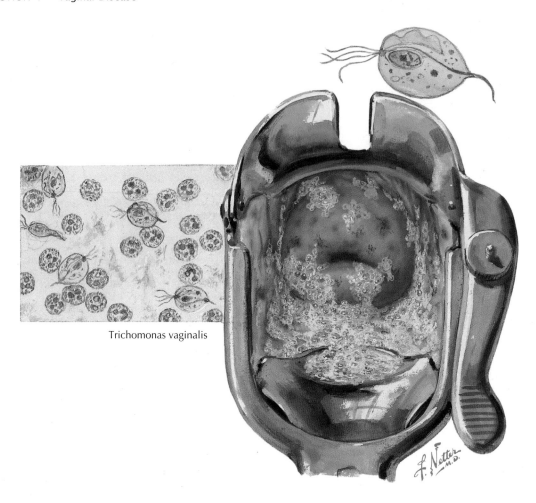

Trichomonas vaginalis

Prevention/Avoidance: Sexual monogamy, condom use for intercourse.

Possible Complications: Cystitis, infections of Skene's or Bartholin's glands, increased risk of pelvic inflammatory disease, pelvic pain, infertility, and other sequelae of sexually transmitted infections.

Expected Outcome: Resistance to metronidazole is uncommon. Most treatment failures are actually caused by reinfection or failure to comply with treatment.

MISCELLANEOUS

Pregnancy Considerations: Vaginal infections are associated with an increased risk of prematurity and premature rupture of the membranes.

ICD-9-CM Codes: 131.01.

REFERENCES

Level I

Lossick JG: Single-dose metronidazole treatment for vaginal trichomoniasis. Obstet Gynecol 1980;56:508.

Level II

Forna F, Gulmezoglu AM: Interventions for treating trichomoniasis in women. Cochrane Database Syst Rev 2003;2:CD000218.

Okun N, Gronau KA, Hannah ME: Antibiotics for bacterial vaginosis or *Trichomonas vaginalis* in pregnancy: a systematic review. Obstet Gynecol 2005;105:857.

Level III

American College of Obstetricians and Gynecologists: Vaginitis. ACOG Practice Bulletin 72. Obstet Gynecol 2006;107:1195.

Anderson MR, Klink K, Cohrssen A: Evaluation of vaginal complaints. JAMA 2004;291:1368.

Centers for Disease Control and Prevention: Sexually transmitted diseases treatment guidelines, 2006. MMWR 2006;55:52.

Eckert LO: Clinical practice. Acute vulvovaginitis. N Engl J Med 2006;355:1244.

Eckert LO, Lentz GM: Infections of the lower genital tract. In Katz VL, Lentz GM, Lobo RA, Gershenson DM: Comprehensive Gynecology, 5th ed. Philadelphia, Mosby/Elsevier, 2007:594.

McLellan R, Spence MR, Brockman M, et al: The clinical diagnosis of trichomoniasis. Obstet Gynecol 1982;60:30.

Mitchell H: Vaginal discharge—Causes, diagnosis, and treatment. BMJ 2004;328:1306.

Thomason JL, Gelbart SM. *Trichomonas vaginalis*. Obstet Gynecol 1989;74:536.

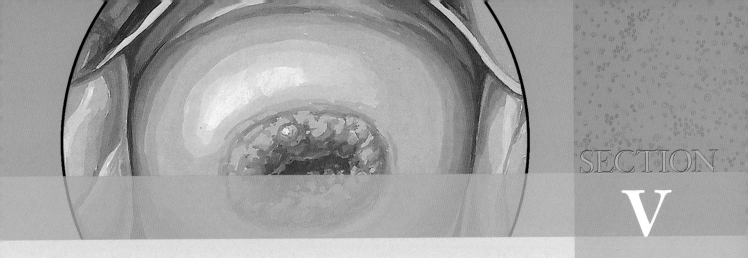

Cervical Disease

INTRODUCTION

Description: One of the most perplexing aspects of management under the Bethesda reporting system is how to interpret smears reported as showing atypical squamous or glandular cells (ASCUS, ASCH, or AGC). The atypical squamous cell (ASC) diagnosis has been developed to describe squamous cell changes that are more severe than reactive changes but not as marked as those found in squamous intraepithelial lesions (SIL, high and low grade). The ACS designation has been subdivided into "atypical squamous cells of undetermined significance" (ASCUS) and "atypical squamous cells cannot exclude HSIL" (ASCH). The latter includes those cytologic changes suggestive of HSIL but insufficient for a definitive diagnosis. The category of atypical glandular cells (AGC) includes a range of findings from benign reactive changes in endocervical or endometrial cells to adenocarcinoma.

Prevalence: ASC—approximately 3% to 5% of all Pap tests; AGC—0.2% to 0.4% of all Pap tests.

Predominant Age: Reproductive.

Genetics: No genetic pattern.

ETIOLOGY AND PATHOGENESIS

Causes: Most, if not all, of the changes that are seen result from infection by the human papillomavirus (HPV). The AGC diagnosis reflects benign reactive changes in endocervical or endometrial cells, endometrial hyperplasia, or adenocarcinoma.

Risk Factors: ASC—exposure to human papillomavirus (HPV). AGC—none known, except for those affecting possible pathologic causes (e.g., unopposed estrogen therapy as a risk factor for endometrial carcinoma).

CLINICAL CHARACTERISTICS

Signs and Symptoms

- Asymptomatic

DIAGNOSTIC APPROACH

Differential Diagnosis

- ASC—inflammatory change (cervicitis)
- Low-grade squamous intraepithelial lesion (LGSIL) change
- AGC—benign reactive changes in endocervical or endometrial cells
- Endometrial hyperplasia or adenocarcinoma
- Endometritis secondary to an intrauterine contraceptive device
- Tuberculous endometritis
- Tubal carcinoma

Associated Conditions: ASC—HPV infection, vaginitis, cervicitis. AGC—dysfunctional uterine bleeding (may be present but is most often absent).

Workup and Evaluation

Laboratory: No evaluation indicated.

Imaging: No imaging indicated.

Special Tests: HPV serotyping followed by colposcopy if high-risk subtypes are found. (In adolescents with high-risk subtypes, a repeat Pap test in 6 and 12 months or high-risk HPV test alone in 12 months is an acceptable alternative.) If low-risk serotypes are the only finding, a repeat cervical cytology (Pap test) should be performed in 12 months. Ultrasonography (including sonohysterography using saline infusion into the uterine cavity) may be considered for the evaluation of Pap test results classified as AGC.

Diagnostic Procedures: Colposcopy, with or without cervical biopsy and endocervical curettage, should be considered if high-risk HPV serotypes are identified, high-risk factors are present, or the abnormality is persistent or recurrent. Endocervical or endometrial biopsy and/or hysteroscopy may be indicated for AGC results because between 9% and 38% of patients will have significant neoplasia eventually found (varying with age).

Pathologic Findings

Minimal gross findings, mildly elevated numbers of nucleated squamous cells with varying degrees of maturation when ASC is present.

MANAGEMENT AND THERAPY

Nonpharmacologic

General Measures: Evaluation of comments made by the cytopathologist. Increased frequency of Pap tests until the abnormality is resolved or further diagnosis is established. (For a follow-up Pap test result to be "negative," it must have normal or benign findings, but it also must be "satisfactory for interpretation.")

Specific Measures: Treatment of infection or inflammation (if present). Treatment of atrophic change (if present). If the cytology report accompanying the AGC test indicates a probability of carcinoma, the endocervical canal and endometrial cavity should be evaluated. Cone biopsy, hysteroscopy, or both, may be required to adequately evaluate these patients.

Diet: No specific dietary changes indicated.

Activity: No restriction.

Patient Education: Reassurance; American College of Obstetricians and Gynecologists Patient Education Pamphlet AP085 (The Pap Test), AP073 (Human Papillomavirus Infection).

Drug(s) of Choice

Based on specific indications.

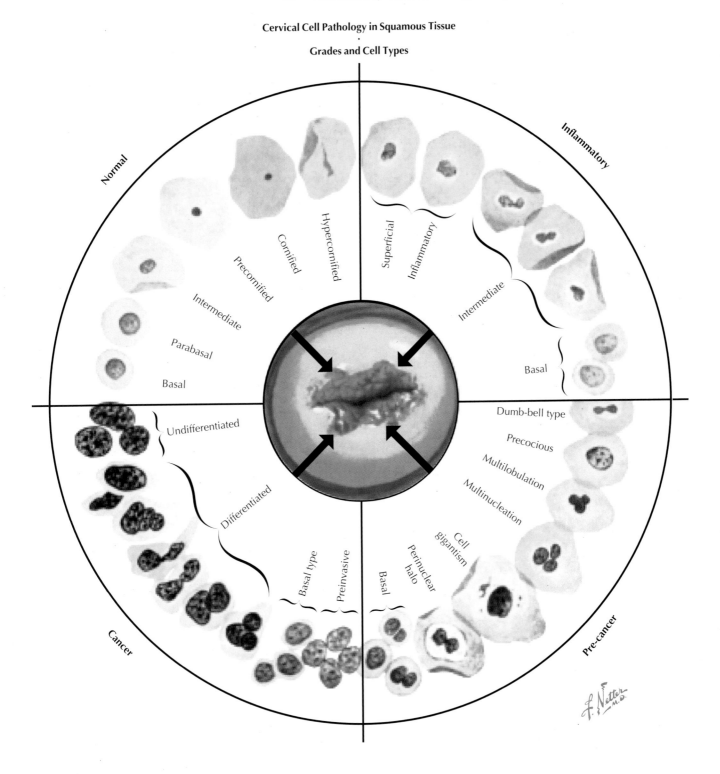

Cervical Cell Pathology in Squamous Tissue

Grades and Cell Types

FOLLOW-UP

Patient Monitoring: Normal health maintenance, increased frequency of Pap tests. If only low-risk serotypes are found, normal schedules for cervical cytology may be followed.

Prevention/Avoidance: Avoidance of HPV infection (ASC).

Possible Complications: Progression to more severe squamous abnormalities or occult disease unless a diagnosis is established and treatment is instituted. (Data suggest that for adolescents, virtually all ASC- and low-grade HPV-mediated changes are transitory and that regression to normal is to be expected without intervention.)

Expected Outcome: Most patients with ASC experience a spontaneous return to normal, as seen if their Pap tests are closely followed (the average length of detectable HPV is 13 months, >90% will clear the infection within 24 months). When a treatable condition is identified, this response rate is even better.

MISCELLANEOUS

Pregnancy Considerations: No effect on pregnancy. The likelihood of significant pathologic changes with ASC abnormalities is small enough that no proscription against pregnancy during the evaluation process is necessary. Although the possibility of significant complications is small in AGC, the underlying causes may be of sufficient concern to mitigate against pregnancy until a diagnosis is established.

ICD-9-CM Codes: 795.0 (ASC), 622.1 (Cervical atypia), 795.0 (AGC).

REFERENCES

Level I

ASCUS-LSIL Triage Study (ALTS) Group: Results of a randomized trial on the management of cytology interpretations of atypical squamous cells of undetermined significance. Am J Obstet Gynecol 2003;188:1383.

ASCUS-LSIL Triage Study (ALTS) Group: A randomized trial on the management of low-grade squamous intraepithelial lesion cytology interpretations. Am J Obstet Gynecol 2003;188:1393.

Level II

Higgins RV, Hall JB, McGee JA, et al: Appraisal of the modalities used to evaluate an initial abnormal Papanicolaou smear. Obstet Gynecol 1994;84:174.

Levi AW, Kelly DP, Rosenthal DL, Ronnett BM: Atypical squamous cells of undetermined significance in liquid-based cytologic specimens: results of reflex human papillomavirus testing and histologic follow-up in routine practice with comparison of interpretive and probabilistic reporting methods. Cancer 2003;99:191.

Montz FJ, Bradley JM, Fowler JM, Nguyen L: Natural history of the minimally abnormal Papanicolaou smear. Obstet Gynecol 1992;80:385.

Toon PG, Arrand JR, Wilson LP, Sharp DS: Human papillomavirus infection of the uterine cervix of women without cytological signs of neoplasia. BMJ 1986;293:1261.

Level III

American College of Obstetricians and Gynecologists: Cervical cytology screening. ACOG Practice Bulletin 45. Obstet Gynecol 2003;102:417.

American College of Obstetricians and Gynecologists: Cervical cancer screening in adolescents. ACOG Committee Opinion 300. Obstet Gynecol 2004;104:885.

American College of Obstetricians and Gynecologists: Management of abnormal cervical cytology and histology. ACOG Practice Bulletin 66. Obstet Gynecol 2005;106:645.

American College of Obstetricians and Gynecologists: Evaluation and management of abnormal cervical cytology and histology in the adolescent. ACOG Committee Opinion 330. Obstet Gynecol 2006;107:963.

Apgar BS, Zoschnick L, Wright TC Jr: The 2001 Bethesda System terminology. Am Fam Physician 2003;68:1992.

Bose J, Kannan V, Kline TS: Abnormal endocervical cells: really abnormal? Really endocervical? Am J Clin Pathol 1994;101:708.

Dehn D, Torkko KC, Shroyer KR: Human papillomavirus testing and molecular markers of cervical dysplasia and carcinoma. Cancer 2007;111:1.

Goff BA, Atanasoff P, Brown E, et al: Endocervical glandular atypia in Papanicolaou smears. Obstet Gynecol 1992;79:101.

Klinkhamer PJ, Meerding WJ, Rosier PF, Hanselaar AG: Liquid-based cervical cytology. Cancer 2003;99:263.

Noller KL: Intraepithelial neoplasia of the lower genital tract (cervix, vulva). In Katz VL, Lentz GM, Lobo RA, Gershenson DM: Comprehensive Gynecology, 5th ed. Philadelphia, Mosby/Elsevier, 2007:746.

Safaeian M, Solomon D, Wacholder S, et al: Risk of precancer and follow-up management strategies for women with human papillomavirus-negative atypical squamous cells of undetermined significance. Obstet Gynecol 2007;109:1325.

Wright TC Jr: Cervical cancer screening in the 21st century: is it time to retire the PAP smear? Clin Obstet Gynecol 2007;50:313.

INTRODUCTION

Description: Low-grade squamous intraepithelial lesions (LGSIL) encompass changes associated with human papillomavirus (HPV), mild dysplasia, and cervical intraepithelial neoplasia (CIN) I. High-grade squamous intraepithelial lesions (HGSIL) include CIN II and III and carcinoma in situ (CIS).

Prevalence: Less than 5% of Pap tests for low-grade and 2% for high-grade abnormalities.

Predominant Age: Reproductive.

Genetics: No genetic pattern.

ETIOLOGY AND PATHOGENESIS

Causes: HPV appears to be responsible for the development of cervical dysplasia. Although as many as 70% of invasive cervical cancers have HPV serotypes 16 or 18 present, these types may be detected in patients with LGSIL as well. Normal patients have HPV prevalence rates that vary from 10% to 50%, depending on the study technique and population evaluated.

Risk Factors: Exposure to HPV and other sexually transmitted disease; smoking is associated with a higher risk.

CLINICAL CHARACTERISTICS

Signs and Symptoms

- Asymptomatic

DIAGNOSTIC APPROACH

Differential Diagnosis

- LGSIL—inflammatory change (cervicitis)
- Cervical carcinoma
- HGSIL—cervical CIS
- Invasive cervical carcinoma

Associated Conditions: HPV infection, vaginitis, cervicitis, cervical dysplasia, carcinoma in situ, invasive carcinoma of the cervix, endocervical adenocarcinoma.

Workup and Evaluation

Laboratory: No evaluation indicated.

Imaging: No imaging indicated.

Special Tests: High prevalence, a poor correlation with later risk, and the cost of screening have resulted in the general recommendation that routine HPV screening or serotyping not be carried out.

Diagnostic Procedures: For many patients with LGSIL, colposcopy, colposcopically directed biopsy, and endocervical curettage are appropriate to establish the source of the cytologic abnormality. (For compliant adolescents, a repeat Pap test in 6 and 12 months or high-risk HPV test alone in 12 months are acceptable alternatives.) If colposcopy is inadequate to delineate lesions present or the entire transformation zone cannot be seen, diagnostic conization may be needed. Colposcopy, colposcopically directed biopsy, and endocervical curettage should be used to evaluate all patients with HGSIL.

Pathologic Findings

Acetowhite areas on colposcopy, early vascular changes leading to mosaicism and punctation. Microscopic—loss of normal maturation, increased nuclear/cytoplasmic ratio, nuclear atypia (mild). Vascular changes leading to mosaicism and punctation (severe) are more typical of HGSIL. Nuclear atypia (moderate to severe) is also a feature of HGSIL.

MANAGEMENT AND THERAPY

Nonpharmacologic

General Measures: Evaluation of comments made by the cytopathologist. Increased frequency of Pap tests until the abnormality is resolved or further diagnosis is established. (For a follow-up Pap test to be "negative," it must have normal or benign findings, but it also must be "satisfactory for interpretation.")

Specific Measures: Compliant patients with LGSIL who are at low risk for HPV, sexually transmitted disease, and malignant progression of the lesion (e.g., smokers) may be followed by serial Pap tests. If colposcopy is adequate and the histologic abnormality found is mild, obtaining follow-up Pap tests at 4- to 6-month intervals for 2 years or three normal tests is suitable. When HGSIL is present, the evaluation determines therapy: cryotherapy, electrocautery, electrosurgical loop excision, laser ablation, or conization. Treatment must be based on an accurate diagnosis and the extent of the lesion involved. (Treatment of CIN 1 in women younger than age 21 is not recommended, even if the lesion persists. Virtually all are manifestations of a transient HPV infection and will resolve, although complete resolution may take up to 36 months.)

Diet: No specific dietary changes indicated.

Activity: No restriction.

Patient Education: Reassurance; American College of Obstetricians and Gynecologists Patient Education Pamphlet AP085 (The Pap Test), AP073 (Human Papillomavirus Infection).

Drug(s) of Choice

Based on specific indications, most therapy is surgical or ablative in nature.

FOLLOW-UP

Patient Monitoring: Normal health maintenance, increased frequency of Pap tests.

Prevention/Avoidance: Avoidance of HPV infection.

Cervical Intraepithelial Neoplasia (CIN)

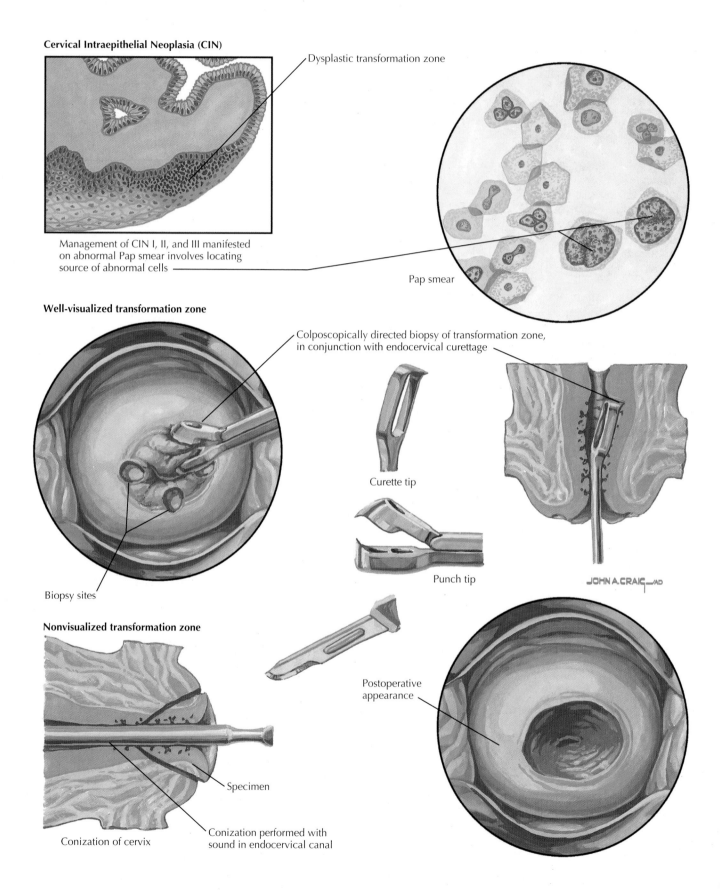

Dysplastic transformation zone

Management of CIN I, II, and III manifested on abnormal Pap smear involves locating source of abnormal cells

Pap smear

Well-visualized transformation zone

Colposcopically directed biopsy of transformation zone, in conjunction with endocervical curettage

Curette tip

Punch tip

Biopsy sites

JOHN A. CRAIG—AD

Nonvisualized transformation zone

Postoperative appearance

Specimen

Conization of cervix

Conization performed with sound in endocervical canal

Possible Complications: Progression to more severe squamous abnormalities. (Data suggest that for adolescents, virtually all atypical squamous cells of undetermined significance [ASCUS] and low-grade HPV-mediated changes are transitory and that regression to normal is to be expected without intervention.)

Expected Outcome: Of patients with these findings, 60% or more undergo spontaneous regression of the underlying process, resulting in a return to normal Pap test results. Only 15% of patients with LGSIL progress to HGSIL. HGSIL abnormalities are more likely to progress and warrant more aggressive evaluation and treatment.

MISCELLANEOUS

Pregnancy Considerations: No effect on pregnancy. Because of the potential significance of the HGSIL abnormality and the pathologic conditions that cause it, a delay in pregnancy while evaluation is ongoing may be advisable.

ICD-9-CM Codes: 622.1 (LGSIL), 233.1 (HGSIL, includes carcinoma in situ).

REFERENCES

Level I

Brewster WR, Hubbell FA, Largent J, et al: Feasibility of management of high-grade cervical lesions in a single visit: a randomized controlled trial. JAMA 2005;294:2182.

Level II

Dehn D, Torkko KC, Shroyer KR: Human papillomavirus testing and molecular markers of cervical dysplasia and carcinoma. Cancer 2007;111:1.

Higgins RV, Hall JB, McGee JA, et al: Appraisal of the modalities used to evaluate an initial abnormal Papanicolaou smear. Obstet Gynecol 1994;84:174.

Nasiell K, Roger V, Nasiell M: Behavior of mild cervical dysplasia during long-term follow-up. Obstet Gynecol 1986;67:665.

Level III

American College of Obstetricians and Gynecologists: Cervical cytology screening. ACOG Practice Bulletin 45. Obstet Gynecol 2003;102:417.

American College of Obstetricians and Gynecologists: Cervical cancer screening in adolescents. ACOG Committee Opinion 300. Obstet Gynecol 2004;104:885.

American College of Obstetricians and Gynecologists: Management of abnormal cervical cytology and histology. ACOG Practice Bulletin 66. Obstet Gynecol 2005;106:645.

American College of Obstetricians and Gynecologists: Evaluation and management of abnormal cervical cytology and histology in the adolescent. ACOG Committee Opinion 330. Obstet Gynecol 2006;107:963.

Apgar BS, Zoschnick L, Wright TC Jr: The 2001 Bethesda System terminology. Am Fam Physician 2003;68:1992.

Brinton LA, Hamman RF, Huggins GR, et al: Sexual and reproductive risk factors for invasive squamous cell cervical cancer. J Natl Cancer Inst 1987;79:23.

Carmichael JA, Maskens PD: Cervical intraepithelial neoplasia: examination, treatment and follow-up: review. Obstet Gynecol Surg 1985;40:545.

Dehn D, Torkko KC, Shroyer KR: Human papillomavirus testing and molecular markers of cervical dysplasia and carcinoma. Cancer 2007;111:1.

Klinkhamer PJ, Meerding WJ, Rosier PF, Hanselaar AG: Liquid-based cervical cytology. Cancer 2003;99:263.

Noller KL: Intraepithelial neoplasia of the lower genital tract (cervix, vulva). In Katz VL, Lentz GM, Lobo RA, Gershenson DM: Comprehensive Gynecology, 5th ed. Philadelphia, Mosby/Elsevier, 2007:752.

INTRODUCTION

Description: Carcinoma in situ of the cervix is characterized by morphologic alteration of the cervical epithelium in which the full thickness of the epithelium is replaced with dysplastic cells (cervical intraepithelial neoplasia [CIN] III). This change is generally associated either spatially or temporally with invasive carcinoma.

Prevalence: Less than 2% of Pap tests.

Predominant Age: Early 30s (peak approximately age 32).

Genetics: No genetic pattern.

ETIOLOGY AND PATHOGENESIS

Causes: Unknown, strongly linked to some serotypes of human papillomavirus (HPV; 99.7% of cancers contain high-risk HPV serotypes).

Risk Factors: Infection by HPV, herpes virus, or cytomegalovirus; early sexual activity; multiple sexual partners; cigarette smoking (1.5 times risk); oral contraceptive use (2 to 4 times risk); early childbearing; intrauterine diethylstilbestrol exposure; immunosuppression.

CLINICAL CHARACTERISTICS

Signs and Symptoms

- Asymptomatic
- Abnormal cervical cytology
- Abnormal colposcopy

DIAGNOSTIC APPROACH

Differential Diagnosis

- Moderate dysplasia
- Microinvasive and invasive carcinoma

Associated Conditions: HPV infection, condyloma acuminata.

Workup and Evaluation

Laboratory: No evaluation indicated.

Imaging: No imaging indicated.

Special Tests: Colposcopy, colposcopically directed biopsy, and endocervical curettage.

Diagnostic Procedures: Cervical cytologic examination, colposcopy, and biopsy.

Pathologic Findings

The entire thickness of the epithelium is replaced with abnormal (dysplastic) cells, but there is no invasion of the underlying stroma.

MANAGEMENT AND THERAPY

Nonpharmacologic

General Measures: Evaluation of comments made by the cytopathologist.

Specific Measures: Cervical conization and endocervical curettage to confirm the absence of invasion or a more extensive lesion. In those wishing to preserve fertility,

this may be curative; in others, standard hysterectomy may be considered. Ablative therapy can be considered only when the entire lesion is visible and invasion has been ruled out.

Diet: No specific dietary changes indicated.

Activity: No restriction.

Patient Education: Reassurance; American College of Obstetricians and Gynecologists Patient Education Pamphlet AP085 (The Pap Test), AP073 (Human Papillomavirus Infection), AP110 (Loop Electrosurgical Excision Procedure).

Drug(s) of Choice

None.

FOLLOW-UP

Patient Monitoring: Follow-up cervical cytologic examination at 6 and 12 months or high-risk HPV test at 12 months, colposcopy for any abnormality.

Prevention/Avoidance: Reduction or avoidance of known risk factors.

Possible Complications: Advancement of disease or recurrence. Untreated disease is anticipated to progress to invasive carcinoma over the course of 12 to 86 months in 15% to 40% of patients.

Expected Outcome: Low recurrence rates (<10%) for most therapies. When recurrence is found, 75% occur in 21 months.

MISCELLANEOUS

Pregnancy Considerations: No effect on pregnancy. The presence of pregnancy complicates both the diagnosis and treatment: endocervical curettage is generally omitted and definitive therapy is delayed until after delivery; colposcopy is usually repeated every 6 to 10 weeks until term. In the absence of invasion, vaginal delivery is appropriate.

ICD-9-CM Codes: 233.1.

REFERENCES

Level II

An HJ, Cho NH, Lee SY, et al: Correlation of cervical carcinoma and precancerous lesions with human papillomavirus (HPV) genotypes detected with the HPV DNA chip microarray method. Cancer 2003;97:1672.

Andersen, Husth M: Cryosurgery for cervical intraepithelial neoplasia: 10-year follow-up. Gynecol Oncol 1992;40:240.

Coupe VM, Berkhof J, Verheijen RH, Meijer CJ: Cost-effectiveness of human papillomavirus testing after treatment for cervical intraepithelial neoplasia. BJOG 2007;114:416.

Level III

American College of Obstetricians and Gynecologists: Cervical cytology screening. ACOG Practice Bulletin 45. Obstet Gynecol 2003;102:417.

American College of Obstetricians and Gynecologists: Cervical cancer screening in adolescents. ACOG Committee Opinion 300. Obstet Gynecol 2004;104:885.

Colposcopic Views of Abnormal Cervical Changes

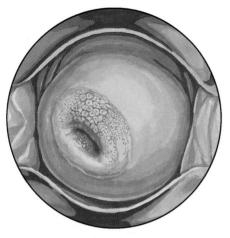

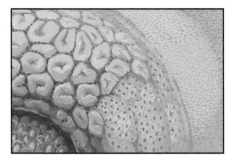

Coarse mosaicism and punctation in transformation zone

JOHN A.CRAIG—AD

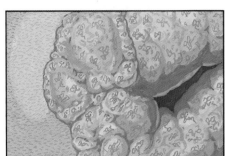

Papilloma of cervix. Some papillomas may predispose to cervical malignancy

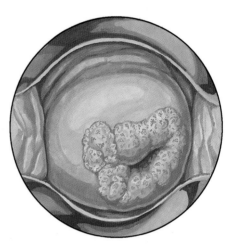

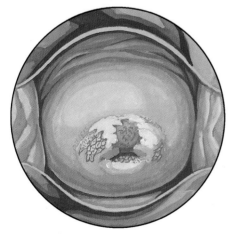

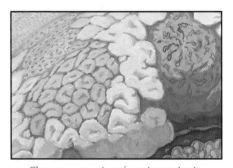

Changes suggestive of carcinoma in situ. Abnormal vasculature with leukoplakia, mosaicism, and punctation

American College of Obstetricians and Gynecologists: Management of abnormal cervical cytology and histology. ACOG Practice Bulletin 66. Obstet Gynecol 2005;106:645.

American College of Obstetricians and Gynecologists: Evaluation and management of abnormal cervical cytology and histology in the adolescent. ACOG Committee Opinion 330. Obstet Gynecol 2006;107:963.

Apgar BS, Zoschnick L, Wright TC Jr: The 2001 Bethesda System terminology. Am Fam Physician 2003;68:1992.

Brinton LA, Hamman RF, Huggins GR, et al: Sexual and reproductive risk factors for invasive squamous cell cervical cancer. J Natl Cancer Inst 1987;79:23.

Carmichael JA, Maskens PD: Cervical intraepithelial neoplasia: examination, treatment and follow-up: review. Obstet Gynecol Surg 1985;40:545.

McIndoe WA, McLean MR, Jones RW, Mullins PR: The invasive potential of carcinoma in situ of the cervix. Obstet Gynecol 1991;77:715.

Noller KL: Intraepithelial neoplasia of the lower genital tract (cervix, vulva). In Katz VL, Lentz GM, Lobo RA, Gershenson DM: Comprehensive Gynecology, 5th ed. Philadelphia, Mosby/Elsevier, 2007:753.

Walboomers JM, Jacobs MV, Manos MM, et al: Human papillomavirus is a necessary cause of invasive cervical cancer worldwide. J Pathol 1999;189:12.

Management of Carcinoma in Situ (CIN III)

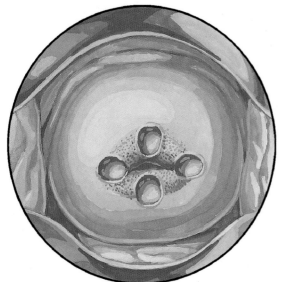

Colposcopy showing biopsy sites
in transformation zone

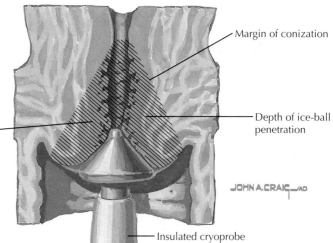

Biopsy specimen showing changes of carcinoma
in situ in transformation zone

Treatment must eradicate transformation
zone and penetrate to a minimal depth
of 5 mm in order to destroy metaplastic
or dysplastic extensions into gland crypts

Treatment modalities include cryosurgery,
CO_2 laser, and radical electrocautery, as
well as conization and hysterectomy

Margin of conization

Depth of ice-ball
penetration

JOHN A. CRAIG—AD

Insulated cryoprobe

Laser burns in
transformation zone

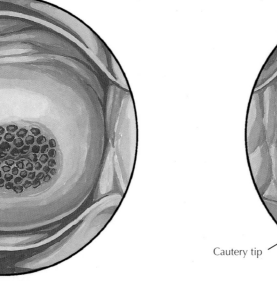

CO_2 laser therapy

Electrocautery burns

Cautery tip

Radical electrocautery

INTRODUCTION

Description: Almost all cancers of the cervix are carcinomas—85% to 90% are squamous carcinoma and 10% to 15% are adenocarcinoma.

Prevalence: 11,150 cases, 3,670 deaths annually (2007 estimates). Lifetime risk: 1 in 135.

Predominant Age: 40s to 60s, median age 52.

Genetics: No genetic pattern.

ETIOLOGY AND PATHOGENESIS

Causes: Strongly linked to some serotypes of human papillomavirus (HPV; 99.7% of all cancers have oncogenic HPV DNA detectable) and associated with early sexual activity and multiple partners.

Risk Factors: Early sexual activity, multiple sexual partners, HPV, African-American race, smoking, immunocompromise, minimal or neglected medical care (Pap test screening) associated with advance disease.

CLINICAL CHARACTERISTICS

Signs and Symptoms

- None until late in the disease
- Abnormal Pap test result
- Late: vaginal bleeding, dark vaginal discharge, postcoital bleeding, ureteral obstruction, back pain, loss of appetite, weight loss
- Exophytic, friable, bleeding lesion

- Late: supraclavicular or inguinal lymph nodes, leg swelling, ascites, pleural effusion, hepatomegaly

DIAGNOSTIC APPROACH

Differential Diagnosis

- Cervical eversion
- Cervical erosion
- Cervical polyp
- Condyloma acuminata
- Nabothian cyst

Associated Conditions: HPV, condyloma acuminata, abnormal vaginal bleeding.

Workup and Evaluation

Laboratory: An assessment of renal function is appropriate if ureteral compromise is suspected (advanced disease).

Imaging: Chest radiograph, intravenous pyelogram, and computed tomographic or magnetic resonance imaging (MRI) scans are used to assess extent of disease and to assist in staging. (As experience grows, magnetic resonance imaging is displacing other imaging modalities because of its ability to assess lymph nodes [72% to 93% accuracy] and possible tumor spread.) Staging is currently clinical and relies primarily on clinical examination and the status of the ureters.

Special Tests: Colposcopy and cervical biopsy (conization preferred), biopsy of vaginal or paracervical tissues may be required to assess extent of disease.

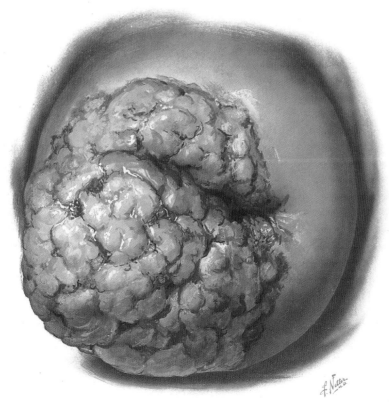

Advanced carcinoma

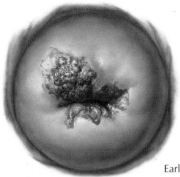

Very early squamous cell cancer starting at squamocolumnar junction

Early carcinoma

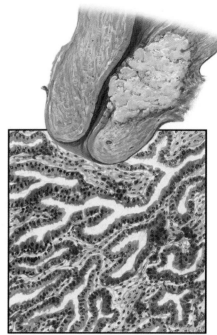

Adenocarcinoma (endocervical)

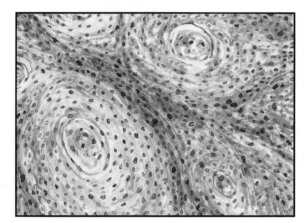

Squamous cell cancer showing pearl formation

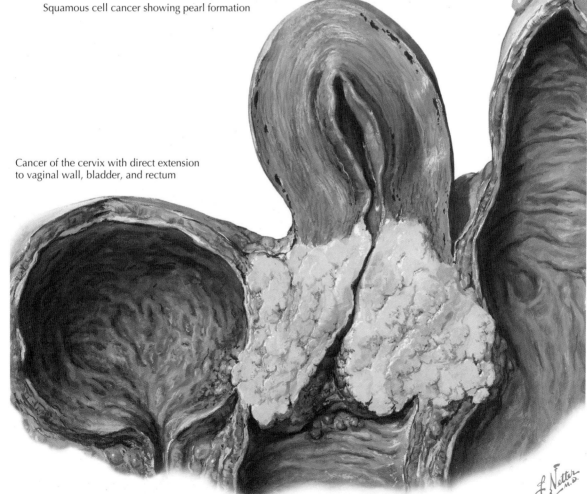

Cancer of the cervix with direct extension to vaginal wall, bladder, and rectum

Diagnostic Procedures: History, physical examination, and histologic diagnosis. Barium enema, flexible sigmoidoscopy or cystoscopy (or both) may be performed in the cases of large tumors or for those who may receive radiation therapy.

Pathologic Findings

Squamous cell carcinomas (large cell [keratinizing or nonkeratinizing], small cell, verrucous), adenocarcinoma (endocervical, endometrioid, clear cell, adenoid cystic, adenoma malignum), mixed carcinomas (adenosquamous, glassy cell).

MANAGEMENT AND THERAPY

Nonpharmacologic

General Measures: Timely evaluation and treatment.

Specific Measures: Therapy is based on stage of disease. Radical surgery is used for selected patients with stage I and II disease. Radiation therapy (brachytherapy, teletherapy) is used for stage IB and IIA disease or greater. Postoperative radiation therapy reduces the risk of recurrence by almost 50%.

Diet: No specific dietary changes indicated.

Activity: No restriction except those imposed by therapies.

Patient Education: American College of Obstetricians and Gynecologists Patient Education Pamphlet AP163 (Cancer of the Cervix), AP0073 (Human Papillomavirus Infections), AP085 (The Pap Test), AP110 (Loop Electrosurgical Excision Procedure).

Drug(s) of Choice

Chemotherapy does not produce long-term cures, but response rates of up to 50% have been obtained with multiagent combinations (cisplatin, doxorubicin, and etoposide; other combinations have also been successful).

FOLLOW-UP

Patient Monitoring: Normal health maintenance, 90% of recurrences occur in the first 5 years.

Prevention/Avoidance: None. Adherence to screening guidelines allows diagnosis and treatment of premalignant changes.

Possible Complications: Risk of nodal involvement is based on stage of disease—pelvic nodes: stage I, 15%; stage II, 29%; stage III, 47%; para-aortic nodes: stage I, 6%; stage II, 19%; stage III, 33%.

Expected Outcome: Survival is based on stage of disease— stage IA, 99% 5 year; stage IB, 85% to 90%; stage IIA, 73% to 80%; stage IIB, 68%; stage IIIA, 45%; stage IIIB, 36%; stage IVA, 15%; stage IVB, 2%. One third of patients develop recurrences, half within 3 years after primary therapy (best prognosis for later recurrences). Short-term serious complications will occur in 1% to 5% of surgical cases.

MISCELLANEOUS

Pregnancy Considerations: Rare in pregnancy. Pregnancy and vaginal delivery do not appear to alter the course of disease, although delivery is associated with hemorrhage. Early stages diagnosed late in pregnancy may be watched until after delivery. Advanced disease may require early delivery or interruption of pregnancy to allow aggressive therapy to begin.

ICD-9-CM Codes: 239.5 (unspecified stage; others based on stage).

REFERENCES

Level I
Garipagaoglu M, Kayikcioglu F, Kose MF, et al: Adding concurrent low dose continuous infusion of cisplatin to radiotherapy in locally advanced cervical carcinoma: a prospective randomized pilot study. Br J Radiol 2004;77:581.

Level II
Dayes IS, Abuzallouf S: Local tumour control in women with carcinoma of the cervix treated with the addition of nitroimidazole agents to radiotherapy: a meta-analysis. Br J Radiol 2005;78:777.

Hacker NF, Berek JS, Lagasse LD: Carcinoma of the cervix associated with pregnancy. Obstet Gynecol 1982;59:735.

Westermann AM, Jones EL, Schem BC, et al: First results of triple-modality treatment combining radiotherapy, chemotherapy, and hyperthermia for the treatment of patients with stage IIB, III, and IVA cervical carcinoma. Cancer 2005;104:763.

Level III
Akin O, Mironov S, Pandit-Taskar N, Hann LE: Imaging of uterine cancer. Radiol Clin North Am 2007;45:167.

American College of Obstetricians and Gynecologists: Diagnosis and treatment of cervical carcinomas. ACOG Practice Bulletin 35. Obstet Gynecol 2002;99:855.

Basen-Engquist K, Paskett ED, Buzaglo J, et al: Cervical cancer. Cancer 2003;98:2009.

Clement PB, Scully RE: Carcinoma of the cervix: histologic types. Semin Oncol 1982;9:251.

Farthing A: Conserving fertility in the management of gynaecological cancers. BJOG 2006;113:129.

Fielding JR: MR imaging of the female pelvis. Radiol Clin North Am 2003;41:179.

Jhingran A, Levenback C: Malignant diseases of the cervix. In Katz VL, Lentz GM, Lobo RA, Gershenson DM: Comprehensive Gynecology, 5th ed. Philadelphia, Mosby/Elsevier, 2007:765.

Kumar R, Alavi A: PET imaging in gynecologic malignancies. Radiol Clin North Am 2004;42:1155, ix.

Leminen A, Paavonen J, Forss M, et al: Adenocarcinoma of the uterine cervix. Cancer 1990;65:53.

Moore DH: Cervical cancer. Obstet Gynecol 2006;107:1152.

Pannu HK, Fishman EK: Evaluation of cervical cancer by computed tomography: current status. Cancer 2003;98:2039.

Schiffman M: Integration of human papillomavirus vaccination, cytology, and human papillomavirus testing. Cancer 2007;111:145.

Schiffman M, Castle PE: The promise of global cervical-cancer prevention. N Engl J Med 2005;353:2101.

Schiffman M, Castle PE: When to test women for human papillomavirus. BMJ 2006;332:61.

Stewart AJ, Viswanathan AN: Current controversies in high-dose-rate versus low-dose-rate brachytherapy for cervical cancer. Cancer 2006;107:908.

Waggoner SE: Cervical cancer. Lancet 2003;361:2217.

Walboomers JM, Jacobs MV, Manos MM, et al: Human papillomavirus is a necessary cause of invasive cervical cancer worldwide. J Pathol 1999;189:12.

Weiss RS, Lucas WE: Adenocarcinoma of the cervix. Cancer 1986;57:1996.

Wolf JK, Franco EL, Arbeit JM, et al: Innovations in understanding the biology of cervical cancer. Cancer 2003;98:2064.

Wright TC Jr: Cervical cancer screening in the 21st century: is it time to retire the PAP smear? Clin Obstet Gynecol 2007; 50:313.

INTRODUCTION

Description: Cervical erosion is loss of the epithelial surface on the vaginal portion of the cervix, resulting in the exposure of the underlying cervical stroma. Cervical eversion (exposing the dark-red columnar epithelium of the endocervix) is often mistaken for or incorrectly labeled as cervical erosion.

Prevalence: Uncommon.

Predominant Age: Reproductive.

Genetics: No genetic pattern.

ETIOLOGY AND PATHOGENESIS

Causes: Generally traumatic. May occur through sexual trauma (fingernail, sexual appliances), iatrogenic process (diaphragm, pessary, biopsy, or other instrumentation), tampon use, or pelvic organ prolapse resulting in exposure of the cervix outside the introitus.

Risk Factors: None known.

CLINICAL CHARACTERISTICS

Signs and Symptoms

- Irregularly shaped, depressed lesion with a red base and sharp borders
- Bleeding generally absent, although tissues may bleed when touched, resulting in postcoital spotting
- Increased mucoid (clear) discharge may be present

DIAGNOSTIC APPROACH

Differential Diagnosis

- Cervical eversion (ectopy)
- Herpes simplex cervicitis
- Carcinoma under the surface of the epithelium (barrel lesion)
- Syphilis (primary lesion)
- Chronic cervicitis
- Cervical polyp
- *Chlamydia trachomatis* infection

Associated Conditions: Chronic cervicitis.

Workup and Evaluation

Laboratory: No evaluation indicated.

Imaging: No imaging indicated.

Special Tests: Colposcopy can be used to confirm the diagnosis but is seldom indicated.

Diagnostic Procedures: Inspection of the cervix.

Pathologic Findings

Loss of surface epithelium. Evidence of inflammation is often present during the healing phase.

MANAGEMENT AND THERAPY

Nonpharmacologic

General Measures: Evaluation and reassurance.

Specific Measures: The use of acidifying agents and topical antibiotics is controversial and generally not necessary.

Diet: No specific dietary changes indicated.

Activity: No restriction.

Patient Education: Reassurance.

Drug(s) of Choice

None.

FOLLOW-UP

Patient Monitoring: Normal health maintenance.

Prevention/Avoidance: None.

Possible Complications: Both overdiagnosis and underdiagnosis; treatment and intervention are generally not warranted and may create additional problems; failure to recognize a more sinister process (cancer) may lead to a delay in treatment.

Expected Outcome: Spontaneous and complete healing is the rule.

MISCELLANEOUS

Pregnancy Considerations: No effect on pregnancy.

ICD-9-CM Codes: 622.0, 616.0 (With chronic cervicitis).

REFERENCES

Level III

American College of Obstetricians and Gynecologists: Pelvic organ prolapse. ACOG Practice Bulletin 79. Obstet Gynecol 2007;109:461.

Barrett KF, Bledsoe S, Greer BE, Droegemueller W: Tampon-induced vaginal or cervical ulceration. Am J Obstet Gynecol 1977;127:332.

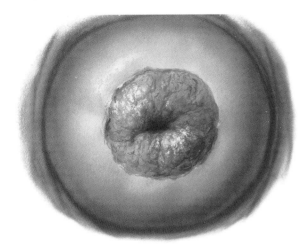

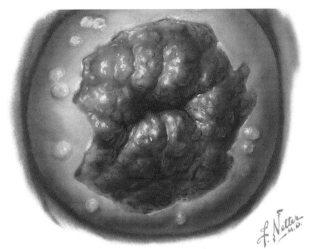

Congenital erosion
in nulliparous cervix

Extensive erosion with proliferation
(papillary erosion); also nabothian cysts

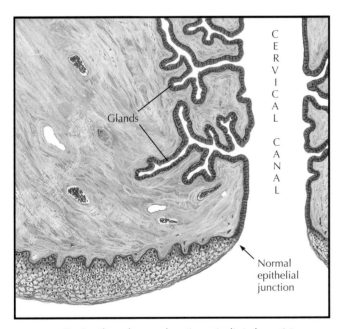

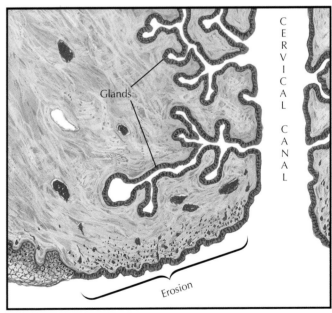

Section through normal portio vaginalis (schematic)

Section through portio vaginalis showing erosion (schematic)

INTRODUCTION

Description: Cervical eversion is a turning outward of the endocervical canal so that it is visible and appears as a red, inflamed mass at the cervical opening.

Prevalence: Common.

Predominant Age: Reproductive.

Genetics: No genetic pattern.

ETIOLOGY AND PATHOGENESIS

Causes: Chronic cervicitis, estrogen exposure (oral contraceptives, pregnancy). (In parous women, the external cervix is sometimes sufficiently patulous to give the false appearance of eversion when the vaginal apex is widely opened during speculum examination.)

Risk Factors: Cervicitis, increased estrogen.

CLINICAL CHARACTERISTICS

Signs and Symptoms

- Generally asymptomatic
- Intermenstrual or postcoital bleeding

DIAGNOSTIC APPROACH

Differential Diagnosis

- Endocervical polyp
- Endocervical cancer
- Cervicitis
- *Chlamydia trachomatis* infection

Associated Conditions: Cervicitis, intermenstrual and postcoital bleeding.

Workup and Evaluation

Laboratory: No evaluation indicated.

Imaging: No imaging indicated.

Special Tests: Colposcopy confirms the diagnosis but is not required.

Diagnostic Procedures: History and speculum inspection of the cervix.

Pathologic Findings

Normal columnar endocervical epithelium.

MANAGEMENT AND THERAPY

Nonpharmacologic

General Measures: Evaluation and reassurance.

Specific Measures: No therapy required once diagnosis is established.

Diet: No specific dietary changes indicated.

Activity: No restriction.

Patient Education: Reassurance.

Drug(s) of Choice

None.

FOLLOW-UP

Patient Monitoring: Normal health maintenance.

Prevention/Avoidance: None.

Possible Complications: Cervicitis, postcoital bleeding.

Expected Outcome: Normal function without therapy.

MISCELLANEOUS

Pregnancy Considerations: No effect on pregnancy.

ICD-9-CM Codes: 622.0, 616.0 (With chronic cervicitis).

Variations in Location of Transformation Zone

Prepubertal

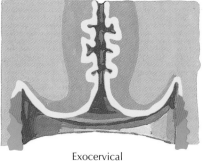

Exocervical

Reproductive

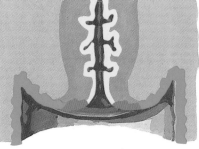

Exocervical

Postmenopausal

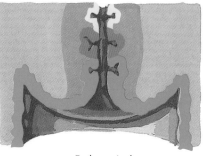

Endocervical

JOHN A. CRAIG—MD

INTRODUCTION

Description: Cervical polyps are benign fleshy tumors that arise from the cells of the endocervical canal (most common) or the ectocervix.

Prevalence: Four percent of gynecologic patients, most common benign growth of the cervix.

Predominant Age: 40s to 50s (multiparous women). (Ectocervical polyps predominate in postmenopausal women.)

Genetics: No genetic pattern.

ETIOLOGY AND PATHOGENESIS

Causes: Thought to arise as a result of inflammation and the focal hyperplasia and proliferation that it causes.

Risk Factors: More common in multiparous women, history of cervical infection, oral contraceptive use.

CLINICAL CHARACTERISTICS

Signs and Symptoms

- Asymptomatic (found on routine examination)
- Intermenstrual spotting
- Postcoital spotting
- Smooth, soft, reddish-purple to cherry-red, friable mass at the cervical os, varying from a few mm to 4 cm in size; may bleed when touched
- Leukorrhea (uncommon)

DIAGNOSTIC APPROACH

Differential Diagnosis

- Endometrial polyp
- Cervical cancer
- Prolapsed leiomyomata (3% to 8% of myomas are cervical)
- Cervical eversion
- Cervical erosion
- Retained products of conception

Associated Conditions: Intramenstrual bleeding, postcoital bleeding, leukorrhea.

Workup and Evaluation

Laboratory: No evaluation indicated.
Imaging: No imaging indicated.
Special Tests: None indicated.
Diagnostic Procedures: Physical examination.

Pathologic Findings

Polypoid growth with a surface epithelium made up of columnar or squamous epithelial cells. The stalk is made up of edematous, loose, often inflamed connective tissue with rich vascularization. The surface may be ulcerated (leading to bleeding). Six histologic types have been described: adenomatous (80%), cystic, fibrous, vascular, inflammatory, and fibromyomatous. Malignant degeneration of an endocervical polyp is extremely rare (<1 in 200).

MANAGEMENT AND THERAPY

Nonpharmacologic

General Measures: Evaluation, Pap test.

Specific Measures: Removal of polyp by gentle traction, twisting, or excision. The base of the polyp may then be treated with chemical cautery, electrocautery, or cryocautery. A polyp may also be cauterized with chemical agents ($AgNO_3$), cryosurgery, or a loop electrosurgical excision procedure. Curettage of the endocervical canal should be considered to rule out a coexisting hyperplasia or cancer. For women older than age 40, endometrial sampling to rule out additional pathology (present in approximately 5% of patients) should be considered.

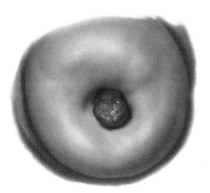

Small cervical polyp

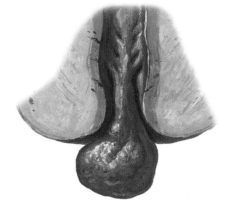

Section showing endocervical origin of a polyp

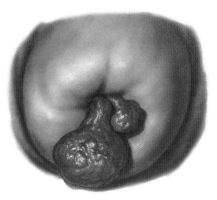

Large and small cervical polyps

Diet: No specific dietary changes indicated.

Activity: No restriction.

Patient Education: Reassurance; American College of Obstetricians and Gynecologists Patient Education Pamphlet AP095 (Abnormal Uterine Bleeding).

Drug(s) of Choice

None.

FOLLOW-UP

Patient Monitoring: Normal health maintenance, no change in Pap test recommendations.

Prevention/Avoidance: None.

Possible Complications: Malignant change is extremely rare.

Expected Outcome: Excision or cautery is curative.

MISCELLANEOUS

Pregnancy Considerations: No effect on pregnancy.

ICD-9-CM Codes: 622.7.

REFERENCES

Level II

Duckman S, Suarez JR, Sese LQ: Giant cervical polyp. Am J Obstet Gynecol 1988;159:852.

Kerner H, Lichtig C: Müllerian adenosarcoma presenting as cervical polyps: a report of seven cases and review of the literature. Obstet Gynecol 1993;81:655.

Pradhan S, Chenoy R, O'Brien PMS: Dilatation and curettage in patients with cervical polyps: a retrospective analysis. Br J Obstet Gynaecol 1995;102:415.

Level III

Katz VL: Benign gynecologic lesions. In Katz VL, Lentz GM, Lobo RA, Gershenson DM: Comprehensive Gynecology, 5th ed. Philadelphia, Mosby/Elsevier, 2007:436.

INTRODUCTION

Description: Cervical stenosis is a narrowing of the cervical canal, either congenital or acquired, which may result in complete or partial obstruction. Stenosis occurs most often in the region of the internal cervical os.

Prevalence: Uncommon.

Predominant Age: 30 to 70.

Genetics: No genetic pattern.

ETIOLOGY AND PATHOGENESIS

Causes: Operative damage (cone biopsy, electrocautery, cryocautery), radiation, infection, neoplasia, atrophy, congenital (rare).

Risk Factors: Operative therapy (cone biopsy, cautery), radiation, chronic infection, neoplasia, untreated menopause.

CLINICAL CHARACTERISTICS

Signs and Symptoms

Premenopausal

- Dysmenorrhea, abnormal bleeding, amenorrhea, infertility
- Boggy uterine enlargement

Postmenopausal

- Asymptomatic
- Hematometra, hydrometra, or pyometra

DIAGNOSTIC APPROACH

Differential Diagnosis

- Endocervical cancer
- Endometrial cancer
- Uterine leiomyomata

Associated Conditions: Endometriosis, dysmenorrhea, chronic pelvic pain, and infertility.

Workup and Evaluation

Laboratory: Ultrasonography may demonstrate uterine enlargement or hematometra.

Imaging: No imaging indicated.

Special Tests: Inability to pass a 1- to 2-mm probe beyond the inner cervical os.

Diagnostic Procedures: History, physical examination, sounding of the endocervical canal with a small probe.

Pathologic Findings

None.

MANAGEMENT AND THERAPY

Nonpharmacologic

General Measures: Evaluation, analgesics (nonsteroidal anti-inflammatory drugs) for dysmenorrhea.

Specific Measures: Dilation of the cervix with progressive dilators under ultrasound guidance. Placement of a cervical stent for several days after dilation has been advocated but is not universally accepted.

Diet: No specific dietary changes indicated.

Activity: No restriction.

Patient Education: American College of Obstetricians and Gynecologists Patient Education Pamphlet AP062 (Dilation and Curettage [D&C]), AP046 (Dysmenorrhea).

Drug(s) of Choice

Symptomatic therapy until definitive surgical dilation.

FOLLOW-UP

Patient Monitoring: Normal health maintenance.

Prevention/Avoidance: Care with surgical technique when cone biopsy or cautery of the cervix is used.

Possible Complications: Retrograde menstruation with the subsequent development of endometriosis, infertility, and chronic pelvic pain. In older patients, the development of hematometra or pyometra.

Expected Outcome: The risk of recurrence is small after dilation (based on causation).

MISCELLANEOUS

Pregnancy Considerations: No effect on pregnancy.

ICD-9-CM Codes: 622.4, 654.6 (Complicating labor), 752.49 (Congenital).

REFERENCES

Level II

Baggish MS, Baltoyannis P: Carbon dioxide laser treatment of cervical stenosis. Fertil Steril 1987;48:24.

Barbierie RL, Callery M, Perez SE: Directionality of menstrual flow: cervical os diameter as a determinant of retrograde menstruation. Fertil Steril 1992;57:727.

Pradhan S, Chenoy R, O'Brien PMS: Dilatation and curettage in patients with cervical polyps: a retrospective analysis. Br J Obstet Gynaecol 1995;102:415.

Level III

Katz VL: Benign gynecologic lesions. In Katz VL, Lentz GM, Lobo RA, Gershenson DM: Comprehensive Gynecology, 5th ed. Philadelphia, Mosby/Elsevier, 2007:438.

Pinsonneault O, Goldstein DP: Obstructing malformations of the uterus and vagina. Fertil Steril 1985;44:241.

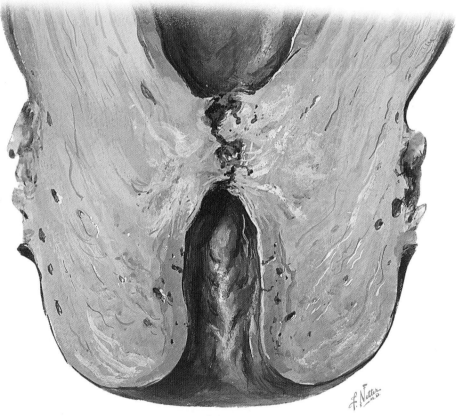

Stricture

Cervicitis

INTRODUCTION

Description: Cervicitis is inflammation (acute or chronic) of the endocervical glands or the ectocervix.
Prevalence: Ten percent to 40% of women.
Predominant Age: Reproductive, greatest rate in adolescents to early 20s.
Genetics: No genetic pattern.

ETIOLOGY AND PATHOGENESIS

Causes: Endocervical—*Chlamydia trachomatis* (up to 60% of cases in some studies), *Neisseria gonorrhoeae*. (Almost 50% of patients will not have an identifiable infection.) Ectocervical—herpes simplex, human papillomavirus (HPV), *Mycoplasma* species (*Mycoplasma hominis*, *Ureaplasma urealyticum*), *Trichomonas vaginalis*.
Risk Factors: Exposure to sexually transmitted infections (multiple sexual partners), postpartum period.

CLINICAL CHARACTERISTICS

Signs and Symptoms

May be asymptomatic (60%)
Mucopurulent discharge (yellow discharge with 10 or more white blood cells at magnification ×1000)
Cervical erythema or edema, ulceration, and friability
Deep-thrust dyspareunia

DIAGNOSTIC APPROACH

Differential Diagnosis

- Vaginitis
- Cervical neoplasia
- Cervical metaplasia
- Cervical erosion
- Cervical eversion

Associated Conditions: Cervical neoplasia, dyspareunia, postcoital bleeding, pelvic inflammatory disease, premature rupture of the membranes in pregnancy, premature labor, and prematurity.

Workup and Evaluation

Laboratory: Cervical culture, Gram stain of cervical material, enzyme-linked immunosorbent assay (ELISA) or fluorescent monoclonal antibody testing for *Chlamydia*. Consider serum testing for other sexually transmitted infections.
Imaging: No imaging indicated.
Special Tests: None indicated.
Diagnostic Procedures: Inspection, Gram stain, culture, ELISA, or fluorescent monoclonal antibody testing. Colposcopy may be of assistance in selected cases. Nucleic acid activation tests are rapidly becoming the method of choice for detecting *C. trachomatis* or *N. gonorrhoeae*.

Pathologic Findings

Diffuse inflammatory changes, koilocytic changes with human papillomavirus infection. Chronic inflammatory changes are extremely common during the reproductive years and, by themselves, are not indicative of a pathologic state.

MANAGEMENT AND THERAPY

Nonpharmacologic

General Measures: Diagnosis and management of causal agent.
Specific Measures: In rare patients with consistently negative cultures, cryosurgery of the cervix has been advocated, although this could result in cervical stricture or other postsurgical complications.
Diet: No specific dietary changes indicated.
Activity: No restriction. (Sexual continence for 7 days after single-day therapy or the completion of 7 days of treatments.)
Patient Education: Infectious nature of the problem, need for partner evaluation, avoidance of sexually transmitted infection; American College of Obstetricians and Gynecologists Patient Education Pamphlet AP009 (How to Prevent Sexually Transmitted Diseases), AP071 (Gonorrhea and Chlamydia), AP073 (Human Papillomavirus Infection), AP028 (Vaginitis: Causes and Treatments).

Drug(s) of Choice

Without gonorrhea—azithromycin 1 g PO (single dose) or doxycycline 100 mg PO twice a day for 7 days
With gonorrhea—ceftriaxone 125 mg IM or (cefixime 400 mg PO or ciprofloxacin 500 mg PO or ofloxacin 400 mg PO) as single dose plus doxycycline 100 mg PO twice a day for 7 days.
Contraindications: Known or suspected allergy to medication. Doxycycline should not be used during pregnancy or nursing.
Precautions: Doxycycline should not be taken with milk, antacids, or iron-containing preparations.
Interactions: Doxycycline may interact with warfarin or oral contraceptives to reduce their effectiveness.

Alternative Drugs

Without gonorrhea—ofloxacin 300 mg PO twice a day for 7 days or erythromycin ethylsuccinate 800 mg PO four times a day for 7 days.

FOLLOW-UP

Patient Monitoring: Repeat cultures for test of cure, annual Pap tests.
Prevention/Avoidance: Use of condoms to reduce the risk of infection.
Possible Complications: Cervical atypia and neoplasia.
Expected Outcome: With treatment, good.

MISCELLANEOUS

Pregnancy Considerations: No effect on pregnancy.
ICD-9-CM Codes: 616.0 (Cervicitis), 098.15 (Acute gonococcal cervicitis), 079.8 (*Chlamydia* infection).

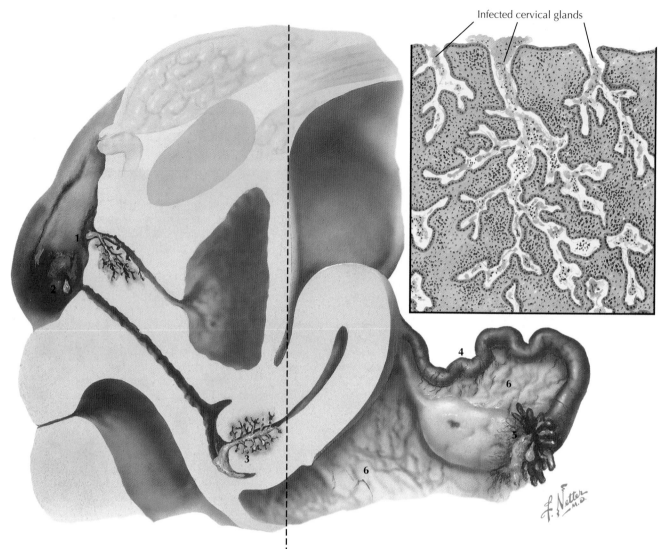

Infected cervical glands

Primary sites of infection
1. Urethra and Skene's gland
2. Bartholin's gland
3. Cervix and cervical glands

Subsequent sites of infection
4. Fallopian tubes (salpingitis)
5. Emergence from tubal ostium (tubo-ovarian abscess and peritonitis)
6. Lymphatic spread to broad ligaments and surrounding tissues (frozen pelvis)

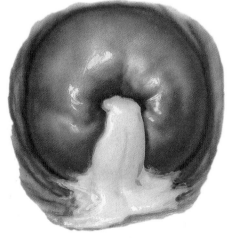

Appearance of cervix
in acute infection

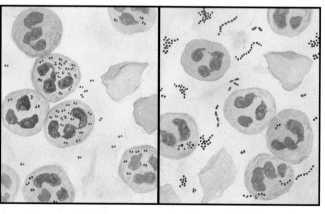

Gonorrheal infection
(Gram stain)

Non-specific infection
(Gram stain)

REFERENCES

Level I

Adair CD, Gunter M, Stovall TG, et al: Chlamydia in pregnancy: a randomized trial of azithromycin and erythromycin. Obstet Gynecol 1998;91:165.

Martin DH, Mroczkowski TF, Dalu ZA, et al: A controlled trial of a single dose of azithromycin for the treatment of chlamydial urethritis and cervicitis: the azithromycin for Chlamydial Infections Study Group. N Engl J Med 1992;327:921.

Paavonen J, Roberts PL, Stevens CE, et al: Randomized treatment of mucopurulent cervicitis with doxycycline or amoxicillin. Am J Obstet Gynecol 1989;161:128.

Romanowski B, Talbot H, Stadnyk M, et al: Minocycline compared with doxycycline in the treatment of nongonococcal urethritis and mucopurulent cervicitis. Ann Intern Med 1993;119:16.

Level II

Amortegui AJ, Meyer MP: Enzyme immunoassay for detection of *Chlamydia trachomatis* from the cervix. Obstet Gynecol 1985; 65:523.

Bush MR, Rosa C: Azithromycin and erythromycin in the treatment of cervical chlamydial infection during pregnancy. Obstet Gynecol 1994;84:61.

Campbell WF, Dodson MG: Clindamycin therapy for *Chlamydia trachomatis* in women. Am J Obstet Gynecol 1990;162:343.

Faro S, Martens MG, Maccato M, et al: Effectiveness of ofloxacin in the treatment of *Chlamydia trachomatis* and *Neisseria gonorrhoeae* cervical infection. Am J Obstet Gynecol 1991;164:1380.

Hawkinson JA, Schulman H: Prematurity associated with cervicitis and vaginitis during pregnancy. Am J Obstet Gynecol 1966; 94:898.

Manhart LE, Critchlow CW, Holmes KK, et al: Mucopurulent cervicitis and Mycoplasma genitalium. J Infect Dis 2004;187:650.

Marrazzo JM, Handsfield HH, Whittington WLH: Predicting chlamydial and gonococcal cervical infection: implications for management of cervicitis. Obstet Gynecol 2002;100:579.

Marrazzo JM, Wiesenfeld HC, Murray PJ, et al: Risk factors for cervicitis among women with bacterial vaginosis. J Infect Dis 2006; 193:617.

McClelland RS, Wang CC, Mandaliya K, et al: Treatment of cervicitis is associated with decreased cervical shedding of HIV-1. AIDS 2001;15:105.

Schwebke JR, Weiss HL: Interrelationships of bacterial vaginosis and cervical inflammation. Sex Transmit Dis 2002;29:59.

Level III

Brunham RC, Kuo CC, Stevens CE, Holmes KK: Therapy of cervical chlamydial infection. Ann Intern Med 1982;97:216.

Centers for Disease Control and Prevention: Sexually transmitted diseases treatment guidelines, 2006. MMWR 2006;55:37.

Eckert LO, Lentz GM: Infections of the lower genital tract. In Katz VL, Lentz GM, Lobo RA, Gershenson DM: Comprehensive Gynecology, 5th ed. Philadelphia, Mosby/Elsevier, 2007:598.

Faro S: *Chlamydia trachomatis:* female pelvic infection. Am J Obstet Gynecol 1991;164:1767.

Majeroni BA: Chlamydial cervicitis: complications and new treatment options. Am Fam Physician 1994;49:1825, 1832.

Rosenfeld WD, Clark J: Vulvovaginitis and cervicitis. Pediatr Clin North Am 1989;36:489.

INTRODUCTION

Description: Nabothian cysts are retention cysts of the cervix made up of endocervical columnar cells and resulting from closure of a gland opening, tunnel, or cleft by the process of squamous metaplasia.
Prevalence: Normal feature of the adult cervix.
Predominant Age: Reproductive.
Genetics: No genetic pattern.

ETIOLOGY AND PATHOGENESIS

Causes: A cervical gland opening, tunnel, or cleft that becomes covered by the process of squamous metaplasia.
Risk Factors: Chronic inflammation of the cervix.

CLINICAL CHARACTERISTICS

Signs and Symptoms

- Asymptomatic
- Translucent or opaque, white to blue to yellow, raised bumps on the ectocervix (3 mm to 3 cm in diameter)

DIAGNOSTIC APPROACH

Differential Diagnosis

- Cervical cancer (barrel or undermining type) uncommon

Associated Conditions: None.

Workup and Evaluation

Laboratory: No evaluation indicated.
Imaging: No imaging indicated.
Special Tests: None indicated.
Diagnostic Procedures: Pelvic (speculum) examination.

Pathologic Findings

Mucus-filled cysts lined with columnar epithelium.

MANAGEMENT AND THERAPY

Nonpharmacologic

General Measures: Evaluation and reassurance.
Specific Measures: None necessary.
Diet: No specific dietary changes indicated.
Activity: No restriction.
Patient Education: Reassurance.

Drug(s) of Choice

None.

FOLLOW-UP

Patient Monitoring: Normal health maintenance.
Prevention/Avoidance: None.
Possible Complications: Distortion or enlargement of the cervix is possible but unlikely.

MISCELLANEOUS

Pregnancy Considerations: No effect on pregnancy.
ICD-9-CM Codes: 616.0.

REFERENCES

Level III
Farrar HK, Nedoss BR: Benign tumors of the uterine cervix. Am J Obstet Gynecol 1961;81:124.
Katz VL: Benign gynecologic lesions. In Katz VL, Lentz GM, Lobo RA, Gershenson DM: Comprehensive Gynecology, 5th ed. Philadelphia, Mosby/Elsevier, 2007:437.
Stepto RC: Treatment of the Nabothian cyst. Am Fam Physician 1971;4:82.

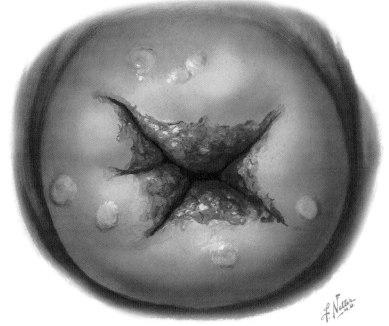

Stellate laceration with nabothian cysts

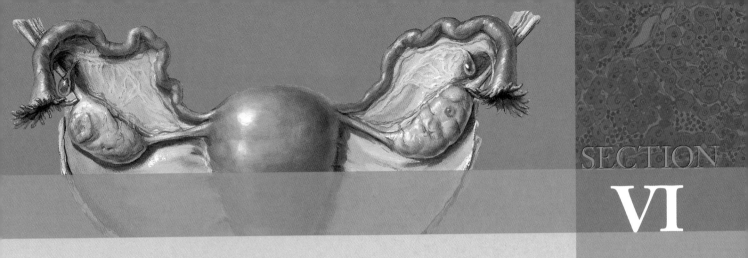

Uterine Pathology

INTRODUCTION

Description: Adenomyosis is characterized by endometrial glands and stroma found in the uterine wall (myometrium).

Prevalence: Ten percent to 15% of women; may be 60% in women 40 to 50 years old.

Predominant Age: 35 to 50.

Genetics: Familial predisposition (polygenic or multifactorial inheritance pattern).

ETIOLOGY AND PATHOGENESIS

Causes: Adenomyosis is derived from aberrant glands of the basalis layer of the endometrium. These grow by direct extension into the myometrium.

Risk Factors: High levels of estrogen (postulated), high parity, postpartum endometritis (postulated). Local endometrial invasion may be seen following cesarean delivery, myomectomy, or curettage.

CLINICAL CHARACTERISTICS

Signs and Symptoms

* Asymptomatic (40%)
* Menorrhagia (40% to 50%) often increasing in severity
* Dysmenorrhea
* Symmetric "woody" enlargement of the uterus (up to two to three times normal)
* Uterine tenderness that varies with the cycle (worst just before menstruation)

DIAGNOSTIC APPROACH

Differential Diagnosis

* Uterine leiomyomata (most often resulting in asymmetric uterine changes)
* Endometrial polyp
* Endometrial hyperplasia
* Endometrial cancer
* Endometriosis (when pain is predominant symptom)

Associated Conditions: Coexistent endometriosis (15%), uterine leiomyomata, dyspareunia, salpingitis isthmica nodosa.

Workup and Evaluation

Laboratory: No evaluation indicated, complete blood count if anemia is suspected.

Imaging: No imaging indicated except to rule out other possible pathologic conditions. Either transvaginal ultrasonography or magnetic resonance imaging (MRI) may demonstrate abnormalities. (On ultrasound, the uterus will have a heterogeneous texture, without focal abnormalities.) MRI (T2-weighted or contrast-enhanced T1-weighted) will be more specific than ultrasonography.

Special Tests: Endometrial biopsy is seldom of help in establishing the diagnosis of adenomyosis, although it may be useful to rule out a possible endometrial cancer when that is a consideration.

Diagnostic Procedures: The characteristic history of painful, heavy periods, accompanied by a generous, symmetrical, firm or "woody" uterus suggests, but does not confirm, the diagnosis. Only histologic examination can confirm the diagnosis.

Pathologic Findings

In adenomyosis, endometrial implants (glands and stroma) develop deep within the myometrial wall. Adenomyosis is, therefore, the intramural equivalent of extrauterine endometriosis. Diagnostic criteria require glands to be identified more than 2.5 mm below the basalis layer of the endometrium.

MANAGEMENT AND THERAPY

Nonpharmacologic

General Measures: Analgesics (nonsteroidal anti-inflammatory drugs), cyclic hormone therapy, gonadotropin-releasing hormone (GnRH) agonists.

Specific Measures: Hysterectomy is the definitive treatment for adenomyosis. Uterine artery embolization has been suggested but remains experimental.

Diet: No specific dietary changes indicated.

Activity: No restriction.

Patient Education: Reassurance; American College of Obstetricians and Gynecologists Patient Education Pamphlet AP013 (Endometriosis), AP046 (Dysmenorrhea).

Drug(s) of Choice

There is no satisfactory medical treatment for adenomyosis. All medical therapy is aimed at ameliorating the symptoms or delaying the progression of the condition. Symptoms generally resolve with the loss of ovarian function.

FOLLOW-UP

Patient Monitoring: Normal health maintenance.

Prevention/Avoidance: None.

Possible Complications: Progressive menorrhagia, anemia, chronic pelvic pain. Some studies have suggested that these patients have a higher level of antiphospholipid autoantibodies, but the clinical significance of this is unknown.

Expected Outcome: Unless associated with endometriosis, surgical therapy (hysterectomy) is curative. Symptoms resolve with the loss of menstrual function at menopause.

MISCELLANEOUS

Pregnancy Considerations: No effect on pregnancy.

ICD-9-CM Codes: 617.0.

Possible Locations of Endometrial Implants

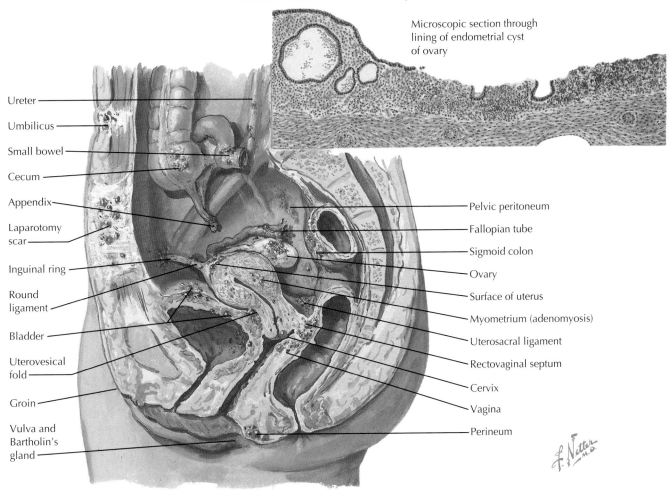

Microscopic section through lining of endometrial cyst of ovary

Ureter

Umbilicus

Small bowel

Cecum

Appendix

Laparotomy scar

Inguinal ring

Round ligament

Bladder

Uterovesical fold

Groin

Vulva and Bartholin's gland

Pelvic peritoneum

Fallopian tube

Sigmoid colon

Ovary

Surface of uterus

Myometrium (adenomyosis)

Uterosacral ligament

Rectovaginal septum

Cervix

Vagina

Perineum

REFERENCES

Level I

Johnson NP, Farquhar CM, Crossley S, et al: A double-blind randomised controlled trial of laparoscopic uterine nerve ablation for women with chronic pelvic pain. BJOG 2004;111:950.

Level II

Arnold LL, Ascher SM, Simon JA: Familial adenomyosis: a case report. Fertil Steril 1994;60:1165.

Byun JY, Kim SE, Choi BG, et al: Diffuse and focal adenomyosis: MR imaging findings. Radiographics 1999;19:S161.

Carter JE, Kong II: Adenomyosis as a major cause for laparoscopic-assisted vaginal hysterectomy for chronic pelvic pain. J Am Assoc Gynecol Laparosc 1994;1:S6.

Fedele L, Bianchi S, Dorta M, et al: Transvaginal ultrasonography in the diagnosis of diffuse adenomyosis. Fertil Steril 1992;58:94.

Hirata JD, Moghissi KS, Ginsburg KA: Pregnancy after medical therapy of adenomyosis with a gonadotropin-releasing hormone agonist. Fertil Steril 1993;59:444.

Kim MD, Kim S, Kim NK, et al: Long-term results of uterine artery embolization for symptomatic adenomyosis. AJR Am J Roentgenol 2007;188:176.

Ota H, Maki M, Shidara Y, et al: Effects of danazol at the immunologic level in patients with adenomyosis, with special reference to autoantibodies: a multi-center cooperative study. Am J Obstet Gynecol 1992;167:481.

Popp LW, Schwiedessen JP, Gaetje R: Myometrial biopsy in the diagnosis of adenomyosis uteri. Am J Obstet Gynecol 1993;169:546.

Raju GC, Naraynsingh V, Woo J, Jankey N: Adenomyosis uteri: a study of 416 cases. Aust N Z J Obstet Gynaecol 1988;28:72.

Reinhold C, Tafazoli F, Mehio A, et al: Uterine adenomyosis: endovaginal US and MR imaging features with histopathologic correlation. Radiographics 1999;19:S147.

Vercellini P, Parazzini F, Oldani S, et al: Adenomyosis at hysterectomy: a study on frequency distribution and patient characteristics. Hum Reprod 1995;10:1160.

Level III

American College of Obstetricians and Gynecologists: Medical management of endometriosis. ACOG Practice Bulletin 11. Washington, DC, ACOG, 1999.

American College of Obstetricians and Gynecologists: Chronic pelvic pain. ACOG Practice Bulletin 51. Obstet Gynecol 2004;103:589.

Arnold LL, Ascher SM, Schruefer JJ, Simon JA: The nonsurgical diagnosis of adenomyosis. Obstet Gynecol 1995;86:461.

Azziz R: Adenomyosis: current perspectives. Obstet Gynecol Clin North Am 1989;16:221.

Outwater EK, Siegelman ES, Van Deerlin V: Adenomyosis: current concepts and imaging considerations. AJR Am J Roentgenol 1998;170:437.

Siegler AM, Camilien L: Adenomyosis. J Reprod Med 1994;39:841.

INTRODUCTION

Description: Asherman's syndrome is characterized by scarring or occlusion of the uterine cavity after curettage, especially when performed after septic abortion or in the immediate postpartum period. (Although the same changes occur following therapeutic endometrial ablation, the term is generally not applied in that setting.)

Prevalence: Rare.

Predominant Age: Reproductive.

Genetics: No genetic pattern.

ETIOLOGY AND PATHOGENESIS

Causes: Endometrial damage (excessive curettage, curettage when infection is present or in the immediate postpartum period—some intrauterine adhesions form in 30% of patients treated by curettage for missed abortion), endometrial infection (tuberculosis or schistosomiasis), scarring after myomectomy or metroplasty. A severe pelvic infection unrelated to surgery may also lead to Asherman's syndrome.

Risk Factors: Instrumentation of the uterine cavity complicated by infection. Endometrial infection unrelated to instrumentation, such as tuberculosis or schistosomiasis.

CLINICAL CHARACTERISTICS

Signs and Symptoms

* Amenorrhea or hypomenorrhea

DIAGNOSTIC APPROACH

Differential Diagnosis

* Amenorrhea (primary or secondary)
* Cervical stenosis

Associated Conditions: Amenorrhea, infertility.

Workup and Evaluation

Laboratory: No evaluation indicated.

Imaging: Sonohysterography or hysterosalpingography.

Special Tests: None indicated.

Diagnostic Procedures: Hysteroscopy.

Pathologic Findings

Intrauterine scarring.

MANAGEMENT AND THERAPY

Nonpharmacologic

General Measures: Evaluation and support.

Specific Measures: Resection of intrauterine scars under hysteroscopic control, followed by intrauterine contraceptive device (IUCD) insertion and estrogen therapy.

Diet: No specific dietary changes indicated.

Activity: No restriction.

Patient Education: Reassurance; American College of Obstetricians and Gynecologists Patient Education Pamphlet AP062 (Dilation and Curettage [D&C]).

Drug(s) of Choice

Estrogen for 1 to 2 months.

Oral—conjugated estrogen 1.25 mg daily, diethylstilbestrol 1 mg daily, esterified estrogens 1.25 mg daily, ethinyl estradiol 0.05 mg daily, micronized estradiol 1 mg daily, piperazine estrone sulfate, estropipate 1.25 mg daily.

Topical—17β-estradiol 0.1 mg per day.

Contraindications: Undiagnosed vaginal bleeding.

FOLLOW-UP

Patient Monitoring: Normal health maintenance.

Prevention/Avoidance: Avoidance of excessive curettage, prompt treatment of endometritis after dilation and curettage.

Possible Complications: Hematocolpos, infertility.

Expected Outcome: Return to normal fertility and menstrual function after treatment.

MISCELLANEOUS

Pregnancy Considerations: Once treated, no effect on future pregnancy.

ICD-9-CM Codes: 621.5.

REFERENCES

Level II

Cohen MA, Sauer MV, Keltz M, Lindheim SR: Utilizing routine sonohysterography to detect intrauterine pathology before initiating hormone replacement therapy. Menopause 1999;6:68.

Hare AA, Olah KS: Pregnancy following endometrial ablation: a review article. J Obstet Gynaecol 2005;25:108.

Level III

Al-Inany H: Intrauterine adhesions. An update. Acta Obstet Gynecol Scand 2001;80:986.

Gambone JC, Munro MG: Office sonography and office hysteroscopy. Curr Opin Obstet Gynecol 1993;5:733.

Gimpelson RJ: Office hysteroscopy. Clin Obstet Gynecol 1992;35:270.

Lancet M, Kessler I: A review of Asherman's syndrome, and results of modern treatment. Int J Fertil 1988;33:14.

Magos A: Hysteroscopic treatment of Asherman's syndrome. Reprod Biomed Online 2002;4:46.

March CM, Israel R, March AD: Hysteroscopic management of intrauterine adhesions. Am J Obstet Gynecol 1978;130:653.

McComb PF, Wagner BL: Simplified therapy for Asherman's syndrome. Fertil Steril 1997;68:1047.

Siegler AM, Valle RF: Therapeutic hysteroscopic procedures. Fertil Steril 1988;50:685.

Asherman's Syndrome (Uterine Synechiae)

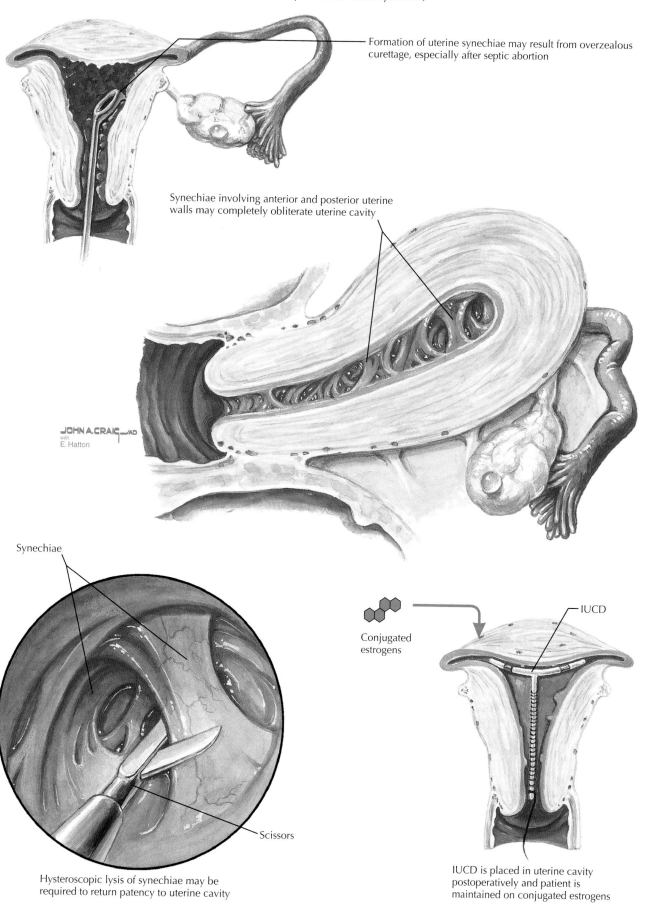

Formation of uterine synechiae may result from overzealous curettage, especially after septic abortion

Synechiae involving anterior and posterior uterine walls may completely obliterate uterine cavity

JOHN A. CRAIG—AD
with
E. Hatton

Synechiae

Scissors

Hysteroscopic lysis of synechiae may be required to return patency to uterine cavity

Conjugated estrogens

IUCD

IUCD is placed in uterine cavity postoperatively and patient is maintained on conjugated estrogens

Dysfunctional Uterine Bleeding

INTRODUCTION

Description: Dysfunctional uterine bleeding is irregular or intermenstrual bleeding with no clinically identifiable underlying cause.

Prevalence: Ten percent to 15% of all gynecologic visits involve menstrual disturbances.

Predominant Age: Reproductive, greatest in adolescents and patients experiencing climacteric changes.

Genetics: No genetic pattern.

ETIOLOGY AND PATHOGENESIS

Causes: Anovulatory patients—chemotherapy, chronic illness, climacteric changes, endometrial carcinoma, endometrial hyperplasia, hormonal contraception (oral, injectable, intrauterine), iatrogenic (anticoagulation, hormone replacement), idiopathic, medications (anticholinergic agents, monamine oxidase inhibitors, morphine, phenothiazines, reserpine), nutritional disruption (anorexia, bulimia, excess physical activity), obesity, pituitary–hypothalamic–ovarian axis immaturity, pituitary tumor, polycystic ovary syndrome, stress, systemic disease (hepatic, renal, thyroid). Ovulatory patients—anatomic lesions (adenomyosis, cervical neoplasia, cervical polyps, endometrial carcinoma, endometrial polyps, leiomyomata, sarcoma), bleeding at ovulation, coagulopathies (natural or iatrogenic), endometritis, fallopian tube disease (infection, tumor), foreign body (IUCD, pessary, tampon), idiopathic, ingested substances (estrogens, ginseng), leukemia, luteal phase dysfunction, pelvic inflammatory disease (including tuberculosis), pregnancy related (abortion, ectopic, hydatidiform mole, retained products of conception), repeated trauma, systemic disease (hepatic, renal, thyroid).

Risk Factors: Prolonged anovulation.

CLINICAL CHARACTERISTICS

Signs and Symptoms

- Intermenstrual bleeding (painless)
- Irregular menstrual cycles (typically prolonged interval)

DIAGNOSTIC APPROACH

Differential Diagnosis

- Pregnancy
- Climacteric changes
- Anovulation
- Endometrial polyps
- Uterine leiomyomata
- Endometrial cancer
- Endometriosis
- Nonuterine sources of bleeding (e.g., cervical, vaginal, vulvar, or perineal)
- Iatrogenic causes (hormones, oral contraceptives)

Associated Conditions: Anovulation, infertility, endometrial cancer, endometrial polyps or carcinoma, uterine leiomyomata, obesity.

Workup and Evaluation

Laboratory: Testing should be chosen on the basis of the differential diagnoses under consideration.

Imaging: Pelvic ultrasonography or sonohysterography may be of assistance in selected patients.

Special Tests: A menstrual calendar helps document the timing and character of the patient's bleeding. Endometrial biopsy, curettage, or hysteroscopy may be indicated.

Diagnostic Procedures: The diagnosis of dysfunctional uterine bleeding is one of exclusion. History and physical examination often point to possible causes for further evaluation.

Pathologic Findings

Proliferation of the endometrial tissues with irregular shedding evident in some patients; in other patients the endometrium is thin and atrophic.

MANAGEMENT AND THERAPY

Nonpharmacologic

General Measures: Evaluation.

Specific Measures: Focused on underlying causation and desires of patient. If anovulation is the cause and fertility is not desired, periodic progestin therapy may be used to stabilize menstrual cycles and suppress intermenstrual bleeding. Suppression of menstrual cycling (gonadotropin-releasing hormone agonists, long-acting progestin), endometrial ablation, or hysterectomy may be required for a small number of patients.

Diet: No specific dietary changes indicated.

Activity: No restriction.

Patient Education: Reassurance; American College of Obstetricians and Gynecologists Patient Education Pamphlet AP095 (Abnormal Uterine Bleeding), AP049 (Menstruation [Especially for Teens]), AP147 (Endometrial Hyperplasia), AP162 (Menopausal Bleeding).

Drug(s) of Choice

Medroxyprogesterone acetate 5 to 10 mg for 1 to 14 days each month. (In roughly 85% of patients who have ovulated in the past, a single cycle provides adequate response.)

Contraindications: Undiagnosed amenorrhea or bleeding.

Precautions: Progestins should not be used until pregnancy has been ruled out.

Alternative Drugs

Norethindrone acetate 5 to 10 mg for 10 to 14 days each month. The levonorgestrel intrauterine system (a polydimethylsiloxane sleeve containing 52 mg of levonorgestrel on the stem that releases 20 µg of levonorgestrel daily) may be inserted or combination oral contraceptives may be used.

Steroid Withdrawal Bleeding

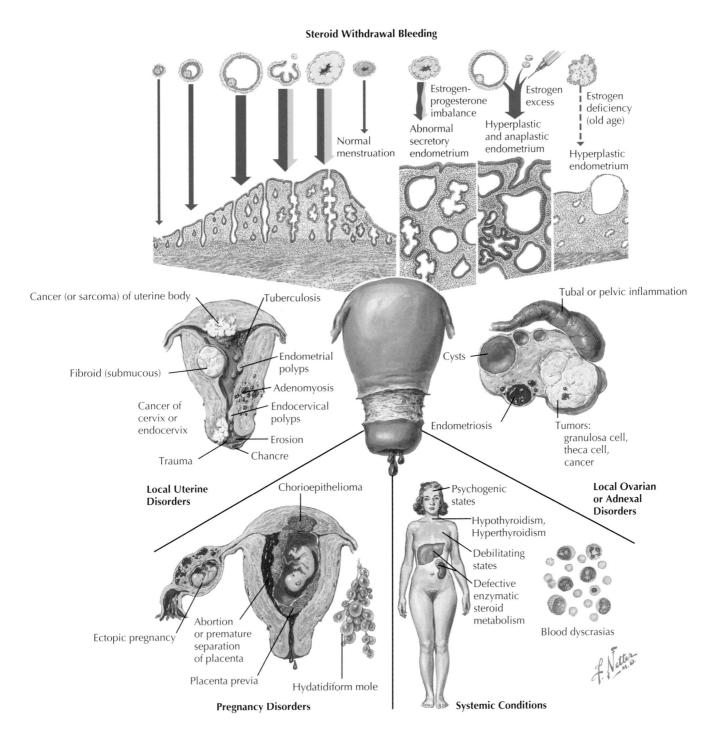

Normal menstruation

Estrogen-progesterone imbalance → Abnormal secretory endometrium

Estrogen excess → Hyperplastic and anaplastic endometrium

Estrogen deficiency (old age) → Hyperplastic endometrium

Cancer (or sarcoma) of uterine body

Tuberculosis

Fibroid (submucous)

Endometrial polyps

Adenomyosis

Cancer of cervix or endocervix

Endocervical polyps

Erosion

Trauma

Chancre

Local Uterine Disorders

Tubal or pelvic inflammation

Cysts

Endometriosis

Tumors: granulosa cell, theca cell, cancer

Local Ovarian or Adnexal Disorders

Chorioepithelioma

Ectopic pregnancy

Abortion or premature separation of placenta

Placenta previa

Hydatidiform mole

Pregnancy Disorders

Psychogenic states

Hypothyroidism, Hyperthyroidism

Debilitating states

Defective enzymatic steroid metabolism

Blood dyscrasias

Systemic Conditions

F. Netter M.D.

FOLLOW-UP

Patient Monitoring: Normal health maintenance.

Prevention/Avoidance: None.

Possible Complications: Anemia, endometrial hyperplasia or carcinoma if anovulation or simple hypertrophy is left untreated.

Expected Outcome: Return to normal menstrual pattern with correction of underlying pathologic condition or periodic progestin therapy.

MISCELLANEOUS

Pregnancy Considerations: No effect on pregnancy aside from that resulting from causative conditions.

ICD-9-CM Codes: 626.8, 626.4 (Irregular menstrual cycle).

REFERENCES

Level I

Aberdeen Endometrial Ablation Trials Group: A randomized trial of endometrial ablation versus hysterectomy for the treatment of dysfunctional uterine bleeding: outcome at four years. Br J Obstet Gynaecol 1999;106:360.

Crosignani PG, Vercellini P, Mosconi P, et al: Levonorgestrel-releasing intrauterine device versus hysteroscopic endometrial resection in the treatment of dysfunctional uterine bleeding. Obstet Gynecol 1997;90:257.

DeVore GR, Owens O, Kase N: Use of intravenous Premarin in the treatment of dysfunctional uterine bleeding—A double-blind randomized controlled study. Obstet Gynecol 1982;59:285.

Pinion SB, Parkin DE, Abramovich DR, et al: Randomised trial of hysterectomy, endometrial laser ablation, and transcervical endometrial resection for dysfunctional uterine bleeding. BMJ 1994;309:979.

Level II

Brooks PG, Clouse J, Morris LS: Hysterectomy vs. resectoscopic endometrial ablation for the control of abnormal uterine bleeding. A cost-comparative study. J Reprod Med 1994;39:755.

Brumsted JR, Blackman JA, Badger GJ, Riddick DH: Hysteroscopy versus hysterectomy for the treatment of abnormal uterine bleeding: a comparison of cost. Fertil Steril 1996;65:310.

Falcone T, Desjardins C, Bourque J, et al: Dysfunctional uterine bleeding in adolescents. J Reprod Med 1994;39:761.

Level III

Aksel S, Jones GS: Etiology and treatment of dysfunctional uterine bleeding. Obstet Gynecol 1974;44:1.

Albers JR, Hull SK, Wesley RM: Abnormal uterine bleeding. Am Fam Physician 2004;69:1915.

American College of Obstetricians and Gynecologists: Management of anovulatory bleeding. ACOG Practice Bulletin 14. Washington, DC, ACOG, 2000.

American College of Obstetricians and Gynecologists: Noncontraceptive uses of the levonorgestrel intrauterine system. ACOG Committee Opinion 337. Obstet Gynecol 2006;107:1479.

Bayer RL, DeCherney AH: Clinical manifestations and treatment of dysfunctional uterine bleeding. JAMA 1993;269:1823.

Cowan BD, Morrison JC: Management of abnormal genital bleeding in girls and women. N Engl J Med 1991;324:1710.

Pitkin J: Dysfunctional uterine bleeding. BMJ 2007;334:1110.

INTRODUCTION

Description: Endometrial cancer is characterized by malignant change of the endometrial tissues. These are generally of the adenocarcinoma, adenosquamous, clear cell, or papillary serous cell types.

Prevalence: Two percent to 3% lifetime risk, the most frequent malignancy of the female reproductive tract, roughly 39,000 cases per year in the United States (2007 estimate); 7400 deaths each year (2007), eighth leading site of cancer-related death among American women.

Predominant Age: 55 to 65.

Genetics: No genetic pattern known except for such conditions as hereditary nonpolyposis colorectal cancer (HNPCC; Lynch II syndrome). (Cancers found in younger women are associated with mutations in the K-*ras*, PTEN, or MLH1 genes.)

ETIOLOGY AND PATHOGENESIS

Causes: Unopposed (without progestins) estrogen stimulation (polycystic ovary syndrome, obesity, chronic anovulation, and estrogen replacement therapy without concomitant progestin) in 90% of cases. Selective estrogen receptor modulators with uterine activity (tamoxifen).

Risk Factors: Unopposed estrogen stimulation of the uterus (chronic anovulation, estrogen therapy, and obesity), tamoxifen use, early menarche, late menopause, nulliparity, breast or colon cancer, diabetes.

CLINICAL CHARACTERISTICS

Signs and Symptoms

- Postmenopausal bleeding (90%)
- Abnormal glandular cells on Pap test (Cervical cytologic tests detect only about 20% of known endometrial carcinomas.)

DIAGNOSTIC APPROACH

Differential Diagnosis

- Endometrial hyperplasia (complex, atypical)
- Cervical cancer
- Endometrial or cervical polyp
- Ovarian cancer metastatic to the endometrium
- Metachronous Müllerian tumor
- Endometriosis
- Early pregnancy (younger women)
- Granulosa cell tumors

Associated Conditions: Obesity, irregular menstrual bleeding, infertility, breast or colon cancer.

Workup and Evaluation

Laboratory: No evaluation indicated, except for preoperative screening.

Imaging: Chest radiograph (for metastases), transvaginal ultrasonography or sonohysterography may be useful (although concerns have been raised about the possibility of extrauterine spread induced by tubal spill of fluid during sonohysterography).

Special Tests: Endometrial biopsy (90% accurate).

Diagnostic Procedures: History, physical examination, and endometrial biopsy.

Pathologic Findings

Atypical, hyperplastic glands with little or no stroma. Mitosis common. (See table for staging.)

MANAGEMENT AND THERAPY

Nonpharmacologic

General Measures: Evaluation and staging.

Specific Measures: Surgical exploration with hysterectomy, bilateral salpingo-oophorectomy, cytologic examination of the abdomen and diaphragm, para-aortic node sampling. Radiation to the vaginal cuff reduces local recurrence. Distant metastatic disease is treated with high-dose progestins, cisplatin, and doxorubicin (Adriamycin). The use of adjuvant radiation therapy in women with disease limited to the uterus based on systematic surgical staging is controversial.

Diet: No specific dietary changes indicated except as dictated by surgical therapy.

Activity: No restriction except as dictated by surgical therapy.

Patient Education: American College of Obstetricians and Gynecologists Patient Education Pamphlet AP097 (Cancer of the Uterus), AP008 (Hysterectomy), AP080 (Preparing for Surgery), AP095 (Abnormal Uterine Bleeding).

Drug(s) of Choice

Hyperplasia and distant metastatic disease: megestrol (Megace) 160 mg PO daily for 3 months. This is generally followed by curettage or other evaluation to assess response.

Doxorubicin (Adriamycin) or cisplatin chemotherapy.

Contraindications: See individual agents.

Precautions: High-dose progestins should be used with caution in patients with congestive heart failure because they may cause fluid retention.

Interactions: See individual agents.

FOLLOW-UP

Patient Monitoring: Follow-up Pap tests from vaginal cuff every 3 months for 2 years, then every 6 months for 3 years, then yearly. Chest radiograph annually.

Prevention/Avoidance: Correction of unopposed estrogen states or the addition of progestin.

Possible Complications: Distant spread with progression to death.

Expected Outcome: Five-year survival based on stage and grade—stage I, 85%; stage II, 60%; stage III, 30%; stage IV, 10%.

MISCELLANEOUS

Pregnancy Considerations: Generally not a consideration because they are unlikely to coexist.

ICD-9-CM Codes: Specific to cell type and location.

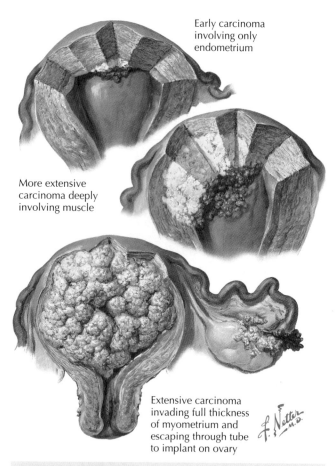

Early carcinoma
involving only
endometrium

More extensive
carcinoma deeply
involving muscle

Extensive carcinoma
invading full thickness
of myometrium and
escaping through tube
to implant on ovary

REFERENCES

Level I

Malur S, Possover M, Michels W, Schneider A: Laparoscopic-assisted vaginal versus abdominal surgery in patients with endometrial cancer—A prospective randomized trial. Gynecol Oncol 2001;80:239.

Level II

Creasman WT, Odicino F, Maisonneuve P, et al: Carcinoma of the corpus uteri. Int J Gynaecol Obstet 2003;83:79.

Cushing KL, Weiss NS, Voigt LF, et al: Risk of endometrial cancer in relation to use of low-dose, unopposed estrogens. Obstet Gynecol 1998;91:35.

Davies JL, Rosenshein NB, Antunes CMF, Stolley PD: A review of the risk factors for endometrial carcinoma. Obstet Gynecol Surv 1981;36:107.

Gallup DG, Stock RJ: Adenocarcinoma of the endometrium in women 40 years or younger. Obstet Gynecol 1984;64:417.

Kalogiannidis I, Lambrechts S, Amant F, et al: Laparoscopy-assisted vaginal hysterectomy compared with abdominal hysterectomy in clinical stage I endometrial cancer: safety, recurrence, and long-term outcome. Am J Obstet Gynecol 2007;196:248.e1.

Level III

Akin O, Mironov S, Pandit-Taskar N, Hann LE: Imaging of uterine cancer. Radiol Clin North Am 2007;45:167.

Amant F, Moerman P, Neven P, et al: Endometrial cancer. Lancet 2005;366:491.

American College of Obstetricians and Gynecologists: Selective estrogen receptor modulators. ACOG Practice Bulletin 39. Obstet Gynecol 2002;100:835.

American College of Obstetricians and Gynecologists: Ovarian, endometrial, and colorectal cancers. Obstet Gynecol 2004;104:77S.

American College of Obstetricians and Gynecologists: Management of endometrial cancer. ACOG Practice Bulletin 65. Obstet Gynecol 2005;106:413.

American College of Obstetricians and Gynecologists: Tamoxifen and uterine cancer. ACOG Committee Opinion 336. Obstet Gynecol 2006;107:1475.

American College of Obstetricians and Gynecologists: Noncontraceptive uses of the levonorgestrel intrauterine system. ACOG Committee Opinion 337. Obstet Gynecol 2006;107:1479.

Boronow RC, Morrow CP, Creasman WT, et al: Surgical staging in endometrial cancer: clinical-pathologic findings of a prospective study. Obstet Gynecol 1984;63:825.

Kodama S, Kase H, Tanaka K, Matsui K: Multivariate analysis of prognostic factors in patients with endometrial cancer. Int J Gynaecol Obstet 1996;53:23.

Lu K, Slomivitz BM: Neoplastic diseases of the uterus. In Katz VL, Lentz GM, Lobo RA, Gershenson DM: Comprehensive Gynecology, 5th ed. Philadelphia, Mosby/Elsevier, 2007:819.

Reid PC, Brown VA, Fothergill DJ: Outpatient investigation of postmenopausal bleeding. Br J Obstet Gynaecol 1993;100:498.

Endometrial Hyperplasia: Simple and Complex

INTRODUCTION

Description: Endometrial hyperplasia is caused by abnormal proliferation of both the glandular and stromal elements of the endometrium with characteristic alteration in the histologic architecture of the tissues. It is this architectural change that differentiates hyperplasia from normal endometrial proliferation. Simple hyperplasia represents the least significant form of alteration. Complex hyperplasia represents the most significant form of alteration.

Prevalence: Five percent of patients with postmenopausal bleeding have endometrial hyperplasia.

Predominant Age: Late reproductive and early menopausal.

Genetics: No genetic pattern.

ETIOLOGY AND PATHOGENESIS

Causes: Unknown.

Risk Factors: Unopposed estrogen stimulation of the uterus (chronic anovulation, estrogen therapy [4-fold to 8-fold risk], obesity [3-fold risk]), nulliparity (2-fold to 3-fold risk), diabetes (2-fold to 3-fold risk), polycystic ovarian syndrome, tamoxifen use.

CLINICAL CHARACTERISTICS

Signs and Symptoms

- Asymptomatic
- Intermenstrual bleeding
- Menorrhagia
- Postmenopausal bleeding

DIAGNOSTIC APPROACH

Differential Diagnosis

- Endometrial adenocarcinoma
- Endocervical or endometrial polyps
- Endocervical carcinoma

Associated Conditions: Endocervical or endometrial polyps, squamous metaplasia, endometrial carcinoma. When nuclear atypia is present, more than 40% of patients will have a coexisting endometrial cancer.

Workup and Evaluation

Laboratory: No evaluation indicated.

Imaging: Ultrasonography may detect thickening of the endometrial stripe. (No standard has emerged for a threshold of endometrial thickness that carries ideal positive and negative predictive values. It does not take the place of histologic evaluation.) Magnetic resonance imaging may also diagnose endometrial thickening, but cost and low specificity argue against its use as a diagnostic tool.

Special Tests: Endometrial biopsy, hysteroscopy, or dilation and curettage.

Diagnostic Procedures: Endometrial biopsy.

Pathologic Findings

Simple hyperplasia—proliferation of both glandular and stromal elements with no atypia. The glands form simple tubules with wide variations in size from small to large cysts. There is little or no outpouching of the epithelium lining the cysts. Complex hyperplasia—proliferation of both glandular and stromal elements. Cellular atypia (characterized by disordered maturation, high nuclear/cytoplasmic ratio, nuclear pleomorphism, mitoses) may be present or absent. Glands are crowded with a "back-to-back" appearance. May be found with coexisting adenocarcinoma (17% to 52% in various studies). Outpouching in glands is common. (It should be noted that the reliability of histologic diagnosis of these two conditions has recently been called into question.)

MANAGEMENT AND THERAPY

Nonpharmacologic

General Measures: Prompt evaluation.

Specific Measures: Simple hyperplasia—medical therapy (progestin) is generally adequate. Many use dilation and curettage by itself or in combination with progestin therapy. Complex hyperplasia—for patients with hyperplasia without atypia or for selected patients who wish to preserve fertility, high-dose prolonged progestin therapy may be used. All others are treated by hysterectomy (with bilateral salpingo-oophorectomy).

Diet: No specific dietary changes indicated.

Activity: No restriction.

Patient Education: Reassurance; American College of Obstetricians and Gynecologists Patient Education Pamphlet AP147 (Endometrial Hyperplasia), AP095 (Abnormal Uterine Bleeding), AP097 (Cancer of the Uterus), AP062 (Dilation and Curettage [D&C]).

Drug(s) of Choice

Simple hyperplasia—medroxyprogesterone acetate (Provera, Cycrin) 10 mg PO daily for 10 days each month, norethindrone acetate (Aygestin) 10 mg PO daily for 10 days each month.

Complex hyperplasia—depot medroxyprogesterone acetate (Depo-Provera) up to 200 to 1000 mg IM weekly for 5 weeks, followed by 100 to 400 mg IM monthly, megestrol acetate (Megace) 40 to 80 mg PO daily for 6 to 12 weeks. (Some authors have advocated therapy for up to 48 months.) Estrogen replacement therapy may be given safely to those treated by hysterectomy.

Contraindications: Undiagnosed vaginal bleeding, thrombophlebitis, markedly impaired liver function, known or suspected breast cancer.

Precautions: Progestins should not be used during the first trimester of pregnancy.

Alternative Drugs

Combination oral contraceptives also may be used for simple hyperplasia.

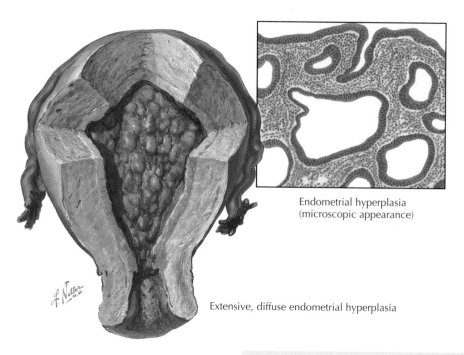

Endometrial hyperplasia
(microscopic appearance)

Extensive, diffuse endometrial hyperplasia

FOLLOW-UP

Patient Monitoring: With simple hyperplasia or for complex hyperplasia managed medically, a follow-up endometrial sampling must be performed after 3 months, then every 6 to 12 months thereafter.

Prevention/Avoidance: None.

Possible Complications: Progression is uncommon with simple hyperplasia (1% to cancer, 3% to complex hyperplasia). A slight risk is associated with endometrial sampling (infection, perforation). Complex hyperplasia, especially with atypia, is associated with coexistent malignancy or the risk of progression to malignant changes (75% of patients). The more atypical the cellular architecture, the greater the risk of malignancy; without atypia, 25% of hyperplasia will progress and 50% will persist.

Expected Outcome: Good response to medical therapy can be anticipated for patients with simple hyperplasia. Progression and recurrence are uncommon.

MISCELLANEOUS

Pregnancy Considerations: No effect on pregnancy.
ICD-9-CM Codes: 621.3.

REFERENCES

Level I
Steiner AZ, Xiang M, Mack WJ, et al: Unopposed estradiol therapy in postmenopausal women: results from two randomized trials. Obstet Gynecol 2007;109:581.

Level II
Clark TJ, Voit D, Gupta JK, et al: Accuracy of hysteroscopy in the diagnosis of endometrial cancer and hyperplasia: a systematic quantitative review. JAMA 2002;288:1610.

Grady D, Ettinger B, Moscarelli E, et al; Multiple Outcomes of Raloxifene Evaluation Investigators: Safety and adverse effects associated with raloxifene: multiple outcomes of raloxifene evaluation. Obstet Gynecol 2004;104:837.

Horn LC, Schnurrbusch U, Bilek K, et al: Risk of progression in complex and atypical endometrial hyperplasia: clinicopathologic analysis in cases with and without progestogen treatment. Int J Gynecol Cancer 2004;14:348.

Janicek MF, Rosenshein NB: Invasive endometrial cancer in uteri resected for atypical endometrial hyperplasia. Gynecol Oncol 1994;52:373.

Kurman RJ, Kaminski PF, Norris HJ: The behavior of endometrial hyperplasia—A long-term study of "untreated" hyperplasia in 170 patients. Cancer 1985;56:403.

Pettersson B, Adami HO, Lindgren A, et al: Endometrial polyps and hyperplasia as risk factors for endometrial carcinoma. Acta Obstet Gynecol Scand 1985;64:653.

Trimble CL, Kauderer J, Zaino R, et al: Concurrent endometrial carcinoma in women with a biopsy diagnosis of atypical endometrial hyperplasia: a Gynecologic Oncology Group study. Cancer 2006;106:812.

Wang J, Wieslander C, Hansen G, et al: Thin endometrial echo complex on ultrasound does not reliably exclude type 2 endometrial cancers. Gynecol Oncol 2006;101:120.

Zaino RJ, Kauderer J, Trimble CL, et al: Reproducibility of the diagnosis of atypical endometrial hyperplasia: a Gynecologic Oncology Group study. Cancer 2006;106:804.

Level III
American College of Obstetricians and Gynecologists: Management of anovulatory bleeding. ACOG Practice Bulletin 14. Washington, DC, ACOG, 2000.

American College of Obstetricians and Gynecologists: Selective estrogen receptor modulators. ACOG Practice Bulletin 39. Obstet Gynecol 2002;100:835.

American College of Obstetricians and Gynecologists: Management of endometrial cancer. ACOG Practice Bulletin 65. Obstet Gynecol 2005;106:413.

American College of Obstetricians and Gynecologists: Tamoxifen and uterine cancer. ACOG Committee Opinion 336. Obstet Gynecol 2006;107:1475.

American College of Obstetricians and Gynecologists: Noncontraceptive uses of the levonorgestrel intrauterine system. ACOG Committee Opinion 337. Obstet Gynecol 2006;107:1479.

Copenhaver EH: Atypical endometrial hyperplasia. Obstet Gynecol 1959;13:264.

Eichner E, Abellera M: Endometrial hyperplasia treated by progestins. Obstet Gynecol 1971;38:739.

Gusberg SB, Chen SY, Cohen CJ: Endometrial cancer: factors influencing the choice of treatment. Gynecol Oncol 1974;2:308.

Wentz WB: Progestin therapy in endometrial hyperplasia. Gynecol Oncol 1974;2:362.

INTRODUCTION

Description: Endometrial polyps are fleshy tumors that arise as local overgrowths of endometrial glands and stroma and project beyond the surface of the endometrium. These are most common in the fundus of the uterus but may occur anywhere in the endometrial cavity. They are generally small (a few millimeters) but may enlarge to fill the entire cavity.

Prevalence: Up to 10% of women (autopsy studies), 20% of uteruses removed because of cancer.

Predominant Age: 40 to 50, infrequent after menopause.

Genetics: No genetic pattern.

ETIOLOGY AND PATHOGENESIS

Causes: Unknown. A role for unopposed estrogen is hypothesized.

Risk Factors: Unopposed estrogen use, tamoxifen therapy.

CLINICAL CHARACTERISTICS

Signs and Symptoms

- Asymptomatic (most)
- Abnormal bleeding (most common intermenstrual bleeding and menorrhagia, perimenopausal bleeding). One fourth of women with abnormal bleeding patterns have an endometrial polyp.
- Polyps with long pedicles may protrude from the cervix.

DIAGNOSTIC APPROACH

Differential Diagnosis

- Endocervical polyp
- Endometrial cancer
- Prolapsed leiomyomata
- Retained products of conception
- Retained (and forgotten) intrauterine contraceptive device

Associated Conditions: Endometrial cancer (2-fold increase).

Workup and Evaluation

Laboratory: No evaluation indicated.

Imaging: Sonohysterography generally identifies the polyp. (Special attention should be directed to the fundus, where most polyps arise.)

Special Tests: None indicated.

Diagnostic Procedures: History, physical examination, endometrial sampling, hysteroscopy, or curettage. (Often not diagnosed until the uterus is removed for other reasons.)

Pathologic Findings

Velvety surface with a rich central vascular core. Endometrial glands, stroma, and vascular channels are present with epithelium identified on three sides to establish the pedunculated nature. The endometrial glands are often immature in appearance with a "Swiss cheese" cystic character that is independent of the phase of the cycle. Infection or metaplasia may be present.

MANAGEMENT AND THERAPY

Nonpharmacologic

General Measures: Evaluation.

Specific Measures: Removal by curettage or operative hysteroscopy. (All polyps removed should be examined histologically.)

Diet: No specific dietary changes indicated.

Activity: No restriction.

Patient Education: Reassurance: American College of Obstetricians and Gynecologists Patient Education Pamphlet AP095 (Abnormal Uterine Bleeding), AP062 (Dilation and Curettage [D&C]).

Drug(s) of Choice

None.

FOLLOW-UP

Patient Monitoring: Normal health maintenance.

Prevention/Avoidance: Evaluation and treatment of prolonged amenorrhea, treatment of unopposed estrogen states.

Possible Complications: Up to 0.5% of polyps undergo malignant transformation (low grade and stage).

Expected Outcome: Removal is generally curative even when malignant transformation is present.

MISCELLANEOUS

Pregnancy Considerations: No effect on pregnancy.

ICD-9-CM Codes: 621.0.

REFERENCES

Level I

Marsh FA, Rogerson LJ, Duffy SR: A randomised controlled trial comparing outpatient versus daycase endometrial polypectomy. BJOG 2006;113:896. Epub 2006 Jun 2.

Level II

Davidson KG, Dubinsky TJ: Ultrasonographic evaluation of the endometrium in postmenopausal vaginal bleeding. Radiol Clin North Am 2003;41:769.

Maia H Jr, Maltez A, Studart E, et al: Ki-67, Bcl-2 and p53 expression in endometrial polyps and in the normal endometrium during the menstrual cycle. BJOG 2004;111:1242.

Level III

American College of Obstetricians and Gynecologists: Management of anovulatory bleeding. ACOG Practice Bulletin 14. Washington, DC, ACOG, 2000.

American College of Obstetricians and Gynecologists: Tamoxifen and uterine cancer. ACOG Committee Opinion 336. Obstet Gynecol 2006;107:1475.

Armenia CC: Sequential relationship between endometrial polyps and carcinoma of the endometrium. Obstet Gynecol 1967;30:524.

Katz VL: Benign gynecologic lesions. In Katz VL, Lentz GM, Lobo RA, Gershenson DM: Comprehensive Gynecology, 5th ed. Philadelphia, Mosby/Elsevier, 2007:438.

Peterson WF, Novak ER: Endometrial polyps. Obstet Gynecol 1956;8:40.

Salm R: The incidence and significance of early carcinomas in endometrial polyps. J Pathol 1972;108:47.

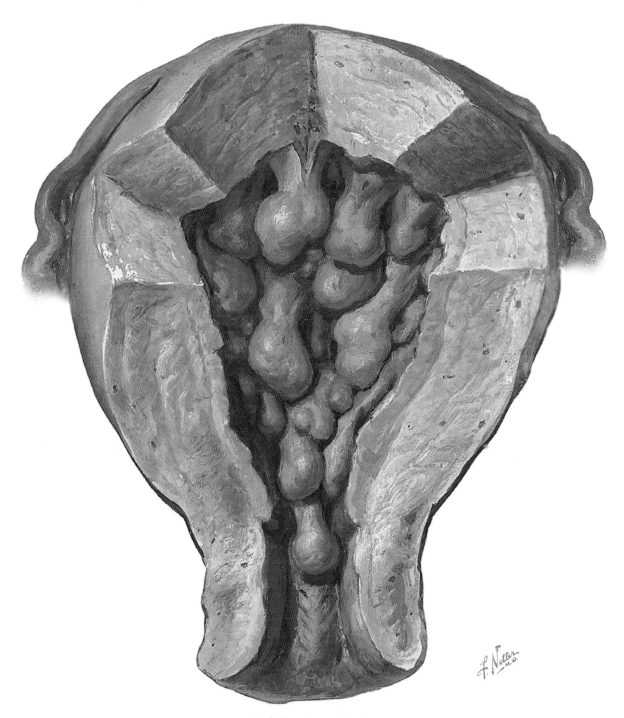

Multiple endometrial polyps

INTRODUCTION

Description: Endometritis is an acute or chronic inflammation, usually of infectious origin, of the lining of the uterus. This is a general term that is used for this condition in either nonpregnant or recently pregnant patients; chorioamnionitis or endomyometritis are the terms commonly used for pregnant patients. Chronic endometritis is often characterized as an intermediate state in ascending infections.

Prevalence: Seventy-five percent of patients with pelvic inflammatory disease, 40% of patients with mucopurulent cervicitis.

Predominant Age: Reproductive.

Genetics: No genetic pattern.

ETIOLOGY AND PATHOGENESIS

Causes: Aseptic inflammation of the endometrium is commonly found in users of intrauterine contraceptive devices (IUCDs). Infection by organisms ascending from the cervix and lower tract are common (most often *Chlamydia trachomatis*, *Neisseria gonorrhoeae*, *Ureaplasma urealyticum*, and *Streptococcus agalactiae)*. Less common are infections by *Actinomyces israelii* or tuberculosis.

Risk Factors: IUCD use, intrauterine instrumentation (biopsy, hysterosalpingography), cervicitis, sexually transmitted disease (STD), retained products of conception.

CLINICAL CHARACTERISTICS

Signs and Symptoms

- Asymptomatic
- Dysfunctional uterine bleeding (typically intermenstrual)
- Postcoital bleeding
- Foul-smelling cervical/vaginal discharge
- Pelvic inflammatory disease
- Chronic pelvic pain
- Tubo-ovarian abscess
- Infertility (rare cause)

DIAGNOSTIC APPROACH

Differential Diagnosis

- Accidents of pregnancy
- Trophoblastic disease
- Endometrial cancer
- Estrogen-producing tumors or exogenous estrogen
- Leiomyomata
- Cervical lesion/cervicitis
- Forgotten IUCD

Associated Conditions: Chronic pelvic pain, tubo-ovarian abscess, cervicitis, and STD.

Workup and Evaluation

Laboratory: Complete blood count, cervical cultures for *C. trachomatis* and *N. gonorrhoeae*. (Tests for other STDs as indicated.)

Imaging: No imaging indicated. Ultrasonography with saline contrast may demonstrate a thickened endometrium but risks spreading an infection to the fallopian tubes, ovaries, and peritoneal cavity. Consequently, this should be reserved until the possibility of active infection has been evaluated.

Special Tests: Endometrial biopsy is generally confirmatory.

Diagnostic Procedures: Endometrial biopsy and culture.

Pathologic Findings

Inflammatory infiltrates (monocytes and plasma cells) in the basal layers and stroma of the endometrium. Sulfur granules may be present in *Actinomyces* infections.

MANAGEMENT AND THERAPY

Nonpharmacologic

General Measures: Evaluation, counseling about STDs (cervicitis).

Specific Measures: Antibiotic therapy (see later), removal of IUCD (if present).

Diet: No specific dietary changes indicated.

Activity: Pelvic rest (no tampons, douches, or intercourse) until therapy has been completed.

Patient Education: American College of Obstetricians and Gynecologists Patient Education Pamphlet AP095 (Abnormal Uterine Bleeding), AP099 (Pelvic Pain), AP077 (Pelvic Inflammatory Disease).

Drug(s) of Choice

Doxycycline (Vibramycin) 200 mg PO initially, 100 mg PO daily for 10 days. If *Actinomyces* is found in a tubo-ovarian abscess, oral penicillin therapy should be continued for 12 weeks.

Contraindications: Known or suspected allergy to tetracycline. Doxycycline is contraindicated in the last half of pregnancy.

Precautions: Photosensitivity may occur in patients taking doxycycline.

Interactions: Doxycycline may enhance the effect of warfarin. Doxycycline absorption is inhibited by most antacids and bismuth subsalicylate (Pepto-Bismol).

Alternative Drugs

Metronidazole or erythromycin may be substituted for doxycycline.

FOLLOW-UP

Patient Monitoring: Normal health maintenance, screening for STDs as needed.

Prevention/Avoidance: Reduce risk of cervicitis or STDs, asepsis during intrauterine procedures.

Possible Complications: Ascending infection resulting in salpingitis, tubo-ovarian abscesses, hydrosalpinx, peritonitis, and chronic pelvic pain.

Expected Outcome: Good with treatment.

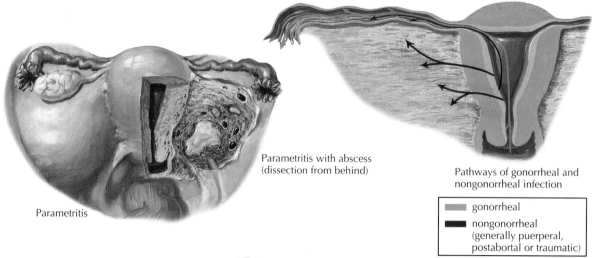

Parametritis

Parametritis with abscess
(dissection from behind)

Pathways of gonorrheal and
nongonorrheal infection

▬	gonorrheal
▬	nongonorrheal (generally puerperal, postabortal or traumatic)

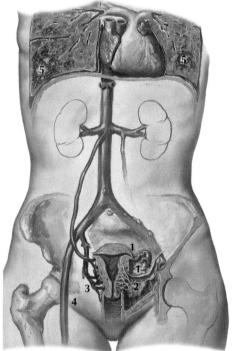

Dissemination of septic endometritis:
(1) Peritonitis
(2) Parametritis (via lymphatics)
(3) Pelvic thrombophlebitis
(4) Femoral thrombophlebitis
(5) Pulmonary infarct or abscess (septic embolus)

MISCELLANEOUS

Pregnancy Considerations: Generally not applicable. *Ureaplasma urealyticum* infection has been implicated as a rare cause of early pregnancy loss.

ICD-9-CM Codes: 615.0 (Acute), 615.1 (Chronic), 670 (Following delivery, excludes pregnancy, abortion, ectopic and molar pregnancies).

REFERENCES

Level I

Starr RV, Zurawski J, Ismail M: Preoperative vaginal preparation with povidone-iodine and the risk of postcesarean endometritis. Obstet Gynecol 2005;105:1024.

Sullivan SA, Smith T, Chang E, et al: Administration of cefazolin prior to skin incision is superior to cefazolin at cord clamping in preventing postcesarean infectious morbidity: a randomized, controlled trial. Am J Obstet Gynecol 2007;196:455.e1.

Level II

Ness RB, Hillier SL, Kip KE, et al: Bacterial vaginosis and risk of pelvic inflammatory disease. Obstet Gynecol 2004;104:761.

Level III

American College of Obstetricians and Gynecologists: Prophylactic antibiotics in labor and delivery. ACOG Practice Bulletin 47. Obstet Gynecol 2003;102:875.

American College of Obstetricians and Gynecologists: Antibiotic prophylaxis for gynecologic procedures. ACOG Practice Bulletin 74. Obstet Gynecol 2006;108:225.

Casey BM, Cox SM: Chorioamnionitis and endometritis. Infect Disease Clin North Am 1997;11:203.

Crossman SH: The challenge of pelvic inflammatory disease. Am Fam Physician 2006;73:859.

Michels TC: Chronic endometritis. Am Fam Physician 1995;52:217.

Pastorek JG 2nd: Postcesarean endometritis. Compr Ther 1995;21:249.

INTRODUCTION

Description: Hematometra is a collection of blood in the body (cavity) of the uterus resulting from obstruction of the normal outflow tract. This obstruction may result from congenital abnormalities, acquired cervical stenosis, or obstruction by neoplasia.

Prevalence: Uncommon.

Predominant Age: Early reproductive and postmenopausal most common.

Genetics: No genetic pattern.

ETIOLOGY AND PATHOGENESIS

Causes: Obstruction or atresia of the uterine outflow tract (congenital malformation; most common are imperforate hymen and transverse vaginal septum, acquired causes; cervical stenosis from senile atrophy of the endocervix and endometrium, scarring by synechiae, scarring after surgery, endometrial ablation, radiation, cryocautery, electrocautery, neoplasia).

Risk Factors: Previous cervical surgery (cone biopsy, cryocoagulation, or electrocautery), menopausal atrophy, cervical neoplasia, incomplete endometrial ablation.

CLINICAL CHARACTERISTICS

Signs and Symptoms

- Asymptomatic (especially in postmenopausal women)
- Uterine enlargement (often soft and slightly tender)
- Dysmenorrhea, abnormal bleeding, amenorrhea and infertility in premenopausal women
- Cyclic abdominal pain

DIAGNOSTIC APPROACH

Differential Diagnosis

- Endometrial hyperplasia/cancer
- Endocervical cancer
- Pyometra
- Leiomyomata
- Ovarian neoplasia

Associated Conditions: Cervical cancer, endometrial cancer, tubo-ovarian abscess, and endometriosis.

Workup and Evaluation

Laboratory: No evaluation indicated.

Imaging: Ultrasonography can confirm uterine enlargement and the presence of fluid but cannot define the character of the fluid. The presence of a cervical mass may occasionally be confirmed.

Special Tests: Endometrial biopsy or hysteroscopic evaluation of the uterine cavity should be considered. Gentle probing with a 1- to 2-mm probe confirms cervical obstruction or stenosis.

Diagnostic Procedures: History, physical examination, ultrasonography, cervical dilation or probing.

Pathologic Findings

Based on cause.

MANAGEMENT AND THERAPY

Nonpharmacologic

General Measures: Evaluation.

Specific Measures: Cervical dilation with or without curettage provides drainage, although it may have to be repeated several times. Antibiotic should be provided to protect against possible colonization by *Bacteroides*, anaerobic *Staphylococcus* and *Streptococcus*, and aerobic coliform bacteria. A mushroom or Foley catheter may be placed to facilitate drainage but may itself become a source of infection. Definitive therapy is based on cause.

Diet: No specific dietary changes indicated.

Activity: No restriction.

Patient Education: American College of Obstetricians and Gynecologists Patient Education Pamphlet AP095 (Abnormal Uterine Bleeding), AP097 (Cancer of the Uterus), AP062 (Dilation and Curettage [D&C]), AP084 (Hysteroscopy).

Drug(s) of Choice

None. Therapy is based on cause and clinical situation. Antibiotic treatment if infection is suspected. (The antibiotic chosen should provide protection against possible colonization by *Bacteroides*, anaerobic *Staphylococcus* and *Streptococcus*, and aerobic coliform bacteria.)

Contraindications: See individual agents.

Precautions: See individual agents.

Interactions: See individual agents.

FOLLOW-UP

Patient Monitoring: Normal health maintenance and periodic reassessment of the cervix and uterus.

Prevention/Avoidance: Avoid unnecessary cervical procedures and limit the scope of therapy when such procedures are necessary. Some authors suggest cervical sounding after such procedures to assess patency, although this has not been shown to reduce the incidence of stenosis.

Possible Complications: Infection (leading to pyometra), progression of underlying disease.

Expected Outcome: Based on cause.

MISCELLANEOUS

Pregnancy Considerations: Incompatible with pregnancy.

ICD-9-CM Codes: 621.4.

REFERENCES

Level II

Gurtcheff SE, Sharp HT: Complications associated with global endometrial ablation: the utility of the MAUDE database. Obstet Gynecol 2003;102:1278.

Kinjo K, Kasai T, Ogawa K: Hematometra and ruptured hematosalpinx with ipsilateral renal agenesis presenting as diffuse peritonitis: a case report. Intens Care Med 1977;23:354.

Hematocolpos with
hematometra and hematosalpinx

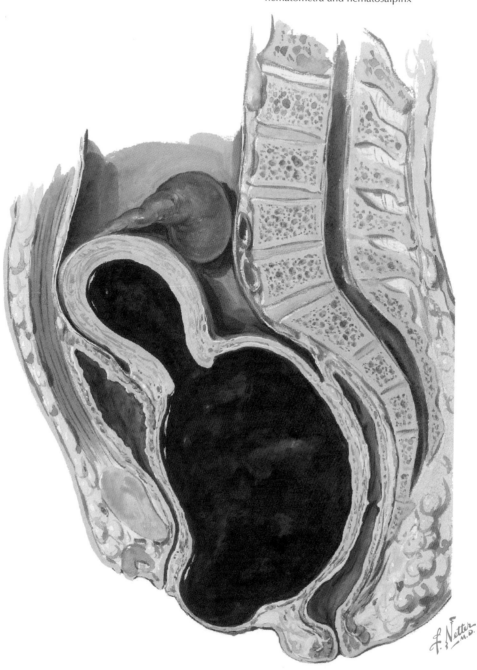

Scheerer LJ, Bartolucci L: Transvaginal sonography in the evaluation of hematometra. A report of two cases. J Reprod Med
1996;41:205.

Sheih CP, Liao YJ, Liang WW, Lu WT: Sonographic presentation
of unilateral hematometra: report of two cases. J Ultrasound Med
1995;14:695.

Vernooij CB, Kruitwagen RF, Rodrigus P, et al: Hematometra after
radiotherapy for cervical carcinoma. Gynecol Oncol 1997;67:325.

Level III

American College of Obstetricians and Gynecologists: Endometrial
ablation. ACOG Practice Bulletin 81. Obstet Gynecol
2007;109:1233.

Jayasinghe Y, Rane A, Stalewski H, Grover S: The presentation and
early diagnosis of the rudimentary uterine horn. Obstet Gynecol
2005;105:1456.

Katz VL: Benign gynecologic lesions. In Katz VL, Lentz GM, Lobo
RA, Gershenson DM: Comprehensive Gynecology, 5th ed. Philadelphia, Mosby/Elsevier, 2007:440.

INTRODUCTION

Description: Bleeding between otherwise normal menstrual cycles is called intermenstrual bleeding.
Prevalence: Ten percent to 15% of all gynecologic visits involve menstrual disturbances.
Predominant Age: Reproductive, greatest in adolescents and patients who are climacteric.
Genetics: No genetic pattern.

ETIOLOGY AND PATHOGENESIS

Causes: Uterine (pregnancy, endometrial polyps, endometrial hyperplasia, endometrial carcinoma, leiomyomata), cervical (polyps, cervicitis, cervical erosion, cervical dysplasia/neoplasia), vaginal (trauma, infection, atrophy), perineal (vulvar lesions, hemorrhoids).
Risk Factors: None known. (The purported relationship to surgical sterilization has been disproved.)

CLINICAL CHARACTERISTICS
Signs and Symptoms

- Intermenstrual bleeding (painless)
- Bleeding after intercourse (common)

DIAGNOSTIC APPROACH
Differential Diagnosis

- Pregnancy
- Climacteric changes
- Anovulation
- Endometrial polyps
- Uterine leiomyomata
- Cervical polyps, lesions, or cervicitis
- Endometrial cancer
- Endometriosis
- Nonuterine sources of bleeding (e.g., vaginal, vulvar, or perineal)
- Coagulopathy (congenital or acquired)
- Iatrogenic (intrauterine device use, medications)

Associated Conditions: Endometrial hyperplasia, endometrial cancer, endometrial polyps, endocervical polyps or carcinoma, uterine leiomyomata.

Workup and Evaluation

Laboratory: Testing should be chosen on the basis of diagnoses being considered.
Imaging: No imaging indicated.
Special Tests: A menstrual calendar helps to document the timing and character of the patient's bleeding. Endometrial biopsy, curettage, or hysteroscopy may be indicated.
Diagnostic Procedures: History and physical examination often point to possible causes for further evaluation.

Pathologic Findings

Based on underlying pathologic conditions.

MANAGEMENT AND THERAPY
Nonpharmacologic

General Measures: Evaluation.
Specific Measures: Focused on underlying causation, age of the patient, and contraceptive needs.
Diet: No specific dietary changes indicated.
Activity: No restriction.
Patient Education: Reassurance; American College of Obstetricians and Gynecologists Patient Education Pamphlet AP095 (Abnormal Uterine Bleeding), AP049 (Menstruation [Especially for Teens]), AP162 (Menopausal Bleeding), AP163 (Cancer of the Cervix).

Drug(s) of Choice

Based on cause. Hormonal agents that produce endometrial thinning (such as combination contraceptives or long-acting progestins) can be useful in selected patients when conception is not desired.

FOLLOW-UP

Patient Monitoring: Normal health maintenance.
Prevention/Avoidance: None.
Possible Complications: Anemia.
Expected Outcome: Return to normal menstrual pattern with correction of underlying pathologic condition or periodic progestin therapy.

MISCELLANEOUS

Pregnancy Considerations: No effect on pregnancy aside from that resulting from causative conditions.
ICD-9-CM Codes: 626.6, 626.7 (Postcoital bleeding).

REFERENCES

Level II
Peterson HB, Jeng G, Folger SG, et al; U.S. Collaborative Review of Sterilization Working Group: The risk of menstrual abnormalities after tubal sterilization. U.S. Collaborative Review of Sterilization Working Group. N Engl J Med 2000;343:1681.

Level III
American College of Obstetricians and Gynecologists: Management of anovulatory bleeding. ACOG Practice Bulletin 14. Washington, DC, ACOG, 2000.
American College of Obstetricians and Gynecologists: Noncontraceptive uses of the levonorgestrel intrauterine system. ACOG Committee Opinion 337. Obstet Gynecol 2006;107:1479.
Bayer RL, DeCherney AH: Clinical manifestations and treatment of dysfunctional uterine bleeding. JAMA 1993;269:1823.
Cowan BD, Morrison JC: Management of abnormal genital bleeding in girls and women. N Engl J Med 1991;324:1710.
Field CS: Dysfunctional uterine bleeding. Primary Care 1988;15:561.
Neese RE: Managing abnormal vaginal bleeding. Postgrad Med 1991;89:205.
Pitkin J: Dysfunctional uterine bleeding. BMJ 2007;334:1110.
Smith RP: Gynecology in primary care. Baltimore, Williams & Wilkins, 1997:375.
Thorneycroft IH: Cycle control with oral contraceptives: a review of the literature. Am J Obstet Gynecol 1999;180:280.
Wathen PI, Henderson MC, Witz CA: Abnormal uterine bleeding. Med Clin North Am 1995;79:329.

Intermenstrual Bleeding

Normal
Cyclic
Bleeding ▶

Days 28 14 28 14 28 14 28

Condition defined as bleeding between otherwise normal menstrual cycles.

Clinical Considerations in Intermenstrual Bleeding

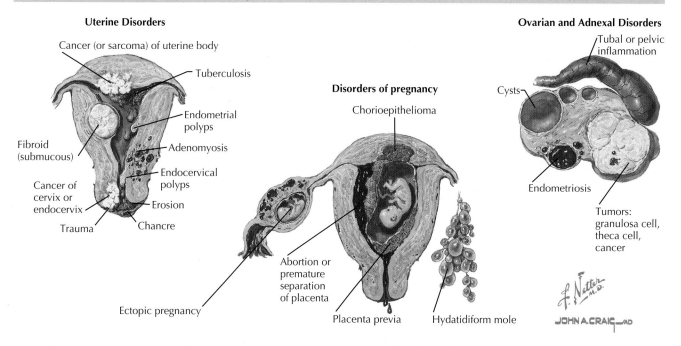

Uterine Disorders

Cancer (or sarcoma) of uterine body

Tuberculosis

Endometrial polyps

Fibroid (submucous)

Adenomyosis

Endocervical polyps

Cancer of cervix or endocervix

Erosion

Trauma

Chancre

Disorders of pregnancy

Chorioepithelioma

Abortion or premature separation of placenta

Ectopic pregnancy

Placenta previa

Hydatidiform mole

Ovarian and Adnexal Disorders

Tubal or pelvic inflammation

Cysts

Endometriosis

Tumors: granulosa cell, theca cell, cancer

Management Flow Chart for Intermenstrual Bleeding

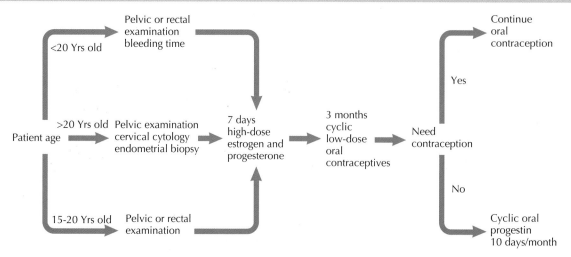

<20 Yrs old → Pelvic or rectal examination bleeding time

Patient age

>20 Yrs old → Pelvic examination cervical cytology endometrial biopsy

15-20 Yrs old → Pelvic or rectal examination

→ 7 days high-dose estrogen and progesterone

→ 3 months cyclic low-dose oral contraceptives

→ Need contraception

Yes → Continue oral contraception

No → Cyclic oral progestin 10 days/month

INTRODUCTION

Description: Menstrual cycles that do not follow a rhythmic pattern or with a pattern differing significantly from that expected as "normal" are considered irregular.

Prevalence: Ten percent to 15% of all gynecologic visits.

Predominant Age: Reproductive, greatest in adolescents and patients who are experiencing climacteric changes.

Genetics: No genetic pattern.

ETIOLOGY AND PATHOGENESIS

Causes: Anovulation or oligo-ovulation, climacteric or menopause, hypogonadism (including exercise induced: excessive, associated with low body weight and anovulation), excess estrogen (obesity, polycystic ovary disease, exogenous estrogen), elevated prolactin, psychosocial conditions (anorexia, bulimia, stress), chronic illness, renal or hepatic failure, thyroid disease.

Risk Factors: Those associated with possible causes.

CLINICAL CHARACTERISTICS

Signs and Symptoms

- Irregular menstrual interval
- Variable character of menstrual flow

DIAGNOSTIC APPROACH

Differential Diagnosis

- Climacteric changes
- Anovulation
- Pregnancy
- Ovarian tumors (rare)

Associated Conditions: Anovulation, infertility, and obesity.

Workup and Evaluation

Laboratory: Testing should be chosen on the basis of the different diagnoses under consideration.

Imaging: No imaging indicated.

Special Tests: A menstrual calendar helps to document the timing and character of the patient's bleeding. Endometrial biopsy, curettage, or hysteroscopy may be indicated in selected patients.

Diagnostic Procedures: History and physical examination often point to possible causes for further evaluation.

Pathologic Findings

Endometrial biopsy may indicate anovulation.

MANAGEMENT AND THERAPY

Nonpharmacologic

General Measures: Evaluation.

Specific Measures: Focused on underlying causation and desires of patient. If anovulation is the cause and fertility is not desired, periodic progestin therapy may be used to stabilize the cycles and suppress intermenstrual bleeding.

Diet: No specific dietary changes indicated.

Activity: No restriction.

Patient Education: Reassurance; American College of Obstetricians and Gynecologists Patient Education Pamphlet AP095 (Abnormal Uterine Bleeding), AP049 (Menstruation [Especially for Teens]), AP162 (Menopausal Bleeding).

Drug(s) of Choice

Medroxyprogesterone acetate 5 to 10 mg for 1 to 14 days each month.

Contraindications: Undiagnosed amenorrhea or bleeding.

Precautions: Progestins should not be used until pregnancy has been ruled out.

Alternative Drugs

Norethindrone acetate 5 to 10 mg for 10 to 14 days each month. Combination oral contraceptives may also be used.

FOLLOW-UP

Patient Monitoring: Normal health maintenance.

Prevention/Avoidance: None.

Possible Complications: Endometrial hyperplasia or carcinoma if anovulation is left untreated.

Expected Outcome: Return to normal menstrual pattern with correction of underlying pathologic condition or periodic progestin therapy.

MISCELLANEOUS

Pregnancy Considerations: No effect on pregnancy once pregnancy is achieved.

ICD-9-CM Codes: 626.4.

REFERENCES

Level II

Adams Hillard PJ, Deitch HR: Menstrual disorders in the college age female. Pediatr Clin North Am 2005;52:179, ix.

Fraiser IS: Treatment of ovulatory and anovulatory dysfunctional uterine bleeding with oral progestogens. Aust N Z J Obstet Gynaecol 1990;30:353.

Hannoun AB, Nassar AH, Usta IM, et al: Effect of war on the menstrual cycle. Obstet Gynecol 2007;109:929.

Level III

American College of Obstetricians and Gynecologists: Management of anovulatory bleeding. ACOG Practice Bulletin 14. Washington, DC, ACOG, 2000.

Cowan BD, Morrison JC: Management of abnormal genital bleeding in girls and women. N Engl J Med 1991;324:1710.

Diddle AW: Athletic activity and menstruation. South Med J 1983;76:619.

Field CS: Dysfunctional uterine bleeding. Primary Care 1988;15:561.

Neese RE: Managing abnormal vaginal bleeding. Postgrad Med 1991;89:205.

Thorneycroft IH: Cycle control with oral contraceptives: a review of the literature. Am J Obstet Gynecol 1999;180:280.

Van Voorhis BJ: Genitourinary symptoms in the menopausal transition. Am J Med 2005;118:47.

Neuroendocrine Regulation of Menstrual Cycle

Hypothalamic regulation of pituitary gonadotropin production and release

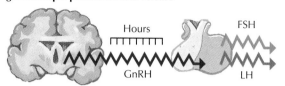

Pulsed release of GnRH by hypothalamus (1 pulse/1–2 hr) permits anterior pituitary production and release of FSH and LH (normal)

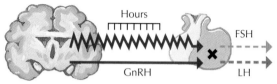

Continuous, excessive, absent, or more frequent GnRH release inhibits FSH and LH production and release (downloading)

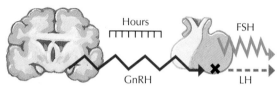

Decreased pulsed release of GnRH decreases LH secretion but increases FSH secretion (slow-pulsing model)

Ovarian feedback modulation of pituitary gonadotropin production and release

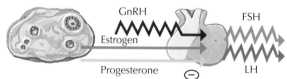

Presence of pulsed GnRH and low estrogen and progesterone levels result in increased levels of pulsed LH and FSH (negative feedback)

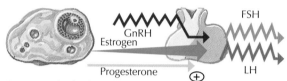

Presence of pulsed GnRH, rapidly increasing levels of estrogen, and small amounts of progesterone results in high pulsed LH and moderately increased pulsed FSH levels (positive feedback)

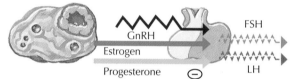

Presence of pulsed GnRH and high levels of estrogen and progesterone results in decreased LH and FSH levels (negative feedback)

Correlation of serum gonadotrophic and ovarian hormone levels and feedback mechanisms

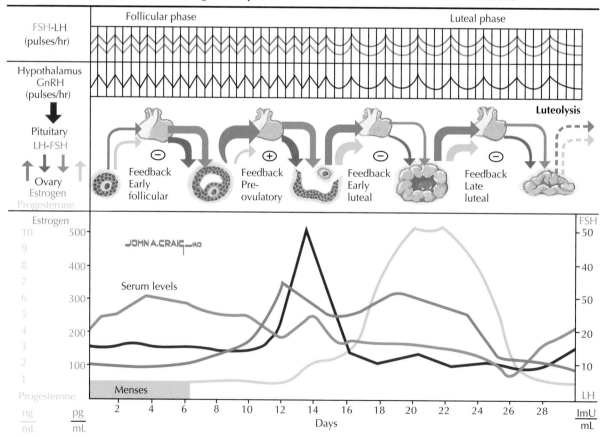

FSH, follicle-stimulating hormore; GnRH, gonadotropin-releasing hormone; LH, luteinizing hormone.

INTRODUCTION

Description: Menorrhagia—heavy menstrual flow—is generally divided into primary and secondary. Secondary is caused by (secondary to) some clinically identifiable cause; primary is caused by a disturbance of prostaglandin production. Menorrhagia is generally distinguished from acute vaginal bleeding (most often associated with pregnancy and pregnancy complications).

Prevalence: Ten percent to 15% of women experience excessive menstrual flow.

Predominant Age: Reproductive.

Genetics: No genetic pattern.

ETIOLOGY AND PATHOGENESIS

Causes: Secondary—see differential diagnosis following. Primary—overproduction, or an imbalance in the relative ratios of uterine prostaglandins (prostaglandin E_2, prostaglandin I_2, and thromboxane A_2). Some evidence suggests that patients with primary menorrhagia may also have increased fibrinolysis, further enhancing a tendency to bleed.

Risk Factors: Diabetes, obesity, or chronic anovulation (which place the patient at higher risk for endometrial hyperplasia or malignancy), systemic disease, or metabolic disturbances associated with bleeding dyscrasias.

CLINICAL CHARACTERISTICS

Signs and Symptoms

- Menstrual loss of greater than 80 mL, which may result in anemia
- Excessive soiling or numbers of menstrual hygiene products used (objective studies have shown a poor correlation with the actual measured blood loss)
- Anemia (in the absence of other causes of anemia, anemia is diagnostic for menstrual volumes of greater than 80 mL per cycle)

DIAGNOSTIC APPROACH

Differential Diagnosis

- Uterine leiomyomata (one third of patients will have menorrhagia)
- Adenomyosis (40% to 50% have menorrhagia)
- Endometrial or cervical polyp(s)
- Endometrial hypertrophy or hyperplasia
- Endometrial cancer
- Cervical lesions (including cancer)
- Infection (cervicitis, chronic endometritis)
- Intrauterine contraceptive device use
- Chronic anovulation
- Nongynecologic causes include blood dyscrasia or coagulopathy, hypothyroidism, leukemia, hepatic or renal disease, systemic lupus erythematosus, thyroid disease
- Benign or malignant tumors of ovary (rare)

Associated Conditions: Anemia, toxic shock syndrome (prolonged tampon use).

Workup and Evaluation

Laboratory: Complete blood count, pregnancy test, clotting profile (as indicated).

Imaging: Pelvic ultrasonography (based on diagnosis being considered—limited to the detection of secondary sources).

Special Tests: None indicated.

Diagnostic Procedures: History, physical, and laboratory evaluation.

Pathologic Findings

Based on cause.

MANAGEMENT AND THERAPY

Nonpharmacologic

General Measures: Evaluation, nutritional support.

Specific Measures: Based on cause. Nonsteroidal anti-inflammatory agents have been shown to reduce menstrual loss in primary menorrhagia. When taken for this indication, they must be taken continuously for the duration of flow. In patients with intractable menorrhagia or patients being prepared for extirpative surgery or endometrial ablation, therapy with gonadotropin-releasing hormone (GnRH) agonists may be considered. Uterine artery embolization has been advocated for selected patients.

Diet: No specific dietary changes indicated. Iron supplementation if indicated (either ferrous sulfate or gluconate, 300 mg PO two to three times a day).

Activity: No restriction.

Patient Education: American College of Obstetricians and Gynecologists Patient Education Pamphlet AP095 (Abnormal Uterine Bleeding), AP116 (Menstrual Hygiene Products), AP046 (Dysmenorrhea).

Drug(s) of Choice

Conjugated estrogen (20 to 25 mg IV) or intramuscular progestins have been widely advocated for acute bleeding.

Oral estrogen (conjugated estrogen 2.5 mg, micronized estradiol 3 to 6 mg) may be given acutely every 2 hours until the bleeding slows or stops. Estrogen therapy is then maintained for 20 to 25 additional days, with a progestin added for the last 10 days of treatment.

Combination oral contraceptives containing estradiol and norgestrel (Ovral, four tablets a day for 3 to 5 days or until bleeding stops, followed by one daily for the duration of the pack or four tablets the first day, followed by three for 1 day, two the next day, and then one daily for the remainder of the package).

For long-term therapy, levonorgestrel-releasing intrauterine devices have been shown to be effective in reducing menstrual blood loss.

Contraindications: Therapy should not be instituted until the possibility of pregnancy has been evaluated and a working diagnosis has been established.

Precautions: See individual agents.

Interactions: See individual agents.

Alternative Drugs

When the endometrium is reasonably intact, high-dose progestin may be used to stop acute uterine bleeding (medroxyprogesterone acetate 10 mg PO three times a day or IM depot medroxyprogesterone acetate, 150 to 300 mg). Nonsteroidal anti-inflammatory agents have been shown to reduce menstrual loss 30% to 50% when

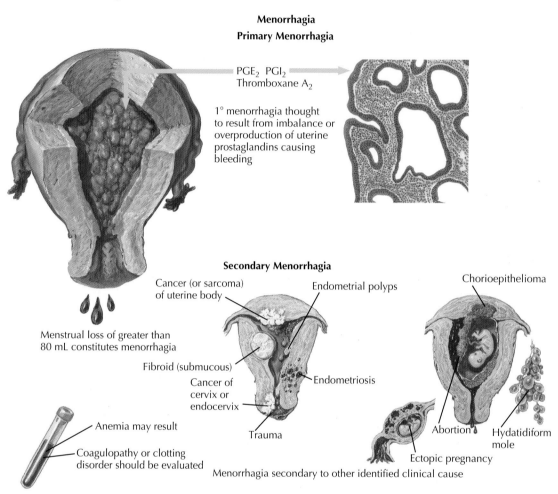

Menorrhagia

Primary Menorrhagia

PGE_2 PGI_2
Thromboxane A_2

1° menorrhagia thought to result from imbalance or overproduction of uterine prostaglandins causing bleeding

Secondary Menorrhagia

Menstrual loss of greater than 80 mL constitutes menorrhagia

Cancer (or sarcoma) of uterine body

Endometrial polyps

Chorioepithelioma

Fibroid (submucous)

Endometriosis

Cancer of cervix or endocervix

Trauma

Anemia may result

Coagulopathy or clotting disorder should be evaluated

Abortion

Ectopic pregnancy

Hydatidiform mole

Menorrhagia secondary to other identified clinical cause

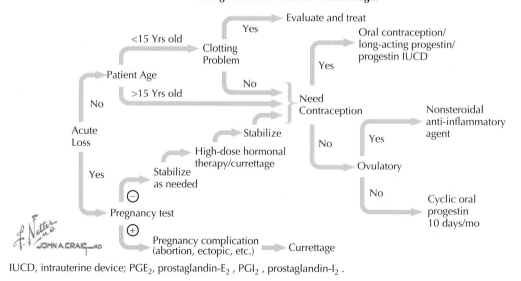

Management Flowchart for Menorrhagia

Patient Age

<15 Yrs old

>15 Yrs old

Clotting Problem

Yes → Evaluate and treat

No

Need Contraception

Yes → Oral contraception/ long-acting progestin/ progestin IUCD

No

Ovulatory

Yes → Nonsteroidal anti-inflammatory agent

No → Cyclic oral progestin 10 days/mo

Acute Loss

No

Yes

Stabilize

High-dose hormonal therapy/currettage

Stabilize as needed

Pregnancy test

⊖

⊕

Pregnancy complication (abortion, ectopic, etc.) → Currettage

IUCD, intrauterine device; PGE_2, prostaglandin-E_2 , PGI_2 , prostaglandin-I_2 .

taken for the duration of flow (e.g., meclofenamate sodium 100 mg PO three times a day during flow, mefenamic acid [Ponstel] 250 mg PO three times a day during flow). Levonorgestrel-releasing intrauterine devices have been shown to provide a comparable reduction in menstrual blood loss.

FOLLOW-UP

Patient Monitoring: Normal health maintenance. Watch for anemia. Patients who are at risk for endometrial hyperplasia or neoplasia, or those who do not respond to initial therapy, may require endometrial biopsy, hysteroscopy, or diagnostic curettage.

Prevention/Avoidance: Based on cause. If contraception is desired, oral combination contraceptives, or continuously dosed progestins (orally, by injection, or as a medicated intrauterine device), or oral contraceptives (either monophasic or polyphasic) are reasonable options. In patients with intractable menorrhagia or in patients being prepared for extirpative surgery or endometrial ablation, therapy with gonadotropin-releasing hormone agonists may be considered for a maximum of 6 months. Cost and side effects limit this approach.

Possible Complications: Anemia, hypovolemia (acute loss).

Expected Outcome: Based on cause; most patients respond to conservative therapy. The most successful therapy is directed at the underlying cause. Once acute control has been gained, cyclic estrogen/progestin therapy should be continued for an additional 3 months. During this interval, additional diagnostic studies may be considered and plans may be laid for long-term management, should it be necessary.

MISCELLANEOUS

Pregnancy Considerations: No effect on pregnancy.
ICD-9-CM Codes: 626.2, 626.3 (Pubertal), 627.0 (Premenopausal).

REFERENCES

Level I
Anderson ABM, Haynes PJ, Cuillebaud J, et al: Reduction of menstrual blood loss by prostaglandin synthetase inhibitors. Lancet 1976;1:774.
Bhattacharya S, Cameron IM, Parkin DE, et al: A pragmatic randomised comparison of transcervical resection of the endometrium with endometrial laser ablation for the treatment of menorrhagia. Br J Obstet Gynaecol 1997;104:601.
Gannon MJ, Holt EM, Fairbank J, et al: A randomised trial comparing endometrial resection and abdominal hysterectomy for the treatment of menorrhagia. BMJ 1991;303:1362.
Halmesmaki K, Hurskainen R, Teperi J, et al: The effect of hysterectomy or levonorgestrel-releasing intrauterine system on sexual functioning among women with menorrhagia: a 5-year randomised controlled trial. BJOG 2007;114:563.
Hehenkamp WJ, Volkers NA, Donderwinkel PF, et al: Uterine artery embolization versus hysterectomy in the treatment of symptomatic uterine fibroids (EMMY trial): peri- and postprocedural results from a randomized controlled trial. Am J Obstet Gynecol 2005;193:1618.
Showstack J, Lin F, Learman LA, et al; Ms Research Group: Randomized trial of medical treatment versus hysterectomy for abnormal uterine bleeding: resource use in the Medicine or Surgery (Ms) trial. Am J Obstet Gynecol 2006;194:332.

Level II
Amso NN, Stabinsky SA, McFaul P, et al: Uterine thermal balloon therapy for the treatment of menorrhagia: the first 300 patients from a multi-centre study. International Collaborative Uterine Thermal Balloon Working Group. Br J Obstet Gynaecol 1998;105:517.
Brown PM, Farquhar CM, Lethaby A, et al: Cost-effectiveness analysis of levonorgestrel intrauterine system and thermal balloon ablation for heavy menstrual bleeding. BJOG 2006;113:797.
Busfield RA, Farquhar CM, Sowter MC, et al: A randomised trial comparing the levonorgestrel intrauterine system and thermal balloon ablation for heavy menstrual bleeding. BJOG 2006;113:257.
Chullapram T, Song JY, Fraser IS: Medium-term follow-up of women with menorrhagia treated by rollerball endometrial ablation. Obstet Gynecol 1996;88:71.
Garside R, Stein K, Wyatt K, Round A: Microwave and thermal balloon ablation for heavy menstrual bleeding: a systematic review. BJOG 2005;112:12.
Goldenberg M, Sivan E, Bider D, et al: Endometrial resection vs. abdominal hysterectomy for menorrhagia. Correlated sample analysis. J Reprod Med 1996;41:333.
Hald K, Klow NE, Qvigstad E, Istre O: Laparoscopic occlusion compared with embolization of uterine vessels: a randomized controlled trial. Obstet Gynecol 2007;109:20.
Khaund A, Moss JG, McMillan N, Lumsden MA: Evaluation of the effect of uterine artery embolisation on menstrual blood loss and uterine volume. BJOG 2004;111:700.
Meyer WR, Walsh BW, Grainger DA, et al: Thermal balloon and rollerball ablation to treat menorrhagia: a multicenter comparison. Obstet Gynecol 1998;92:98.
Rauramo I, Elo I, Istre O: Long-term treatment of menorrhagia with levonorgestrel intrauterine system versus endometrial resection. Obstet Gynecol 2004;104:1314.
Reid PC, Virtanen-Kari S: Randomised comparative trial of the levonorgestrel intrauterine system and mefenamic acid for the treatment of idiopathic menorrhagia: a multiple analysis using total menstrual fluid loss, menstrual blood loss and pictorial blood loss assessment charts. BJOG 2005;112:1121.

Level III
American College of Obstetricians and Gynecologists: Management of anovulatory bleeding. ACOG Practice Bulletin 14. Washington, DC, ACOG, 2000.
American College of Obstetricians and Gynecologists: Surgical alternatives to hysterectomy in the management of leiomyomas. ACOG Practice Bulletin 16. Washington, DC, ACOG, 2000.
American College of Obstetricians and Gynecologists: Noncontraceptive uses of the levonorgestrel intrauterine system. ACOG Committee Opinion 337. Obstet Gynecol 2006;107:1479.
Cohen BJB, Gibor J: Anemia and menstrual blood loss. Obstet Gynecol Surv 1980;35:597.
Duncan KM, Hart LL: Nonsteroidal antiinflammatory drugs in menorrhagia. Ann Pharmacother 1993;27:1353.
Fraser IS: Hysteroscopy and laparoscopy in women with menorrhagia. Am J Obstet Gynecol 1990;165:1264.
Higham JM: The medical management of menorrhagia. Br J Hosp Med 1991;45:19.
Liddell H: Menorrhagia. N Z Med J 1993;106:255.
Long CA, Gast MJ: Menorrhagia. Obstet Gynecol Clin North Am 1990;17:343.
Sharp HT: Assessment of new technology in the treatment of idiopathic menorrhagia and uterine leiomyomata. Obstet Gynecol 2006;108:990.
Shaw RW: Treating the patient with menorrhagia. Br J Obstet Gynaecol 1994;101:1.
Sowter MC: New surgical treatments for menorrhagia. Lancet 2003;361:1456.

INTRODUCTION

Description: As a symptom only, postmenopausal bleeding—vaginal bleeding that occurs in women who have passed menopause—requires evaluation to rule out processes that may threaten the long-term health of the patient.

Prevalence: Common.

Predominant Age: 50 or older.

Genetics: No genetic pattern.

ETIOLOGY AND PATHOGENESIS

Causes: Systemic—estrogen, estrogen/progesterone, thrombocytopenia. Uterine—endometrial cancer, endometrial hyperplasia, endometritis, submucous leiomyomata. Cervical sources—carcinoma, cervical eversion, cervicitis, condyloma, polyps. Vaginal sources—adenosis, atrophic change, carcinoma, foreign bodies (condom, pessary, tampon), infection, lacerations (coital injury, trauma). Vulvar and extragenital sources—atrophy, condyloma, cystitis/urethritis, gastrointestinal (cancer, diverticulitis, inflammatory bowel disease), hematuria, hemorrhoids, infection, labial varices, neoplasm, trauma, urethral caruncle, urethral diverticula, urethral prolapse/eversion.

Risk Factors: Estrogen replacement therapy, others based on specific pathologic conditions.

CLINICAL CHARACTERISTICS

Signs and Symptoms

- Painless vaginal bleeding (spontaneous or iatrogenic)
- Pink or dark discharge noted on the underwear or when wiping after urination

DIAGNOSTIC APPROACH

Differential Diagnosis

- Pregnancy (in the climacteric period or early menopause)
- Iatrogenic bleeding (estrogen, estrogen/progestin)
- Endometrial cancer
- Endometrial disease (hyperplasia, endometritis)
- Vaginal atrophy
- Endometrial polyps
- Cervicitis or cervical lesions (including polyps and cancer)
- Vaginitis
- Retained intrauterine contraceptive device
- Nongynecologic sources of bleeding (e.g., perineal or rectal)

Associated Conditions: See differential diagnosis.

Workup and Evaluation

Laboratory: No evaluation indicated.

Imaging: Saline infusion ultrasonography (sonohysterography) may allow measurement of endometrial thickness and the possibility of endometrial polyps. Transvaginal ultrasonography may be used to assess endometrial thickness. (No standard has emerged for a threshold of endometrial thickness that carries ideal positive and negative predictive values. Recently published data suggest that when the endometrial thickness is less than 5 mm, endometrial biopsy is not required.)

Special Tests: Endometrial biopsy should be strongly considered to evaluate the cause and to check for the possibility of a malignancy.

Diagnostic Procedures: History and physical examination, cervical cytologic examination, endometrial sampling.

Pathologic Findings

Varies with cause.

MANAGEMENT AND THERAPY

Nonpharmacologic

General Measures: Evaluation.

Specific Measures: Based on cause identified.

Diet: No specific dietary changes indicated.

Activity: No restriction.

Patient Education: Reassurance; American College of Obstetricians and Gynecologists Patient Education Pamphlet AP162 (Menopausal Bleeding), AP025 (Ultrasound Exams), AP047 (The Menopause Years), AP066 (Hormone Therapy).

Drug(s) of Choice (Based on Pathophysiologic Condition Present)

In many cases of postmenopausal bleeding, the endometrium is thin and atrophic. This endometrium is prone to irregular slough, resulting in erratic, although generally light, bleeding. Because the endometrial tissue is so denuded, it does not respond well to progestational agents. Estrogen, alone initially or in combination with progestin therapy, is required to induce initial growth and the development of progestin receptors to effect endometrial stabilization.

FOLLOW-UP

Patient Monitoring: Postmenopausal bleeding should be presumed to indicate the presence of a malignancy, until proved otherwise. The only exception to this is the withdrawal bleeding that occurs as a part of cyclic estrogen–progesterone hormone therapy.

Prevention/Avoidance: None.

Possible Complications: Progression of undiagnosed malignancy.

Expected Outcome: If diagnosis is prompt and appropriate therapy is instituted, the outcome should be excellent.

MISCELLANEOUS

Pregnancy Considerations: Not applicable.

ICD-9-CM Codes: 627.1.

Postmenopausal Bleeding
Evaluation of Postmenopausal Bleeding

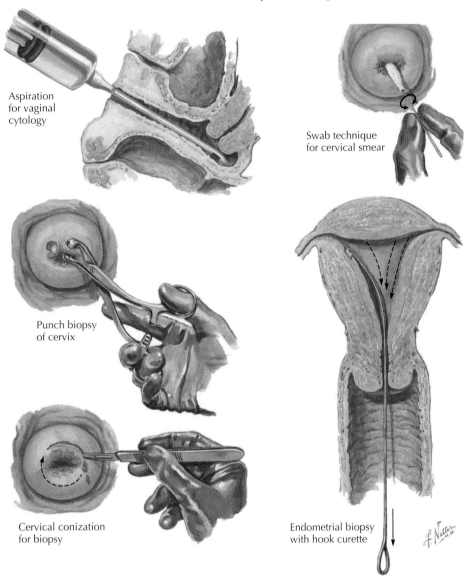

Aspiration
for vaginal
cytology

Swab technique
for cervical smear

Punch biopsy
of cervix

Cervical conization
for biopsy

Endometrial biopsy
with hook curette

REFERENCES

Level I
Steiner AZ, Xiang M, Mack WJ, et al: Unopposed estradiol therapy in postmenopausal women: results from two randomized trials. Obstet Gynecol 2007;109:581.

Level II
Clark TJ, Voit D, Gupta JK, et al: Accuracy of hysteroscopy in the diagnosis of endometrial cancer and hyperplasia: a systematic quantitative review. JAMA 2002;288:1610.

de Kroon CD, de Bock GH, Dieben SW, Jansen FW: Saline contrast hysterosonography in abnormal uterine bleeding: a systematic review and meta-analysis. BJOG 2003;110:938.

Feldman S, Berkowitz RS, Tosteson ANA: Cost-effectiveness of strategies to evaluate postmenopausal bleeding. Obstet Gynecol 1993;81:968.

Ferry J, Farnsworth A, Webster M, Wren B: The efficacy of the Pipelle endometrial biopsy in detecting endometrial carcinoma. Aust N Z J Obstet Gynaecol 1993;33:76.

Goldschmit R, Katz Z, Blickstein I, et al: The accuracy of endometrial Pipelle sampling with and without sonographic measurement of endometrial thickness. Obstet Gynecol 1993;82:727.

Goldstein SR: Use of ultrasono-hysterography for triage of perimenopausal patients with unexplained uterine bleeding. Am J Obstet Gynecol 1994;170:565.

van Dongen H, de Kroon CD, Jacobi CE, et al: Diagnostic hysteroscopy in abnormal uterine bleeding: a systematic review and meta-analysis. BJOG 2007;114:664.

Level III
Davidson KG, Dubinsky TJ: Ultrasonographic evaluation of the endometrium in postmenopausal vaginal bleeding. Radiol Clin North Am 2003;41:769.

Langlois JP, Nashelsky J: Clinical inquiries. How useful is ultrasound to evaluate patients with postmenopausal bleeding? J Fam Pract 2004;53:1005.

Lentz GM: Differential diagnosis of major gynecologic problems by age group. In Katz VL, Lentz GM, Lobo RA, Gershenson DM: Comprehensive Gynecology, 5th ed. Philadelphia, Mosby/Elsevier, 2007:157.

Opmeer BC, van Doorn HC, Heintz AP, et al: Improving the existing diagnostic strategy by accounting for characteristics of the women in the diagnostic work up for postmenopausal bleeding. BJOG 2007;114:51.

Reid PC, Brown VA, Fothergill DJ: Outpatient investigation of postmenopausal bleeding. Br J Obstet Gynaecol 1993;100:498.

INTRODUCTION

Description: Uterine sarcoma is characterized by sarcomatous change in the tissues of the Müllerian system including the endometrial stroma and myometrium. Mixed Müllerian sarcomas may include elements not native to the genital tract such as cartilage or bone (heterologous type).

Prevalence: Less than 5% of uterine malignancies, 1 of 800 smooth muscle tumors, 0.67 of 100,000 women older than age 20.

Predominant Age: 40 to 60, mean age 52.

Genetics: No genetic pattern. Seen more often in African-American women, although there is no racial predisposition.

ETIOLOGY AND PATHOGENESIS

Causes: Etiology unknown.

Risk Factors: Leiomyomata, estrogen and obesity have also been proposed; oral contraceptive use is associated with a reduced risk.

CLINICAL CHARACTERISTICS

Signs and Symptoms

- Bleeding and passage of tissue
- Lower abdominal pain and mass
- Rapid enlargement of the uterus
- Uterine growth after menopause

DIAGNOSTIC APPROACH

Differential Diagnosis

- Benign leiomyomata
- Cervical cancer
- Ovarian cancer metastatic to the endometrium
- Metachronous Müllerian tumor

Associated Conditions: Breast or colon cancer.

Workup and Evaluation

Laboratory: No evaluation indicated except for preoperative screening.

Imaging: Chest radiograph (for metastases), transvaginal ultrasonography, or sonohysterography may be useful.

Special Tests: None. (Endometrial biopsy results are rarely positive.)

Diagnostic Procedures: Diagnosis rarely made before surgery.

Pathologic Findings

Based on cell type and tissue involved. Most often soft fleshy tumors with a gray–yellow or pink character. Areas of necrosis and hemorrhage are common (75%). Vascular invasion is present in 10% to 20% of patients. Higher mitotic rates are associated with greater atypia.

MANAGEMENT AND THERAPY

Nonpharmacologic

General Measures: Evaluation and staging.

Specific Measures: Surgical exploration with hysterectomy, bilateral salpingo-oophorectomy, cytologic examination of the abdomen and diaphragm, and para-aortic node sampling. Radiation to the vaginal cuff reduces local recurrence (although objective evidence of improved survival is lacking).

Diet: No specific dietary changes indicated except as dictated by surgical therapy.

Activity: No restriction except as dictated by surgical therapy.

Patient Education: American College of Obstetricians and Gynecologists Patient Education Pamphlet AP097 (Cancer of the Uterus), AP008 (Hysterectomy), AP080 (Preparing for Surgery), AP095 (Abnormal Uterine Bleeding), AP074 (Uterine Fibroids).

Drug(s) of Choice

None. (Adjuvant chemotherapy [vincristine, actinomycin D, and cyclophosphamide or doxorubicin (Adriamycin)] has been advocated but an improvement in prognosis has not been demonstrated.) Temozolomide (an imidazotetrazine derivative) has been explored as an additional option.

FOLLOW-UP

Patient Monitoring: Follow-up Pap tests from vaginal cuff every 3 months for 2 years, then every 6 months for 3 years, then yearly. Chest radiograph annually.

Prevention/Avoidance: None.

Possible Complications: Distant spread.

Expected Outcome: Depends on stage of tumor and number of mitotic figures present. Overall survival is approximately 20% at 5 years; patients with stage I and II disease have survival rates of up to 40%.

MISCELLANEOUS

Pregnancy Considerations: Generally not a consideration because they are unlikely to coexist.

ICD-9-CM Codes: Specific to cell type and location.

REFERENCES

Level II

Aaro LA, Symmonds RE, Dockerty MB: Sarcoma of the uterus. A clinical and pathologic study of 177 cases. Am J Obstet Gynecol 1966;94:101.

Barter JF, Smith EB, Szpak CA, et al: Leiomyosarcoma of the uterus: clinicopathologic study of 21 cases. Gynecol Oncol 1985;21:220.

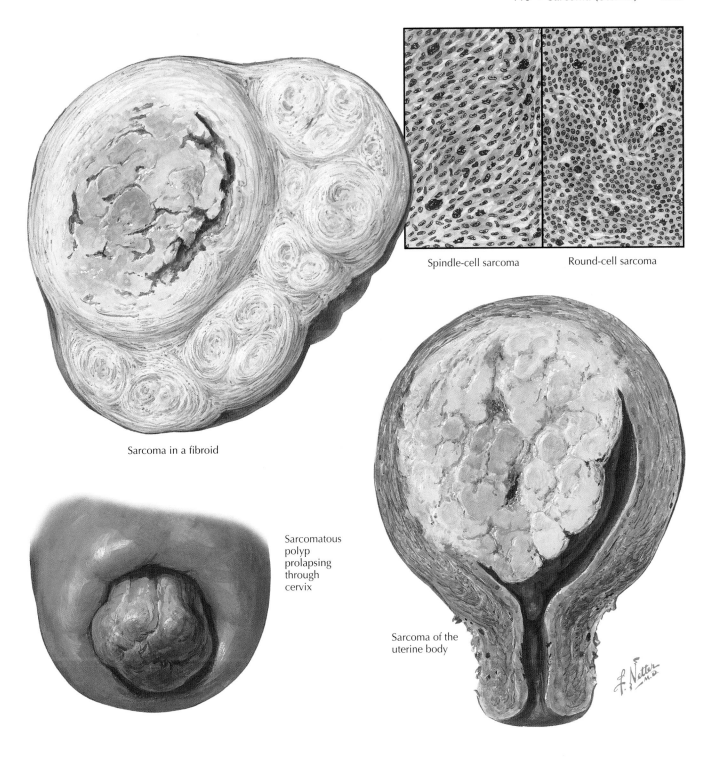

Spindle-cell sarcoma

Round-cell sarcoma

Sarcoma in a fibroid

Sarcomatous
polyp
prolapsing
through
cervix

Sarcoma of the
uterine body

Gallup DG, Cordray DR: Leiomyosarcoma of the uterus: case report and a review. Obstet Gynecol Surv 1979;34:300.

Shakfeh AM, Woodruff JD: Primary ovarian sarcomas: report of 46 cases and review of literature. Obstet Gynecol 1987;42:331.

Talbot SM, Keohan ML, Hesdorffer M, et al: A phase II trial of temozolomide in patients with unresectable or metastatic soft tissue sarcoma. Cancer 2003;98:1942.

Level III

Kempson RL, Bari W: Uterine sarcomas. Classification, diagnosis, and prognosis. Hum Pathol 1970;1:331.

Lu K, Slomivitz BM: Neoplastic diseases of the uterus. In Katz VL, Lentz GM, Lobo RA, Gershenson DM: Comprehensive Gynecology, 5th ed. Philadelphia, Mosby/Elsevier, 2007:829.

INTRODUCTION

Description: Uterine abnormalities are characterized by incomplete formation of the uterus resulting in one or two separate halves or horns or a single uterus with a central septum. (The central septum may divide the uterine cavity either partially or completely. The two resulting halves may be of unequal size or volume.) In its most extensive form, duplication of the cervix and vaginal canal also may occur. These abnormalities are associated with renal agenesis and blind vaginal pouches that may become filled with menstrual fluid after puberty, resulting in a painful mass.

Prevalence: Estimated to be 0.1% of female births. Septate or arcuate uterine anomalies may be present in up to 3% of women.

Predominant Age: Congenital.

Genetics: May be transmitted by polygenic or multifactorial pattern.

ETIOLOGY AND PATHOGENESIS

Causes: Failure of the fusion of the Müllerian ducts, which normally takes place near the beginning of the 10th week of gestation. This may vary from septation of the uterus to complete duplication of the uterus, cervix, and vaginal canal. Most septations are due to a failure of the normal processes of development of the Müllerian system between the 10th and 13th week of gestation when the lower portion of the median septum of the uterus is resorbed, or between the 13th and 20th week when the upper septum (in the uterine body) is resorbed. In utero exposure to diethylstilbestrol has been associated with a T-shaped uterine cavity similar to the arcuate form of a septate uterus. A unicornuate uterus may result from a failure of the normal formation or the destruction of one the Müllerian ducts. This may occur if there is a lack of development of the mesonephric system on the affected side resulting in a failure of the associated Müllerian system. (In these patients, the ipsilateral kidney and ureter are usually absent.)

Risk Factors: None known.

CLINICAL CHARACTERISTICS

Signs and Symptoms

- Asymptomatic
- Recurrent abortion (15% to 25% of patients with recurrent abortions have uterine abnormalities; there is a 50% risk of pregnancy loss when the uterus is unicornuate)
- Premature labor (20% risk for unicornuate uterus)
- Uterine pain or rupture in early pregnancy
- Abnormal presentation in labor (breech or transverse position)
- Inability to stop menstrual flow using tampons (when there is duplication of the vagina as well)
- When outflow is obstructed—hematometra
- Dysmenorrhea, abdominal pain, pelvic mass, abrupt blood discharge

DIAGNOSTIC APPROACH

Differential Diagnosis

- Leiomyomata
- Adnexal mass
- Endometriosis
- Chromosomal abnormality resulting in recurrent abortion

Associated Conditions: Endometriosis (75% when outflow obstruction is present), pelvic adhesions, recurrent abortion, infertility, dysmenorrhea, dyspareunia, hematocolpos, and renal anomalies (contralateral pelvic, horseshoe, or absent kidney).

Workup and Evaluation

Laboratory: No evaluation indicated.

Imaging: Hysterosalpingography, ultrasonography, or sonohysterography. Magnetic resonance imaging may be used, but expense and availability limit its utility.

Special Tests: Hysteroscopy or laparoscopy may be required to complete the evaluation.

Diagnostic Procedures: Physical examination, imaging, and direct observation by hysteroscopy, laparoscopy, or both. Differentiation between septate and bicornuate uterine anomalies requires visualization of the uterine fundus.

Pathologic Findings

In patients with an unicornuate uterus, a normal ovary and tube are generally present. A normal ovary may be present on the opposite side as well. The septate uterus is characterized by the presence of a fibrous septum of variable length with poor vascularization.

MANAGEMENT AND THERAPY

Nonpharmacologic

General Measures: Evaluation and education.

Specific Measures: Patients with nonobstructive abnormalities require no therapy. Patients with recurrent fetal wastage may be considered for uterine reunification (metroplasty) procedures or the excision of any septum, usually by operative hysteroscopy. Patients with a unicornuate deformity and recurrent fetal wastage should be counseled about adoption or the possibilities of in vitro fertilization with implantation into a host uterus.

Diet: No specific dietary changes indicated.

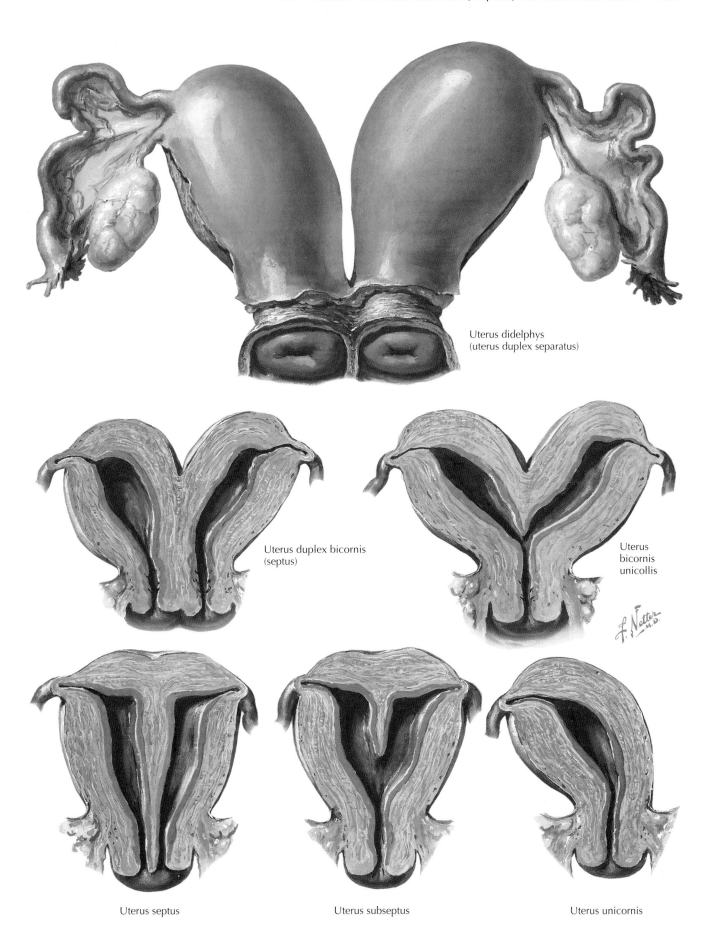

Uterus didelphys
(uterus duplex separatus)

Uterus duplex bicornis
(septus)

Uterus
bicornis
unicollis

Uterus septus

Uterus subseptus

Uterus unicornis

Activity: No restriction.

Patient Education: Reassurance; American College of Obstetricians and Gynecologists Patient Education Pamphlet AP079 (If Your Baby Is Breech), AP100 (Repeated Miscarriage), AP090 (Early Pregnancy Loss: Miscarriage and Molar Pregnancy), AP143 (Hysterosalpingography).

Drug(s) of Choice

None. (Estrogen therapy is often given for 1 to 2 months after resection of a uterine septum, although the need for this is still debated.)

FOLLOW-UP

Patient Monitoring: Normal health maintenance.

Prevention/Avoidance: None.

Possible Complications: Obstruction of the outflow of menstrual blood is associated with a 75% chance of endometriosis with resultant pelvic scarring and infertility. There is an increased risk of ectopic pregnancy and early pregnancy loss (33% to 35%).

Expected Outcome: Normal reproduction is frequently possible without intervention (25% of cases) for patients with a bicornuate uterus; metroplasty is associated with an increased likelihood of success when pregnancy failures have occurred (80% to 90%). When the only abnormality is a uterine septum, normal reproduction is generally possible without intervention (85% success). For patients with a unicornuate uterus, a live birth rate of 40% may be expected; outcomes are not statistically different from those experienced by women with didelphic uteri.

MISCELLANEOUS

Pregnancy Considerations: Increased risk of pregnancy loss, premature delivery, or fetal malpresentation. The risk of ectopic pregnancy is increased for patients with a unicornuate uterus.

ICD-9-CM Codes: 752.2 (Unicornuate or bicornuate uterus), 752.3 (Septate uterus).

REFERENCES

Level II

Lin PC: Reproductive outcomes in women with uterine anomalies. J Womens Health (Larchmt) 2004;13:33.

Moutos DM, Damewood MD, Schlaff WD, Rock JA: A comparison of the reproductive outcome between women with a unicornuate uterus and women with a didelphic uterus. Fertil Steril 1992;58:88.

Reinhold C, Hricak H, Forstner R, et al: Primary amenorrhea: evaluation with MR imaging. Radiology 1997;203:383.

Rock JA, Jones HJ: The double uterus associated with an obstructed hemivagina and ipsilateral renal agenesis. Am J Obstet Gynecol 1980;138:339.

Toaff ME, Lev-Toaff AS, Toaff R: Communicating uteri: review and classification with introduction of two previously unrecorded types. Fertil Steril 1984;41:661

Level III

Buttram VC: Müllerian anomalies and their management. Fertil Steril 1983;40:159.

Doyle MB: Magnetic resonance imaging in mullerian fusion defects. J Reprod Med 1992;37:33.

Golan A, Langer R, Bukovsky I, Caspi E: Congenital anomalies of the mullerian system. Fertil Steril 1989;51:747.

Grimbizis GF, Camus M, Tarlatzis BC, et al: Clinical implications of uterine malformations and hysteroscopic treatment results. Hum Reprod Update 2001;7:161.

Hay D: Uterus unicornis and its relationship to pregnancy. J Obstet Gynecol Br Emp 1961;68:371.

Jayasinghe Y, Rane A, Stalewski H, Grover S: The presentation and early diagnosis of the rudimentary uterine horn. Obstet Gynecol 2005;105:1456.

Jones HW: Reproductive impairment and the malformed uterus. Fertil Steril 1981;36:137.

Katz VL, Lentz GM: Congenital abnormalities of the female reproductive tract. In Katz VL, Lentz GM, Lobo RA, Gershenson DM: Comprehensive Gynecology, 5th ed. Philadelphia, Mosby/Elsevier, 2007:250.

Markham SM, Waterhouse TB: Structural anomalies of the reproductive tract. Curr Opin Obstet Gynecol 1992;4:867.

Mayo-Smith WW, Lee MJ: MR imaging of the female pelvis. Clin Radiol 1995;50:667.

Nahum GG: Uterine anomalies. How common are they, and what is their distribution among subtypes? J Reprod Med 1998;43:877.

Pinsonneault O, Goldstein DP: Obstructing malformations of the uterus and vagina. Fertil Steril 1985;44:241.

Woodward PJ, Sohaey R, Wagner BJ: Congenital uterine malformations. Curr Probl Diagn Radiol 1995;24:178.

Woodward PJ, Wagner BJ, Farley TE: MR imaging in the evaluation of female infertility. Radiographics 1993;13:293.

INTRODUCTION

Description: Uterine leiomyomata is a benign connective tissue tumor found in or around the uterus, which may be disseminated in rare cases.

Prevalence: Thirty percent of all women, 40% to 50% of women older than 50 (one study has demonstrated a rate of more than 80% in African Americans older than 50), leiomyomata account for approximately 30% of all hysterectomies.

Predominant Age: 35 to 50 or older.

Genetics: No genetic pattern.

ETIOLOGY AND PATHOGENESIS

Causes: Unknown; thought to arise from a single smooth muscle cell (of vascular origin) resulting in tumors that are each monoclonal. Estrogen, progesterone, and epidermal growth factor all thought to stimulate growth.

Risk Factors: Nulliparity, early menarche, African Americans (4- to10-fold increase in risk), increasing age, obesity, high-fat diet (proposed).

CLINICAL CHARACTERISTICS

Signs and Symptoms: (30% to 50% Symptomatic)

- Uterine enlargement and distortion
- Pelvic or abdominal heaviness, low back pain
- Pressure on bowel or bladder (i.e., frequency, infrequently causing urinary retention or rarely hydroureter to develop)
- Dysmenorrhea, menorrhagia, intermenstrual bleeding (30% to 40% of patients)
- Acute pain (with torsion or degeneration)
- Submucous fibroids may prolapse through the cervix
- Recurrent pregnancy loss

DIAGNOSTIC APPROACH

Differential Diagnosis

- Pregnancy
- Adnexal mass
- Other pelvic or abdominal tumor
- Pelvic kidney
- Urachal cyst
- Urinary retention

Associated Conditions: Dysmenorrhea, menorrhagia, miscarriage, and infertility (rare).

Workup and Evaluation

Laboratory: No evaluation indicated, hemoglobin or hematocrit if anemia suspected.

Imaging: Ultrasonography only when the diagnosis is uncertain.

Special Tests: None indicated.

Diagnostic Procedures: Pelvic examination is generally sufficient and may be augmented by ultrasonography but generally is not required.

Pathologic Findings

Localized proliferation of smooth muscle cells surrounded by a pseudocapsule of compressed muscle fibers. Of uterine fibroids, 70% to 80% are found within the wall of the uterus, with 5% to 10% lying below the endometrium and less than 5% arising in or near the cervix. Multiple fibroids are found in up to 85% of patients. Myomas may weigh up to 100 pounds.

MANAGEMENT AND THERAPY

Nonpharmacologic

General Measures: Reassurance, observation.

Specific Measures: Surgical therapy (hysterectomy or myomectomy) for uncontrollable symptoms, rapid growth, or uncertain diagnosis. Medical therapy with gonadotropin-releasing hormone (GnRH) agonists may be used temporarily to prepare for surgery, pregnancy, or menopause. Uterine artery embolization may be used for patients who are not surgical candidates or those who wish to preserve fertility. (Successful pregnancy is possible, but uterine embolization has been associated with a number of both short- and long-term complications, making its role limited.)

Diet: No specific dietary changes indicated.

Activity: No restriction.

Patient Education: Reassurance; American College of Obstetricians and Gynecologists Patient Education Pamphlet AP074 (Uterine Fibroids) or AP008 (Understanding Hysterectomy).

Drug(s) of Choice

Gonadotropin-releasing hormone agonists (therapy limited to 6 months)—buserelin (Depo-Lupron 3.75 mg IM monthly or Depo-Lupron 3-month 22.5 mg IM every 3 months), goserelin (Zoladex 3.6 mg implant SC monthly or Zoladex 3-month implant SC every 3 months).

Contraindications: Pregnancy or possible pregnancy.

Precautions: Must exclude possibility of pregnancy before medical therapy. Gonadotropin-releasing hormone agonists may produce significant symptoms of estrogen withdrawal (menopause).

Interactions: None known.

Alternative Drugs

Synarel nasal solution 2 mg/mL one spray in alternate nostril in AM and PM (not labeled for the treatment of leiomyomata).

Nonsteroidal antiinflammatory drugs may be used to reduce menorrhagia.

Medroxyprogesterone acetate (depot) 100 to 300 mg IM every 1 to 3 months may be used to suppress menstruation.

FOLLOW-UP

Patient Monitoring: Watch for development of symptoms. Monitor uterine size.

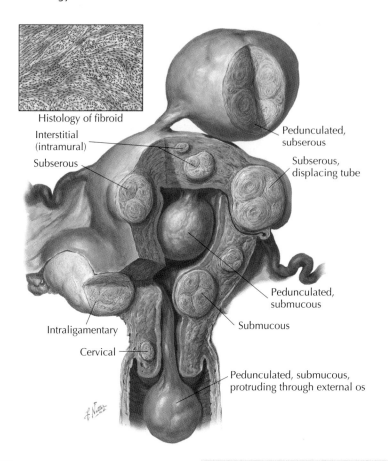

Histology of fibroid

Interstitial
(intramural)

Subserous

Pedunculated,
subserous

Subserous,
displacing tube

Pedunculated,
submucous

Submucous

Intraligamentary

Cervical

Pedunculated, submucous,
protruding through external os

Prevention/Avoidance: None.

Possible Complications: Possibility of bone loss with prolonged gonadotropin-releasing hormone therapy. Leiomyomata may undergo degeneration (hyaline; 65%, myxomatous; 15%, calcific; 10%), rarely causing acute symptoms of pain.

Expected Outcome: Leiomyomata generally stop growing after menopause (even with estrogen replacement). Recurrence after myomectomy is common (25%).

MISCELLANEOUS

Pregnancy Considerations: May (rarely) interfere with early pregnancy or obstruct delivery. Fibroids may grow rapidly or undergo hemorrhage or necrosis and may occasionally even be a cause for disseminated intravascular coagulopathy. Cesarean delivery should be considered for subsequent deliveries if the endometrial cavity is entered during myomectomy.

ICD-9-CM Codes: 218.0 (Submucous), 218.1 (Intramural), 218.2 (Subserous), 218.9 (Unspecified).

REFERENCES

Level I
Fiscella K, Eisinger SH, Meldrum S, et al: Effect of mifepristone for symptomatic leiomyomata on quality of life and uterine size: a randomized controlled trial. Obstet Gynecol 2006;108:1381.

Hald K, Klow NE, Qvigstad E, Istre O: Laparoscopic occlusion compared with embolization of uterine vessels: a randomized controlled trial. Obstet Gynecol 2007;109:20.

Level II
Aungst M, Wilson M, Vournas K, McCarthy S: Necrotic leiomyoma and gram-negative sepsis eight weeks after uterine artery embolization. Obstet Gynecol 2004;104:1161.

Pron G, Mocarski E, Bennett J, et al; Ontario UFE Collaborative Group: Pregnancy after uterine artery embolization for leiomyomata: the Ontario multicenter trial. Obstet Gynecol 2005; 105:67.

Spies JB, Myers ER, Worthington-Kirsch R, et al; FIBROID Registry Investigators: The FIBROID Registry: Symptom and quality-of-life status 1 year after therapy. Obstet Gynecol 2005;106:1309.

Steinauer J, Pritts EA, Jackson R, Jacoby AF: Systematic review of mifepristone for the treatment of uterine leiomyomata. Obstet Gynecol 2004;103:1331.

Level III
American College of Obstetricians and Gynecologists: Surgical alternatives to hysterectomy in the management of leiomyomas. ACOG Practice Bulletin 16. Washington, DC, ACOG, 2000.

American College of Obstetricians and Gynecologists: Uterine artery embolization. ACOG Committee Opinion 293. Obstet Gynecol 2004;103:403.

Cramer SF, Horiszny JA, Leppert P: Epidemiology of uterine leiomyomas. J Reprod Med 1995;40:595.

Katz VL: Benign gynecologic lesions. In Katz VL, Lentz GM, Lobo RA, Gershenson DM: Comprehensive Gynecology, 5th ed. Philadelphia, Mosby/Elsevier, 2007:441.

Myers ER, Barber MD, Gustilo-Ashby T, et al: Management of uterine leiomyomata: what do we really know? Obstet Gynecol 2002;100:8.

Reiter RC, Wagner PL, Gambone JC: Routine hysterectomy for large asymptomatic uterine leiomyomata: a reappraisal. Obstet Gynecol 1992;79:481.

Sharp HT: Assessment of new technology in the treatment of idiopathic menorrhagia and uterine leiomyomata. Obstet Gynecol 2006;108:990.

Stewart EA, Morton CC: The genetics of uterine leiomyomata: what clinicians need to know. Obstet Gynecol 2006;107:917.

Vollenhoven BJ, Lawrence AS, Healy DL: Uterine fibroids: a clinical review. Br J Obstet Gynaecol 1990;97:285.

INTRODUCTION

Description: Uterine prolapse is loss of the normal support mechanism resulting in descent of the uterus down the vaginal canal. In the extreme, this may result in the uterus descending beyond the vulva to a position outside the body (procidentia).

Prevalence: Some degree of uterine descent is common in parous women.

Predominant Age: Late reproductive and beyond; incidence increases with the loss of estrogen.

Genetics: No genetic pattern.

ETIOLOGY AND PATHOGENESIS

Causes: Loss of normal structural support as a result of trauma (childbirth), surgery, chronic intra-abdominal pressure elevation (such as obesity, chronic cough, or heavy lifting), or intrinsic weakness. Most common sites of injury are the cardinal and uterosacral ligaments and the levator ani muscles that form the pelvic floor, which may relax or rupture. Rarely, increased intra-abdominal pressure from a pelvic mass or ascites may weaken pelvic support and result in prolapse. Injury to or neuropathy of the S_1 to S_4 nerve roots may also result in decreased muscle tone and pelvic relaxation.

Risk Factors: Birth trauma, chronic intra-abdominal pressure elevation (such as obesity, chronic cough, or heavy lifting), intrinsic tissue weakness, or atrophic changes resulting from estrogen loss.

CLINICAL CHARACTERISTICS

Signs and Symptoms

- Pelvic pressure or heaviness (a sense of "falling out")
- Mass or protrusion at or beyond the vaginal entrance
- New onset or paradoxical resolution of urinary incontinence
- Drying, thickening, chronic inflammation, and ulceration of the exposed tissues, which may result in bleeding, discharge, or odor

DIAGNOSTIC APPROACH

Differential Diagnosis

- Cystocele
- Urethrocele
- Rectocele
- Enterocele
- Prolapsed uterine leiomyomata
- Bartholin's cyst
- Vaginal cyst or tumor
- Cervical hypertrophy (with normal uterine support)

Associated Conditions: Urinary incontinence, pelvic pain, dyspareunia, intermenstrual or postmenopausal bleeding. Almost always associated with a cystocele, rectocele, and enterocele.

Workup and Evaluation

Laboratory: No evaluation indicated.
Imaging: No imaging indicated.

Special Tests: Urodynamics testing may be considered if voiding or continence is altered.

Diagnostic Procedures: History and physical examination.

Pathologic Findings

Tissue change is common because of mechanical trauma and desiccation.

MANAGEMENT AND THERAPY

Nonpharmacologic

General Measures: Weight reduction, modification of activity (lifting), addressing factors such as chronic cough.

Specific Measures: Minimal prolapse does not require therapy. For those with more severe prolapse or symptoms, pessary therapy (Smith-Hodge, doughnut, cube, or inflatable ball), surgical repair, or hysterectomy (with colporrhaphy) should be considered. Postmenopausal women should receive estrogen and progesterone replacement therapy for at least 30 days before pessary fitting or surgical repair.

Diet: No specific dietary changes indicated.
Activity: No restriction.
Patient Education: Reassurance: American College of Obstetricians and Gynecologists Patient Education Pamphlet AP012 (Pelvic Support Problems), AP081 (Urinary Incontinence).

Drug(s) of Choice

Estrogen and progesterone therapy (for postmenopausal patients) improves tissue tone and healing and is often prescribed before surgical repair or as an adjunct to pessary therapy.

Contraindications: Estrogen therapy should not be used if undiagnosed vaginal bleeding is present.

FOLLOW-UP

Patient Monitoring: Normal health maintenance. If a pessary is used, frequent follow-up (both initially and long term) is required. (Most recommend monthly checks of the vaginal epithelium for lesions and to reassess pessary placement and fit.)

Prevention/Avoidance: Maintenance of normal weight, avoidance of known (modifiable) risk factors.

Possible Complications: Thickening or ulceration of the vaginal tissues and cervix, urinary incontinence, kinking of the ureters, obstipation.

Expected Outcome: Uterine descent tends to worsen with time. If uncorrected, complete prolapse is associated with vaginal and cervical skin changes, ulceration, and bleeding.

MISCELLANEOUS

Pregnancy Considerations: No effect on pregnancy, though these conditions rarely coexist.

ICD-9-CM Codes: 618.1 (codes 618.2 to 618.4 are used when cystocele, urethrocele, or rectocele is present).

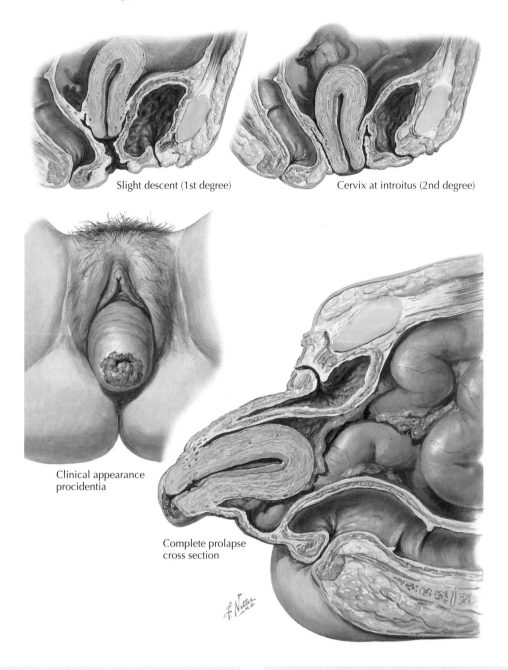

Slight descent (1st degree)

Cervix at introitus (2nd degree)

Clinical appearance
procidentia

Complete prolapse
cross section

REFERENCES

Level I

Cundiff GW, Amundsen CL, Bent AE, et al: The PESSRI study: Symptom relief outcomes of a randomized crossover trial of the ring and Gellhorn pessaries. Am J Obstet Gynecol 2007;196:405. e1.

Level II

Swift S, Woodman P, O'Boyle A, et al: Pelvic Organ Support Study (POSST): The distribution, clinical definition, and epidemiologic condition of pelvic organ support defects. Am J Obstet Gynecol 2005;192:795.

Thomas AG, Brodman ML, Dottino PR, et al: Manchester procedure vs vaginal hysterectomy for uterine prolapse: a comparison. J Reprod Med 1995;40:299.

Level III

Altman D, Falconer C: Perioperative morbidity using transvaginal mesh in pelvic organ prolapse repair. Obstet Gynecol 2007;109: 303.

American College of Obstetricians and Gynecologists: Urinary incontinence in women. ACOG Practice Bulletin 63. Obstet Gynecol 2005;105:1533.

American College of Obstetricians and Gynecologists: Pelvic organ prolapse. ACOG Practice Bulletin 79. Obstet Gynecol 2007;109:461.

Beecham CT: Classification of vaginal relaxation. Am J Obstet Gynecol 1980;136:957.

Bump RC, Mattiasson A, Bo K, et al: The standardization of terminology of female pelvic organ prolapse and pelvic floor dysfunction. Am J Obstet Gynecol 1996;175:10.

DeLancey JO: The hidden epidemic of pelvic floor dysfunction: achievable goals for improved prevention and treatment. Am J Obstet Gynecol 2005;192:1488.

Jelovsek JE, Maher C, Barber MD: Pelvic organ prolapse. Lancet 2007;369:1027.

Lentz GM: Anatomic defects of the abdominal wall and pelvic floor. In Katz VL, Lentz GM, Lobo RA, Gershenson DM: Comprehensive Gynecology, 5th ed. Philadelphia, Mosby/Elsevier, 2007:513.

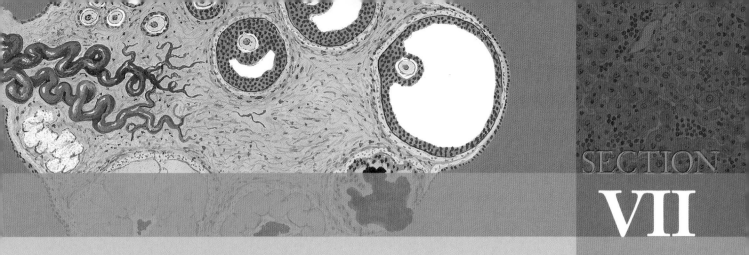

Adnexal Disease

INTRODUCTION

Description: An adenofibroma is an epithelial tumor that consists of glandular elements and large amounts of stromal (fibrous) elements. Adenofibromas are most commonly found as ovarian masses. They may also occur in the cervix or uterine body. Adenofibromas are closely related to cystadenofibromas, which have cystic areas but still contain more than 25% fibrous connective tissue.

Prevalence: Uncommon.

Predominant Age: Perimenopausal and postmenopausal.

Genetics: No genetic pattern.

ETIOLOGY AND PATHOGENESIS

Causes: Unknown.

Risk Factors: None known.

CLINICAL CHARACTERISTICS

Signs and Symptoms

- Asymptomatic (often an incidental finding after oophorectomy)
- Adnexal mass (adenofibromas are bilateral in 25% of cases)
- Fibrous cervical or endometrial polyp
- Acute abdominal pain if torsion occurs (rare)

DIAGNOSTIC APPROACH

Differential Diagnosis

- Thecoma (fibroma)
- Stromal and germ cell tumors
- Brenner tumor
- Endometrioma
- Benign cystic teratoma
- Serous or mucinous cystadenoma
- Metastatic tumors
- Pedunculated leiomyomata
- Endocervical polyp

Associated Conditions: None.

WORKUP AND EVALUATION

Laboratory: No specific evaluation indicated; evaluate as with other adnexal or cervical masses.

Imaging: Ultrasonography may suggest a solid tumor.

Special Tests: None indicated.

Diagnostic Procedures: Histopathology.

Pathologic Findings

Fibrous and epithelial elements make up this tumor. The epithelial components may be serous, mucinous, clear cell, or endometrioid. Epithelial or fibrous elements may predominate, changing the gross character of the tumor. Size is generally 1 to 15 cm in diameter.

MANAGEMENT AND THERAPY

Nonpharmacologic

General Measures: Evaluation and diagnosis.

Specific Measures: Simple surgical excision. Adenofibromas that are borderline or of low malignant potential do exist. These tumors must be treated on the basis of their size, location, and histologic evaluation, but they may require more extensive surgical therapy.

Diet: No specific dietary changes indicated.

Activity: No restriction.

Patient Education: Reassurance; American College of Obstetricians and Gynecologists Patient Education Pamphlet AP075 (Ovarian Cysts), AP096 (Cancer of the Ovary).

Drug(s) of Choice

None.

FOLLOW-UP

Patient Monitoring: Normal health maintenance.

Prevention/Avoidance: None.

Possible Complications: Torsion of solid ovarian tumors. Adenofibromas that are borderline or of low malignant potential may spread or recur.

Expected Outcome: Surgical excision is generally curative.

MISCELLANEOUS

Pregnancy Considerations: No effect on pregnancy.

ICD-9-CM Codes: Based on location and predominant cell type.

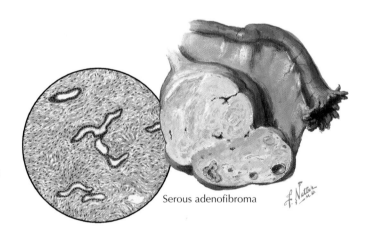

Serous adenofibroma

REFERENCES

Level III

Fleischer AC: Transabdominal and transvaginal sonography of ovarian masses. Clin Obstet Gynecol 1991;34:433.

Herman JR, Locher GW, Goldhirsch A: Sonographic patterns of ovarian tumors: prediction of malignancy. Obstet Gynecol 1987;69:777.

Katz VL: Benign gynecologic lesions. In Katz VL, Lentz GM, Lobo RA, Gershenson DM: Comprehensive Gynecology, 5th ed. Philadelphia, Mosby/Elsevier, 2007:462.

INTRODUCTION

Description: A clear cell carcinoma is an ovarian tumor made up of cells containing large amounts of glycogen, giving them a clear or "hobnailed" appearance. These tumors may also arise in the endocervix, endometrium, and vagina. Cervical and vaginal tumors have been linked to in utero exposure to diethylstilbestrol (DES).

Prevalence: Five percent to 11% of ovarian cancers.

Predominant Age: 40 to 78.

Genetics: No genetic pattern.

ETIOLOGY AND PATHOGENESIS

Causes: Unknown. May arise from mesonephric or Müllerian elements.

Risk Factors: None known.

CLINICAL CHARACTERISTICS

Signs and Symptoms

- Asymptomatic
- Pelvic mass (up to 30 cm)—partially cystic with yellow, gray, and hemorrhagic areas
- Papillary projections generally present, giving the mass a velvety appearance; 40% of tumors are bilateral

DIAGNOSTIC APPROACH

Differential Diagnosis

- Benign adnexal masses (corpus luteum, follicular cyst)
- Nongynecologic pelvic masses
- Hepatic, renal, or cardiac disease resulting in weight loss and ascites
- Endometriosis
- Hydrosalpinx
- Ectopic pregnancy (reproductive-age women)
- Pedunculated leiomyomata
- Pelvic or horseshoe kidney
- Gastrointestinal malignancy

Associated Conditions: None.

Workup and Evaluation

Laboratory: As indicated before surgery. (Serum testing for tumor markers, such as CA-125, lipid-associated sialic acid, carcinoembryonic antigen, α-fetoprotein, and others, should be reserved for following the progress of patients with known malignancies and not for prognostic evaluation.)

Imaging: No imaging indicated.

Special Tests: A frozen-section histologic evaluation should be considered for any ovarian mass that appears suspicious for malignancy.

Diagnostic Procedures: History, physical examination, and imaging. Final diagnosis is established by histologic evaluation.

Pathologic Findings

Usually found as a malignant tumor. Despite the presence of hobnail cells that are similar to those seen in the endo-metrium, cervix, and vagina of women exposed to diethylstilbestrol in utero, there is no evidence that diethylstilbestrol has a role in clear cell ovarian tumors.

MANAGEMENT AND THERAPY

Nonpharmacologic

General Measures: Evaluation, supportive therapy based on symptoms.

Specific Measures: Requires surgical exploration and extirpation, including the uterus and contralateral ovary. Adjunctive chemotherapy (platinum-based and paclitaxel [Taxol]) or radiation therapy is often included, based on the location and stage of the disease.

Diet: No specific dietary changes indicated, except those imposed by advanced disease.

Activity: No restriction except that imposed by advanced disease.

Patient Education: American College of Obstetricians and Gynecologists Patient Education Pamphlet AP096 (Cancer of the Ovary), AP075 (Ovarian Cysts).

Drug(s) of Choice

None, except as adjunctive or symptomatic therapy. Preoperative bowel cleansing (mechanical or with antibiotics) is often recommended as a precaution should bowel resection become necessary at the time of surgical staging and resection.

Contraindications: See individual agents.

Precautions: Alkylating agents are associated with an increased risk of future leukemia (10% by 8 years after therapy).

Interactions: See individual agents.

FOLLOW-UP

Patient Monitoring: Careful follow-up for recurrent pelvic disease or enlargement of the remaining ovary (if any). This is generally performed by pelvic examination, augmented with ultrasonography in selected patients. In those suspected of having recurrent disease and other selected patients, second-look surgery may be desirable to assess progress and discover occult disease.

Prevention/Avoidance: None.

Possible Complications: Rapid spread and progressive deterioration of the patient's condition.

Expected Outcome: Typically aggressive course with rapid disease progression and spread. Clear cell ovarian carcinoma has the worst prognosis of all ovarian malignancies, with a 5-year survival rate of <40%. (The 5-year survival rate is modified by stage of disease at diagnosis: limited to one ovary, 80%; higher stage disease, 11%).

MISCELLANEOUS

Pregnancy Considerations: No direct effect on pregnancy. (Generally not an issue.)

ICD-9-CM Codes: M8310/3.

Clear Cell Carcinoma of Ovary

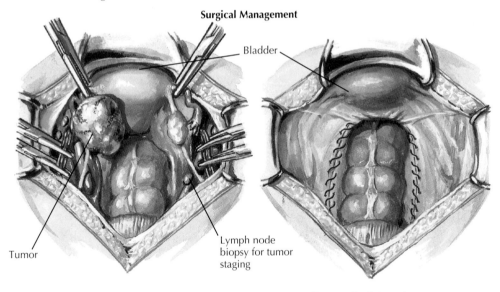

Pelvic mass (up to 30 cm)
Partially cystic 40% bilateral
predominantly

Papillary
projections

Glycogen-containing cells create
"hobnailed" histologic appearance.
Similar tumors occur in endocervix,
vagina, and endometrium.

JOHN A. CRAIG___AD
D. Mascaro

Surgical Management

Bladder

Tumor

Lymph node
biopsy for tumor
staging

Total abdominal hysterectomy
with bilateral salpingo-oophorectomy

Closure of pelvic peritoneum
postoperative appearance

REFERENCES

Level II

Eastwood J: Mesonephroid (clear cell) carcinoma of the ovary and endometrium: a comparative prospective clinico-pathological study and review of literature. Cancer 1978;41:1911.

Level III

American College of Obstetricians and Gynecologists: The role of the generalist obstetrician–gynecologist in the early detection of ovarian cancer. ACOG Committee Opinion 280. Obstet Gynecol 2002;100:1413.

Coleman RL, Gershenson DM: Neoplastic diseases of the ovary. In Katz VL, Lentz GM, Lobo RA, Gershenson DM: Comprehensive Gynecology, 5th ed. Philadelphia, Mosby/Elsevier, 2007:845, 852.

Fleischer AC: Transabdominal and transvaginal sonography of ovarian masses. Clin Obstet Gynecol 1991;34:433.

Hameed K, Burslem MRG, Tupper WRC: Clear cell carcinoma of the ovary. Cancer 1969;24:452.

Sugiyama T, Kamura T, Kigawa J, et al: Clinical characteristics of clear cell carcinoma of the ovary: a distinct histologic type with poor prognosis and resistance to platinum-based chemotherapy. Cancer 2000;88:2584.

INTRODUCTION

Description: The most common ovarian tumor in young, reproductive-age women is the cystic teratoma, or dermoid, which originates from a germ cell and contains elements from all three germ cell layers. These tumors may be benign or malignant (1% to 2% malignant, usually in women older than 40). These tumors account for 20% to 25% of all ovarian tumors and one third of all benign tumors.

Prevalence: Fifteen percent to 25% of ovarian tumors.

Predominant Age: 20s to 30s (75%), most younger than 40.

Genetics: No genetic pattern.

ETIOLOGY AND PATHOGENESIS

Causes: Unknown. Thought to arise from a single germ cell during the first meiotic division at roughly 13 weeks of fetal life. They routinely have a chromosomal makeup of 46,XX.

Risk Factors: None known.

CLINICAL CHARACTERISTICS

Signs and Symptoms

- Asymptomatic (50% to 60%)
- Adnexal mass (<10 cm in diameter in 80% of patients; bilateral in 10% to 15% of patients)—the contents of cystic teratomas are of low density; they are often found "floating" anterior to the uterus or broad ligament, displacing the uterus posteriorly
- May present with pain secondary to torsion (approximately 10%) or bleeding into the cyst, a sense of pelvic heaviness, or dysmenorrhea
- Thyroid storm (when thyroid tissue predominates: struma ovarii) or carcinoid syndrome (rare)

DIAGNOSTIC APPROACH

Differential Diagnosis

- Functional cysts (follicle, corpus luteum)
- Epithelial tumors (cystic or solid)
- Ectopic pregnancy
- Tubo-ovarian abscess
- Endometrioma
- Hydrosalpinx
- Paratubal cyst
- Appendiceal abscess

Associated Conditions: None.

WORKUP AND EVALUATION

Laboratory: No evaluation indicated.

Imaging: Ultrasonography (abdominal or transvaginal may be of assistance but usually is not required; when used, it has a 95% positive predictive value). Of teratomas, 30% to 50% have calcifications and may be detected by radiographic examination.

Special Tests: None indicated.

Diagnostic Procedures: History, physical examination, imaging. May be found incidentally at laparotomy or laparoscopy.

Pathologic Findings

These tumors are derived from primary germ cells and include tissues from all three embryonic germ layers (ectoderm, mesoderm, and endoderm). Consequently, these often contain hair, sebaceous material, cartilage, bone, teeth, or neural tissue. On some occasions, functional thyroid tissue may be present (up to 12% of cases). Cystic teratomas contain malignant elements in only about 1% to 2% of cases.

MANAGEMENT AND THERAPY

Nonpharmacologic

General Measures: Evaluation, support for acute symptoms.

Specific Measures: Surgical exploration and resection.

Diet: No specific dietary changes indicated.

Activity: No restriction.

Patient Education: Reassurance; American College of Obstetricians and Gynecologists Patient Education Pamphlet AP075 (Ovarian Cysts).

Drug(s) of Choice

None.

FOLLOW-UP

Patient Monitoring: Normal health maintenance.

Prevention/Avoidance: None.

Possible Complications: Most common—torsion (3% to 12%). Possible—infection, rupture, and malignant transformation (squamous carcinoma, 1% to 2%). (The risk of malignant transformation is greatest when these tumors are found in postmenopausal women.) Recurrence of teratomas is as high as 3.4% in some studies. Rupture of a dermoid cyst can result in an intense chemical peritonitis and is a surgical emergency. Slow leakage may mimic disseminated carcinoma.

Expected Outcome: Based on the size and location of the tumor, it is often possible to conserve some or most of the ovary while the tumor itself is resected.

MISCELLANEOUS

Pregnancy Considerations: No effect on pregnancy. Of teratomas, 10% are diagnosed during pregnancy and account for 20% to 40% of ovarian tumors found during pregnancy. Rupture of the cyst, although rare, is more common during pregnancy.

ICD-9-CM Codes: M9084/0.

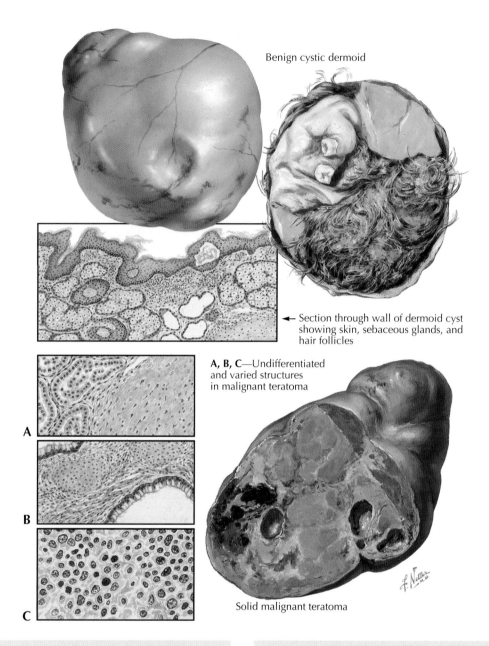

Benign cystic dermoid

◄— Section through wall of dermoid cyst showing skin, sebaceous glands, and hair follicles

A, B, C—Undifferentiated and varied structures in malignant teratoma

A

B

C

Solid malignant teratoma

REFERENCES

Level I
Wang PH, Lee WL, Juang CM, et al: Excision of mature teratoma using culdotomy, with and without laparoscopy: a prospective randomized trial. BJOG 2001;108:91.

Level II
Emoto M, Obama H, Horiuchi S, et al: Transvaginal color Doppler ultrasonic characterization of benign and malignant ovarian cystic teratomas and comparison with serum squamous cell carcinoma antigen. Cancer 2000;88:2298.

Howard FM: Surgical management of benign cystic teratoma: laparoscopy vs. laparotomy. J Reprod Med 1995;40:495.

Koonings PP, Campbell K, Mishell DR Jr, et al: Relative frequency of primary ovarian neoplasms: a 10-year review. Obstet Gynecol 1989;74:921.

Lakkis WG, Martin MC, Gelfand MM: Benign cystic teratoma of the ovary: a 6-year review. Can J Surg 1985;28:244.

Mais V, Ajossa S, Mallarini G, et al: No recurrence of mature ovarian teratomas after laparoscopic cystectomy. BJOG 2003;110:624.

Mais V, Guerriero S, Ajossa S, et al: Transvaginal ultrasonography in the diagnosis of cystic teratoma. Obstet Gynecol 1995;85:48.

Pantoja E, Noy MA, Axtmayer RW, et al: Ovarian dermoids and their complications: comprehensive historical review. Obstet Gynecol Surv 1975;30:1.

Level III
Fleischer AC: Transabdominal and transvaginal sonography of ovarian masses. Clin Obstet Gynecol 1991;34:433.

Gallion H, van Nagell JR Jr, Donaldson ES, et al: Immature teratoma of the ovary. Am J Obstet Gynecol 1983;146:361.

Katz VL: Benign gynecologic lesions. In Katz VL, Lentz GM, Lobo RA, Gershenson DM: Comprehensive Gynecology, 5th ed. Philadelphia, Mosby/Elsevier, 2007:457.

Linder D, McCau BK, Hecht F: Parthenogenic origin of benign ovarian teratomas. N Engl J Med 1975;292:63.

Parazzini F, La Vecchia C, Negri E, et al: Risk factors for benign ovarian teratomas. Br J Cancer 1995;71:664.

Petersen WF, Prevost EC, Edmunds FT, et al: Benign cystic teratomas of the ovary. Am J Obstet Gynecol 1955;70:368.

Vergote IB, Abeler VM, Kjorstad KE, et al: Management of malignant ovarian immature teratoma. Role of adriamycin. Cancer 1990;66:882.

INTRODUCTION

Description: A dysgerminoma is an ovarian tumor made up of germ cells and stroma that appears analogous in structure to the seminomas found in the male testes. Although rare, these tumors are the most common malignant germ cell tumors.

Prevalence: Rare, 1% to 2% of ovarian malignancies.

Predominant Age: Older than 30 (10% in prepubertal girls).

Genetics: No genetic pattern.

ETIOLOGY AND PATHOGENESIS

Causes: Unknown. (May differentiate from primitive germ cells.)

Risk Factors: None known.

CLINICAL CHARACTERISTICS

Signs and Symptoms

- Asymptomatic
- Adnexal mass (bilateral in 5% to 10%), lobulated, solid and soft or firm, with a gray–white or cream-colored cut surface.

DIAGNOSTIC APPROACH

Differential Diagnosis

- Benign adnexal masses (corpus luteum, follicular cyst)
- Endometriosis
- Hydrosalpinx
- Paratubal cyst
- Appendiceal abscess
- Ectopic pregnancy
- Pedunculated leiomyomata
- Pelvic or horseshoe kidney
- Nongynecologic pelvic masses

Associated Conditions: None.

WORKUP AND EVALUATION

Laboratory: As indicated before surgery. β-Human chorionic gonadotropin is often elevated (several thousand units), as is lactic dehydrogenase. (Serum testing for tumor markers, such as CA-125, lipid-associated sialic acid, carcinoembryonic antigen, α-fetoprotein, and others, should be reserved for following the progress of patients with known malignancies and not for prognostic evaluation.)

Imaging: Preoperative evaluation (computed tomography [CT] or ultrasonography) for possible lymph node enlargement or intra-abdominal spread is indicated for patients for whom malignancy is a significant possibility.

Special Tests: None indicated.

Diagnostic Procedures: History, physical examination, and imaging. Final diagnosis is established by histologic evaluation.

Pathologic Findings

Primitive germ cells with stroma infiltrated by lymphocytes (analogous to seminomas in the testes). Areas of malignant cells are found in 10% to 15% of tumors.

MANAGEMENT AND THERAPY

Nonpharmacologic

General Measures: Evaluation, supportive therapy based on symptoms.

Specific Measures: Surgical exploration and resection. When the tumor is confined to one ovary, preservation of the uterus and other ovary is possible to preserve fertility. These tumors are very sensitive to radiation therapy, which may be used as an adjunct or to treat recurrent disease. Multiagent chemotherapy has fewer side effects and is often the preferred adjunct.

Diet: No specific dietary changes indicated, except those imposed by advanced disease.

Activity: No restriction except that imposed by advanced disease.

Patient Education: American College of Obstetricians and Gynecologists Patient Education Pamphlet AP096 (Cancer of the Ovary), AP075 (Ovarian Cysts).

Drug(s) of Choice

Adjunctive or symptomatic therapy. Combination chemotherapy in selected patients (vincristine, actinomycin D, and cyclophosphamide or bleomycin, etoposide, and cisplatin).

FOLLOW-UP

Patient Monitoring: Careful follow-up for recurrent pelvic disease or enlargement of the remaining ovary (if any). This is generally performed by pelvic examination, augmented with ultrasonography in selected patients. In patients suspected of having recurrent disease and other selected patients, second-look surgery may be desirable to assess progress and discover occult disease.

Prevention/Avoidance: None.

Possible Complications: Tumor progression or growth. These tumors tend to spread by lymphatic channels. Recurrence of tumor is found in 20% of patients, but recurrent disease generally responds well to additional surgery, chemotherapy, or radiation.

Expected Outcome: The prognosis is good for patients with pure dysgerminomas less than 15 cm in size. With limited disease and no indication of spread at the time of surgery (stage I) there is a >90% 5-year survival.

MISCELLANEOUS

Pregnancy Considerations: No effect on pregnancy. May be discovered during pregnancy.

ICD-9-CM Codes: Specific to cell type and location.

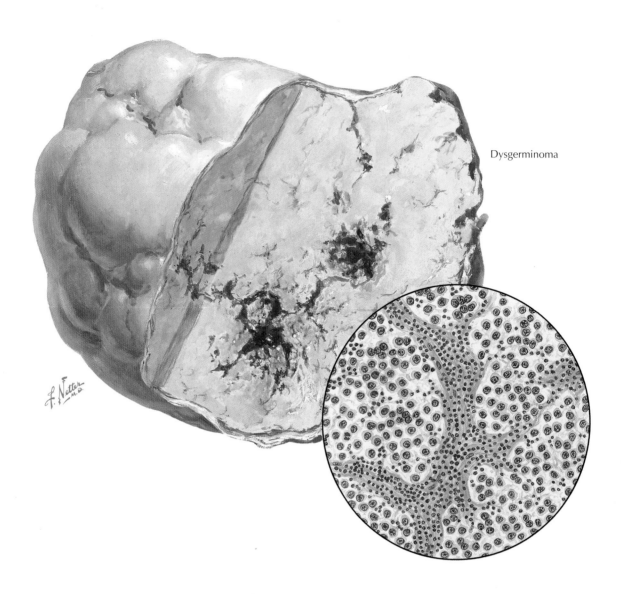

Dysgerminoma

REFERENCES

Level I
Williams SD, Blessing JA, Moore DH, et al: Cisplatin, vinblastine, and bleomycin in advanced and recurrent ovarian germ-cell tumors. A trial of the Gynecologic Oncology Group. Ann Intern Med 1989;111:22.

Level II
Assadourian LA, Taylor HB: Dysgerminoma: an analysis of 105 cases. Obstet Gynecol 1969;33:370.

Gallion HH, van Nagell JR Jr, Donaldson ES, Powell DE: Ovarian dysgerminoma: report of seven cases and review of the literature. Am J Obstet Gynecol 1988;158:591.

Level III
Barber HR. Ovarian cancer. CA Cancer J Clin 1986;36:149.

Coleman RL, Gershenson DM: Neoplastic diseases of the ovary. In Katz VL, Lentz GM, Lobo RA, Gershenson DM: Comprehensive Gynecology, 5th ed. Philadelphia, Mosby/Elsevier, 2007: 867.

Fleischer AC: Transabdominal and transvaginal sonography of ovarian masses. Clin Obstet Gynecol 1991;34:433.

Gershenson DM: Update on malignant ovarian germ cell tumors. Cancer 1993;71:1581.

Thomas GM, Dembo AJ, Hacker NF, et al: Current therapy for dysgerminoma of the ovary. Obstet Gynecol 1987;70: 268.

INTRODUCTION

Description: An ectopic pregnancy is one that implants outside of the endometrial cavity (fallopian tube, ovary, abdominal cavity, or cervix).

Prevalence: Ten to 15 of 1000 pregnancies; varies with age, race, and location (highest in Jamaica and Vietnam).

Predominant Age: 25 to 34 (>50%).

Genetics: No genetic pattern.

ETIOLOGY AND PATHOGENESIS

Causes: Tubal damage or altered motility that causes the fertilized egg to be improperly transported, resulting in implantation outside the uterine cavity. The most common cause is acute salpingitis (50%). In the majority of the remaining patients (40%), no risk factor is apparent. Abnormal embryonic development may play a role.

Risk Factors: Tubal damage (pelvic infections; 6-fold increased risk), prior ectopic pregnancy (10-fold increased risk), prior female sterilization, age (age 35 to 44, 3-fold greater rate of extrauterine gestations than for women aged 15 to 24), nonwhite race (1.5-fold increased risk), assisted reproduction, cigarette smoking (30+/day: 3- to 5-fold increased risk), intrauterine contraceptive device (IUCD) use, and endometriosis. More than half of cases occur in women who have been pregnant three or more times.

CLINICAL CHARACTERISTICS

Signs and Symptoms

- Normal signs and symptoms of pregnancy (amenorrhea, uterine softening)
- Acute abdominal pain (dull, crampy, or colicky)
- Evidence of intra-abdominal bleeding including hypotension and collapse
- Adnexal mass (with or without tenderness)
- Vaginal bleeding
- Signs of peritoneal irritation
- Absence of a gestational sac on ultrasonography with β-human chorionic gonadotropin (β-hCG) level >2500 mIU/mL
- Abdominal pregnancy may be asymptomatic until near term

DIAGNOSTIC APPROACH

Differential Diagnosis

- Appendicitis
- Degenerating fibroid
- Dysfunctional uterine bleeding
- Endometriosis
- Gastroenteritis
- Mesenteric thrombosis
- Ovulation
- Ruptured corpus luteum cyst
- Salpingitis
- Septic abortion (fever >38°C or a white blood count >20,000 WBC/dL are rare in patients with ectopic pregnancies; the presence of either should suggest the possibility of a pelvic infection, including septic abortion)
- Threatened or incomplete abortion
- Torsion of an adnexal mass

Associated Conditions: Pelvic inflammatory disease, infertility, and recurrent abortion.

Workup and Evaluation

Laboratory: Serial quantitative β-hCG levels (if patient's condition permits). (Levels are lower than 3000 mIU/mL in about half of cases.) Serum progesterone (low) may be of diagnostic help if <6 weeks gestation. (Almost 90% of patients with an ectopic pregnancy have levels less than 30 nM/L [10 ng/mL].) A hematocrit level of less than 30% is found in about one fourth of women with ruptured ectopic pregnancy.

Imaging: Ultrasonography (transvaginal preferred) may be augmented by color-flow Doppler studies.

Special Tests: Culdocentesis has largely been replaced by ultrasonography.

Diagnostic Procedures: History and physical examination, serum β-hCG level and ultrasonography. (When laparoscopy is used as a diagnostic tool, there is a 2% to 5% chance of a false-positive or false-negative diagnosis.)

Pathologic Findings

Placental villi invading tissue other than the endometrium. Most ectopic pregnancies are tubal, with the ampulla (approximately 80%) and isthmus (12%) being the most common locations with 5% in the fimbrial region.

MANAGEMENT AND THERAPY

Nonpharmacologic

General Measures: Rapid assessment and general support when intra-abdominal bleeding is present.

Specific Measures: Expeditious diagnosis. (Diagnostic delay is a factor in approximately half of all deaths associated with ectopic pregnancy; 50% of patients have had one or more visits to a health care provider before the diagnosis is made in even nonfatal cases.) Surgical intervention generally is required for symptomatic patients (salpingostomy, salpingectomy). Medical therapy may be considered for asymptomatic or mildly symptomatic patients.

Diet: In acute rupture, nothing by mouth in anticipation of possible surgical intervention. If medical therapy is used, avoid folate supplements and folate-containing preparations (e.g., multivitamins, prenatal vitamins).

Activity: No restriction except those dictated by the patient's status.

Patient Education: Reassurance; American College of Obstetricians and Gynecologists Patient Education

Sites of Ectopic Implantation

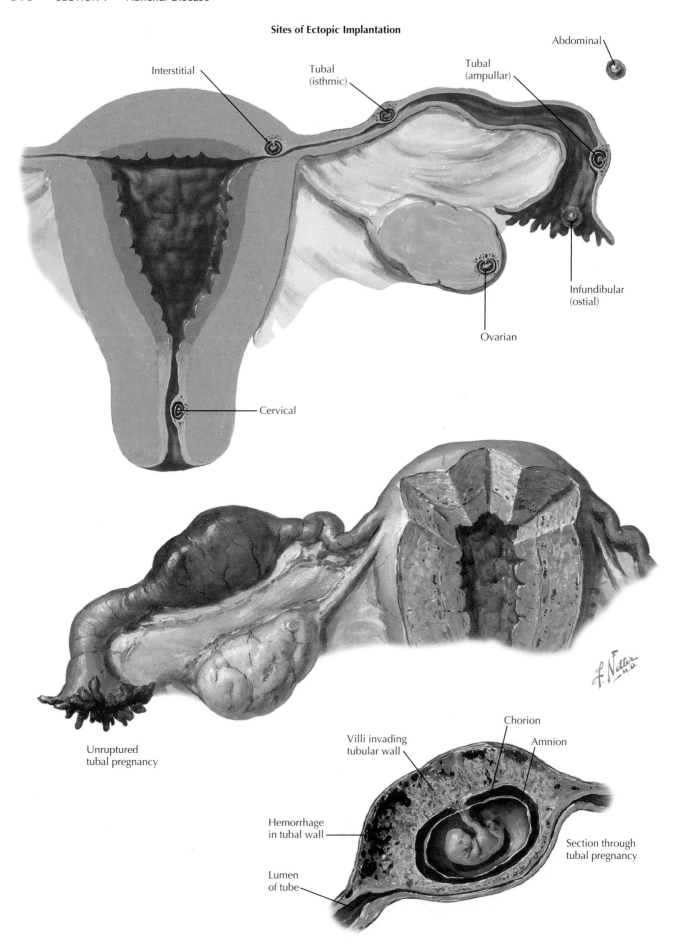

Interstitial

Tubal (isthmic)

Tubal (ampullar)

Abdominal

Infundibular (ostial)

Ovarian

Cervical

Unruptured tubal pregnancy

Villi invading tubular wall

Chorion

Amnion

Hemorrhage in tubal wall

Lumen of tube

Section through tubal pregnancy

Diagnosis of Ectopic Pregnancy

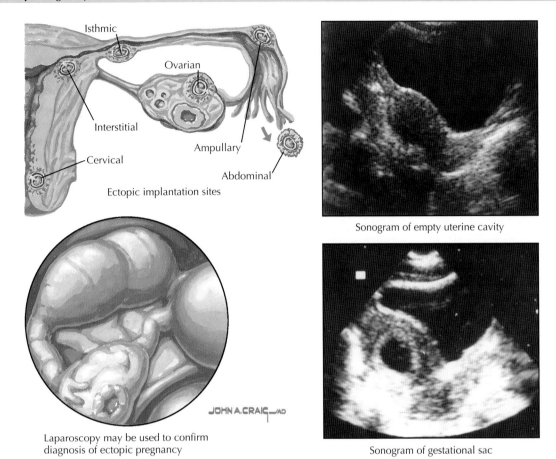

Ectopic implantation sites

Sonogram of empty uterine cavity

JOHN A. CRAIG—MD

Laparoscopy may be used to confirm
diagnosis of ectopic pregnancy

Sonogram of gestational sac

Pregnancy Monitoring with Serial Sonograms and β-HCG Determinations

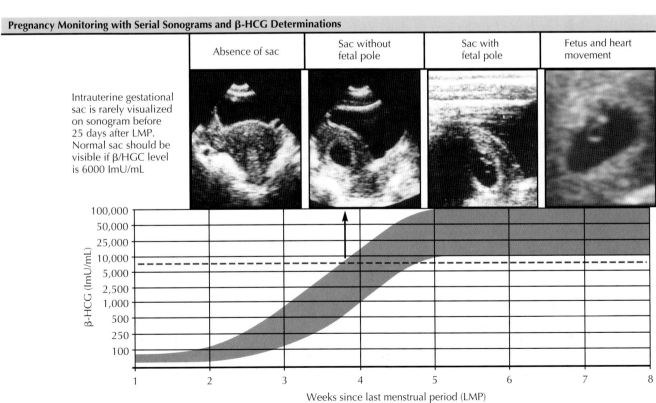

Intrauterine gestational
sac is rarely visualized
on sonogram before
25 days after LMP.
Normal sac should be
visible if β/HGC level
is 6000 ImU/mL

| Absence of sac | Sac without fetal pole | Sac with fetal pole | Fetus and heart movement |

β-HCG (ImU/mL)

Weeks since last menstrual period (LMP)

HCG, human choriocnic gonadotropin

Pamphlet AP077 (Pelvic Inflammatory Disease [PID]), American Society for Reproductive Medicine, *Ectopic Pregnancy: A Guide for Patients*, 1996.

Drug(s) of Choice

Methotrexate IM 50 mg/m^2 surface area with a maximum of 80 mg.

Contraindications: Methotrexate should not be used if the β-hCG level is greater than 15,000 mIU/mL, the adnexal mass is greater than 3 cm, or the patient's hemodynamic status is unstable. Patients with a history of active hepatic or renal disease, fetal cardiac activity demonstrated in the ectopic gestation, active ulcer disease, or significant alterations in blood count (white blood cell count <3000, platelet count of <100,000) are not candidates for this therapy.

All women with ectopic pregnancies who are Rh-negative and unsensitized should receive Rh immunoglobulin at a dosage of 50 μg if the gestation is of less than 12 weeks duration and 300 μg if it is beyond 12 weeks.

Precautions: A transient increase in abdominal symptoms is often encountered 48 to 72 hours after methotrexate therapy. Approximately 5% to 10% of patients managed medically experience complications before medical therapy can be effective, necessitating surgical intervention.

Interactions: If patients are receiving methotrexate therapy, they should not take multivitamins with folic acid (e.g., prenatal vitamins) because this counteracts the effects of the methotrexate.

FOLLOW-UP

Patient Monitoring: Follow-up assessment of serum β-hCG level to confirm a decline toward normal.

Prevention/Avoidance: Reduce modifiable risk factors, such as pelvic infections.

Possible Complications: Rupture of an ectopic pregnancy dooms the pregnancy and may result in catastrophic intra-abdominal bleeding that jeopardizes the life of the mother. (It is the most common cause of maternal death in the first half of pregnancy.) Maternal mortality from ectopic pregnancy has declined with earlier detection made possible by laboratory and ultrasonography diagnosis. Current statistics suggest a rate of 3.8 of 10,000 patients (varies with age and race—African Americans have a 5-fold greater risk). Maternal death is most often associated with blood loss and delay in diagnosis.

Expected Outcome: With prompt diagnosis, the prognosis for the patient is good, although infertility rates are high (40%) and the likelihood of a successful pregnancy is reduced (50%). The prognosis for the current pregnancy is uniformly bad. Methotrexate therapy is associated with a roughly 90% efficacy rate.

MISCELLANEOUS

Pregnancy Considerations: Poor outcomes for future pregnancy including increased risk of subsequent ectopic implantation and spontaneous pregnancy loss.

ICD-9-CM Codes: 633.1 (Tubal), 633.0 (Abdominal), 633.2 (Ovarian), 633.8 (Other site such as cervical or cornual).

REFERENCES

Level I
Ness RB, Trautmann G, Richter HE, et al: Effectiveness of treatment strategies of some women with pelvic inflammatory disease: a randomized trial. Obstet Gynecol 2005;106:573.

Stovall TG, Ling FW, Buster JE: Outpatient chemotherapy of unruptured ectopic pregnancy. Fertil Steril 1989;51:435.

Level II
Barnhart KT, Gosman G, Ashby R, Sammel M: The medical management of ectopic pregnancy: a meta-analysis comparing "single dose" and "multidose" regimens. Obstet Gynecol 2003;101:778.

Bickell NA, Bodian C, Anderson RM, Kase N: Time and the risk of ruptured tubal pregnancy. Obstet Gynecol 2004;104:789.

Jeng CJ, Ko ML, Shen J: Transvaginal ultrasound-guided treatment of cervical pregnancy. Obstet Gynecol 2007;109:1076.

Khan KS, Wojdyla D, Say L, et al: WHO analysis of causes of maternal death: a systematic review. Lancet 2006;367:1066.

Shalev E, Yarom I, Bustan M, et al: Transvaginal sonography as the ultimate diagnostic tool for the management of ectopic pregnancy: experience with 840 cases. Fertil Steril 1998;69:62.

Shannon C, Brothers LP, Philip NM, Winikoff B: Ectopic pregnancy and medical abortion. Obstet Gynecol 2004;104:161.

Level III
American College of Obstetricians and Gynecologists: Medical Management of Tubal Pregnancy. ACOG Practice Bulletin 3. Washington, DC, ACOG, 1998.

American College of Obstetricians and Gynecologists: Avoiding inappropriate clinical decisions based on false-positive human chorionic gonadotropin test results. ACOG Committee Opinion 278. Obstet Gynecol 2002;100:1057.

Ankum WM, Van der Veen F, Hamerlynck JVTH, Lammes FB: Suspected ectopic pregnancy: what to do when human chorionic gonadotropin levels are below the discrimination zone. J Reprod Med 1995;40:525.

Farquhar CM: Ectopic pregnancy. Lancet 2005;366:583.

Lobo RA: Ectopic pregnancy. In Katz VL, Lentz GM, Lobo RA, Gershenson DM: Comprehensive Gynecology, 5th ed. Philadelphia, Mosby/Elsevier, 2007:389.

Reich H, Freifeld ML, McGlynn F, Reich E: Laparoscopic treatment of tubal pregnancy. Obstet Gynecol 1987;69:275.

Russell JB: The etiology of ectopic pregnancy. Clin Obstet Gynecol 1987;30:181.

Seeber BE, Barnhart KT: Suspected ectopic pregnancy. Obstet Gynecol 2006;107:399.

INTRODUCTION

Description: Endometriosis is a benign but progressive condition characterized by endometrial glands and stroma found in locations other than the endometrium.

Prevalence: Five percent to 15% of women, 20% of gynecologic laparotomies, 30% of patients with chronic pain, 30% to 50% of patients experiencing infertility.

Predominant Age: Third and fourth decades of life, 5% diagnosed after menopause.

Genetics: Familial predisposition (polygenic or multifactorial inheritance pattern).

ETIOLOGY AND PATHOGENESIS

Causes: Endometriosis may arise by one of several proposed mechanisms—lymphatic spread, metaplasia of celomic epithelium or Müllerian rests, seeding by retrograde menstruation, or direct hematogenous spread. Instances of presumed iatrogenic spread (surgical) have been reported. A role for an immunologic defect is debated but remains to be conclusively established.

Risk Factors: Obstructive anomalies such as an unrecognized double uterus or a cervical and/or vaginal outflow-tract obstruction. (Approximately 10% of teenagers diagnosed with endometriosis have associated congenital outflow obstruction.)

CLINICAL CHARACTERISTICS

Signs and Symptoms

- Asymptomatic (up to 30%)
- Cyclic pelvic pain or dyspareunia (both worst 36 to 48 hours before menses), premenstrual and menstrual pain, dyschezia, midcycle (ovulatory) pain—often the pain reported by patients seems inversely proportional to the amount of disease; small implants seem to be exquisitely painful, and large endometriomata may be asymptomatic
- Infertility
- Intermenstrual bleeding (15% to 20%)
- Anovulation (15%)
- Intermittent constipation or diarrhea
- Adnexal mass(es)
- Uterine retroversion, scarring and nodularity of the posterior cul-de-sac

DIAGNOSTIC APPROACH

Differential Diagnosis

- Pelvic adhesive disease (secondary to pelvic infection, surgery)
- Uterine fibroids
- Gastrointestinal, urologic, or musculoskeletal problems
- Corpus luteum cysts
- Ovarian neoplasia

- Adenocarcinoma of the large bowel (endometrial implants my be difficult to differentiate grossly from a primary neoplasm of the large bowel)

Associated Conditions: Infertility, nulliparity, pelvic pain, dyspareunia (deep thrust), uterine retroversion, premenstrual and menstrual pain, intermenstrual bleeding, and adenomyosis (20% of these patients).

WORKUP AND EVALUATION

Laboratory: No evaluation indicated (CA-125 is not useful for screening or follow-up).

Imaging: No imaging indicated; pelvic or transvaginal ultrasonography, or magnetic resonance imaging (MRI) may demonstrate endometriomas or signs of scarring (nonspecific, a detection ratio and specificity of around 78% for implants, sensitivity and specificity of approximately 91% to 95%).

Special Tests: None indicated.

Diagnostic Procedures: The ultimate diagnosis of endometriosis rests on direct inspection of the involved area (laparoscopy or laparotomy), supported by histologic confirmation.

Pathologic Findings

Endometriosis is characterized by endometrial glands and stroma found in locations other than the endometrium. Nests of endometrial glands and stroma may occur in many distant locations throughout the body, although they are most common in the pelvis (60% on the surfaces of the ovaries). Vulva implants occur in 1 in 500 patients with endometriosis, generally at the site of an episiotomy or obstetric laceration. Evidence of old hemorrhage (hemosiderin-laden macrophages) is often present.

MANAGEMENT AND THERAPY

Nonpharmacologic

General Measures: Analgesics (nonsteroidal anti-inflammatory drugs), modification of periods (oral contraceptives), suppression of periods (gonadotropin-releasing hormone [GnRH] agonists, danazol sodium, oral progestins, long-acting progestins, continuous oral contraceptives).

Specific Measures: The selection of therapy depends on many factors—reliability of diagnosis, the extent of disease and symptoms, the patient's desire for fertility, and degree of involvement with other organs. Endometriomata of greater than 5 cm require surgical therapy. Surgical therapy may be conservative (resection of lesions) or definitive (hysterectomy, oophorectomy).

Diet: No specific dietary changes indicated.

Activity: No restriction.

Patient Education: Reassurance; American College of Obstetricians and Gynecologists Patient Education Pamphlet AP013 (Endometriosis), AP136 (Evaluating Infertility), AP137 (Treating Infertility).

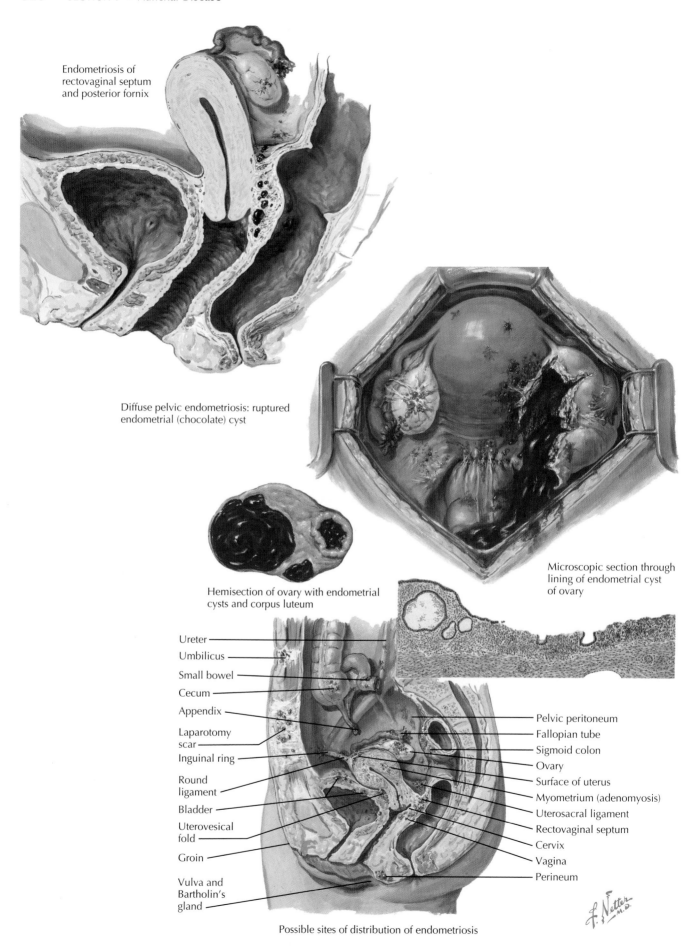

Endometriosis of rectovaginal septum and posterior fornix

Diffuse pelvic endometriosis: ruptured endometrial (chocolate) cyst

Microscopic section through lining of endometrial cyst of ovary

Hemisection of ovary with endometrial cysts and corpus luteum

Ureter

Umbilicus

Small bowel

Cecum

Appendix

Laparotomy scar

Inguinal ring

Round ligament

Bladder

Uterovesical fold

Groin

Vulva and Bartholin's gland

Pelvic peritoneum

Fallopian tube

Sigmoid colon

Ovary

Surface of uterus

Myometrium (adenomyosis)

Uterosacral ligament

Rectovaginal septum

Cervix

Vagina

Perineum

Possible sites of distribution of endometriosis

Drug(s) of Choice

GnRH agonists for 6 months: leuprolide acetate (Lupron) 3.75 mg IM monthly; nafarelin acetate (Synarel) 200 µg intranasal in morning and in opposite nostril at bedtime; goserelin acetate (Zoladex) 3.6 mg implant monthly.

Contraindications: Known or suspected pregnancy, breastfeeding, undiagnosed vaginal bleeding.

Precautions: A decrease in bone mass of 5% to 7% during a 6-month course of therapy with GnRH agonists has been documented. This is believed to be reversible.

Add-Back Therapy: Progestins, low-dose estrogens, or both may be used to suppress bothersome side effects without reducing efficacy.

Alternative Drugs

Danazol sodium 200 mg PO four times a day for 6 to 9 months (80% of patients experience side effects, 10% to 20% discontinue therapy because of them) or

Continuous combination oral contraceptives (monophasic or long-cycle formulation) taken daily for 6 to 9 months (if breakthrough bleeding occurs, the dose is doubled for 5 days) or

Medroxyprogesterone acetate 30 mg PO daily or 150 mg IM every 3 months for 6 to 9 months.

FOLLOW-UP

Patient Monitoring: Any therapy must be reevaluated at no less than 6-month intervals. History and physical evaluations are usually sufficient.

Prevention/Avoidance: None.

Possible Complications: Pelvic scarring, chronic pelvic pain, erosion into bowel or urinary tract resulting in hematochezia or hematuria.

Expected Outcome: Endometriosis is never considered to be "cured." Symptoms may be resolved and progression of the disease may be halted through medical or surgical therapy, although 5% to 15% of patients have a recurrence after 1 year and 40% to 50% have a recurrence by 5 years. The success of therapy and the risk of recurrence are proportional to the extent of the initial disease. Up to 40% of patients may eventually conceive with therapy. Endometriosis generally regresses after menopause (natural or surgically induced).

MISCELLANEOUS

Pregnancy Considerations: No effect on pregnancy once pregnancy is achieved. Pregnancy may actually resolve symptoms of endometriosis and promote regression of implants in some patients.

ICD-9-CM Codes: 617.9 (Codes 617.0–617.8 used for specific sites).

REFERENCES

Level I
Zullo F, Palomba S, Zupi E, et al: Effectiveness of presacral neurectomy in women with severe dysmenorrhea caused by endometriosis who were treated with laparoscopic conservative surgery: a 1-year prospective randomized double-blind controlled trial. Am J Obstet Gynecol 2003;189:5.

Level II
Friedman AJ, Hornstein MD: Gonadotropin-releasing hormone agonist plus estrogen-progestin "add-back" therapy for endometriosis-related pelvic pain. Fertil Steril 1993;60:236.

Hughes EG, Fedorkow DM, Collins JA: A quantitative overview of controlled trials in endometriosis-associated infertility. Fertil Steril 1993;59:963.

Waller KG, Shaw RW: GnRH analogs in the treatment of endometriosis: long-term follow-up. Fertil Steril 1993;59:511.

Wright S, Valdes CT, Dunn RC, Franklin RR: Short-term Lupron or Danazol therapy for pelvic endometriosis. Fertil Steril 1995;63:504.

Level III
American College of Obstetricians and Gynecologists: Medical management of endometriosis. ACOG Practice Bulletin 11. Washington, DC, ACOG, 1999.

American College of Obstetricians and Gynecologists: Chronic pelvic pain. ACOG Practice Bulletin 51. Obstet Gynecol 2004;103:589.

American College of Obstetricians and Gynecologists: Endometriosis in adolescents. ACOG Committee Opinion 310. Obstet Gynecol 2005;105:921.

Appleyard TL, Mann CH, Khan KS: Guidelines for the management of pelvic pain associated with endometriosis: a systematic appraisal of their quality. BJOG 2006;113:7497.

Barbieri RL: Etiology and epidemiology of endometriosis. Am J Obstet Gynecol 1990;162:565.

Cook AS, Rock JA: The role of laparoscopy in the treatment of endometriosis. Fertil Steril 1991;55:663.

Farquhar C: Endometriosis. BMJ 2007;334:249.

Giudice LC, Kao LC: Endometriosis. Lancet 2004;364:1789.

Lobo RA: Endometriosis. In Katz VL, Lentz GM, Lobo RA, Gershenson DM: Comprehensive Gynecology, 5th ed. Philadelphia, Mosby/Elsevier, 2007:473.

Winkel CA: Evaluation and management of women with endometriosis. Obstet Gynecol 2003;102:397.

INTRODUCTION

Description: The most common type of ovarian tumors (65% of ovarian tumors, 85% of ovarian malignancies), endometrial stromal tumors are derived from the surface (celomic) epithelium and the ovarian stroma and include serous (20% to 50%), mucinous (15% to 25%), endometrioid (5%), clear cell (<5%), and Brenner (2% to 3%) types. Epithelial tumors are categorized as benign (adenoma), malignant (adenocarcinoma), or of an intermediate form (borderline malignant adenocarcinoma or tumors of low malignant potential).

Prevalence: Two of three ovarian tumors and 85% of ovarian malignancies, 14.3 of 100,000 women.

Predominant Age: Benign tumors—age 20 to 29, malignant tumors—one half are in women older than 50.

Genetics: No genetic pattern.

ETIOLOGY AND PATHOGENESIS

Causes: Unknown.

Risk Factors: Family history, high-fat diet, advanced age, nulliparity, early menarche, late menopause, white race, higher economic status, cigarette smoking (mucinous type only). Oral contraception, high parity, and breastfeeding reduce risk.

CLINICAL CHARACTERISTICS

Signs and Symptoms

- Asymptomatic
- Weight loss
- Increasing abdominal girth despite constant or reduced caloric intake
- Ascites
- Adnexal mass (multilocular or partly solid masses in patients older than 40 are likely to be malignant; the risk of a mass being malignant is one in three for women older than 45, versus <1% for women 20 to 45 years of age)
- Vague lower abdominal discomfort

DIAGNOSTIC APPROACH

Differential Diagnosis

- Functional cyst (corpus luteum, follicular)
- Endometriosis
- Hydrosalpinx
- Paratubal cyst
- Appendiceal abscess
- Ectopic pregnancy
- Pedunculated leiomyomata
- Pelvic or horseshoe kidney
- Gastrointestinal malignancy (colon, stomach)

Associated Conditions: None. In patients with advanced malignant disease, bowel obstruction, ascites, and inanition are common.

WORKUP AND EVALUATION

Laboratory: As indicated before surgery. β-Human chorionic gonadotropin or α-fetoprotein levels may be elevated in some tumors. (The CA-125 level may be useful for monitoring disease response to treatment or progression, but it is not a good prognostic test. Only 80% of epithelial ovarian tumors express CA-125, and many benign and other malignant processes [lung, breast, and pancreas] may cause CA-125 to become higher than normal.)

Imaging: Preoperative evaluation (computed tomography or ultrasonography) for possible lymph node enlargement or intra-abdominal spread is indicated for patients in whom malignancy is a significant possibility.

Special Tests: A frozen-section histologic evaluation (intraoperative consultation) should be considered for any ovarian mass that appears suspicious for malignancy.

Diagnostic Procedures: History, physical examination, and imaging. Final diagnosis is established by histologic evaluation.

Pathologic Findings

Varies with cell type. Malignant epithelial tumors are more likely to be bilateral than are benign epithelial neoplasms.

MANAGEMENT AND THERAPY

Nonpharmacologic

General Measures: Evaluation, supportive therapy based on symptoms.

Specific Measures: Generally requires surgical exploration and extirpation. In benign disease or tumors of borderline malignant potential, the uterus and other ovary generally may be spared. Adjunctive chemotherapy (platinum-based and paclitaxel [Taxol]) or radiation therapy is often included, based on the location and stage of the disease. It currently is not recommended that a grossly normal opposite ovary be bisected to look for a contralateral mass.

Diet: No specific dietary changes indicated, except those imposed by advanced disease.

Activity: No restriction, except that imposed by advanced disease.

Patient Education: American College of Obstetricians and Gynecologists Patient Education Pamphlet AP096 (Cancer of the Ovary), AP075 (Ovarian Cysts).

Drug(s) of Choice

None, except as adjunctive or symptomatic therapy. Preoperative bowel cleansing (mechanical or with antibiosis) is often recommended as a precaution should bowel resection become necessary at the time of surgical staging and resection.

Contraindications: See individual agents.

Precautions: Alkylating agents are associated with an increased risk of future leukemia (10% by 8 years after therapy).

Interactions: See individual agents.

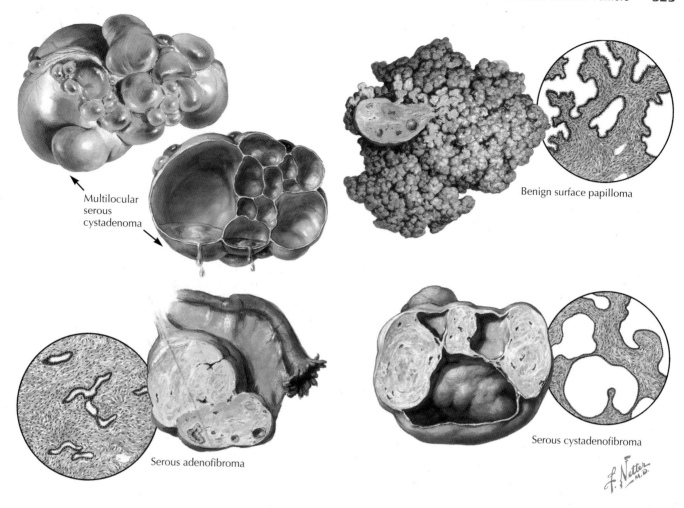

Multilocular serous cystadenoma

Benign surface papilloma

Serous adenofibroma

Serous cystadenofibroma

FOLLOW-UP

Patient Monitoring: Careful follow-up for recurrent pelvic disease or enlargement of the remaining ovary (if any). This is generally performed by pelvic examination, augmented with ultrasonography in selected patients. In patients suspected of having recurrent disease and other selected patients, second-look surgery may be desirable to assess progress and discover occult disease. Estrogen therapy does not have a negative influence on the disease-free interval and overall survival in women who have had ovarian carcinoma.

Prevention/Avoidance: None.

Possible Complications: Spread and advancement of malignant tumors.

Expected Outcome: Generally good.

MISCELLANEOUS

Pregnancy Considerations: No effect on pregnancy.
ICD-9-CM Codes: Based on cause and type.

REFERENCES

Level I
Guidozzi F, Daponte A: Estrogen replacement therapy for ovarian carcinoma survivors: a randomized controlled trial. Cancer 1999;86:1013.
Rufford BD, Jacobs IJ, Menon U: Feasibility of screening for ovarian cancer using symptoms as selection criteria. BJOG 2007;114:59.

Level II
Bostwick DG, Tazelaar HD, Ballon SC, et al: Ovarian epithelial tumors of borderline malignancy: clinical and pathologic study of 109 cases. Cancer 1986;58:2052.
Koonings PP, Campbell K, Mishell DR Jr, Grimes DA: Relative frequency of primary ovarian neoplasms: a 10-year review. Obstet Gynecol 1989;74:921.
Marchbanks PA, Wilson H, Bastos E, et al: Cigarette smoking and epithelial ovarian cancer by histologic type. Obstet Gynecol 2000;95:255.
Simpson JL, Michael H, Roth LM: Unclassified sex cord-stromal tumors of the ovary: a report of eight cases. Arch Pathol Lab Med 1998;122:52.

Level III
Abu-Rustum NR, Chi DS, Curtin JP: Epithelial ovarian cancer. Curr Probl Surg 1999;36:1.
American College of Obstetricians and Gynecologists: Prophylactic oophorectomy. ACOG Practice Bulletin 7. Washington, DC, ACOG, 1999.
Bhoola S, Hoskins WJ: Diagnosis and management of epithelial ovarian cancer. Obstet Gynecol 2006;107:1399.
Fleischer AC: Transabdominal and transvaginal sonography of ovarian masses. Clin Obstet Gynecol 1991;34:433.
Kristensen GB, Trope C: Epithelial ovarian carcinoma. Lancet 1997;349:113.
Partridge EE, Barnes MN: Epithelial ovarian cancer: prevention, diagnosis, and treatment. CA Cancer J Clin 1999;49:297.
Pretorius RG, Matory WE Jr, LaFontaine D: Management of massive ovarian tumors. Surg Gynecol Obstet 1989;169:532.
Schwarts PE, Smith JP: Treatment of ovarian stromal tumors. Am J Obstet Gynecol 1976;125:402.

INTRODUCTION

Description: The second most common type of ovarian tumor, germ cell tumors contain cells that echo the three layers of embryonic tissue (ectoderm, mesoderm, and endoderm) or extraembryonic elements.

Prevalence: Second most frequent ovarian neoplasm (25% of tumors), most common ovarian tumor in women younger than age 30.

Predominant Age: Younger than 30, most common malignancy of women in their teens and 20s.

Genetics: No genetic pattern.

ETIOLOGY AND PATHOGENESIS

Causes: Unknown (may differentiate from primitive germ cells).

Risk Factors: None known.

CLINICAL CHARACTERISTICS

Signs and Symptoms

- Asymptomatic
- Ovarian enlargement (Ovarian masses in premenarchal girls are most often germ cell tumors.)

DIAGNOSTIC APPROACH

Differential Diagnosis

- Benign adnexal masses (corpus luteum, follicular cyst)
- Endometriosis
- Hydrosalpinx
- Paratubal cyst
- Appendiceal abscess
- Ectopic pregnancy
- Pedunculated leiomyomata
- Pelvic or horseshoe kidney
- Nongynecologic pelvic masses

Associated Conditions: Varies with cell type.

WORKUP AND EVALUATION

Laboratory: As indicated before surgery. β-Human chorionic gonadotropin or α-fetoprotein may be elevated in some tumors (dysgerminoma, primary choriocarcinoma). (The CA-125 level may be useful for monitoring disease response to treatment or progression, but it is not a good prognostic test. Only 80% of epithelial ovarian tumors express CA-125, and many benign and other malignant tumors [lung, breast, and pancreas] may also cause CA-125 to become higher than normal.)

Imaging: Preoperative evaluation (computed tomography or ultrasonography) for possible lymph node enlargement or intra-abdominal spread is indicated for patients in whom malignancy is a significant possibility.

Special Tests: None indicated.

Diagnostic Procedures: History, physical examination, imaging. Final diagnosis is established by histologic evaluation.

Pathologic Findings

Germ cell tumors include dysgerminoma (45% of malignant germ cell tumors), endodermal sinus tumors (10%), embryonal carcinoma, choriocarcinoma, teratomas (immature, mature, solid and cystic, struma ovarii, carcinoid) and mixed forms. Roughly one third of germ cell tumors in women younger than age 21 are malignant.

MANAGEMENT AND THERAPY

Nonpharmacologic

General Measures: Evaluation, supportive therapy based on symptoms.

Specific Measures: Surgical exploration and resection (often with salvage of the ovary in the case of teratomas). Immature (malignant) teratomas are often treated with adjunctive chemotherapy (vincristine, actinomycin D, and cyclophosphamide); endodermal sinus tumors should all be treated with chemotherapy after surgical resection.

Diet: No specific dietary changes indicated, except those imposed by advanced disease.

Activity: No restriction, except that imposed by advanced disease.

Patient Education: American College of Obstetricians and Gynecologists Patient Education Pamphlet AP096 (Cancer of the Ovary), AP075 (Ovarian Cysts).

Drug(s) of Choice

Vincristine (1.5 mg/m² IV weekly for 12 weeks), actinomycin D, and cyclophosphamide (0.5 mg of actinomycin D + 5 to 7 mg/kg/day cyclophosphamide, IV daily for 5 days every 4 weeks).

Adjunctive or symptomatic therapy. Preoperative bowel cleansing (mechanical or with antibiosis) is often recommended as a precaution should bowel resection become necessary at the time of surgical staging and resection.

Contraindications: See individual agents.

Precautions: Alkylating agents are associated with an increased risk of future leukemia (10% by 8 years after therapy).

Interactions: See individual agents.

Alternative Drugs

Chemotherapy for endodermal sinus tumors may alternately include actinomycin D, 5-fluorouracil, and cyclophosphamide.

FOLLOW-UP

Patient Monitoring: Careful follow-up for recurrent pelvic disease or enlargement of the remaining ovary (if any). This is generally performed by pelvic examination, augmented with ultrasonography in selected patients. In patients suspected of recurrent disease and other selected patients, second-look surgery may be desirable to assess progress and discover occult disease.

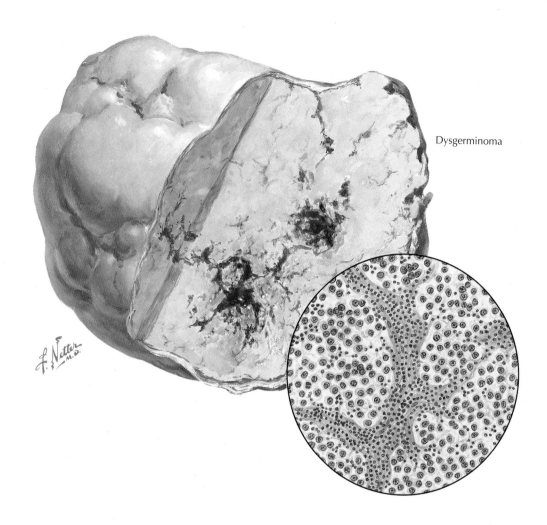

Dysgerminoma

Prevention/Avoidance: None.
Possible Complications: Spread and advancement in the case of malignant tumors.
Expected Outcome: Generally good.

MISCELLANEOUS

Pregnancy Considerations: No effect on pregnancy.
ICD-9-CM Codes: Based on cause and type.

REFERENCES

Level II

Koonings PP, Campbell K, Mishell DR Jr, Grimes DA: Relative frequency of primary ovarian neoplasms: a 10-year review. Obstet Gynecol 1989;74:921.

Mais V, Ajossa S, Mallarini G, et al: No recurrence of mature ovarian teratomas after laparoscopic cystectomy. BJOG 2003;110:624.

Peccatori F, Bonazzi C, Chiari S, et al: Surgical management of malignant ovarian germ-cell tumors: 10 years' experience of 129 patients. Obstet Gynecol 1995;86:367.

Level III

Coleman RL, Gershenson DM: Neoplastic diseases of the ovary. In Katz VL, Lentz GM, Lobo RA, Gershenson DM: Comprehensive Gynecology, 5th ed. Philadelphia, Mosby/Elsevier, 2007:865.

Creasman WT, Soper JT: Assessment of the contemporary management of germ cell malignancy. Am J Obstet Gynecol 1985;153:828.

Fleischer AC: Transabdominal and transvaginal sonography of ovarian masses. Clin Obstet Gynecol 1991;34:433.

Kurman RJ, Norris HJ: Malignant germ cell tumors of the ovary. Hum Pathol 1977;8:551.

INTRODUCTION

Description: A granulosa cell tumor is a sex cord stromal tumor of the ovary made up of granulosa cells (sex cord) and stromal cells (thecal cells or fibroblasts). The tumor often secretes estrogen.

Prevalence: Six percent of ovarian neoplasms and the majority of hormonally active tumors.

Predominant Age: Any, 5% before puberty, most before age 40.

Genetics: No genetic pattern.

ETIOLOGY AND PATHOGENESIS

Causes: Unknown.

Risk Factors: None known.

CLINICAL CHARACTERISTICS

Signs and Symptoms

* Asymptomatic
* Enlarging or ruptured adnexal mass (may present with acute pain and an acute abdomen with hemoperitoneum, 6%); 10% to 15% are not palpable; tumors are bilateral in <2% of cases.
* Ascites (10%)
* Precocious (pseudoprecocious) puberty in young children (5%) (granulosa tumors are responsible of 10% of precocious puberty cases)
* Abnormal menstrual patterns, menorrhagia, amenorrhea
* Postmenopausal bleeding

DIAGNOSTIC APPROACH

Differential Diagnosis

* Benign adnexal masses (corpus luteum, follicular cyst)
* Endometriosis
* Hydrosalpinx
* Paratubal cyst
* Appendiceal abscess
* Pedunculated leiomyomata
* Pelvic or horseshoe kidney
* Nongynecologic pelvic masses
* Hepatic, renal, or cardiac disease resulting in weight loss and ascites
* Ectopic pregnancy (reproductive-age women)
* Gastrointestinal malignancy (colon, stomach)

Associated Conditions: Evidence of increased estrogen (e.g., breast tenderness, menstrual disturbances, isosex-

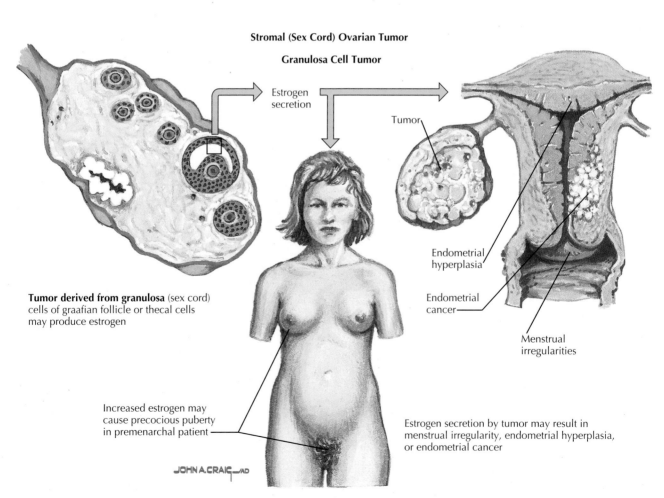

Stromal (Sex Cord) Ovarian Tumor

Granulosa Cell Tumor

Estrogen secretion

Tumor

Endometrial hyperplasia

Endometrial cancer

Menstrual irregularities

Tumor derived from granulosa (sex cord) cells of graafian follicle or thecal cells may produce estrogen

Increased estrogen may cause precocious puberty in premenarchal patient

Estrogen secretion by tumor may result in menstrual irregularity, endometrial hyperplasia, or endometrial cancer

JOHN A.CRAIG—AD

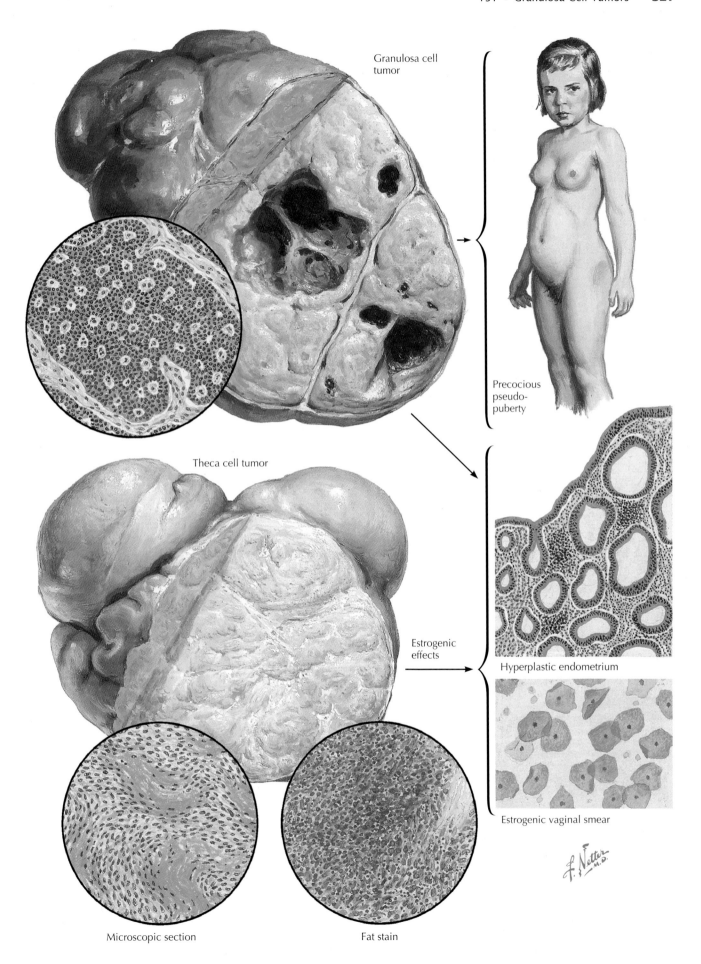

Granulosa cell tumor

Precocious pseudo-puberty

Theca cell tumor

Estrogenic effects

Hyperplastic endometrium

Estrogenic vaginal smear

Microscopic section

Fat stain

ual pseudoprecocity, endometrial cancer [5%]). Virilization rarely occurs.

WORKUP AND EVALUATION

Laboratory: As indicated before surgery. (Serum testing for tumor markers, such as CA-125, lipid-associated sialic acid, carcinoembryonic antigen, α-fetoprotein, and others, should be reserved for following the progress of patients with known malignancies and not for prognostic evaluation.)

Imaging: Preoperative evaluation (computed tomography or ultrasonography) for possible lymph node enlargement or intra-abdominal spread is indicated for patients in whom malignancy is a significant possibility.

Special Tests: None indicated.

Diagnostic Procedures: History, physical examination, and imaging. Final diagnosis is established by histologic evaluation.

Pathologic Findings

Derived from the sex cords of the ovary and the stroma of the developing gonad, these tumors have a predominance of granulosa cells. Classically, these tumors contain eosinophilic bodies surrounded by granulosa cells (Call-Exner bodies). Poorly differentiated tumors may be confused with adenocarcinomas (especially small cell carcinoma).

MANAGEMENT AND THERAPY
Nonpharmacologic

General Measures: Evaluation, supportive therapy based on symptoms.

Specific Measures: Surgical exploration and resection. Because <5% of these tumors are bilateral, conservative surgery is generally indicated for tumors at stage IA or lower. Chemotherapy (cisplatin, doxorubicin) and radiation have been used for recurrent disease.

Diet: No specific dietary changes indicated, except those imposed by advanced disease.

Activity: No restriction, except that imposed by advanced disease.

Patient Education: American College of Obstetricians and Gynecologists Patient Education Pamphlet AP096 (Cancer of the Ovary), AP075 (Ovarian Cysts).

Drug(s) of Choice

Adjunctive (unproved benefit) or symptomatic therapy. Preoperative bowel cleansing (mechanical or with antibiosis) is often recommended as a precaution should bowel resection become necessary at the time of surgical staging and resection.

Contraindications: See individual agents.

Precautions: Alkylating agents are associated with an increased risk of future leukemia (10% by 8 years after therapy).

Interactions: See individual agents.

Alternative Drugs

Chemotherapy with alternative use of actinomycin D, 5-fluorouracil, and cyclophosphamide.

FOLLOW-UP

Patient Monitoring: Careful follow-up for recurrent pelvic disease or enlargement of the remaining ovary (if any). This is generally performed by pelvic examination, augmented with ultrasonography in selected cases. In those suspected of having recurrent disease and other selected patients, second-look surgery may be desirable to assess progress and discover occult disease.

Prevention/Avoidance: None.

Possible Complications: Recurrences are frequent even 5 years after initial therapy. In 10% of patients the tumor is diagnosed when it ruptures, causing pain or intraperitoneal bleeding.

Expected Outcome: Prognosis does not correlate with the histologic pattern of the tumor: 90% of tumors found are stage I and the prognosis is good (90% 10-year survival); a poorer prognosis is found with tumors >15 cm that have ruptured or that have a high mitotic rate or aneuploidy.

MISCELLANEOUS

Pregnancy Considerations: No effect on pregnancy.

ICD-9-CM Codes: Specific to cell type and location.

REFERENCES

Level II

Colombo N, Sessa C, Landoni F, et al: Cisplatin, vinblastine, and bleomycin, combination chemotherapy in metastatic granulosa cell tumor of the ovary. Obstet Gynecol 1986;67:265.

Lack EE, Perez-Atayde AR, Murthy AS, et al: Granulosa theca cell tumors in premenarcheal girls: a clinical and pathological study of 10 cases. Cancer 1981;48:1846.

Swanson SA, Norris HJ, Kelsten ML, Wheeler JE: DNA content of juvenile granulosa tumors determined by flow cytometry. Int J Gynecol Pathol 1990;9:101.

Level III

Bjorkholm E, Silfversward C: Prognostic factors in granulosa cell tumor. Gynecol Oncol 1981;11:261.

Coleman RL, Gershenson DM: Neoplastic diseases of the ovary. In Katz VL, Lentz GM, Lobo RA, Gershenson DM: Comprehensive Gynecology, 5th ed. Philadelphia, Mosby/Elsevier, 2007:845, 871.

Segal R, DePetrillo AD, Thomas G: Clinical review of adult granulosa cell tumors of the ovary. Gynecol Oncol 1995;56:338.

Hydrosalpinx (Chronic Pelvic Inflammatory Disease)

INTRODUCTION

Description: Recurrent or chronic adnexal infections may result in a cystic dilation of the fallopian tube (hydrosalpinx), which may present as an adnexal mass.

Prevalence: Forty percent of female infertility is the result of tubal damage, including the most severe form, hydrosalpinx.

Predominant Age: 15 to 25.

Genetics: No genetic pattern.

ETIOLOGY AND PATHOGENESIS

Causes: Recurrent or chronic adnexal infection. This is the end-stage condition of pyosalpinx.

Risk Factors: Early (age) sexual activity, multiple sexual partners, pelvic inflammatory disease, sexually transmitted diseases (STDs; *Chlamydia*, gonorrhea), uterine instrumentation (hysterosalpingography, intrauterine contraceptive device placement, endometrial biopsy, dilation and curettage), and douching.

CLINICAL CHARACTERISTICS

Signs and Symptoms

* Asymptomatic (most common)
* Vague lower abdominal pressure or chronic pelvic pain
* Infertility
* Unilateral or bilateral cystic masses (often elongated or sausage-shaped)

(Data indicate that a clinical diagnosis of symptomatic pelvic inflammatory disease has a positive predictive value for salpingitis of only 65%.)

DIAGNOSTIC APPROACH

Differential Diagnosis

* Functional cysts (follicle, corpus luteum)
* Epithelial tumors (cystic or solid)
* Ovarian cysts
* Paratubal or paraovarian cysts
* Uterine leiomyomata
* Ectopic pregnancy
* Tubo-ovarian abscess
* Endometrioma
* Appendiceal abscess

Associated Conditions: Pelvic pain, infertility, and STDs.

WORKUP AND EVALUATION

Laboratory: Complete blood count or erythrocyte sedimentation rate if active infection is suspected. Screening for coexistent STDs should be strongly considered.

Imaging: Ultrasonography (abdominal or transvaginal), computed tomography (CT) or magnetic resonance imaging (MRI) may be used but are more expensive without providing greater specificity.

Special Tests: None indicated.

Diagnostic Procedures: History, physical examination, and ultrasonography.

Pathologic Findings

Chronic induration and inflammation with cystic dilation of the fallopian tube and flattening and atrophy of the epithelial lining. The fluid found is generally sterile.

MANAGEMENT AND THERAPY

Nonpharmacologic

General Measures: Evaluation, including screening for other STDs.

Specific Measures: Generally requires surgical evaluation and therapy (laparoscopy or laparotomy).

Diet: No specific dietary changes indicated.

Activity: No restriction.

Patient Education: American College of Obstetricians and Gynecologists Patient Education Pamphlet AP077 (Pelvic Inflammatory Disease), AP009 (How to Prevent Sexually Transmitted Diseases), AP099 (Pelvic Pain), AP071 (Gonorrhea, Chlamydia, and Syphilis), AP136 (Evaluating Infertility), AP137 (Treating Infertility), AP020 (Pain During Intercourse).

Drug(s) of Choice

Broad-spectrum antibiotics if active infection is suspected. (Most hydrosalpinx are sterile and are the inactive end-stage disease.)

FOLLOW-UP

Patient Monitoring: Normal health maintenance, periodic surveillance for other STDs.

Prevention/Avoidance: Avoidance of STDs (barrier contraception, "safe sex"), screening for those at risk, and aggressive treatment.

Possible Complications: Chronic pelvic pain, infertility, increased risk of hysterectomy, and oophorectomy.

Expected Outcome: Surgical therapy (salpingectomy or salpingo-oophorectomy) is curative. Neosalpingostomy may be considered when fertility is to be maintained, but the success of this procedure is inversely proportional to the size of the hydrosalpinx and is generally less than 15%. More often, in vitro fertilization, bypassing the damaged tubes, is recommended, although the success rates are lower in these patients.

MISCELLANEOUS

Pregnancy Considerations: Successful pregnancy is much less likely because of the increased risk of infertility and ectopic pregnancy.

ICD-9-CM Codes: 614.1.

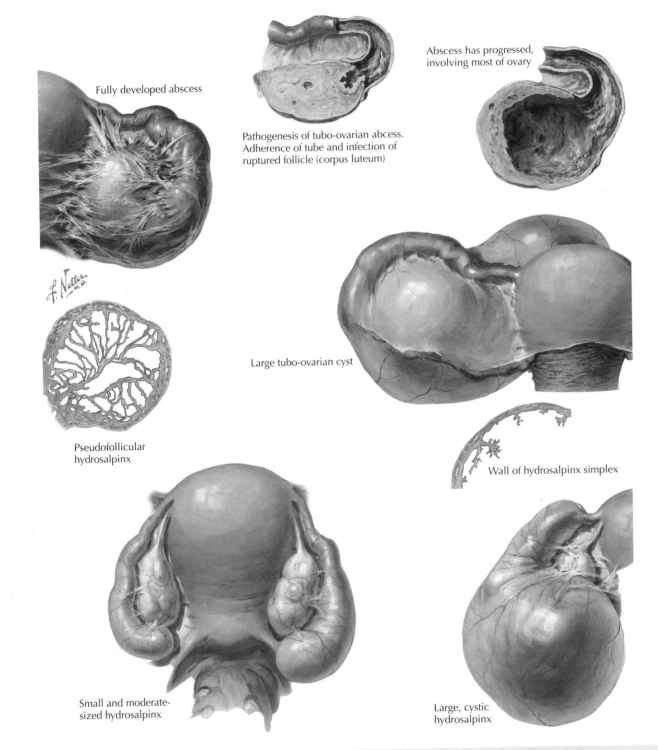

Fully developed abscess

Pathogenesis of tubo-ovarian abcess. Adherence of tube and infection of ruptured follicle (corpus luteum)

Abscess has progressed, involving most of ovary

Large tubo-ovarian cyst

Pseudofollicular hydrosalpinx

Wall of hydrosalpinx simplex

Small and moderate-sized hydrosalpinx

Large, cystic hydrosalpinx

REFERENCES

Level I
Ness RB, Trautmann G, Richter HE, et al: Effectiveness of treatment strategies of some women with pelvic inflammatory disease: a randomized trial. Obstet Gynecol 2005;106:573.

Level II
Ness RB, Hillier SL, Kip KE, et al: Bacterial vaginosis and risk of pelvic inflammatory disease. Obstet Gynecol 2004;104:761.

Level III
American College of Obstetricians and Gynecologists: Chronic pelvic pain. ACOG Practice Bulletin 51. Obstet Gynecol 2004;103:589.

Ault KA, Faro S: Pelvic inflammatory disease. Current diagnostic criteria and treatment guidelines. Postgrad Med 1993;93:85, 89.

Centers for Disease Control and Prevention: Sexually Transmitted Diseases Treatment Guidelines, 2006. MMWR 2006;55:56.

Centers for Disease Control and Prevention: Updated recommended treatment regimens for gonococcal infections and associated conditions—United States, April 2007. Available at: http://www.cdc.gov/std/treatment/2006/GonUpdateApril2007.pdf. Accessed May 31, 2007.

Eckert LO, Lentz GM: Neoplastic diseases of the ovary. In Katz VL, Lentz GM, Lobo RA, Gershenson DM: Comprehensive Gynecology, 5th ed. Philadelphia, Mosby/Elsevier, 2007:608.

INTRODUCTION

Description: A Krukenberg tumor is a metastatic tumor (generally from the gastrointestinal tract) that is characterized by large signet-ring cells. The most common site or origin is the stomach or large intestine.
Predominant Age: Postmenopausal.
Genetics: No genetic pattern.

ETIOLOGY AND PATHOGENESIS

Causes: Metastatic spread of carcinoma from the gastrointestinal tract (most commonly the stomach or colon). Metastatic breast cancer may appear similar histologically.
Risk Factors: None known.

CLINICAL CHARACTERISTICS

Signs and Symptoms

- Asymptomatic
- Adnexal enlargement (bilateral solid adnexal masses in an older patient should always suggest the possibility of a gastrointestinal tract source)
- Metastatic tumors from the gastrointestinal tract to the ovary can be associated with sex hormone production, usually estrogen.

DIAGNOSTIC APPROACH

Differential Diagnosis

- Benign adnexal masses (corpus luteum, follicular cyst)
- Endometriosis
- Hydrosalpinx
- Paratubal cyst
- Appendiceal abscess
- Ectopic pregnancy
- Pedunculated leiomyomata
- Pelvic or horseshoe kidney
- Nongynecologic pelvic masses
- Breast cancer
- Lung cancer

Associated Conditions: Gastrointestinal or breast malignancy.

WORKUP AND EVALUATION

Laboratory: As indicated before surgery.
Imaging: Preoperative evaluation (computed tomography or ultrasonography) for possible lymph node enlargement or intra-abdominal spread is indicated for patients in whom malignancy is a significant possibility. Radiographic evaluation of the gastrointestinal tract. Mammography as indicated based on differential diagnosis and routine screening needs.
Special Tests: Esophagoscopy, gastroscopy, sigmoidoscopy, or colonoscopy should be considered as a part of the evaluation when a gastrointestinal source is being sought.

Diagnostic Procedures: History, physical examination, and imaging. Final diagnosis is established by histologic evaluation.

Pathologic Findings

Nests of mucin-filled signet-ring cells in a cellular stroma.

MANAGEMENT AND THERAPY

Nonpharmacologic

General Measures: Evaluation, establishment of location of primary tumor (most often stomach or large intestine).
Specific Measures: Therapy of the original tumor.
Diet: No specific dietary changes indicated except those dictated by the original tumor and its therapy.
Activity: No restrictions except those dictated by the original tumor and its therapy.
Patient Education: American College of Obstetricians and Gynecologists Patient Education Pamphlet AP096 (Cancer of the Ovary), AP075 (Ovarian Cysts).

Drug(s) of Choice

None (based on primary tumor and its therapy).

FOLLOW-UP

Patient Monitoring: Based on primary tumor.
Prevention/Avoidance: None.
Possible Complications: Progression and spread of the primary tumor is generally well under way when the ovarian sites are discovered.
Expected Outcome: Generally poor, with 5-year survival unlikely.

MISCELLANEOUS

Pregnancy Considerations: Does not directly threaten pregnancy except by the jeopardy caused to the mother.
ICD-9-CM Codes: 198.6.

REFERENCES

Level II
de Palma P, Wronski M, Bifernino V, Bovani I: Krukenberg tumor in pregnancy with virilization. A case report. Eur J Gynaecol Oncol 1995;16:59.
Kakushima N, Kamoshida T, Hirai S, et al: Early gastric cancer with Krukenberg tumor and review of cases of intramucosal gastric cancers with Krukenberg tumor. J Gastroenterol 2003; 38:1176.
Kuhlman JE, Hruban RH, Fishman EK: Krukenberg tumors: CT features and growth characteristics. South Med J 1989;82: 1215.

Level III
Al-Agha OM, Nicastri AD: An in-depth look at Krukenberg tumor: an overview. Arch Pathol Lab Med 2006;130:1725.

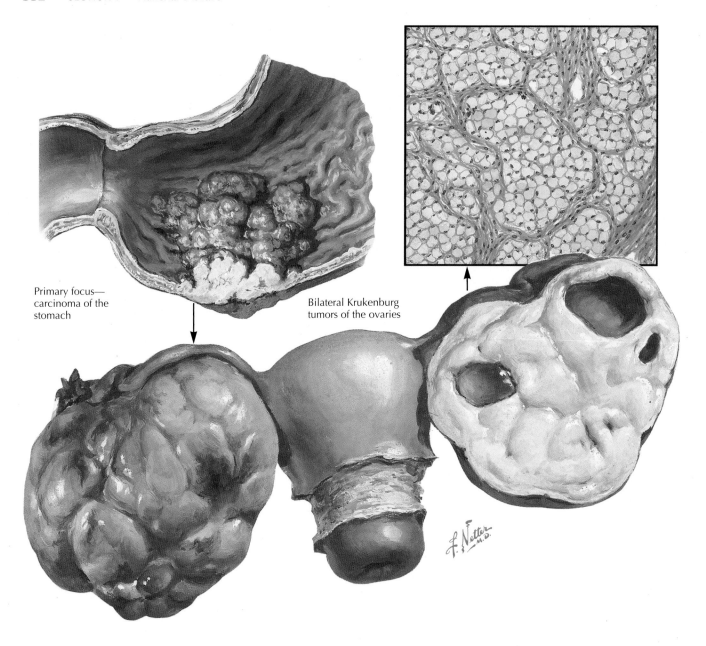

Primary focus—carcinoma of the stomach

Bilateral Krukenburg tumors of the ovaries

Coleman RL, Gershenson DM: Neoplastic diseases of the ovary. In Katz VL, Lentz GM, Lobo RA, Gershenson DM: Comprehensive Gynecology, 5th ed. Philadelphia, Mosby/Elsevier, 2007:874.

Fleischer AC: Transabdominal and transvaginal sonography of ovarian masses. Clin Obstet Gynecol 1991;34:433.

Young RH: From Krukenberg to today: the ever present problems posed by metastatic tumors in the ovary: Part I. Historical perspective, general principles, mucinous tumors including the Krukenberg tumor. Adv Anat Pathol 2006;13:205.

Young RH: From Krukenberg to today: the ever present problems posed by metastatic tumors in the ovary. Part II. Adv Anat Pathol 2007;14:149.

INTRODUCTION

Description: A group of benign and malignant epithelial tumors of the ovary that are characterized by the secretion of mucin. These tumors tend to be the largest types of ovarian masses encountered and may be 30 cm or greater in size.

Prevalence: Fifteen percent to 25% of ovarian cysts, 6% to 10% of ovarian cancers. Although ovarian cysts are common in younger women, mucinous cysts account for about 50% of those that do occur in women older than 20 years.

Predominant Age: Reproductive (benign), 30 to 60 (malignant tumors).

Genetics: No genetic pattern.

ETIOLOGY AND PATHOGENESIS

Causes: Unknown. May represent a monomorphic endodermal differentiation of a teratoma or a tumor of Müllerian origin.

Risk Factors: Family history, high-fat diet, advanced age, nulliparity, early menarche and late menopause, white race, higher economic status. Oral contraception, high parity, and breastfeeding reduce risk.

CLINICAL CHARACTERISTICS

Signs and Symptoms

- Asymptomatic
- Vague lower abdominal symptoms
- Adnexal mass (bilateral in 5% of benign and 10% to 20% of malignant lesions) up to 50 cm in diameter (average 15 to 30 cm)

DIAGNOSTIC APPROACH

Differential Diagnosis

- Benign adnexal masses (corpus luteum, follicular cyst)
- Endometriosis
- Hydrosalpinx
- Paratubal cyst
- Appendiceal abscess
- Ectopic pregnancy
- Pedunculated leiomyomata
- Pelvic or horseshoe kidney
- Nongynecologic pelvic masses

Associated Conditions: Pseudomyxoma peritonei.

WORKUP AND EVALUATION

- **Laboratory:** As indicated before surgery. (CA-125 levels may be useful for the monitoring of disease response to treatment or progression, but this is not a good prognostic test. Only 80% of epithelial ovarian tumors express CA-125, and many benign and other malignant processes [lung, breast, and pancreas] may also cause CA-125 to become higher than normal.)
- **Imaging:** No imaging Oindicated.

- **Special Tests:** A frozen-section histologic evaluation should be considered for any ovarian mass that appears suspicious for malignancy.
- **Diagnostic Procedures:** History, physical examination, and imaging. Final diagnosis is established by histologic evaluation.

Pathologic Findings

Gross—smooth translucent cyst wall with infrequent papillary areas. Microscopic—epithelial cells filled with mucin that resemble cells of the endocervix or intestinal epithelium. Mucinous tumors have a higher chance of being of borderline malignant potential (grade 0) than do other epithelial tumors.

MANAGEMENT AND THERAPY

Nonpharmacologic

General Measures: Evaluation, supportive therapy based on symptoms.

Specific Measures: Generally require surgical exploration and extirpation. In benign disease or tumors of borderline malignant potential, the uterus and other ovary generally may be spared. Adjunctive chemotherapy (platinum-based and paclitaxel [Taxol]) or radiation therapy is often included, based on the location and stage of malignant disease.

Diet: No specific dietary changes indicated, except those imposed by advanced disease.

Activity: No restriction, except that imposed by advanced disease.

Patient Education: American College of Obstetricians and Gynecologists Patient Education Pamphlet AP096 (Cancer of the Ovary), AP075 (Ovarian Cysts).

Drug(s) of Choice

None, except as adjunctive or symptomatic therapy. Preoperative bowel cleansing (mechanical or with antibiosis) is often recommended as a precaution should bowel resection become necessary at the time of surgical staging and resection.

Contraindications: See individual agents.

Precautions: Alkylating agents are associated with an increased risk of future leukemia (10% by 8 years after therapy).

Interactions: See individual agents.

FOLLOW-UP

Patient Monitoring: Careful follow-up for recurrent pelvic disease or enlargement of the remaining ovary (if any). This is generally performed by pelvic examination, augmented with ultrasonography in selected patients. In those suspected of having recurrent disease and other selected patients, second-look surgery may be desirable to assess progress and discover occult disease.

Prevention/Avoidance: None.

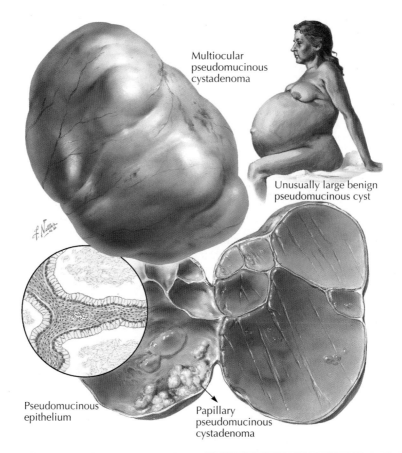

Multiocular pseudomucinous cystadenoma

Unusually large benign pseudomucinous cyst

Pseudomucinous epithelium

Papillary pseudomucinous cystadenoma

Possible Complications: Perforation of the tumor capsule with rupture, which may lead to the seeding of the peritoneal cavity (pseudomyxoma peritonei, 2% to 5% of patients).

Expected Outcome: Tumors with borderline malignant potential tend to grow slowly, and patients have prolonged survival with these tumors (40% 20-year survival with stage III disease). Of ovarian malignancies, mucinous cystadenocarcinoma has one of the best 5-year survival rates (40%).

MISCELLANEOUS

Pregnancy Considerations: No effect on pregnancy. More than 10% of tumors with borderline malignant potential are discovered during pregnancy.

ICD-9-CM Codes: Specific to cell type and location.

REFERENCES

Level I
Carmo-Pereira J, Costa FO, Henriques E, Ricardo JA: Advanced ovarian carcinoma: a prospective and randomized clinical trial of cyclophosphamide versus combination cytotoxic chemotherapy (Hexa-CAF). Cancer 1981;48:1947.

Level II
Barlow JJ, Lele SB, Emrich LJ: Long-term survival rates with various chemotherapeutic regimens in stages III and IV ovarian adenocarcinoma. The influence of optimum pretreatment surgical resection. Am J Obstet Gynecol 1985;152:310.
Bostwick DG, Tazelaar HD, Ballon SC, et al: Ovarian epithelial tumors of borderline malignancy: clinical and pathologic study of 109 cases. Cancer 1986;58:2052.
Chaitin BA, Gershenson DM, Evans HL: Mucinous tumors of the ovary: a clinicopathologic study of 70 cases. Cancer 1985;55:1958.

Chao A, Chao A, Yen YS, Huang CH: Abdominal compartment syndrome secondary to ovarian mucinous cystadenoma. Obstet Gynecol 2004;104:1180.
Hreshchyshyn MM, Park RC, Blessing JA, et al: The role of adjuvant therapy in Stage I ovarian cancer. Am J Obstet Gynecol 1980;138:139.
Koonings PP, Campbell K, Mishell DR Jr, Grimes DA: Relative frequency of primary ovarian neoplasms: a 10-year review. Obstet Gynecol 1989;74:921.
van Dessel T, Hameeteman TM, Wagenaar SS: Mucinous cystadenocarcinoma in pregnancy. Case report. Br J Obstet Gynaecol 1988;95:527.

Level III
Acs G: Serous and mucinous borderline (low malignant potential) tumors of the ovary. Am J Clin Pathol 2005;123:S13.
Bhoola S, Hoskins WJ: Diagnosis and management of epithelial ovarian cancer. Obstet Gynecol 2006;107:1399.
Carter J, Carson LF, Moradi MM, et al: Pseudomyxoma peritonei: a review. Int J Gynecol Cancer 1991;1:243.
Coleman RL, Gershenson DM: Neoplastic diseases of the ovary. In Katz VL, Lentz GM, Lobo RA, Gershenson DM: Comprehensive Gynecology, 5th ed. Philadelphia, Mosby/Elsevier, 2007:844.
Crissman JD, Azoury RS, Barnes AE, Schellhas HF: Endometrial carcinoma in women 40 years of age or younger. Obstet Gynecol 1981;57:699.
Fleischer AC: Transabdominal and transvaginal sonography of ovarian masses. Clin Obstet Gynecol 1991;34:433.
Hein DJ, Kellerman RD, Abbott G: Ovarian mucinous cystadenoma: evaluating the pelvic mass. Am Fam Physician 1993;48:818.
Lentz GM: Differential diagnosis of major gynecologic problems by age group. In Katz VL, Lentz GM, Lobo RA, Gershenson DM: Comprehensive Gynecology, 5th ed. Philadelphia, Mosby/Elsevier, 2007:167.
Link CJ Jr, Reed E, Sarosy G, Kohn EC: Borderline ovarian tumors. Am J Med 1996;101:217.
Massad LS Jr, Hunter VJ, Szpak CA, et al: Epithelial ovarian tumors of low malignant potential. Obstet Gynecol 1991;78:1027.
Pretorius RG, Matory WE Jr, LaFontaine D: Management of massive ovarian tumors. Surg Gynecol Obstet 1989;169:532.
Scully RE: Ovarian tumors. A review. Am J Pathol 1977;87:686.

INTRODUCTION

Description: Ovarian cancer is a malignancy arising in the ovary, generally of epithelial origin. This represents the second most common malignancy of the genital tract (after endometrial cancer), but it is the most common fatal gynecologic cancer.

Prevalence: Annually: 22,430 cases (estimated for 2007); 15,280 deaths (estimated for 2007). Ovarian cancer is the most common cause of gynecologic cancer death. The lifetime risk of developing ovarian cancer is approximately 1 in 70.

Predominant Age: Postmenopausal (50%), average 59, highest rate 60 to 64 years. Only one fourth to one third of ovarian tumors in postmenopausal women are malignant.

Genetics: Family pattern recognized in a small percentage of cases. Association with abnormalities of the breast cancer gene (BRCA1 and BRCA2). Hereditary ovarian cancers are rare but usually fatal; 95% of ovarian cancers are sporadic.

ETIOLOGY AND PATHOGENESIS

Causes: Unknown.

Risk Factors: Family history (greatest risk in those few women with an inheritable cancer syndrome, such as Lynch II), high-fat diet, advanced age, nulliparity, early menarche, late menopause, white race, higher economic status, and the use of talc on the perineum. More than 95% of patients with ovarian cancer have no risk factor. Oral contraception, high parity, tubal ligation, hysterectomy, and breastfeeding reduce risk.

CLINICAL CHARACTERISTICS

Signs and Symptoms

- Asymptomatic until late in the disease (most diagnosed at stage III or IV)
- Weight loss
- Increasing abdominal girth despite constant or reduced caloric intake
- Ascites
- Adnexal mass (multilocular or partly solid masses in patients older than age 40 likely to be malignant; ovarian masses in premenarchal girls are most often germ cell tumors)
- Vague lower abdominal discomfort (severe pain uncommon)

DIAGNOSTIC APPROACH

Differential Diagnosis

- Benign adnexal masses (corpus luteum, follicular cyst)
- Nongynecologic pelvic masses
- Hepatic, renal, or cardiac disease resulting in weight loss and ascites
- Endometriosis
- Hydrosalpinx
- Ectopic pregnancy (reproductive-age women)
- Pedunculated leiomyomata
- Pelvic or horseshoe kidney
- Gastrointestinal malignancy

Associated Conditions: Breast cancer, endometrial cancer.

WORKUP AND EVALUATION

Laboratory: Serum testing for tumor markers, such as CA-125, lipid-associated sialic acid, carcinoembryonic antigen, α-fetoprotein, lactate dehydrogenase (LDH) and others, should be reserved for following the progress of patients with known malignancies and not for prognostic evaluation.

Imaging: Ultrasonography, magnetic resonance imaging (MRI), and computed tomography (CT) are helpful in evaluating patients suspected of having ovarian cancer. (The normal postmenopausal ovary is typically 1.5 to 2 cm in size.) Asymptomatic simple cysts of less than 5 cm diameter can generally be followed conservatively. (Routing screening using transvaginal ultrasonography has not been shown to be cost effective without the presence of significant risk factors or symptoms.)

Special Tests: A frozen-section histologic evaluation (intraoperative consultation) should be considered for any ovarian mass that appears suspicious for malignancy. Flow cytometry may be of prognostic value.

Diagnostic Tests: History, physical examination, and imaging. Final diagnosis is established by histologic evaluation.

Pathologic Findings

More than 90% of ovarian cancer is of the epithelial cell type, thought to arise from pluripotential mesothelial cells of the visceral peritoneum of the ovarian capsule. Lymphatic spread occurs in roughly 20% of tumors that appear grossly confined to the ovary.

MANAGEMENT AND THERAPY

Nonpharmacologic

General Measures: Evaluation, supportive therapy based on symptoms.

Specific Measures: Ovarian cancer is a disease that requires surgical exploration and extirpation (generally including the uterus and contralateral ovary). Adjunctive chemotherapy (platinum-based and paclitaxel [Taxol]) or radiation therapy is often included based on the location and stage of the disease.

Diet: No changes except those imposed by advanced disease. Parenteral nutrition may be required before or after surgery in advanced disease.

Activity: No restriction, except that imposed by advanced disease.

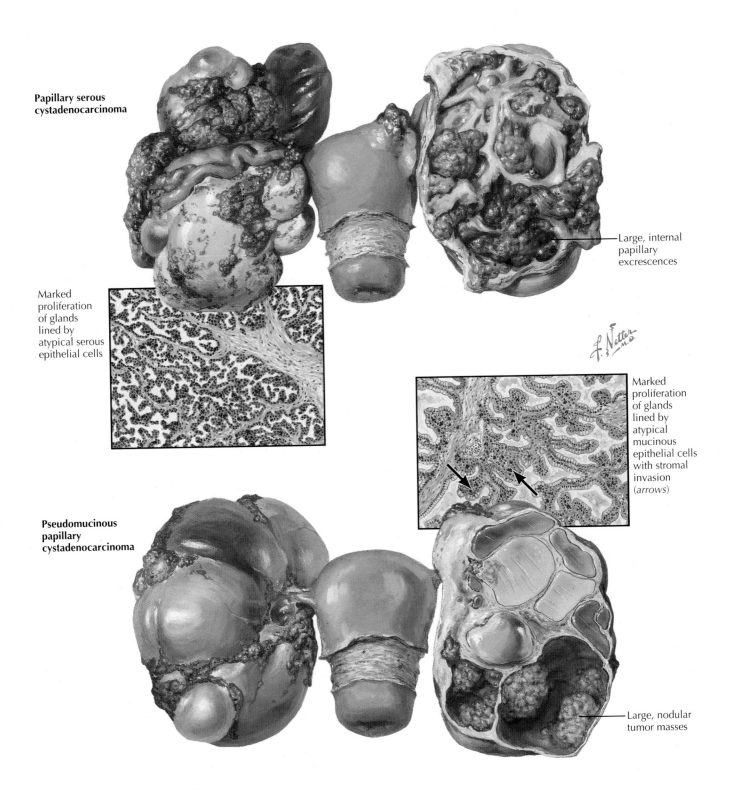

Papillary serous cystadenocarcinoma

Marked proliferation of glands lined by atypical serous epithelial cells

Large, internal papillary excrescences

Marked proliferation of glands lined by atypical mucinous epithelial cells with stromal invasion (*arrows*)

Pseudomucinous papillary cystadenocarcinoma

Large, nodular tumor masses

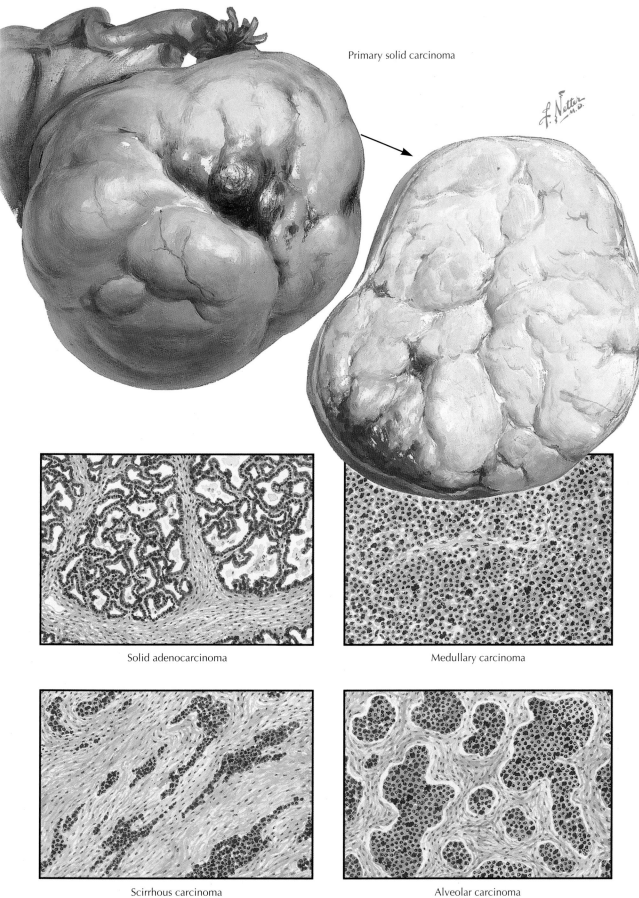

Primary solid carcinoma

Solid adenocarcinoma

Medullary carcinoma

Scirrhous carcinoma

Alveolar carcinoma

Patient Education: Reassurance; American College of Obstetricians and Gynecologists Patient Education Pamphlet AP096 (Cancer of the Ovary), AP075 (Ovarian Cysts).

Drug(s) of Choice

None, except as adjunctive therapy. Preoperative bowel cleansing (mechanical or with antibiosis) is often recommended as a precaution should bowel resection become necessary at the time of surgical staging and resection.

Precautions: Alkylating agents are associated with an increased risk of future leukemia (10% by 8 years after therapy).

FOLLOW-UP

Patient Monitoring: As yet, there are no effective screening tools for the early detection of primary ovarian cancer. Ultrasonography, magnetic resonance imaging, computed tomography, and biochemical markers such as CA 125, which are useful for evaluating a suspicious mass or following the progress of treatment, are not of value for mass screening. In those suspected of having recurrent disease and other selected patients, second-look surgery may be desirable to assess progress and discover occult disease. (When second look surgery is negative, the associated 5-year survival is approximately 50%.)

Prevention/Avoidance: For those few patients at truly high risk (familial cancer syndromes), prophylactic oophorectomy after childbearing is completed is preferable to any attempt at prolonged surveillance with current technology. Even this aggressive step does not preclude the development of "ovarian" cancer; up to 10% of ovarian cancers are found in women who have had bilateral oophorectomies.

Possible Complications: Ascites, pulmonary effusion, small bowel obstruction, disease progression, and death.

Expected Outcome: Ovarian cancer has the highest mortality of any gynecologic cancer, resulting in more deaths annually than cervical and endometrial cancer combined. If discovered early in the process and treated with aggressive surgical resection and adjunctive therapy, disease-free survival is possible. Survival is affected by stage, grade, cell type, and residual tumor after surgical resection. Survival (5-year) by stage: stage I, 80%; stage II, 60%; stage III, 25%; stage, IV 15%. Serous adenocarcinoma has the poorest prognosis of the epithelial types.

MISCELLANEOUS

Pregnancy Considerations: Does not threaten pregnancy except by the jeopardy caused to the mother.
ICD-9-CM Codes: Based on type and stage.

REFERENCES

Level II

Averette HE, Nguyen HN: The role of prophylactic oophorectomy in cancer prevention. Gynecol Oncol 1994;55:S38.

Bell R, Petticrew M, Sheldon T: The performance of screening tests for ovarian cancer: results of a systematic review. Br J Obstet Gynaceol 1998;105:1136.

Elit L, Oliver TK, Covens A, et al: Intraperitoneal chemotherapy in the first-line treatment of women with stage III epithelial ovarian cancer: a systematic review with metaanalyses. Cancer 2007;109:692.

Jamal A, Siegel R, Ward E, et al: Cancer statistics, 2007. CA Cancer J Clin 2007;57:43.

Lacey JV Jr, Greene MH, Buys SS, et al: Ovarian cancer screening in women with a family history of breast or ovarian cancer. Obstet Gynecol 2006;108:1176.

Randall TC, Rubin SC: Cytoreductive surgery for ovarian cancer. Surg Clin North Am 2001;81:871.

Rufford BD, Jacobs IJ, Menon U: Feasibility of screening for ovarian cancer using symptoms as selection criteria. BJOG 2007;114:59.

Schildkraut JM, Cooper GS, Halabi S, et al: Age at natural menopause and the risk of epithelial ovarian cancer. Obstet Gynecol 2001;98:85.

van Nagell JR Jr, DePriest PD, Ueland FR, et al: Ovarian cancer screening with annual transvaginal sonography: findings of 25,000 women screened. Cancer 2007;109:1887.

Level III

American College of Obstetricians and Gynecologists: Prophylactic oophorectomy. ACOG Practice Bulletin 7. Washington, DC, ACOG, 1999.

American College of Obstetricians and Gynecologists: The role of the generalist obstetrician–gynecologist in the early detection of ovarian cancer. ACOG Committee Opinion 280. Obstet Gynecol 2002;100:1413.

American College of Obstetricians and Gynecologists: Ovarian, endometrial, and colorectal cancers. Obstet Gynecol 2004;104:77S.

American College of Obstetricians and Gynecologists: Routine cancer screening. ACOG Committee Opinion 356. Obstet Gynecol 2006;108:1611.

Bhoola S, Hoskins WJ. Diagnosis and management of epithelial ovarian cancer. Obstet Gynecol 2006;107:1399.

Boente MP, Godwin AK, Hogan WM: Screening, imaging and early diagnosis of ovarian cancer. Clin Obstet Gynecol 1994;37:377.

Cannistra SA: Cancer of the ovary. N Engl J Med 2004;351:2519.

Coleman RL, Gershenson DM: Neoplastic diseases of the ovary. In Katz VL, Lentz GM, Lobo RA, Gershenson DM: Comprehensive Gynecology, 5th ed. Philadelphia, Mosby/Elsevier, 2007:839.

Farthing A: Conserving fertility in the management of gynaecological cancers. BJOG 2006;113:129.

Lynch HT, Watson P, Conway T, Lynch J: Hereditary ovarian cancer: natural history, surveillance, management, and genetic counseling. Hematol/Oncol Ann 1994;2:107.

Marth C, Walker JL, Barakat RR, et al: Results of the 2006 Innsbruck International Consensus Conference on intraperitoneal chemotherapy in patients with ovarian cancer. Cancer 2007;109:645.

U.S. Preventive Services Task Force: Screening for ovarian cancer: recommendation statement. U.S. Preventive Services Task Force. Am Fam Physician 2005;71:759.

van Nagell JR, DePriest PD: Management of adnexal masses in postmenopausal women. Am J Obstet Gynecol 2005;193:30.

Wooster R, Weber BL: Breast and ovarian cancer. N Engl J Med 2003;348:2339.

THE CHALLENGE

Description: An ovarian cyst is a cystic growth within the ovary, generally arising from epithelial components and most often benign.

Scope of the Problem: Benign ovarian tumors are most frequently diagnosed at the time of routine examination and are asymptomatic. When symptoms do occur, they generally are either catastrophic (as when bleeding, rupture, or torsion occur) or indolent and nonspecific (such as a vague sense of pressure or fullness).

Objectives of Management: The most important objective of the management of an ovarian cyst is the timely diagnosis of its type and origin. Subsequent therapy and assessment of risk is based on the correctness of the diagnosis. For acutely symptomatic cysts, rapid evaluation and intervention may be necessary.

TACTICS

Relevant Pathophysiology: Approximately 90% of ovarian tumors encountered in younger women are benign and metabolically inactive. More than 75% of the benign adnexal masses are functional. Functional cysts are not true neoplasms; rather, they are anatomic variants resulting from the normal function of the ovary. Follicular cysts occur when ovulation fails to take place, leaving the developing follicle to continue beyond its normal time. In a similar manner, the corpus luteum may persist or, through internal bleeding, enlarge and become symptomatic. Approximately 25% of ovarian enlargements in reproductive-age women represent true neoplasia, with only approximately 10% being malignant. The largest group of benign ovarian tumors is those that arise from the epithelium of the ovary and its capsule. Despite the diversity of tumors with epithelial beginnings, the most common ovarian tumor in young reproductive-age women is the cystic teratoma, or dermoid, which is germ cell in origin. These tumors are derived from primary germ cells and include tissues from all three embryonic germ layers (ectoderm, mesoderm, and endoderm).

Strategies: History and physical examination are generally sufficient to establish the presence of the mass. No laboratory tests are of specific help in the global diagnosis of ovarian cysts. Laboratory investigations may support specific diagnoses. Ultrasonography, computed tomography, and magnetic resonance imaging are of limited value in evaluating asymptomatic masses in young patients. Exceptions to this are patients in whom clinical assessment is impractical or inadequate (e.g., massive obesity) or those in whom malignancy is suspected. Serum testing for tumor markers, such as CA-125, lipid-associated sialic acid, carcinoembryonic antigen, α-fetoprotein, lactate dehydrogenase (LDH), and others, should be reserved for following the progress of patients with known malignancies and not for prognostic evaluation.

Patient Education: Reassurance; American College of Obstetricians and Gynecologists Patient Education Pamphlet AP075 (Ovarian Cysts).

IMPLEMENTATION

Special Considerations: Some authors favor giving young patients with small, presumably benign, cystic masses ovulation suppression therapy, such as oral contraceptives, to hasten the process of regression. Regression rates of 65% to 75% are often cited for this approach, but this strategy is largely a matter of personal choice because definitive studies are lacking. Physiologic ovarian enlargements, including follicular or corpus luteum cysts, should not be present if a patient is using oral contraceptives. For this reason, patients who are already using oral contraceptives and develop adnexal masses are more likely to have pathologic conditions that will not regress, increasing the possibility that eventual surgical exploration may be required. Perimenopausal and postmenopausal patients may still have benign processes as a cause of an adnexal mass, but the likelihood of a malignant process is much increased (up to one third of cases), altering management. In these patients, masses larger than 6 cm generally prompt surgical exploration and excision. The availability of transvaginal ultrasonography to measure and track masses has allowed smaller masses that once would have required exploration to be followed conservatively. As in younger patients, the size, shape, mobility, and consistency of the mass should be estimated. Irregular, immobile, or mixed-character masses (solid and cystic) are more likely to be malignant and deserve immediate consultation with a surgeon for exploration. The final diagnosis of ovarian cancer must be made surgically.

REFERENCES

Level II

Geomini PM, Kluivers KB, Moret E, et al: Evaluation of adnexal masses with three-dimensional ultrasonography. Obstet Gynecol 2006;108:1167.

Rufford BD, Jacobs IJ, Menon U: Feasibility of screening for ovarian cancer using symptoms as selection criteria. BJOG 2007;114:59.

Simpkins F, Zahurak M, Armstrong D, et al: Ovarian malignancy in breast cancer patients with an adnexal mass. Obstet Gynecol 2005;105:507.

Whitecar MP, Turner S, Higby MK: Adnexal masses in pregnancy: a review of 130 cases undergoing surgical management. Am J Obstet Gynecol 1999;181:19.

Level III

Coleman RL, Gershenson DM: Neoplastic diseases of the ovary. In Katz VL, Lentz GM, Lobo RA, Gershenson DM: Comprehensive Gynecology, 5th ed. Philadelphia, Mosby/Elsevier, 2007:846.

Fleischer AC: Transabdominal and transvaginal sonography of ovarian masses. Clin Obstet Gynecol 1991;34:433.

Gallup DG, Talledo E: Management of the adnexal mass in the 1990s. South Med J 1997;90:972.

Patel MD. Practical approach to the adnexal mass. Radiol Clin North Am 2006;44:879.

Petersen WF, Prevost EC, Edmunds FT, et al: Benign cystic teratomas of the ovary. Am J Obstet Gynecol 1955;70:368.

Russell DJ: The female pelvic mass. Diagnosis and management. Med Clin North Am 1995;79:1481.

Differential Diagnosis

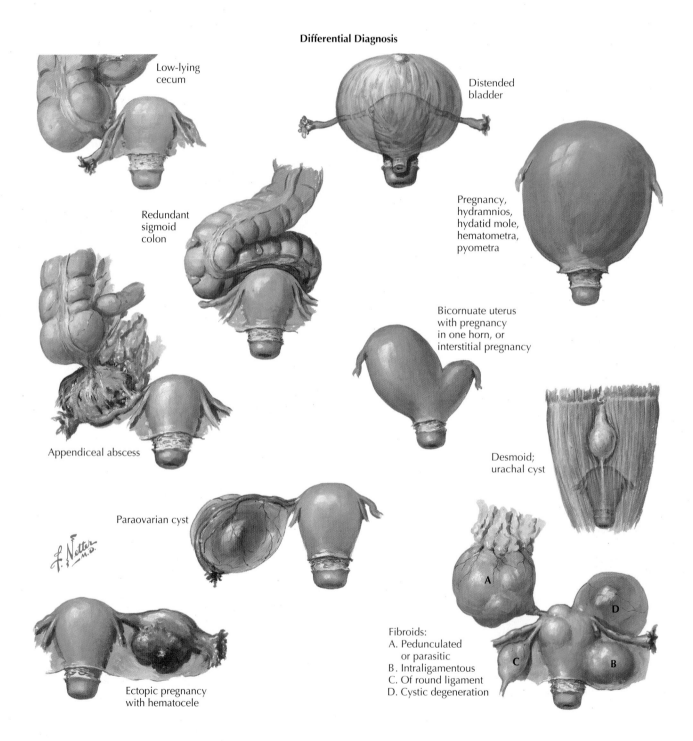

Low-lying cecum

Distended bladder

Redundant sigmoid colon

Pregnancy, hydramnios, hydatid mole, hematometra, pyometra

Bicornuate uterus with pregnancy in one horn, or interstitial pregnancy

Appendiceal abscess

Desmoid; urachal cyst

Paraovarian cyst

Ectopic pregnancy with hematocele

Fibroids:
A. Pedunculated or parasitic
B. Intraligamentous
C. Of round ligament
D. Cystic degeneration

137

Ovarian Fibroma

INTRODUCTION

Description: The most common benign ovarian tumor, an ovarian fibroma is composed of stromal cells (fibroblasts). Although benign, these tumors are sometimes associated with ascites and hydrothorax (Meigs, syndrome, 1% of patients).

Prevalence: Four percent of all ovarian tumors, most common solid tumor.

Predominant Age: Any, most common in perimenopausal and menopausal women, average: 48, <10% younger than 30.

Genetics: No genetic pattern with the exception of Gorlin syndrome.

ETIOLOGY AND PATHOGENESIS

Causes: Unknown.
Risk Factors: None known.

CLINICAL CHARACTERISTICS

Signs and Symptoms

- Asymptomatic (may grow to a large size without detection)
- Adnexal mass (average size 6 cm, may weigh as much as 50 pounds)
- Ascites (40% if the tumor is >10 cm)
- Hydrothorax (Meigs' syndrome, regresses after removal of the tumor)
- Estrogen secretion (when theca cells predominate)
- Bilateral masses in <10% of patients

DIAGNOSTIC APPROACH

Differential Diagnosis

- Benign adnexal masses (corpus luteum, follicular cyst)
- Endometriosis
- Hydrosalpinx
- Paratubal cyst
- Appendiceal abscess
- Ectopic pregnancy
- Pedunculated leiomyomata
- Pelvic or horseshoe kidney
- Nongynecologic pelvic masses
- Fibromatosis
- Stromal hyperplasia
- Fibrosarcoma

Associated Conditions: Ascites, hydrothorax, basal cell nevus syndrome (Gorlin's syndrome—early basal cell carcinomas, keratosis of the jaw, calcification of the dura, mesenteric cysts, and bilateral ovarian fibromas).

WORKUP AND EVALUATION

Laboratory: As indicated before surgery.
Imaging: Preoperative evaluation (computed tomography or ultrasonography) for possible lymph node enlargement or intra-abdominal spread is indicated for patients in whom malignancy is a significant possibility.
Special Tests: None fïndicated.

Diagnostic Tests: History, physical examination, and imaging. Final diagnosis is established by histologic evaluation.

Pathologic Findings

These tumors contain fibroblasts and spindle cells and may grow to a large size without detection. The cut surface reveals hard, flat, chalky-white surfaces with a whorled appearance. Small cyst formation is relatively common.

MANAGEMENT AND THERAPY

Nonpharmacologic

General Measures: Evaluation, supportive therapy based on symptoms.
Specific Measures: Surgical exploration and resection is adequate. In older women, hysterectomy and removal of the contralateral ovary is generally performed. Fibromas of low malignant potential are rare.
Diet: No specific dietary changes indicated.
Activity: No restriction.
Patient Education: American College of Obstetricians and Gynecologists Patient Education Pamphlet AP096 (Cancer of the Ovary), AP075 (Ovarian Cysts).

Drug(s) of Choice

Adjunctive or symptomatic therapy.

FOLLOW-UP

Patient Monitoring: Normal health maintenance.
Prevention/Avoidance: None.
Possible Complications: Uncommon. Torsion or bleeding may occur. Fibromas of low malignant potential that are adherent or that are ruptured may recur.
Expected Outcome: Simple surgical excision is generally curative.

MISCELLANEOUS

Pregnancy Considerations: No effect on pregnancy. Hormonally active tumors (thecoma) may disrupt menstrual patterns and ovulation, leading to reduced fertility.
ICD-9-CM Codes: 220 (Benign neoplasm of ovary).

REFERENCES

Level II

Brun JL: Demons syndrome revisited: a review of the literature. Gynecol Oncol 2007;105:796. Epub 2007 Apr 11.

Leung SW, Yuen PM: Ovarian fibroma: a review on the clinical characteristics, diagnostic difficulties, and management options of 23 cases. Gynecol Obstet Invest 2006;62:1. Epub 2006 Feb 22.

Onderoglu LS, Gultekin M, Dursun P, et al: Bilateral ovarian fibromatosis presenting with ascites and hirsutism. Gynecol Oncol 2004;94:223.

Timmerman D, Moerman P, Vergote I: Meigs' syndrome with elevated serum CA 125 levels: two case reports and review of the literature. Gynecol Oncol 1995;59:405.

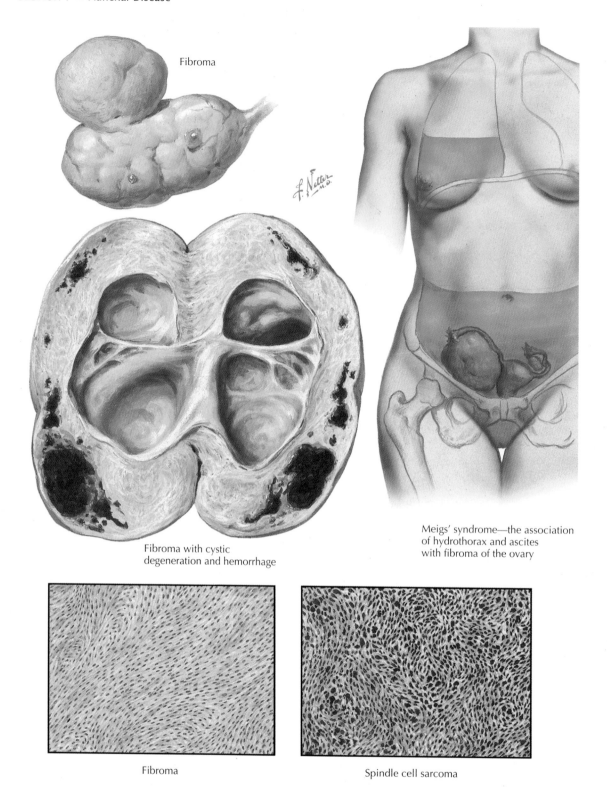

Fibroma

Fibroma with cystic
degeneration and hemorrhage

Meigs' syndrome—the association
of hydrothorax and ascites
with fibroma of the ovary

Fibroma

Spindle cell sarcoma

Level III

Burket RL, Rauh JL: Gorlin's syndrome. Ovarian fibromas at adolescence. Obstet Gynecol 1976;47:43s.

Fleischer AC: Transabdominal and transvaginal sonography of ovarian masses. Clin Obstet Gynecol 1991;34:433.

Gorlin RJ: Nevoid basal-cell carcinoma syndrome. Medicine (Baltimore) 1987;66:98.

Meigs JV: Fibroma of the ovary with ascites and hydrothorax. Meigs' syndrome. Am J Obstet Adynecol 1954;67:962.

Meigs JV, Armstrong SH, Hamilton HH: A further contribution to the syndrome of fibroma of the ovary with fluid in the abdomen and chest, Meigs' syndrome. Am J Obstet Gynecol 1943;46:19.

Roth LM: Recent advances in the pathology and classification of ovarian sex cord-stromal tumors. Int J Gynecol Pathol 2006; 25:199.

Scully RE: Ovarian tumors. A review. Am J Pathol 1977;87:686.

138

Ovarian Torsion

INTRODUCTION

Description: Ovarian torsion involves the twisting of part or all of the adnexa on its mesentery, resulting in tissue ischemia and frank infarction. This usually involves the ovary but may include the fallopian tube as well.

Prevalence: Uncommon; 2% to 3% of gynecologic operative emergencies.

Predominant Age: Mid-20s.

Genetics: No genetic pattern.

ETIOLOGY AND PATHOGENESIS

Causes: Spontaneous twisting of the ovary on its mesentery, generally associated with ovarian enlargement (50% to 60% have an ovarian tumor or cyst).

Risk Factors: Torsion of the adnexa is usually associated with the presence of an ovarian, tubal, or paratubal mass. Risk of torsion is higher during pregnancy or after ovulation induction.

CLINICAL CHARACTERISTICS

Signs and Symptoms

- Pain (generally abrupt, intense, and unilateral—the pain of adnexal torsion generally comes and goes with a periodicity that varies from hours to days or longer; this is in contrast to the variable pain caused by obstruction of the bowel, ureter, or common bile duct, which is more regular and frequent)
- Nausea and vomiting (60% to 70%)
- Unilateral palpable (tender) mass (90% of patients)

DIAGNOSTIC APPROACH

Differential Diagnosis

- Ectopic pregnancy
- Bleeding into an ovarian cyst
- Ruptured corpus luteum
- Adnexal abscess
- Acute appendicitis
- Small bowel obstruction

Associated Conditions: Adnexal mass.

WORKUP AND EVALUATION

Laboratory: Pregnancy test to evaluate the possibility of an ectopic pregnancy.

Imaging: Ultrasonography may demonstrate a cystic adnexal mass, but the acute character and intensity of symptoms usually encountered mean that the diagnosis is most often made at the time of surgery.

Special Tests: None indicated.

Diagnostic Tests: History, physical examination, and imaging (if the patient's condition permits).

Pathologic Findings

Ischemia and infarction in ovarian or tubal tissues, other pathologic conditions based on a coexistent mass (50% to 60% of patients have a mass).

MANAGEMENT AND THERAPY

Nonpharmacologic

General Measures: Evaluation, stabilization (when acute symptoms are present).

Specific Measures: Surgical exploration (conservative operative management may be possible in up to 75% of patients).

Diet: Nothing by mouth pending surgical exploration.

Activity: Bed rest.

Patient Education: American College of Obstetricians and Gynecologists Patient Education Pamphlet AP075 (Ovarian Cysts).

Drug(s) of Choice

Analgesics (based on patient condition).

Contraindications: No analgesics should be given until the diagnosis is established and the patient's condition is stabilized.

FOLLOW-UP

Patient Monitoring: Normal health maintenance as follow-up.

Prevention/Avoidance: None.

Possible Complications: Complete loss of the involved ovary.

Expected Outcome: Part or all of the ovary may be salvaged in some patients if intervention takes place early enough in the process.

MISCELLANEOUS

Pregnancy Considerations: Twenty percent of cases occur during pregnancy.

ICD-9-CM Codes: 620.5.

REFERENCES

Level II
Gittleman AM, Price AP, Goffner L, Katz DS: Ovarian torsion: CT findings in a child. J Pediatr Surg 2004;39:1270.

Gordon JD, Hopkins KL, Jeffrey RB, Giudice LC: Adnexal torsion: color Doppler diagnosis and laparoscopic treatment. Fertil Steril 1994;61:383.

Oelsner G, Bider D, Goldenberg M, et al: Long-term follow-up of the twisted ischemic adnexa managed by detorsion. Fertil Steril 1993;60:976.

Rody A, Jackisch C, Klockenbusch W, et al: The conservative management of adnexal torsion—A case-report and review of the literature. Eur J Obstet Gynecol Reprod Biol 2002;101:83.

Level III
American College of Obstetricians and Gynecologists: Management of adnexal masses ACOG Practice Bulletin 83. Obstet Gynecol 2007; 110:201.

Bayer AI, Wiskind AK: Adnexal torsion: can the adnexa be saved? Am J Obstet Gynecol 1994;171:1506.

Bider D, Maschiach S, Dulitzky M, et al: Clinical, surgical and pathologic findings of adnexal torsion in pregnant and nonpregnant women. Surg Gynecol Obstet 1991;173:363.

Breech LL, Hillard PJ: Adnexal torsion in pediatric and adolescent girls. Curr Opin Obstet Gynecol 2005;17:483.

Clinical Findings

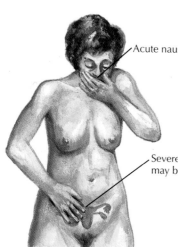

Acute nausea and vomiting

Severe lower-quadrant abdominal pain, may be confused with ruptured ovarian cyst

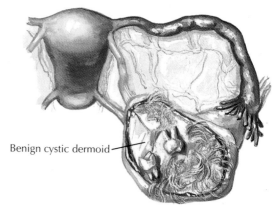

Benign cystic dermoid

Up to 50% of torsion cases may be associated with a medium-sized (10–12 cm) mass

Mechanism of Torsion

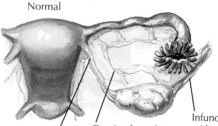

Normal

Ovarian ligament

Ovarian branches of uterine vessels

Infundibulopelvic ligament with ovarian vessels

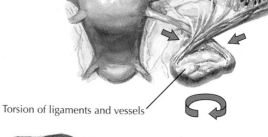

Torsion

Torsion of ligaments and vessels

Torsion of ligaments and vessels

Torsion of ovary causes twisting of suspensory ligaments and vascular pedicles resulting in venous occlusion and congestion and, in severe cases, arterial occlusion and ischemia

Venous congestion and hemorrhage

JOHN A. CRAIG—AD
D. Mascaro

Cass DL: Ovarian torsion. Semin Pediatr Surg 2005;14:1486.

Giuntoli RL 2nd, Vang RS, Bristow RE: Evaluation and management of adnexal masses during pregnancy. Clin Obstet Gynecol 2006;49:492.

Hibbard LT: Adnexal torsion. Am J Obstet Gynecol 1985;152:456.

Katz VL: Benign gynecologic lesions. In Katz VL, Lentz GM, Lobo RA, Gershenson DM: Comprehensive Gynecology, 5th ed. Philadelphia, Mosby/Elsevier, 2007:462.

Nichols DH, Julian PJ: Torsion of the adnexa. Clin Obstet Gynecol 1985;28:375.

Oelsner G, Shashar D: Adnexal torsion. Clin Obstet Gynecol 2006;49:459.

Schiller VL, Grant EG: Doppler ultrasonography of the pelvis. Radiol Clin North Am 1992;30:735.

Strickland JL: Ovarian cysts in neonates, children and adolescents. Curr Opin Obstet Gynecol 2002;14:459.

Zweizig S, Perron J, Grubb D, Mishell DR Jr: Conservative management of adnexal torsion. Am J Obstet Gynecol 1993;168:1791.

INTRODUCTION

Description: Pelvic inflammatory disease (PID) is a serious, diffuse, frequently multiorganism infection of the pelvic organs that results in significant morbidity.

Prevalence: One percent to 3% of women; most common gynecologic reason for emergency visits for women aged 15 to 44. Roughly 168,000 cases and approximately 70,000 hospitalizations annually.

Predominant Age: 16 to 25; 85% of cases found in sexually active women of menstrual age.

Genetics: No genetic pattern.

ETIOLOGY AND PATHOGENESIS

Causes: In roughly one third of cases the causative organism is *Neisseria gonorrhoeae* alone. One third of cases involve infection with *N. gonorrhoeae* and additional "mixed" infections with other organisms. The last third of infections result from mixed aerobic and anaerobic bacteria, including respiratory pathogens such as *Haemophilus influenzae*, *Streptococcus pneumoniae*, and *Streptococcus pyogenes* found in up to 5% of patients. Polymicrobial infections are present in more than 40% of patients with laparoscopically proven salpingitis, with one study reporting an average of 6.8 bacterial types per patient. Only approximately 15% of women with cervical *N. gonorrhoeae* infections develop acute pelvic infections. Orgasmic uterine contractions or the attachment of *N. gonorrhoeae* to sperm may provide transportation to the upper genital tract. *Chlamydia* is involved in roughly 20% of patients, with this rate increasing to roughly 40% among hospitalized patients. Infection of the upper genital tract by *Chlamydia* causes a milder form of salpingitis with more insidious symptoms.

Risk Factors: Multiple sexual partners, uterine or cervical instrumentation, douching. Because many of the anaerobic bacteria found in mixed infections mimic those found in the vagina of patients with bacterial vaginosis, bacterial vaginosis has been considered a risk factor for the development of pelvic infections, but recently published studies suggest that this is not the case. Of cases, 15% occur after instrumentation such as endometrial biopsy, hysterosalpingography, intrauterine contraceptive device placement, or the like.

CLINICAL CHARACTERISTICS

Signs and Symptoms

- Pelvic pain and tenderness (100%), muscular guarding, or rebound tenderness
- Fever (up to 39.5°C, 40%) or chills
- Elevated white blood cell count
- Irregular vaginal bleeding or discharge
- Tachycardia, nausea, and vomiting
- Purulent cervical discharge is often demonstrated (should be sampled for Gram staining and culture)

DIAGNOSTIC APPROACH

Differential Diagnosis

- Ectopic pregnancy
- Adnexal accident (torsion, bleeding)
- Appendicitis
- Endometriosis
- Cholecystitis
- Enteritis
- Septic incomplete abortion
- Diverticular abscess

Associated Conditions: Tubal factor infertility, ectopic pregnancy, and chronic abdominal pain.

WORKUP AND EVALUATION

Laboratory: Complete blood count, including differential, white blood cell count, and erythrocyte sedimentation rate. Cervical culture (although there is only a 50% correlation between cervical culture and upper-tract organisms) and Gram staining.

Imaging: Ultrasonography may demonstrate free fluid in the posterior cul-de-sac (supportive but not diagnostic).

Special Tests: Confirmation by laparoscopy should be considered for any patient who does not respond in a timely manner or for whom the diagnosis is uncertain. In 35% of patients no infection is found. (Data indicate that a clinical diagnosis of symptomatic PID has a positive predictive value [PPV] for salpingitis of 65% to 90% compared with laparoscopy.)

Diagnostic Tests: History, physical examination, and ultrasonography. Diagnostic criteria are shown in the following box. (Empiric treatment of PID should be started in sexually active women at risk for STDs if they are experiencing pelvic or lower abdominal pain, if no cause for the illness other than PID can be identified, and if they have cervical motion or cervical or uterine tenderness.)

Pathologic Findings

Inflammation of the fallopian tubes, ovaries, and surrounding peritoneal surfaces.

Diagnostic Criteria for Pelvic Inflammatory Disease

Must Have All Three:
- Abdominal tenderness
- Adnexal tenderness
- Cervical tenderness

Must Have at Least One:
- Positive Gram stain
- Temperature >38°C
- White blood cell count >10,000
- Pus on culdocentesis or laparoscopy
- Tubo-ovarian abscess

MANAGEMENT AND THERAPY
Nonpharmacologic

General Measures: Rapid evaluation, cervical cultures, supportive therapy (fluids, analgesics, and antipyretics).

Specific Measures: Aggressive antibiotic therapy. For some, hysterectomy may be required. Rupture of a tubo-ovarian abscess, with subsequent septic shock, may be life threatening.

Diet: No specific dietary changes indicated.

Activity: Pelvic rest. Ambulatory care is possible with early mild infections; hospitalization may be required.

Patient Education: American College of Obstetricians and Gynecologists Patient Education Pamphlet AP077 (Pelvic Inflammatory Disease), AP009 (How to Prevent Sexually Transmitted Diseases), AP099 (Pelvic Pain), AP071 (Gonorrhea, Chlamydia, and Syphilis), AP020 (Pain During Intercourse).

Drug(s) of Choice

Ambulatory care—ceftriaxone (250 mg IM in a single dose) plus doxycycline (100 mg PO twice a day for 14 days) with or without metronidazole (500 mg twice a day for 14 days), or cefoxitin (2 g IM) plus probenecid (1 g PO) combined with a 14-day course of doxycycline (100 mg, twice a day) or a combination of ceftriaxone (250 mg IM) plus the 14-day course of doxycycline both with or without metronidazole (500 mg twice a day for 14 days). (Fluoroquinolone-resistant gonorrhea is now widespread in the United States, making this class of antibiotics no longer appropriate for the treatment of gonorrhea and, hence, PID.)

Hospitalized patients—cefotetan (2 g IV every 12 hours) or cefoxitin (2 g IV every 6 hours) with doxycycline (100 mg every 12 hours PO or IV) is recommended. For mixed infections, clindamycin (900 mg IV every 8 hours) plus an aminoglycoside such as gentamicin (2 mg/kg loading doses, then 1.5 mg/kg every 8 hours) will give better protection.

After discharge—doxycycline (100 mg PO twice a day) or clindamycin (450 mg four times a day) for 14 days.

Contraindications: See individual agents.
Precautions: See individual agents.
Interactions: See individual agents.

Alternative Drugs

Spectinomycin 2 g in a single intramuscular dose. Augmentin (500 mg three times a day for 10 days) may also be used with similar results. Excellent results have been reported with the combination of clindamycin and aztreonam (2 g IM every 8 hours). Piperacillin (4 g) combined with tazobactam (500 mg) given IV every 8 hours may also be used but has given cure rates of only 90% (5% improved). Amoxicillin/clavulanic acid and doxycycline were effective in obtaining short-term clinical response in a single clinical trial; however, gastrointestinal symptoms limit compliance.

FOLLOW-UP

Patient Monitoring: Hospitalized care is indicated when differential diagnosis includes ectopic pregnancy or appendicitis, human immunodeficiency virus, immunosuppression, intrauterine contraceptive device use, nulliparity, paralytic ileus, peritonitis or toxicity, pregnancy, previous treatment failure, significant gastrointestinal symptoms, significant morbidity, temperature >39°C, tubo-ovarian abscess, uncertain or complicated differential diagnosis, unreliable patient, or white blood cell count >20,000 or <4000.

Prevention/Avoidance: Prevention of these sequelae is based on prevention of infection (barrier contraception, "safe sex"), screening for those at risk, and aggressive treatment. As with most sexually transmitted diseases, the partners of patients with PID should be screened for gonococcal, chlamydial, or human immunodeficiency virus infections and treated accordingly.

Possible Complications: Roughly one in four women with acute PID experiences medical sequelae. PID leads

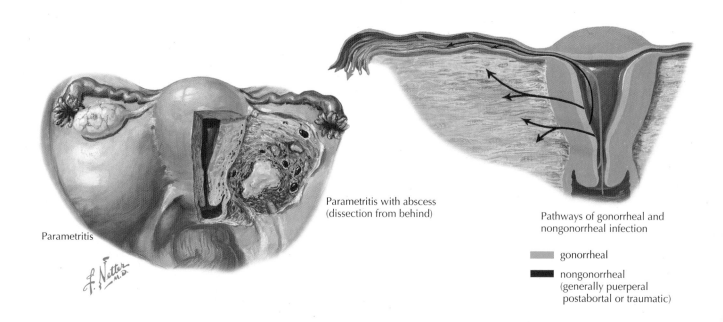

Parametritis

Parametritis with abscess
(dissection from behind)

Pathways of gonorrheal and
nongonorrheal infection

■ gonorrheal

■ nongonorrheal
(generally puerperal
postabortal or traumatic)

to tubal factor infertility, ectopic pregnancy, and chronic abdominal pain in a high percentage of patients. The risk of infertility roughly doubles with each subsequent episode, resulting in a 40% rate of infertility after only three episodes. Women with documented salpingitis have a 4-fold increase in their rate of ectopic pregnancy, and 5% to 15% of women require surgery because of damage caused by PID. Peritoneal involvement may spread to include perihepatitis (Fitz-Hugh–Curtis syndrome). Rupture of a tubo-ovarian abscess, with subsequent septic shock, may be life threatening. Death from pelvic infections or their complications (for women aged 15 to 45) is reported to be 0.29 of 100,000.

Expected Outcome: Early, aggressive therapy is generally associated with resolution, but the possibility of recurrence or sequelae is significant.

MISCELLANEOUS

Pregnancy Considerations: Often associated with reduced fertility and an increased risk of ectopic pregnancy. Once pregnancy is established, the risk of new infection is reduced because of obstruction of the upper genital tract by the gestation. Scarring from previous infections may cause pain when stretched by the enlarging uterus.

ICD-9-CM Codes: 614.3 (others based on chronicity, structures involved, and relation to pregnancy).

REFERENCES

Level I

Ness RB, Trautmann G, Richter HE, et al: Effectiveness of treatment strategies of some women with pelvic inflammatory disease: a randomized trial. Obstet Gynecol 2005;106:573.

Pastorek JG 2nd, Cole C, Aldridge KE, Crapanzano JC: Aztreonam plus clindamycin as therapy for pelvic infections in women. Am J Med 1985;78:47.

Level II

Dodson MG: Antibiotic regimens for treating acute pelvic inflammatory disease: an evaluation. J Reprod Med 1994;39:285.

Gaitán H, Angel E, Diaz R, et al: Accuracy of five different diagnostic techniques in mild-to-moderate pelvic inflammatory disease. Infect Dis Obstet Gynecol 2002;10:171.

Hager WE, Eschenbach DA, Spence MR, Sweet RL: Criteria for diagnosis and grading of salpingitis. Obstet Gynecol 1983;61:113.

Latthe P, Mignini L, Gray R, et al: Factors predisposing women to chronic pelvic pain: systematic review. BMJ 2006;332:749. Epub 2006 Feb 16.

Ledger WJ: Laparoscopy in the diagnosis and management of patients with suspected salpingo-oophoritis. Am J Obstet Gynecol 1980; 138:1012.

Ness RB, Hillier SL, Kip KE, et al: Bacterial vaginosis and risk of pelvic inflammatory disease. Obstet Gynecol 2004;104:761.

Peipert JF, Ness RB, Blume J, et al: Clinical predictors of endometritis in women with symptoms and signs of pelvic inflammatory disease. Am J Obstet Gynecol 2001;184:856.

Tapp A, Wise B, Cardozo L: Efficacy and safety of piperacillin/tazobactam in gynecologic infections. J Antimicrob Chemother 1993; Suppl B:61.

Washington AE, Cates W, Zaidi AA: Hospitalization for pelvic inflammatory disease. JAMA 1984;25:2529.

Level III

American College of Obstetricians and Gynecologists: Chronic pelvic pain. ACOG Practice Bulletin 51. Obstet Gynecol 2004;103:589.

American College of Obstetricians and Gynecologists: Intrauterine device. ACOG Practice Bulletin 59. Obstet Gynecol 2005;105: 223.

Centers for Disease Control and Prevention: Sexually Transmitted Diseases Treatment Guidelines, 2006. MMWR 2006;55:56.

Centers for Disease Control and Prevention: Updated recommended treatment regimens for gonococcal infections and associated conditions—United States, April 2007. MMWR 2007;56;332.

Crossman SH: The challenge of pelvic inflammatory disease. Am Fam Physician 2006;73:859.

Eckert LO, Lentz GM: Infections of the upper genital tract. In Katz VL, Lentz GM, Lobo RA, Gershenson DM: Comprehensive Gynecology, 5th ed. Philadelphia, Mosby/Elsevier, 2007:608.

Jacobson LJ: Differential diagnosis of acute pelvic inflammatory disease. Am J Obstet Gynecol 1980;138:1006.

INTRODUCTION

Description: Pseudomyxoma peritonei is the intraperitoneal spread of a mucin-secreting tumor (either a mucinous cystadenoma or carcinoma), which results in recurrent abdominal masses, often massive ascites, and multiple bowel obstructions. Frequently, this tumor may begin in the appendix.

Prevalence: Two of 10,000 laparotomies, 2% to 5% of ovarian mucinous tumors (16% in mucinous cystadenocarcinomas).

Predominant Age: Middle to late reproductive.

Genetics: No genetic pattern.

ETIOLOGY AND PATHOGENESIS

Causes: Spread, rupture, spill, or leakage of a primary appendiceal tumor or other gastrointestinal or ovarian tumor. Recent histologic studies suggest that in the majority of patients the appendix is the primary tumor source. In rare cases, metaplasia by the cells of the peritoneal surface may account for this tumor.

Risk Factors: Rupture or leakage of an ovarian mucinous tumor at the time of surgical resection. (This role has been debated in recent literature.)

CLINICAL CHARACTERISTICS

Signs and Symptoms

- Accumulation of large amounts of mucinous material in the peritoneal cavity
- Recurrent bowel obstruction
- Implants of tumor on the omentum, undersurface of the diaphragm, pelvis, right retrohepatic space, left abdominal gutter, and ligament of Treitz (the peritoneal surface of the bowel is generally spared [in contrast to carcinoma]; metastasis outside the peritoneal cavity does not occur)

DIAGNOSTIC APPROACH

Differential Diagnosis

- Disseminated ovarian cancer
- Metastatic colon cancer
- Disseminated leiomyomata
- Ascites

Associated Conditions: Gastrointestinal tumors, bowel obstruction.

WORKUP AND EVALUATION

Laboratory: As indicated before surgery. (Serum testing for tumor markers, such as CA-125, lipid-associated sialic acid, carcinoembryonic antigen, α-fetoprotein, and others, should be reserved for following the progress of patients with known malignancies and not for prognostic evaluation.)

Imaging: Ultrasonography or computed tomography may be helpful in determining the extent of disease.

Special Tests: None indicated.

Diagnostic Tests: History, physical examination, and imaging. Final diagnosis is established by histologic evaluation.

Pathologic Findings

Perforation of the capsule of a mucinous tumor with rupture and seeding of the peritoneal cavity. Most often associated with malignant tumors, although benign mucinous neoplasms may perforate and result in pseudomyxoma peritonei as well. Tumors of the ovary and appendix may be synchronous, making the determination of origin difficult or impossible.

MANAGEMENT AND THERAPY

Nonpharmacologic

General Measures: Evaluation, supportive therapy based on symptoms.

Specific Measures: Surgical exploration and extirpation. Extensive bowel resection is often required because of diffuse peritoneal implants of tumor.

Diet: No specific dietary changes indicated, except those imposed by advanced disease.

Activity: No restriction, except that imposed by advanced disease.

Patient Education: Reassurance; American College of Obstetricians and Gynecologists Patient Education Pamphlet AP075 (Ovarian Cysts), AP096 (Cancer of the Ovary), AP080 (Preparing for Surgery).

Drug(s) of Choice

None, except as adjunctive or symptomatic therapy. Chemotherapy (systemic or intraperitoneal alkylating agents) and mucolytic agents have not been shown to be effective. A recent publication has advocated intraperitoneal hyperthermic perfusion. Preoperative bowel cleansing (mechanical or with antibiosis) is often recommended as a precaution should bowel resection become necessary at the time of surgical staging and resection.

Precautions: Alkylating agents are associated with an increased risk of future leukemia (10% by 8 years after therapy).

FOLLOW-UP

Patient Monitoring: Careful follow-up for recurrent pelvic disease or enlargement of the remaining ovary (if any). This is generally performed by pelvic examination, augmented with ultrasonography in selected patients.

Prevention/Avoidance: Care in the handling and surgical removal of ovarian masses.

Possible Complications: Generally follows an indolent course with progressive bowel dysfunction, intercurrent infection, inanition, and death.

Expected Outcome: The prognosis is better for the patient when the tumor arises from adenomas (appendiceal or ovarian) than if it comes from a carcinoma.

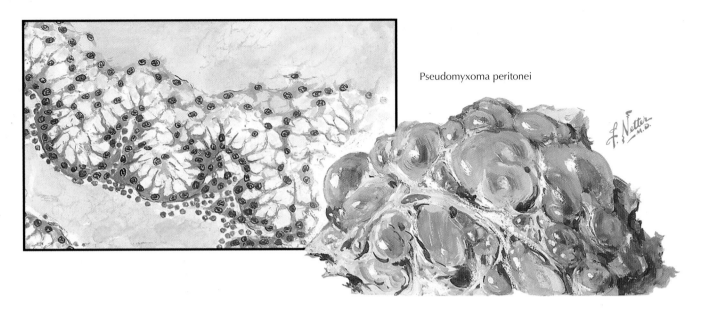

Pseudomyxoma peritonei

MISCELLANEOUS

Pregnancy Considerations: No effect on pregnancy.
ICD-9-CM Codes: 197.6.

REFERENCES

Level II

Geisinger KR, Levine EA, Shen P, et al: Pleuropulmonary involvement in pseudomyxoma peritonei: morphologic assessment and literature review. Am J Clin Pathol 2007;127:135.

Kusamura S, Younan R, Baratti D, et al: Cytoreductive surgery followed by intraperitoneal hyperthermic perfusion: analysis of morbidity and mortality in 209 peritoneal surface malignancies treated with closed abdomen technique. Cancer 2006;106:1144.

Ronnett BM, Kurman RJ, Zahn CM, et al: Pseudomyxoma peritonei in women: a clinicopathologic analysis of 30 cases with emphasis on site of origin, prognosis, and relationship to ovarian mucinous tumors of low malignant potential. Hum Pathol 1995;26:509.

Wertheim I, Fleischhacker D, McLachlin CM, et al: Pseudomyxoma peritonei: a review of 23 cases. Obstet Gynecol 1994;84:17.

Yan TD, Links M, Xu ZY, et al: Cytoreductive surgery and perioperative intraperitoneal chemotherapy for pseudomyxoma peritonei from appendiceal mucinous neoplasms. Br J Surg 2006;93:1270.

Level III

Acs G: Serous and mucinous borderline (low malignant potential) tumors of the ovary. Am J Clin Pathol 2005;123:S13.

Jones DH: Pseudomyxoma peritonei. Br J Clin Pract 1965;19:675.

Rutgers JL, Baergen RN: Mucin histochemistry of ovarian borderline tumors of mucinous and mixed-epithelial types. Mod Pathol 1994;7:825.

INTRODUCTION

Description: Serous ovarian cysts are a group of benign and malignant epithelial tumors of the ovary that are characterized as serous cells. These tumors are the most commonly encountered epithelial ovarian tumors. When malignant, these tumors tend to be high grade and virulent.

Prevalence: Twenty percent of all benign ovarian neoplasms.

Predominant Age: Reproductive.

Genetics: No genetic pattern.

ETIOLOGY AND PATHOGENESIS

Causes: Unknown.

Risk Factors: Family history, high-fat diet, advanced age, nulliparity, early menarche and late menopause, white race, higher economic status. Oral contraception, high parity, and breastfeeding reduce risk.

CLINICAL CHARACTERISTICS

Signs and Symptoms

- Asymptomatic
- Vague lower abdominal symptoms
- Adnexal mass (bilateral in 10% of benign and in 33% to 66% of malignant lesions), cystic and filled with a clear serous fluid. Benign tumors tend to be unilocular and smooth; malignant tumors are more often multilocular with papillary projections over much of the surface.

DIAGNOSTIC APPROACH

Differential Diagnosis

- Benign adnexal masses (corpus luteum, follicular cyst)
- Endometriosis
- Hydrosalpinx
- Paratubal cyst
- Appendiceal abscess
- Ectopic pregnancy
- Pedunculated leiomyomata
- Pelvic or horseshoe kidney
- Nongynecologic pelvic masses

Associated Conditions: None.

WORKUP AND EVALUATION

Laboratory: As indicated before surgery. (CA-125 levels may be useful for the monitoring of disease response to treatment or progression, but this is not a good prognostic test. Only 80% of epithelial ovarian tumors express CA-125, and many benign and other malignant processes [lung, breast, and pancreas] may also cause CA-125 to become higher than normal.)

Imaging: No imaging indicated.

Special Tests: A frozen-section histologic evaluation should be considered for any ovarian mass that appears suspicious for malignancy.

Diagnostic Tests: History, physical examination, and imaging. Final diagnosis is established by histologic evaluation.

Pathologic Findings

Serous tumors are more likely to be found with poorer differentiation and are more likely to be discovered late in the disease process. Papillary surface carcinomas of the ovary are most likely to be serous in type. The diagnosis is made on the basis of the histologic analysis of the cyst wall, not the character of the cyst fluid.

MANAGEMENT AND THERAPY

Nonpharmacologic

General Measures: Evaluation, supportive therapy based on symptoms.

Specific Measures: Generally require surgical exploration and extirpation. In benign disease or tumors of borderline malignant potential, the uterus and other ovary generally may be spared. Adjunctive chemotherapy (platinum-based and paclitaxel [Taxol]) or radiation therapy is often included, based on the location and stage of the disease.

Diet: No specific dietary changes indicated, except those imposed by advanced disease.

Activity: No restriction, except that imposed by advanced disease.

Patient Education: American College of Obstetricians and Gynecologists Patient Education Pamphlet AP096 (Cancer of the Ovary), AP075 (Ovarian Cysts).

Drug(s) of Choice

None, except as adjunctive or symptomatic therapy. Preoperative bowel cleansing (mechanical or with antibiosis) is often recommended as a precaution should bowel resection become necessary at the time of surgical staging and resection.

Precautions: Alkylating agents are associated with an increased risk of future leukemia (10% by 8 years after therapy).

FOLLOW-UP

Patient Monitoring: Careful follow-up for recurrent pelvic disease or enlargement of the remaining ovary (if any). This is generally performed by pelvic examination, augmented with ultrasonography in selected patients. In those suspected of having recurrent disease and other selected patients, second-look surgery may be desirable to assess progress and discover occult disease.

Prevention/Avoidance: None.

Possible Complications: Torsion, hemorrhage, progression, and spread of malignant disease.

Expected Outcome: Generally good for benign tumors; the prognosis for malignant tumors is based on stage. Overall, 5-year survival for malignant serous carcinomas

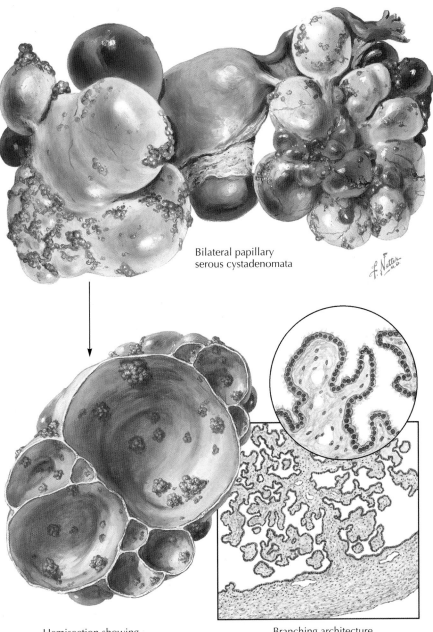

Bilateral papillary
serous cystadenomata

Hemisection showing
internal papillary excrescences

Branching architecture
of papillary growth

is roughly 20%. Of malignant serous carcinomas, 75% are at an advanced stage at the time of diagnosis.

MISCELLANEOUS

Pregnancy Considerations: No effect on pregnancy.
ICD-9-CM Codes: Specific to cell type and location.

REFERENCES

Level II

Flynn MK, Niloff JM: Outpatient minilaparotomy for ovarian cysts. J Reprod Med 1999;44:399.

Rufford BD, Jacobs IJ, Menon U: Feasibility of screening for ovarian cancer using symptoms as selection criteria. BJOG 2007; 114:59.

Timmerman D, Testa AC, Bourne T, et al; International Ovarian Tumor Analysis Group: Logistic regression model to distinguish between the benign and malignant adnexal mass before surgery: a multicenter study by the International Ovarian Tumor Analysis Group. J Clin Oncol 2005;23:8794.

Vuento MH, Pirhonen JP, Makinen JI, et al: Evaluation of ovarian findings in asymptomatic postmenopausal women with color Doppler ultrasound. Cancer 1995;76:1214.

Level III

American College of Obstetricians and Gynecologists: Management of adnexal masses. ACOG Practice Bulletin 83. Obstet Gynecol 2007;110:201.

Fleischer AC: Transabdominal and transvaginal sonography of ovarian masses. Clin Obstet Gynecol 1991;34:433.

Fromm GL, Gershenson DM, Silva EG: Papillary serous carcinoma of the peritoneum. Obstet Gynecol 1990;75:89.

Fromm GL, Silva EG: Metastatic serous ovarian tumors of low malignant potential. Cancer 1990;65:578.

Lentz GM: Differential diagnosis of major gynecologic problems by age group. In Katz VL, Lentz GM, Lobo RA, Gershenson DM: Comprehensive Gynecology, 5th ed. Philadelphia, Mosby/Elsevier, 2007:166.

INTRODUCTION

Description: A Sertoli-Leydig cell tumor is a rare sex cord tumor of the ovary that carries male elements and may be associated with virilization. Tumors vary in size but generally are 5 to 15 cm in diameter.

Prevalence: Very rare (<0.5% of ovarian tumors).

Predominant Age: Older than 30 (70%), <10% older than 50.

Genetics: No genetic pattern.

ETIOLOGY AND PATHOGENESIS

Causes: Unknown.

Risk Factors: None known.

CLINICAL CHARACTERISTICS

Signs and Symptoms

- Asymptomatic
- Adnexal enlargement (1.5% bilateral)
- Abdominal swelling or pain
- Ascites (4%)
- Oligomenorrhea or amenorrhea
- Loss of female secondary sex characteristics (breast atrophy, loss of body contours)
- Virilization or masculinization (one third of patients; acne, hirsutism, temporal balding, deepening of voice, clitoral enlargement)

DIAGNOSTIC APPROACH

Differential Diagnosis

- Adrenal virilizing tumors
- Benign adnexal masses (corpus luteum, follicular cyst)
- Endometriosis
- Hydrosalpinx
- Paratubal cyst
- Appendiceal abscess
- Ectopic pregnancy
- Pedunculated leiomyomata
- Pelvic or horseshoe kidney
- Nongynecologic pelvic masses

Associated Conditions: Virilization, hirsutism, clitoral enlargement.

WORKUP AND EVALUATION

Laboratory: As indicated before surgery. Plasma levels of testosterone, androstenedione, and other androgens may be elevated; urinary 17-ketosteroid values are usually normal. (Androgen secretion by the tumor may result in erythrocytosis.) Laboratory studies cannot reliably differentiate between virilization caused by adrenal tumors and virilization caused by ovarian sources.

Imaging: Preoperative evaluation (computed tomography or ultrasonography) for possible lymph node enlargement or intra-abdominal spread is indicated for patients in whom malignancy is a significant possibility.

Special Tests: None indicated.

Diagnostic Tests: History, physical examination, and imaging. Final diagnosis is established by histologic evaluation.

Pathologic Findings

Variable gross appearance. Sex cord (Sertoli) cells and stromal (Leydig) cells are present in varying proportion, but tubular patterns predominate. Individual cells may appear immature. Lipochrome pigments (crystalloids of Reinke) are present in 20% of tumors. These tumors may be hard to differentiate from granulosa cell tumors and may mimic endometrioid or Krukenberg tumors. Eighty percent of tumors are stage IA at discovery.

MANAGEMENT AND THERAPY

Nonpharmacologic

General Measures: Evaluation, supportive therapy based on symptoms.

Specific Measures: Surgical exploration and resection. Young patients with stage IA disease may be treated with unilateral salpingo-oophorectomy. Undifferentiated tumors or advanced-stage disease require more aggressive surgical resection and may be treated with adjunctive chemotherapy (vincristine, actinomycin D, and cyclophosphamide) or radiation.

Diet: No specific dietary changes indicated.

Activity: No restriction.

Patient Education: American College of Obstetricians and Gynecologists Patient Education Pamphlet AP096 (Cancer of the Ovary), AP075 (Ovarian Cysts).

Drug(s) of Choice

Vincristine (1.5 mg/m^2 IV weekly for 12 weeks), actinomycin D, and cyclophosphamide (0.5 mg of actinomycin D + 5 to 7 mg/kg/day of cyclophosphamide, IV daily for 5 days every 4 weeks). Adjunctive or symptomatic therapy as required.

Precautions: Alkylating agents are associated with an increased risk of future leukemia (10% by 8 years after therapy).

FOLLOW-UP

Patient Monitoring: Careful follow-up and normal health maintenance.

Prevention/Avoidance: None.

Possible Complications: Disease progression or spread (<20%). In advanced-stage disease, recurrence within 1 year in two thirds of patients.

Expected Outcome: These tumors behave as low-grade malignancies and have 5-year survival rates of 70% to 90%. Survival is poorer for higher stage and poorly differentiated tumors. Menses may be anticipated to return approximately 4 weeks after removal of the tumor. Excessive hair often regresses but does not disappear; clitoral enlargement and voice changes (if present) are unlikely to reverse.

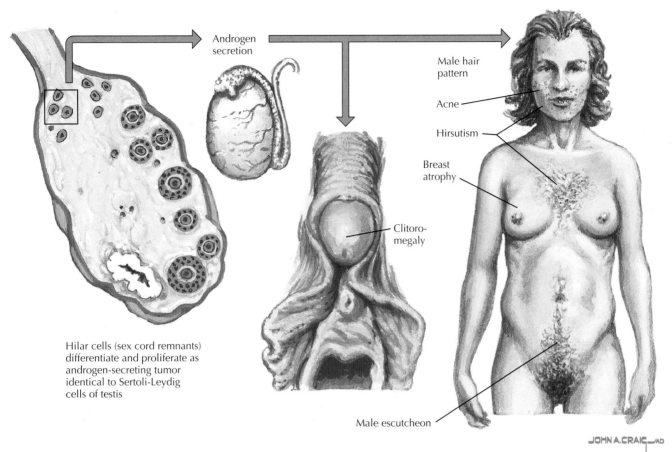

Androgen secretion

Male hair pattern

Acne

Hirsutism

Breast atrophy

Clitoro-megaly

Male escutcheon

Hilar cells (sex cord remnants) differentiate and proliferate as androgen-secreting tumor identical to Sertoli-Leydig cells of testis

JOHN A.CRAIG—AD

Excessive androgen production results in loss of female secondary sex characteristics

MISCELLANEOUS

Pregnancy Considerations: Pregnancy unlikely in the presence of these tumors. No direct effect on the pregnancy, if they coexist. (Hormonal effects on the fetus could be postulated, but tumors with significant hormonal function generally preclude pregnancy.)

ICD-9-CM Codes: Based on location and tumor character.

REFERENCES

Level II

Gheorghisan-Galateanu A, Fica S, Terzea DC, et al: Sertoli-Leydig cell tumor—A rare androgen secreting ovarian tumor in postmenopausal women. Case report and review of literature. J Cell Mol Med 2003;7:461.

Motoyama I, Watanabe H, Gotoh A, et al: Ovarian Sertoli-Leydig cell tumor with elevated serum alpha-fetoprotein. Cancer 1989; 63:2047.

Takeuchi S, Ishihara N, Ohbayashi C, et al: Stromal Leydig cell tumor of the ovary. Case report and literature review. Int J Gynecol Pathol 1999;18:178.

Tomlinson MW, Treadwell MC, Deppe G: Platinum based chemotherapy to treat recurrent Sertoli-Leydig cell ovarian carcinoma during pregnancy. Eur J Gynaecol Oncol 1997;18:44.

Young RH: Sertoli-Leydig cell tumors of the ovary: review with emphasis on historical aspects and unusual variants. Int J Gynecol Pathol 1993;12:141.

Young RH, Scully RE: Ovarian Sertoli-Leydig cell tumors. A clinicopathological analysis of 207 cases. Am J Surg Pathol 1985; 9:543.

Level III

Borer JG, Tan PE, Diamond DA: The spectrum of Sertoli cell tumors in children. Urol Clin North Am 2000;27:529.

Fleischer AC: Transabdominal and transvaginal sonography of ovarian masses. Clin Obstet Gynecol 1991;34:433.

Roth LM: Recent advances in the pathology and classification of ovarian sex cord-stromal tumors. Int J Gynecol Pathol 2006; 25:199.

Young RH, Scully RE: Ovarian sex cord-stromal tumours: recent advances and current status. Clin Obstet Gynaecol 1984;11:93.

INTRODUCTION

Description: A transitional cell (Brenner) tumor is an epithelial tumor that is made up of cells that resemble urothelium and Walthard's cell nests, intermixed with the ovarian stroma. Most are benign.

Prevalence: One percent to 3% of ovarian tumors.

Predominant Age: 40 to 80, average 50.

Genetics: No genetic pattern.

ETIOLOGY AND PATHOGENESIS

Causes: Unknown. Most are derived from ovarian surface epithelium that undergoes metaplasia to form the typical urothelial-like components.

Risk Factors: None known.

CLINICAL CHARACTERISTICS

Signs and Symptoms

* Asymptomatic (often an incidental finding after oophorectomy)
* Adnexal mass, generally solid, most smaller than 2 cm, bilateral in 6% (unilateral lesions are more common in the left ovary)
* Abdominal pain and swelling, with abnormal uterine bleeding (20%) if malignant disease (malignant masses are more likely to be large [10 to 30 cm] and contain cystic areas; when the ovary is palpably enlarged, the risk of malignancy is approximately 5%)

DIAGNOSTIC APPROACH

Differential Diagnosis

* Thecoma (fibroma)
* Stromal and germ cell tumors
* Endometrioma
* Benign cystic teratoma
* Serous or mucinous cystadenoma
* Metastatic tumors
* Pedunculated leiomyomata

Associated Conditions: Malignant tumors are associated with endometrial hyperplasia.

WORKUP AND EVALUATION

Laboratory: No specific evaluation indicated.

Imaging: No imaging indicated. Ultrasonography may be used to differentiate solid and cystic adnexal masses, but it does not establish the diagnosis.

Special Tests: None indicated.

Diagnostic Tests: Histopathologic evaluation.

Pathologic Findings

Cells that resemble transitional epithelium of the bladder and Walthard's cells of the ovary with abundant stroma. The cut surface of the tumor is generally whorled or lobulated. The nests of cells often demonstrate nuclei with obvious nucleoli-containing longitudinal grooves, giving them a "coffee-bean" appearance. Atypia and mitoses are rare. Occasionally, small transitional cell tumors may be found in the walls of otherwise-typical mucinous cystademonas. Atypical or malignant forms may be associated with similar bladder tumors.

MANAGEMENT AND THERAPY

Nonpharmacologic

General Measures: Evaluation and diagnosis.

Specific Measures: Simple surgical excision. When changes associated with borderline malignant potential are present, bilateral oophorectomy with hysterectomy is sufficient, and unilateral oophorectomy may be considered in younger patients.

Diet: No specific dietary changes indicated.

Activity: No restriction.

Patient Education: Reassurance; American College of Obstetricians and Gynecologists Patient Education Pamphlet AP075 (Ovarian Cysts), AP096 (Cancer of the Ovary).

Drug(s) of Choice

None.

FOLLOW-UP

Patient Monitoring: Normal health maintenance.

Prevention/Avoidance: None.

Possible Complications: The rare malignant form has a poor prognosis despite surgical therapy. Chemotherapy has not been proved to be effective.

Expected Outcome: Most Brenner tumors are benign and are cured by simple oophorectomy.

MISCELLANEOUS

Pregnancy Considerations: No effect on pregnancy.

ICD-9-CM Codes: 220, 236.2 (Borderline or proliferative), 183.0 (Malignant).

REFERENCES

Level II

de Lima GR, de Lima OA, Baracat EC, et al: Virilizing Brenner tumor of the ovary: case report. Obstet Gynecol 1989;73:895.

Rufford BD, Jacobs IJ, Menon U: Feasibility of screening for ovarian cancer using symptoms as selection criteria. BJOG 2007;114:59.

Silverberg SG: Brenner tumor of the ovary. A clinicopathologic study of 60 tumors in 54 women. Cancer 1971;28:588.

Yang DM, Heller DS, Ganesh V, Gittens L: Brenner tumor of the ovary with extensive stromal luteinization presenting in pregnancy: report of a case and review of the literature. J Matern Fetal Neonatal Med 2002;12:281.

Yoshida M, Obayashi C, Tachibana M, Minami R: Coexisting Brenner tumor and struma ovarii in the right ovary: case report and review of the literature. Pathol Int 2004;54:793.

Level III

Austin RM, Norris HJ: Malignant Brenner tumors and transitional cell carcinoma of the ovary. Int J Gynecol Pathol 1987;6:29.

Chen KT, Hoffmann KD: Malignant Brenner tumor of the ovary. J Surg Oncol 1988;39:260.

Hampton HL, Huffman HT, Meeks GR: Extraovarian Brenner tumor. Obstet Gynecol 1992;79:844.

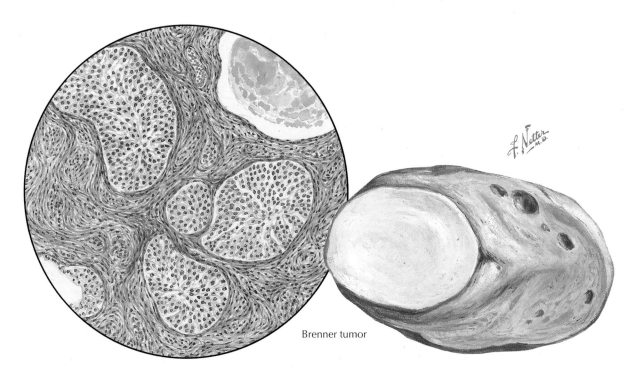

Brenner tumor

Miles PA, Norris HJ: Proliferative and malignant Brenner tumors of the ovary. Cancer 1972;30:174.

Oùtwater EK, Siegelman ES, Kim B, et al: Ovarian Brenner tumors: MR imaging characteristics. Magn Reson Imaging 1998;16:1147.

Roth LM, Czernobilsky B: Ovarian Brenner tumors. II: Malignant. Cancer 1985;56:592.

Roth LM, Dallenbach-Hellweg G, Czernobilsky B: Ovarian Brenner tumors. I: Metaplastic, proliferating and of low malignant potential. Cancer 1985;56:582.

Roth LM, Gersell DJ, Ulbright TM: Ovarian Brenner tumors and transitional cell carcinoma: recent developments. Int J Gynecol Pathol 1993;12:128.

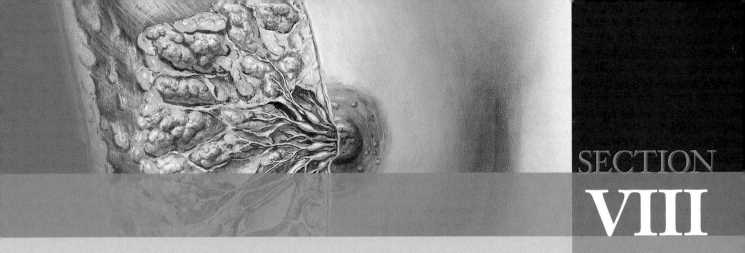

Breast Diseases and Conditions

INTRODUCTION

Description: Accessory nipples are supernumerary nipples found along defined developmental lines known as the "milk lines."

Prevalence: Seen in 0.22% to 2.5% of women and in up to 5% to 6% of Asian women.

Predominant Age: Congenital in origin.

Genetics: No genetic pattern.

ETIOLOGY AND PATHOGENESIS

Causes: Developmental abnormality.

Risk Factors: More common in males and in African Americans.

CLINICAL CHARACTERISTICS

Signs and Symptoms

- Asymptomatic
- Most commonly found below a normal left breast. It is more common to have one or more extra nipples (polythelia) than to have true accessory breasts (polymastia).

DIAGNOSTIC APPROACH

Differential Diagnosis

- Skin papilloma
- Nevis

Associated Conditions: Polymastia, duplicate renal arteries.

WORKUP AND EVALUATION

Laboratory: No evaluation indicated.

Imaging: No imaging indicated.

Special Tests: None indicated.

Diagnostic Procedures: History, physical examination.

Pathologic Findings

None.

MANAGEMENT AND THERAPY

Nonpharmacologic

General Measures: Evaluation and reassurance.

Specific Measures: None.

Diet: No specific dietary changes indicated.

Activity: No restriction.

Patient Education: Reassurance, instruction on monthly breast self-examination; American College of Obstetricians and Gynecologists Patient Education Pamphlet AP026 (Detecting and Treating Breast Problems).

Drug(s) of Choice

None.

FOLLOW-UP

Patient Monitoring: Normal health maintenance.

Prevention/Avoidance: None.

MISCELLANEOUS

Pregnancy Considerations: No effect on pregnancy, although occasionally accessory nipples undergo hypertrophy during pregnancy.

ICD-9-CM Codes: 757.6.

REFERENCES

Level II

Brown J, Schwartz RA: Supernumerary nipples and renal malformations: a family study. J Cutan Med Surg 2004;8:170. Epub 2004 May 13.

Casey HD, Chasan PE, Chick LR: Familial polythelia without associated anomalies. Ann Plast Surg 1996;36:101.

Level III

American College of Obstetricians and Gynecologists: Breast concerns in the adolescent. ACOG Committee Opinion 350. Obstet Gynecol 2006;108:1329.

Newman M: Supernumerary nipples. Am Fam Physician 1988;38: 183.

Smith RP: Gynecology in primary care. Baltimore, Williams & Wilkins, 1997, p319.

Valea FA, Katz VL: Breast diseases. In Katz VL, Lentz GM, Lobo RA, Gershenson DM. Comprehensive Gynecology, 5th ed. Philadelphia, Mosby/Elsevier, 2007:330.

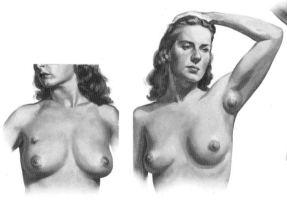

Polythelia   Polymastia   The milk lines

INTRODUCTION

Description: Breast cancer is a malignant neoplasm of the breast classified by cell type, location, and degree of invasion. Breast cancer is the most common malignancy of women, accounting for almost one third of all women's malignancies. Breast cancer accounts for approximately 18% of cancer deaths and results in about the same number of deaths per year as auto accidents.

Prevalence: Lifetime risk of 1 in 8 by age 90, >212,000 new cases, lifetime risk of death of 1 in 28, >40,000 deaths annually (2006). Roughly one new case of breast cancer is diagnosed every 3 minutes, and every 13 minutes there is a breast cancer death.

Predominant Age: Of all breast cancer cases, 85% occur after age 40 and 75% occur after age 50.

Genetics: Women with BRCA1 mutations have a 60% lifetime risk of breast cancer (BRCA2 mutations carry an 85% risk of breast cancer and up to 20% risk of ovarian cancer). Only 20% of patients with breast cancer have a family history of breast cancer. African-American women have a lower incidence of breast cancer (119.4/100,000 versus 141.1/100,000 for white women) but they have a higher mortality rate (34.7/100,000 versus 25.9/100,000).

ETIOLOGY AND PATHOGENESIS

Causes: Unknown.

Risk Factors: First-degree relative with breast cancer (relative risk [RR] = 2.3, RR = 10.5 with bilateral disease), moderate alcohol use (>3 to 5 drinks/day, RR = 1.41), early menarche, late menopause, nulliparity or late first pregnancy (>30 years), prior history of breast cancer (5%/year), estrogen use (RR = 1.12). Only 21% of patients with breast cancer age 30 to 54 years are identified by risk factors.

CLINICAL CHARACTERISTICS

Signs and Symptoms

- Palpable mass (55%), 60% located in the upper outer quadrant of the breast
- Abnormal mammogram without a palpable mass (35%)
- Skin change—color or dimpling (peau d'orange)
- Nipple retraction (nipple discharge [bloody or otherwise], skin changes, or ulceration are late occurrences and portend a bad prognosis)
- Axillary mass
- Breast pain is present in <10% of women with early breast cancer

DIAGNOSTIC APPROACH

Differential Diagnosis

- Benign breast disease (abscess, fat necrosis, fibrocystic disease, fibroadenomas).
- **Associated Conditions:** Metastatic spread to other organs (bone, brain, and ovaries).

Workup and Evaluation

Laboratory: Complete blood count and assessment of liver and bone enzymes after diagnosis is made.

Imaging: Mammography (detects 80% of all tumors), ultrasonography (may help to differentiate between solid and cystic masses), bone scan, and chest radiograph after diagnosis is established. Recent evidence suggests that for women with a lifetime risk that exceeds 20%, magnetic resonance imaging (MRI) screening may be beneficial. Digital radiography, thermal imaging (thermography), transillumination, mammoscintigraphy, ductography, and other techniques have not been shown to be comparable or superior to mammography.

Special Tests: Fine needle aspiration (FNA) of cells from a breast mass can provide histologic confirmation of malignancy and help direct definitive therapy.

Diagnostic Procedures: One fourth of all breast cancers are found during routine examination. Excisional biopsy with or without radiographic control provides the only definitive diagnosis.

Pathologic Findings

Based on cell type. At the time of diagnosis, 70% of breast cancers show signs of invasion. Ductal carcinoma is the most common type, accounting for 65% to 85% of cases.

MANAGEMENT AND THERAPY

Nonpharmacologic

General Measures: Evaluation and staging. If surgical treatment affects pectoralis muscles, physical or occupational therapy may speed return to function.

Specific Measures: Surgical resection with or without adjunctive chemotherapy.

Diet: Moderation in alcohol use recommended to reduce risk.

Activity: No restriction.

Patient Education: Instruction on monthly breast self-examination; American College of Obstetricians and Gynecologists Patient Education Pamphlet AP145 (Breast Self-Examination), AP026 (Detecting and Treating Breast Problems), AP076 (Mammography). (Despite a lack of definitive data for or against breast self-examination, its use has the potential to detect palpable breast cancer and can be recommended.)

Drug(s) of Choice

Adjuvant chemotherapy considered for stage I and II disease (cyclophosphamide, methotrexate, fluorouracil, anthracyclines, or taxanes, single agent or in combination).

Contraindications: Strict guidelines for hepatic and renal function before chemotherapy.

Precautions: Increased risk of infection during chemotherapy.

ALTERNATIVE THERAPY

Adjunctive or palliative radiation therapy is often recommended. Agents that suppress cancer growth by interfering with surface proteins that are involved with cell division are under evaluation. An example of this approach is trastuzumab (Herceptin), approved by the U.S. Food and Drug Administration (FDA) in 1998.

A number of studies suggest that estrogen therapy (for other indications) may actually reduce the mortality of patients who are being treated for breast cancer.

FOLLOW-UP

Patient Monitoring: Watch for recurrence (60% risk in first 5 years).

Prevention/Avoidance: Reduced dietary fat and alcohol have been suggested, but effects are unproven. Routine mammography. Prophylactic use of tamoxifen was approved by the Food and Drug Administration late in 1998 for use in women at high risk. Selective estrogen receptor modulators (SERMs) have been effective in reducing the incidence of recurrence or the development of primary lesions for those at increased risk.

Possible Complications: Postoperative lymphedema, seroma, wound infections, or breakdown. Chemotherapy associated with nausea, vomiting, alopecia, leukopenia, stomatitis, fatigue, and infections. Tamoxifen therapy associated with hot flashes, menstrual irregularity, endometrial hyperplasia, or carcinoma. Radiation therapy associated with fibrosis and scarring, brachial neuropathy, and pulmonary fibrosis.

Expected Outcome: Breast cancer disseminates by vascular and lymphatic routes, in addition to direct infiltration. There is also a growing trend to view breast cancer as a multifocal disease. Breast cancer survival depends less on cell type than it does on the size of the tumor and stage of disease. Ten-year survival based on stage: stage I, 95%; stage II, 40%; stage III, 15%; and stage IV (metastatic), 0%.

MISCELLANEOUS

Pregnancy Considerations: Breast cancer occurs infrequently during pregnancy, accounting for only 2% to 3% of all cancers: no effect on pregnancy. Pregnancy often results in a delay in diagnosis but does not appreciably affect clinical course.

ICD-9-CM Codes: 174.

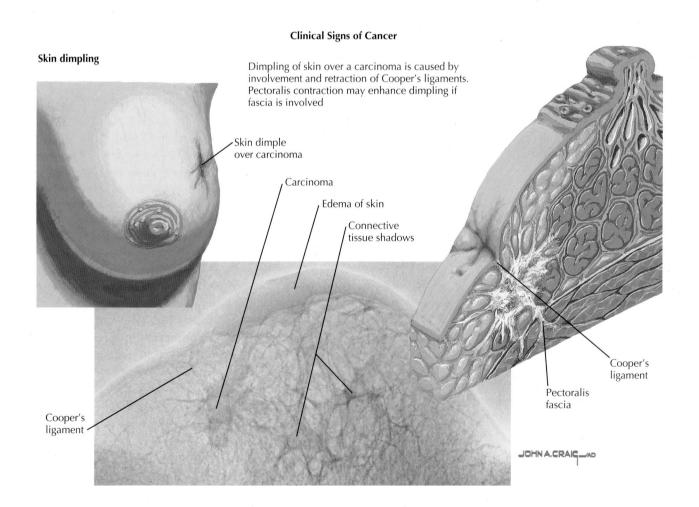

Clinical Signs of Cancer

Skin dimpling

Dimpling of skin over a carcinoma is caused by involvement and retraction of Cooper's ligaments. Pectoralis contraction may enhance dimpling if fascia is involved

Skin dimple over carcinoma

Carcinoma

Edema of skin

Connective tissue shadows

Cooper's ligament

Cooper's ligament

Pectoralis fascia

JOHN A. CRAIG—AD

Needle Biopsy

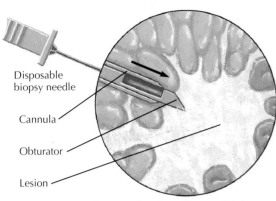
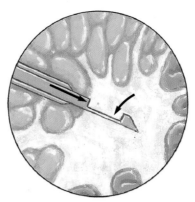
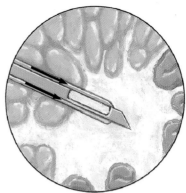

Disposable biopsy needle

Cannula

Obturator

Lesion

1. Closed needle assembly is advanced to edge of lesion

2. Obturator tip is advanced into lesion. Tissue prolapses into open specimen notch

3. Cannula is advanced over obturator, entrapping tissue specimen within notch. Needle is withdrawn

Vascular signs

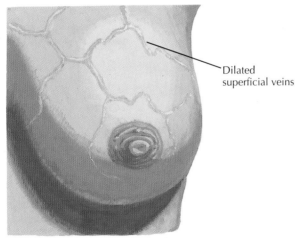

Dilated superficial veins

Fast-growing tumor with large vascular demand may cause dilation of superficial veins, creating prominent vascular pattern over breast

Skin edema

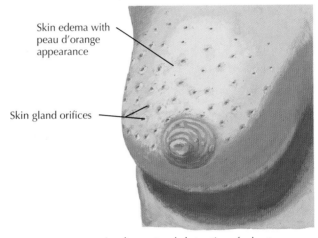

Skin edema with peau d'orange appearance

Skin gland orifices

Involvement and obstruction of subcutaneous lymphatics by tumor result in lymphatic dilation and lymph accumulation in the skin. Resultant edema creates "orange peel" appearance because of prominence of skin gland orifices

JOHN A.CRAIG—AD

REFERENCES

Level I

Butler JA, Vargas HI, Worthen N, Wilson SE: Accuracy of combined clinical-mammographic-cytologic diagnosis of dominant breast masses: a prospective study. Arch Surg 1990;125:893.

Geyer CE, Forster J, Lindquist D, et al: Lapatinib plus capecitabine for HER2-positive advanced breast cancer. N Engl J Med 2006;355:2733.

Moss SM, Cuckle H, Evans A, et al; Trial Management Group: Effect of mammographic screening from age 40 years on breast cancer mortality at 10 years' follow-up: a randomised controlled trial. Lancet 2006;368:2053.

Pritchard KI, Shepherd LE, O'Malley FP, et al; National Cancer Institute of Canada Clinical Trials Group: HER2 and responsiveness of breast cancer to adjuvant chemotherapy. N Engl J Med 2006;354:2103.

Stefanick ML, Anderson GL, Margolis KL, et al; WHI Investigators: Effects of conjugated equine estrogens on breast cancer and mammography screening in postmenopausal women with hysterectomy. JAMA 2006;295:1647.

Vogel VG, Costantino JP, Wickerham DL, et al; National Surgical Adjuvant Breast and Bowel Project (NSABP): Effects of tamoxifen vs raloxifene on the risk of developing invasive breast cancer and other disease outcomes: the NSABP Study of Tamoxifen and Raloxifene (STAR) P-2 trial. JAMA 2006;295:2727. Epub 2006 Jun 5.

Level II

Armstrong K, Moye E, Williams S, et al: Screening mammography in women 40 to 49 years of age: a systematic review for the American College of Physicians. Ann Intern Med 2007;146:516.

Coombs NJ, Taylor R, Wilcken N, Boyages J: Hormone replacement therapy and breast cancer: estimate of risk. BMJ 2005;331:347.

Lacey JV Jr, Greene MH, Buys SS, et al: Ovarian cancer screening in women with a family history of breast or ovarian cancer. Obstet Gynecol 2006;108:1176.

Lehman CD, Gatsonis C, Kuhl CK, et al; ACRIN Trial 6667 Investigators Group: MRI evaluation of the contralateral breast in women with recently diagnosed breast cancer. N Engl J Med 2007;356:1295. Epub 2007 Mar 28.

Punglia RS, Morrow M, Winer EP, Harris JR: Local therapy and survival in breast cancer. N Engl J Med 2007;356:2399.

Ries LAG, Harkins D, Krapcho M, et al: SEER Cancer Statistics Review, 1975–2003. Bethesda, MD, National Cancer Institute, 2006.

Schell MJ, Yankaskas BC, Ballard-Barbash R, et al: Evidence-based target recall rates for screening mammography. Radiology 2007;243:681.

Level III

American College of Obstetricians and Gynecologists: Breast cancer screening. ACOG Practice Bulletin 42. Obstet Gynecol 2003;101:821.

American College of Obstetricians and Gynecologists: Role of the obstetrician–gynecologist in the screening and diagnosis of breast masses. ACOG Committee Opinion 334. Obstet Gynecol 2005;106:1141.

Bartella L, Smith CS, Dershaw DD, Liberman L: Imaging breast cancer. Radiol Clin North Am 2007;45:45.

Barthelmes L, Davidson LA, Gaffney C, Gateley CA: Pregnancy and breast cancer. BMJ 2005;330:1375.

Elmore JG, Armstrong K, Lehman CD, Fletcher SW: Screening for breast cancer. JAMA 2005;293:1245.

Fletcher SW, Black W, Harris R, et al: Report of the International Workshop on Screening for Breast Cancer. Bethesda, MD, National Cancer Institute, 1993.

Hayes DF: Clinical practice. Follow-up of patients with early breast cancer. N Engl J Med 2007;356:2505.

Loibl S, von Minckwitz G, Gwyn K, et al: Breast carcinoma during pregnancy. International recommendations from an expert meeting. Cancer 2006;106:237.

Saslow D, Boetes C, Burke W, et al; American Cancer Society Breast Cancer Advisory Group: American Cancer Society guidelines for breast screening with MRI as an adjunct to mammography. CA Cancer J Clin 2007;57:75.

Smith I, Chua S: Medical treatment of early breast cancer. III: Chemotherapy. BMJ 2006;332:161.

Smith I, Chua S: Medical treatment of early breast cancer. IV: Neoadjuvant treatment. BMJ 2006;332:223.

Valea FA, Katz VL: Breast diseases. In Katz VL, Lentz GM, Lobo RA, Gershenson DM. Comprehensive Gynecology, 5th ed. Philadelphia, Mosby/Elsevier, 2007. p 334.

Veronesi U, Boyle P, Goldhirsch A, et al: Breast cancer. Lancet 2005;365:1727.

THE CHALLENGE

Cystic breast masses are frequently encountered in the clinical care of women. Sorting out those that represent a threat from those that may be followed conservatively is the challenge posed by the presence of breast cysts.

Scope of the Problem: Some authors estimate that cysts form in the breasts of roughly 50% of women during their reproductive years. Roughly one in four women requires medical attention for some form of breast problem; often this takes the form of a palpable mass. The most common cause of a palpable breast cyst is fibrocystic change, which is estimated to be found in one third to three fourths of all women. Dilation of ducts and complications of breastfeeding (galactoceles, abscess) may also cause cysts.

Objectives: To appropriately diagnose and treat patients with a cystic breast, to allay fear, and to protect health.

TACTICS

Relevant Pathophysiology: The pathogenesis is not clear for the most common types of cystic change (those associated with fibrocystic change). Cyclic changes in hormones induce stromal and epithelial changes that may lead to fibrosis and cyst formation. Cysts may be single or in clusters, with some as large as 4 cm in diameter. Small cysts have a firm character and are filled with clear fluid, giving the cyst a bluish cast. Larger cysts may have a brown color resulting from hemorrhage into the cyst. Inspissated secretions or milk may form a cystic dilation of ducts (galactocele, ductal ectasia) that may be palpable as a cystic mass. Variable degrees of fibrosis and inflammation may be seen in the surrounding stroma. (Leakage of cyst fluid into the surrounding tissue induces an inflammatory response that may alter physical findings and imitate cancer.) The microscopic findings associated with breast cysts depend on the pathophysiologic changes involved.

Strategies: The diagnosis and management of cystic masses in the breast are based on history, physical examination, and aspiration, with the occasional adjunctive use of mammography and ultrasonography. (Ultrasonography is useful in differentiating solid and cystic breast masses but it has limited spatial resolution and cannot be used to differentiate benign and malignant tissues.) Needle aspiration with a 22- to 25-gauge needle may be both diagnostic and therapeutic. If the cyst disappears completely and does not re-form by 1-month follow-up examination, no further therapy is required. Fluid aspirated from patients with fibrocystic changes is customarily straw colored. Fluid that is dark brown or green occurs in cysts that have been present for a long time, but it is innocuous. Bloody fluid requires further evaluation. Cytologic evaluation of the fluid obtained is of little value. After aspiration of a cyst, the patient should be rechecked in 2 to 4 weeks. Recurrence of the cyst or the presence of a palpable mass should prompt additional evaluation, such as fine needle aspiration (FNA) or open biopsy.

Patient Education: Instruction on monthly breast self-examination; American College of Obstetricians and Gynecologists Patient Education Pamphlet AP026 (Detecting and Treating Breast Problems), AP145 (Breast Self-Examination), AP076 (Mammography).

IMPLEMENTATION

Special Considerations: Whereas most cystic changes in the breast are not associated with malignancy and are not premalignant, the presence of atypia in any of the cellular components requires special attention because this is associated with a roughly 5-fold increased risk for malignancy. In women older than 35 years, mammography before aspiration should be considered because of the increased incidence of malignancy. Once aspiration has been attempted, mammography should be delayed several weeks because of artifactual changes induced by the manipulation, making mammograms difficult to interpret. Patients with a history of multiple cysts or diffuse fibrocystic change or a strong family history of breast disease should have close follow-up, including mammography, to delve for other occult lesions.

REFERENCES

Level II
Devitt JE, To T, Miller AB: Risk of breast cancer in women with breast cysts. CMAJ 1992;147:45.

Level III
American College of Obstetricians and Gynecologists: Role of the obstetrician–gynecologist in the screening and diagnosis of breast masses. ACOG Committee Opinion 334. Obstet Gynecol 2005;106:1141.

American College of Obstetricians and Gynecologists: Breast concerns in the adolescent. ACOG Committee Opinion 350. Obstet Gynecol 2006;108:1329.

Donegan WL: Evaluation of a palpable breast mass. N Engl J Med 1992;327:937.

Ferguson CM, Powel RW: Breast masses in young women. Arch Surg 1989;124:1338.

Lucas JH, Cone DL: Breast cyst aspiration. Am Fam Physician 2003;68:1983.

Morrow M: The evaluation of common breast problems. Am Fam Physician 2000;61:2371, 2385.

Santen RJ, Mansel R: Benign breast disorders. N Engl J Med 2005;353:275.

Seltzer MH, Skiles MS: Disease of the breast in young women. Surg Gynecol Obstet 1980;150:360.

Smith RP. Gynecology in primary care. Baltimore, Williams & Wilkins, 1997:319.

Smith RP, Ling FW: Procedures in women's health. Baltimore, Williams & Wilkins, 1997, p 37.

Valea FA, Katz VL: Breast diseases. In Katz VL, Lentz GM, Lobo RA, Gershenson DM. Comprehensive Gynecology, 5th ed. Philadelphia, Mosby/Elsevier, 2007, p 330.

Aspiration

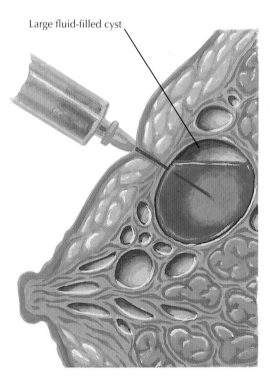

Large fluid-filled cyst

A 22- or 25-gauge needle is advanced
into cyst. Fluid is aspirated and sent
for cytologic examination

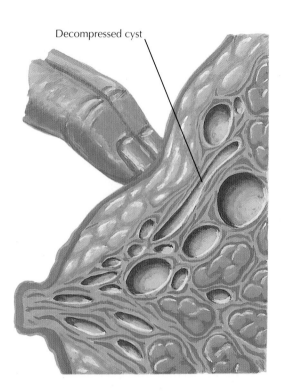

Decompressed cyst

Aspiration should decompress the
cyst unless wall is exceedingly thick

JOHN A.CRAIG⌐ᴀᴅ

INTRODUCTION

Description: Duct ectasia is dilation of the ducts of the breast with inspissation of normal secretions, arising from chronic intraductal and periductal inflammation.

Prevalence: Relatively common in asymptomatic form.

Predominant Age: Older than 50.

Genetics: No genetic pattern.

ETIOLOGY AND PATHOGENESIS

Causes: Chronic intraductal and periductal inflammation.

Risk Factors: Mastitis, breast abscess.

CLINICAL CHARACTERISTICS

Signs and Symptoms

- Thick gray to black nipple discharge
- Pain and nipple tenderness
- Thickening often present; may be difficult to distinguish from cancer (firm, rounded, and fixed, with skin retraction)
- Nipple retraction common (ductal ectasia is the most common cause of an acquired nipple inversion)

DIAGNOSTIC APPROACH

Differential Diagnosis

- Galactocele
- Lipoma
- Fibrocystic change
- Fibroadenoma
- Breast abscess

Associated Conditions: Mastitis, galactocele, and nipple discharge.

Workup and Evaluation

Laboratory: No evaluation indicated.

Imaging: No imaging indicated.

Special Tests: None indicated.

Diagnostic Procedures: History and physical examination; biopsy confirms the diagnosis. (The characteristic discharge may easily be demonstrated during clinical examination.)

Pathologic Findings

Dilation of the ducts with atrophy of the epithelium, thickening of the underlying wall, and inflammatory reaction in the duct wall and surrounding tissue.

MANAGEMENT AND THERAPY

Nonpharmacologic

General Measures: Evaluation and reassurance.

Specific Measures: No further therapy is needed unless warranted by the patient's symptoms. When therapy is required, surgical excision with a cone of tissue surrounding the duct is curative.

Diet: No specific dietary changes indicated.

Activity: No restriction.

Patient Education: Instruction on monthly breast self-examination; American College of Obstetricians and Gynecologists Patient Education Pamphlet AP026 (Detecting and Treating Breast Problems), AP145 (Breast Self-Examination), AP076 (Mammography).

Drug(s) of Choice

None.

FOLLOW-UP

Patient Monitoring: Normal health maintenance.

Prevention/Avoidance: None.

Possible Complications: Secondary infection and abscess formation.

Expected Outcome: Gradual resolution of symptoms, complete resolution with surgical excision.

MISCELLANEOUS

Pregnancy Considerations: No effect on pregnancy.

ICD-9-CM Codes: 610.4.

REFERENCES

Level II

Duchesne N, Skolnik S, Bilmer S: Ultrasound appearance of chronic mammary duct ectasia. Can Assoc Radiol J 2005;56:297.

Rahal RM, de Freitas-Junior R, Paulinelli RR: Risk factors for duct ectasia. Breast J 2005;11:262.

Richards T, Hunt A, Courtney S, Umeh H: Nipple discharge: a sign of breast cancer? Ann R Coll Surg Engl 2007;89:124.

Level III

Dixon JM: Periductal mastitis/duct ectasia. World J Surg 1989;13:715.

Hamed H, Fentiman IS: Benign breast disease. Int J Clin Pract 2001;55:461.

Hughes LE: Non-lactational inflammation and duct ectasia. Br Med Bull 1991;47:272.

Santen RJ, Mansel R: Benign breast disorders. N Engl J Med 2005;353:275.

Seltzer MH, Skiles MS: Disease of the breast in young women. Surg Gynecol Obstet 1980;150:360.

Mammary Duct Ectasia

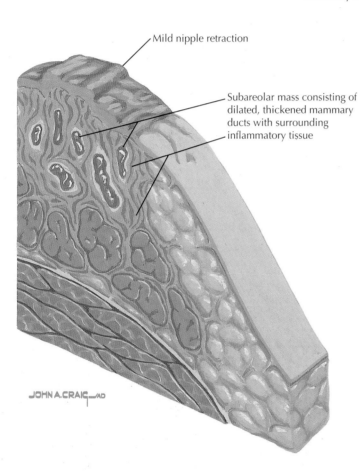

Mild nipple retraction

Subareolar mass consisting of dilated, thickened mammary ducts with surrounding inflammatory tissue

JOHN A. CRAIG—AD

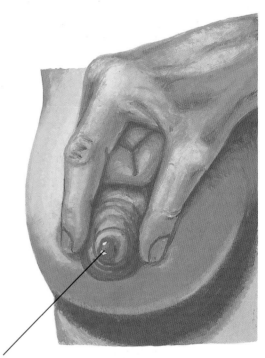

Thick, sticky, green to greenish-black discharge suggests mammary duct ectasia. Associated subareolar mass and/or nipple retraction may also be present. Treatment requires major mammary duct excision, including the surrounding inflammatory tissue

INTRODUCTION

Description: Trauma to the breast may result in necrosis of fatty tissues, leading to an ill-defined mass that can mimic cancer.
Prevalence: Uncommon.
Predominant Age: Reproductive.
Genetics: No genetic pattern.

ETIOLOGY AND PATHOGENESIS

Causes: Fat necrosis is most often the result of trauma, although the causative event cannot be identified (or recalled) in roughly one half of patients. May also follow surgical intervention in the breast, such as biopsy or augmentation.
Risk Factors: Trauma to the breast.

CLINICAL CHARACTERISTICS

Signs and Symptoms

- Solitary, irregular, ill-defined, tender mass that is easily confused with cancer
- Skin retraction sometimes present
- Fine, stippled calcification and stellate or infiltrative fibrosis often seen on mammograms

DIAGNOSTIC APPROACH

Differential Diagnosis

- Cancer
- Lipoma

Associated Conditions: Mastalgia.

Workup and Evaluation

Laboratory: No evaluation indicated.
Imaging: Mammography findings mimic cancer.
Special Tests: Open biopsy often required to establish the diagnosis.
Diagnostic Procedures: Even with a history of trauma, the commonality of findings between fat necrosis and cancer with physical examination, mammography, and ultrasonography generally mandates further evaluation and biopsy.

Pathologic Findings

Diffuse changes consistent with necrosis and fibrosis of tissue. Hemorrhage and cystic spaces are common. Calcification of older lesions may occur. Histiocytic foam cells with mitotic figures and pleomorphism are common.

MANAGEMENT AND THERAPY

Nonpharmacologic

General Measures: Evaluation.
Specific Measures: Excisional biopsy.
Diet: No specific dietary changes indicated.
Activity: No restriction.
Patient Education: Instruction on monthly breast self-examination; American College of Obstetricians and Gynecologists Patient Education Pamphlet AP026 (Detecting and Treating Breast Problems), AP145 (Breast Self-Examination), AP076 (Mammography).

Drug(s) of Choice

None.

FOLLOW-UP

Patient Monitoring: Normal health maintenance, periodic mammography screening.
Prevention/Avoidance: Minimize the risk of trauma.
Possible Complications: An occult malignancy may be missed if a mass is presumed to be fat necrosis without tissue evaluation for confirmation.
Expected Outcome: With excision, complete resolution.

MISCELLANEOUS

Pregnancy Considerations: No effect on pregnancy.
ICD-9-CM Codes: 611.3.

REFERENCES

Level II
Chala LF, de Barros N, de Camargo Moraes P, et al: Fat necrosis of the breast: mammographic, sonographic, computed tomography, and magnetic resonance imaging findings. Curr Probl Diagn Radiol 2004;33:106.
Gatta G, Pinto A, Romano S, et al: Clinical, mammographic and ultrasonographic features of blunt breast trauma. Eur J Radiol 2006;59:327. Epub 2006 Jun 19.

Level III
Osuch JR: Benign lesions of the breast other than fibrocystic change. Obstet Gynecol Clin North Am 1987;14:703.
Santen RJ, Mansel R: Benign breast disorders. N Engl J Med 2005;353:275.
Seltzer MH, Skiles MS: Disease of the breast in young women. Surg Gynecol Obstet 1980;150:360.
Tan PH, Lai LM, Carrington EV, et al: Fat necrosis of the breast—A review. Breast 2006;15:313. Epub 2005 Sep 29.

Fat Necrosis of Breast

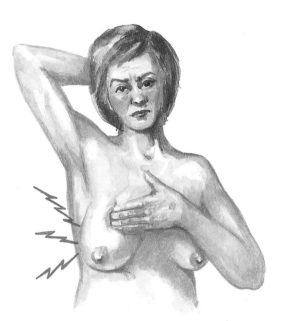

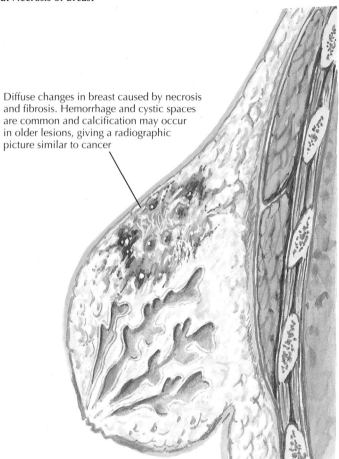

Diffuse changes in breast caused by necrosis and fibrosis. Hemorrhage and cystic spaces are common and calcification may occur in older lesions, giving a radiographic picture similar to cancer

Trauma to breast may result in fat necrosis, an ill-defined, irregular, tender mass that may be confused with cancer both clinically and radiographically

JOHN A. CRAIG—MD

D. Mascaro

Excision Biopsy for Fat Necrosis

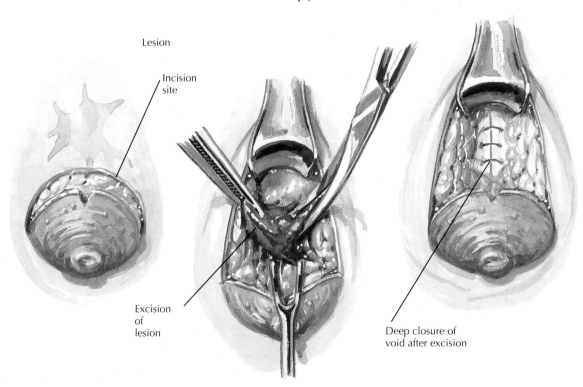

Lesion

Incision site

Excision of lesion

Deep closure of void after excision

Excisional biopsy indicated to confirm diagnosis and rule out cancer

INTRODUCTION

Description: Fibroadenomas are the second most common form of breast disease and the most common breast mass.

Prevalence: Two percent to three percent of women (some state as many as 25% of all women).

Predominant Age: 21 to 25, most younger than 30.

Genetics: No genetic pattern.

ETIOLOGY AND PATHOGENESIS

Causes: Unknown.

Risk Factors: Twice as common in African-American women (30% of breast complaints), patients with high hormone states (adolescence, pregnancy), and patients receiving unopposed estrogen therapy.

CLINICAL CHARACTERISTICS

Signs and Symptoms

- Firm, painless, mobile, rubbery, solitary breast mass (may grow rapidly during adolescence or in high-estrogen states [pregnancy, estrogen therapy])
- Generally discovered incidentally or during breast self-examination and average 2 to 3 cm in diameter; fibroadenomas may grow to as large as 6 to 10 cm
- Multiple fibroadenomas in 15% to 20% of patients; bilateral in 10% to 20% of patients
- Generally undergo no cyclic change

DIAGNOSTIC APPROACH

Differential Diagnosis

- Fibrocystic change
- Solitary cyst

Associated Conditions: None.

Workup and Evaluation

Laboratory: No evaluation indicated.

Imaging: Mammography is generally avoided but can be diagnostic if needed. Breast ultrasonography can distinguish between solid and cystic masses, although it is often not required.

Special Tests: Fine needle aspiration (FNA) of the mass may be performed in the office.

Diagnostic Procedures: History and physical examination.

Pathologic Findings

Centrifugal nodule with sharply circumscribed, fleshy, and homogeneous character, usually spherical or ovoid in shape. Pink or tan–white fibrous whorls bulge from the surface when cut. Hemorrhagic infarcts are common.

MANAGEMENT AND THERAPY

Nonpharmacologic

General Measures: Reassurance and observation may be sufficient for small, asymptomatic tumors.

Specific Measures: Primary therapy is surgical excision, although tamoxifen and danazol have been used. Cyroablative therapy has been evaluated but has not displaced surgery as the primary management.

Diet: No specific dietary changes indicated.

Activity: No restriction.

Patient Education: Instruction on monthly breast self-examination; American College of Obstetricians and Gynecologists Patient Education Pamphlet AP026 (Detecting and Treating Breast Problems), AP145 (Breast Self-Examination), AP076 (Mammography).

Drug(s) of Choice

Danazol sodium 50 to 200 mg PO twice a day (therapy should start during menstruation or pregnancy must be ruled out). Side effects may be significant and recurrence is likely after therapy is discontinued.

Contraindications: Danazol sodium is contraindicated in pregnancy (category X drug). It may also worsen epilepsy, migraine headaches, and cardiac or renal function.

Interactions: Danazol sodium may prolong prothrombin time in patients receiving warfarin.

Alternative Drugs

Tamoxifen has been advocated in some studies.

FOLLOW-UP

Patient Monitoring: Normal health maintenance.

Prevention/Avoidance: Combination oral contraceptives provide some protection when taken for longer than 1 year.

Possible Complications: Hemorrhage into the fibroadenoma may result in pain or rapid growth of the tumor. Malignant change is extremely rare.

Expected Outcome: Lesions tend to grow over time without treatment. Prognosis with surgical excision is excellent and fair with medical therapy. After menopause, fibroadenomas tend to regress and become hyalinized, but they may remain unchanged or grow with estrogen replacement therapy.

MISCELLANEOUS

Pregnancy Considerations: No effect on pregnancy; fibroadenomas may grow rapidly during pregnancy.

ICD-9-CM Codes: 217.

REFERENCES

Level II

Alle KM, Moss J, Venegas RJ, et al: Conservative management of fibroadenoma of the breast. Br J Surg 1996;83:992.

El-Wakeel H, Umpleby HC: Systematic review of fibroadenoma as a risk factor for breast cancer. Breast 2003;12:302.

Littrup PJ, Freeman-Gibb L, Andea A, et al: Cryotherapy for breast fibroadenomas. Radiology 2005;234:63. Epub 2004 Nov 18.

Nurko J, Mabry CD, Whitworth P, et al: Interim results from the FibroAdenoma Cryoablation Treatment Registry. Am J Surg 2005;190:647.

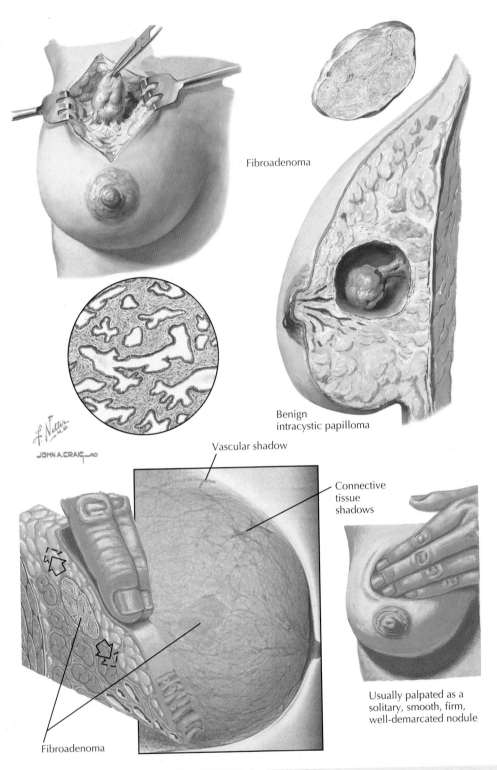

Fibroadenoma

Benign
intracystic papilloma

Vascular shadow

Connective
tissue
shadows

Fibroadenoma

Usually palpated as a
solitary, smooth, firm,
well-demarcated nodule

Yoshida Y, Takaoka M, Fukumoto M: Carcinoma arising in fibroadenoma: case report and review of the world literature. J Surg Oncol
1985;29:132.

Level III

American College of Obstetricians and Gynecologists: Breast con-
cerns in the adolescent. ACOG Committee Opinion 350. Obstet
Gynecol 2006;108:1329.
Dent DM, Cant PJ: Fibroadenoma. World J Surg 1989;13:706.
Greydanus DE, Matytsina L, Gains M: Breast disorders in children
and adolescents. Prim Care 2006;33:455.

Hamed H, Fentiman IS: Benign breast disease. Int J Clin Pract
2001;55:461.
Hindle WH: Other benign breast problems. Clin Obstet Gynecol
1994;37:916.
Houssami N, Cheung MN, Dixon JM: Fibroadenoma of the breast.
Med J Aust 2001;174:185.
Seltzer MH, Skiles MS: Disease of the breast in young women. Surg
Gynecol Obstet 1980;150:360.
Valea FA, Katz VL: Breast diseases. In Katz VL, Lentz GM,
Lobo RA, Gershenson DM. Comprehensive Gynecology, 5th ed.
Philadelphia, Mosby/Elsevier, 2007, p 333.
Zylstra S: Office management of benign breast disease. Clin Obstet
Gynecol 1999;42:234.

INTRODUCTION

Description: Fibrocystic breast changes are characterized by stromal and ductal proliferation that results in cyst formation, diffuse thickening, cyclic pain, and tenderness. The term fibrocystic change encompasses a multitude of different processes and older terms, including fibrocystic disease. It is the most common of all benign breast conditions, accounting for its linguistic demotion to "change" from the designation "disease."

Prevalence: Sixty percent to seventy-five percent of all women.

Predominant Age: Most common between 30 and 50, 10% of women younger than 21.

Genetics: A family history of fibrocystic change is often present, but causality is difficult to establish.

ETIOLOGY AND PATHOGENESIS

Causes: The cause or causes of fibrocystic change are unknown, but it is postulated to arise from an exaggerated response to hormones. A role for progesterone has been suggested based on the common occurrence of premenstrual breast swelling and tenderness. Other proposed sources for fibrocystic changes are altered ratios of estrogen and progesterone or an increased rate of prolactin secretion, but none of these have been conclusively established.

Risk Factors: Methylxanthine intake has been proposed, but hard data are lacking. There is no evidence that oral contraceptive use increases the risk of these changes.

CLINICAL CHARACTERISTICS

Signs and Symptoms

- Asymptomatic (50%)
- Cyclic, diffuse, bilateral pain and engorgement, with the worst symptoms occurring just before menses (the pain associated with fibrocystic change often radiates to the shoulders or upper arms)
- Multiple cysts and nodules intermixed with scattered bilateral nodularity typical, ropy thickening, especially in the upper outer quadrants of the breast

DIAGNOSTIC APPROACH

Differential Diagnosis

- Fibroadenoma
- Carcinoma
- Fat necrosis
- Lipoma
- Radiculitis (Tietze's syndrome)

Associated Conditions: Mastalgia, fibroadenoma.

Workup and Evaluation

Laboratory: No evaluation indicated.

Imaging: Mammography may be used to assist with the diagnosis or to provide a baseline, but it is not necessary for diagnosis. Mammography is more difficult in the younger women who predominantly have these complaints. Ultrasonography may be of more help when imaging is deemed necessary.

Special Tests: If the patient has a cystic breast mass, needle aspiration with a 22- to 25-gauge needle may be both diagnostic and therapeutic. Fine needle aspiration (FNA) or core biopsy may be required if malignancy is suspected.

Diagnostic Procedures: Diagnosis is based on symptoms and physical findings rather than histologic evaluation.

Pathologic Findings

Fibrocystic changes appear in three steps: (1) proliferation of stroma, especially in the upper outer quadrants of the breast, is seen; (2) proliferation of the ducts and alveolar cells occurs, adenosis ensues, and cysts are formed; and (3) larger cysts are found and pain generally decreases. Proliferative changes may be extensive (although usually benign) in any of the involved tissues.

MANAGEMENT AND THERAPY

Nonpharmacologic

General Measures: Mechanical support (a well-fitting brassiere worn day and night), analgesics, and reassurance. Cold compresses or ice may be helpful for acute exacerbations.

Specific Measures: Diuretics (such as spironolactone or hydrochlorothiazide given before menstrual periods) and nonsteroidal anti-inflammatory agents (NSAIDs) for analgesia may be necessary; for severe symptoms, danazol, bromocriptine, tamoxifen, or gonadotropin-releasing hormone (GnRH) agonists may be needed. Rarely, patients with intractable pain refractory to medical management may require subcutaneous mastectomy.

Diet: Reduction in methylxanthine intake is often beneficial. Premenstrual restriction of salt or fluids is useful for selected patients. The role of vitamins A and E is unknown.

Activity: No restriction. To reduce discomfort, good breast support is recommended during vigorous activity.

Patient Education: Instruction on monthly breast self-examination; American College of Obstetricians and Gynecologists Patient Education Pamphlet AP145 (Breast Self-Examination), AP026 (Detecting and Treating Breast Problems), AP076 (Mammography).

Drug(s) of Choice

Combination oral contraceptives (70% to 90% success).

Spironolactone (50 mg PO twice a day given 7 to 10 days before periods).

Danazol sodium 200 mg PO twice a day (therapy should start during menstruation or pregnancy must be ruled out); side effects may be significant, and recurrence is likely after therapy is discontinued.

Bromocriptine 2.5 mg PO daily (with food), may be increased after 3 to 7 days if needed.

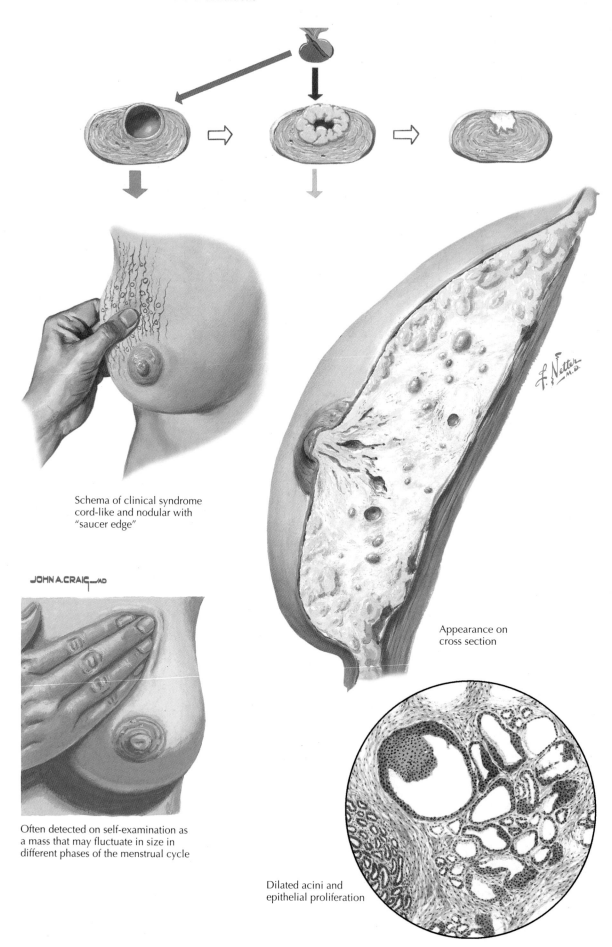

Schema of clinical syndrome
cord-like and nodular with
"saucer edge"

JOHN A. CRAIG—AD

Often detected on self-examination as
a mass that may fluctuate in size in
different phases of the menstrual cycle

Appearance on
cross section

Dilated acini and
epithelial proliferation

Contraindications: Spironolactone is contraindicated in the presence of anuria, renal insufficiency, or hyperkalemia. Danazol sodium is contraindicated in pregnancy (category X). It may also worsen epilepsy, migraine headaches, and cardiac or renal function. Bromocriptine is contraindicated in patients with uncontrolled hypertension or in those known to be sensitive to ergot alkaloids.

Precautions: Diuretics must be used with care to avoid fluid and electrolyte disturbances. Bromocriptine may cause hypotension during the first several days of therapy. Care should also be used with patients who have compromised hepatic or renal function.

Interactions: Spironolactone enhances the action of other diuretics and increases digoxin levels. Danazol sodium may prolong prothrombin time in patients receiving warfarin.

Alternative Drugs

Hydrochlorothiazide 25 mg PO at bedtime for 7 to 10 days before menses. Gonadotropin-releasing hormone agonists (Lupron 3.75 mg IM monthly for no more than 6 months).

Tamoxifen has had up to a 70% response rate in some trials.

FOLLOW-UP

Patient Monitoring: Patients with mastalgia but no dominant mass may be safely rechecked at a different portion of the next menstrual cycle. After aspiration of a cyst (yielding clear fluid and complete loss of the mass), the patient should be rechecked in 2 to 4 weeks. Recurrence of the cyst or the presence of a palpable mass should prompt additional evaluation, such as fine needle aspiration or open biopsy.

Prevention/Avoidance: None.

Possible Complications: When atypia is found in hyperplastic ducts or apocrine cells, there is a 5-fold increase in the risk of development of carcinoma in the future.

Expected Outcome: Symptomatic relief can generally be achieved with a combination of diet changes, analgesics, and specific medications. The underlying pathologic features remain unchanged or progress.

MISCELLANEOUS

Pregnancy Considerations: No effect on pregnancy. The hormonal changes of pregnancy may worsen symptoms.

ICD-9-CM Codes: 610.1.

REFERENCES

Level I

Ernster VL, Mason L, Goodson WH 3rd, et al: Effects of caffeine-free diet on benign breast disease: a randomized trial. Surgery 1982;91:263.

Level II

Boyle CA, Berkowitz GS, LiVolsi VA, et al: Caffeine consumption and fibrocystic breast disease: a case control epidemiologic study. J Natl Cancer Inst 1984;72:1015.

Level III

American College of Obstetricians and Gynecologists: Breast concerns in the adolescent. ACOG Committee Opinion 350. Obstet Gynecol 2006;108:1329.

American College of Obstetricians and Gynecologists: Use of hormonal contraception in women with coexisting medical conditions. ACOG Practice Bulletin 73. Obstet Gynecol 2006:107:1453.

Donegan WL: Evaluation of a palpable breast mass. N Engl J Med 1992;327:937.

Drukker BH: Fibrocystic change of the breast. Clin Obstet Gynecol 1994;37:903.

Drukker BH, deMendonca WC: Fibrocystic change and fibrocystic disease of the breast. Obstet Gynecol Clin North Am 1987;14:685.

Ferguson CM, Powel RW: Breast masses in young women. Arch Surg 1989;124:1338.

Maddox PR, Mansel RE: Management of breast pain and nodularity. World J Surg 1989;13:699.

Seltzer MH, Skiles MS: Disease of the breast in young women. Surg Gynecol Obstet 1980;150:360.

Valea FA, Katz VL: Breast diseases. In Katz VL, Lentz GM, Lobo RA, Gershenson DM. Comprehensive Gynecology, 5th ed. Philadelphia, Mosby/Elsevier, 2007, p 331.

INTRODUCTION

Description: Galactocele is cystic dilation of a duct or ducts, with inspissated milk and desquamated epithelial cells, that may become infected, resulting in acute mastitis or an abscess.

Prevalence: Common in asymptomatic form.

Predominant Age: Reproductive.

Genetics: No genetic pattern.

ETIOLOGY AND PATHOGENESIS

Causes: Ductal obstruction and inflammation during or soon after lactation may lead to cystic dilation of a duct or ducts and the subsequent development of a galactocele. Galactocele is generally associated with breastfeeding, but it may on rare occasions be associated with galactorrhea or oral contraceptive use.

Risk Factors: Breastfeeding, mastitis, galactorrhea, and abrupt weaning.

CLINICAL CHARACTERISTICS

Signs and Symptoms

* Painless mass palpable in the central portion of the breast

DIAGNOSTIC APPROACH

Differential Diagnosis

* Duct ectasia
* Lipoma
* Fibrocystic change
* Fibroadenoma
* Breast abscess

Associated Conditions: Mastitis, ductal ectasia, and nipple discharge.

Workup and Evaluation

Laboratory: No evaluation indicated.

Imaging: No imaging indicated.

Special Tests: Aspiration produces thick, creamy material.

Diagnostic Procedures: History and physical examination, needle aspiration.

Pathologic Findings

Cystic dilation of ducts with milky-white material made of lipid-rich foam cells and ductal epithelial cells, granular eosinophilic secretions, and lipids.

MANAGEMENT AND THERAPY

Nonpharmacologic

General Measures: Evaluation and reassurance.

Specific Measures: No specific therapy is required for a galactocele, and the mass will subside in a few weeks. When uncomplicated by infection, needle aspiration or drainage by gentle pressure is diagnostic and decompression is curative. Excision may be required for recurrences.

Diet: No specific dietary changes indicated.

Activity: No restriction.

Patient Education: Instruction on monthly breast self-examination; American College of Obstetricians and Gynecologists Patient Education Pamphlet AP145 (Breast Self-Examination), AP026 (Detecting and Treating Breast Problems), AP029 (Breastfeeding Your Baby), AP076 (Mammography).

Drug(s) of Choice

None.

FOLLOW-UP

Patient Monitoring: Normal health maintenance.

Prevention/Avoidance: None.

Possible Complications: Secondary infection and abscess formation.

Expected Outcome: The mass will subside in a few weeks with no therapy.

MISCELLANEOUS

Pregnancy Considerations: No effect on pregnancy.

ICD-9-CM Codes: 611.5.

REFERENCES

Level III

Santen RJ, Mansel R: Benign breast disorders. N Engl J Med 2005;353:275.

Seltzer MH, Skiles MS: Disease of the breast in young women. Surg Gynecol Obstet 1980;150:360.

Smith RP: Gynecology in primary care. Baltimore, Williams & Wilkins, 1997, p 319.

Winker JM: Galactocele of the breast. Am J Surg 1964;108:357.

Galactocele

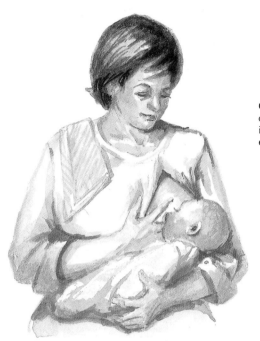

Ductal obstruction resulting in galactocele formation usually occurs during or soon after lactation or abrupt weaning

JOHN A.CRAIG—AD
D. Mascaro

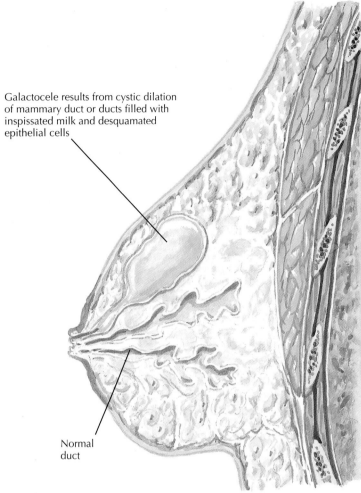

Galactocele results from cystic dilation of mammary duct or ducts filled with inspissated milk and desquamated epithelial cells

Normal duct

Clinical Findings

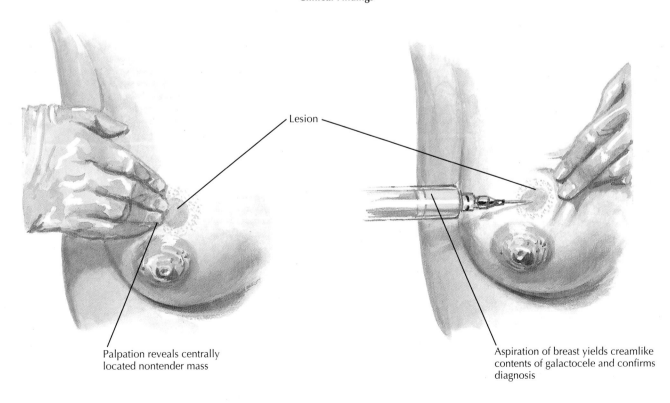

Lesion

Palpation reveals centrally located nontender mass

Aspiration of breast yields creamlike contents of galactocele and confirms diagnosis

INTRODUCTION

Description: Intraductal papilloma involves polypoid fibrovascular tumors covered by benign ductal epithelium that arise in the ducts of the breast.

Prevalence: Found in 0.4% of the general population and up to 20% of women older than age 70.

Predominant Age: Median 40, most common just before menopause.

Genetics: No genetic pattern.

ETIOLOGY AND PATHOGENESIS

Causes: Unknown.

Risk Factors: None known.

CLINICAL CHARACTERISTICS

Signs and Symptoms

- Spontaneous, intermittent, bloody, serous, or cloudy unilateral nipple discharge (roughly 50% to 75% of patients), varying from a few drops to a few milliliters of fluid; serosanguineous or bloody nipple discharge is associated with malignancy in between 7% and 17% of cases, but the color or clarity of the fluid cannot diagnose or rule out carcinoma
- Sense of fullness below the nipple, relieved by passage of discharge
- Mass rare—tumors from 2 to 5 mm in diameter typically are not palpable

DIAGNOSTIC APPROACH

Differential Diagnosis

- Breast cancer
- Galactocele
- Ductal ectasia
- Fibrocystic change

Associated Conditions: Fibrocystic change, fibroadenoma.

Workup and Evaluation

Laboratory: No evaluation indicated.

Imaging: Ductogram or galactogram is diagnostic.

Special Tests: Cytologic evaluation of the nipple discharge is associated with a false-negative result rate of almost 20% and is therefore of little value.

Diagnostic Procedures: History, physical examination, and excisional biopsy.

Pathologic Findings

A pedunculated proliferation of duct epithelium that generally arises within 1 cm of the areola and rarely is greater than 5 mm in size. The associated duct is generally dilated.

The epithelium is friable with a delicate villus structure made up of fibrovascular tissue covered by epithelial cells. Intraductal papilloma is difficult to differentiate from papillary carcinoma, especially on frozen section.

MANAGEMENT AND THERAPY

Nonpharmacologic

General Measures: Evaluation and reassurance.

Specific Measures: Intraductal papillomas are most often benign, but the similarity of symptoms to those of a carcinoma and a sometimes-confusing histologic picture mandate excisional biopsy for most patients.

Diet: No specific dietary changes indicated.

Activity: No restriction.

Patient Education: Instruction on monthly breast self-examination; American College of Obstetricians and Gynecologists Patient Education Pamphlet AP145 (Breast Self-Examination), AP026 (Detecting and Treating Breast Problems), AP076 (Mammography).

Drug(s) of Choice

None.

FOLLOW-UP

Patient Monitoring: Normal health maintenance.

Prevention/Avoidance: None.

Possible Complications: Atypia of the epithelial cells may occur and increases the possibility of malignancy.

Expected Outcome: Surgical excision is both diagnostic and therapeutic.

MISCELLANEOUS

Pregnancy Considerations: No effect on pregnancy.

ICD-9-CM Codes: 611.9.

REFERENCES

Level III

American College of Obstetricians and Gynecologists: Breast concerns in the adolescent. ACOG Committee Opinion 350. Obstet Gynecol 2006;108:1329.

Devitt JE: Benign disorders of the breast in older women. Surg Gynecol Obstet 1986;162:340.

Drukker BH: Breast disease: a primer on diagnosis and management. Int J Fertil Womens Med 1997;42:278.

Ganesan S, Karthik G, Joshi M, Damodaran V: Ultrasound spectrum in intraductal papillary neoplasms of breast. Br J Radiol 2006;79:843. Epub 2006 Apr 26.

Santen RJ, Mansel R: Benign breast disorders. N Engl J Med 2005;353:275.

Vargas HI, Romero L, Chlebowski RT: Management of bloody nipple discharge. Curr Treat Options Oncol 2002;3:157.

Solitary Intraductal Papilloma

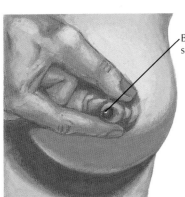

Blood-tinged or brownish nipple discharge suggests intraductal papilloma

Palpation will often reveal a mass near the nipple. Duct opening can be cannulated with a fine probe, and only involved duct need be excised

Single large papilloma located within a dilated mammary duct

JOHN A.CRAIG—AD

INTRODUCTION

Description: Mondor's disease, or superficial angiitis, is a superficial thrombophlebitis of the breast.
Prevalence: Uncommon.
Predominant Age: 30 to 60.
Genetics: No genetic pattern.

ETIOLOGY AND PATHOGENESIS

Causes: Phlebitis is most often linked to recent pregnancy, trauma, or operative procedures but may occur spontaneously. It most often involves the thoracoepigastric veins of the breast.
Risk Factors: Pregnancy, trauma or operative procedures, thrombophilias.

CLINICAL CHARACTERISTICS

Signs and Symptoms

- Pain (acute, generally upper outer quadrant)
- Dimpling of the skin or a distinct cord with erythematous margins
- Shallow groove seen extending upward toward the axilla when the arm is raised

DIAGNOSTIC APPROACH

Differential Diagnosis

- Breast abscess
- Duct ectasia
- Carcinoma (may be distinguished from inflammatory cancer of the breast by the presence of sudden pain, early skin adherence, and progressive improvement)
- Mastitis
- Fat necrosis
- Scarring from previous surgery (biopsy, augmentation, or reduction)

Associated Conditions: Mastitis.

Workup and Evaluation

Laboratory: No evaluation indicated.
Imaging: Mammography may be required to rule out other processes, but the diagnosis is generally established by examination and history.
Special Tests: On rare occasions, biopsy may be required to establish the diagnosis.
Diagnostic Procedures: History and physical examination. (Accentuation of dimpling, or the formation of a groove over the affected vein, often occurs when the ipsilateral arm is raised during physical examination.)

Pathologic Findings

Thrombophlebitis of the superficial veins.

MANAGEMENT AND THERAPY

Nonpharmacologic

General Measures: Evaluation and reassurance, symptomatic therapy.
Specific Measures: Analgesics and heat reduce symptoms. The condition generally resolves in 2 to 3 weeks, but it may take 6 weeks or longer.
Diet: No specific dietary changes indicated.
Activity: No restriction. Good mechanical support improves comfort during vigorous activity.
Patient Education: Instruction on monthly breast self-examination; American College of Obstetricians and Gynecologists Patient Education Pamphlet AP145 (Breast Self-Examination), AP026 (Detecting and Treating Breast Problems), AP029 (Breastfeeding Your Baby), AP076 (Mammography).

Drug(s) of Choice

Nonsteroidal anti-inflammatory agents (NSAIDs). (Antibiotics and anticoagulants have little effect on the course of the disease and are not indicated.)

FOLLOW-UP

Patient Monitoring: Normal health maintenance.
Prevention/Avoidance: Avoidance of breast trauma.
Possible Complications: Unlikely.
Expected Outcome: Mondor's disease is self-limited, although full resolution may take 8 to 10 weeks.

MISCELLANEOUS

Pregnancy Considerations: No effect on pregnancy.
ICD-9-CM Codes: 451.89.

REFERENCES

Level III
Camiel MR: Mondor's disease in the breast. Am J Obstet Gynecol 1985;152:879.
Duff P: Mondor's disease in pregnancy. Obstet Gynecol 1981;58:117.
Fiorica JV: Special problems. Mondor's disease, macrocysts, trauma, squamous metaplasia, miscellaneous disorders of the nipple. Obstet Gynecol Clin North Am 1994;21:479.
Oldfield MC: Mondor's disease. A superficial phlebitis of the breast. Lancet 1962;1:994.
Pugh CM, DeWitty RL: Mondor's disease. J Natl Med Assoc 1996;88:359.
Samlaska CP, James WD: Superficial thrombophlebitis. II. Secondary hypercoagulable states. J Am Acad Dermatol 1990;23:1.
Seltzer MH, Skiles MS: Disease of the breast in young women. Surg Gynecol Obstet 1980;150:360.

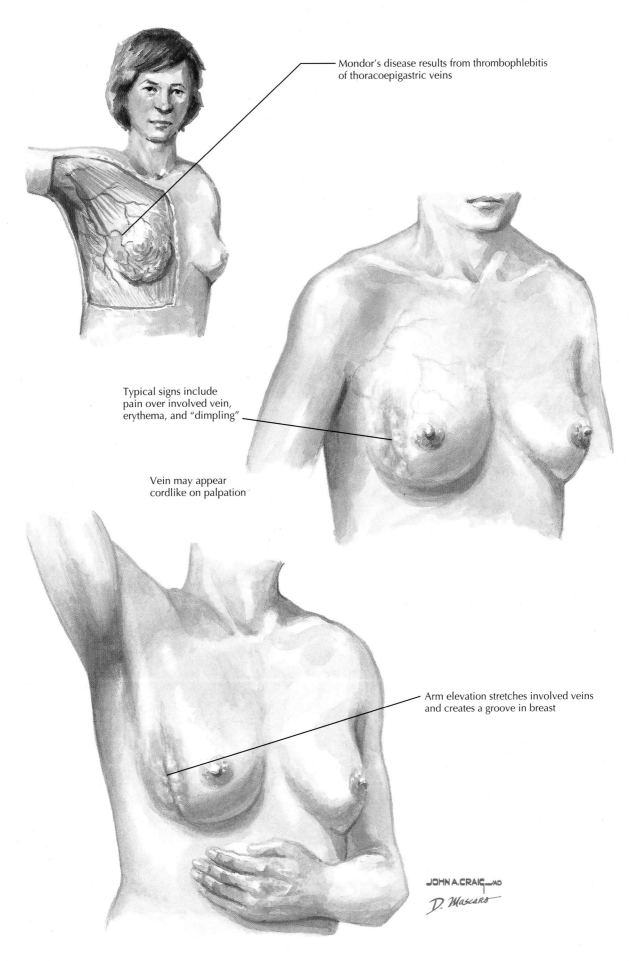

Mondor's disease results from thrombophlebitis of thoracoepigastric veins

Typical signs include pain over involved vein, erythema, and "dimpling"

Vein may appear cordlike on palpation

Arm elevation stretches involved veins and creates a groove in breast

JOHN A. CRAIG—AD

D. Mascaro

INTRODUCTION

Description: Nipple discharge is a distressing symptom that accounts for roughly 5% of breast complaints.

Prevalence: Three percent to five percent of breast problems, 5% of women who are not lactating, >50% of women can express secretions.

Predominant Age: Reproductive (based on pathophysiologic changes).

Genetics: No genetic pattern.

ETIOLOGY AND PATHOGENESIS

Causes: Based on underlying pathophysiologic changes.

Risk Factors: See individual pathologic conditions.

CLINICAL CHARACTERISTICS

Signs and Symptoms

- Spontaneous, continuous, or intermittent release of fluid from one or both breasts that may be milky, bloody, serous, serosanguineous, or cloudy; most physiologic discharge is white or green, clear, or yellow; serosanguineous or bloody nipple discharge is associated with malignancy in 7% to 17% of cases, but the color or clarity of the fluid cannot diagnose or rule out carcinoma.

DIAGNOSTIC APPROACH

Differential Diagnosis

- Breast cancer
- Intraductal papilloma
- Galactocele
- Ductal ectasia (associated with burning, itching, or local discomfort in older patients)
- Fibrocystic change
- Mastitis

Associated Conditions: Fibrocystic change, fibroadenoma.

Workup and Evaluation

Laboratory: Cytologic evaluation of the nipple discharge is associated with a false-negative result rate of almost 20% and is therefore of little value. A simple fat stain of the discharge confirms the physiologic character of the discharge (milk).

Imaging: Ductogram or galactogram may be diagnostic; mammography may be of assistance in evaluation. Ductoscopy has been advocated but does not have widespread availability or acceptance.

Special Tests: Surgical excision of the involved duct may be required for diagnosis and treatment. Approximately 25% of patients who undergo operations are found to have a malignancy.

Diagnostic Procedures: History and physical examination often differentiate between physiologic discharge and breast disease.

Pathologic Findings

Based on the pathophysiologic condition involved. Multiple papillomas or atypia suggest an increased risk for cancer.

MANAGEMENT AND THERAPY

Nonpharmacologic

General Measures: Evaluation and reassurance.

Specific Measures: Surgical excision of the affected duct or other pathologic process.

Diet: No specific dietary changes indicated.

Activity: No restriction.

Patient Education: Instruction on monthly breast self-examination; American College of Obstetricians and Gynecologists Patient Education Pamphlet AP145 (Breast Self-Examination), AP026 (Detecting and Treating Breast Problems), AP076 (Mammography).

Drug(s) of Choice

None.

FOLLOW-UP

Patient Monitoring: Normal health maintenance.

Prevention/Avoidance: None.

Possible Complications: Failure to consider the possibility of significant disease may result in delay of diagnosis and treatment.

Expected Outcome: Surgical excision of the involved duct may be required for diagnosis and treatment.

MISCELLANEOUS

Pregnancy Considerations: No effect on pregnancy.

ICD-9-CM Codes: 611.79.

REFERENCES

Level III

American College of Obstetricians and Gynecologists: Breast concerns in the adolescent. ACOG Committee Opinion 350. Obstet Gynecol 2006;108:1329.

Devitt JE: Benign disorders of the breast in older women. Surg Gynecol Obstet 1986;162:340.

Drukker BH: Breast disease: a primer on diagnosis and management. Int J Fertil Womens Med 1997;42:278.

Escobar PF, Crowe JP, Matsunaga T, Mokbel K: The clinical applications of mammary ductoscopy. Am J Surg 2006;191:211.

Falkenberry SS: Nipple discharge. Obstet Gynecol Clin North Am 2002;29:21.

Fentiman IS, Hamed H: Assessment of breast problems. Int J Clin Pract 2001;55:458.

Fiorica JV: Nipple discharge. Obstet Gynecol Clin North Am 1994;21:453.

Hamed H, Fentiman IS: Benign breast disease. Int J Clin Pract 2001;55:461.

Hussain AN, Policarpio C, Vincent MT: Evaluating nipple discharge. Obstet Gynecol Surv 2006;61:278.

Isaacs JH: Other nipple discharge. Clin Obstet Gynecol 1994; 37:898.

Clinical Considerations

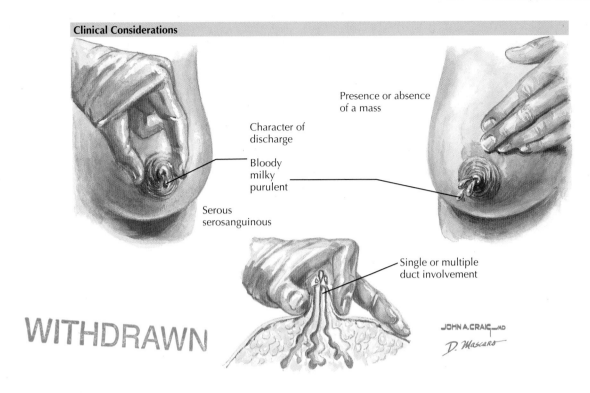

Character of discharge

Bloody
milky
purulent

Serous
serosanguinous

Presence or absence of a mass

Single or multiple duct involvement

WITHDRAWN

JOHN A. CRAIG—MD
D. Mascaro

Management Algorithm For Nipple Discharge

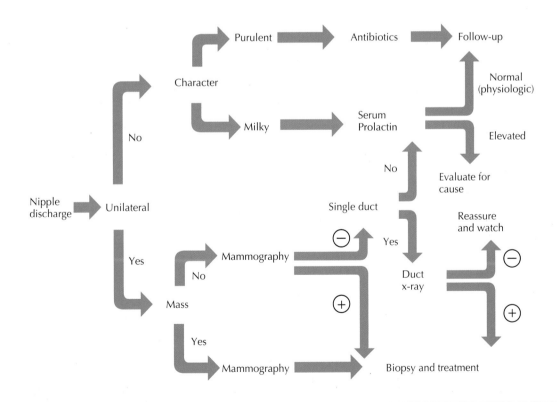

Leis HP Jr: Management of nipple discharge. World J Surg 1989;13:736.

Masood S, Khalbuss WE: Nipple fluid cytology. Clin Lab Med 2005;25:787, vii.

Sakorafas GH: Nipple discharge: current diagnostic and therapeutic approaches. Cancer Treat Rev 2001;27:275.

Santen RJ, Mansel R: Benign breast disorders. N Engl J Med 2005;353:275.

Seltzer MH, Skiles MS: Disease of the breast in young women. Surg Gynecol Obstet 1980;150:360.

Vargas HI, Romero L, Chlebowski RT: Management of bloody nipple discharge. Curr Treat Options Oncol 2002;3:157.

INTRODUCTION

Description: Mastalgia is the nonspecific term used for breast pain of any etiology.

Prevalence: Most women experience breast pain at some point in their lives (may be transient).

Predominant Age: Reproductive.

Genetics: No genetic pattern.

ETIOLOGY AND PATHOGENESIS

Causes: Fibrocystic change. Rapid hormonal change (especially a change that involves an increase in estrogen levels, such as starting birth control pills or hormone replacement or during early pregnancy). In the absence of obvious pathologic changes, mastalgia has been attributed to caffeine consumption and high-fat diets, but hard data are lacking. Nongynecologic causes—dorsal radiculitis or inflammatory changes in the costochondral junction (Tietze's syndrome), sclerosing adenosis, chest wall muscle spasms, costochondritis, neuritis, fibromyalgia, and referred pain.

Risk Factors: Pregnancy, hormone therapy. Caffeine consumption and high-fat diets have been suggested but remain unconfirmed causes.

CLINICAL CHARACTERISTICS

Signs and Symptoms

- Diffuse breast pain, often with radiation to the shoulders or upper arms, which may or may not be related to the menstrual cycle. Unilateral or localized pain suggests a pathologic process.

DIAGNOSTIC APPROACH

Differential Diagnosis

- Fibrocystic change (most commonly presents as cyclic, diffuse, bilateral pain and engorgement, with the worst symptoms occurring just before menses)
- Mastitis or breast abscess
- Trauma
- Chest wall abnormalities (herpes zoster, costochondritis, radicular pain)
- Breast cancer (breast pain is a presenting complaint in less than 10% of patients with breast cancer)
- Mondor's disease

Associated Conditions: Fibrocystic change, fibroadenoma, and mastitis.

Workup and Evaluation

Laboratory: No evaluation indicated.

Imaging: Mammography may be indicated for other reasons but seldom directly assists in the evaluation of mastalgia.

Special Tests: None indicated.

Diagnostic Procedures: History and physical examination. The presence of scattered bilateral nodularity suggests fibrocystic change.

Pathologic Findings

Based on pathophysiologic changes present.

MANAGEMENT AND THERAPY

Nonpharmacologic

General Measures: Analgesics, mechanical support (a well-fitting brassiere worn day and night), local heat, reassurance.

Specific Measures: Caffeine restriction, medical treatment of underlying pathophysiologic changes (e.g., fibrocystic change).

Diet: A reduction in methylxanthine intake is often beneficial. Premenstrual restriction of salt or fluids is recommended for selected patients. The role of vitamins A and E is unknown.

Activity: No restriction. To reduce discomfort, good mechanical breast support is recommended during vigorous activity.

Patient Education: Instruction on monthly breast self-examination; American College of Obstetricians and Gynecologists Patient Education Pamphlet AP145 (Breast Self-Examination), AP026 (Detecting and Treating Breast Problems), AP076 (Mammography).

Drug(s) of Choice

Combination oral contraceptives (70% to 90% success).

Spironolactone 50 mg PO twice a day given 7 to 10 days before periods.

Danazol sodium 200 mg PO twice a day (therapy should start during menstruation or pregnancy must be ruled out); side effects may be significant and recurrence is likely after therapy is discontinued.

Bromocriptine 2.5 mg PO daily (with food), may be increased after 3 to 7 days if needed.

Contraindications: Spironolactone is contraindicated in the presence of anuria, renal insufficiency, or hyperkalemia. Danazol sodium is contraindicated in pregnancy (category X). It may also worsen epilepsy, migraine headaches, and cardiac or renal function. Bromocriptine is contraindicated in patients with uncontrolled hypertension or in patients known to be sensitive to ergot alkaloids.

Precautions: Diuretics must be used with care to avoid fluid and electrolyte disturbances. Bromocriptine may cause hypotension during the first several days of therapy. Care should also be exercised with patients who have compromised hepatic or renal function.

Interactions: Spironolactone enhances the action of other diuretics and increases digoxin levels. Danazol sodium may prolong prothrombin time in patients receiving warfarin.

Alternative Drugs

Hydrochlorothiazide 25 mg PO at bedtime for 7 to 10 days before menses.

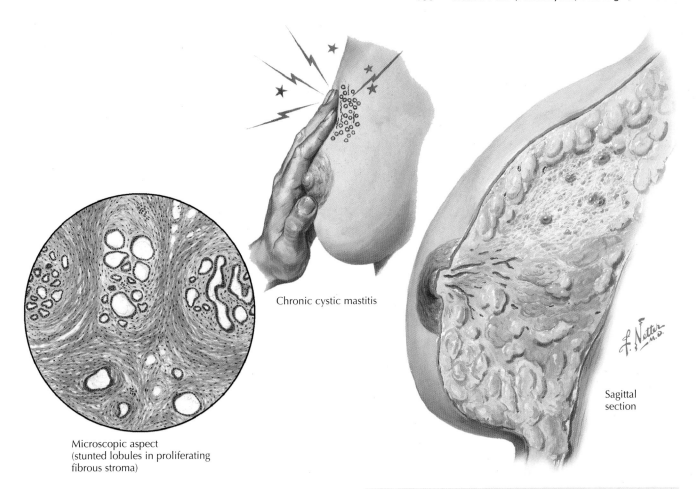

Chronic cystic mastitis

Sagittal section

Microscopic aspect
(stunted lobules in proliferating
fibrous stroma)

Gonadotropin-releasing hormone agonists (GnRH; leu-prolide acetate [Lupron] 3.75 mg IM monthly for no more than 6 months).

Evening primrose and chastberry have shown efficacy in limited trials, but standardization of both therapy and active ingredients in varying preparations limits the ability to fully evaluate these as therapeutic options.

FOLLOW-UP

Patient Monitoring: Patients with mastalgia but no dominant mass may be safely rechecked at a different portion of the next menstrual cycle.

Prevention/Avoidance: None.

Expected Outcome: Symptomatic relief can generally be achieved with a combination of diet changes, analgesics, and specific medications.

MISCELLANEOUS

Pregnancy Considerations: No effect on pregnancy, although pregnancy may induce mastalgia.

ICD-9-CM Codes: 611.71.

REFERENCES

Level I

Doberl A, Tobiassen T, Rasmussen T: Treatment of recurrent cyclical mastodynia in patients with fibrocystic breast disease. A double-blind placebo-controlled study—The Hjorring project. Acta Obstet Gynecol Scand Suppl 1984;123:177.

Gorins A, Perret F, Tournant B, et al: A French double-blind cross-over study (danazol versus placebo) in the treatment of severe fibrocystic breast disease. Eur J Gynaecol Oncol 1984;5:85-.

Ioannidou-Mouzaka L, Niagassas M, Galanos A, Kalovidouris A: Pilot study on the treatment of cyclical mastodynia with Quinagolide. Eur J Gynaecol Oncol 1999;20:117.

Parlati E, Polinari U, Salvi G, et al: Bromocriptine for treatment of benign breast disease. A double-blind clinical trial versus placebo. Acta Obstet Gynecol Scand 1987;66:483.

Level II

Andersch B: Bromocriptine and premenstrual symptoms: a survey of double blind trials. Obstet Gynecol Surv 1983;38:643.

Boyle CA, Berkowitz GS, LiVolsi VA, et al: Caffeine consumption and fibrocystic breast disease: a case control epidemiologic study. J Natl Cancer Inst 1984;72:1015.

Winkler UH, Schindler AE, Brinkmann US, et al: Cyclic progestin therapy for the management of mastopathy and mastodynia. Gynecol Endocrinol 2001;15:37.

Level III

American College of Obstetricians and Gynecologists: Use of botanicals for management of menopausal symptoms. ACOG Practice Bulletin 28. Washington, DC, ACOG, 2001.

Anonymous: Mastodynia. Lancet 1982;2:590.

BeLieu RM: Mastodynia. Obstet Gynecol Clin North Am 1994; 21:461.

Carranza-Lira S, Garduno-Hernandez MP, Caisapanta DA, Aparicio H: Evaluation of mastodynia in postmenopausal women taking hormone therapy. Int J Gynaecol Obstet 2005;89:158.

Ferguson CM, Powel RW: Breast masses in young women. Arch Surg 1989;124:1338.

Lurie S, Borenstein R: The premenstrual syndrome. Obstet Gynecol Surv 1990;45:220.

Seltzer MH, Skiles MS: Disease of the breast in young women. Surg Gynecol Obstet 1980;150:360.

INTRODUCTION

Description: Spontaneous, bilateral nipple discharge (milky fluid only) is called galactorrhea.

Prevalence: Uncommon, but reports vary from 1% to 30%, depending on the population studied.

Predominant Age: Reproductive.

Genetics: No genetic pattern.

ETIOLOGY AND PATHOGENESIS

Causes: Pituitary adenoma, disruptions in thyroid or prolactin hormone levels, pharmacologic (most often those drugs that affect dopamine or serotonin), autoimmune disease (sarcoid, lupus), Cushing's disease, herpes zoster, chest wall/breast stimulation or irritation, physiologic changes during pregnancy or after childbirth and/or breastfeeding, specific foods (licorice).

Risk Factors: None known.

CLINICAL CHARACTERISTICS

Signs and Symptoms

- Bilateral, spontaneous, milky discharge from both breasts
- Often symptoms of underlying pathologic condition (e.g., hypothyroidism, Cushing's disease, or pituitary enlargement)
- Amenorrhea common

DIAGNOSTIC APPROACH

Differential Diagnosis

- Pregnancy
- Breast cancer
- Chronic nipple stimulation
- Hypothyroidism
- Sarcoidosis
- Lupus
- Cirrhosis or hepatic disease

Associated Conditions: One third of patients with an elevated prolactin level experience amenorrhea or infertility. Prolonged amenorrhea is associated with an increased risk of osteoporosis, vaginal and genital atrophic changes, dyspareunia, and libidinal dysfunction.

Workup and Evaluation

Laboratory: Pregnancy should always be considered if menses are absent. There is a poor correlation between serum prolactin levels and the size or detectability of a pituitary lesion.

Imaging: Computed tomography or magnetic resonance imaging (preferred) frequently are indicated.

Special Tests: Testing of visual fields may be indicated.

Pathologic Findings

None.

MANAGEMENT AND THERAPY

Nonpharmacologic

General Measures: When prolactin levels are low and a coned-down view of the sella turcica is normal, observation alone may be sufficient. If observation is chosen, periodic re-evaluation is required to check for the emergence of slow-growing tumors.

Specific Measures: Treatment with bromocriptine is recommended for patients who desire pregnancy or for those with distressing degrees of galactorrhea or to suppress intermediate-sized pituitary tumors. Rapidly growing tumors, tumors that are large at the time of discovery, or those that do not respond to bromocriptine therapy may require surgical therapy.

Diet: No specific dietary changes indicated.

Activity: No restriction.

Patient Education: Reassurance, discuss treatment options; American College of Obstetricians and Gynecologists Patient Education Pamphlet AP102 (Infertility), AP029 (Breastfeeding Your Baby), AP145 (Breast Self-Examination).

Drug(s) of Choice

If the prolactin level is elevated—bromocriptine (Parlodel) 2.5 mg daily increased gradually to three times a day.

Contraindications: Uncontrolled hypertension, pregnancy.

Precautions: With medical therapy—nausea, orthostatic hypotension, drowsiness, syncope, hypertension, or seizures.

Interactions: Medical therapy may interact with phenothiazines or butyrophenones.

Alternative Drugs

Intravaginal bromocriptine.

Dopamine agonists (cabergoline) may become available.

FOLLOW-UP

Patient Monitoring: Normal health maintenance. If a pituitary adenoma is present, periodic assessment of visual fields should be considered.

Prevention/Avoidance: None.

Possible Complications: Visual field loss; symptoms may return after medication is discontinued.

Expected Outcome: Generally good depending on cause. Prolactin levels should be measured every 6 to 12 months, and visual fields should be reassessed yearly. The pituitary should be re-evaluated every 2 to 5 years, based on initial diagnosis.

MISCELLANEOUS

Pregnancy Considerations: No effect on pregnancy, although pregnancy may cause adenomas to grow rapidly.

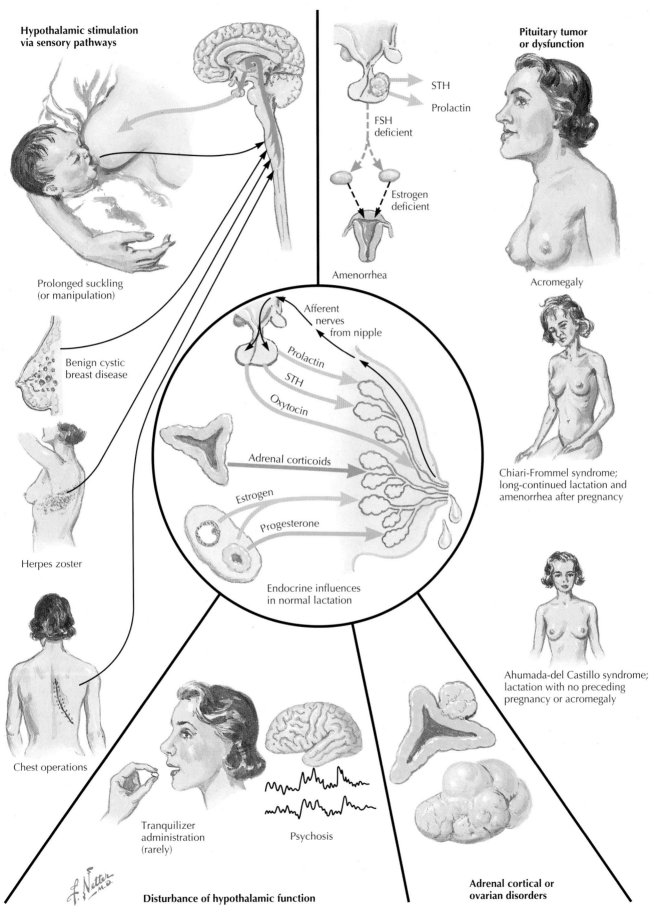

Hypothalamic stimulation via sensory pathways

Prolonged suckling (or manipulation)

Benign cystic breast disease

Herpes zoster

Chest operations

Pituitary tumor or dysfunction

STH

Prolactin

FSH deficient

Estrogen deficient

Amenorrhea

Acromegaly

Afferent nerves from nipple

Prolactin

STH

Oxytocin

Adrenal corticoids

Estrogen

Progesterone

Endocrine influences in normal lactation

Chiari-Frommel syndrome; long-continued lactation and amenorrhea after pregnancy

Ahumada-del Castillo syndrome; lactation with no preceding pregnancy or acromegaly

Tranquilizer administration (rarely)

Psychosis

Disturbance of hypothalamic function

Adrenal cortical or ovarian disorders

FSH, follicle-stimulating hormone; STH, somatotropic hormone.

ICD-9-CM Codes: 611.6, 626.0 (Amenorrhea), 676.6 (Galactorrhea) should only be used in conjunction with pregnancy and breastfeeding.

REFERENCES

Level I
Kletzky OA, Borenstein R, Mileikowsky GN: Pergolide and bromocriptine for the treatment of patients with hyperprolactinemia. Am J Obstet Gynecol 1986;154:431.

Level II
Cuellar FG: Bromocriptine mesylate (Parlodel) in the management of amenorrhea/galactorrhea associated with hyperprolactinemia. Obstet Gynecol 1980;55:278.

Schlechte J, Dolan K, Sherman B, et al: The natural history of untreated hyperprolactinemia: a prospective analysis. J Clin Endocrinol Metab 1989;68:412.

Level III
American College of Obstetricians and Gynecologists: Breast concerns in the adolescent. ACOG Committee Opinion 350. Obstet Gynecol 2006;108:1329.

Besser GM, Edwards CR: Galactorrhoea. Br Med J 1972;2:280.

Chang RJ, Keye WR, Young JR, et al: Detection, evaluation, and treatment of pituitary microadenomas in patients with galactorrhea and amenorrhea. Am J Obstet Gynecol 1977;128:356.

Molitch ME: Medication-induced hyperprolactinemia. Mayo Clin Proc 2005;80:1050.

Parkes D: Drug therapy: bromocriptine. N Engl J Med 1979;301:873.

Santen RJ, Mansel R: Benign breast disorders. N Engl J Med 2005;353:275.

Schlechte JA: Clinical practice. Prolactinoma. N Engl J Med 2003;349:2035.

Zacur HA, Chapanis NP, Lake CR, et al: Galactorrhea-amenorrhea: psychological interaction with neuroendocrine function. Am J Obstet Gynecol 1976;125:859.

THE CHALLENGE

To improve the use of breast imaging to detect occult disease.

Scope of the Problem: Widespread use of mammography has been credited with reducing the mortality rate from breast cancer by up to 30%. Unfortunately, not all women receive appropriate screening on a regular basis. One study indicated that only 39% of women aged 50 to 59 and 36% of women aged 60 to 69 had had a mammogram in the preceding year. In another study, only 24% of women older than age 65 followed the current recommendations for annual examinations. It has been estimated that breast cancer mortality could be reduced by as much as one half if all women older than 40 received annual screening. In one study, 6 cancers per 1000 screening mammograms were found, and 3 additional cancers per 1000 annual repeat studies were detected.

Objectives: To appropriately use mammography for the evaluation of breast complaints and to improve compliance with screening guidelines.

TACTICS

Relevant Pathophysiology: Mammography is the best mode of screening for early lesions currently available. Mammography localizes, documents, objectifies, and identifies other occult pathologic changes. Approximately 85% of breast cancers found by mammography are early-stage lesions versus 54% to 70% found by physicians and 38% to 64% of tumors found by the patient herself during breast self-examination. Approximately 35% of breast cancers are found with an abnormal mammogram, without a palpable mass present. Mammography can identify small lesions (1 to 2 mm), calcifications, or other changes suspicious for malignancy about 2 years before a lesion is clinically palpable. Ten-year disease-free survival for patients with these lesions is 90% to 95%. The average lesion found on breast self-examination is 2.5 cm, and half of these patients have nodal involvement. For these patients, 10-year survival falls to between 50% and 70%. More than one third of occult breast cancers have calcifications, making the otherwise-undetected tumors visible through mammography.

Strategies: The American Cancer Society guidelines for mammographic screening are the following:

- Mammography every 1 to 2 years from age 40 to 49.
- Annual mammogram from age 50 on. (If the patient has a first-degree relative with premenopausal breast cancer, screening should begin about 5 years before the age at which the relative's cancer was diagnosed.)
- For patients at increased risk for breast cancer (strong family history or genetic abnormality such as mutations of BRCA1 or BRCA2) mammography should be augmented by magnetic resonance imaging (MRI) studies.

Patient Education: Instruction on need for and timing of mammography; American College of Obstetricians and Gynecologists Patient Education Pamphlet AP026 (Detecting and Treating Breast Problems), AP076 (Mammography), AP145 (Breast Self-Examination).

IMPLEMENTATION

Special Considerations: Mammography in younger women is more difficult to interpret than in older women because of the greater tissue density present during the reproductive years. Whereas the increasing ability to diagnose cancer in older women parallels their increasing risk, breast cancers in younger women are more easily missed. This diagnostic difficulty and the relatively higher rate of false-positive study results that necessitate further evaluation have raised questions about routine screening of women younger than age 50. The finding of clusters of calcification that often are associated with cancer is nonspecific. Of calcification clusters found on mammography, 75% result from benign disease. Overall, mammography is approximately 85% accurate in diagnosing malignancy, with a 10% to 15% false-negative rate. For this reason, it provides an adjunct to clinical impressions and the definitive procedure of biopsy, but it does not replace them. Approximately 10% of mammographic studies require additional views. Between 1% and 2% of screening studies necessitate histologic evaluation to establish a diagnosis. Mammographic radiation exposure is minimal (less than 1 rad). Based on this level of exposure, mammography might induce up to 5 new lifetime cancers for every 1 million women of age 40 to 44 screened and less than 1 per 1 million for women aged 60 to 64 (background risk is 115 and 292 for these age groups, respectively). Therefore, the risk of death caused by radiation exposure is roughly equivalent to the risk of death encountered by driving a car 220 miles, riding a bicycle for 10 miles, or smoking 1.5 cigarettes.

REFERENCES

Level I

Alexander FE, Anderson TJ, Brown HK, et al: 14 years of follow-up from the Edinburgh randomised trial of breast-cancer screening. Lancet 1999;353:1903.

Level II

Armstrong K, Moye E, Williams S, et al: Screening mammography in women 40 to 49 years of age: a systematic review for the American College of Physicians. Ann Intern Med 2007;146:516.

Fenton JJ, Taplin SH, Carney PA, et al: Influence of computer-aided detection on performance of screening mammography. N Engl J Med 2007;356:1399.

Lazarus E, Mainiero MB, Schepps B, et al: BI-RADS lexicon for US and mammography: interobserver variability and positive predictive value. Radiology 2006;239:385.

Mandelblatt J, Saha S, Teutsch S, et al; Cost Work Group of the U.S. Preventive Services Task Force: The cost-effectiveness of screening mammography beyond age 65 years: a systematic review for the U.S. Preventive Services Task Force. Ann Intern Med 2003;139:835.

Mammography

Position for craniocaudad projection

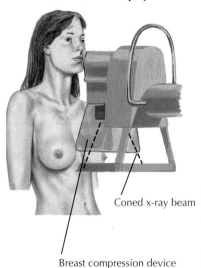

Coned x-ray beam

Breast compression device

Usually two exposures at right angles (craniocaudad and lateral) are made of each breast

Position for lateral projection

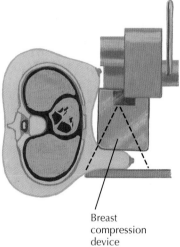

Breast compression device

When additional breast and rib detail is needed, a mediolateral exposure is also made

Position for mediolateral projection

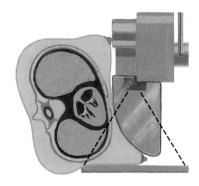

JOHN A. CRAIG—AD

Translucent fatty tissue

Connective tissue shadows

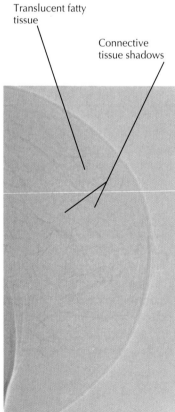

Craniocaudad projection of normal fatty breast

Prominent ducts and glandular elements

Vascular shadows

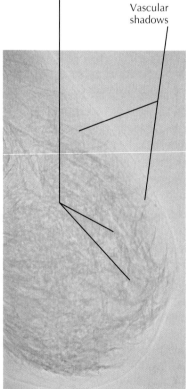

Lateral projection of normal dense glandular breast

Rib detail shown in this projection

Connective tissue shadows

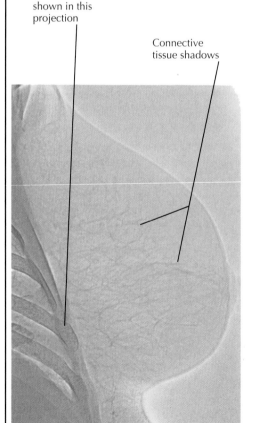

Mediolateral projection of normal breast

Meeson S, Young KC, Wallis MG, et al: Image features of true positive and false negative cancers in screening mammograms. Br J Radiol 2003;76:13.

Moss SM, Cuckle H, Evans A, et al; Trial Management Group: Effect of mammographic screening from age 40 years on breast cancer mortality at 10 years' follow-up: a randomised controlled trial. Lancet 2006;368:2053.

Level III

American College of Obstetricians and Gynecologists: Follow-up of abnormal screening mammography. ACOG Committee Opinion 272. Obstet Gynecol 2002;99:869.

American College of Obstetricians and Gynecologists: Breast cancer screening. ACOG Practice Bulletin 42. Obstet Gynecol 2003;101:821.

American College of Obstetricians and Gynecologists: Role of the obstetrician–gynecologist in the screening and diagnosis of breast masses. ACOG Committee Opinion 334. Obstet Gynecol 2005;106:1141.

American College of Obstetricians and Gynecologists: Routine cancer screening. ACOG Committee Opinion 356. Obstet Gynecol 2006;108:1611.

American College of Radiology: Breast Imaging Reporting and Data System (BI-RADS), 4th ed. Reston, VA, American College of Radiology, 2003.

Blamey RW, Wilson AR, Patnick J: ABC of breast diseases: screening for breast cancer. BMJ 2000;321:689.

Breast cancer screening guidelines agreed on by AMA, other medically related organizations [medical news and perspectives]. JAMA 1989;262:1155.

Elmore JG, Armstrong K, Lehman CD, Fletcher SW: Screening for breast cancer. JAMA 2005;293:1245.

Farria DM, Monsees B: Screening mammography practice essentials. Radiol Clin North Am 2004;42:831, vi.

Fletcher SW, Black W, Harris R, et al: Report of the International Workshop on Screening for Breast Cancer. Bethesda, MD, National Cancer Institute, 1993.

Fletcher SW, Elmore JG: Clinical practice. Mammographic screening for breast cancer. N Engl J Med 2003;348:1672.

Jackson VP: Diagnostic mammography. Radiol Clin North Am 2004;42:853, vi.

Lewin JM, D'Orsi CJ, Hendrick RE: Digital mammography. Radiol Clin North Am 2004;42:871, vi.

Lisby MD: Screening mammography in women 40 to 49 years of age. Am Fam Physician 2004;70:1750.

Pisano ED, Yaffe MJ: Digital mammography. Radiology 2005;234:353.

Qaseem A, Snow V, Sherif K, et al; Clinical Efficacy Assessment Subcommittee of the American College of Physicians: Screening mammography for women 40 to 49 years of age: a clinical practice guideline from the American College of Physicians. Ann Intern Med 2007;146:511.

Saslow D, Boetes C, Burke W, et al; American Cancer Society Breast Cancer Advisory Group: American Cancer Society guidelines for breast screening with MRI as an adjunct to mammography. CA Cancer J Clin. 2007;57:75.

Thornton H, Edwards A, Baum M: Women need better information about routine mammography. BMJ 2003;327:101.

Valea FA, Katz VL: Breast diseases. In Katz VL, Lentz GM, Lobo RA, Gershenson DM. Comprehensive Gynecology, 5th ed. Philadelphia, Mosby/Elsevier, 2007, p 340.

INTRODUCTION

Description: Mastitis is an infection of one or more ductal complexes of the breast, generally associated with breast-feeding and potentially causing significant morbidity if not recognized and treated aggressively.

Prevalence: Two percent to 3% of women who are breast-feeding after delivery.

Predominant Age: Reproductive, 2 to 4 weeks after delivery.

Genetics: No genetic pattern.

ETIOLOGY AND PATHOGENESIS

Causes: Infection comes from organisms carried in the nose and mouth of the nursing infant, most commonly *Staphylococcus aureus* and Streptococcus species. Common agents include β-hemolytic streptococci, *Haemophilus influenzae*, *Haemophilus parainfluenzae*, *Escherichia coli*, and *Klebsiella pneumoniae*.

Risk Factors: Diabetes, steroid use, heavy cigarette smoking, and retracted (inverted) nipples.

CLINICAL CHARACTERISTICS

Signs and Symptoms

- Firm, sore, red, and tender portion of the breast, most commonly in the upper outer quadrant
- High fever, tachycardia, headaches, anorexia, and malaise
- Axillary nodes tender or enlarged
- In patients who are not breastfeeding, a palpable, recurrent mass, accompanied by a multicolored discharge from the nipple or adjacent to a Montgomery's follicle

DIAGNOSTIC APPROACH

Differential Diagnosis

- Breast abscess
- Blocked (plugged) duct
- Breast engorgement
- Galactocele

Associated Conditions: Breast engorgement.

Workup and Evaluation

Laboratory: A complete blood count documents an elevated white blood cell count but is not required for diagnosis. Cultures of the mother's milk and the infant's nose and mouth may be helpful but are not required.

Imaging: No imaging indicated.

Special Tests: None indicated.

Diagnostic Procedures: History and physical examination combined with knowledge of the condition of the breast at or before delivery.

Pathologic Findings

Swelling and obstruction of the involved ducts with inflammation. When present in nonpregnant and postmenopausal women, it may be accompanied by squamous metaplasia. When well established, ductal thickening may lead to nipple retraction.

MANAGEMENT AND THERAPY

Nonpharmacologic

General Measures: Mild fluid restriction, analgesics, ice packs, and support (well-fitting brassiere). In mild cases, it is not necessary to cease breastfeeding.

Specific Measures: Prompt and aggressive antibiotic therapy is indicated. Breastfeeding from the opposite side or pumping or expression of the involved breast may be helpful. If tenderness or fever do not decrease promptly, abscess must be suspected and prompt surgical drainage, usually under general anesthesia, is required.

Diet: No specific dietary changes indicated.

Activity: No restriction.

Patient Education: Reassurance, support, specific suggestions; American College of Obstetricians and Gynecologists Patient Education Pamphlet AP029 (Breastfeeding Your Baby).

Drug(s) of Choice

Penicillin G or erythromycin (250 to 500 mg PO four times a day, erythromycin ethylsuccinate [EES] 400 mg PO four times a day) for 10 days. First-generation oral cephalosporins (cephalexin 500 mg PO twice a day, cefaclor 250 mg PO three times a day, or amoxicillin/clavulanate [Augmentin] 250 mg PO three times a day) may also be used. The level of erythromycin achieved in milk is very high.

Contraindications: Known or suspected allergy.

Precautions: If response to therapy is not prompt, surgical drainage is required.

Alternative Drugs

Dicloxacillin may be required for penicillin-resistant strains or severe infections.

FOLLOW-UP

Patient Monitoring: Normal health maintenance. Watch for development of an abscess.

Prevention/Avoidance: Attention to normal hygiene practices during breastfeeding (hand washing, avoid drying agents). Avoid cracking or fissuring of nipples. Use of breast or nipple shield when cracked nipples are present.

Possible Complications: Progression of infection, abscess formation, scarring, squamous metaplasia, ductal ectasia. Abscesses may form even while a patient is receiving antibiotic therapy.

Expected Outcome: Generally good with aggressive therapy.

MISCELLANEOUS

Pregnancy Considerations: No effect on pregnancy.

ICD-9-CM Codes: 675.2.

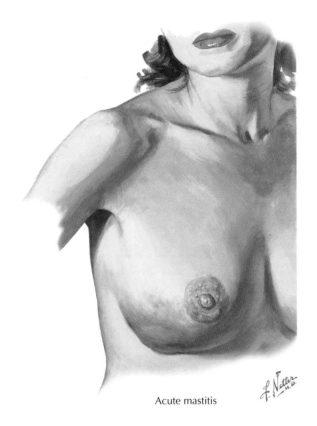

Acute mastitis

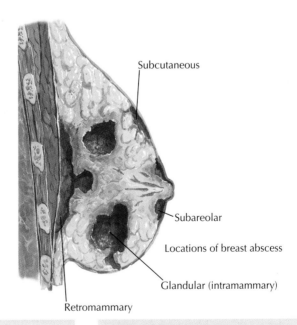

Subcutaneous

Subareolar

Locations of breast abscess

Glandular (intramammary)

Retromammary

REFERENCES

Level II

Amir LH, Forster D, McLachlan H, Lumley J: Incidence of breast abscess in lactating women: report from an Australian cohort. BJOG 2004;111:1378.

Peters F, Flick-Fillies D: Hand disinfection to prevent puerperal mastitis. Lancet 1991;338:831.

Level III

American College of Obstetricians and Gynecologists: Breast concerns in the adolescent. ACOG Committee Opinion 350. Obstet Gynecol 2006;108:1329.

Melnikow J, Bedinghaus JM: Management of common breast-feeding problems. J Fam Pract 1994;39:56.

Michie C, Lockie F, Lynn W: The challenge of mastitis. Arch Dis Child 2003;88:818.

Scott-Conner CE, Schorr SJ: The diagnosis and management of breast problems during pregnancy and lactation. Am J Surg 1995;170:401.

INTRODUCTION

Description: Paget's disease of the breast is a malignant process that involves the nipple and areola. Rarely, it may also involve the skin of the vulva.

Prevalence: Two percent of breast cancers.

Predominant Age: Menopausal and perimenopausal.

Genetics: No genetic pattern.

ETIOLOGY AND PATHOGENESIS

Causes: Thought to arise in the dermoepidermal junction from multipotent cells that can differentiate into either glandular or squamous cells.

Risk Factors: None known.

CLINICAL CHARACTERISTICS

Signs and Symptoms

- Pruritic, red, eczematoid skin lesion, often associated with bleeding and crusting
- Almost always associated with infiltrating or intraductal carcinoma in deeper parts of the breast

DIAGNOSTIC APPROACH

Differential Diagnosis

- Eczema of the nipple
- Inflammatory breast cancer
- Chronic nipple irritation (jogger's nipples)

Associated Conditions: Infiltrating or intraductal carcinoma.

Workup and Evaluation

Laboratory: No evaluation indicated.

Imaging: Mammography to detect deeper lesions and lesions in the contralateral breast.

Special Tests: A touch smear obtained by softening the crust with saline and gently scraping the surface often demonstrates the characteristic Paget's cells.

Diagnostic Procedures: History, physical examination, and biopsy.

Pathologic Findings

Dermal infiltrates of large neoplastic cells (Paget's cells). These cells have abundant clear cytoplasm with mucin and irregular prominent nucleoli. Most often, these cells arise from infiltrating ductal carcinoma.

MANAGEMENT AND THERAPY

Nonpharmacologic

General Measures: Evaluation, mammography.

Specific Measures: Therapy is focused on treatment of the underlying malignancy. When limited to the nipple, breast conservation may be possible.

Diet: No specific dietary changes indicated.

Activity: No restriction.

Patient Education: Instruction on monthly breast self-examination; American College of Obstetricians and Gynecologists Patient Education Pamphlet AP026 (Detecting and Treating Breast Problems), AP076 (Mammography), AP145 (Breast Self-Examination).

Drug(s) of Choice

None. Adjunctive chemotherapy is often recommended based on cell type and stage.

FOLLOW-UP

Patient Monitoring: Increased surveillance for recurrence or the development of tumors in the contralateral breast.

Prevention/Avoidance: None.

Possible Complications: Progression and spread of the underlying malignancy. Local skin erosion with bleeding and discharge.

Expected Outcome: Local recurrence is common.

MISCELLANEOUS

Pregnancy Considerations: Generally not a consideration. No direct effect on pregnancy.

ICD-9-CM Codes: Based on location and severity of disease.

REFERENCES

Level I
Bijker N, Rutgers EJ, Duchateau L, et al; EORTC Breast Cancer Cooperative Group: Breast-conserving therapy for Paget disease of the nipple: a prospective European Organization for Research and Treatment of Cancer study of 61 patients. Cancer 2001;91:472.

Level II
Davis AB, Patchefsky AS: Basal cell carcinoma of the nipple: case report and review of the literature. Cancer 1977;40:1780.

Marshall JK, Griffith KA, Haffty BG, et al: Conservative management of Paget disease of the breast with radiotherapy: 10- and 15-year results. Cancer 2003;97:2142.

Level III
Dixon JM, Sainsbury JR, Rodger A: ABC of breast diseases. Breast cancer: treatment of elderly patients and uncommon conditions. BMJ 1994;309:1292.

Jamali FR, Ricci A Jr, Deckers PJ: Paget's disease of the nipple-areola complex. Surg Clin North Am 1996;76:365.

Lloyd J, Flanagan AM: Mammary and extramammary Paget's disease. J Clin Pathol 2000;53:742.

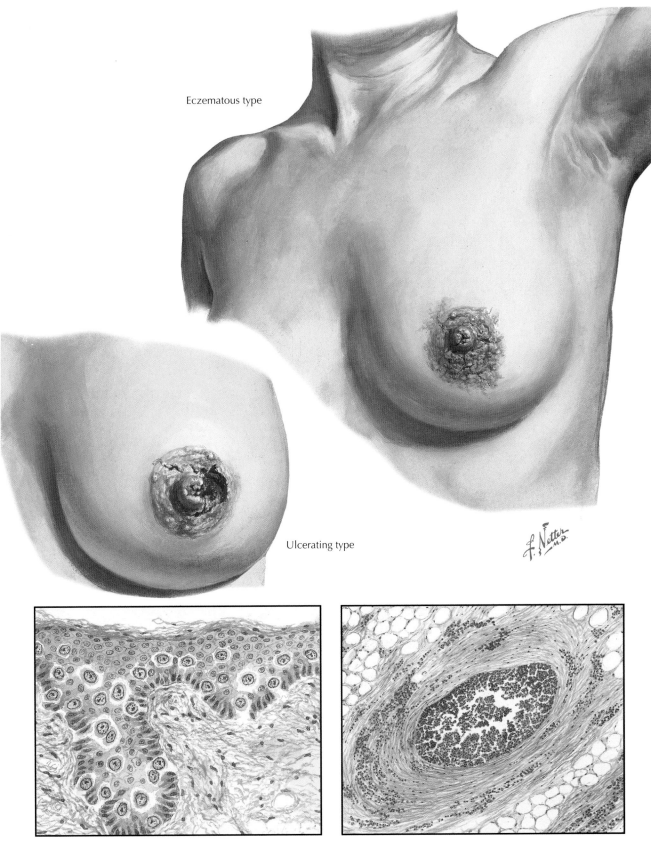

Eczematous type

Ulcerating type

Paget cells in epidermis

Duct invasion

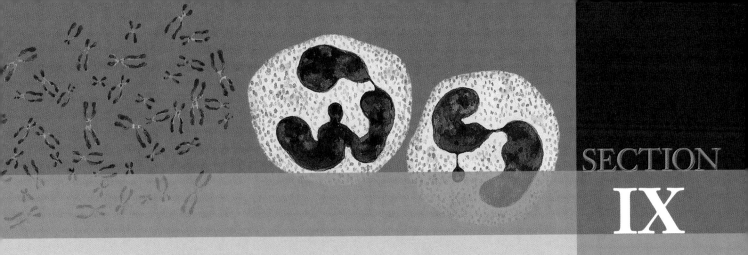

Reproductive, Genetic, and Endocrine Conditions

INTRODUCTION

Description: When a woman has had two consecutive or three total first-trimester spontaneous pregnancy losses it is considered recurrent abortion.

Prevalence: Found in 0.4% to 0.8% of women.

Predominant Age: Reproductive.

Genetics: No genetic pattern.

ETIOLOGY AND PATHOGENESIS

Causes: Chromosomal abnormalities. When the losses occur early in gestation, there is a greater likelihood that a chromosomal abnormality is the cause, whereas for later abortions a maternal cause such as a uterine anomaly is more likely. Although most chromosomal abnormalities result from disorders of meiosis in gamete formation or in mitosis after fertilization, 5% of couples who experience recurrent abortion have a detectable parental chromosomal abnormality, surgically correctable uterine abnormalities, an incompetent cervix, or intrauterine synechiae. Uterine anomalies are found in 15% to 25% of women with recurrent abortion. The possibility of immunologic factors as a cause of recurrent losses should also be evaluated (e.g., lupus anticoagulant). Two thirds of recurrent abortions occur after 12 weeks of gestation, suggesting that maternal or environmental factors play a large role in this process.

Risk Factors: Those associated with spontaneous abortion, including increasing maternal and paternal age and autoimmune disorders.

CLINICAL CHARACTERISTICS

Signs and Symptoms

- Two consecutive or three total first-trimester spontaneous pregnancy losses.

DIAGNOSTIC APPROACH

Differential Diagnosis

- Uterine anomalies (fibroids, incompetent cervix, intra-uterine synechiae, developmental abnormalities such as a septum or duplication)
- Chromosomal abnormality (maternal [more likely] or paternal)
- Immunologic causes (such as lupus anticoagulant)
- Endocrinopathy (such as hypothyroidism)
- Coagulopathy or thrombophilia

Associated Conditions: None.

Workup and Evaluation

Laboratory: Screening for immunologic or endocrine abnormality; coagulopathy or thrombophilia as indicated.

Imaging: Ultrasonography of the pelvis or hysterosalpingography may be of assistance when a uterine anomaly is suspected.

Special Tests: Karyotyping of both parents is recommended when recurrent early abortions have occurred. Karyotyping of the abortus may be helpful but requires fresh tissue, specialized transport media, and laboratory capabilities.

Diagnostic Procedures: Hysteroscopy may be of limited value (indicated only when a uterine factor is strongly considered).

Pathologic Findings

None.

MANAGEMENT AND THERAPY

Nonpharmacologic

General Measures: Support and evaluation.

Specific Measures: Those with parental chromosomal anomalies may be offered donor oocytes or artificial insemination with donor sperm. Uterine anomalies or submucous fibroids may be treated, although care must be taken to recognize the possibility of continued failure for other reasons and the possible impact of future delivery options.

Diet: No specific dietary changes indicated.

Activity: No restriction.

Patient Education: Reassurance; American College of Obstetricians and Gynecologists Patient Education Pamphlet AP100 (Repeated Miscarriage), AP090 (Early Pregnancy Loss: Miscarriage, Ectopic Pregnancy, and Molar Pregnancy).

Drug(s) of Choice

None. Progesterone and thyroid supplements have not been shown to reduce the risk of pregnancy loss. When immunologic factors are present, the use of low-dose aspirin and subcutaneous heparin (5000 units twice daily) has reduced the rate of subsequent loss.

FOLLOW-UP

Patient Monitoring: Normal health maintenance.

Prevention/Avoidance: None.

Expected Outcome: Based on underlying pathologic condition.

MISCELLANEOUS

Pregnancy Considerations: When due to correctable factors, future pregnancies will not be affected.

ICD-9-CM Codes: 646.3.

REFERENCES

Level I

Dolitzky M, Inbal A, Segal Y, et al: A randomized study of thromboprophylaxis in women with unexplained consecutive recurrent miscarriages. Fertil Steril 2006;86:362. Epub 2006 Jun 12.

Level II

Franssen MT, Korevaar JC, van der Veen F, et al: Reproductive outcome after chromosome analysis in couples with two or more miscarriages: index [corrected]-control study. BMJ 2006;332:759. Epub 2006 Feb 22.

Goel N, Tuli A, Choudhry R: The role of aspirin versus aspirin and heparin in cases of recurrent abortions with raised anticardiolipin antibodies. Med Sci Monit 2006;12:CR132. Epub 2006 Feb 23.

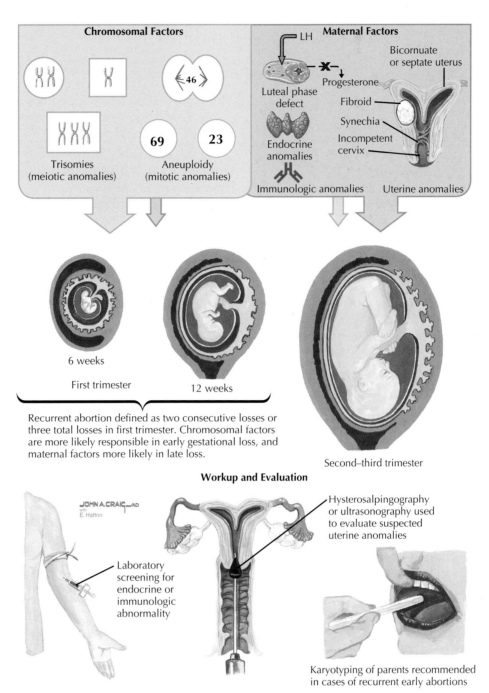

Chromosomal Factors

Trisomies
(meiotic anomalies)

Aneuploidy
(mitotic anomalies)

Maternal Factors

LH

Progesterone

Luteal phase
defect

Endocrine
anomalies

Immunologic anomalies

Bicornuate
or septate uterus

Fibroid

Synechia

Incompetent
cervix

Uterine anomalies

6 weeks

First trimester

12 weeks

Recurrent abortion defined as two consecutive losses or
three total losses in first trimester. Chromosomal factors
are more likely responsible in early gestational loss, and
maternal factors more likely in late loss.

Second–third trimester

Workup and Evaluation

JOHN A. CRAIG—MD
with
E. Hatton

Laboratory
screening for
endocrine or
immunologic
abnormality

Hysterosalpingography
or ultrasonography used
to evaluate suspected
uterine anomalies

Karyotyping of parents recommended
in cases of recurrent early abortions

LH, luteinizing hormone

Noori M, Helmig RB, Hein M, Steer PJ: Could a cervical occlusion suture be effective at improving perinatal outcome? BJOG 2007;114:532.

Sotiriadis A, Makrigiannakis A, Stefos T, et al: Fibrinolytic defects and recurrent miscarriage: a systematic review and meta-analysis. Obstet Gynecol 2007;109:1146.

Level III

American College of Obstetricians and Gynecologists: Perinatal viral and parasitic infections. ACOG Practice Bulletin 20. Washington, DC, ACOG, 2000.

American College of Obstetricians and Gynecologists: Management of recurrent early pregnancy loss. ACOG Practice Bulletin 24. Washington, DC, ACOG, 2001.

American College of Obstetricians and Gynecologists: Cervical insufficiency. ACOG Practice Bulletin 48. Obstet Gynecol 2003; 102:1091.

American College of Obstetricians and Gynecologists: Antiphospholipid syndrome. ACOG Practice Bulletin 68. Obstet Gynecol 2005;106:1113.

Carrington B, Sacks G, Regan L: Recurrent miscarriage: pathophysiology and outcome. Curr Opin Obstet Gynecol 2005;17:591.

Kujovich JL: Thrombophilia and pregnancy complications. Am J Obstet Gynecol 2004;191:412.

Petri M, Qazi U: Management of antiphospholipid syndrome in pregnancy. Rheum Dis Clin North Am 2006;32:591.

Price M, Kelsberg G, Safranek S, Damitz B: Clinical inquiries. What treatments prevent miscarriage after recurrent pregnancy loss? J Fam Pract 2005;54:892, 894.

Rai R, Regan L: Recurrent miscarriage. Lancet 2006;368:601.

Wu S, Stephenson MD: Obstetrical antiphospholipid syndrome. Semin Reprod Med 2006;24:40.

INTRODUCTION

Description: Primary amenorrhea is the absence of normal menstruation in a patient without previously established cycles.

Prevalence: Uncommon.

Predominant Age: Mid to late teens.

Genetics: One third caused by chromosomal abnormalities such as 45,XO, 46,XY gonadal dysgenesis, or 46,XX q5 X long-arm deletion.

ETIOLOGY AND PATHOGENESIS

Causes: Gonadal abnormalities (failure, 60% of patients)—autoimmune ovarian failure (Blizzard syndrome), gonadal dysgenesis, pure gonadal dysgenesis, 45,XO (Turner's syndrome), 46,XY gonadal dysgenesis (Swyer syndrome), 46,XX q5 X chromosome long-arm deletion, mixed or mosaic, follicular depletion, autoimmune disease, infection (e.g., mumps), infiltrative disease processes (e.g., tuberculosis, galactosemia), iatrogenic ovarian failure (e.g., alkylating chemotherapy, irradiation), ovarian insensitivity syndrome (resistant ovary [Savage's] syndrome), 17α-hydroxylase deficiency, chronic anovulation of pubertal onset. Extragonadal anomalies (40%)—congenital absence of uterus and vagina (15%) (Müllerian agenesis), constitutional delay, imperforate hymen, male pseudohermaphroditism (testicular feminization syndrome), pituitary–hypothalamic dysfunction, transverse vaginal septum.

Risk Factors: None known.

CLINICAL CHARACTERISTICS

Signs and Symptoms

- No period by age 14 with no secondary sex changes
- No period by age 16 regardless of secondary sex changes
- No period by 2 years after the start of secondary sex changes

Evaluation should not be delayed any time there is the suggestion of a chromosomal abnormality or an obstructed genital tract.

DIAGNOSTIC APPROACH

Differential Diagnosis

- Pregnancy before first cycle
- Obstructed outflow tract (making menstruation cryptic)
- Gonadal dysgenesis
- Uterine agenesis
- Androgen insensitivity syndrome
- Mayer-Rokitansky-Küster-Hauser syndrome

Associated Conditions: Infertility, abnormal stature (short or tall), and cardiac changes in some congenital syndromes; hypertension and hypokalemic alkalosis in 17α-hydroxylase deficiency, virilization, or hirsutism; and cyclic pelvic pain with outflow obstruction. Renal and skeletal abnormalities may also occur. Prolonged amenorrhea is associated with an increased risk of osteoporosis.

Workup and Evaluation

Laboratory: The development of sexual hair or breasts provides an outward sign of androgen and estrogen production, respectively.

Imaging: Based on conditions being considered.

Special Tests: Based on conditions being considered.

Diagnostic Procedures: Laparoscopy to evaluate internal organs and gonads may be required.

Pathologic Findings

None.

MANAGEMENT AND THERAPY

Nonpharmacologic

General Measures: Determination of underlying cause(s).

Specific Measures: Based on the diagnosis and specific needs of the patient.

Diet: No specific dietary changes indicated.

Activity: No restriction.

Patient Education: Reassurance; American College of Obstetricians and Gynecologists Patient Education Pamphlet AP049 (Menstruation [Especially for Teens]) or AP041 (Growing Up [Especially for Teens]).

Drug(s) of Choice

Based on underlying cause. Hormone replacement may be required or desirable for many patients.

FOLLOW-UP

Patient Monitoring: Normal health maintenance.

Prevention/Avoidance: None.

Possible Complications: Risk of gonadal malignancy is increased if a Y chromosome is present. Risk of osteoporosis is present if the patient is hypoestrogenic and does not receive replacement therapy. Extensive damage to the upper tract may occur if obstruction is not corrected.

Expected Outcome: Menstruation and fertility may be restored for many of these patients if there are no structural or chromosomal conditions that preclude the possibility (uterine agenesis, androgen insensitivity syndrome, gonadal dysgenesis).

MISCELLANEOUS

Pregnancy Considerations: Infertility common. If pregnancy is achieved, there are no effects except those imposed by underlying cause.

ICD-9-CM Codes: 626.0.

Neuroendocrine Regulation of Menstrual Cycle

Hypothalamic regulation of pituitary gonadotropin production and release

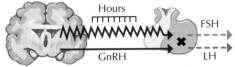

Pulsed release of GnRH by hypothalamus (1 pulse/1–2 hr) permits anterior pituitary production and release of FSH and LH (normal)

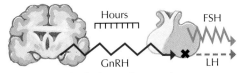

Continuous, excessive, absent, or more frequent GnRH release inhibits FSH and LH production and release (downloading)

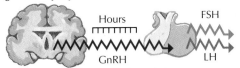

Decreased pulsed release of GnRH decreases LH secretion but increases FSH secretion (slow-pulsing model)

Ovarian feedback modulation of pituitary gonadotropin production and release

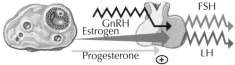

Presence of pulsed GnRH and low estrogen and progesterone levels result in increased levels of pulsed LH and FSH (negative feedback)

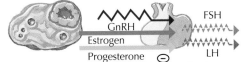

Presence of pulsed GnRH, rapidly increasing levels of estrogen, and small amounts of progesterone results in high pulsed LH and moderately increased pulsed FSH levels (positive feedback)

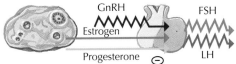

Presence of pulsed GnRH and high levels of estrogen and progesterone results in decreased LH and FSH levels (negative feedback)

Correlation of serum gonadotrophic and ovarian hormone levels and feedback mechanisms

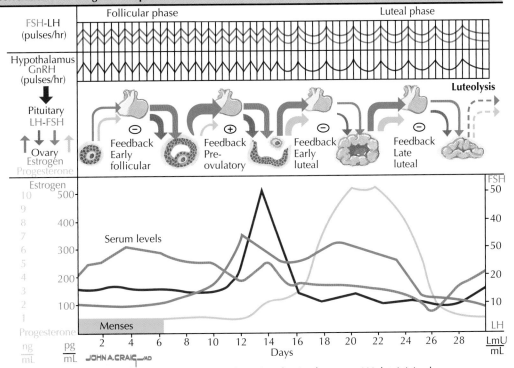

FSH, follicle-stimulating hormone; GnRH, gonadotropin-releasing hormone; LH, luteinizing hormone.

REFERENCES

Level III

American Academy of Pediatrics, American College of Obstetricians and Gynecologists: Menstruation in girls and adolescents: using the menstrual cycle as a vital sign. ACOG Committee Opinion 349. Obstet Gynecol 2006;108:1323.

American College of Obstetricians and Gynecologists: Vaginal agenesis: diagnosis, management, and routine care. ACOG Committee Opinion 355. Obstet Gynecol 2006;108:1605.

Lobo RA: Primary and secondary amenorrhea and precocious puberty. In Katz VL, Lentz GM, Lobo RA, Gershenson DM: Comprehensive Gynecology, 5th ed. Philadelphia, Mosby/Elsevier, 2007, p 937.

Master-Hunter T, Heiman DL: Amenorrhea: evaluation and treatment. Am Fam Physician 2006;73:1374.

Pletcher JR, Slap GB: Menstrual disorders. Amenorrhea. Pediatr Clin North Am 1999;46:505.

van Niekerk WA: Chromosomes and the gynecologist. Am J Obstet Gynecol 1978;130:862.

INTRODUCTION

Description: Secondary amenorrhea is the absence of normal menstruation in a patient with previously established cycles.

Prevalence: Common.

Predominant Age: Reproductive (menarche to menopause).

Genetics: No genetic pattern.

ETIOLOGY AND PATHOGENESIS

Causes: Most common—pregnancy. Other causes—end organ: Asherman's syndrome, outflow obstruction; ovarian: menopause, resistant ovary [Savage's] syndrome, toxin exposure, surgery, autoimmune disease; central, behavioral, and others: anorexia, obesity, athletics (overtraining), drugs/medications, nutritional deprivation, psychogenic (stress); medical: adenoma, craniopharyngioma, Sheehan's syndrome, tuberculosis, sarcoid, empty sella syndrome; virilizing syndromes: polycystic ovary syndrome, adrenal hyperplasia, virilizing tumors.

Risk Factors: Unprotected intercourse, exposure to toxins or radiation, surgery, overtraining, eating disorders, psychosocial stress.

CLINICAL CHARACTERISTICS

Signs and Symptoms

- Absent menstruation—may be associated with symptoms that suggest the cause.

DIAGNOSTIC APPROACH

Differential Diagnosis

- Pregnancy
- Menopause (natural or premature)
- Exogenous hormone use
- Virilization
- Metabolically active ovarian tumor
- Lactational amenorrhea

Associated Conditions: Endometrial hyperplasia, osteoporosis in hypoestrogenic states.

Workup and Evaluation

Laboratory: A pregnancy test is always indicated.

Imaging: Based on conditions being considered.

Special Tests: Women who are younger than age 30 who have ovarian failure should have a karyotype performed.

Diagnostic Procedures: Based on conditions being considered.

Pathologic Findings

None.

MANAGEMENT AND THERAPY

Nonpharmacologic

General Measures: Determination of underlying cause(s). If a pathologic condition has been ruled out and pregnancy is not desired, reassurance only. Evaluation should not be delayed any time there is the suggestion of an abnormality or pregnancy.

Specific Measures: Periodic (every 3 to 6 months) progestin withdrawal to prevent endometrial hyperplasia and to re-evaluate status. Specific therapy is based on the underlying cause (such as estrogen/progestin therapy for menopause). Treatment is focused on restoring or inducing ovulation if pregnancy is desired.

Diet: No specific dietary changes indicated.

Activity: No restriction.

Patient Education: Reassurance; American College of Obstetricians and Gynecologists Patient Education Pamphlet AP049 (Menstruation [Especially for Teens]) or AP041 (Growing Up [Especially for Teens]), AP121 (Polycystic Ovary Syndrome), AP047 (The Menopause Years).

Drug(s) of Choice

Based on diagnosis (e.g., thyroid replacement for hypothyroidism, estrogen and progestin therapy for ovarian failure, periodic progestin therapy [oral or transvaginal] or ovulation induction for anovulation).

Contraindications: All medical interventions are contraindicated until pregnancy has been ruled out.

FOLLOW-UP

Patient Monitoring: Normal health maintenance. Watch for changing status or intercurrent pregnancy.

Prevention/Avoidance: None (contraception).

Possible Complications: Endometrial hyperplasia with continued estrogen (unopposed) exposure.

Expected Outcome: Most causes of secondary amenorrhea may be successfully treated with return of menstruation.

MISCELLANEOUS

Pregnancy Considerations: Pregnancy must be ruled out.

ICD-9-CM Codes: 626.0.

REFERENCES

Level II

Warren MP, Biller BM, Shangold MM: A new clinical option for hormone replacement therapy in women with secondary amenorrhea: effects of cyclic administration of progesterone from the sustained-release vaginal gel Crinone (4% and 8%) on endometrial morphologic features and withdrawal bleeding. Am J Obstet Gynecol 1999;180:42.

Level III

American Academy of Pediatrics, American College of Obstetricians and Gynecologists: Menstruation in girls and adolescents: using the menstrual cycle as a vital sign. ACOG Committee Opinion 349. Obstet Gynecol 2006;108:1323.

American College of Obstetricians and Gynecologists: Management of anovulatory bleeding. ACOG Practice Bulletin 14. Washington, DC, ACOG, 2000.

American College of Obstetricians and Gynecologists: Management of infertility caused by ovulatory dysfunction. ACOG Practice Bulletin 34. Obstet Gynecol 2002;99:347.

Causes of Ovulatory Dysfunction

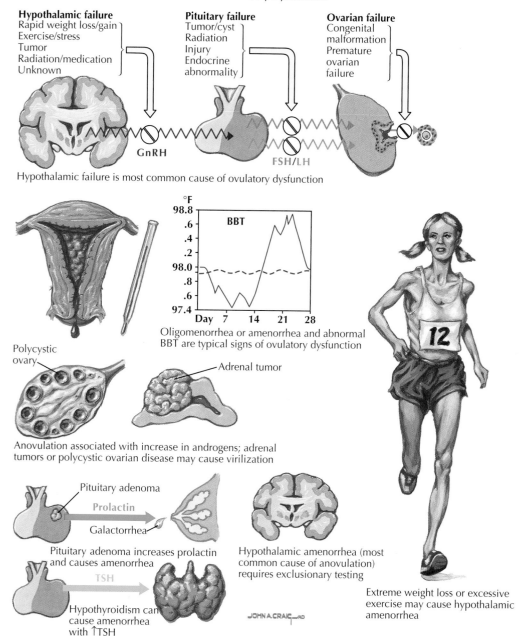

Hypothalamic failure
Rapid weight loss/gain
Exercise/stress
Tumor
Radiation/medication
Unknown

Pituitary failure
Tumor/cyst
Radiation
Injury
Endocrine
abnormality

Ovarian failure
Congenital
malformation
Premature
ovarian
failure

GnRH

FSH/LH

Hypothalamic failure is most common cause of ovulatory dysfunction

°F
98.8
.6
.4
.2
98.0
.8
.6
97.4
Day 7   14   21   28

BBT

Oligomenorrhea or amenorrhea and abnormal BBT are typical signs of ovulatory dysfunction

Polycystic ovary

Adrenal tumor

Anovulation associated with increase in androgens; adrenal tumors or polycystic ovarian disease may cause virilization

Pituitary adenoma
Prolactin
Galactorrhea

Pituitary adenoma increases prolactin and causes amenorrhea

TSH

Hypothyroidism can cause amenorrhea with ↑TSH

Hypothalamic amenorrhea (most common cause of anovulation) requires exclusionary testing

JOHN A. CRAIG—AD

Extreme weight loss or excessive exercise may cause hypothalamic amenorrhea

BBT, basal body temperature; FSH, follicle-stimulating hormone; SnRTT, gonadotropin-releasing hormone; LH, luteinizing hormone; TSH, thyroid-stimulating hormone.

American College of Obstetricians and Gynecologists: Polycystic ovary syndrome. ACOG Practice Bulletin 41. Obstet Gynecol 2002;100:1389.

Bloomfield D. Secondary amenorrhea. Pediatr Rev 2006;27: 113.

Diddle AW: Athletic activity and menstruation. South Med J 1983;76:619.

Haller E: Eating disorders. A review and update. West J Med 1992;157:658.

Hull MG, Savage PE, Jacobs HS: Investigation and treatment of amenorrhoea resulting in normal fertility. Br Med J 1979; 1:1257.

Lobo RA: Primary and secondary amenorrhea and precocious puberty. In Katz VL, Lentz GM, Lobo RA, Gershenson DM: Comprehensive Gynecology, 5th ed. Philadelphia, Mosby/Elsevier, 2007, p 942.

Master-Hunter T, Heiman DL: Amenorrhea: evaluation and treatment. Am Fam Physician 2006;73:1374.

Perkins RB, Hall JE, Martin KA: Neuroendocrine abnormalities in hypothalamic amenorrhea: spectrum, stability, and response to neurotransmitter modulation. J Clin Endocrinol Metab 1999;84:1905.

Pletcher JR, Slap GB: Menstrual disorders. Amenorrhea. Pediatr Clin North Am 1999;46:505.

Practice Committee of the American Society for Reproductive Medicine: Current evaluation of amenorrhea. Fertil Steril 2006;86: S148.

Sabatini S: The female athlete triad. Am J Med Sci 2001;322:193.

Schwabe AD, Lippe BM, Chang RJ, et al: Anorexia nervosa. Ann Intern Med 1981;94:371.

Walshe JM, Denduluri N, Swain SM: Amenorrhea in premenopausal women after adjuvant chemotherapy for breast cancer. J Clin Oncol 2006;24:5769. Epub 2006 Nov 27.

Warren MP: Clinical review 77: evaluation of secondary amenorrhea. J Clin Endocrinol Metab 1996;81:437.

White CM, Hergenroeder AC: Amenorrhea, osteopenia, and the female athlete. Pediatr Clin North Am 1990;37:1125.

INTRODUCTION

Description: Patients with androgen insensitivity have a normal male karyotype but a genetic alteration that results in somatic cells that cannot recognize or respond to testosterone. This results in a normal female phenotype, absent uterus, and scant (or absent) body hair. The syndrome was known at one time as "testicular feminization."

Prevalence: Uncommon, 10% of patients with primary amenorrhea (third most common cause).

Predominant Age: Generally discovered in middle to late teens.

Genetics: Absence of an X-chromosome gene that encodes for cytoplasmic or nuclear testosterone receptor protein, X-linked recessive.

ETIOLOGY AND PATHOGENESIS

Causes: Testosterone and gonadotropin levels are essentially normal (there may be a slight increase in luteinizing hormone [LH]), but the testosterone is biologically ineffective because of the body's inability to use it. Consequently, masculinization does not take place, and the normal production of Müllerian-inhibiting factor results in regression of the upper genital tract and a blind vaginal pouch.

Risk Factors: None known.

CLINICAL CHARACTERISTICS

Signs and Symptoms

- Amenorrhea
- Tall stature
- Normal breast development with immature nipples and hypopigmented areolae
- Short or absent blind vaginal pouch
- Scant or no pubic or axillary hair
- Gonads (testes) may be palpable in the inguinal canal or labioscrotal folds
- Inguinal hernia (50%)

DIAGNOSTIC APPROACH

Differential Diagnosis

- Pregnancy before first cycle
- Obstructed outflow tract (making menstruation cryptic)
- Gonadal dysgenesis
- Uterine agenesis
- Complete lack of Müllerian development (Mayer-Rokitansky-Küster-Hauser syndrome)

Associated Conditions: Infertility, amenorrhea, mildly impaired visual–spatial ability, horseshoe kidney.

Workup and Evaluation

Laboratory: Measurement of gonadotropins, estrogen, and testosterone (not required for diagnosis).

Imaging: Ultrasonography may be used to confirm the absence of the uterus, although it is not required for diagnosis.

Special Tests: Chromosomal analysis confirms the diagnosis.

Diagnostic Procedures: History and physical examination should provide the suggestion, confirmed by chromosomal analysis.

Pathologic Findings

The presence of testicular tissue in the labioscrotal folds.

MANAGEMENT AND THERAPY

Nonpharmacologic

General Measures: Evaluation and reassurance.

Specific Measures: Surgical extirpation of the gonads must be performed because of a 25% to 30% risk of malignant gonadal tumor formation. This should not be performed until complete breast development has occurred and there has been epiphyseal closure (age 18). Genetic counseling should be offered to siblings.

Diet: No specific dietary changes indicated.

Activity: No restriction.

Patient Education: Frank discussion about the syndrome and its effects (infertility and amenorrhea). Patients should be informed that they carry an abnormal sex chromosome without mentioning the Y chromosome specifically because of the "male" connotations this carries. In addition, the term gonads should be used rather than testes when discussing the need for removal. Refer patients to the Androgen Insensitivity Syndrome Support Group (www.aissg.org)

Drug(s) of Choice

None. (Estrogen replacement therapy is generally not necessary after removal of the gonads; the insensitivity of the peripheral tissues to the effects of circulating androgens results in unopposed estrogen effects from the low levels of estrogen that come from adrenal and peripheral conversion sources.)

FOLLOW-UP

Patient Monitoring: Normal health maintenance once the diagnosis is established and the gonads are removed (at the appropriate time).

Prevention/Avoidance: None.

Possible Complications: There is a 25% to 30% risk of malignant gonadal tumor formation if the testes are not removed (rare before age 25).

Expected Outcome: These patients are phenotypically, behaviorally, and psychologically female and continue to lead normal lives with the exception of infertility and amenorrhea.

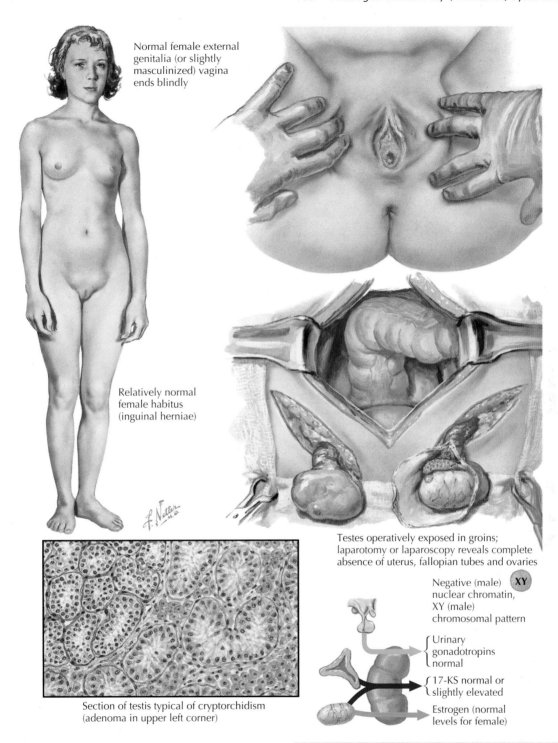

Normal female external genitalia (or slightly masculinized) vagina ends blindly

Relatively normal female habitus (inguinal herniae)

Testes operatively exposed in groins; laparotomy or laparoscopy reveals complete absence of uterus, fallopian tubes and ovaries

Negative (male) nuclear chromatin, XY (male) chromosomal pattern   **XY**

Urinary gonadotropins normal

17-KS normal or slightly elevated

Estrogen (normal levels for female)

Section of testis typical of cryptorchidism (adenoma in upper left corner)

MISCELLANEOUS

Pregnancy Considerations: These patients are infertile.
ICD-9-CM Codes: 257.8.

REFERENCES

Level III

American College of Obstetricians and Gynecologists: Vaginal agenesis: diagnosis, management, and routine care. ACOG Committee Opinion 355. Obstet Gynecol 2006;108:1605.

Evans BA, Hughes IA, Bevan CL, et al: Phenotypic diversity in siblings with partial androgen insensitivity syndrome. Arch Dis Child 1997;76:529.

Golditch IM: Vaginal aplasia. Surg Gynecol Obstet 1969;129: 361.

Griffin JE, Wilson JD: The syndromes of androgen resistance. N Engl J Med 1980;302:198.

Hyun G, Kolon TF: A practical approach to intersex in the newborn period. Urol Clin North Am 2004;31:435, viii.

Lentz SS, Cappellari JO: Postmenopausal diagnosis of testicular feminization. Am J Obstet Gynecol 1998;179:268.

Lobo RA: Primary and secondary amenorrhea and precocious puberty. In Katz VL, Lentz GM, Lobo RA, Gershenson DM: Comprehensive Gynecology, 5th ed. Philadelphia, Mosby/Elsevier, 2007, p 937.

Savage MO, Grant DB: The incomplete male. Arch Dis Child 1978;53:701.

INTRODUCTION

Description: Anovulation is characterized by absence of ovulation in women of reproductive age.

Prevalence: Up to 30% of couples who are infertile.

Predominant Age: Reproductive.

Genetics: No genetic pattern, some chromosomal abnormalities are associated with premature ovarian failure (deletions on the X chromosome).

ETIOLOGY AND PATHOGENESIS

Causes: Physiologic—menopause (normal or premature), pregnancy; hormonal—elevated prolactin, hypothyroidism; functional—exercise (excessive), malnutrition, obesity, weight loss; drug-induced—alkylating chemotherapy, hormonal contraception, marijuana, tranquilizers; neoplasia—craniopharyngioma, hypothalamic hamartoma, pituitary adenoma (prolactin-secreting), small cell carcinoma of lung; psychogenic—anorexia nervosa, anxiety, pseudocyesis, stress; other—adrenal androgenization, central nervous system trauma, chronic medical illness, hemochromatosis, histiocytosis X, internal carotid artery aneurysms, irradiation, juvenile diabetes mellitus, polycystic ovary syndrome, Sheehan's syndrome (postpartum ischemic necrosis), syphilitic gummas, tuberculosis, uremia.

Risk Factors: Factors noted in previous section.

CLINICAL CHARACTERISTICS

Signs and Symptoms

- Amenorrhea (primary or secondary)
- Absence of premenstrual molimina (prodromal symptoms)

DIAGNOSTIC APPROACH

Differential Diagnosis

- Pregnancy must always be considered
- Menopause
- Congenital abnormality of the outflow tract causing amenorrhea
- Cervical stenosis resulting in amenorrhea

Associated Conditions: Infertility, dysfunctional uterine bleeding, endometrial hyperplasia, and endometrial cancer.

Workup and Evaluation

Laboratory: Follicle-stimulating hormone (FSH), prolactin, thyroid function studies (e.g., sensitive thyroid-stimulating hormone [TSH]), others as indicated clinically.

Imaging: No imaging indicated.

Special Tests: Basal body temperature charting may be used to detect ovulation, but other laboratory tests are more specific for establishing the cause.

Diagnostic Procedures: Endometrial biopsy performed during the presumed luteal phase.

Pathologic Findings

Endometrial—proliferative changes only, hyperplasia possible with prolonged anovulation.

MANAGEMENT AND THERAPY

Nonpharmacologic

General Measures: Evaluation.

Specific Measures: If pregnancy is desired, induction of ovulation. If pregnancy is not desired, periodic progestin therapy.

Diet: No specific dietary changes indicated.

Activity: No restriction.

Patient Education: Reassurance; American College of Obstetricians and Gynecologists Patient Education Pamphlet AP136 (Evaluating Infertility), AP137 (Treating Infertility), AP095 (Abnormal Uterine Bleeding), AP121 (Polycystic Ovary Syndrome), AP047 (The Menopause Years).

Drug(s) of Choice

Ovulation induction—clomiphene citrate 50 mg PO daily on days 5 to 10 of the menstrual cycle, may be increased to 100 mg PO daily on days 5 to 10 of the menstrual cycle if ovulation does not occur. Metformin (1500 mg/day) as an adjunctive treatment for ovulation induction (considered now as first-line therapy for polycystic ovary syndrome).

Progestin withdrawal—medroxyprogesterone acetate 5 to 10 mg for 1 to 14 days each month.

Contraindications: Undiagnosed amenorrhea or bleeding.

Precautions: Progestins should not be used until pregnancy has been ruled out.

Alternative Drugs

Aromatase inhibitors are efficacious as primary agents for ovulation induction (e.g., letrozole; 2.5 mg or 5 mg administered for 5 days, beginning on cycle days 3 to 5.).

Norethindrone acetate 5 to 10 mg for 10 to 14 days each month for progestin withdrawal.

FOLLOW-UP

Patient Monitoring: Normal health maintenance.

Prevention/Avoidance: None.

Possible Complications: Infertility, dysfunctional uterine bleeding, endometrial hyperplasia.

Expected Outcome: For many patients, normal ovulation and fertility may be restored.

MISCELLANEOUS

Pregnancy Considerations: No effect on pregnancy once pregnancy is achieved.

ICD-9-CM Codes: 628.0.

Assessment of Ovulation

Ovulatory phase
Hormonal and physical findings indicate ovulation occurred

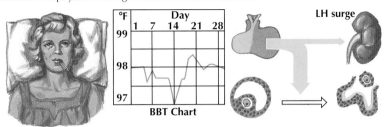

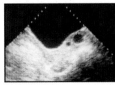

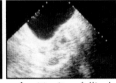

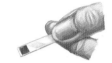

LH surge

Basal body temperature (BBT). Detects signs of ovulation

Preovulatory follicle   Ruptured follicle

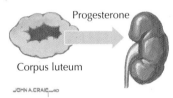

Serial follicular ultrasonography. Monitors follicular rupture

Ovulation detection kit. Detects urinary metabolites of luteinizing hormone (LH)

Luteal phase
Hormonal and physical findings indicate functioning corpus luteum

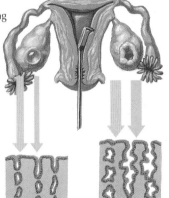

Progesterone

Corpus luteum

JOHN A.CRAIG—AD

Endometrial biopsy and dating. Provides evidence of functioning corpus luteum and end organ response

Proliferative phase   Secretory phase

REFERENCES

Level I
Eisenhardt S, Schwarzmann N, Henschel V, et al: Early effects of metformin in women with polycystic ovary syndrome: a prospective randomized, double-blind, placebo-controlled trial. J Clin Endocrinol Metab 2006;91:946. Epub 2005 Dec 13.

Palomba S, Orio F Jr, Falbo A, et al: Prospective parallel randomized, double-blind, double-dummy controlled clinical trial comparing clomiphene citrate and metformin as the first-line treatment for ovulation induction in nonobese anovulatory women with polycystic ovary syndrome. J Clin Endocrinol Metab 2005;90:4068. Epub 2005 Apr 19.

Level II
Lord JM, Flight IH, Norman RJ: Metformin in polycystic ovary syndrome: systematic review and meta-analysis. BMJ 2003; 327:951.

Level III
American Academy of Pediatrics, American College of Obstetricians and Gynecologists: Menstruation in girls and adolescents: using the menstrual cycle as a vital sign. ACOG Committee Opinion 349. Obstet Gynecol 2006;108:1323.

American College of Obstetricians and Gynecologists: Management of anovulatory bleeding. ACOG Practice Bulletin 14. Washington, DC, ACOG, 2000.

American College of Obstetricians and Gynecologists: Management of infertility caused by ovulatory dysfunction. ACOG Practice Bulletin 34. Obstet Gynecol 2002;99:347.

American College of Obstetricians and Gynecologists: Polycystic ovary syndrome. ACOG Practice Bulletin 41. Obstet Gynecol 2002;100:1389.

Casper RF, Mitwally MF: Review: Aromatase inhibitors for ovulation induction. J Clin Endocrinol Metab 2006;91:760. Epub 2005 Dec 29.

Chang RJ: A practical approach to the diagnosis of polycystic ovary syndrome. Am J Obstet Gynecol 2004;191:713.

Davis CH 3rd, Hall MN, Kaufman L, Danis P: Clinical inquiries. what is the best way to evaluate secondary infertility? J Fam Pract 2007;56:573.

Guzick DS: Polycystic ovary syndrome. Obstet Gynecol 2004; 103:181.

Hamilton-Fairley D, Taylor A: Anovulation. BMJ 2003;327:546.

Hardiman P, Pillay OC, Atiomo W: Polycystic ovary syndrome and endometrial carcinoma. Lancet 2003;361:1810.

Healy DL, Trounson AO, Andersen AN: Female infertility: causes and treatment. Lancet 1994;343:1539.

Lobo RA, Carmina E: The importance of diagnosing the polycystic ovary syndrome. Ann Intern Med 2000;132:989.

Lobo RA: Primary and secondary amenorrhea and precocious puberty. In Katz VL, Lentz GM, Lobo RA, Gershenson DM: Comprehensive Gynecology, 5th ed. Philadelphia, Mosby/Elsevier, 2007, p 942.

Lobo RA: Infertility. In Katz VL, Lentz GM, Lobo RA, Gershenson DM: Comprehensive Gynecology, 5th ed. Philadelphia, Mosby/Elsevier, 2007, p 1013.

Setji TL, Brown AJ: Polycystic ovary syndrome: diagnosis and treatment. Am J Med 2007;120:128.

THE CHALLENGE

To use advanced reproductive technology to assist couples who experience difficulty conceiving through normal means.

Scope of the Problem: Ten percent to fifteen percent of couples who are infertile require or benefit from assisted reproductive technologies.

Objectives of Management: To achieve a successful pregnancy (carried to term) with minimal intervention. The treatment of an infertile couple is based on identifying the impediment to fertility and overcoming or bypassing it to achieve pregnancy. A number of techniques are available to accomplish this end. Most are less exotic than their acronyms suggest (see Table). Among infertile couples seeking treatment, 85% to 90% can be treated with conventional medical and surgical procedures and do not require assisted reproductive technologies such as in vitro fertilization.

TACTICS

Relevant Pathophysiology: The success of treatment depends to a great extent on the identified cause of infertility because some problems are more easily overcome than others. It must be recognized that success is also a function of the age of the woman. It is also true that the rate of spontaneous pregnancy loss increases rapidly after age 35, adversely affecting success.

ABBREVIATIONS FOR TECHNIQUES

Abbreviation	Technique
AID	Artificial insemination, donor (using donor sperm, occasionally referred to as TDI or therapeutic donor insemination)
AIH	Artificial insemination, homologous (using the partner's sperm)
BT	Basal body temperature
GIFT	Gamete intrafallopian transfer (gametes placed in the fallopian tube for fertilization)
HSG	Hysterosalpingogram or uterine cavity radiograph
ICSI	Intracytoplasmic sperm injection
IUI	Intrauterine insemination (placement of either donor or husband sperm directly into the uterine cavity)
IVF/ET	In vitro fertilization with embryo transfer
PCT	Postcoital test or Huhner-Sims test
SPA	Sperm penetration assay (also known as a hamster egg test or zona-free egg penetration test)
ZIFT	Zygote intrafallopian transfer (fertilization takes place in vitro and the zygote is transferred to the fallopian tube to be transported into the uterine cavity)

Strategies: Often a good starting point in the treatment of infertility is a frank and open discussion about sexuality and the physiology of conception. When couples have intercourse four or more times per week, more than 80% achieve pregnancy in the first 6 months of trying. By contrast, only about 15% of couples conceive when intercourse happens less than once a week. Intercourse should be maintained on an every-other-day cycle for the period from 3 to 4 days before the presumed ovulation until 2 to 3 days after that time. When ovulation disorders are encountered, ovulation induction or control may be used to enhance the likelihood of pregnancy. Tubal factor infertility may be addressed by either surgical repair of the damage or by bypassing the tubes completely through in vitro fertilization and embryo transfer (IVF/ET). According to 2004 statistics, in vitro fertilization techniques account for only about 5% of infertility services and are associated with a roughly 32% live delivery rate per egg retrieval. Success rates for surgical repair, including the reversal of previous sterilization procedure, are highly variable. Technologies such as intracellular sperm injection may allow fertility with as few as one sperm per oocyte.

Patient Education: Reassurance; American College of Obstetricians and Gynecologists Patient Education Pamphlet AP136 (Evaluating Infertility), AP137 (Treating Infertility).

IMPLEMENTATION

Special Considerations: Patients experiencing infertility are usually extremely motivated, following to the letter any suggestion made by the health care team. For this reason, care must be taken that during the evaluation and treatment of infertility the couple's relationship is not destroyed in the process. In the end, there is no guarantee that efforts will result in a conception, so the health care team must not damage what is present in the quest of something that may not be. Couples should be reminded that "If you miss having intercourse at the 'right time' in a given month, remember that ovulations are like commuter trains—there is probably another one on its way." If the couple is in the mood for "making love," in any of its myriad forms, they should not worry about what the temperature chart is doing. To do otherwise is the fodder of cinematic comedy and divorce lawyers. Because infertility does not threaten life or health, many insurance providers do not cover the cost of its evaluation or treatment. A frank and open discussion about the time and expense involved in infertility evaluation allows the couple to make informed choices and avoids unnecessary financial or emotional hardship in the future.

All types of assisted reproductive technologies involving ovarian stimulation are associated with an increased incidence of multiple gestations (40%): The majority of these pregnancies are twins (25%), and 5% are higher-order gestations.

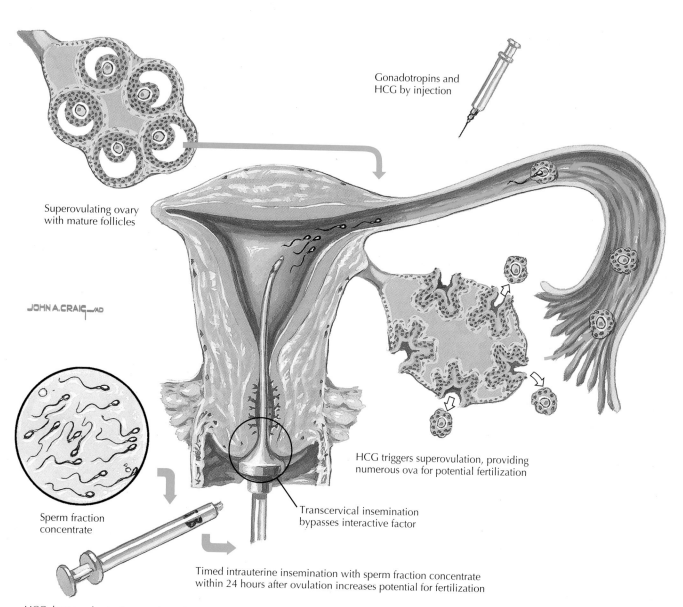

Gonadotropins and
HCG by injection

Superovulating ovary
with mature follicles

JOHN A.CRAIG—AD

HCG triggers superovulation, providing
numerous ova for potential fertilization

Sperm fraction
concentrate

Transcervical insemination
bypasses interactive factor

Timed intrauterine insemination with sperm fraction concentrate
within 24 hours after ovulation increases potential for fertilization

HCG, human chorionic gonadotropin.

In Vitro Fertilization

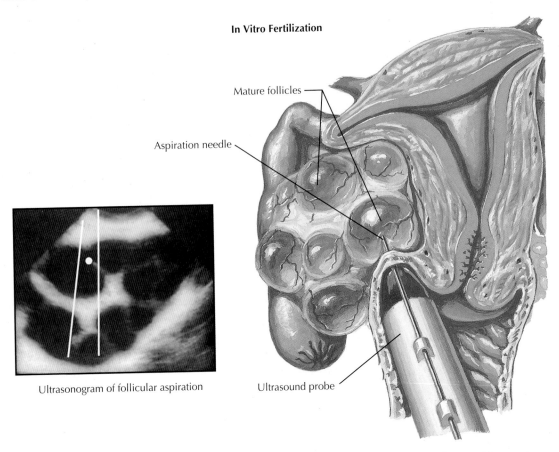

Mature follicles

Aspiration needle

Ultrasonogram of follicular aspiration

Ultrasound probe

In superovulating ovary, ova harvested from mature follicles transvaginally with ultrasound-guided needle

JOHN A. CRAIG—AD

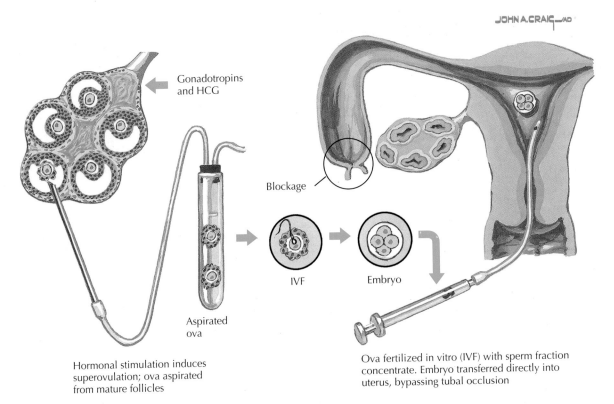

Gonadotropins and HCG

Blockage

Aspirated ova

IVF

Embryo

Hormonal stimulation induces superovulation; ova aspirated from mature follicles

Ova fertilized in vitro (IVF) with sperm fraction concentrate. Embryo transferred directly into uterus, bypassing tubal occlusion

HCG, human chorionic gonadotropin.

Gamete Intrafallopian Transfer (GIFT) and Zygote Intrafallopian Transfer (ZIFT)

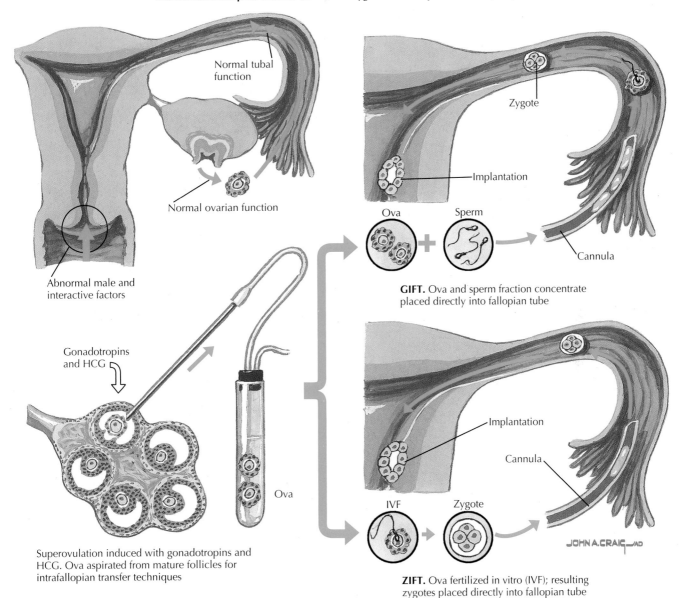

Normal tubal function

Normal ovarian function

Abnormal male and interactive factors

Gonadotropins and HCG

Superovulation induced with gonadotropins and HCG. Ova aspirated from mature follicles for intrafallopian transfer techniques

Ova

Zygote

Implantation

Ova

Sperm

Cannula

GIFT. Ova and sperm fraction concentrate placed directly into fallopian tube

Implantation

Cannula

IVF

Zygote

JOHN A. CRAIG—AD

ZIFT. Ova fertilized in vitro (IVF); resulting zygotes placed directly into fallopian tube

HCG, human chorionic gonadotropin.

REFERENCES

Level III

American College of Obstetricians and Gynecologists: Management of infertility caused by ovulatory dysfunction. ACOG Practice Bulletin 34. Obstet Gynecol 2002;99:347.

American College of Obstetricians and Gynecologists: Polycystic ovary syndrome. ACOG Practice Bulletin 41. Obstet Gynecol 2002;100:1389.

American College of Obstetricians and Gynecologists: Perinatal risks associated with assisted reproductive technology. ACOG Committee Opinion 324. Obstet Gynecol 2005;106:1143.

American College of Obstetricians and Gynecologists: Using preimplantation embryos for research. ACOG Committee Opinion 347. Obstet Gynecol 2006;108:1305.

American College of Obstetricians and Gynecologists: Adoption. ACOG Committee Opinion 368. Obstet Gynecol 2007;109:1507.

Braude P, Rowell P: Assisted conception. II—In vitro fertilisation and intracytoplasmic sperm injection. BMJ 2003;327:852.

Braude P, Rowell P: Assisted conception. III—Problems with assisted conception. BMJ 2003;327:920.

Lobo RA: Infertility. In Katz VL, Lentz GM, Lobo RA, Gershenson DM: Comprehensive Gynecology, 5th ed. Philadelphia, Mosby/Elsevier, 2007, p 1030.

Rowell P, Braude P: Assisted conception. I—General principles. BMJ 2003;327:799.

INTRODUCTION

Description: Down syndrome is characterized by physical and mental symptoms that have their origin in the presence of extra genetic material from chromosome 21. This may be due to errors of duplication or the translocation of genetic material that results in effective duplication. Patients with Down syndrome exhibit a spectrum of changes that range from mild to profound.

Prevalence: Based on maternal age, from about 1 in 1250 at age 25 to about 1 in 100 at age 40. Overall incidence 1 in 733 live births (United States, 2006)

Predominant Age: Most patients with Down syndrome are identified at birth; their life span is generally shorter than average (usually 50 to 60 years).

Genetics: Ninety percent caused by nondisjunction resulting in an extra chromosome 21, 5% caused by translocation, 5% caused by mosaicism.

ETIOLOGY AND PATHOGENESIS

Causes: Nondisjunction of chromosome 21, resulting in two copies from one parent and one from the other, with a net of three. Balanced translocation of chromosome 21q material onto another chromosome (most often 12, 13, or 15) in 90% of patients. During cell division, this is inherited independently from the normal chromosome 21s, resulting in extra genetic material. Roughly one half of these duplications are new occurrences; one half have a parental carrier. Mosaicism of two cell lines: one normal and one with trisomy 21. This is generally associated with milder clinical manifestations.

Risk Factors: Maternal age, known carrier state (translocation), prior chromosomal abnormality. Screening based on age identifies only 25% of all cases (the remainder are born to mothers considered to be at low risk).

CLINICAL CHARACTERISTICS

Signs and Symptoms

- Brachycephaly (100%)
- Hypotonia at birth (80%)
- Posterior third fontanel
- Small or low-set ears
- Prominent epicanthal folds, mongoloid eyes (90%)
- Enlarged tongue (75%)
- Depressed nasal bridge
- Cardiac murmur (50%)
- Mental retardation (IQ 40 to 45)
- Abnormal dermatoglyphics (single palmar crease, absent plantar whorl)

DIAGNOSTIC APPROACH

Differential Diagnosis

Familial structural mimics (mongoloid faces).

Associated Conditions: Renal and cardiac anomalies, mental retardation, bowel obstruction, Hirschsprung's disease, and thyroid disease.

Workup and Evaluation

Laboratory: Maternal serum α-fetoprotein (MSAFP) screening between 15 and 22 weeks of gestation (16 to 18 optimal) may be abnormally low, suggesting the presence of an infant with Down syndrome.

Imaging: Ultrasonographic studies that measure fetal nasal bones or nuchal translucency show promise as diagnostic tools, but they require very specific training or experience and have not gained wide acceptance or availability. Imaging of the urinary tract should be considered to look for anomalies.

Special Tests: Karyotyping should be performed to look for translocation—useful for genetic counseling of parents. Chorionic villus sampling or amniocentesis may be performed for antenatal diagnosis.

Diagnostic Procedures: History, physical examination, chromosomal analysis (antenatal or after birth). (The presence of a whorl on the ball of the foot generally indicates a normal child, not a trisomy.)

Pathologic Findings

Physical changes as noted. Alzheimer's plaques common after age 20.

MANAGEMENT AND THERAPY

Nonpharmacologic

General Measures: Genetic and cardiac evaluation and counseling. Assessment of abilities and assistance with activities of daily living as appropriate.

Specific Measures: Based on the needs of the individual. Parental support and counseling are vital.

Diet: No specific dietary changes indicated.

Activity: No restriction, except if cardiac abnormalities are present.

Patient Education: American College of Obstetricians and Gynecologists Patient Education Pamphlet AP094 (Genetic Disorders), AP060 (Later Childbearing).

Drug(s) of Choice

None.

FOLLOW-UP

Patient Monitoring: Normal health maintenance, monitor for renal or cardiac complications.

Prevention/Avoidance: Recurrence rate is 1% for true trisomy, 16% to 20% for translocation, 100% for trisomy involving chromosome 12.

Possible Complications: Congenital heart disease (50%), bowel obstruction (10%), Hirschsprung's disease (3%), thyroid disease (5% to 8%), and Alzheimer's disease.

Expected Outcome: One third of patients have normal development during the first year of life; growth, language, and mental development slow thereafter. Life expectancy is reduced by cardiac and other associated anomalies. Life potential varies from ability to live and

Down (Trisomy 21) Syndrome

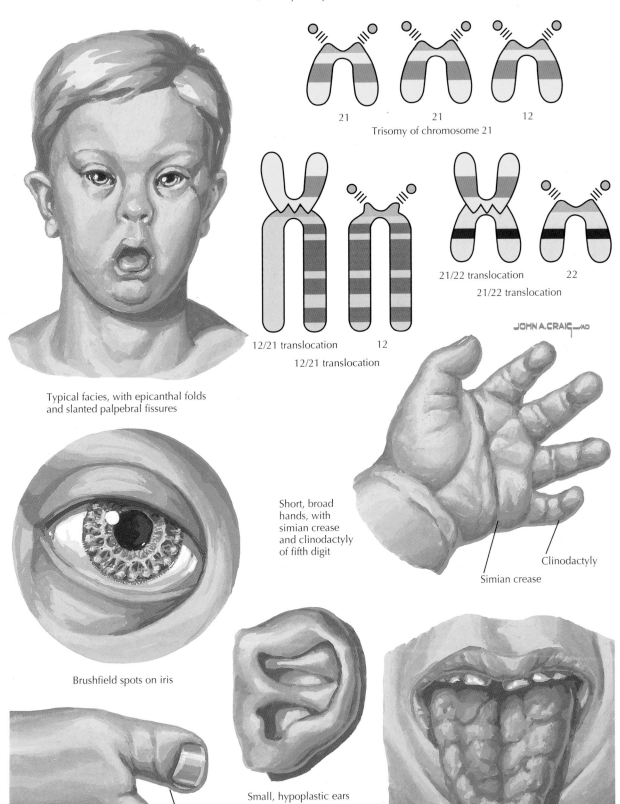

Trisomy of chromosome 21

21/22 translocation
21/22 translocation

12/21 translocation   12
12/21 translocation

JOHN A. CRAIG—AD

Typical facies, with epicanthal folds
and slanted palpebral fissures

Short, broad
hands, with
simian crease
and clinodactyly
of fifth digit

Clinodactyly

Simian crease

Brushfield spots on iris

Wide gap between
first and second toes

Small, hypoplastic ears

Fissured tongue in adults

work within sheltered environment to profound restriction. Premature aging is common, with life expectancy of 50 to 60 years.

MISCELLANEOUS

Pregnancy Considerations: Chorionic villus sampling (9 to 10 weeks) or amniocentesis (13 to 15 weeks) should be offered for patients at risk by age or other factors. Maternal serum α-fetoprotein (low) or triple screening (maternal serum α-fetoprotein, β-human chorionic gonadotropin, estriol) should be performed at 14 to 16 weeks. Pregnancy is possible for patients with Down syndrome; recurrence rate is 50%.

ICD-9-CM Codes: 758.0.

REFERENCES

Level I

Bahado-Singh RO, Wapner R, Thom E, et al; First Trimester Maternal Serum Biochemistry and Fetal Nuchal Translucency Screening Study Group: Elevated first-trimester nuchal translucency increases the risk of congenital heart defects. Am J Obstet Gynecol 2005;192:1357.

Canick JA, Lambert-Messerlian GM, Palomaki GE, et al; First and Second Trimester Evaluation of Risk (FASTER) Trial Research Consortium: Comparison of serum markers in first-trimester Down syndrome screening. Obstet Gynecol 2006;108:1192.

Crossley JA, Aitken DA, Cameron AD, et al: Combined ultrasound and biochemical screening for Down's syndrome in the first trimester: a Scottish multicentre study. BJOG 2002;109:667.

Evans MI, Krantz DA, Hallahan TW, Galen RS: Meta-analysis of first trimester Down syndrome screening studies: free beta-human chorionic gonadotropin significantly outperforms intact human chorionic gonadotropin in a multimarker protocol. Am J Obstet Gynecol 2007;196:198.

Malone FD, Canick JA, Ball RH, et al; First- and Second-Trimester Evaluation of Risk (FASTER) Research Consortium: First-trimester or second-trimester screening, or both, for Down's syndrome. N Engl J Med 2005;353:2001.

Malone FD, D'Alton ME; Society for Maternal-Fetal Medicine: First-trimester sonographic screening for Down syndrome. Obstet Gynecol 2003;102:1066.

Rozenberg P, Bussieres L, Chevret S, et al: Screening for Down syndrome using first-trimester combined screening followed by second-trimester ultrasound examination in an unselected population. Am J Obstet Gynecol 2006;195:1379. Epub 2006 May 24.

Level II

Freeman SB, Allen EG, Oxford-Wright CL, et al: The National Down Syndrome Project: Design and implementation. Public Health Rep 2007;122:62.

Haddow JE, Palomaki GE, Knight GJ, et al: Screening of maternal serum for fetal Down's syndrome in the first trimester. N Engl J Med 1998;338:955.

Mikic TS, Johnson P: Second trimester maternal serum beta human chorionic gonadotrophin and pregnancy outcome. Br J Obstet Gynaecol 1999;106:598.

Mol BW, Lijmer JG, van der Meulen J, et al: Effect of study design on the association between nuchal translucency measurement and Down syndrome. Obstet Gynecol 1999;94:864.

Smith-Bindman R, Hosmer W, Feldstein VA, et al: Second-trimester ultrasound to detect fetuses with Down syndrome: a meta-analysis. JAMA 2001;285:1044.

Sonek JD, Cicero S, Neiger R, Nicolaides KH: Nasal bone assessment in prenatal screening for trisomy 21. Am J Obstet Gynecol 2006;195:1219. Epub 2006 Apr 17.

Level III

American College of Obstetricians and Gynecologists: Ultrasonography in pregnancy. ACOG Practice Bulletin 58. Obstet Gynecol 2004;104:1449.

American College of Obstetricians and Gynecologists: Screening for fetal chromosomal abnormalities. ACOG Practice Bulletin 77. Obstet Gynecol 2007;109:217.

Baliff JP, Mooney RA: New developments in prenatal screening for Down syndrome. Am J Clin Pathol 2003;120:S14.

Nicolaides KH: Nuchal translucency and other first-trimester sonographic markers of chromosomal abnormalities. Am J Obstet Gynecol 2004;191:45.

Reddy UM, Mennuti MT: Incorporating first-trimester Down syndrome studies into prenatal screening: executive summary of the National Institute of Child Health and Human Development workshop. Obstet Gynecol 2006;107:167.

Roizen NJ, Patterson D: Down's syndrome. Lancet 2003;361:1281.

INTRODUCTION

Description: Gonadal dysgenesis is a developmental abnormality of patients who do not carry the stigmata of Turner's syndrome but still have absent menarche because of chromosomal abnormalities. These patients generally are tall (>150 cm), are more normal in appearance, and are a chromosomally heterogeneous group (46,XX, 46,XY, or mosaic X/XY karyotypes).

Prevalence: Appears in 1 of 2500 female births.

Predominant Age: Present at birth, may not be detected until puberty is delayed.

Genetics: Sporadic, loss of part or all of one X chromosome (amenorrhea more common with long arm loss; short stature with short arm loss).

ETIOLOGY AND PATHOGENESIS

Causes: Pure gonadal dysgenesis—45,XO (Turner's syndrome); 46,XY gonadal dysgenesis (Swyer syndrome); 46,XX q5 X chromosome long-arm deletion, mixed or mosaic.

Risk Factors: Translocations involving the X chromosome (rare).

CLINICAL CHARACTERISTICS

Signs and Symptoms

(Based on the amount of chromatin lost.)

- Primary amenorrhea and infertility (the most common cause of failure to begin menstruation is gonadal dysgenesis; in approximately 60% of women with primary amenorrhea, an abnormality of gonadal differentiation or function has occurred during the fetal or neonatal period)
- Absent or grossly abnormal gonad development

DIAGNOSTIC APPROACH

Differential Diagnosis

- Polycystic ovary syndrome
- Hypothyroidism
- Growth hormone deficiency or glucocorticoid excess
- Androgen insensitivity syndrome (male pseudohermaphroditism, testicular feminization)
- Intersex abnormality
- Enzymatic defects (such as 17α-hydroxylase deficiency)
- Structural genital tract abnormalities (uterine and/or vaginal agenesis or an imperforate hymen)
- Ovarian insensitivity syndrome (resistant ovary [Savage's] syndrome)
- Follicular depletion (autoimmune disease, infection [mumps], infiltrative disease processes [tuberculosis, galactosemia])

Associated Conditions: Amenorrhea, infertility, incomplete or abnormal external genitalia, and premature menopause.

Workup and Evaluation

Laboratory: Follicle-stimulating hormone (FSH) and luteinizing hormone (LH) levels are high (nonspecific). (Follicle-stimulating hormone is usually elevated in gonadal dysgenesis.) Assessment of thyroid function, prolactin, or growth hormone if indicated by the differential diagnosis being considered.

Imaging: Pelvic ultrasound studies to evaluate the presence and condition of upper genital tract organs.

Special Tests: Karyotype.

Diagnostic Procedures: History, physical examination, karyotyping.

Pathologic Findings

Abnormal karyotype. Germ cell involution occurs soon after they migrate into the undifferentiated gonad. This results in fibrous streak gonads that are hormonally inactive.

MANAGEMENT AND THERAPY

Nonpharmacologic

General Measures: Evaluation, screening for associated defects, counseling about menstrual and fertility issues.

Specific Measures: Hormone replacement therapy. When there is a mosaicism involving a Y chromosome, surgical extirpation of the gonads must be performed because of a 25% to 30% risk of malignant gonadal tumors. Timing of gonadal removal in patients with a Y chromosome is controversial: removal as soon as the diagnosis is made versus delaying removal until pubertal changes are complete.

Diet: No specific dietary changes indicated.

Activity: No restriction.

Patient Education: Extensive counseling about sexual maturation and fertility.

Drug(s) of Choice

Adolescents are much more sensitive to the effects of estrogen than are postmenopausal women, allowing doses in the range of 0.3 mg of conjugated estrogen, 0.5 mg of estradiol, or their equivalent, daily. After 6 to 12 months of therapy at this level, the dose should be doubled and a progestin (e.g., medroxyprogesterone acetate, 10 mg for the first 12 days of the month) should be added, or the patient's treatment should be switched to combination oral contraceptives. This generally results in regular menstruation, and normal pubertal development proceeds on its own when the patient reaches a bone age of 13.

Contraindications: Undiagnosed amenorrhea.

FOLLOW-UP

Patient Monitoring: Normal health maintenance.

Prevention/Avoidance: Prenatal chromosomal analysis for those known to carry translocations (detection only, not prevention, although the couple may choose not to continue the pregnancy based on the findings).

Possible Complications: Gonadal malignancy or virilization in those with Y chromatin present. Others based on cause.

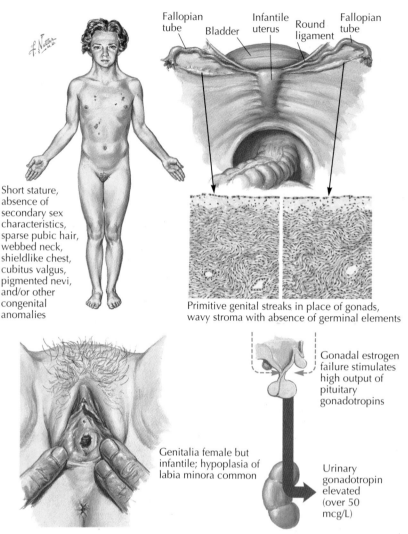

Short stature, absence of secondary sex characteristics, sparse pubic hair, webbed neck, shieldlike chest, cubitus valgus, pigmented nevi, and/or other congenital anomalies

Fallopian tube · Bladder · Infantile uterus · Round ligament · Fallopian tube

Primitive genital streaks in place of gonads, wavy stroma with absence of germinal elements

Genitalia female but infantile; hypoplasia of labia minora common

Gonadal estrogen failure stimulates high output of pituitary gonadotropins

Urinary gonadotropin elevated (over 50 mcg/L)

Expected Outcome: Reasonably normal lives with the exception of fertility.

MISCELLANEOUS

Pregnancy Considerations: These patients may be infertile. In pure gonadal dysgenesis and XX/XY mosaicism, a uterus is present. Consequently, some patients may achieve pregnancy. Pregnancy is associated with a 50% chance of aneuploidy.

ICD-9-CM Codes: 752.0.

REFERENCES

Level II
Gravholt CH, Fedder J, Naeraa RW, Muller J: Occurrence of gonado-blastoma in females with Turner syndrome and Y chromosome material: a population study. J Clin Endocrinol Metab 2000;85:3199.

Ogata T, Muroya K, Matsuo N, et al: Turner syndrome and Xp deletions: clinical and molecular studies in 47 patients. J Clin Endocrinol Metab 2001;86:5498.

Level III
American Academy of Pediatrics, American College of Obstetricians and Gynecologists: Menstruation in girls and adolescents: using the menstrual cycle as a vital sign. ACOG Committee Opinion 349. Obstet Gynecol 2006;108:1323.

American College of Obstetricians and Gynecologists: Vaginal agenesis: diagnosis, management, and routine care. ACOG Committee Opinion 355. Obstet Gynecol 2006;108:1605.

Bondy CA; Turner Syndrome Study Group. Care of girls and women with Turner syndrome: a guideline of the Turner Syndrome Study Group. J Clin Endocrinol Metab 2007;92:10. Epub 2006 Oct 17.

Federman DD: Disorders of sexual development. N Engl J Med 1967;277:351.

Hall JG, Gilchrist DM: Turner syndrome and its variants. Pediatr Clin North Am 1990;37:1421.

Lobo RA: Primary and secondary amenorrhea and precocious puberty. In Katz VL, Lentz GM, Lobo RA, Gershenson DM: Comprehensive Gynecology, 5th ed. Philadelphia, Mosby/Elsevier, 2007, p 937.

Master-Hunter T, Heiman DL: Amenorrhea: evaluation and treatment. Am Fam Physician 2006;73:1374.

Park SY, Jameson JL: Minireview: transcriptional regulation of gonadal development and differentiation. Endocrinology 2005;146:1035. Epub 2004 Dec 16.

Pletcher JR, Slap GB: Menstrual disorders. Amenorrhea. Pediatr Clin North Am 1999;46:505.

Ranke MB, Saenger P: Turner's syndrome. Lancet 2001;358:309.

Saenger P: Turner's syndrome. N Engl J Med 1996;335:1749.

Styne DM, Kaplan SL: Normal and abnormal puberty in the female. Pediatr Clin North Am 1979;26:123.

Sybert VP, McCauley E: Turner's syndrome. N Engl J Med 2004;351:1227.

van Niekerk WA: Chromosomes and the gynecologist. Am J Obstet Gynecol 1978;130:862.

INTRODUCTION

Description: Hirsutism refers to increased or excessive hair growth only. It may be idiopathic (hypertrichosis) or caused by androgen-stimulated excessive growth. Hypertrichosis involves increased hair on the extremities and tends to be ethnic, racial, or familial in origin. This is not considered hirsutism.

Prevalence: Five percent to twenty-five percent of women, variable within ethnic groups, 60% of women with Cushing's disease.

Predominant Age: After puberty.

Genetics: Influenced by the number of hair follicles present, a function of race and ethnicity.

ETIOLOGY AND PATHOGENESIS

Causes: Familial, idiopathic, increased hair follicle androgens (5α-reductase). Increased androgen production—ovarian (polycystic ovary syndrome, hilus cell hyperplasia/tumor, arrhenoblastoma, adrenal rest), adrenal (congenital adrenal hyperplasia [10% to 15% of women with hirsutism], Cushing's disease, virilizing carcinoma or adenoma). Drugs (minoxidil, androgens [including Danocrine], phenytoin, diazoxide). Other (hypothyroidism, hyperprolactinemia).

Risk Factors: Androgen use, danazol sodium, minoxidil, phenytoin, and diazoxide.

CLINICAL CHARACTERISTICS
Signs and Symptoms

- Increased or excessive hair growth, primarily along the angle of the jaw, upper lip, and chin. (For most patients, hirsutism dates from puberty.)
- Menstrual irregularity or amenorrhea (60%)
- Acne (40%)

DIAGNOSTIC APPROACH
Differential Diagnosis

- Virilization (especially when hirsutism is in a male pattern)
- Familial hypertrichosis
- Cushing's disease (truncal obesity, facial rounding, cervicodorsal fat deposition [buffalo hump], and red or purple striae are often not fully developed)
- Polycystic ovary syndrome
- Iatrogenic hirsutism (patients may use steroids for a number of reasons, legal and otherwise, and may not recognize the possibility of virilizing side effects; the use of danazol sodium [e.g., for endometriosis therapy] also may be associated with increased hair growth)
- Acromegaly
- Hypothyroidism
- Hyperprolactinemia
- Anorexia nervosa

Associated Conditions: Obesity, menstrual irregularity, amenorrhea, infertility, acne, oily skin, increased libido, alopecia, acanthosis nigricans.

Workup and Evaluation

Laboratory: Evaluation for possible virilizing process (prolactin, dehydroepiandrosterone sulfate [DHEA-s], follicle-stimulating hormone [FSH], thyroid screening). (Patients suspected of having adrenal sources of hyperandrogenicity may be screened by measuring 24-hour urinary-free cortisol, by performing adrenocorticotropic hormone [ACTH] stimulation tests, or by performing an overnight dexamethasone suppression test.) Circulating testosterone is generally normal or only mildly elevated (>1.5 ng/mL). Of patients with idiopathic hirsutism, 80% have elevated levels of 3α-diol-G (metabolite of 5α-reductase).

Imaging: No imaging indicated, except as indicated by physical or laboratory findings.

Special Tests: Clitoral index may be useful if virilization is suspected. (The clitoral index is defined as the vertical dimension times the horizontal dimension, in millimeters. The normal range is from 9 to 35 mm, with borderline values in the range of 36 to 99 mm. Values of more than 100 mm indicate severe hyperandrogenicity and should prompt aggressive evaluation and referral.) Hirsutism may be quantified using the Ferriman-Gallwey scoring system.

Diagnostic Procedures: History and physical examination, Ferriman-Gallwey score greater than 8.

Pathologic Findings

Based on underlying pathophysiologic conditions.

MANAGEMENT AND THERAPY
Nonpharmacologic

General Measures: Evaluation, shaving, depilatories, or electrolysis. Topical treatment of acne (if present). Weight reduction if obesity is present.

Specific Measures: Suppressive therapies reduce the growth of new hair, but once a hair follicle is induced, or turned on, it continues to grow. For this reason, shaving, depilatories, or electrolysis may be required. These are satisfactory only if combined with other therapies to reduce new growth.

Diet: No specific dietary changes indicated.

Activity: No restriction.

Patient Education: Instruction on management of unwanted hair; American College of Obstetricians and Gynecologists Patient Education Pamphlet AP121 (Polycystic Ovary Syndrome).

Drug(s) of Choice

5α-Reductase inhibitors (finasteride 5 mg PO daily).

Polycystic ovary syndrome—combination oral contraceptives: spironolactone (100 to 200 mg PO daily), medroxyprogesterone acetate (Depo-Provera 150 to 300 mg IM every 3 months), metformin (1500 mg/day), or other insulin sensitizers. Aromatase inhibitors may be used if ovulation induction is desired (e.g., letrozole; 2.5 mg or 5 mg administered for 5 days, beginning on cycle days 3 to 5).

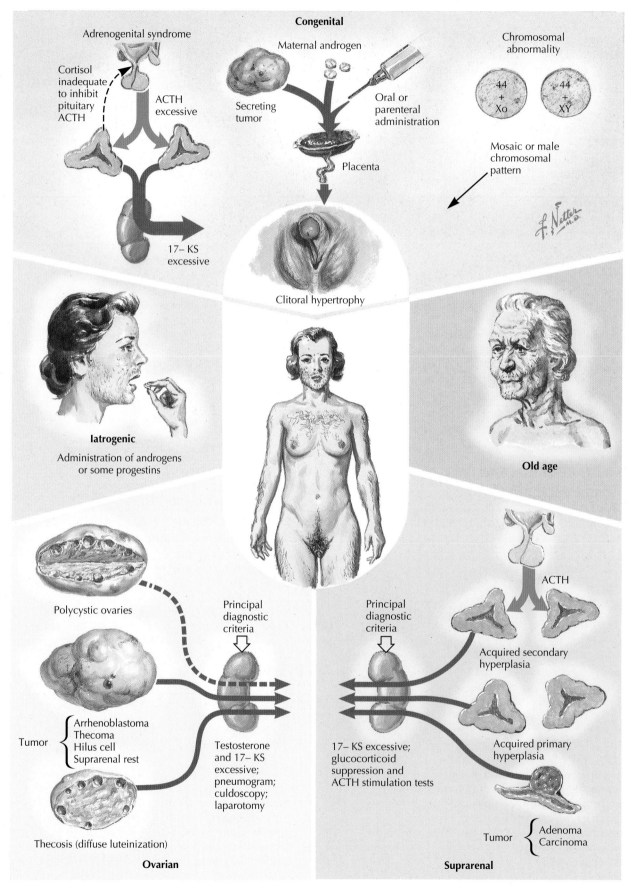

Congenital

Adrenogenital syndrome

Cortisol inadequate to inhibit pituitary ACTH

ACTH excessive

17– KS excessive

Maternal androgen

Secreting tumor

Oral or parenteral administration

Placenta

Clitoral hypertrophy

Chromosomal abnormality

44 + Xo   44 + XY

Mosaic or male chromosomal pattern

Iatrogenic

Administration of androgens or some progestins

Old age

Polycystic ovaries

Principal diagnostic criteria

Tumor { Arrhenoblastoma
Thecoma
Hilus cell
Suprarenal rest

Testosterone and 17– KS excessive; pneumogram; culdoscopy; laparotomy

Thecosis (diffuse luteinization)

Ovarian

Principal diagnostic criteria

ACTH

Acquired secondary hyperplasia

Acquired primary hyperplasia

17– KS excessive; glucocorticoid suppression and ACTH stimulation tests

Tumor { Adenoma
Carcinoma

Suprarenal

ACTH, adrenocorticotropic hormone.

Hyperandrogenicity of adrenal origin—cortisol administration. If DHEA-s is elevated, dexamethasone (0.25 to 0.5 mg PO every bedtime) may be added.

Contraindications: Pregnancy. (Spironolactone and finasteride are category X drugs; patients using them and able to become pregnant must use reliable contraception.)

FOLLOW-UP

Patient Monitoring: Normal health maintenance once a diagnosis is established. Contraception and weight maintenance should also be addressed. There is an increased risk of diabetes for patients with polycystic ovaries.

Prevention/Avoidance: None.

Possible Complications: Permanent induction of hair changes. Chronic anovulation is associated with increased risk of endometrial hyperplasia and cancer.

Expected Outcome: Approximately 70% response after 1 year of therapy may be expected.

MISCELLANEOUS

Pregnancy Considerations: No effect on pregnancy, although some metabolic causes of hirsutism may result in reduced fertility or virilization of a fetus.

ICD-9-CM Codes: 704.1. Chiromegaly, 642.2 (excludes that found in endocrine disorders 255.2, 256.1).

REFERENCES

Level I

Azziz R, Ehrmann D, Legro RS, et al; PCOS/Troglitazone Study Group: Troglitazone improves ovulation and hirsutism in the polycystic ovary syndrome: a multicenter, double blind, placebo-controlled trial. J Clin Endocrinol Metab 2001;86:1626.

Azziz R, Ochoa TM, Bradley EL Jr, et al: Leuprolide and estrogen versus oral contraceptive pills for the treatment of hirsutism: a prospective randomized study. J Clin Endocrinol Metab 1995;80:3406.

Moghetti P, Tosi F, Tosti A, et al: Comparison of spironolactone, flutamide, and finasteride efficacy in the treatment of hirsutism: a randomized, double blind, placebo-controlled trial. J Clin Endocrinol Metab 2000;85:89.

Wong IL, Morris RS, Chang L, et al: A prospective randomized trial comparing finasteride to spironolactone in the treatment of hirsute women. J Clin Endocrinol Metab 1995;80:233.

Level II

Guido M, Romualdi D, Giuliani M, et al: Drospirenone for the treatment of hirsute women with polycystic ovary syndrome: a clinical, endocrinological, metabolic pilot study. J Clin Endocrinol Metab 2004;89:2817.

Harborne L, Fleming R, Lyall H, et al: Metformin or antiandrogen in the treatment of hirsutism in polycystic ovary syndrome. J Clin Endocrinol Metab 2003;88:4116.

Ibanez L, Lopez-Bermejo A, del Rio L, et al: Combined low-dose pioglitazone, flutamide, and metformin for women with androgen excess. J Clin Endocrinol Metab 2007;92:1710. Epub 2007 Feb 13.

Ibanez L, Potau N, Marcos MV, de Zegher F: Treatment of hirsutism, hyperandrogenism, oligomenorrhea, dyslipidemia, and hyperinsulinism in nonobese, adolescent girls: effect of flutamide. J Clin Endocrinol Metab 2000;85:3251.

Ibanez L, Valls C, Potau N, et al: Sensitization to insulin in adolescent girls to normalize hirsutism, hyperandrogenism, oligomenorrhea, dyslipidemia, and hyperinsulinism after precocious pubarche. J Clin Endocrinol Metab 2000;85:3526.

Level III

American College of Obstetricians and Gynecologists: Polycystic ovary syndrome. ACOG Practice Bulletin 41. Obstet Gynecol 2002;100:1389.

Azziz R: The evaluation and management of hirsutism. Obstet Gynecol 2003;101:995.

Bailey-Pridham DD, Sanfilippo JS: Hirsutism in the adolescent female. Pediatr Clin North Am 1989;36:581.

Bergfeld WF: Hirsutism in women. Effective therapy that is safe for long-term use. Postgrad Med 2000;107:93, 99.

Conn JJ, Jacobs HS: Managing hirsutism in gynaecological practice. Br J Obstet Gynaecol 1998;105:687.

Curran DR, Moore C, Huber T: Clinical inquiries. What is the best approach to the evaluation of hirsutism? J Fam Pract 2005;54:465.

Ferriman D, Gallwey JD: Clinical assessment of body hair growth in women. J Clin Endocrin 1961;21:1440.

Ginsburg J, White MC: Hirsutism and virilisation. Br Med J 1980;280:369.

Lobo RA: Hyperandrogenism. In Katz VL, Lentz GM, Lobo RA, Gershenson DM: Comprehensive Gynecology, 5th ed. Philadelphia, Mosby/Elsevier, 2007, p 979.

Marshburn PB, Carr BR: Hirsutism and virilization. A systematic approach to benign and potentially serious causes. Postgrad Med 1995;97:99, 105.

Rosenfield RL: Clinical practice. Hirsutism. N Engl J Med 2005;353:2578.

Sakiyama R: Approach to patients with hirsutism. West J Med 1996;165:386.

Setji TL, Brown AJ: Polycystic ovary syndrome: diagnosis and treatment. Am J Med 2007;120:128.

INTRODUCTION

Description: Hyperprolactinemia is the pathologic elevation of serum prolactin levels. The finding of elevated levels of prolactin is nonspecific as to cause, requiring careful clinical evaluation.

Prevalence: Uncommon; reports vary from 1% to 30% depending on the population studied.

Predominant Age: Reproductive.

Genetics: No genetic pattern.

ETIOLOGY AND PATHOGENESIS

Causes: Pituitary adenoma (most common), pharmacologic (most often those that affect dopamine or serotonin: major tranquilizers [phenothiazines], trifluoperazine [Stelazine], and haloperidol [Haldol]; some antipsychotic medications; metoclopramide [Reglan], less often, α-methyldopa and reserpine), herpes zoster, chest wall/breast stimulation or irritation, physiologic during pregnancy, or after childbirth and/or breastfeeding.

Risk Factors: Exposure to known pharmacologic agents, specific disease processes (see Table).

CLINICAL CHARACTERISTICS

Signs and Symptoms

- Asymptomatic
- Bilateral, spontaneous milky discharge from both breasts (75%)
- Amenorrhea (30%)
- Large adenoma, clinical appearance of impingement on the optic nerve or adjacent structures

DIAGNOSTIC APPROACH

Differential Diagnosis

- Pregnancy
- Breast cancer
- Chronic nipple stimulation
- Hypothyroidism
- Sarcoidosis
- Lupus
- Cirrhosis or hepatic disease
- Radiculopathy (herpetic)

Associated Conditions: One third of patients with elevated prolactin levels experience amenorrhea or infertility. Prolonged amenorrhea is associated with an increased risk of osteoporosis.

Workup and Evaluation

Laboratory: Serum prolactin level. Pregnancy should always be considered if menses are absent.

Imaging: Computed tomography (CT) or magnetic resonance imaging (MRI) to evaluate the pituitary and surrounding bony structures; magnetic resonance imaging now is preferred.

Special Tests: Assessment of visual fields may be indicated.

Diagnostic Procedures: History, physical examination, and laboratory determination of prolactin levels.

Pathologic Findings

None.

MANAGEMENT AND THERAPY

Nonpharmacologic

General Measures: When prolactin levels are low and a coned-down view of the sella turcica is normal, observation alone may be sufficient. If observation is chosen, periodic re-evaluation is required to check for the emergence of slow-growing tumors.

Specific Measures: Treatment with a dopamine receptor agonist (bromocriptine, pergolide, or cabergoline) is recommended for patients who desire pregnancy or for those with distressing degrees of galactorrhea or to suppress intermediate-sized pituitary tumors. Rapidly growing tumors, tumors that are large at the time of discovery, or those that do not respond to bromocriptine therapy may have to be treated surgically.

Diet: No specific dietary changes indicated.

Activity: No restriction.

Patient Education: American College of Obstetricians and Gynecologists Patient Education Pamphlet AP136 (Evaluating Infertility), AP137 (Treating Infertility).

Drug(s) of Choice

Bromocriptine (Parlodel) 2.5 mg daily increased gradually to three times a day.

Contraindications: Uncontrolled hypertension, pregnancy.

Precautions: With medical therapy—may experience nausea, orthostasis, drowsiness, or syncope; rarely may produce hypertension or seizures.

Interactions: Medical therapy may interact with phenothiazines or butyrophenones.

Alternative Drugs

Intravaginal bromocriptine (associated with lower rates of side effects).

Cabergoline may also be used.

FOLLOW-UP

Patient Monitoring: Normal health maintenance. If a pituitary adenoma is present, periodic assessment of visual fields should be considered.

Prevention/Avoidance: None.

Possible Complications: Visual field loss, symptoms may return after medication is discontinued. Chronic anovulation is associated with an increased risk of endometrial hyperplasia and cancer.

Hyperprolactinemia

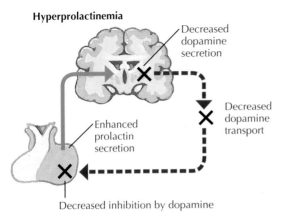

Decreased dopamine secretion

Decreased dopamine transport

Enhanced prolactin secretion

Decreased inhibition by dopamine

Conditions in which normal dopamine short-loop inhibition is blocked or prolactin secretion is enhanced cause clinically evident hyperprolactinemia

Estrogen

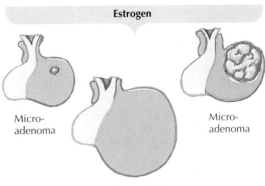

Micro-adenoma

Hyperplasia

Micro-adenoma

Conditions that increase estrogen levels may cause pituitary hyperplasia and induce growth of adenomas, causing hyperprolactinemia

Conditions associated with hyperprolactinemia

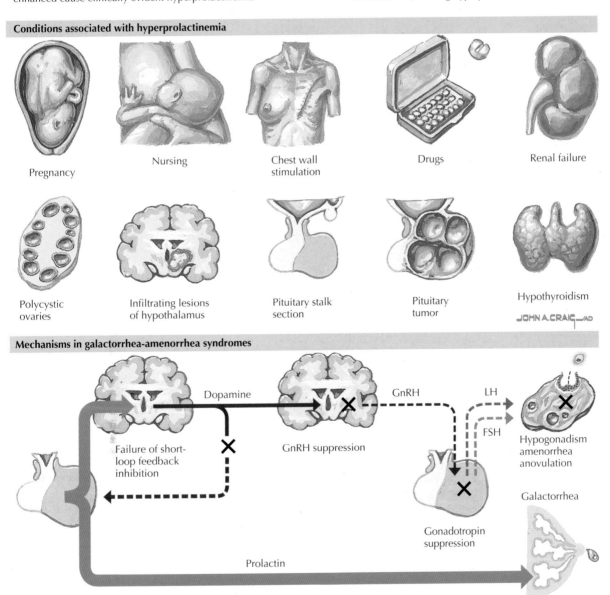

Pregnancy

Nursing

Chest wall stimulation

Drugs

Renal failure

Polycystic ovaries

Infiltrating lesions of hypothalamus

Pituitary stalk section

Pituitary tumor

Hypothyroidism

JOHN A. CRAIG—AD

Mechanisms in galactorrhea-amenorrhea syndromes

Dopamine

GnRH

LH

Failure of short-loop feedback inhibition

GnRH suppression

FSH

Hypogonadism amenorrhea anovulation

Galactorrhea

Gonadotropin suppression

Prolactin

Galactorrhea results from direct effect of prolactin on breast; amenorrhea and hypogonadism result from secondary prolactin effects (via dopamine) on GnRH and gonadotropin production and release

FSH, follicle-stimulating hormone; GnRH, gonadotropin-releasing hormone; LH, luteinizing hormone.

SOURCES OF ELEVATED PROLACTIN LEVELS

Pharmacologic (Examples)	Pathophysiologic Causes
Anesthetics	Central Nervous System
Central nervous system: dopamine-depleting agents	Cavernous sinus thrombosis
α-Methyldopa	Infection
Monoamine oxidase inhibitors	Neurofibromas
Reserpine	Temporal arteritis
Dopamine receptor blocking agents	Tumors and cysts (all types)
Domperidone	Hypothalamic
Haloperidol	Craniopharyngioma
Metoclopramide	Glioma
Phenothiazines	Granulomas
Pimozide	Histiocytosis disease
Sulpiride	Sarcoid
Dopamine reuptake blockers	Tuberculosis
Nomifensine	Irradiation damage
Histamine H2-receptor antagonists	Pituitary stalk transaction
Cimetidine	Surgical
Hormones	Traumatic
Estrogens	Pseudocyesis (functional)
Oral contraceptives	Pituitary lesions
Thyrotropin-releasing hormone	Acromegaly
Opiates	Mixed growth hormone or adrenocorticotropic
Stimulators of serotoninergic inhibitors	hormone–prolactin-secreting adenoma
Amphetamines	Prolactinoma
Hallucinogens	Somatic sources
	Breast augmentation or reduction
	Bronchogenic carcinoma
	Chest wall trauma
	Chronic nipple stimulation
	Cushing syndrome
	Herpes zoster
	Hypernephroma
	Hypothyroidism
	Pregnancy
	Renal failure
	Upper abdominal surgery

Expected Outcome: Generally good depending on cause. Prolactin levels should be measured every 6 to 12 months, and visual fields should be reassessed yearly. The pituitary should be re-evaluated every 2 to 5 years, based on initial diagnosis. Approximately 10% of patients receiving oral therapy will not experience return of prolactin to normal level.

MISCELLANEOUS

Pregnancy Considerations: No effect on pregnancy. Pregnancy may cause adenomas to grow rapidly.

ICD-9-cm Codes: 253.1.

REFERENCES

Level I
Webster J, Piscitelli G, Polli A, et al: A comparison of cabergoline and bromocriptine in the treatment of hyperprolactinemic amenorrhea. Cabergoline Comparative Study Group. N Engl J Med 1994;331:904.

Level II
Vermesh M, Fossum GT, Kletzky OA: Vaginal bromocriptine: pharmacology and effect on serum prolactin in normal women. Obstet Gynecol 1988;72:693.

Level III
American College of Obstetricians and Gynecologists: Polycystic ovary syndrome. ACOG Practice Bulletin 41. Obstet Gynecol 2002;100:1389.

Besser GM, Edwards CR: Galactorrhoea. Br Med J 1972;2:280.

Cuellar FG: Bromocriptine mesylate (Parlodel) in the management of amenorrhea/galactorrhea associated with hyperprolactinemia. Obstet Gynecol 1980;55:278.

Frantz AG: Prolactin. N Engl J Med 1978;298:201.

Hartog M, Hull MG: Hyperprolactinaemia. BMJ 1988;297:701.

Lobo RA: Hyperprolactinemia, galactorrhea, and pituitary adenomas. In Katz VL, Lentz GM, Lobo RA, Gershenson DM: Comprehensive Gynecology, 5th ed. Philadelphia, Mosby/Elsevier, 2007, p 963.

Molitch ME: Medication-induced hyperprolactinemia. Mayo Clin Proc 2005;80:1050.

Rosenfield RL: Hyperandrogenism in peripubertal girls. Pediatr Clin North Am 1990;37:1333.

Schlechte JA: Clinical practice. Prolactinoma. N Engl J Med 2003;349:2035.

Serri O, Chik CL, Ur E, Ezzat S: Diagnosis and management of hyperprolactinemia. CMAJ 2003;169:575.

INTRODUCTION

Description: Infertility is the inability to conceive or bear a child despite more than 1 year of trying. Under ordinary circumstances, 80% to 90% of normal couples conceive during 1 year of attempting pregnancy. Infertility may be further subdivided into primary and secondary types based on the patient's past reproductive history: patients who are infertile and nulligravid are in the primary infertility group and those who have become pregnant more than 1 year previously, regardless of the outcome of that pregnancy, are in the secondary infertility group. Slightly more than one half of patients experiencing infertility fall into the primary group.

Prevalence: Eight percent to eighteen percent of the American population; slightly higher for couples who have never conceived and slightly lower for couples who have conceived before. Roughly 6.1 million women in the United States.

Predominant Age: Reproductive. The prevalence of infertility increases with the age of the woman. Age-related infertility is becoming more common because about 20% of American women delay their attempts at pregnancy to after age 35.

Genetics: No specific genetic pattern. Some chromosomal abnormalities are associated with reduced or absent fertility.

ETIOLOGY AND PATHOGENESIS

Causes: Approximately 35% to 50% of infertility is due to a male factor such as azoospermia. Female factors, such as tubal disease (20% to 30%), ovulation disorders (10% to 15%), and cervical factors (5%), contribute to the roughly 50% to 60% of female causes. The remaining 10% to 20% of couples have no identifiable cause for their infertility (idiopathic). Couples experiencing primary infertility are more likely to have idiopathic or chromosomal causes than are couples who have conceived previously.

Risk Factors: Factors that increase the risk of anovulation (obesity, athletic overtraining, exposure to drugs or toxins), pelvic adhesive disease (infection, surgery, endometriosis), impaired sperm production (mumps, varicocele), or sperm delivery (ejaculatory dysfunction).

CLINICAL CHARACTERISTICS
Signs and Symptoms

Inability to conceive after 1 year of attempts.

DIAGNOSTIC APPROACH
Differential Diagnosis

- Recurrent pregnancy loss
- Primary infertility—chromosomal abnormality (e.g., 45,XO [Turner's syndrome], 46,XY gonadal dysgenesis [Swyer syndrome], 46,XX q5 X chromosome long-arm deletion)
- Congenital abnormality of the genital tract (either partner)

Associated Conditions: Based on the pathologic condition causing the infertility.

Workup and Evaluation

Laboratory: Based on diagnoses being considered.
Imaging: Based on diagnoses being considered.
Special Tests: Half of all women found to have tubal factor infertility have no history of antecedent infections or surgery, supporting the need to evaluate tubal patency in patients regardless of their past history.
Diagnostic Procedures: Based on diagnoses being considered.

Pathologic Findings

None.

MANAGEMENT AND THERAPY
Nonpharmacologic

General Measures: Support—because infertility involves both members of the couple and intrudes on the most intimate aspects of their relationship, all with no promise of success, a great deal of support is vital.

Specific Measures: The treatment of a couple experiencing infertility is based on identifying the impediment to fertility and overcoming or bypassing it to achieve pregnancy. Most couples can be successfully treated with conventional therapies (e.g., medications or surgery) rather than advanced assisted reproductive technologies. In vitro fertilization techniques account for only about 5% of infertility services and are associated with a roughly 32% live delivery rate per egg retrieval (2004).

Diet: No specific dietary changes indicated.

Activity: No restriction, unless athletic activities are thought to be adversely affecting fertility (exercise-induced amenorrhea). While the evaluation of infertility proceeds, couples should be instructed to continue attempting pregnancy through intercourse timed to the most fertile days of the cycle.

Patient Education: Reassurance; American College of Obstetricians and Gynecologists Patient Education Pamphlet AP136 (Evaluating Infertility), AP137 (Treating Infertility).

Drug(s) of Choice

(Based on diagnosis of cause.)
Secondary infertility (ovulation induction)—clomiphene citrate 50 mg PO daily on days 5 to 10 of the menstrual cycle; may be increased to 100 mg PO daily on days 5 to 10 of the menstrual cycle if ovulation does not occur. Metformin (1500 mg/day) as an adjunctive treatment for

Infertility

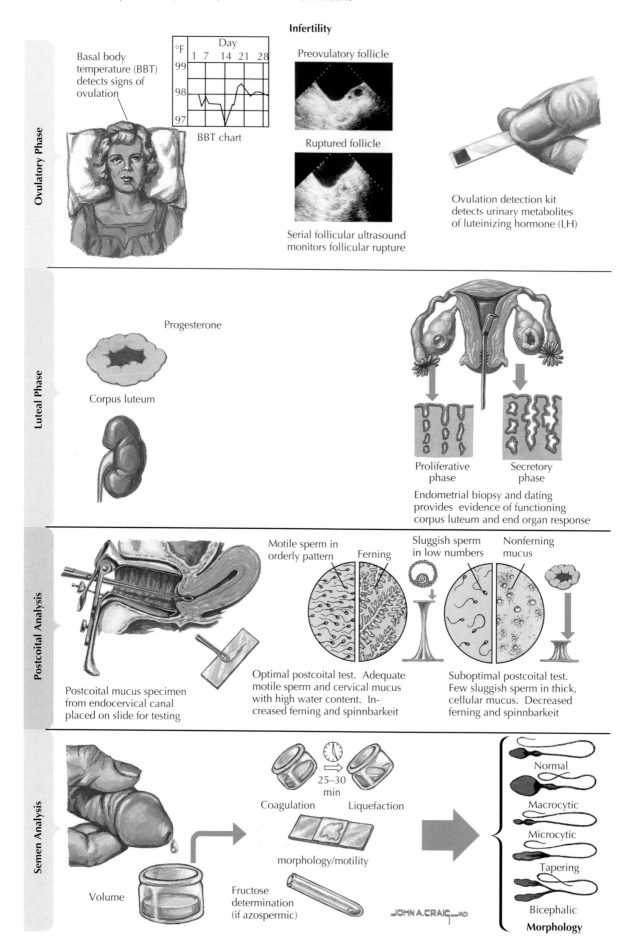

Ovulatory Phase

Basal body temperature (BBT) detects signs of ovulation

°F
Day
BBT chart

Preovulatory follicle

Ruptured follicle

Serial follicular ultrasound monitors follicular rupture

Ovulation detection kit detects urinary metabolites of luteinizing hormone (LH)

Luteal Phase

Progesterone

Corpus luteum

Proliferative phase

Secretory phase

Endometrial biopsy and dating provides evidence of functioning corpus luteum and end organ response

Postcoital Analysis

Postcoital mucus specimen from endocervical canal placed on slide for testing

Motile sperm in orderly pattern

Ferning

Sluggish sperm in low numbers

Nonferning mucus

Optimal postcoital test. Adequate motile sperm and cervical mucus with high water content. Increased ferning and spinnbarkeit

Suboptimal postcoital test. Few sluggish sperm in thick, cellular mucus. Decreased ferning and spinnbarkeit

Semen Analysis

Volume

Coagulation

25–30 min

Liquefaction

morphology/motility

Fructose determination (if azospermic)

Normal

Macrocytic

Microcytic

Tapering

Bicephalic

Morphology

JOHN A. CRAIG—AD

ovulation induction (considered now as first-line therapy for polycystic ovary syndrome).

Contraindications: Undiagnosed infertility.

Precautions: The possibility of ovarian hyperstimulation must be considered and close follow-up should be maintained if ovulation induction is attempted.

Alternative Drugs

Gonadotropin-releasing hormone (GnRH) agonists may be used to control the hormonal environment during ovulation induction. Human gonadotropins may be used to induce ovulation but are associated with an increased risk of multiple ovulations and multiple gestations if pregnancy ensues.

FOLLOW-UP

Patient Monitoring: Normal health maintenance.

Prevention/Avoidance: None.

Expected Outcome: Less than 40% of couples with primary infertility conceive after 6 years of therapy compared with more than 50% of secondary infertility couples who conceive by 3 years.

MISCELLANEOUS

Pregnancy Considerations: No effect on pregnancy once pregnancy is achieved. Some causes of impaired fertility are associated with a greater risk of early pregnancy loss.

ICD-9-CM Codes: 628.9 (other more specific classifications based on cause).

REFERENCES

Level I

Steures P, van der Steeg JW, Hompes PG, et al; Collaborative Effort on the Clinical Evaluation in Reproductive Medicine: Intrauterine insemination with controlled ovarian hyperstimulation versus expectant management for couples with unexplained subfertility and an intermediate prognosis: a randomised clinical trial. Lancet 2006;368:216.

Level II

Legro RS, Barnhart HX, Schlaff WD, et al; Cooperative Multicenter Reproductive Medicine Network: Clomiphene, metformin, or both for infertility in the polycystic ovary syndrome. N Engl J Med 2007;356:551.

Reddy UM, Wapner RJ, Rebar RW, Tasca RJ: Infertility, assisted reproductive technology, and adverse pregnancy outcomes: executive summary of a National Institute of Child Health and Human Development workshop. Obstet Gynecol 2007;109:967.

Level III

American College of Obstetricians and Gynecologists: Management of infertility caused by ovulatory dysfunction. ACOG Practice Bulletin 34. Obstet Gynecol 2002;99:347.

American College of Obstetricians and Gynecologists: Adoption. ACOG Committee Opinion 368. Obstet Gynecol 2007;109:1507.

Bagshawe A, Taylor A: ABC of subfertility. Counselling. BMJ 2003;327:1038.

Bagshawe A, Taylor A: Intractable infertility. BMJ 2003;327:1098.

Braude P, Rowell P: Assisted conception. II—In vitro fertilisation and intracytoplasmic sperm injection. BMJ 2003;327:852.

Braude P, Rowell P: Assisted conception. III—Problems with assisted conception. BMJ 2003;327:920.

Cahill DJ, Wardle PG: Management of infertility. BMJ 2002;325:28.

Evers JL: Female subfertility. Lancet 2002;360:151.

Frey KA, Patel KS: Initial evaluation and management of infertility by the primary care physician. Mayo Clin Proc 2004;79:1439.

Hamilton-Fairley D, Taylor A: Anovulation. BMJ 2003;327:546.

Hart R: Unexplained infertility, endometriosis, and fibroids. BMJ 2003;327:721.

Khalaf Y: ABC of subfertility. Tubal subfertility. BMJ 2003;327:610.

Makar RS, Toth TL: The evaluation of infertility. Am J Clin Pathol 2002;117:S95.

Pickering S, Braude P: Further advances and uses of assisted conception technology. BMJ 2003;327:1156.

Rowell P, Braude P: Assisted conception. I—General principles. BMJ 2003;327:799.

Setji TL, Brown AJ: Polycystic ovary syndrome: diagnosis and treatment. Am J Med 2007;120:128.

Smith S, Pfeifer SM, Collins JA: Diagnosis and management of female infertility. JAMA 2003;290:1767.

Taylor A: ABC of subfertility: extent of the problem. BMJ 2003;327:434.

Taylor A: ABC of subfertility. Making a diagnosis. BMJ 2003;327:494.

Van Voorhis BJ: Outcomes from assisted reproductive technology. Obstet Gynecol 2006;107:183.

Van Voorhis BJ: Clinical practice. In vitro fertilization. N Engl J Med 2007;356:379.

INTRODUCTION

Description: Menopause is an endocrinopathy caused by the loss of normal ovarian steroidogenesis because of age, chemotherapy, radiation, or surgical therapy. (An endocrinopathy is the loss of an endocrine function with adverse health consequences.)

Prevalence: Of postmenopausal women who do not receive estrogen replacement, 100%.

Predominant Age: Median 51.5, 95% between 44 and 55 (or after surgical menopause).

Genetics: Loss of genetic material from the long arm of the X chromosome is associated with premature menopause.

ETIOLOGY AND PATHOGENESIS

Causes: Loss of estrogen production because of surgery, chemotherapy (alkylating agents), radiation, or natural cessation of ovarian function (menopause).

Risk Factors: Menopause may occur at a younger age in smokers, those with poor nutrition or chronic illness, or those who have a loss of genetic material from the long arm of the X chromosome.

CLINICAL CHARACTERISTICS

Signs and Symptoms

- Absence of menstruation (with a normal uterus and outflow tract)
- Hot flashes, flushes, and night sweats
- Vaginal atrophy
- Dysuria, urgency, and urgency incontinence; urinary frequency; nocturia; and an increased incidence of stress urinary incontinence
- Decrease in libido
- Irregular bleeding common during the climacteric (perimenopausal) period

DIAGNOSTIC APPROACH

Differential Diagnosis

- Pregnancy
- Hypothyroidism
- Polycystic ovary syndrome
- Prolactin-secreting tumor
- Hypothalamic dysfunction
- Hypothyroidism

Associated Conditions: Dyspareunia, vulvodynia, atrophic vulvitis, osteoporosis, increased risk of cardiovascular disease, hot flashes and flushes, sleep disturbances, stress urinary incontinence, and others.

WORKUP AND EVALUATION

Laboratory: Usually not necessary. When the diagnosis of ovarian failure must be confirmed, measurement of serum follicle-stimulating hormone (FSH) is sufficient. Levels of greater than 100 mIU/mL are diagnostic, although lower levels (40 to 50 mIU/mL) may be sufficient to establish a diagnosis when symptoms are also present. Serum estradiol levels may be determined (generally less than 15 pg/mL) but are less reliable as a marker of ovarian failure. A pregnancy test is always indicated in women who are perimenopausal and sexually active and not using contraception.

Imaging: No imaging indicated. Standard imaging does not document bone loss of less than 30%.

Special Tests: A vaginal maturation index may be obtained but is generally not required for diagnosis. Bone densitometry may be indicated for those at special risk. When noncyclic bleeding occurs in these patients, endometrial biopsy should be strongly considered. Women younger than age 30 years who have ovarian failure should have a karyotype performed.

Pathologic Findings

Vaginal, vulvar, and endometrial atrophy. Thinned ovarian stroma with few, inactive oocytes. Accelerated calcium loss from bone.

MANAGEMENT AND THERAPY

Nonpharmacologic

General Measures: Health maintenance, annual mammogram, annual pelvic and rectal examinations, thyroid and cholesterol screening every 5 years or as indicated, tetanus booster shot every 10 years, pneumococcus vaccine as indicated.

Specific Measures: For symptom relief: systemic estrogen (estrogen/progestin) therapy. (Less than 1% of women do not benefit from therapy.) Topical estrogen supplements.

Diet: Adequate dietary calcium (1000 to 1500 mg/day).

Activity: No restriction, weightbearing activity to promote bone health, cardiovascular fitness training/maintenance.

Patient Education: Reassurance; American College of Obstetricians and Gynecologists Patient Education Pamphlet AP047 (The Menopause Years), AP066 (Hormone Replacement Therapy), AP158 (Herbal Products for Menopause), AP048 (Preventing Osteoporosis), AP028 (Vaginitis: Causes and Treatments).

Drug(s) of Choice

(Most common drug doses shown.)

Oral estrogens—conjugated equine estrogens (0.625 to 1.25 mg/day), diethylstilbestrol, esterified estrogens (0.625 to 1.25 mg/day), ethinyl estradiol (0.05 mg/day), micronized estradiol (0.5 to 1 mg/day), piperazine estrone sulfate, estropipate, quinestrol.

Injectable estrogens—conjugated equine estrogens, estradiol benzoate, estradiol cypionate, estradiol valerate (oil), estrone (aqueous), ethinyl estradiol, polyestradiol phosphate.

Topical estrogens—17β-estradiol (transdermal) (0.05 to 0.10 mg/day), conjugated equine estrogens (0.625 mg/g), estradiol (0.1 mg/g), estropipate (1.5 mg/g).

Pituitary and Ovarian Hormone Changes in Menopause

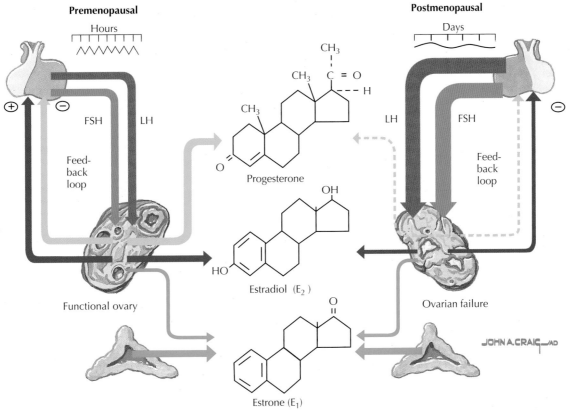

Premenopausal

Hours

FSH   LH

Feed-
back
loop

Functional ovary

Postmenopausal

Days

LH   FSH

Feed-
back
loop

Ovarian failure

Progesterone

Estradiol (E$_2$)

Estrone (E$_1$)

JOHN A. CRAIG—AD

Hormone levels increase and decrease cyclically during menstrual cycle. Modulation occurs by pulsatile releases of gonadotropins and positive and negative feedback loops

In postmenopausal period, gonadotropin levels increase and ovarian hormone levels decrease secondary to ovarian failure. Endogenous estrogen is primarily of adrenal origin, and E$_1$ to E$_2$ ratio is reversed

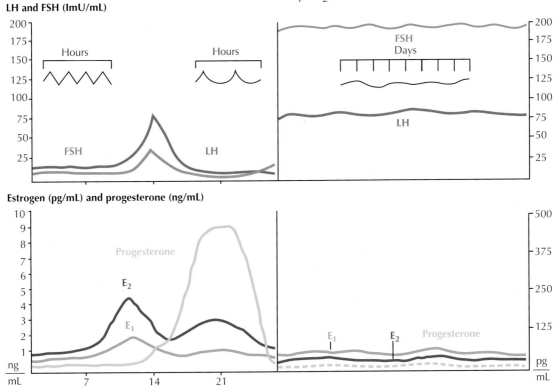

LH and FSH (lmU/mL)

Hours   Hours

FSH   LH

FSH
Days

LH

Estrogen (pg/mL) and progesterone (ng/mL)

Progesterone

E$_2$

E$_1$

E$_1$ E$_2$ Progesterone

FSH, follicle-stimulating hormone; LH, luteinizing hormone.

Contraindications: Systemic therapy: active liver disease, carcinoma of the breast (current), chronic liver damage (impaired function), endometrial carcinoma (current), recent thrombosis (with or without emboli), unexplained vaginal bleeding. Relative contraindications/special considerations—endometriosis, familial hyperlipidemia, gallbladder disease, hypertension (uncontrolled), migraine headaches, seizure disorders, thrombophlebitis (unknown risk), uterine leiomyomas. Topical use—known sensitivity to vehicle.

Precautions: Continuous estrogen exposure without periodic or concomitant progestins increases the risk of endometrial carcinoma 6-fold to 8-fold. Continuous estrogen/progestin therapy frequently results in random vaginal bleeding, but biopsy or other investigation is still warranted. Patients receiving cyclic estrogen/progestin therapy should experience vaginal bleeding only after withdrawal of the progestin; biopsy or other investigation is warranted for other bleeding.

Interactions: Raloxifene should not be used with cholestyramine. Most therapies alter the effects of warfarin therapy.

Alternative Drugs

Raloxifene (Evista) 60 mg PO daily—no relief for hot flashes or vaginal dryness, but does reduce breast cancer risk.

Progestin therapy (oral, vaginal, or injectable)—effective for hot flashes, may reduce bone loss, but has no effect on coronary artery disease or urogenital atrophy.

Clonidine (oral or transdermal).

Bellergal-S (phenobarbital, ergotamine tartrate, belladonna).

Alendronate (Fosamax)—for osteoporosis.

Topical moisturizers for atrophic vaginitis.

(Botanical agents have not been shown to be efficacious for most menopausal symptoms or for osteoporosis prevention.)

FOLLOW-UP

Patient Monitoring: Normal health maintenance. Serious consideration should be given to a trial of therapy discontinuation after 2 or more years.

Prevention/Avoidance: Estrogen replacement therapy at menopause. The use of progestins is required if the patient retains her uterus to reduce the risk of iatrogenic endometrial hyperplasia or cancer. Therapy may be oral (such as medroxyprogesterone acetate [Provera] 5 to 10 mg PO daily for 12 to 14 days per month or 2.5 mg PO daily) or vaginal (progesterone bioadhesive gel [Crinone] 4% to 8%, 45 mg [1.125 g] intravaginally every other day for six doses per month).

Possible Complications: Endometrial hyperplasia if the uterus is present and progestins not used, vaginal bleeding (predictable or otherwise).

Expected Outcome: Reversal of symptoms, reestablishment of normal physiology with treatment. Selective estrogen receptor modulators (also called SERMS or tissue-specific estrogens) may provide protection against cardiac, bone, and colon cancer and Alzheimer's disease with reduced rates of risk for both breast and endometrial cancer.

MISCELLANEOUS

Pregnancy Considerations: Menopause is associated with the loss of fertility.

ICD-9-CM Codes: 627.2 (Menopause or female climacteric states), 256.3 (Premature), 256.2 (Premature: post irradiation or surgical), 627.4 (Surgical).

REFERENCES

Level I

Newton KM, Reed SD, LaCroix AZ, et al: Treatment of vasomotor symptoms of menopause with black cohosh, multibotanicals, soy, hormone therapy, or placebo: a randomized trial. Ann Intern Med 2006;145:869.

Rapp SR, Espeland MA, Shumaker SA, et al; WHIMS Investigators: Effect of estrogen plus progestin on global cognitive function in postmenopausal women: The Women's Health Initiative Memory Study: a randomized controlled trial. JAMA 2003;289:2663.

Reddy SY, Warner H, Guttuso T Jr, et al: Gabapentin, estrogen, and placebo for treating hot flushes: a randomized controlled trial. Obstet Gynecol 2006;108:41.

Shumaker SA, Legault C, Rapp SR, et al; WHIMS Investigators: Estrogen plus progestin and the incidence of dementia and mild cognitive impairment in postmenopausal women: The Women's Health Initiative Memory Study: a randomized controlled trial. JAMA 2003;289:2651.

Simon JA, Bouchard C, Waldbaum A, et al: Low dose of transdermal estradiol gel for treatment of symptomatic postmenopausal women: a randomized controlled trial. Obstet Gynecol 2007;109:588.

Steiner AZ, Xiang M, Mack WJ, et al: Unopposed estradiol therapy in postmenopausal women: results from two randomized trials. Obstet Gynecol 2007;109:581.

Level II

Anderson GL, Limacher M, Assaf AR, et al; Women's Health Initiative Steering Committee: Effects of conjugated equine estrogen in postmenopausal women with hysterectomy: The Women's Health Initiative randomized controlled trial. JAMA 2004;291:1701.

Bath PM, Gray LJ: Association between hormone replacement therapy and subsequent stroke: a meta-analysis. BMJ 2005;330:342. Epub 2005 Jan 7.

Cauley JA, Robbins J, Chen Z, et al; Women's Health Initiative Investigators: Effects of estrogen plus progestin on risk of fracture and bone mineral density: The Women's Health Initiative randomized trial. JAMA 2003;290:1729.

Cheong JM, Martin BR, Jackson GS, et al: Soy isoflavones do not affect bone resorption in postmenopausal women: a dose-response study using a novel approach with 41Ca. J Clin Endocrinol Metab 2007;92:577. Epub 2006 Dec 5.

Cushman M, Kuller LH, Prentice R, et al; Women's Health Initiative Investigators: Estrogen plus progestin and risk of venous thrombosis. JAMA 2004;292:1573.

Hendrix SL, Wassertheil-Smoller S, Johnson KC, et al; WHI Investigators: Effects of conjugated equine estrogen on stroke in the Women's Health Initiative. Circulation 2006;113:2425. Epub 2006 May 15.

Hsia J, Langer RD, Manson JE, et al; Women's Health Initiative Investigators: Conjugated equine estrogens and coronary heart disease: The Women's Health Initiative. Arch Intern Med 2006;166:357.

Magliano DJ, Rogers SL, Abramson MJ, Tonkin AM: Hormone therapy and cardiovascular disease: a systematic review and meta-analysis. BJOG 2006;113:5.

Manson JE, Allison MA, Rossouw JE, et al; WHI and WHI-CACS Investigators: Estrogen therapy and coronary-artery calcification. N Engl J Med 2007;356:2591.

Nedrow A, Miller J, Walker M, et al: Complementary and alternative therapies for the management of menopause-related symptoms: a systematic evidence review. Arch Intern Med 2006;166:1453.

Nelson HD: Commonly used types of postmenopausal estrogen for treatment of hot flashes: scientific review. JAMA 2004;291:1610.

Nelson HD, Vesco KK, Haney E, et al: Nonhormonal therapies for menopausal hot flashes: systematic review and meta-analysis. JAMA 2006;295:2057.

Rossouw JE, Anderson GL, Prentice RL, et al; Writing Group for the Women's Health Initiative Investigators: Risks and benefits of estrogen plus progestin in healthy postmenopausal women: principal results from the Women's Health Initiative randomized controlled trial. JAMA 2002;288:321.

Rossouw JE, Prentice RL, Manson JE, et al: Postmenopausal hormone therapy and risk of cardiovascular disease by age and years since menopause. JAMA 2007;297:1465.

Wassertheil-Smoller S, Hendrix SL, Limacher M, et al; WHI Investigators: Effect of estrogen plus progestin on stroke in postmenopausal women: The Women's Health Initiative: a randomized trial. JAMA 2003;289:2673.

Level III

American College of Obstetricians and Gynecologists: Use of botanicals for management of menopausal symptoms. ACOG Practice Bulletin 28. Washington, DC, ACOG, 2001.

American College of Obstetricians and Gynecologists: Selective estrogen receptor modulators. ACOG Practice Bulletin 39. Obstet Gynecol 2002;100:835.

American College of Obstetricians and Gynecologists: Osteoporosis. ACOG Practice Bulletin 50. Obstet Gynecol 2004;103:203.

American College of Obstetricians and Gynecologists: Compounded bioidentical hormones. ACOG Committee Opinion 322. Obstet Gynecol 2005; 106:1139.

Cheung AM, Feig DS, Kapral M, et al; Canadian Task Force on Preventive Health Care: Prevention of osteoporosis and osteoporotic fractures in postmenopausal women: recommendation statement from the Canadian Task Force on Preventive Health Care. CMAJ 2004;170:1665.

Creasman WT, Hoel D, Disaia PJ: WHI: Now that the dust has settled: a commentary. Am J Obstet Gynecol 2003;189:621.

Grady D: Clinical practice. Management of menopausal symptoms. N Engl J Med 2006;355:2338.

Grimes DA, Lobo RA: Perspectives on the Women's Health Initiative trial of hormone replacement therapy. Obstet Gynecol 2002; 100:1344.

Hickey M, Davis SR, Sturdee DW: Treatment of menopausal symptoms: what shall we do now? Lancet 2005;366:409.

National Institutes of Health: National Institutes of Health State-of-the-Science Conference statement: Management of menopause-related symptoms. Ann Intern Med 2005;142:1003. Epub 2005 May 27.

Roberts H: Managing the menopause. BMJ 2007;334:736.

Sahdev A: Imaging the endometrium in postmenopausal bleeding. BMJ 2007;334:635.

Santoro N: The menopausal transition. Am J Med 2005;118:8.

Warren MP: Historical perspectives in postmenopausal hormone therapy: defining the right dose and duration. Mayo Clin Proc 2007;82:219.

INTRODUCTION

Description: Polycystic ovary syndrome (PCOS) consists of amenorrhea, hirsutism, insulin resistance, and obesity in association with enlarged, multicystic ovaries.

Prevalence: Up to 5% of women, 30% of secondary amenorrhea. The most common hormonal disorder among women of reproductive age.

Predominant Age: Begins at menarche.

Genetics: No genetic pattern established, suggestion of increased family tendency.

ETIOLOGY AND PATHOGENESIS

Causes: The exact pathophysiology of polycystic ovary syndrome is not well established, but increased amplitude of gonadotropin-releasing hormone (GnRH) pulsation and abnormal secretion of follicle-stimulating hormone (FSH) and luteinizing hormone (LH) during puberty are thought to result in androgen excess. Elevated levels of LH persist and may be used to help establish the diagnosis. Insulin resistance is a prominent aspect of this syndrome.

Risk Factors: Borderline adrenal hyperplasia, occult hypothyroidism, and childhood obesity.

CLINICAL CHARACTERISTICS

Signs and Symptoms

- Anovulation and amenorrhea (75% to 80%)
- Infertility (75%)
- Excessive hair growth, primarily along the angle of the jaw, upper lip, and chin (70%)
- Obesity (50%) ("apple-shaped" obesity centered around the lower half of the torso)
- Acanthosis nigricans
- Acne

DIAGNOSTIC APPROACH

Differential Diagnosis

- Virilization (especially when hirsutism is in a male pattern)
- Familial hypertrichosis
- Cushing's disease (truncal obesity, facial rounding, cervicodorsal fat deposition [buffalo hump], and red or purple striae are often not fully developed)

Associated Conditions: Increased risk of cardiovascular disease (adverse lipid profiles), diabetes (insulin resistance in 50% of patients), hypertension, and infertility.

Workup and Evaluation

Laboratory: Elevated levels of luteinizing hormone may be used to help establish the diagnosis. (A two-to-one ratio of luteinizing hormone to follicle-stimulating hormone is considered diagnostic.) Evaluation for possible virilizing process (prolactin, follicle-stimulating hormone, thyroid screening). (Patients suspected of having adrenal sources of hyperandrogenicity may be screened by measuring 24-hour urinary-free cortisol, by performing adrenocorticotropin hormone [ACTH]

stimulation tests, or an overnight dexamethasone suppression test.) Serum testosterone (total) is generally 70 to 120 ng/mL and androstenedione is 3 to 5 ng/mL. Dehydroepiandrosterone sulfate (DHEA-s) is elevated in approximately 50% of patients.

Imaging: Ultrasonography (abdominal or transvaginal) may identify ovarian enlargement or the presence of multiple small follicles. Magnetic resonance imaging (MRI) or computed tomography (CT) may be used to evaluate the adrenal glands.

Special Tests: None indicated.

Diagnostic Procedures: History, physical examination, imaging and laboratory evaluations. May be confirmed at laparoscopy, but seldom required for diagnosis.

Pathologic Findings

The ovaries are enlarged with a thickened white capsule. They contain multiple follicles in varying stages of development. Luteinization of theca cells may be present.

MANAGEMENT AND THERAPY

Nonpharmacologic

General Measures: Evaluation. Weight loss is often associated with resolution of symptoms and a return of menstrual function in patients with mild or early polycystic ovary syndrome.

Specific Measures: Medical therapy has replaced surgical treatment. Treatment depends on desire for pregnancy; if pregnancy is desired, then ovulation induction may be required.

Diet: No specific dietary changes indicated; weight loss or control desirable.

Activity: No restriction.

Patient Education: American College of Obstetricians and Gynecologists Patient Education Pamphlet AP121 (Polycystic Ovary Syndrome).

Drug(s) of Choice

Combination oral contraceptives (less than 50-mg formulation and a progestin other than norgestrel).

If DHEA-s is elevated, dexamethasone (0.25 to 0.5 mg PO every bedtime) may be added to oral contraceptives.

Spironolactone (100 to 200 mg PO daily).

Metformin (1500 mg/day) as an adjunctive treatment for ovulation induction (considered now as first-line therapy for polycystic ovary syndrome).

Contraindications: Pregnancy. (Spironolactone is a category X drug; patients using it and able to become pregnant must use reliable contraception.)

Alternative Drugs

Gonadotropin-releasing hormone analogues and clomiphene citrate may be used.

FOLLOW-UP

Patient Monitoring: Normal health maintenance once diagnosis and management have been implemented. There is an increased risk of diabetes in patients with

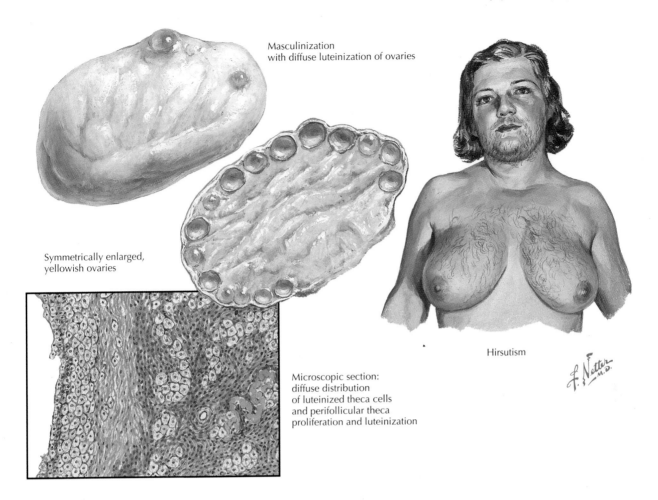

Masculinization with diffuse luteinization of ovaries

Symmetrically enlarged, yellowish ovaries

Microscopic section: diffuse distribution of luteinized theca cells and perifollicular theca proliferation and luteinization

Hirsutism

polycystic ovaries. Weight control and contraception should also be addressed.

Prevention/Avoidance: Role of normalized weight debated.

Possible Complications: Chronic anovulation is associated with osteoporosis and endometrial hyperplasia or carcinoma.

Expected Outcome: Generally good response to medical therapy.

MISCELLANEOUS

Pregnancy Considerations: No effect on pregnancy, although fertility is often reduced.

ICD-9-CM Codes: 256.4.

2003 Rotterdam Criteria

Patient must have two or more of the following:
1. Oligo-ovulation and/or anovulation
2. Excess androgen activity
3. Polycystic ovaries (by gynecologic ultrasound)

Data based on Welt CK, Gudmundsson JA, Arason G, et al: Characterizing discrete subsets of polycystic ovary syndrome as defined by the Rotterdam Criteria: the impact of weight on phenotype and metabolic features. J Clin Endocrinol Metab 2006;91:4842.

REFERENCES

Level I

Azziz R, Ehrmann D, Legro RS, et al; PCOS/Troglitazone Study Group: Troglitazone improves ovulation and hirsutism in the polycystic ovary syndrome: a multicenter, double blind, placebo-controlled trial. J Clin Endocrinol Metab 2001;86:1626.

Bridger T, MacDonald S, Baltzer F, Rodd C: Randomized placebo-controlled trial of metformin for adolescents with polycystic ovary syndrome. Arch Pediatr Adolesc Med 2006;160:241.

Eisenhardt S, Schwarzmann N, Henschel V, et al: Early effects of metformin in women with polycystic ovary syndrome: a prospective randomized, double-blind, placebo-controlled trial. J Clin Endocrinol Metab 2006;91:946. Epub 2005 Dec 13.

Legro RS, Zaino RJ, Demers LM, et al: The effects of metformin and rosiglitazone, alone and in combination, on the ovary and endometrium in polycystic ovary syndrome. Am J Obstet Gynecol 2007;196:402.e1.

Moll E, Bossuyt PM, Korevaar JC, et al: Effect of clomifene citrate plus metformin and clomifene citrate plus placebo on induction of ovulation in women with newly diagnosed polycystic ovary syndrome: randomised double blind clinical trial. BMJ 2006;332:1485. Epub 2006 Jun 12.

Level II

Legro RS, Barnhart HX, Schlaff WD, et al; Cooperative Multicenter Reproductive Medicine Network: Clomiphene, metformin, or both for infertility in the polycystic ovary syndrome. N Engl J Med 2007;356:551.

Lord JM, Flight IH, Norman RJ: Metformin in polycystic ovary syndrome: systematic review and meta-analysis. BMJ 2003; 327:951.

Pasquali R, Gambineri A, Pagotto U: The impact of obesity on reproduction in women with polycystic ovary syndrome. BJOG 2006;113:1148. Epub 2006 Jul 7. Review.

Level III

American College of Obstetricians and Gynecologists: Management of anovulatory bleeding. ACOG Practice Bulletin 14. Washington, DC, ACOG, 2000.

American College of Obstetricians and Gynecologists: Management of infertility caused by ovulatory dysfunction. ACOG Practice Bulletin 34. Obstet Gynecol 2002;99:347.

American College of Obstetricians and Gynecologists: Polycystic ovary syndrome. ACOG Practice Bulletin 41. Obstet Gynecol 2002; 100:1389.

American College of Obstetricians and Gynecologists: The overweight adolescent: prevention, treatment, and obstetric–gynecologic implications. ACOG Committee Opinion 351. Obstet Gynecol 2006;108:1337.

Barbieri RL: Metformin for the treatment of polycystic ovary syndrome. Obstet Gynecol 2003;101:785.

Berga SL: The obstetrician-gynecologist's role in the practical management of polycystic ovary syndrome. Am J Obstet Gynecol 1998;179:S109.

Bloomfield D: Secondary amenorrhea. Pediatr Rev 2006;27:113.

Carmina E, Lobo RA: Polycystic ovary syndrome (PCOS): arguably the most common endocrinopathy is associated with significant morbidity in women. J Clin Endocrinol Metab 1999;84:1897.

Chang RJ: A practical approach to the diagnosis of polycystic ovary syndrome. Am J Obstet Gynecol 2004;191:713.

Ehrmann DA: Polycystic ovary syndrome. N Engl J Med 2005; 352:1223.

Franks S: Polycystic ovary syndrome. N Engl J Med 1995;333:853.

Guzick DS: Polycystic ovary syndrome. Obstet Gynecol 2004; 103:181.

Hopkinson ZE, Sattar N, Fleming R, Greer IA: Polycystic ovarian syndrome: the metabolic syndrome comes to gynaecology. BMJ 1998;317:329.

Lakhani K, Seifalian AM, Atiomo WU, Hardiman P: Polycystic ovaries. Br J Radiol 2002;75:9.

Legro RS: Polycystic ovary syndrome: current and future treatment paradigms. Am J Obstet Gynecol 1998;179:S101.

Lobo RA: Primary and secondary amenorrhea and precocious puberty. In Katz VL, Lentz GM, Lobo RA, Gershenson DM: Comprehensive Gynecology, 5th ed. Philadelphia, Mosby/Elsevier, 2007, p 942.

Lobo RA: Hyperandrogenism. In Katz VL, Lentz GM, Lobo RA, Gershenson DM: Comprehensive Gynecology, 5th ed. Philadelphia, Mosby/Elsevier, 2007, p 983.

Lobo RA, Carmina E: The importance of diagnosing the polycystic ovary syndrome. Ann Intern Med 2000;132:989.

Sartor BM, Dickey RP: Polycystic ovarian syndrome and the metabolic syndrome. Am J Med Sci 2005;330:336.

Setji TL, Brown AJ: Polycystic ovary syndrome: diagnosis and treatment. Am J Med 2007;120:128.

Siassakos D, Wardle P: Polycystic ovary syndrome and pregnancy outcome: red herring or red flag? BJOG 2007;114:922.

Slowey MJ: Polycystic ovary syndrome: new perspective on an old problem. South Med J 2001;94:190.

THE CHALLENGE

To evaluate patients who do not experience the normal events of puberty when expected and to provide reassurance with appropriate or timely diagnosis and intervention when more sinister processes are at work. Abnormal (precocious) puberty is estimated to affect roughly 1 in 10,000 girls.

Scope of the Problem: For all patients with precocious puberty (pubertal changes before age 7 or cyclic menstruation before age 10), the possibility of a serious process, either central or peripheral, must be evaluated. (Because of evolving changes in maturation rates, these traditional ages should be adjusted downward by 1 year for African American girls.) Precocious puberty is customarily divided into two classifications: true or gonadotropin-releasing hormone (GnRH)-dependent (70%), and precocious pseudopuberty that is independent of GnRH control. For most girls older than 4 years, no specific cause is discovered for the early development. By contrast, the most common cause of precocious change in girls younger than 4 is a central nervous system lesion, most often hamartomas of the hypothalamus. Even when the sequence of events appears normal, a serious process (such as a slowly progressing brain tumor) must be aggressively sought initially and watched for with long-term continuing follow-up. Delayed puberty is a relatively uncommon problem in girls. When it occurs, the possibility of a genetic or hypothalamic–pituitary abnormality must be considered, along with a moderately large number of other possibilities. Based on the average age and normal variation of puberty, any girl who has not exhibited breast budding by age 13 requires preliminary investigation. Similarly, girls who do not menstruate by age 15 or 16, regardless of other sexual development, should be evaluated. Patients should also be evaluated any time there is a disruption in the normal sequence of puberty or when there is patient or parental concern. Patients with significant abnormalities of either height or weight should be evaluated for chromosomal abnormalities or endocrinopathies.

Objectives of Management: To establish the cause of delayed events of puberty with appropriate speed and care, without adding to the trauma of adolescence.

TACTICS

Relevant Pathophysiology: True precocious puberty, also known as complete, isosexual, or central precocity, is related to early activation of the hypothalamic–pituitary–gonadal axis. In three fourths of patients, there is no indication of how or why the normal processes of puberty are accelerated. In the remaining one fourth, a central nervous system abnormality is the cause. A number of central nervous system pathologic conditions may result in activation of GnRH secretion and the early onset of pubertal changes. Precocious pseudopuberty is also referred to as incomplete or peripheral and may be isosexual or heterosexual. In these patients, there may be secretion of sex steroids or human chorionic gonado-

tropin from sources other than the pituitary. More than 10% of girls with precocious puberty have an ovarian tumor. These tumors are palpable in 80% of patients or may be readily detected by ultrasonography or tomographic studies. Bleeding is heavy and irregular in character, befitting escape from the normal control mechanisms. One of the most common chromosomal causes of absent (delayed) menstruation is the premature ovarian failure found in patients with Turner's syndrome (45,X). The absence of one X chromosome results in accelerated ovarian follicular atresia, to the extent that by the age of puberty, no functionally competent follicles remain. The appearance of these patients is noteworthy for short stature, webbed neck (pterygium colli), a shieldlike chest with widely spaced nipples, and an increased carrying angle of the arms (cubitus valgus). Buccal smears do not demonstrate Barr bodies, and chromosomal analysis confirms the diagnosis. Because these women will not undergo any secondary sexual maturation, referral to a specialist for counseling and management of replacement hormonal manipulations is advisable. Deletions of only a part of the long arm of the X chromosome have been shown to be associated with premature ovarian failure, with the earliest failures associated with the greatest deletions.

Strategies: The evaluation of patients with precocious puberty is focused on detecting possible life-threatening disease and defining the velocity of the process. When the diagnosis of true precocious puberty is established, generally by exclusion, treatment with GnRH agonists usually halts the progression of change. This therapy is expensive and is effective only if the observed changes are under central control. Suppression of GnRH may also be carried out using medroxyprogesterone acetate (Depo-Provera), in doses of 100 to 200 mg given intramuscularly every 2 to 4 weeks. This therapy is less likely to control bone growth abnormalities than is GnRH agonist treatment. (Without any therapy, approximately 50% of girls will not reach 5 feet in height.) The evaluation of patients with delayed pubertal development must begin with a general history, including general health, weight and height records, and family history, including the pubertal experience of others in the family. Physical examination should identify the type and degree of sexual development present. The presence of breast changes generally indicates the production of estrogen, and the development of pubic or axillary hair indicates the production of androgens. Laboratory evaluation should include serum follicle-stimulating hormone (FSH), luteinizing hormone (LH), and prolactin measurements; skull radiographs; and thyroid function studies. Bone age, chromosomal or cytologic studies, and pelvic ultrasonography or other imaging studies may also be indicated. Because of the significance of the potential causes of disordered puberty, most of these patients should be evaluated by or in consultation with a specialist.

Patient Education: Reassurance; American College of Obstetricians and Gynecologists Patient Education

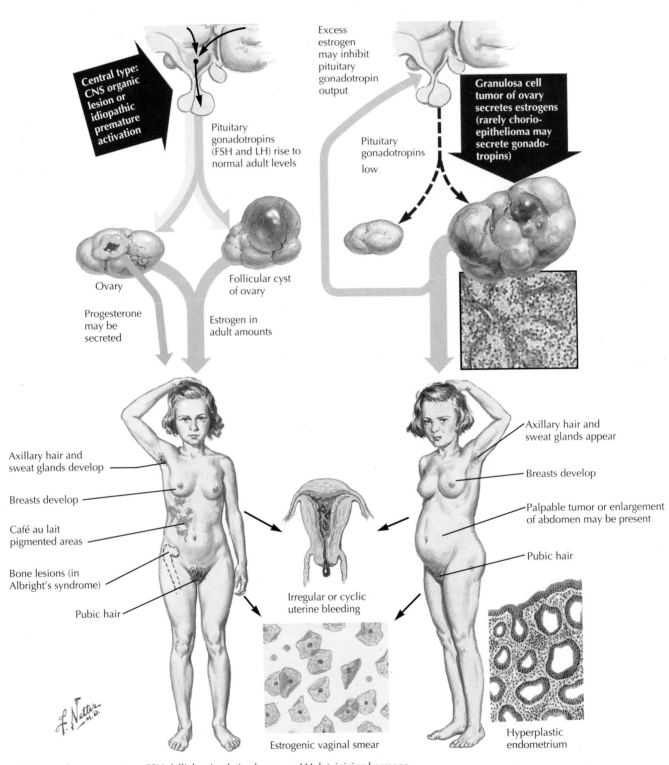

Central type:
CNS organic
lesion or
idiopathic
premature
activation

Excess
estrogen
may inhibit
pituitary
gonadotropin
output

Granulosa cell
tumor of ovary
secretes estrogens
(rarely chorio-
epithelioma may
secrete gonado-
tropins)

Pituitary
gonadotropins
(FSH and LH) rise to
normal adult levels

Pituitary
gonadotropins
low

Ovary

Follicular cyst
of ovary

Progesterone
may be
secreted

Estrogen in
adult amounts

Axillary hair and
sweat glands develop

Breasts develop

Café au lait
pigmented areas

Bone lesions (in
Albright's syndrome)

Pubic hair

Axillary hair and
sweat glands appear

Breasts develop

Palpable tumor or enlargement
of abdomen may be present

Pubic hair

Irregular or cyclic
uterine bleeding

Estrogenic vaginal smear

Hyperplastic
endometrium

CNS, central nervous system; FSH, follicle-stimulating hormone; LH, luteinizing hormone.

Pamphlet AP041 (Growing Up [Especially for Teens]), AP049 (Menstruation [Especially for Teens]).

IMPLEMENTATION

Special Considerations: Although precocious puberty is most often heralded by the sequence of increased growth, thelarche, and adrenarche, these events may occur simultaneously, or menarche itself may be the first indication. Idiopathic or constitutional precocious puberty is associated with a normal reproductive life and normal age of menopause. The greatest risk for abnormality comes from the early closure of the bony growth plates that often leaves these patients with short stature. Therapy is worth considering for young children to achieve adult height and to avoid the social and emotional stresses that early maturation can entail. If the cause of delayed puberty is found to be hypogonadism, hormonal therapy initiates and sustains the development of normal secondary sex characteristics. Hormonal therapy also allows for normal height and bone mass deposition to be achieved. Adolescents require much less hormone therapy than do adults or postmenopausal women. Therapy usually begins with unopposed estrogen at a dose of 0.3 mg of conjugated estrogen, 0.5 mg of estradiol, or their equivalent daily. In 6 to 12 months, this dose is roughly doubled and medroxyprogesterone acetate is added (10 mg for the first 12 days of the month). This combination results in regular menstruation but is insufficient for contraception. Normal puber-tal development generally proceeds when the patient reaches a bone age of 13.

REFERENCES

Level III

American Academy of Pediatrics, American College of Obstetricians and Gynecologists: Menstruation in girls and adolescents: using the menstrual cycle as a vital sign. ACOG Committee Opinion 349. Obstet Gynecol 2006;108:1323.

American College of Obstetricians and Gynecologists: Breast concerns in the adolescent. ACOG Committee Opinion 350. Obstet Gynecol 2006;108:1329.

Gulledge CC, Burow ME, McLachlan JA: Endocrine disruption in sexual differentiation and puberty. What do pseudohermaphroditic polar bears have to do with the practice of pediatrics? Pediatr Clin North Am 2001;48:1223, x.

Lobo RA: Primary and secondary amenorrhea and precocious puberty. In Katz VL, Lentz GM, Lobo RA, Gershenson DM: Comprehensive Gynecology, 5th ed. Philadelphia, Mosby/Elsevier, 2007, p 934, 951.

Loriaux DL: The pathophysiology of precocious puberty. Hosp Pract (Off Ed) 1989;24:55.

Neinstein LS: Menstrual problems in adolescents. Med Clin North Am 1990;74:1181.

Sizonenko PC: Preadolescent and adolescent endocrinology: physiology and physiopathology. II. Hormonal changes during abnormal pubertal development. Am J Dis Child 1978;132:797.

Styne DM: New aspects in the diagnosis and treatment of pubertal disorders. Pediatr Clin North Am 1997;44:505.

Styne DM, Kaplan SL: Normal and abnormal puberty in the female. Pediatr Clin North Am 1979;26:123.

INTRODUCTION

Description: Structural abnormalities present at birth may make the assignment of an appropriate sex of rearing (gender) difficult or impossible (sexual ambiguity). The evaluation of these infants represents both a social and medical emergency because life-threatening conditions may be present.

Prevalence: Less than 1 of 2000 births.

Predominant Age: Present at birth.

Genetics: Some enzymatic defects may be inheritable. A history of a previously affected relative may be present for patients with androgen insensitivity or its variants.

ETIOLOGY AND PATHOGENESIS

Causes: Enzyme defects (5α-reductase, 11β- 17α-, or 21-hydroxylase deficiencies), androgen insensitivity syndrome, intrauterine androgen exposure. (Most patients with ambiguous genitalia prove to be androgenized females with adrenal hyperplasia.) Cases are often placed into one of four categories: female pseudohermaphroditism, male pseudohermaphroditism, dysgenetic gonads (including true hermaphroditism), and true hermaphroditism (rare).

Risk Factors: In utero androgen exposure.

CLINICAL CHARACTERISTICS

Signs and Symptoms

- Incompletely formed or malformed external genitalia (varies from labial adhesion to clitoral hypertrophy and vaginal agenesis based on cause and genetic makeup of the individual)
- Infants—rapid development of vomiting, diarrhea, dehydration, and shock (congenital adrenal hyperplasia)

DIAGNOSTIC APPROACH

Differential Diagnosis

- Congenital adrenal hyperplasia (may be life-threatening—must be first consideration in any newborn with ambiguous genitalia or male babies with cryptorchidism; if gonads are not palpable, adrenal hyperplasia must be presumed, and treated, until disproved).
- Androgen exposure in utero (exogenous, luteoma of pregnancy)
- Vaginal agenesis
- Imperforate hymen
- Other enzymatic defects

Associated Conditions: Premature puberty, infertility, sexual dysfunction, and gender dysphoria.

Workup and Evaluation

Laboratory: Electrolytes, hormonal and enzymatic function.

Imaging: Ultrasonography may be used to assess the internal genitalia, but it is seldom necessary for initial diagnosis.

Special Tests: Karyotyping may be desirable, but a buccal smear to detect Barr bodies is often sufficient.

Diagnostic Procedures: Systematic examination of the genitalia (mons and groin, clitoris/phallus, urethral opening, labioscrotal folds, vaginal opening, posterior fourchette and perineum, anus and anal patency—the penis has a midline frenulum; the clitoris has two lateral folds that extend to the labia minora), karyotype, laboratory testing. A multidisciplinary team may be required to complete the evaluation.

Pathologic Findings

Based on cause.

MANAGEMENT AND THERAPY

Nonpharmacologic

General Measures: Rapid assessment and treatment as if congenital adrenal hyperplasia is present should be instituted until the possibility has been ruled out. (The assignment of gender must be made as soon as possible after delivery but should be delayed until a gender can be established considering all available evidence. Many experts argue against the use of names that are gender ambiguous such as Leslie, Terry, or Jamie.)

Specific Measures: Therapy is medical and surgical—medical therapy to reverse the effects of enzyme defects; surgical therapy for cosmetics and sexual function. Surgery is often delayed until late infancy or adolescence (based on the type of reconstruction planned). If a Y-chromosome cell line is present, removal of the gonads is indicated.

Diet: No specific dietary changes indicated.

Activity: No restriction.

Drug(s) of Choice

For congenital adrenal hyperplasia: cortisol 12 to 18 mg/m^2 or prednisone 3.5 to 5 mg/m^2 or higher to maintain adrenal suppression.

FOLLOW-UP

Patient Monitoring: Normal health maintenance, continuing support for enzymatic defects.

Prevention/Avoidance: Avoidance of agents with androgenic activity during pregnancy (drugs and food supplements).

Possible Complications: Failure to establish a clear, unambiguous gender (sex of rearing) can result in life-long social and psychological problems and may limit future surgical reconstruction and sexual options.

Expected Outcome: With early detection, successful growth and development appropriate to gender may be anticipated. With reconstruction, even severe anatomic deformities can be corrected to provide cosmetic and sexually acceptable results.

MISCELLANEOUS

Pregnancy Considerations: Based on cause—androgenized females are fully fertile and have normal

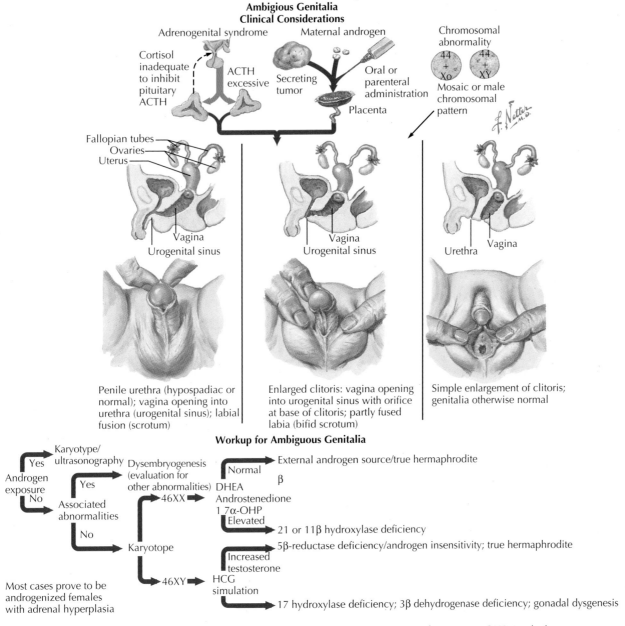

**Ambigious Genitalia
Clinical Considerations**

Adrenogenital syndrome

Maternal androgen

Chromosomal abnormality

Cortisol inadequate to inhibit pituitary ACTH

ACTH excessive

Secreting tumor

Oral or parenteral administration

Placenta

Mosaic or male chromosomal pattern

Fallopian tubes
Ovaries
Uterus

Vagina
Urogenital sinus

Vagina
Urogenital sinus

Urethra   Vagina

Penile urethra (hypospadiac or normal); vagina opening into urethra (urogenital sinus); labial fusion (scrotum)

Enlarged clitoris: vagina opening into urogenital sinus with orifice at base of clitoris; partly fused labia (bifid scrotum)

Simple enlargement of clitoris; genitalia otherwise normal

Workup for Ambiguous Genitalia

Androgen exposure

Yes — Karyotype/ ultrasonography

No

Associated abnormalities

Yes

No

Dysembryogenesis (evaluation for other abnormalities)

46XX

Karyotope

46XY

Normal β

DHEA Androstenedione 1 7α-OHP

Elevated

External androgen source/true hermaphrodite

21 or 11β hydroxylase deficiency

HCG simulation

Increased testosterone

5β-reductase deficiency/androgen insensitivity; true hermaphrodite

17 hydroxylase deficiency; 3β dehydrogenase deficiency; gonadal dysgenesis

Most cases prove to be androgenized females with adrenal hyperplasia

ACTH, adrenocorticotropic hormone; DHEA, dehydroepiandrosterone; HCG, human chorionic gonadotropin; 17α-OHP, 17α hydroxyprogesterone.

pregnancies; males with isolated hypospadias or cryptorchidism may be fertile; all others are sterile.
ICD-9-CM Codes: 752.7.

REFERENCES

Level III
Bidarkar SS, Hutson JM: Evaluation and management of the abnormal gonad. Semin Pediatr Surg 2005;14:118.

Brown J, Warne G: Practical management of the intersex infant. J Pediatr Endocrinol Metab 2005;18:3.

Cunningham FG, Gant NF, Leveno KJ, et al, eds: Williams obstetrics, 21st ed. New York, McGraw-Hill, 2001, p 156.

Haqq CM, Donahoe PK: Regulation of sexual dimorphism in mammals. Physiol Rev 1998;78:1.

Hughes IA: The masculinized female and investigation of abnormal sexual development. Baillieres Clin Endocrinol Metab 1998; 12:157.

Jaaskelainen J, Tiitinen A, Voutilainen R: Sexual function and fertility in adult females and males with congenital adrenal hyperplasia. Horm Res 2001;56:73.

Kirk JM, Perry LA, Shand WS, et al: Female pseudohermaphroditism due to a maternal adrenocortical tumor. J Clin Endocrinol Metab 1990;70:1280.

Low Y, Hutson JM; Murdoch Children's Research Institute Sex Study Group: Rules for clinical diagnosis in babies with ambiguous genitalia. J Paediatr Child Health 2003;39:406.

Miller WL: Disorders of androgen biosynthesis. Semin Reprod Med 2002;20:205.

Reindollar RH, Tho SP, McDonough PG: Abnormalities of sexual differentiation: evaluation and management. Clin Obstet Gynecol 1987;30:697.

Sultan C, Lobaccaro JM, Belon C, et al: Molecular biology of disorders of sex differentiation. Horm Res 1992;38:105.

Vilain E: Anomalies of human sexual development: clinical aspects and genetic analysis. Novartis Found Symp 2002;244:43.

Wiener JS: Insights into causes of sexual ambiguity. Curr Opin Urol 1999;9:507.

INTRODUCTION

Description: Sheehan's syndrome is characterized by loss of pituitary function resulting from damage or necrosis that occurs through anoxia, thrombosis, or hemorrhage. When associated with pregnancy, it is called Sheehan's syndrome; when unrelated to pregnancy it is called Simmonds disease.

Prevalence: Rare, less than 1 of 10,000 deliveries.

Predominant Age: Reproductive.

Genetics: No genetic pattern.

ETIOLOGY AND PATHOGENESIS

Causes: Anoxia, thrombosis, or hemorrhage that results in damage or necrosis of the pituitary gland. (The exact mechanism of pituitary damage is unknown.)

Risk Factors: Postpartum hemorrhage with hypotension.

CLINICAL CHARACTERISTICS

Signs and Symptoms

- Secondary amenorrhea
- Secondary hypothyroidism
- Adrenal insufficiency (the degree of pituitary damage and resultant loss is highly variable; as a result, the reduction of adrenal and thyroid hormone production seen is also variable, from slight to virtually complete loss)
- Postpartum failure of lactation and loss of pubic and axillary hair (lactation following delivery virtually precludes pituitary necrosis)
- Uterine superinvolution

DIAGNOSTIC APPROACH

Differential Diagnosis

- Lactational amenorrhea
- Pregnancy
- Exogenous hormone use
- Metabolically active ovarian tumor
- Other causes of secondary amenorrhea

Associated Conditions: Hypothyroidism, adrenal insufficiency, and postpartum hemorrhage.

Workup and Evaluation

Laboratory: Follicle-stimulating hormone (FSH), luteinizing hormone (LH), thyroid-stimulating hormone (TSH), and adrenocorticotropin hormone (ACTH) levels are diagnostic.

Imaging: Computed tomography (CT) of the pituitary is suggestive but not diagnostic.

Special Tests: None indicated.

Diagnostic Procedures: History and laboratory evaluation.

Pathologic Findings

Necrosis of the pituitary gland.

MANAGEMENT AND THERAPY

Nonpharmacologic

General Measures: Evaluation (rapid, potentially life threatening through loss of adrenal and thyroid hormones).

Specific Measures: Hormone replacement (thyroid, adrenal, and ovarian steroids).

Diet: No specific dietary changes indicated.

Activity: No restriction.

Patient Education: Patients must be carefully instructed in the need for continuing adrenal and thyroid hormone replacement therapy.

Drug(s) of Choice

Hormone replacement (thyroid, adrenal, and ovarian steroids).

FOLLOW-UP

Patient Monitoring: Careful follow-up of thyroid and adrenal function is required.

Prevention/Avoidance: Maintenance of adequate perfusion and oxygenation when postpartum hemorrhage occurs.

Possible Complications: Failure to diagnose the loss of pituitary function can result in life-threatening adrenal insufficiency and hypothyroidism.

Expected Outcome: With timely diagnosis and hormone replacement, normal life and function may be expected.

MISCELLANEOUS

Pregnancy Considerations: Without ovulation induction and assisted reproduction, pregnancy is unlikely.

ICD-9-CM Codes: 253.2.

REFERENCES

Level III

Benvenga S, Campenni A, Ruggeri RM, Trimarchi F: Clinical review 113: hypopituitarism secondary to head trauma. J Clin Endocrinol Metab 2000;85:1353.

Cunningham FG, Gant NF, Leveno KJ, et al, eds. Williams obstetrics, 21st ed. New York, McGraw-Hill, 2001, p 638.

Grimes HG, Brooks MH: Pregnancy in Sheehan's syndrome. Report of a case and review. Obstet Gynecol Surv 1980;35:481.

Lamberts SW, de Herder WW, van der Lely AJ: Pituitary insufficiency. Lancet 1998;352:127.

Miller KK, Biller BM, Hier J, et al: Androgens and bone density in women with hypopituitarism. J Clin Endocrinol Metab 2002; 87:2770.

Roberts DM: Sheehan's syndrome. Am Fam Physician 1988;37: 223.

Schneider HJ, Aimaretti G, Kreitschmann-Andermahr I, et al: Hypopituitarism. Lancet 2007;369:1461.

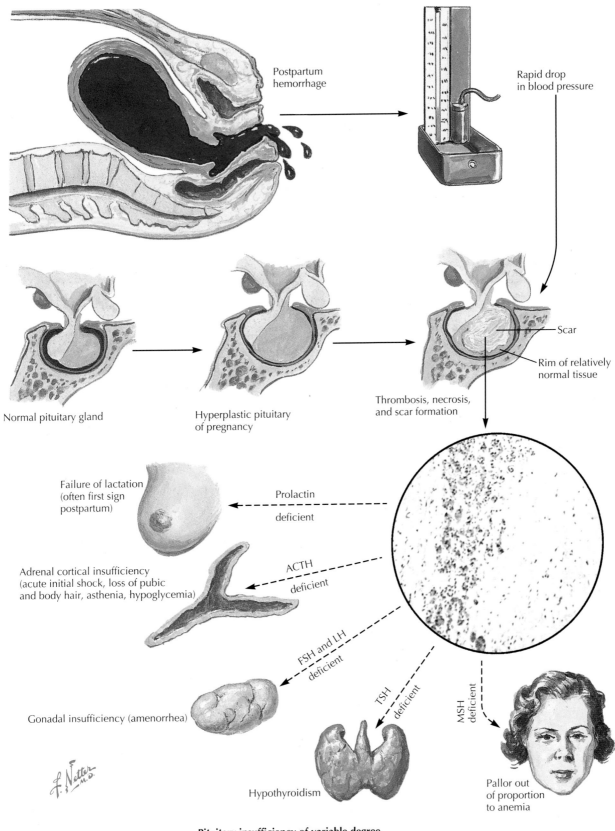

Postpartum hemorrhage

Rapid drop in blood pressure

Scar

Rim of relatively normal tissue

Normal pituitary gland

Hyperplastic pituitary of pregnancy

Thrombosis, necrosis, and scar formation

Failure of lactation (often first sign postpartum)

Prolactin deficient

Adrenal cortical insufficiency (acute initial shock, loss of pubic and body hair, asthenia, hypoglycemia)

ACTH deficient

FSH and LH deficient

Gonadal insufficiency (amenorrhea)

TSH deficient

MSH deficient

Pallor out of proportion to anemia

Hypothyroidism

Pituitary insufficiency of variable degree usually <u>without</u> diabetes insipidus

ACTH, adrenocorticotropic hormone; FSH, follicle-stimulating hormone; LH, luteinizing hormone; MSH, melanocyte-stimulating hormone; TSH, thyroid-stimulating hormone.

INTRODUCTION

Description: Caused by the absence of one X chromosome, Turner's syndrome is a collection of stigmata that includes edema of the hands and feet, webbing of the neck, short stature, left-sided heart or aortic anomalies, and gonadal dysgenesis resulting in primary amenorrhea and infertility. These patients have normal mental abilities but may have difficulty with mathematics, visual–motor coordination, and spatial–temporal processing.

Prevalence: One of 2700 female births.

Predominant Age: Present at birth, may not be detected until puberty is delayed.

Genetics: Sporadic, loss of one X chromosome (45,XO, 60% of cases, others partial losses: amenorrhea with long-arm loss; short stature with short-arm loss). Of conceptuses with only one X chromosome, 98% spontaneously abort in early pregnancy.

ETIOLOGY AND PATHOGENESIS

Causes: Monosomy for the X chromosome.

Risk Factors: Translocations involving the X chromosome (rare).

CLINICAL CHARACTERISTICS

Signs and Symptoms

- Short stature (<150 cm) (98%)
- Gonadal dysgenesis, amenorrhea (95%)
- Short neck; high palate; low hairline; and wide-spaced, hypoplastic nipples (80%)
- Broad (shield) chest, nail hypoplasia (75%)
- Lymphedema, cubitus valgus, prominent anomalous ears, multiple nevi, hearing impairment (70%)
- Webbing of the neck, short fourth metacarpal (65%)
- Renal and cardiac anomalies

DIAGNOSTIC APPROACH

Differential Diagnosis

- Pure gonadal dysgenesis
- Polycystic ovary disease
- Noonan's syndrome
- Hypothyroidism
- Familial short stature
- Growth hormone deficiency or glucocorticoid excess
- Hereditary congenital lymphedema
- Pseudohypoparathyroid

Associated Conditions: Renal and cardiac anomalies, amenorrhea, infertility, short stature, hearing difficulties, Hashimoto's thyroiditis, hypothyroidism (10%), alopecia, vitiligo, and autoimmune disorders. Gonadoblastomas or virilization may occur if the individual is mosaic for 45 X/46 XY.

Workup and Evaluation

Laboratory: Follicle-stimulating (FSH) and luteinizing hormone (LH) levels are high but do not need to be tested to establish the siagnosis (nonspecific).

Imaging: Renal and cardiac ultrasound studies to evaluate the possibility of anomalies. In some studies, up to 87% of Turner's syndrome cases have been detected by measurements of nuchal translucency.

Special Tests: Karyotype (40% of those thought to have Turner's syndrome have a mosaic karyotype or have an abnormal X or Y chromosome), electrocardiogram, blood pressure in each arm or arm and leg (to screen for coarctation of the aorta).

Diagnostic Procedures: Karyotyping, physical examination.

Pathologic Findings

A 45,X karyotype, gonadal dysgenesis (with rudimentary streak gonads), horseshoe kidney or double collecting system (60%), bicuspid aortic valve, coarctation of the aorta, aortic valvular stenosis, and bone dysplasia.

MANAGEMENT AND THERAPY

Nonpharmacologic

General Measures: Evaluation, screening for associated defects, counseling about stature and fertility issues.

Specific Measures: Hormone replacement therapy, growth hormone therapy if diagnosis is established before age 10. Removal of the gonadal tissue in individuals with X/XY mosaic.

Diet: No specific dietary changes indicated. (There is a tendency for obesity.)

Activity: No restriction (based on cardiac and renal status).

Patient Education: Extensive counseling about stature, sexual maturation, and fertility.

Drug(s) of Choice

Adolescents are much more sensitive to the effects of estrogen than are postmenopausal women, allowing doses in the range of 0.3 mg of conjugated estrogen, 0.5 mg of estradiol, or their equivalent daily. After 6 to 12 months of therapy at this level, the dose should be doubled and a progestin (e.g., medroxyprogesterone acetate, 10 mg for the first 12 days of the month) should be added, or the patient's therapy should be switched to combination oral contraceptives. This generally results in regular menstruation, and normal pubertal development proceeds on its own when the patient reaches a bone age of 13. Growth hormone (0.05 mg/kg SC daily) may be effective if given before age 10.

Contraindications: Undiagnosed amenorrhea.

FOLLOW-UP

Patient Monitoring: Screening for cardiac and renal anomalies, periodic hearing and thyroid testing (annual), monitor of growth. Screening of serum lipids and glucose and pelvic examinations to detect gonadal neoplasia should be performed annually.

Prevention/Avoidance: Prenatal chromosomal analysis for those known to carry translocations (detection only,

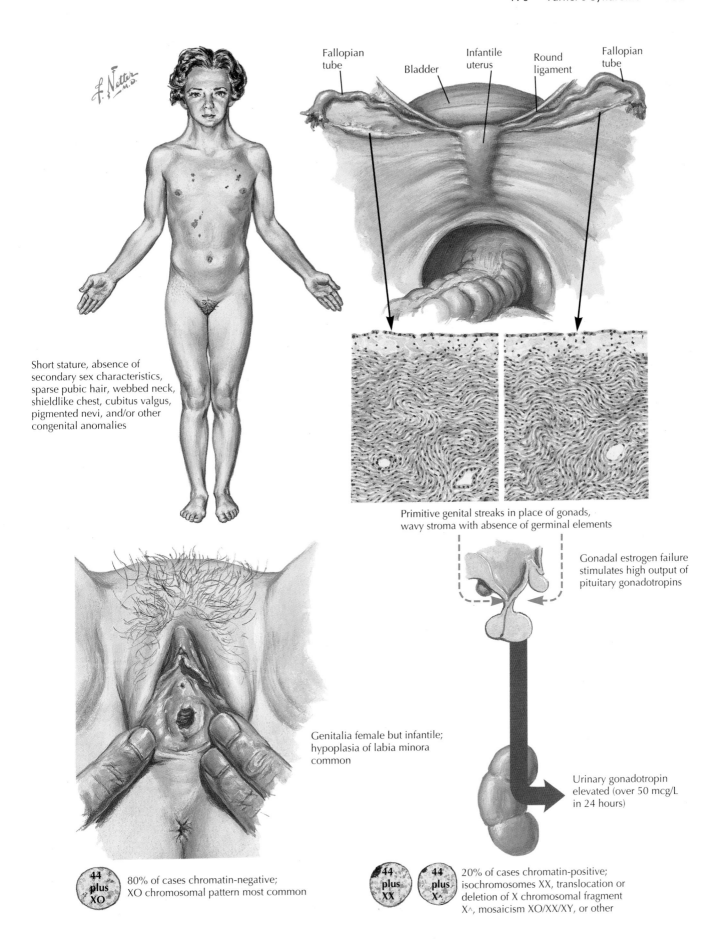

Fallopian tube

Bladder

Infantile uterus

Round ligament

Fallopian tube

Short stature, absence of secondary sex characteristics, sparse pubic hair, webbed neck, shieldlike chest, cubitus valgus, pigmented nevi, and/or other congenital anomalies

Primitive genital streaks in place of gonads, wavy stroma with absence of germinal elements

Gonadal estrogen failure stimulates high output of pituitary gonadotropins

Genitalia female but infantile; hypoplasia of labia minora common

Urinary gonadotropin elevated (over 50 mcg/L in 24 hours)

44 plus XO

80% of cases chromatin-negative; XO chromosomal pattern most common

44 plus XX

44 plus X^

20% of cases chromatin-positive; isochromosomes XX, translocation or deletion of X chromosomal fragment X^, mosaicism XO/XX/XY, or other

not prevention, although the couple may choose not to continue the pregnancy based on the findings).

Possible Complications: Renal or cardiac complications. New-onset breast growth or sexual hair growth should suggest the development of a gonadal tumor.

Expected Outcome: Reasonably normal life with the exception of infertility.

MISCELLANEOUS

Pregnancy Considerations: These patients are infertile. Individuals with a mosaic karyotype may be fertile but pregnancy is associated with a 50% chance of aneuploidy.

ICD-9-CM Codes: 758.6.

REFERENCES

Level I

Blum WF, Crowe BJ, Quigley CA, et al; SHOX Study Group: Growth hormone is effective in treatment of short stature associated with short stature homeobox-containing gene deficiency: two-year results of a randomized, controlled, multicenter trial. J Clin Endocrinol Metab 2007;92:219. Epub 2006 Oct 17.

Sas TC, de Muinck Keizer-Schrama SM, Stijnen T, et al: Normalization of height in girls with Turner syndrome after long-term growth hormone treatment: results of a randomized dose-response trial. J Clin Endocrinol Metab 1999;84:4607.

Level II

Gravholt CH, Fedder J, Naeraa RW, Muller J: Occurrence of gonadoblastoma in females with Turner syndrome and Y chromosome material: a population study. J Clin Endocrinol Metab 2000;85:3199.

Nicolaides KH: Nuchal translucency and other first-trimester sonographic markers of chromosomal abnormalities. Am J Obstet Gynecol 2004;191:45.

Ogata T, Muroya K, Matsuo N, et al: Turner syndrome and Xp deletions: clinical and molecular studies in 47 patients. J Clin Endocrinol Metab 2001;86:5498.

Piippo S, Lenko H, Kainulainen P, Sipila I: Use of percutaneous estrogen gel for induction of puberty in girls with Turner syndrome. J Clin Endocrinol Metab 2004;89:3241.

Sagi L, Zuckerman-Levin N, Gawlik A, et al: Clinical significance of the parental origin of the X chromosome in turner syndrome. J Clin Endocrinol Metab 2007;92:846. Epub 2006 Dec 27.

Level III

American College of Obstetricians and Gynecologists: Screening for fetal chromosomal abnormalities. ACOG Practice Bulletin 77. Obstet Gynecol 2007;109:217.

Bondy CA; Turner Syndrome Study Group: Care of girls and women with Turner syndrome: a guideline of the Turner Syndrome Study Group. J Clin Endocrinol Metab 2007;92:10. Epub 2006 Oct 17.

Chu CE, Connor JM: Molecular biology of Turner's syndrome. Arch Dis Child 1995;72:285.

Donaldson MD, Gault EJ, Tan KW, Dunger DB: Optimising management in Turner syndrome: from infancy to adult transfer. Arch Dis Child 2006;91:513.

Doswell BH, Visootsak J, Brady AN, Graham JM Jr: Turner syndrome: an update and review for the primary pediatrician. Clin Pediatr 2006;45:301. Review.

Hall JG, Gilchrist DM: Turner syndrome and its variants. Pediatr Clin North Am 1990;37:1421.

Linden MG, Bender BG, Robinson A: Intrauterine diagnosis of sex chromosome aneuploidy. Obstet Gynecol 1996;87:468.

Ranke MB, Saenger P: Turner's syndrome. Lancet 2001;358:309.

Saenger P: Growth-promoting strategies in Turner's syndrome. J Clin Endocrinol Metab 1999;84:4345.

Sybert VP, McCauley E: Turner's syndrome. N Engl J Med 2004;351:1227.

INTRODUCTION

Description: Uterine agenesis is failure of the Müllerian system to fuse in the midline to form the uterus. Incomplete variations of this failure result in a didelphic, bicornuate, septate, or arcuate uterus. It is also known as Mayer-Rokitansky-Küster-Hauser syndrome.

Prevalence: One of 4000 to 5000 female births. Second most common (15%) cause of primary amenorrhea.

Predominant Age: Congenital.

Genetics: Isolated developmental defect except for androgen insensitivity syndrome.

ETIOLOGY AND PATHOGENESIS

Causes: Isolated developmental defect in most patients, production of anti-Müllerian hormone by Sertoli's cells in fetal testes (in androgen resistance syndrome). 17α-Hydroxylase deficiency, 17, 20-desmolase deficiency, and agonadism may account for those rare individuals with no breast or uterine development and a male karyotype (vanishing testes syndrome).

Risk Factors: None known.

CLINICAL CHARACTERISTICS

Signs and Symptoms

- Primary amenorrhea (accounts for 15% of primary amenorrhea)
- Shortened or absent vagina
- Breast development may be absent in some syndromes; most often present and normal

DIAGNOSTIC APPROACH

Differential Diagnosis

- Androgen resistance (testicular feminization)—may be ruled out by the presence of normal pubic hair
- Vaginal agenesis
- Imperforate hymen
- Primary amenorrhea

Associated Conditions: Primary amenorrhea, infertility, urinary tract abnormalities (25% to 40%), skeletal abnormalities (12%), congenital rectovaginal fistula, imperforate anus, and hypospadias.

Workup and Evaluation

Laboratory: Serum follicle-stimulating hormone (FSH; to differentiate hypogonadal hypogonadism and gonadal dysgenesis).

Imaging: No imaging indicated. Ultrasonography may be used to assist the diagnosis but is generally not indicated. Intravenous pyelography should be considered.

Special Tests: Measurement of height, weight, and arm span. (A karyotype or buccal smear may be performed but is generally not necessary.)

Diagnostic Procedures: History, physical examination, imaging procedures.

Pathologic Findings

One or both fallopian tubes and some fibrous tissue may be present in the normal location of the uterus. Normal ovaries, with normal cyclic ovarian function, are usually present.

MANAGEMENT AND THERAPY

Nonpharmacologic

General Measures: Evaluation and education.

Specific Measures: Patients may require surgical removal of abnormal gonads (after puberty: age 18) because of an increased risk of malignancy. Fertility may be achieved through in vitro fertilization with implantation into a host uterus.

Diet: No specific dietary changes indicated.

Activity: No restriction.

Patient Education: Frank discussion about the syndrome and its effects (infertility and amenorrhea).

Drug(s) of Choice

None.

FOLLOW-UP

Patient Monitoring: Normal health maintenance.

Prevention/Avoidance: None.

Possible Complications: Renal, skeletal, and cardiac abnormalities are more common in these patients.

Expected Outcome: Normal life expectancy without reproductive capability. (Fertility may be achieved through in vitro fertilization with implantation into a host uterus.)

MISCELLANEOUS

Pregnancy Considerations: Normal pregnancy is not possible.

ICD-9-CM Codes: 752.3.

REFERENCES

Level III

Dwyer PL, Rosamilia A: Congenital urogenital anomalies that are associated with the persistence of Gartner's duct: a review. Am J Obstet Gynecol 2006;195:354. Epub 2006 Apr 21.

Fisher K, Esham RH, Thorneycroft I: Scoliosis associated with typical Mayer-Rokitansky-Küster-Hauser syndrome. South Med J 2000;93:243.

Golditch IM: Vaginal aplasia. Surg Gynecol Obstet 1969;129:361.

Griffin JE, Edwards C, Madden JD, et al: Congenital absence of the vagina. The Mayer-Rokitansky-Kuster-Hauser syndrome. Ann Intern Med 1976;85:224.

Jayasinghe Y, Rane A, Stalewski H, Grover S: The presentation and early diagnosis of the rudimentary uterine horn. Obstet Gynecol 2005;105:1456.

Lobo RA: Primary and secondary amenorrhea and precocious puberty. In Katz VL, Lentz GM, Lobo RA, Gershenson DM: Comprehensive Gynecology, 5th ed. Philadelphia, Mosby/Elsevier, 2007, p 940.

Troiano RN, McCarthy SM: Mullerian duct anomalies: imaging and clinical issues. Radiology 2004;233:19. Epub 2004 Aug 18.

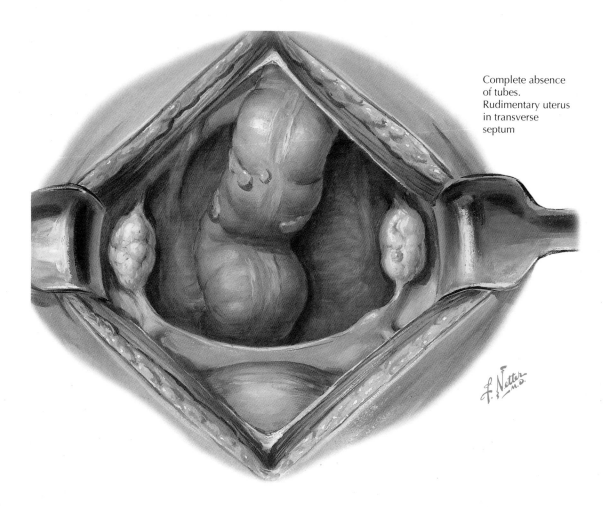

Complete absence
of tubes.
Rudimentary uterus
in transverse
septum

INTRODUCTION

Description: Vaginal agenesis is congenital absence of the vagina, most often associated with an absence of the uterus (Mayer-Rokitansky-Küster-Hauser syndrome).

Prevalence: Reported to vary from 1 of 4000 to 1 of 10,500 female births.

Predominant Age: Generally not diagnosed until puberty, often following a delay of 2 to 3 years or more.

Genetics: No genetic pattern (accident of development), although in some inbred communities there is a suggestion that an autosomal recessive gene is present.

ETIOLOGY AND PATHOGENESIS

Causes: Failure of the endoderm of the urogenital sinus and the epithelium of the vaginal vestibule to fuse and perforate during embryonic development. This process is normally completed by the 21st week of gestation. Patients with a congenital absence of the vagina but with a uterus present represent an extreme form of transverse vaginal septum.

Risk Factors: None known.

CLINICAL CHARACTERISTICS

Signs and Symptoms

- Vaginal obstruction (absence)
- Primary amenorrhea
- Cyclic abdominal pain
- Hematometra (if uterus is present)

DIAGNOSTIC APPROACH

Differential Diagnosis

- Imperforate hymen
- Hermaphroditism
- Androgen insensitivity syndrome (testicular feminization)
- Mayer-Rokitansky-Küster-Hauser syndrome (75% have vaginal agenesis, 25% have shortened vaginal pouch)
- Transverse vaginal septum

Associated Conditions: Endometriosis, infertility, chronic pelvic pain, sexual dysfunction, hematometra (when uterus is present), urologic abnormalities (25% to 40%), and skeletal abnormalities (10% to 15%).

Workup and Evaluation

Laboratory: No evaluation indicated.

Imaging: Ultrasonography, magnetic resonance imaging (MRI), or computed tomography (CT) to determine the presence and status of the upper genital tract structures. Intravenous pyelography should be considered.

Special Tests: Karyotyping or buccal smear should be considered. Laparoscopy may be desirable in some patients to confirm the diagnosis, although this is generally not necessary.

Diagnostic Procedures: History and physical examination (including rectal examination).

Pathologic Findings

The ovaries are usually normal and the fallopian tubes are present.

MANAGEMENT AND THERAPY

Nonpharmacologic

General Measures: Evaluation and reassurance.

Specific Measures: Surgical creation of a vagina if intercourse is desired. May be created by a flap procedure (McIndoe procedure) or progressive perineal pressure techniques (Ingram dilators or bicycle seat). Patients with androgen insensitivity should have their gonads (testes) removed to prevent seminoma; patients with Mayer-Rokitansky-Küster-Hauser syndrome have normal ovaries and should not have them removed.

Diet: No specific dietary changes indicated.

Activity: No restriction.

Drug(s) of Choice

None.

FOLLOW-UP

Patient Monitoring: Normal health maintenance. Patients in whom a neovagina is created must be monitored for narrowing.

Prevention/Avoidance: None.

Possible Complications: Hematocolpos, endometriosis, sexual dysfunction. If a neovagina is created, it will scar and stenose if it is not used frequently or maintained with the use of a dilator.

Expected Outcome: Sexual function can generally be restored through the creation of a neovagina. The presence of a uterus is associated with cyclic pain and often must be removed. Except as an egg donor, fertility is unlikely to be restored.

MISCELLANEOUS

Pregnancy Considerations: Generally not a consideration. Patients may be able to achieve reproduction as egg donors.

ICD-9-CM Codes: 752.49.

REFERENCES

Level II

Ingram JM: The bicycle seat stool in the treatment of vaginal agenesis and stenosis: a preliminary report. Am J Obstet Gynecol 1981;140:867.

Woodhouse CR: The sexual and reproductive consequences of congenital genitourinary anomalies. J Urol 1994;152:645.

Level III

American College of Obstetricians and Gynecologists: Vaginal agenesis: diagnosis, management, and routine care. ACOG Committee Opinion 355. Obstet Gynecol 2006;108:1605.

Dwyer PL, Rosamilia A: Congenital urogenital anomalies that are associated with the persistence of Gartner's duct: a review. Am J Obstet Gynecol 2006;195:354. Epub 2006 Apr 21.

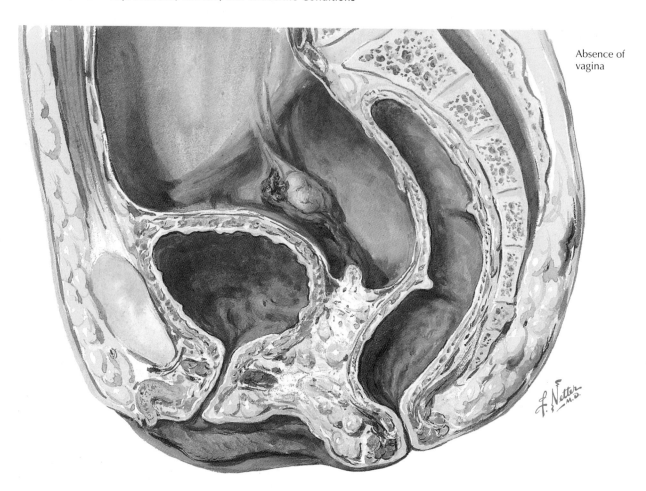

Absence of vagina

Giacalone PL, Laffargue F, Faure JM, Deschamps F: Ultrasound-assisted laparoscopic creation of a neovagina by modification of Vecchietti's operation. Obstet Gynecol 1999;93:446.

Golditch IM: Vaginal aplasia. Surg Gynecol Obstet 1969;129:361.

Griffin JE, Edwards C, Madden JD, et al: Congenital absence of the vagina. The Mayer-Rokitansky-Küster-Hauser syndrome. Ann Intern Med 1976;85:224.

Hensle TW, Chang DT: Vaginal reconstruction. Urol Clin North Am 1999;26:39, vii.

Katz VL, Lentz GM: Congenital abnormalities of the female reproductive tract. In Katz VL, Lentz GM, Lobo RA, Gershenson DM: Comprehensive Gynecology, 5th ed. Philadelphia, Mosby/Elsevier, 2007, p 247.

Lindenman E, Shepard MK, Pescovitz OH: Müllerian agenesis: an update. Obstet Gynecol 1997;90:307.

Tolhurst DE, van der Helm TW: The treatment of vaginal atresia. Surg Gynecol Obstet 1991;172:407.

INTRODUCTION

Description: Virilization refers to the loss of female sexual characteristics such as body contour and the acquisition of masculine qualities such as increased muscle mass, temporal balding, deepening of the voice, and clitoromegaly.

Prevalence: Uncommon.

Predominant Age: Reproductive.

Genetics: No genetic pattern.

ETIOLOGY AND PATHOGENESIS

Causes: Idiopathic ovarian (polycystic ovary syndrome, hilus cell hyperplasia/tumor, arrhenoblastoma, adrenal rest), adrenal (congenital adrenal hyperplasia [10% to 15% of women with hirsutism], Cushing disease, virilizing carcinoma or adenoma), drugs (minoxidil, androgens including danazol [Danocrine], phenytoin, diazoxide), pregnancy (androgen excess of pregnancy, luteoma, or hyperreactio luteinalis).

Risk Factors: None known.

CLINICAL CHARACTERISTICS

Signs and Symptoms

- Amenorrhea (common but not universal)
- Temporal or frontal balding
- Deepening of the voice
- Clitoral enlargement
- Vaginal dryness
- Increased muscle mass
- Male-pattern hair growth

DIAGNOSTIC APPROACH

Differential Diagnosis

- Iatrogenic or exogenous steroid use
- Polycystic ovary syndrome
- Ovarian stromal hyperthecosis
- Ovarian tumors (Sertoli-Leydig tumors)
- Cushing's disease (truncal obesity, facial rounding, cervicodorsal fat deposition [buffalo hump], and red or purple striae are often not fully developed)
- Adrenal tumors
- Congenital adrenal hyperplasia (especially in infants and children)

Associated Conditions: Defeminization, amenorrhea, obesity, menstrual irregularity, amenorrhea, infertility, acne, oily skin, increased libido, and alopecia.

Workup and Evaluation

Laboratory: Prolactin, follicle-stimulating hormone (FSH), thyroid screening. Patients suspected of having adrenal sources of hyperandrogenicity may be screened by measuring 24-hour urinary-free cortisol, by performing adrenocorticotropin hormone (ACTH) stimulation tests, or by performing an overnight dexamethasone suppression test. Dehydroepiandrosterone sulfate (DHEA-s) and testosterone should be measured. The circulating testosterone level is generally ≥2 ng/mL.

Imaging: Despite the ability of transvaginal ultrasonography and computerized tomography (CT) to detect 90% of virilizing tumors, 5% to 10% of tumors may not be detected, necessitating surgical exploration when these are suspected.

Special Tests: Clitoral index. (The clitoral index is defined as the vertical dimension times the horizontal dimension, in millimeters. The normal range is from 9 to 35 mm, with borderline values in the range of 36 to 99 mm. Values greater than 100 mm indicate severe hyperandrogenicity and should prompt aggressive evaluation and referral.)

Diagnostic Procedures: History, physical examination, and laboratory evaluation.

Pathologic Findings

Based on underlying pathophysiologic conditions.

MANAGEMENT AND THERAPY

Nonpharmacologic

General Measures: Evaluation and support, shaving, depilatories, or electrolysis. Topical treatment of acne (if present).

Specific Measures: Patients with polycystic ovary syndrome often do well with oral contraceptive suppression of ovarian function or with the use of spironolactone. Patients with hyperandrogenicity of adrenal origin respond well to cortisol administration, which results in a reduction of the production of androgenic precursors. Tumors require surgical removal.

Diet: No specific dietary changes indicated.

Activity: No restriction.

Drug(s) of Choice

Polycystic ovary syndrome—combination oral contraceptives, spironolactone (100 to 200 mg PO daily), medroxyprogesterone acetate (Depo-Provera 150 to 300 mg IM every 3 months).

Hyperandrogenicity of adrenal origin—cortisol administration.

Contraindications: Pregnancy. (Spironolactone is teratogenic; patients using it and able to become pregnant must use reliable contraception.)

FOLLOW-UP

Patient Monitoring: Normal health maintenance once diagnosis and management have been implemented. There is an increased risk of diabetes in patients with polycystic ovaries.

Prevention/Avoidance: None.

Possible Complications: Permanent loss of feminine attributes and induction of hirsutism, lowering of voice, and others. Chronic anovulation is associated with increased risk of endometrial hyperplasia and cancer.

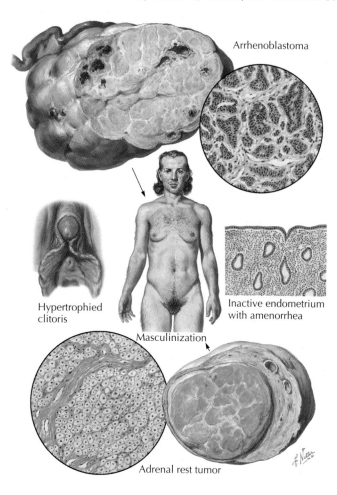

Arrhenoblastoma

Hypertrophied clitoris

Masculinization

Inactive endometrium with amenorrhea

Adrenal rest tumor

Expected Outcome: Good, with appropriate diagnosis and treatment.

MISCELLANEOUS

Pregnancy Considerations: No effect on pregnancy, although some metabolic causes of virilization of the mother may result in reduced fertility or virilization of a fetus.

ICD-9-CM Codes: 255.2 (others based on diagnosis).

REFERENCES

Level I
Azziz R, Ochoa TM, Bradley EL Jr, et al: Leuprolide and estrogen versus oral contraceptive pills for the treatment of hirsutism: a prospective randomized study. J Clin Endocrinol Metab 1995;80:3406.

Moghetti P, Tosi F, Tosti A, et al: Comparison of spironolactone, flutamide, and finasteride efficacy in the treatment of hirsutism: a randomized, double blind, placebo-controlled trial. J Clin Endocrinol Metab 2000;85:89.

Level II
Coonrod DV, Rizkallah TH: Virilizing adrenal carcinoma in a woman of reproductive age: a case presentation and literature review. Am J Obstet Gynecol 1995;172:1912.

Guido M, Romualdi D, Giuliani M, et al: Drospirenone for the treatment of hirsute women with polycystic ovary syndrome: a clinical, endocrinological, metabolic pilot study. J Clin Endocrinol Metab 2004;89:2817.

Ibanez L, Potau N, Marcos MV, de Zegher F: Treatment of hirsutism, hyperandrogenism, oligomenorrhea, dyslipidemia, and hyperinsulinism in nonobese, adolescent girls: effect of flutamide. J Clin Endocrinol Metab 2000;85:3251.

Level III
American College of Obstetricians and Gynecologists: Polycystic ovary syndrome. ACOG Practice Bulletin 41. Obstet Gynecol 2002;100:1389.

Azziz R: The evaluation and management of hirsutism. Obstet Gynecol 2003;101:995.

Bailey-Pridham DD, Sanfilippo JS: Hirsutism in the adolescent female. Pediatr Clin North Am 1989;36:581.

Bergfeld WF: Hirsutism in women. Effective therapy that is safe for long-term use. Postgrad Med 2000;107:93, 99.

Chang RJ: A practical approach to the diagnosis of polycystic ovary syndrome. Am J Obstet Gynecol 2004;191:713.

Conn JJ, Jacobs HS: Managing hirsutism in gynaecological practice. Br J Obstet Gynaecol 1998;105:687.

Curran DR, Moore C, Huber T: Clinical inquiries. What is the best approach to the evaluation of hirsutism? J Fam Pract 2005;54:465.

Ehrmann DA: Polycystic ovary syndrome. N Engl J Med 2005;352:1223.

Ehrmann DA, Rosenfield RL: Clinical review 10: an endocrinologic approach to the patient with hirsutism. J Clin Endocrinol Metab 1990;71:1.

Ginsburg J, White MC: Hirsutism and virilisation. Br Med J 1980;280:369.

Gordon CM: Menstrual disorders in adolescents. Excess androgens and the polycystic ovary syndrome. Pediatr Clin North Am 1999;46:519.

Harborne L, Fleming R, Lyall H, et al: Metformin or antiandrogen in the treatment of hirsutism in polycystic ovary syndrome. J Clin Endocrinol Metab 2003;88:4116.

Karp L, Herrmann WL: Diagnosis and treatment of hirsutism in women. Obstet Gynecol 1973;41:283.

Lobo RA: Hyperandrogenism. In Katz VL, Lentz GM, Lobo RA, Gershenson DM: Comprehensive Gynecology, 5th ed. Philadelphia, Mosby/Elsevier, 2007, p 979.

Marshburn PB, Carr BR: Hirsutism and virilization. A systematic approach to benign and potentially serious causes. Postgrad Med 1995;97:99, 105.

Rosenfield RL: Clinical practice. Hirsutism. N Engl J Med 2005;353:2578.

Tagatz GE, Kopher RA, Nagel TC, Okagaki T: The clitoral index: a bioassay of androgenic stimulation. Obstet Gynecol 1979;54:562.

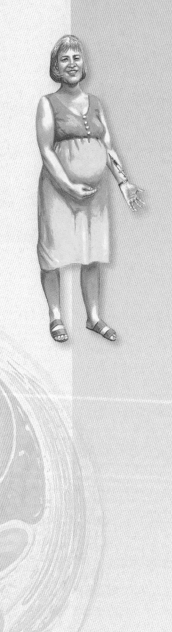

PART 2

OBSTETRICS

SECTION X
Obstetrics: General Considerations

SECTION XI
Obstetric Conditions and Concerns

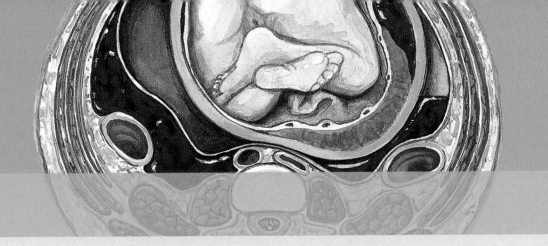

Obstetrics: General Considerations

THE CHALLENGE

In many ways, prenatal care is the prototypical example of preventive medicine. Preconceptional care is directed toward ensuring the optimal health of the prospective mother and doing those things that will remove preventable impediments to a healthy outcome for the pregnancy. The care these women receive during this and the prenatal phase of their lives is critical to both their health and the success of the pregnancy.

Scope of the Problem: In the United States, roughly 4.1 million women give birth each year, and >90% of American women will bear children during their lifetime. Twenty percent or more of women have one or more risk factors that could adversely affect a pregnancy if not addressed. Therefore, women who receive delayed (after 12 weeks of pregnancy) or no prenatal care are at risk for having undetected or preventable complications of pregnancy that can result in significant maternal or fetal morbidity or mortality.

Objectives of Management: To protect the health and well-being of mother, fetus, and neonate through screening and optimizing a woman's health and knowledge before conceiving a pregnancy.

TACTICS

Relevant Pathophysiology: The initiation of folic acid supplementation at least 1 month before pregnancy has been shown to reduce the incidence of neural tube defects such as spina bifida and anencephaly. (Because organogenesis begins early in pregnancy, starting folic acid supplementation after neural tube closure [28 days after conception] has no demonstrated benefit in reducing neural tube defects.) Similarly, adequate glucose control in a woman with diabetes before conception and throughout pregnancy decreases maternal morbidity, spontaneous abortion, fetal malformation, fetal macrosomia, intrauterine fetal death, and neonatal morbidity. Reducing the risk of infectious diseases that can have adverse effects on the mother or fetus if contracted during pregnancy, through vaccination (e.g., rubella) or avoidance (e.g., toxoplasmosis), is a proven preventive strategy.

Strategies: Ideally, obstetric care should commence before pregnancy with a preconception visit, during which a thorough family and medical history for both parents is taken and a physical examination of the prospective mother is performed. Both before and between pregnancies, pre-existing conditions that may affect conception, pregnancy, or both should be identified, and appropriate management plans should be formulated with the goal of a "healthy" subsequent pregnancy. Unfortunately, nearly half of all pregnancies in the United States are unintended, making the challenge of preconception care more difficult. As a result, effective preconceptional care must address pregnancy planning for women who seek care in anticipation of a planned pregnancy and, just as importantly, for all women with childbearing potential.

General evaluations are directed toward establishing optimal maternal health, providing nutritional counseling, and instituting appropriate prophylaxis. This generally takes the form of genetic screening or the detection of maternal diseases that will alter or be altered by the future pregnancy. Based on age, ethnic origin, race, or family history, couples may be identified who are at increased risk of chromosomal or enzymatic abnormalities, such as sickle cell trait, thalassemia, or Tay-Sachs disease carrier state. A family history that is positive for certain diseases, such as cystic fibrosis and congenital hearing loss, indicates the need for additional screening.

The evaluation should focus on many aspects of the woman's life that can adversely influence the outcome of the pregnancy: undiagnosed, untreated, or poorly controlled medical conditions; immunization history; medication use; occupational and environmental exposures; nutritional issues; tobacco and substance use; and any other high-risk behaviors. Social and mental health issues that may affect the woman's ability to access and participate in prenatal care should also be addressed.

Before pregnancy is the optimal time for immunizing against hepatitis B, rubella, and varicella; screening for human immunodeficiency virus and syphilis infections; and, if found, beginning treatment to prevent the transmission of disease to the fetus. The patient should be counseled on ways to prevent infection with toxoplasmosis, cytomegalovirus, and parvovirus. Anemia, hypothyroidism, urinary tract infections, and other conditions may be identified; nutritional counseling and weight reduction may be effected before pregnancy; and admonitions about the risks of using medications, drugs, alcohol, and tobacco and avoidance of chemicals such as solvents and pesticides during early pregnancy may be given.

Patients considering pregnancy in the immediate future should be prescribed prenatal vitamins, folic acid supplements, or both. (Prenatal vitamins should include at least 400 μg of folic acid and 30 mg of elemental iron for patients at average risk. The dosage of folic acid should be increased to 1 mg per day for women with diabetes mellitus, epilepsy, or hemoglobinopathies; patients who have given birth to a child with neural tube defects should take 4 mg of folic acid per day for subsequent pregnancies. Higher levels of supplementation should not be achieved by taking excess multivitamins because of the risk of vitamin A toxicity.)

Patient Education: American College of Obstetricians and Gynecologists Patient Education Booklet AP056 (Good Health Before Pregnancy: Preconceptional Care), AB012 (Planning Your Pregnancy), AP001 (Nutrition During Pregnancy), AP0103 (Having a Baby [Especially for Teens]), AB005 (You and Your Baby: Prenatal Care, Labor and Delivery, and Postpartum Care), AP060 (Later Childbearing), AP104 (Drugs and Pregnancy), AP032 (Especially for Fathers).

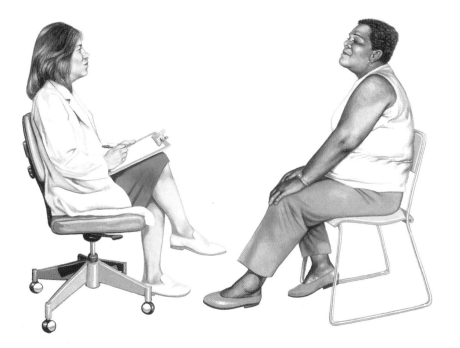

Preconception Visit

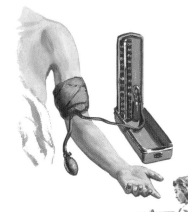

Preconception Nutrition and Health

Prenatal vitamins should include at least 400 µg of folic acid and 30 mg of elemental iron for patients at average risk

Obstetric care should commence before pregnancy with preconception visit, during which a thorough family and medical history for both parents and a physical examination, including blood pressure and weight of the prospective mother, is done.

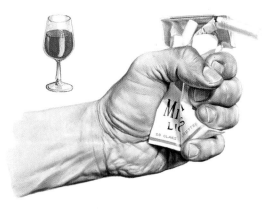

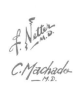

Risks of using medications, drugs, alcohol, tobacco, and chemicals should be provided to patient.

Preconception Tests

·Hepatitis B

·Rubella, varicella

·Human immunodeficiency virus (HIV)

·Syphilis

·Family history may indicate need for additional tests

Nutritional information, including recommendations on weight reduction, should be discussed.

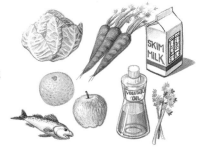

IMPLEMENTATION

Special Considerations: If the patient has significant medical problems, the impact of pregnancy on these problems, and the implications for the pregnancy, may be determined and, where possible, the risks may be reduced before conception. Medications for hypertension, epilepsy, thromboembolism, depression, and anxiety should be reviewed and changed, if necessary, before the patient becomes pregnant.

REFERENCES

Level II

Jack BW, Campanile C, McQuade W, Kogan MD: The negative pregnancy test. An opportunity for preconception care. Arch Fam Med 1995;4:340.

Milunsky A, Jick H, Jick SS, et al: Multivitamin/folic acid supplementation in early pregnancy reduces the prevalence of neural tube defects. JAMA 1989;262:2847.

Level III

American Academy of Pediatrics, American College of Obstetricians and Gynecologists: Guidelines for perinatal care, 5th ed. Elk Grove Village, IL,: AAP, Washington, DC, ACOG, 2002.

American College of Obstetricians and Gynecologists: Perinatal viral and parasitic infections. ACOG Practice Bulletin 20. Washington, DC, ACOG, 2000.

American College of Obstetricians and Gynecologists: Access to women's health care. ACOG Statement of Policy. Washington, DC, ACOG, 2003.

American College of Obstetricians and Gynecologists: Neural tube defects. ACOG Practice Bulletin 44. Obstet Gynecol 2003; 102:203.

American College of Obstetricians and Gynecologists: Prenatal and perinatal human immunodeficiency virus testing: expanded recommendations. ACOG Committee Opinion 304. Obstet Gynecol 2004;104:1119.

American College of Obstetricians and Gynecologists: Pregestational diabetes mellitus. ACOG Practice Bulletin 60. Obstet Gynecol 2005;105:675.

American College of Obstetricians and Gynecologists: The importance of preconception care in the continuum of women's health care. ACOG Committee Opinion 313. Obstet Gynecol 2005; 106:665.

American College of Obstetricians and Gynecologists: Update on carrier screening for cystic fibrosis. ACOG Committee Opinion 325. Obstet Gynecol 2005;106:1465.

American College of Obstetricians and Gynecologists, American College of Medical Genetics: Preconception and prenatal carrier screening for cystic fibrosis. Clinical and laboratory guidelines. Washington, DC, ACOG, 2001.

American Diabetes Association: Preconception care of women with diabetes. Clinical Diabetes 2000;18:124.

Botto LD, Moore CA, Khoury MJ, Erickson JD: Neural-tube defects. N Engl J Med 1999;341:1509.

Centers for Disease Control and Prevention: Entry into prenatal care—United States, 1989–1997. JAMA 2000;283:2924.

Czeizel AE, Dudas I: Prevention of the first occurrence of neural-tube defects by periconceptional vitamin supplementation. N Engl J Med 1992;327:1832.

Henshaw SK: Unintended pregnancy in the United States. Fam Plann Perspect 1998;30:24, 46.

Institute of Medicine: Preventing low birthweight. Washington, DC, Institute of Medicine, National Academy Press, 1985.

Iqbal MM: Prevention of neural tube defects by periconceptional use of folic acid. Pediatr Rev 2000;21:58.

Johnson K, Posner SF, Biermann J, et al: Recommendations to improve preconception health and health care—United States. MMWR Recomm Rep 2006;55:1.

Leuzzi RA, Scoles KS: Preconception counseling for the primary care physician. Med Clin North Am 1996;80:337.

Lu MC, Kotelchuck M, Culhane JF, et al: Preconception care between pregnancies: the content of internatal care. Matern Child Health J 2006;10:107.

Mustard CA, Roos NP: The relationship of prenatal care and pregnancy complications to birthweight in Winnipeg, Canada. Am J Public Health 1994;84:1450.

Prevention of neural tube defects: results of the Medical Research Council Vitamin Study. MRC Vitamin Study Research Group. Lancet 1991;338:131.

THE CHALLENGE

Despite the dramatic and vulnerable changes that the conceptus undergoes in the first 14 weeks of gestation, many patients are unaware of their pregnancy or delay seeking prenatal care. Emerging evidence suggests that it is during this period the foundations of a successful pregnancy and even the future health of the adult individual are set. Although most pregnant women would deliver healthy infants without any prenatal care, obstetric care is designed to promote optimal health throughout the course of normal pregnancy while screening for and managing any complications that may develop.

Scope of the Problem: Roughly one fourth of pregnant women do not receive care during the first trimester.

Objectives of Management: To protect the health and well-being of mother and fetus.

TACTICS

Relevant Pathophysiology: During the first trimester of gestation, the developing embryo implants in the endometrium (except in the case of ectopic pregnancies), the placental attachment to the mother is created, and the major structures and organs of the body are formed. The developing embryo is sensitive to exposures to toxins, medications, and radiation and the effects of maternal conditions that can disrupt this process. Errors in this process may result in major disruptions in structure or function of the fetus or even the complete loss of the pregnancy.

About the 12th week of gestation, the placenta takes over hormonal support for the pregnancy from the corpus luteum. If this transition does not happen smoothly, the pregnancy can be lost.

Strategies: At the first prenatal visit, a comprehensive history should be taken, including previous pregnancy outcome(s), if any, and any medical or surgical conditions that may affect pregnancy. This should include past medical history, information pertinent to genetic screening, and any events in the course of the current pregnancy. Special attention should also be given to diet, tobacco or alcohol use, and any medications or substances used. Routine laboratory studies should be ordered, and the patient should be given instructions concerning routine prenatal care, warning signs of complications, and who to contact with questions or problems. A complete physical examination should be performed, including a Pap test and tests for sexually transmitted diseases.

It is important early in the course of pregnancy to establish an accurate gestational age and estimated date of confinement (EDC, or due date). This information is needed to manage later complications of pregnancy and to determine the timing of evaluations (e.g., neural tube screening, 1-hour glucose challenge testing, Rh prophylaxis). If needed, transvaginal and transabdominal ultrasonographic techniques allow gestational age determination with approximately 7- to 10-day accuracy when performed during the first trimester.

At each visit, the patient should be asked about any problems such as vaginal bleeding, nausea/vomiting, dysuria, or vaginal discharge. Each prenatal visit should include measurements of blood pressure and weight and an assessment for edema. (Blood pressure generally declines at the end of the first trimester, increasing again in the third trimester.) A clean-catch urine sample should be tested (most often by dipstick) for protein and signs of infection. Obstetric assessments should include uterine size by pelvic examination or fundal height measurement and documentation of the presence and rate of fetal heart tones by the use of a fetal Doppler ultrasound device. (The fetal heart may not be routinely detected by a Doppler device until 12 weeks or later.) Patients at low risk may be followed at 4-week intervals until 28 weeks of gestation.

Patient Education: American College of Obstetricians and Gynecologists Patient Education Booklet AP001 (Nutrition During Pregnancy), AB005 (You and Your Baby: Prenatal Care, Labor and Delivery, and Postpartum Care), AP032 (Especially for Fathers), AP060 (Later Childbearing), AP090 (Early Pregnancy Loss: Miscarriage and Molar Pregnancy), AP0103 (Having a Baby [Especially for Teens]), AP104 (Drugs and Pregnancy), AP119 (Exercise During Pregnancy), AP126 (Morning Sickness), AP133 (Routine Tests in Pregnancy), AP156 (How Your Baby Grows During Pregnancy), AP165 (Screening Tests for Birth Defects), CP001 (Cystic Fibrosis Carrier Testing: The Decision Is Yours).

IMPLEMENTATION

Special Considerations: Between 4% and 8% of pregnant women are victims of "battering" and will benefit from counseling or help finding shelters and other social supports. (In the United States, suicide, homicide, and trauma associated with auto accidents where seat belts

Commonly Ordered Initial Laboratory and Other Tests

- Complete blood count
- Urinalysis and urine culture and sensitivity
- Blood group, Rh, antibody screen
- Serologic test for syphilis (rapid plasma reagin [RPR], Venereal Disease Research Laboratory [VDRL])
- Human immunodeficiency virus (HIV) titer by enzyme-linked immunosorbent assay (ELISA); Western blot if HIV+ by ELISA
- Hepatitis B surface antigen
- Rubella titer
- Cervical cytology (Pap test)
- Cervical culture for *Neisseria gonorrhoeae*
- Hemoglobin electrophoresis (selected patients)
- Maternal serum screening for open neural tube defects (triple or quad screen) at 15 to 20 weeks (maternal serum alpha-fetoprotein plus other markers)

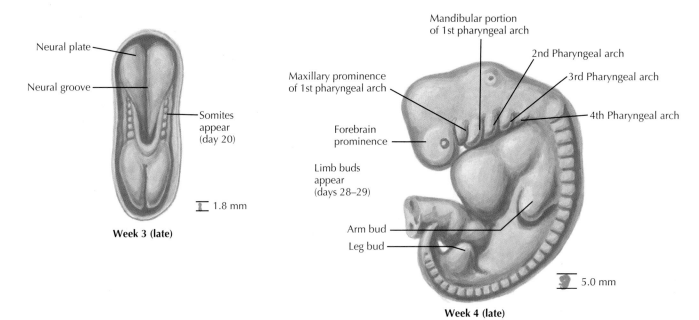

Neural plate

Neural groove

Somites appear (day 20)

1.8 mm

Week 3 (late)

Mandibular portion of 1st pharyngeal arch

2nd Pharyngeal arch

3rd Pharyngeal arch

Maxillary prominence of 1st pharyngeal arch

4th Pharyngeal arch

Forebrain prominence

Limb buds appear (days 28–29)

Arm bud

Leg bud

5.0 mm

Week 4 (late)

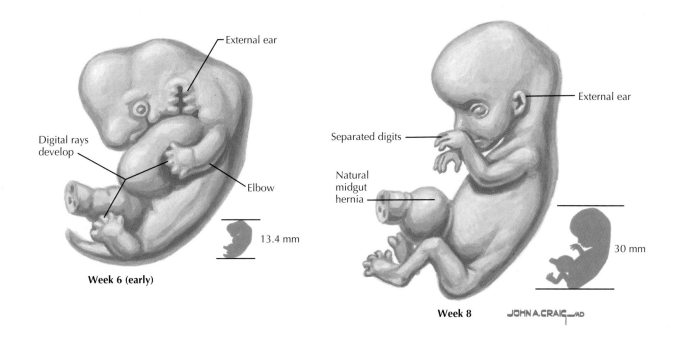

External ear

Digital rays develop

Elbow

13.4 mm

Week 6 (early)

External ear

Separated digits

Natural midgut hernia

30 mm

Week 8   JOHN A.CRAIG╴AD

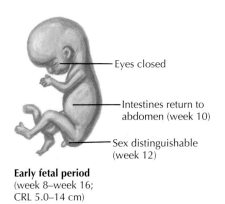

Eyes closed

Intestines return to abdomen (week 10)

Sex distinguishable (week 12)

Early fetal period
(week 8–week 16;
CRL 5.0–14 cm)

CRL, crown-to-rump length.

were not used account for three fourths of maternal mortality. These are all areas in which proactive counseling and assistance can have a positive impact on reducing morbidity or mortality.)

If a genetic evaluation of the fetus is indicated, chorionic villus sampling may be performed between the 10th and 12th week of gestation. Screening for cystic fibrosis should be offered to all patients during either the first or second trimester.

REFERENCES

Level III

American Academy of Pediatrics, American College of Obstetricians and Gynecologists: Guidelines for perinatal care, 5th ed. Elk Grove Village, IL, AAP; Washington, DC, ACOG, 2002.

American College of Obstetricians and Gynecologists: Prevention of Rh D alloimmunization. ACOG Practice Bulletin 4. Washington, DC, ACOG, 1999.

American College of Obstetricians and Gynecologists: Air travel during pregnancy. ACOG Committee Opinion 264. Obstet Gynecol 2001;98:1187.

American College of Obstetricians and Gynecologists: Exercise during pregnancy and the postpartum period. ACOG Committee Opinion 267. Obstet Gynecol 2002;99:171.

American College of Obstetricians and Gynecologists: Guidelines for women's health care. 2nd ed. Washington, DC, ACOG, 2002.

American College of Obstetricians and Gynecologists: Thyroid disease in pregnancy. ACOG Practice Bulletin 37. Obstet Gynecol 2002;100:387.

American College of Obstetricians and Gynecologists: Neural tube defects. ACOG Practice Bulletin 44. Obstet Gynecol 2003; 102:203.

American College of Obstetricians and Gynecologists: Guidelines for diagnostic imaging during pregnancy. ACOG Committee Opinion 299. Obstet Gynecol 2004;104:647.

American College of Obstetricians and Gynecologists: Nausea and vomiting of pregnancy. ACOG Practice Bulletin 52. Obstet Gynecol 2004;103:803.

American College of Obstetricians and Gynecologists: Ultrasonography in pregnancy. ACOG Practice Bulletin 58. Obstet Gynecol 2004;104:1449.

American College of Obstetricians and Gynecologists: Management of alloimmunization during pregnancy. ACOG Practice Bulletin 75. Obstet Gynecol 2006;108:457.

American College of Obstetricians and Gynecologists: Screening for fetal chromosomal abnormalities. ACOG Practice Bulletin 77. Obstet Gynecol 2007;109:217.

Kogan MD, Martin JA, Alexander GR, et al: The changing pattern of prenatal care utilization in the United States, 1981–1995, using different prenatal care indices. JAMA 1998;279:1623.

Mustard CA, Roos NP: The relationship of prenatal care and pregnancy complications to birthweight in Winnipeg, Canada. Am J Public Health 1994;84:1450.

Prevention of neural tube defects: Results of the Medical Research Council Vitamin Study. MRC Vitamin Study Research Group. Lancet 1991;338:131.

Yu SM, Alexander GR, Schwalberg R, Kogan MD: Prenatal care use among selected Asian American groups. Am J Public Health 2001;91:1865.

THE CHALLENGE

During the second trimester (14 to 28 weeks) the fetus continues to grow and develop, organ function becomes more normal, and the growing uterus is more apparent. Prenatal care during this period is directed toward monitoring the progress of the pregnancy and detecting treatable complications.

Scope of the Problem: Despite the relative lack of complications that occur during the second trimester, the early signs of later problems may first appear during this phase of pregnancy. These may be missed without continued vigilance.

Objectives of Management: To protect the health and well-being of mother and fetus.

TACTICS

Relevant Pathophysiology: During the second trimester of gestation, levels of human chorionic gonadotropin plateau and often decline, easing many of the early maladies of pregnancy such as breast tenderness and morning sickness, although the growing uterus may now bring on heartburn and constipation. The risk of early pregnancy loss has passed (except for infrequent cases of cervical incompetence and preterm labor) and the fetus grows from being just 3 inches in length at 14 weeks to weighing roughly 2 pounds by the end of the second trimester. There is an increase in maternal blood volume and cardiac output (20% greater) to feed the needs of the growing pregnancy. The first detectable movements of the baby (quickening) occur during this trimester (generally about 16 to 20 weeks of gestation) and the female fetus has the most egg cells of any point in her life. (Oocytes peak at 6 to 7 million at about 16 to 20 weeks of gestation, declining to about 1 million at birth.) Fetal viability (ability to survive apart from the mother) begins at about 24 weeks, although intact survival at this stage is unlikely. Toward the end of this trimester maternal hemorrhoids and low back pain may occur. Colostrum (the first form of breast milk) is present by 26 weeks of gestation.

Strategies: At each visit, patients should be asked about any problems such as vaginal bleeding, nausea/vomiting, dysuria, or vaginal discharge. Each prenatal visit should include measurements of blood pressure and weight and an assessment for edema. (Blood pressure generally declines at the end of the first trimester, increasing again in the third trimester.) A clean-catch urine sample should be tested (most often by dipstick) for protein and signs of infection. Obstetric assessments should include uterine size by fundal height measurement and documentation of the presence and rate of fetal heart tones by the use of a fetal Doppler ultrasound device.

Screening for open neural tube and other defects (via measurement of maternal serum alpha-fetoprotein and other markers) is generally performed between 15 and 20 weeks.

Toward the end of this trimester, a repeat measurement of hemoglobin is taken, glucose screening (usually 1-hour glucose challenge at 28 weeks for patients at low risk) is performed, and prophylactic treatment with Rh D immune globulin is given for patients who are Rh negative.

Patients at low risk may be followed at 4-week intervals until the end of this trimester. Routine use of ultrasonography to screen low-risk pregnancies in not currently recommended.

Patient Education: American College of Obstetricians and Gynecologists Patient Education Booklet AP001 (Nutrition During Pregnancy), AB005 (You and Your Baby: Prenatal Care, Labor and Delivery, and Postpartum Care), AP060 (Later Childbearing), AP0103 (Having a Baby [Especially for Teens]), AP104 (Drugs and Pregnancy), AP119 (Exercise During Pregnancy), AP133 (Routine Tests in Pregnancy), AP156 (How Your Baby Grows During Pregnancy), CP001 (Cystic Fibrosis Carrier Testing: The Decision Is Yours).

IMPLEMENTATION

Special Considerations: If a genetic evaluation of the fetus is indicated, an amniocentesis may be performed between the 12th and 21st weeks of gestation. Screening for cystic fibrosis should be offered to all patients during either the first or second trimester.

REFERENCES

Level III

American Academy of Pediatrics, American College of Obstetricians and Gynecologists: Guidelines for perinatal care, 5th ed. Elk Grove Village, IL, AAP; Washington, DC, ACOG, 2002.

American College of Obstetricians and Gynecologists: Prevention of Rh D alloimmunization. ACOG Practice Bulletin 4. Washington, DC, ACOG, 1999.

American College of Obstetricians and Gynecologists: Chronic hypertension in pregnancy. ACOG Practice Bulletin 29. Obstet Gynecol 2001;98:177.

American College of Obstetricians and Gynecologists: Air travel during pregnancy. ACOG Committee Opinion 264. Obstet Gynecol 2001;98:1187.

American College of Obstetricians and Gynecologists: Exercise during pregnancy and the postpartum period. ACOG Committee Opinion 267. Obstet Gynecol 2002;99:171.

American College of Obstetricians and Gynecologists: Thyroid disease in pregnancy. ACOG Practice Bulletin 37. Obstet Gynecol 2002;100:387.

American College of Obstetricians and Gynecologists: Perinatal care at the threshold of viability. ACOG Practice Bulletin 38. Obstet Gynecol 2002;100:617.

American College of Obstetricians and Gynecologists: Neural tube defects. ACOG Practice Bulletin 44. Obstet Gynecol 2003; 102:203.

American College of Obstetricians and Gynecologists: Cervical insufficiency. ACOG Practice Bulletin 48. Obstet Gynecol 2003; 102:1091.

American College of Obstetricians and Gynecologists: Guidelines for diagnostic imaging during pregnancy. ACOG Committee Opinion 299. Obstet Gynecol 2004;104:647.

American College of Obstetricians and Gynecologists: Ultrasonography in pregnancy. ACOG Practice Bulletin 58. Obstet Gynecol 2004;104:1449.

American College of Obstetricians and Gynecologists: Management of alloimmunization during pregnancy. ACOG Practice Bulletin 75. Obstet Gynecol 2006;108:457.

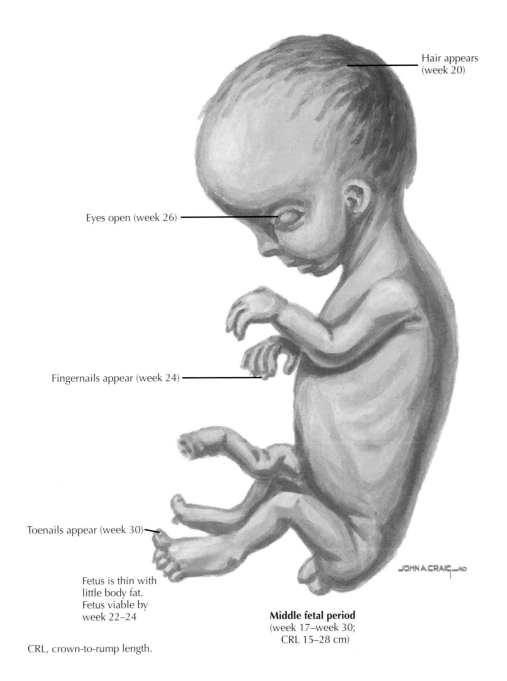

Hair appears
(week 20)

Eyes open (week 26)

Fingernails appear (week 24)

Toenails appear (week 30)

Fetus is thin with
little body fat.
Fetus viable by
week 22–24

CRL, crown-to-rump length.

JOHN A. CRAIG—AD

Middle fetal period
(week 17–week 30;
CRL 15–28 cm)

THE CHALLENGE

During the third trimester (29 to 40+ weeks) the fetus continues to grow and develop with full maturation in organ function being established, maternal physiology continuing to change, and the cervix and uterus preparing for the processes of childbirth. Prenatal care during this period continues to be directed toward monitoring the progress of the pregnancy and detecting treatable complications.

Scope of the Problem: It is during the third trimester that the uterus and fetus prepare for labor and delivery. It is also during this phase of pregnancy that complications such as pre-eclampsia, bleeding, complications of diabetes or hypertension, abnormalities of growth or amniotic fluid, and preterm labor may arise.

Objectives of Management: To protect the health and well-being of mother and fetus.

TACTICS

Relevant Pathophysiology: During the third trimester of gestation, the dramatic growth of the fetus continues as it gains its final birthweight and its organs prepare for full function as an autonomous individual. Maternal blood volume almost doubles, and cardiac output reaches its maximum. By the 29th week, the fetus has 300 bones, although many of them will fuse after birth, leaving the adult total of 206. The fetal presenting part begins to descend into the maternal pelvis in the last month of pregnancy, resulting in a decline in fundal height, improved respiratory and gastric function, and greater pelvic pressure and discomfort. Late in this trimester, changes in the cervix begin the preparations for dilation and effacement during labor and delivery.

Strategies: At each visit, patients continue to be asked about any problems such as vaginal bleeding, nausea/vomiting, dysuria, or vaginal discharge. Each prenatal visit should include measurements of blood pressure and weight and an assessment for edema. A clean-catch urine sample should be tested (most often by dipstick) for protein and signs of infection. Obstetric assessments should include uterine size by fundal height measurement and documentation of the presence and rate of fetal heart tones by the use of a fetal Doppler ultrasound device. (Fundal height in centimeters will generally match the gestational age of the pregnancy up to between 31 and 34 weeks. All measurements should be made with the patient's bladder empty; a full bladder can add up to 3 cm to the measurement.) Vaginal examinations to assess the dilation and effacement of cervix may be indicated for those with a history of premature labor or those experiencing symptoms of labor. (Routine cervical checks near term are not normally necessary.)

For selected patients, "kick counts" may be used to assess the overall health of the fetus. In general, the detection of more than four fetal movements over the course of an hour indicates a healthy fetus. All patients should be encouraged to monitor their baby's activity levels and be evaluated for any prolonged reduction or absence in activity.

At approximately 35 to 37 weeks of gestation a culture for group B streptococcus should be obtained to identify patients who are carriers and will require antibiotic treatment during labor. Some practitioners choose to just treat all patients during labor based on a review of risk factors. Both strategies are equally acceptable.

Planning and preparation for breastfeeding should be undertaken during this trimester. No special physical preparation is needed for successful breastfeeding, but discussion, questions, and the acquisition of needed supplies (e.g., nursing bra) are best taken care of before delivery.

For high-risk pregnancies, antenatal testing (nonstress test, contraction stress test, biophysical profile) should be considered and implemented as indicated.

Patients at low risk may be followed at 2-week intervals until approximately the 36th week, when visits occur at weekly intervals (or more often as dictated by the course of the pregnancy).

Patient Education: American College of Obstetricians and Gynecologists Patient Education Booklet AP001 (Nutrition During Pregnancy), AB005 (You and Your Baby: Prenatal Care, Labor and Delivery, and Postpartum Care), AP060 (Later Childbearing), AP069 (What to Expect After Your Due Date), AP079 (If Your Baby is Breech), AP098 (Special Test for Monitoring Fetal Health), AP0103 (Having a Baby [Especially for Teens]), AP104 (Drugs and Pregnancy), AP119 (Exercise During Pregnancy), AP133 (Routine Tests in Pregnancy), AP156 (How Your Baby Grows During Pregnancy)

IMPLEMENTATION

Special Considerations: Patients at high risk should be rechecked for sexually transmitted diseases (syphilis, gonorrhea, and chlamydia) toward the end of pregnancy.

REFERENCES

Level III

American Academy of Pediatrics, American College of Obstetricians and Gynecologists: Guidelines for perinatal care, 5th ed. Elk Grove Village, IL, AAP; Washington, DC, ACOG, 2002.

American College of Obstetricians and Gynecologists: Chronic hypertension in pregnancy. ACOG Practice Bulletin 29. Obstet Gynecol 2001;98:177.

American College of Obstetricians and Gynecologists: Air travel during pregnancy. ACOG Committee Opinion 264. Obstet Gynecol 2001;98:1187.

American College of Obstetricians and Gynecologists: Exercise during pregnancy and the postpartum period. ACOG Committee Opinion 267. Obstet Gynecol 2002;99:171.

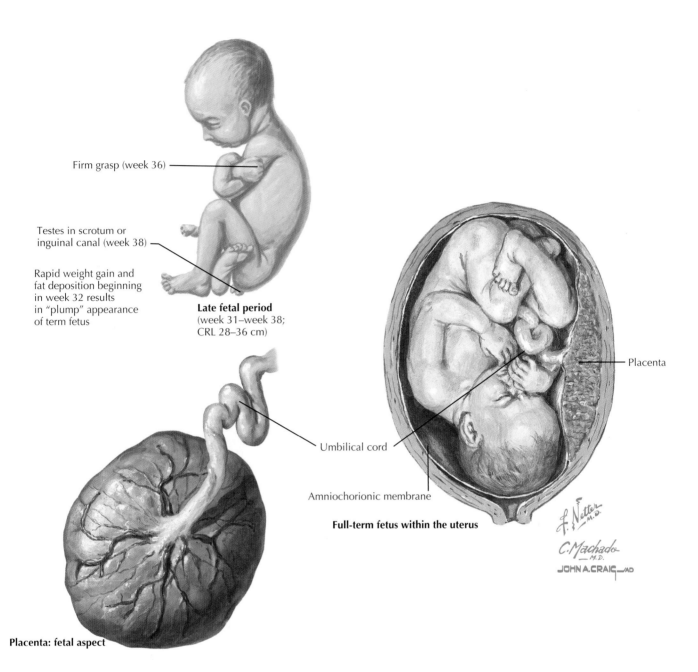

Firm grasp (week 36)

Testes in scrotum or inguinal canal (week 38)

Rapid weight gain and fat deposition beginning in week 32 results in "plump" appearance of term fetus

Late fetal period (week 31–week 38; CRL 28–36 cm)

Placenta

Umbilical cord

Amniochorionic membrane

Full-term fetus within the uterus

Placenta: fetal aspect

CRL, crown-to-rump length.

American College of Obstetricians and Gynecologists: Thyroid disease in pregnancy. ACOG Practice Bulletin 37. Obstet Gynecol 2002;100:387.

American College of Obstetricians and Gynecologists: Guidelines for diagnostic imaging during pregnancy. ACOG Committee Opinion 299. Obstet Gynecol 2004;104:647.

American College of Obstetricians and Gynecologists: Ultrasonography in pregnancy. ACOG Practice Bulletin 58. Obstet Gynecol 2004;104:1449.

American College of Obstetricians and Gynecologists: Management of alloimmunization during pregnancy. ACOG Practice Bulletin 75. Obstet Gynecol 2006;108:457.

THE CHALLENGE

To reduce the risk of fetal demise in those at high risk through the use of noninvasive tests that have acceptably low false-positive and false-negative results.

Scope of the Problem: There are roughly 15 fetal or neonatal deaths for every 1000 births in the United States.

Objectives of Management: To identify those fetuses at high risk and those whose status is deteriorating or non-reassuring so that intervention can take place to prevent mortality. Ultimately, the reduction of fetal morbidity and the improvement of neurologic outcome would be ideal as well, but objective studies to support the effectiveness of antepartum fetal testing are lacking.

TACTICS

Relevant Pathophysiology: The nonstress test (NST) and contraction stress test (CST) are based on the premise that when fetal oxygenation is only marginally adequate, the fetus will not possess the normal ability to modulate heart rate in response to fetal movement or to tolerate the stress of placental ischemia induced by uterine contractions. A normal (reactive) NST has two or more accelerations (15 beats/min for 15 seconds) in a 20-minute period. Acoustic stimulation may also be used to startle the fetus and induce a heart rate increase. In the CST, the occurrence of late decelerations occurring with 50% or more contractions (regardless of frequency) is "positive" and suggests fetal risk. The biophysical profile (BPP) is based on the NST, augmented by measures of fetal breathing movements, fetal activity and tone, and quantitation of amniotic fluid volume rated on a 10-point scale (normal: 8–10/10, equivocal: 6/10, abnormal: ≤5/10). The pulsatile character of fetal blood flow in the umbilical cord or the middle cerebral artery may be used to assess the health of high-risk pregnancies, but these tests require special expertise to both perform and interpret.

Strategies: The most commonly used antepartum fetal tests are the NST, CST, BPP, and movement assessment (kick count and others). These may be used individually, in sequence, or in any combination as the individual case demands. Each has advantages and disadvantages; no single test can be said to be definitive. Some possible indications for the use of antenatal fetal testing are shown.

Patient Education: American College of Obstetricians and Gynecologists Patient Education Pamphlet AP098 (Special Tests for Monitoring Fetal Health), AP015 (Fetal Heart Rate Monitoring During Labor).

IMPLEMENTATION

Special Considerations: The NST is more easily performed than the CST, but it has the highest false-positive rate (up to 90% of positive tests) and the highest risk of a false-negative test result (1.4 of 1000). The CST requires the induction of contractions by intravenous oxytocin or nipple stimulation. There must be ≥3 con-tractions in a 10-minute test period and no late decelerations. The CST has a lower false-positive rate (50%) and a lower risk of a false-negative result (0.4 of 1000). The BPP has the lowest false-positive and false-negative rates (0 to 0.6 of 1000) but is the most expensive and requires the most expertise and equipment. All testing must be viewed in the context of the clinical picture. The choice of timing and test must be made on clinical grounds, degree of risk, and the availability and expertise of those who will perform and interpret the test. Normal test results generally warrant further testing in a few days to a week. Positive or nonreassuring test results may suggest the need for a more invasive test (e.g., NST to CST, CST to BPP) or more direct intervention in the course of the pregnancy (delivery). Despite the extent of study that has accompanied these technologies, all studies must always be interpreted in light of all available clinical factors.

REFERENCES

Level I

Brown VA, Sawers RS, Parsons RJ, et al: The value of antenatal cardiotocography in the management of high-risk pregnancy: a randomized controlled trial. Br J Obstet Gynaecol 1982;89:716.

Chauhan SP, Doherty DD, Magann EF, et al: Amniotic fluid index vs single deepest pocket technique during modified biophysical profile: a randomized clinical trial. Am J Obstet Gynecol 2004;191:661.

Kidd LC, Patel NB, Smith R: Non-stress antenatal cardiotocography—A prospective randomized clinical trial. Br J Obstet Gynaecol 1985;92:1156.

Lumley J, Lester A, Anderson I, et al: A randomized trial of weekly cardiotocography in high-risk obstetric patients. Br J Obstet Gynaecol 1983;90:1018.

Smith CV, Phelan JP, Platt LD, et al: Fetal acoustic stimulation testing. II. A randomized clinical comparison with the nonstress test. Am J Obstet Gynecol 1986;155:131.

Vintzileos AM, Antsaklis A, Varvarigos I, et al: A randomized trial of intrapartum electronic fetal heart rate monitoring versus intermittent auscultation. Obstet Gynecol 1993;81:899.

Level II

Nageotte MP, Towers CV, Asrat T, et al: The value of a negative antepartum test: contraction stress test and modified biophysical profile. Obstet Gynecol 1994;84:231.

Nageotte MP, Towers CV, Asrat T, Freeman RK: Perinatal outcome with the modified biophysical profile. Am J Obstet Gynecol 1994;170:1672.

Reece EA, Hagay Z, Garofalo J, Hobbins JC: A controlled trial of self-nonstress test versus assisted nonstress test in the evaluation of fetal well-being. Am J Obstet Gynecol 1992;166:489.

Level III

American College of Obstetricians and Gynecologists: Antepartum fetal surveillance. ACOG Practice Bulletin 9. Washington, DC, ACOG, 1999. American College of Obstetricians and Gynecologists: Management of postterm pregnancy. ACOG Practice Bulletin 55. Obstet Gynecol 2004;104:639.

Miller DA, Rabello YA, Paul RH: The modified biophysical profile: antepartum testing in the 1990s. Am J Obstet Gynecol 1996;174:812.

Rayburn WF: Clinical implications from monitoring fetal activity. Am J Obstet Gynecol 1982;144:967.

Zimmer EZ, Divon MY: Fetal vibroacoustic stimulation. Obstet Gynecol 1993;81:451.

Noninvasive testing used to identify "high-risk" fetus and to elicit signs of deteriorating status to allow intervention and prevent mortality

Testing based on premise that marginal fetal oxygenation limits fetal ability to modulate fetal heart rate in response to fetal movement or to placental ischemia as a result of uterine contraction. Fetal heart rate should show acceleration to movement or contraction

Nonstress Test (NST)
Contraction Stress Test (CST)
Biophysical Profile (BPP)

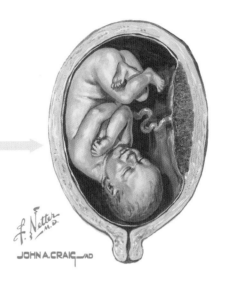

Some Conditions That Suggest Need for Antepartum Testing

Chronic renal disease

Hyperthyroidism

Type 1 diabetes mellitus

Maternal hypertension

Maternal cyanotic heart disease

Intrauterine growth restriction

Reduced fetal movement

Management Flowchart for Antepartum Fetal Testing

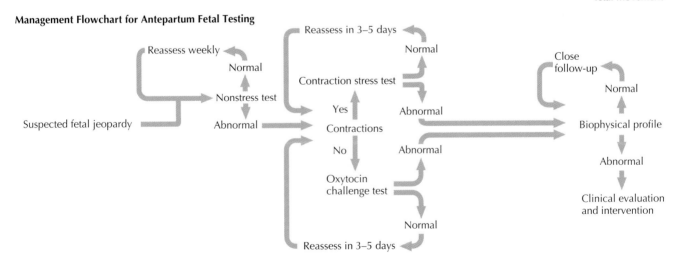

Suspected fetal jeopardy

Reassess weekly

Normal

Nonstress test

Abnormal

Reassess in 3–5 days

Normal

Contraction stress test

Yes

Contractions

No

Oxytocin challenge test

Abnormal

Abnormal

Normal

Reassess in 3–5 days

Close follow-up

Normal

Biophysical profile

Abnormal

Clinical evaluation and intervention

THE CHALLENGE

The biophysical profile is one of several tests used to evaluate fetal health and reserve. Of the tests used for fetal assessment, the biophysical profile is the most technologically intensive and most expensive, but it carries the lowest false-positive and false-negative rates (0.6 to 1/1000).

Scope of the Problem: Of pregnancies, 3% to 12% are at risk because of gestations that extend beyond term and more may be compromised by maternal disease states that affect fetal health or placental function (e.g., hypertension, diabetes), resulting in abnormalities of fetal growth and amniotic fluid volume and other problems.

Objectives of Test: To assess fetal health and reserve.

TACTICS

Relevant Pathophysiology: The biophysical profile is based on fetal heart rate response to activity (as in the nonstress test) but also adds the assessment of fetal tone, activity, and breathing as evaluated by ultrasonography. These parameters of activity often reflect the impact of acute and subacute stress. The volume of amniotic fluid (also measured by ultrasonography) can be indicative of fetal risk in that reductions are often associated with either maternal or fetal compromise (most often reduced fetal urine output in the face of chronic stress).

Strategies: The biophysical profile is made up of five assessments of fetal well-being: the volume of amniotic fluid present, the frequency of fetal breathing movements, fetal tone, gross body movements, and the results of a nonstress test. Each parameter is scored as present or absent (0 or 2 scale) and then scores are totaled. A score of 8 or 10 is considered normal; 6 is equivocal and suggests further evaluation; and a score of 4 or less is abnormal and augurs for immediate intervention. A score of 0 is invariably associated with significant fetal acidemia.

Patient Education: Reassurance; American College of Obstetricians and Gynecologists Patient Education Booklet AP098 (Special Tests for Monitoring Fetal Health).

IMPLEMENTATION

Special Considerations: Approximately 97% of biophysical profiles will be normal. The false-normal rate of biophysical profiles is approximately 1/1000 tests; false-positive test results occur in 1.5% of patients.

Despite the extent of study that has accompanied the biophysical profile, these studies must always be interpreted in light of all available clinical factors.

REFERENCES

Level I

Chauhan SP, Doherty DD, Magann EF, et al: Amniotic fluid index vs single deepest pocket technique during modified biophysical profile: a randomized clinical trial. Am J Obstet Gynecol 2004;191:661.

Lewis DF, Adair CD, Weeks JW, et al: A randomized clinical trial of daily nonstress testing versus biophysical profile in the management of preterm premature rupture of membranes. Am J Obstet Gynecol 1999;181:1495.

Level II

Dayal AK, Manning FA, Berck DJ, et al: Fetal death after normal biophysical profile score: an eighteen-year experience. Am J Obstet Gynecol 1999;181:1231.

Manning FA, Harman CR, Morrison I, et al: Fetal assessment based on fetal biophysical profile scoring. IV. An analysis of perinatal morbidity and mortality. Am J Obstet Gynecol 1990;138:575.

Manning FA, Lange IR, Morrison I, Harman CR: Fetal biophysical profile score and the nonstress test: a comparative trial. Obstet Gynecol 1984;64:326.

Moore TR, Piacquadio K: A prospective evaluation of fetal movement screening to reduce the incidence of antepartum fetal death. Am J Obstet Gynecol 1989;160:1075.

Nageotte MP, Towers CV, Asrat T, et al: The value of a negative antepartum test: contraction stress test and modified biophysical profile. Obstet Gynecol 1994;84:231.

Nageotte MP, Towers CV, Asrat T, Freeman RK: Perinatal outcome with the modified biophysical profile. Am J Obstet Gynecol 1994;170:1672.

Ott WJ, Mora G, Arias F, et al: Comparison of the modified biophysical profile to a "new" biophysical profile incorporating the middle cerebral artery to umbilical artery velocity flow systolic/diastolic ratio. Am J Obstet Gynecol 1998;178:1346.

Platt LD, Walla CA, Paul RH, et al: A prospective trial of the fetal biophysical profile versus the nonstress test in the management of high-risk pregnancies. Am J Obstet Gynecol 1985;153:624.

Yoon BH, Romero R, Roh CR, et al: Relationship between the fetal biophysical profile score, umbilical artery Doppler velocimetry, and fetal blood acid-base status determined by cordocentesis. Am J Obstet Gynecol 1993;169:1586.

Level III

American College of Obstetricians and Gynecologists: Antepartum fetal surveillance. ACOG Practice Bulletin 9. Washington, DC, ACOG, 1999.

American College of Obstetricians and Gynecologists: Management of postterm pregnancy. ACOG Practice Bulletin 55. Obstet Gynecol 2004;104:639.

Magann EF, Doherty DA, Field K, et al: Biophysical profile with amniotic fluid volume assessments. Obstet Gynecol 2004;104:5.

Miller DA, Rabello YA, Paul RH: The modified biophysical profile: antepartum testing in the 1990s. Am J Obstet Gynecol 1996;174:812.

BIOPHYSICAL PROFILE SCORE

Profile Parameter	Normal (= 2 points)	Abnormal (= 0 points)
Amniotic fluid volume	At least 1 pocket of 1 cm in 2 perpendicular planes	No fluid or no pockets >1 cm
Fetal breathing movements (FBM)	≥1 FBM of 30-sec duration in 30 minutes	No FBM of 30-sec duration in 30 minutes
Fetal tone	≥1 episode of active extension and return or hand opening and closing	No or slow extension, poor return or no activity
Gross body movements	≥3 body or limb movements in 30 minutes	≤2 body or limb movements in 30 min
Reactive fetal heart rate	Reactive nonstress test	Nonreactive nonstress test

The biophysical profile score is established by summing the values obtained on each of the five-component tests.

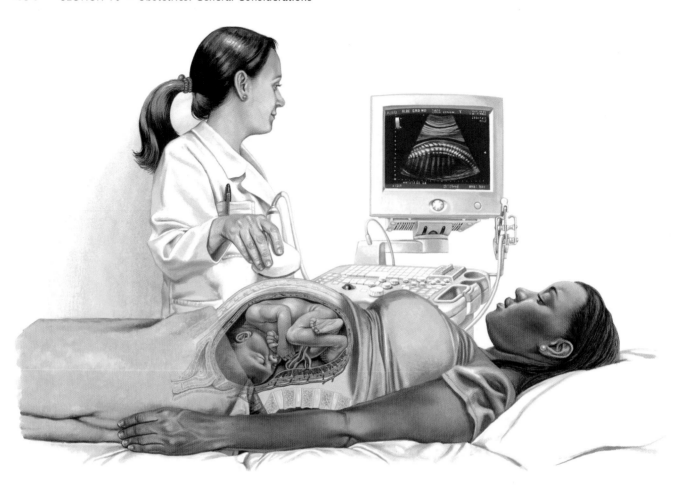

An ultrasound is used for four of the five factors in the biophysical profile (fetal breathing, movement, tone, and fluid volume).

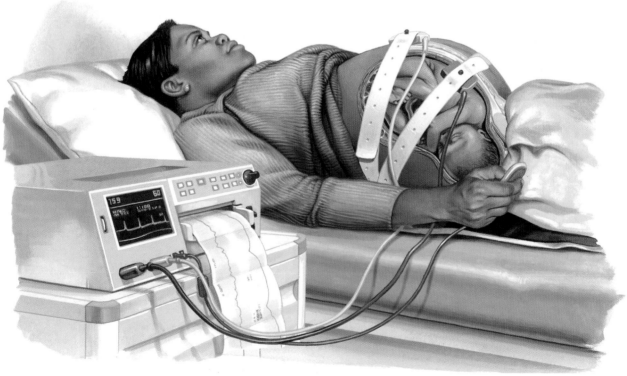

The fifth factor in a biophysical profile is the heart rate response to activity, which is measured by a nonstress test.

THE CHALLENGE

Fetal health may be assessed using the contraction stress test (also called "oxytocin challenge test"). This test is somewhat analogous to an exercise stress test for the evaluation of adult cardiac function in that problems or weaknesses that are normally compensated for at rest may become apparent with stress. In the contraction stress test, the fetal–placental–maternal unit is stressed through uterine contractions. The resulting periodic deprivation of uterine blood flow can be used to evaluate the robustness of the fetal condition.

Scope of the Problem: Of pregnancies, 3% to 12% are at risk because of gestations that extend beyond term. More pregnancies may be compromised by maternal disease states that affect fetal health or placental function (e.g., hypertension, diabetes) resulting in abnormalities of fetal growth and amniotic fluid volume and other problems.

Objectives of the Test: To assess fetal health and reserve.

TACTICS

Relevant Pathophysiology: During uterine contractions, uterine intramural pressure exceeds perfusion pressure, resulting in transient ischemia and loss of blood delivery to the intervillous spaces. When the fetus and placenta are healthy, this loss of blood flow causes no change in fetal tissue oxygenation, and there is no compensatory or reactive change in fetal heart rate. When the fetal–placental or placental–maternal relationships have been degraded, this brief loss of perfusion may be sufficient to cause a reduction in heart rate in the same way as that seen in labor when late decelerations are found.

Strategies: If uterine contractions are occurring spontaneously, the contraction stress test may proceed directly. To perform the oxytocin challenge test there must be no contraindications to the use of oxytocin. Fetal heart rate and uterine activity monitoring are established and contractions are induced using oxytocin or through intermittent nipple stimulation. Contractions must occur at a rate of three per 10 minutes for at least three 10-minute periods. A normal stress test should show normal fetal heart rate variability and the absence of periodic decelerations. Accelerations with fetal activity are reassuring.

Patient Education: Reassurance; American College of Obstetricians and Gynecologists Patient Education Pamphlet 098 (Special Tests for Monitoring Fetal Health), AP015 (Fetal Heart Rate Monitoring During Labor).

IMPLEMENTATION

Special Considerations: If contractions are occurring spontaneously at a rate of at least three every 10 minutes, the term "contraction stress test" is generally used, whereas the term "oxytocin challenge test" is used when contractions must be induced through oxytocin administration. Like most tests of fetal status, the contraction stress test has a moderate false-positive rate. Consequently, the interpretation of a positive test result must be made in the perspective of other information about the mother and fetus, including the results of other tests such as the nonstress test or biophysical profile. (See also "Antepartum Testing.")

REFERENCES

Level I

Freeman RK, Anderson G, Dorchester W: A prospective multi-institutional study of antepartum fetal heart rate monitoring. II. Contraction stress test versus nonstress test for primary surveillance. Am J Obstet Gynecol 1982;143:778–81.

Knox GE, Huddleston JF, Flowers CE Jr: Management of prolonged pregnancy: results of a prospective randomized trial. Am J Obstet Gynecol 1979;134:376.

Lipitz S, Barkai G, Rabinovici J, Mashiach S: Breast stimulation test and oxytocin challenge test in fetal surveillance: a prospective randomized study. Am J Obstet Gynecol 1987;157:1178.

Level II

Nageotte MP, Towers CV, Asrat T, Freeman RK: Perinatal outcome with the modified biophysical profile. Am J Obstet Gynecol 1994;170:1672.

Nageotte MP, Towers CV, Asrat T, et al: The value of a negative antepartum test: contraction stress test and modified biophysical profile. Obstet Gynecol 1994;84:231.

Level III

American College of Obstetricians and Gynecologists: Antepartum fetal surveillance. ACOG Practice Bulletin 9. Washington, DC, ACOG, 1999.

American College of Obstetricians and Gynecologists: Management of postterm pregnancy. ACOG Practice Bulletin 55. Obstet Gynecol 2004;104:639.

Freeman RK: Contraction stress testing for primary fetal surveillance in patients at high risk for uteroplacental insufficiency. Clin Perinatol 1982;9:265.

Miller DA, Rabello YA, Paul RH: The modified biophysical profile: antepartum testing in the 1990s. Am J Obstet Gynecol 1996;174:812.

Contraction Stress Testing

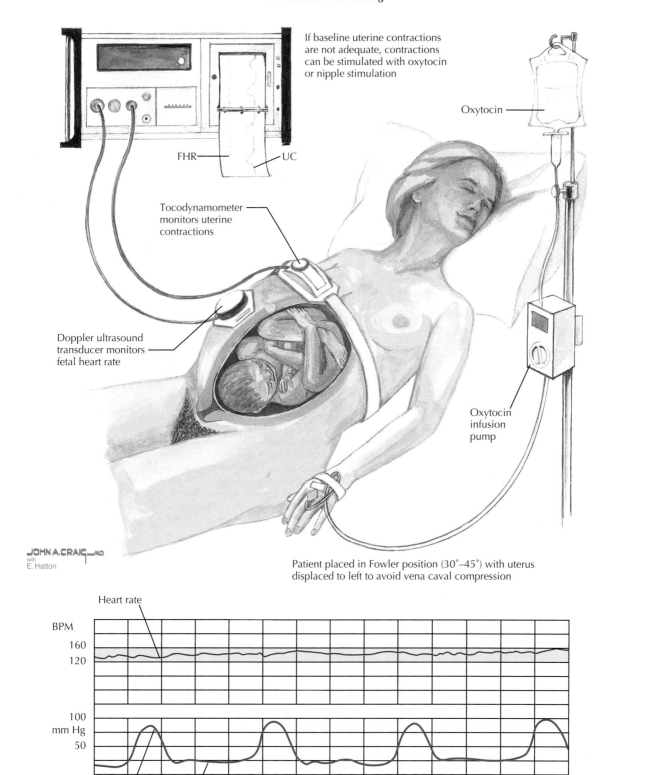

If baseline uterine contractions are not adequate, contractions can be stimulated with oxytocin or nipple stimulation

FHR   UC

Oxytocin

Tocodynamometer monitors uterine contractions

Doppler ultrasound transducer monitors fetal heart rate

Oxytocin infusion pump

JOHN A. CRAIG
with
E. Hatton

Patient placed in Fowler position (30°–45°) with uterus displaced to left to avoid vena caval compression

Heart rate

BPM
160
120

100
mm Hg
50

Uterine contraction   Uterine relaxation   (Contractions must occur at rate of 3/10 min for at least three 10-minute periods)

Portion of a "normal" (negative) contraction stress test exhibiting absence of heart rate decelerations following uterine contractions

BPM, beats per minute; FHR, fetal heart rate; UC, uterine contractions.

THE CHALLENGE

Doppler flow studies (also known as Doppler velocimetry) constitute a group of tests used to evaluate fetal health and reserve through the assessment of blood flow characteristics in the umbilical cord, middle cerebral artery, or other vascular structures. Of the tests used for fetal assessment, Doppler flow studies are technologically intensive, are expensive, and require special expertise to perform and interpret.

Scope of the Problem: Of pregnancies, 3% to 12% are at risk because of gestations that extend beyond term and more may be compromised by maternal disease states that affect fetal health or placental function (e.g., hypertension, diabetes), resulting in abnormalities of fetal growth or amniotic fluid volume and other problems. Current applications of Doppler flow studies are generally limited to cases of fetal growth restriction.

Objectives of Test: To assess fetal health and reserve.

TACTICS

Relevant Pathophysiology: The Doppler principle states that when energy is reflected from a moving boundary, the frequency of the reflected energy varies in relation to the velocity of the moving boundary. In clinical practice, this principle is used to determine the velocity of blood flow in vessels because the frequency of sound reflected from moving blood cells is slightly altered in proportion to the velocity of the blood flow (and the cosine of the angle of incidence).

During the cardiac cycle, blood flow within the fetal circulation is pulsatile, with the difference in flow during systole and diastole gradually declining with gestational age and other factors. In the umbilical artery, this systolic to diastolic (S/D) ratio decreases from about four at 20 weeks, to less than three at 30 weeks, and finally to around two near term. Much of this change is mediated by the health and function of the placenta, and when this is compromised, diastolic flow diminishes. In extreme cases of fetal–placental compromise, diastolic flow may be absent or even show reversal of flow direction. Absent end-diastolic flow is associated with significant fetal compromise. Babies with abnormal umbilical artery Doppler blood flow results have a significantly higher rate of cesarean delivery for fetal distress, longer stays in the neonatal intensive care unit, and increased neonatal morbidity regardless of whether they were of normal size or growth restricted.

When there is fetal anemia, the associated increased cardiac output and relatively lower blood viscosity result in increased blood flow in the middle cerebral artery. This flow can be measured and used to evaluate fetuses with alloimmunization. (Fetuses with blood flow greater than 1.5 times the median [multiples of median, or MoM] are correctly identified with anemia with only a 12% false-positive rate.) Increased middle cerebral artery blood flow has also been proposed as a marker for altered blood flow before other indicators of hypoxemia may be present.

Uterine artery blood flow increases from about 50 mL/min in early gestation to 500 to 750 mL/min by term. Doppler flow studies of the uterine artery have been used in an effort to predict the development of pre-eclampsia and other complications. Unfortunately, uterine artery Doppler flow velocity appears to have limited diagnostic accuracy in predicting pre-eclampsia, intrauterine growth restriction (IUGR), and perinatal death.

Strategies: Doppler flow studies may be used to assess blood flow in the umbilical blood vein and arteries, fetal brain, and fetal heart. A Doppler flow study is often used when a fetus has intrauterine growth restriction or abnormalities of amniotic fluid volume.

Blood flow in the fetal ductus arteriosus can be assessed when the fetus has been exposed to nonsteroidal anti-inflammatory drugs.

Patient Education: Reassurance; American College of Obstetricians and Gynecologists Patient Education Booklet AP098 (Special Tests for Monitoring Fetal Health).

IMPLEMENTATION

Special Considerations: Despite its usefulness in the evaluation of the fetus at risk, intrapartum umbilical artery Doppler velocimetry is a poor predictor of adverse perinatal outcomes.

Recent studies suggest that even such factors as a cholesterol-lowering diet can influence umbilical artery blood-flow patterns.

Notwithstanding the extent of study that has accompanied these technologies, Doppler flow studies must always be interpreted in light of all available clinical factors. Because prenatal Doppler studies have not been proved to benefit pregnancy outcome, many investigators still consider obstetric Doppler velocimetry to be an investigational tool.

REFERENCES

Level I

Giles W, Bisits A, O'Callaghan S, Gill A; DAMP Study Group: The Doppler assessment in multiple pregnancy: randomised controlled trial of ultrasound biometry versus umbilical artery Doppler ultrasound and biometry in twin pregnancy. BJOG 2003;110:593.

Newnham JP, O'Dea MR, Reid KP, Diepeveen DA: Doppler flow velocity waveform analysis in high risk pregnancies: a randomized controlled trial. Br J Obstet Gynaecol 1991;98:956.

Omtzigt AM, Reuwer PJ, Bruinse HW: A randomized controlled trial on the clinical value of umbilical Doppler velocimetry in antenatal care. Am J Obstet Gynecol 1994;170:625.

Trudinger BJ, Cook CM, Giles WB, et al: Umbilical artery flow velocity waveforms in high-risk pregnancy. Randomised controlled trial. Lancet 1987;1:188.

Whittle MJ, Hanretty KP, Primrose MH, Neilson JP: Screening for the compromised fetus: a randomized trial of umbilical artery velocimetry in unselected pregnancies. Am J Obstet Gynecol 1994;170:555.

Williams KP, Farquharson DF, Bebbington M, et al: Screening for fetal well-being in a high-risk pregnant population comparing the nonstress test with umbilical artery Doppler velocimetry: a ran-

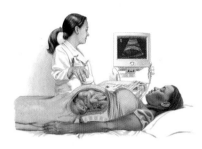

Doppler Flow Studies (Doppler velocimetry)

Doppler flow studies constitute a group of tests used to evaluate fetal health and reserve through the assessment of blood flow characteristics in fetal and uterine vessels and fetal heart. Routinely, though, only the study of umbilical and cerebral blood vessels is of major relevance.

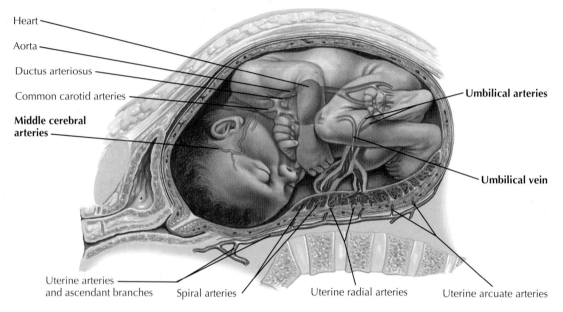

Heart
Aorta
Ductus arteriosus
Common carotid arteries

Middle cerebral arteries

Umbilical arteries

Umbilical vein

Uterine arteries and ascendant branches
Spiral arteries
Uterine radial arteries
Uterine arcuate arteries

Current applications of Doppler flow studies are generally limited to cases of fetal intrauterine growth restriction (IUGR). Babies with abnormal umbilical artery Doppler blood flow results have a significantly higher rate of cesarean section delivery for fetal distress, longer stays in the neonatal intensive care unit, and increased neonatal morbidity regardless of whether they were of normal size or growth restricted.

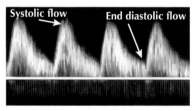

Systolic flow
End diastolic flow

Normal blood flow in umbilical arteries.

C. Machado — M.D.

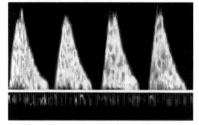

Absent end diastolic flow in umbilical arteries is associated with significant fetal compromise.

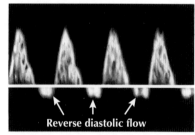

Reverse diastolic flow

Presence of reverse diastolic flow in umbilical arteries indicates extreme case of fetal-placental compromise.

domized controlled clinical trial. Am J Obstet Gynecol 2003; 188:1366–71.

Zimmerman R, Carpenter RJ Jr, Durig P, Mari G: Longitudinal measurement of peak systolic velocity in the fetal middle cerebral artery for monitoring pregnancies complicated by red cell alloimmunisation: a prospective multicentre trial with intention-to-treat. BJOG 2002;109:746.

Level II

Almstrom H, Axelsson O, Cnattingius S, et al: Comparison of umbilical-artery velocimetry and cardiotocography for surveillance of small-for-gestational-age fetuses. Lancet 1992;340:936.

Farrell T, Chien PF, Gordon A: Intrapartum umbilical artery Doppler velocimetry as a predictor of adverse perinatal outcome: a systematic review. Br J Obstet Gynaecol 1999;106:783.

Johnstone FD, Prescott R, Hoskins P, et al: The effect of introduction of umbilical Doppler recordings to obstetric practice. Br J Obstet Gynaecol 1993;100:733.

Karsdorp VH, van Vugt JM, van Geijn HP, et al: Clinical significance of absent or reversed end diastolic velocity waveforms in umbilical artery. Lancet 1994;344:1664.

Khoury J, Haugen G, Tonstad S, et al: Effect of a cholesterol-lowering diet during pregnancy on maternal and fetal Doppler velocimetry: the CARRDIP study. Am J Obstet Gynecol 2007; 196:549.e1.

Konchak PS, Bernstein IM, Capeless EL: Uterine artery Doppler velocimetry in the detection of adverse obstetric outcomes in women with unexplained elevated maternal serum alpha-fetoprotein levels. Am J Obstet Gynecol 1995;173:1115.

Konje JC, Howarth ES, Kaufmann P, Taylor DJ: Longitudinal quantification of uterine artery blood volume flow changes during gestation in pregnancies complicated by intrauterine growth restriction. BJOG 2003;110:301.

Mari G, Deter RL, Carpenter RL, et al: Noninvasive diagnosis by Doppler ultrasonography of fetal anemia due to maternal red-cell alloimmunization. Collaborative Group for Doppler Assessment of the Blood Velocity in Anemic Fetuses. N Engl J Med 2000;342:9.

Ott WJ, Mora G, Arias F, et al: Comparison of the modified biophysical profile to a "new" biophysical profile incorporating the middle cerebral artery to umbilical artery velocity flow systolic/diastolic ratio. Am J Obstet Gynecol 1998;178:1346.

Papageorghiou AT, Yu CK, Erasmus IE, et al: Assessment of risk for the development of pre-eclampsia by maternal characteristics and uterine artery Doppler. BJOG 2005;112:703.

Pietryga M, Brazert J, Wender-Ozegowska E, et al: Abnormal uterine Doppler is related to vasculopathy in pregestational diabetes mellitus. Circulation 2005;112:2496.

Yoon BH, Romero R, Roh CR, et al: Relationship between the fetal biophysical profile score, umbilical artery Doppler velocimetry, and fetal blood acid-base status determined by cordocentesis. Am J Obstet Gynecol 1993;169:1586.

Yu CK, Smith GC, Papageorghiou AT, et al; Fetal Medicine Foundation Second Trimester Screening Group: An integrated model for the prediction of preeclampsia using maternal factors and uterine artery Doppler velocimetry in unselected low-risk women. Am J Obstet Gynecol 2005;193:429.

Level III

American College of Obstetricians and Gynecologists: Antepartum fetal surveillance. ACOG Practice Bulletin 9. Washington, DC, ACOG, 1999.

American College of Obstetricians and Gynecologists: Intrauterine growth restriction. ACOG Practice Bulletin 12. Washington, DC, ACOG, 2000.

American College of Obstetricians and Gynecologists: Management of postterm pregnancy. ACOG Practice Bulletin 55. Obstet Gynecol 2004;104:639.

American College of Obstetricians and Gynecologists: Ultrasonography in pregnancy. ACOG Practice Bulletin 58. Obstet Gynecol 2004;104:1449.

Chan FY, Pun TC, Lam C, et al: Pregnancy screening by uterine artery Doppler velocimetry—Which criterion performs best? Obstet Gynecol 1995;85:596.

Chien PF, Arnott N, Gordon A, et al: How useful is uterine artery Doppler flow velocimetry in the prediction of pre-eclampsia, intrauterine growth retardation and perinatal death? An overview. BJOG 2000;107:196.

Detti L, Johnson SC, Diamond MP, Puscheck EE: First-trimester Doppler investigation of the uterine circulation. Am J Obstet Gynecol 2006;195:1210. Epub 2006 Apr 17.

Divon MY: Umbilical artery Doppler velocimetry: clinical utility in high-risk pregnancies. Am J Obstet Gynecol 1996;174:10.

Karsdorp VH, van Vugt JM, van Geijn HP, et al: Clinical significance of absent or reversed end diastolic velocity waveforms in umbilical artery. Lancet 1994;344:1664.

Pattinson RC, Norman K, Odendaal HJ: The role of Doppler velocimetry in the management of high risk pregnancies. Br J Obstet Gynaecol 1994;101:114.

THE CHALLENGE

Fetal health may be assessed using the nonstress test (NST). This test is the simplest of the antenatal tests to perform and often represents the first line in managing an at-risk pregnancy.

Scope of the Problem: Of pregnancies, 3% to 12% are at risk because of gestations that extend beyond term. More pregnancies may be compromised by maternal disease states that affect fetal health or placental function (e.g., hypertension, diabetes) resulting in abnormalities of fetal growth or amniotic fluid volume and other problems.

Objectives of the Test: To assess fetal health and reserve.

TACTICS

Relevant Pathophysiology: The NST is based on the premise that when fetal oxygenation is only marginally adequate, the fetus will not possess the normal ability to alter heart rate in response to fetal movement. A normal (reactive) NST has two or more accelerations in fetal heart rate that peak at 15 beats/min (although not necessarily remaining at that level), lasting for 15 seconds in a 20-minute period. Loss of reactivity is most often associated with fetal sleep but may result from any cause of central nervous system depression, including fetal acidosis. It may be necessary to continue the tracing for 40 minutes or longer to take into account the fetal sleep–wake cycle. Acoustic stimulation may also be used to startle the fetus and induce a heart rate increase.

Strategies: The NST is considered reactive (normal) if there are two or more fetal heart rate accelerations (as defined previously) within a 20-minute period, with or without fetal movement felt by the mother. Accelerations with fetal activity are reassuring. A nonreactive NST is one that does not meet these criteria (lacks sufficient fetal heart rate accelerations) over a 40-minute period. A reactive NST is a good predictor of adequate fetal oxygenation, and most reactive fetuses do well for at least another week.

Patient Education: Reassurance; American College of Obstetricians and Gynecologists Patient Education Pamphlet 098 (Special Tests for Monitoring Fetal Health), AP015 (Fetal Heart Rate Monitoring During Labor).

IMPLEMENTATION

Special Considerations: To increase the reliability of the NST, the patient should not have smoked recently. The NST is more easily performed than the contraction stress test, but it has the highest false-positive rate (up to 90% of positive tests) and the highest risk of a false-negative test result (1.4 of 1000). (The NST of the healthy preterm fetus is frequently nonreactive: from 24 to 28 weeks of gestation, up to 50% of NSTs may not be reactive, and from 28 to 32 weeks of gestation, 15% of NSTs are not reactive.) Variable decelerations may be observed in up to 50% of NSTs. If sporadic and brief (<30 seconds), they are inconsequential and do not indicate fetal compromise or the need for intervention. (Repetitive variable decelerations [at least three in 20 minutes], even if mild, have been associated with an increased risk of cesarean delivery for fetal indications.) Because of these factors, the interpretation of a nonreactive test must be made in the perspective of other information about the mother and fetus, including the results of other tests such as the contraction stress test or biophysical profile. (See also "Antepartum Testing.")

REFERENCES

Level I
Knox GE, Huddleston JF, Flowers CE Jr: Management of prolonged pregnancy: results of a prospective randomized trial. Am J Obstet Gynecol 1979;134:376.

Level II
Anyaegbunam A, Brustman L, Divon M, Langer O: The significance of antepartum variable decelerations. Am J Obstet Gynecol 1986;155:707.

Bishop EH: Fetal acceleration test. Am J Obstet Gynecol 1981;141:905.

Evertson LR, Gauthier RJ, Schifrin BS, Paul RH: Antepartum fetal heart rate testing. I. Evolution of the nonstress test. Am J Obstet Gynecol 1979;133:29.

Lavin JP Jr, Miodovnik M, Barden TP: Relationship of nonstress test reactivity and gestational age. Obstet Gynecol 1984;63:338.

Meis PJ, Ureda JR, Swain M, et al: Variable decelerations during nonstress tests are not a sign of fetal compromise. Am J Obstet Gynecol 1986;154:586.

Nageotte MP, Towers CV, Asrat T, Freeman RK: Perinatal outcome with the modified biophysical profile. Am J Obstet Gynecol 1994;170:1672.

Pazos R, Vuolo K, Aladjem S, et al: Association of spontaneous fetal heart rate decelerations during antepartum nonstress testing and intrauterine growth retardation. Am J Obstet Gynecol 1982;144:574.

Level III
American College of Obstetricians and Gynecologists: Antepartum fetal surveillance. ACOG Practice Bulletin 9. Washington, DC, ACOG, 1999.

American College of Obstetricians and Gynecologists: Management of postterm pregnancy. ACOG Practice Bulletin 55. Obstet Gynecol 2004;104:639.

Bourgeois FJ, Thiagarajah S, Harbert GM Jr: The significance of fetal heart rate decelerations during nonstress testing. Am J Obstet Gynecol 1984;150:213.

Druzin ML, Fox A, Kogut E, Carlson C: The relationship of the nonstress test to gestational age. Am J Obstet Gynecol 1985;153:386.

Druzin ML, Gratacos J, Keegan KA, Paul RH: Antepartum fetal heart rate testing. VII. The significance of fetal bradycardia. Am J Obstet Gynecol 1981;139:194.

Graca LM, Cardoso CG, Clode N, Calhaz-Jorge C: Acute effects of maternal cigarette smoking on fetal heart rate and fetal body movements felt by the mother. J Perinat Med 1991;19:385.

O'Leary JA, Andrinopoulos GC, Giordano PC: Variable decelerations and the nonstress test: an indication of cord compromise. Am J Obstet Gynecol 1980;137:704.

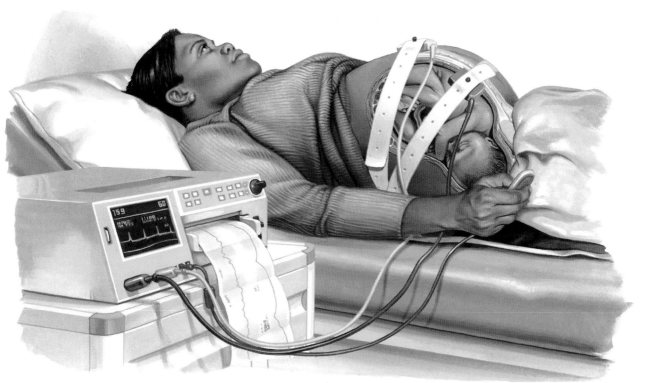

INTRODUCTION

Description: Bradycardia is a decrease in the baseline heart rate (generally below 120 beats per minute [bpm]). Moderate bradycardia is generally defined as 80 to 100 bpm, and severe bradycardia as less than 80 bpm, for more than 3 minutes.

Prevalence: Mild fetal bradycardia is seen during approximately 2% of labors.

Predominant Age: Reproductive.

Genetics: No genetic pattern.

ETIOLOGY AND PATHOGENESIS

Causes: Depressed fetal oxygenation (placental dysfunction, abruption); fetal acidosis. Effects of maternal condition (hypotension, medication, position, significant hypothermia); congenital fetal heart block; paracervical block; head compression (during final descent of the fetus especially in the occiput posterior position).

Risk Factors: Fetal hypoxia, reduced placental perfusion (maternal or fetal side), maternal sedation.

CLINICAL CHARACTERISTICS

Signs and Symptoms

- Baseline heart rate below 120 bpm (110 bpm in some countries or studies)

DIAGNOSTIC APPROACH

Differential Diagnosis

- Capture of maternal heart beat rather than that of the fetus

- Medication effects
- Prolonged deceleration
- Fetal anomaly (cardiac or other)
- Uterine hypertonus or tachysystole (resulting in fetal stress)
- Conduction anesthesia

Associated Conditions: Possible fetal hypoxia, depression, acidosis.

Workup and Evaluation

Laboratory: No evaluation indicated.

Imaging: Ultrasonography may identify abnormalities of the placenta (abruption) but plays a minor role in the evaluation of the fetus with bradycardia.

Special Tests: Fetal scalp pH or pulse oximetry (when available) may be of assistance in determining the fetal status.

Diagnostic Procedures: Clinical evaluation of mother and fetus.

Pathologic Findings

Based on underlying pathophysiologic conditions.

MANAGEMENT AND THERAPY

Nonpharmacologic

General Measures: Maternal hydration, change in maternal position (lateral recumbent), maternal oxygen therapy.

Specific Measures: Aggressive fetal and maternal evaluation, amnioinfusion, tocolytics (when hypertonus is involved), expedited delivery in the face of nonreassuring changes.

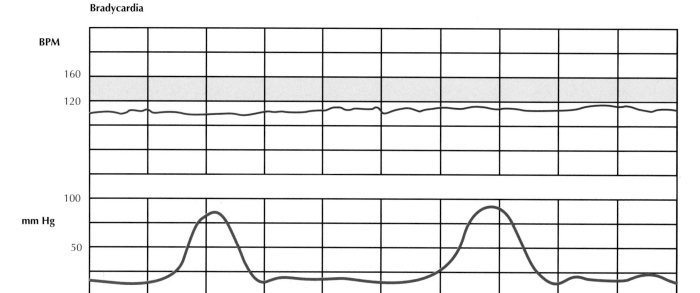

Bradycardia

BPM, beats per minute.

Patient Education: American College of Obstetricians and Gynecologists Patient Education Booklet AP015 (Fetal Heart Rate Monitoring During Labor), AP098 (Special Tests for Monitoring Fetal Health).

Drug(s) of Choice

(Tocolytics may be used if uterine tetany is thought to play a role in fetal stress.)

Contraindications: Tocolytics are relatively contraindicated in the absence of a diagnosis.

FOLLOW-UP

Patient Monitoring: Continued maternal and fetal assessment.

Prevention/Avoidance: Adequate maternal hydration, left lateral recumbent position for labor.

Possible Complications: Progressive deterioration of fetal status unless underlying processes are identified and corrected.

Expected Outcome: With aggressive diagnosis and management, outcome will generally be good.

MISCELLANEOUS

Other Notes: Intrapartum fetal heart rate monitoring is only one part of the overall evaluation of mother and fetus. This modality must be used to augment clinical judgment, not replace it.

REFERENCES

Level I
Rees SG, Thurlow JA, Gardner IC, et al: Maternal cardiovascular consequences of positioning after spinal anaesthesia for Caesarean section: left 15 degree table tilt vs. left lateral. Anaesthesia 2002;57:15.

Level II
Graham EM, Petersen SM, Christo DK, Fox HE: Intrapartum electronic fetal heart rate monitoring and the prevention of perinatal brain injury. Obstet Gynecol 2006;108:656.

Mardirosoff C, Dumont L, Boulvain M, Tramer MR: Fetal bradycardia due to intrathecal opioids for labour analgesia: a systematic review. BJOG 2002;109:274.

Level III
American College of Obstetricians and Gynecologists: Antepartum fetal surveillance. ACOG Practice Bulletin 9. Washington, DC, ACOG, 1999.

American College of Obstetricians and Gynecologists: Intrapartum fetal heart rate monitoring. ACOG Practice Bulletin 70. Obstet Gynecol 2005;106:1453.

Hon EH: Additional observations on "pathologic" bradycardia. Am J Obstet Gynecol 1974;118:428.

National Institute of Child Health and Human Development Research Planning Workshop: Electronic fetal heart rate monitoring: research guidelines for interpretation. Am J Obstet Gynecol 1997;177:1385.

Parer JT, King T: Fetal heart rate monitoring: is it salvageable? Am J Obstet Gynecol 2000;182:982.

Parer JT, Livingston EG: What is fetal distress? Am J Obstet Gynecol 1990;162:1421.

Rosen MA: Paracervical block for labor analgesia: a brief historic review. Am J Obstet Gynecol 2002;186:S127.

Schifrin BS: Fetal heart rate monitoring during labor. JAMA 1972;222:196.

Sweha A, Hacker TW, Nuovo J: Interpretation of the electronic fetal heart rate during labor. Am Fam Physician 1999;59:2487.

INTRODUCTION

Description: Periodic changes in the fetal heart rate in conjunction with uterine contractions may occur. These may indicate fetal stress when they are persistent, are progressively deeper, or become longer lasting. Recurrent decelerations are defined as occurring with ≥50% of contractions during a 20-minute period. In the United States, decelerations in the fetal heart rate are classified by their relationship to uterine activity: early, late, and variable. The shape of the deceleration is also significant in the classification. Accelerations higher than the baseline often accompany fetal movement and are reassuring.

Prevalence: Mild and transient periodic decelerations are not uncommon during the course of normal labor. Accelerations are documented in virtually all normal labors.

Predominant Age: Reproductive.

Genetics: No genetic pattern.

ETIOLOGY AND PATHOGENESIS

Causes:

* Accelerations
  Physiologic response to fetal activity or external stimuli (acoustic stimulation, scalp stimulation, fetal scalp blood sampling). Compensatory accelerations also occur following variable decelerations. These changes reflect an intact neurohormonal cardiovascular control system
* Early decelerations
  Physiologic response to head compression; dural stimulation mediated via the vagus nerve ("diving reflex"); these changes are not associated with hypoxia, academia, or low Apgar scores
* Variable decelerations
  Compensatory response to obstruction of umbilical blood flow
* Late decelerations
  Decreased fetal oxygenation with reflex bradycardia or myocardial depression; this type of deceleration suggests the greatest fetal stress despite the relatively modest change in heart rate

Risk Factors: Early: occiput posterior position, cephalopelvic disproportion. Variable: low amniotic fluid volume, cord prolapse, abnormal lie. Late: placental aging, reduced placental perfusion (maternal disease, vascular spasm, medications).

CLINICAL CHARACTERISTICS

Signs and Symptoms

* Accelerations
  Abrupt increase in fetal heart rate that reaches a maximum within 30 seconds
* Early decelerations

Shallow U-shaped, with gradual onset and resolution, generally (10 to 30 bpm), that reaches a nadir at the peak of uterine activity; rarely associated with heart rates below 100 to 110 bpm
* Variable decelerations
  Slowing with abrupt onset and return, frequently associated with accelerations before, after, or both; variable in depth and duration but coincide with the compression of the umbilical cord during contraction
* Late decelerations
  U-shaped, with gradual onset and resolution, generally shallow (10 to 30 bpm), and reaches a nadir after the peak of uterine activity; often associated with decreased variability

DIAGNOSTIC APPROACH

Differential Diagnosis

Variable Decelerations

* Cord compression
* Cord prolapse
* Head compression (less common, generally results in a more gradual deceleration that is proportional to the strength and duration of the contraction but may reflect maternal expulsive efforts)

Late Decelerations

* Uterine hypertonus or tachysystole
* Conduction anesthesia
* Maternal hypotension
* Placental abruption
* Medication effects

Associated Conditions: Oligohydramnios, preeclampsia, eclampsia, maternal hypertension, transient maternal hypotension, intrauterine growth restriction, placental abruption.

Workup and Evaluation

Laboratory: No evaluation indicated.

Imaging: Ultrasonography may be used to assess possible causes.

Special Tests: Fetal scalp pH or pulse oximetry (when available) may be of assistance in determining the fetal status.

Diagnostic Procedures: Clinical evaluation of mother and fetus.

Pathologic Findings

An elongated umbilical cord or an umbilical cord wrapped around the neck are frequently seen in the presence of variable decelerations. Placental findings often reflect underlying maternal or fetal disease associated with late decelerations.

Periodic changes

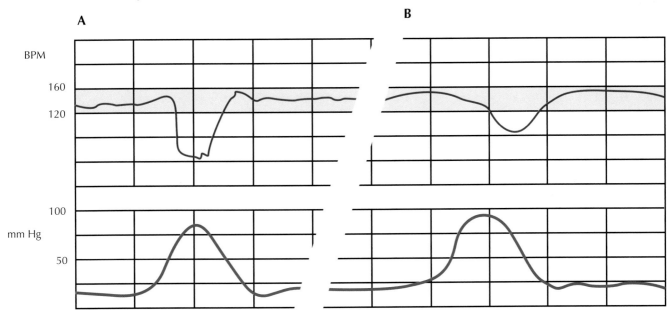

Variable decelerations (A) are generally sharp in contour, coincide with the contraction in a variable manner, and may have associated accelerations before or after. Late decelerations (B) are subtle with their nadir occurring after the peak of the contraction.

BPM, beats per minute.

MANAGEMENT AND THERAPY

Nonpharmacologic

General Measures: Maternal hydration, change in maternal position (lateral recumbent), maternal oxygen therapy.

Specific Measures: Aggressive fetal and maternal evaluation, amnioinfusion, tocolytics (when hypertonus is involved), expedited delivery in the face of nonreassuring changes.

Patient Education: American College of Obstetricians and Gynecologists Patient Education Booklet AP015 (Fetal Heart Rate Monitoring During Labor), AP098 (Special Tests for Monitoring Fetal Health).

Drug(s) of Choice

(Tocolytics may be used if uterine tetany or tachysystole are thought to play a role in fetal stress.)

Contraindications: Tocolytics are relatively contraindicated in the absence of a diagnosis.

FOLLOW-UP

Patient Monitoring: Continued maternal and fetal assessment.

Prevention/Avoidance: Adequate maternal hydration, left lateral recumbent position for labor. Continued assessment of fetal status in postdate pregnancies.

Possible Complications: Progressive deterioration of fetal status unless underlying processes are identified and corrected.

Expected Outcome: With aggressive diagnosis and management, outcome will generally be good.

MISCELLANEOUS

Other Notes: Intrapartum fetal heart rate monitoring is only one part of the overall evaluation of mother and fetus. This modality must be used to augment clinical judgment, not replace it.

REFERENCES

Level I
Ellison PH, Foster M, Sheridan-Pereira M, MacDonald D: Electronic fetal heart monitoring, auscultation, and neonatal outcome. Am J Obstet Gynecol 1991;164:1281.

Rinehart BK, Terrone DA, Barrow JH, et al: Randomized trial of intermittent or continuous amnioinfusion for variable decelerations. Obstet Gynecol 2000;96:571.

Level II
Graham EM, Petersen SM, Christo DK, Fox HE: Intrapartum electronic fetal heart rate monitoring and the prevention of perinatal brain injury. Obstet Gynecol 2006;108:656.

Nielsen PE, Erickson JR, Abouleish EI, et al: Fetal heart rate changes after intrathecal sufentanil or epidural bupivacaine for labor analgesia: incidence and clinical significance. Anesth Analg 1996; 83:742.

Level III
American College of Obstetricians and Gynecologists: Antepartum fetal surveillance. ACOG Practice Bulletin 9. Washington, DC, ACOG, 1999.

American College of Obstetricians and Gynecologists: Intrapartum fetal heart rate monitoring. ACOG Practice Bulletin 70. Obstet Gynecol 2005;106:1453.

Burrus DR, O'Shea TM Jr, Veille JC, Mueller-Heubach E: The predictive value of intrapartum fetal heart rate abnormalities in the extremely premature infant. Am J Obstet Gynecol 1994;171:1128.

Gardiner HM: Fetal echocardiography: 20 years of progress. Heart 2001;86:II12.

Larmay HJ, Strasburger JF: Differential diagnosis and management of the fetus and newborn with an irregular or abnormal heart rate. Pediatr Clin North Am 2004;51:1033.

National Institute of Child Health and Human Development Research Planning Workshop: Electronic fetal heart rate monitoring: research guidelines for interpretation. Am J Obstet Gynecol 1997;177:1385.

Parer JT, King T: Fetal heart rate monitoring: is it salvageable? Am J Obstet Gynecol 2000;182:982.

Parer JT, Livingston EG: What is fetal distress? Am J Obstet Gynecol 1990;162:1421.

Schifrin BS: Fetal heart rate monitoring during labor. JAMA 1972;222:196.

Sweha A, Hacker TW, Nuovo J: Interpretation of the electronic fetal heart rate during labor. Am Fam Physician 1999;59:2487.

INTRODUCTION

Description: Reduced variability is characterized by a reduction in the normal variation in heart rate from beat to beat that may signal fetal stress.

Prevalence: Reduced variability is a common finding when the fetal status is compromised. It also occurs when the fetus is sleeping.

Predominant Age: Reproductive.

Genetics: No genetic pattern.

ETIOLOGY AND PATHOGENESIS

Causes: Fetal hypoxia with neurologic depression (when decelerations are absent, reduced variability is unlikely to result from hypoxia); extreme prematurity; maternal sedation; fetal sleep.

Risk Factors: Prematurity, maternal sedation.

CLINICAL CHARACTERISTICS

Signs and Symptoms

* Reduction in the variation of heart rate to below 3 to 5 beats per minute (most commonly associated with periodic decelerations). This must be differentiated from the sinusoidal patterns of variations that have a smooth sine-wave–like pattern of regular frequency and amplitude.

DIAGNOSTIC APPROACH

Differential Diagnosis

* Uterine hypertonus or tachysystole
* Conduction anesthesia

* Maternal hypotension
* Placental abruption
* Medication effects (magnesium sulfate, sedatives)

Associated Conditions: Prematurity, fetal stress.

Workup and Evaluation

Laboratory: No evaluation indicated

Imaging: Ultrasonography may be used to assess possible causes.

Special Tests: Fetal scalp pH (when available) may be of assistance in determining the fetal status.

Diagnostic Procedures: Clinical evaluation of mother and fetus.

Pathologic Findings

None.

MANAGEMENT AND THERAPY

Nonpharmacologic

General Measures: Maternal hydration, change in maternal position (lateral recumbent), maternal oxygen therapy.

Specific Measures: Aggressive fetal and maternal evaluation, amnioinfusion, tocolytics (when hypertonus is involved), expedited delivery in the face of nonreassuring changes.

Patient Education: American College of Obstetricians and Gynecologists Patient Education Booklet AP015 (Fetal Heart Rate Monitoring During Labor), AP098 (Special Tests for Monitoring Fetal Health).

Reduced variablility

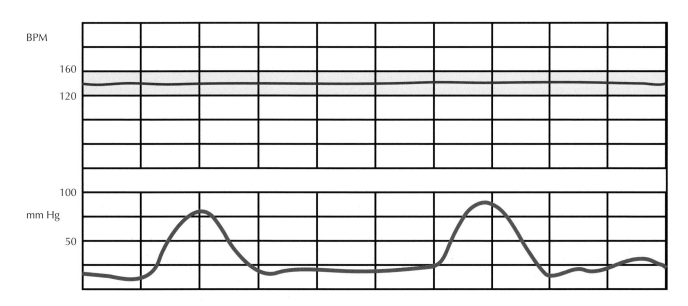

BPM, beats per minute.

Drug(s) of Choice

(Tocolytics may be used if uterine tetany or tachysystole are thought to play a role in fetal stress.)

Contraindications: Tocolytics are relatively contraindicated in the absence of a diagnosis.

FOLLOW-UP

Patient Monitoring: Continued maternal and fetal assessment.

Prevention/Avoidance: Adequate maternal hydration, left lateral recumbent position for labor.

Possible Complications: Progressive deterioration of fetal status unless underlying processes are identified and corrected.

Expected Outcome: With aggressive diagnosis and management, outcome will generally be good.

MISCELLANEOUS

Other Notes: When the fetal heart rate is increased, there is an apparent reduction in beat-to-beat variability based solely on physiologic constraints and does not reflect fetal stress.

Intrapartum fetal heart rate monitoring is only one part of the overall evaluation of mother and fetus. This modality must be used to augment clinical judgment, not replace it.

REFERENCES

Level I

Ellison PH, Foster M, Sheridan-Pereira M, MacDonald D: Electronic fetal heart monitoring, auscultation, and neonatal outcome. Am J Obstet Gynecol 1991;164:1281.

Hallak M, Martinez-Poyer J, Kruger ML, et al: The effect of magnesium sulfate on fetal heart rate parameters: a randomized, placebo-controlled trial. Am J Obstet Gynecol 1999;181:1122.

Level II

Davidson SR, Rankin JHG, Martin CB Jr, Reid DL: Fetal heart rate variability and behavioral state: analysis by poser spectrum. Am J Obstet Gynecol 1992;167:717.

Graham EM, Petersen SM, Christo DK, Fox HE: Intrapartum electronic fetal heart rate monitoring and the prevention of perinatal brain injury. Obstet Gynecol 2006;108:656.

Siira SM, Ojala TH, Vahlberg TJ, et al: Marked fetal acidosis and specific changes in power spectrum analysis of fetal heart rate variability recorded during the last hour of labour. BJOG 2005; 112:418.

Viscomi CM, Hood DD, Melone PJ, Eisenach JC: Fetal heart rate variability after epidural fentanyl during labor. Anesth Analg 1990;71:679.

Level III

American College of Obstetricians and Gynecologists: Antepartum fetal surveillance. ACOG Practice Bulletin 9. Washington, DC, ACOG, 1999.

American College of Obstetricians and Gynecologists: Intrapartum fetal heart rate monitoring. ACOG Practice Bulletin 70. Obstet Gynecol 2005;106:1453.

Burrus DR, O'Shea TM Jr, Veille JC, Mueller-Heubach E: The predictive value of intrapartum fetal heart rate abnormalities in the extremely premature infant. Am J Obstet Gynecol 1994;171:1128.

Gardiner HM. Fetal echocardiography: 20 years of progress. Heart 2001;86:II12.

National Institute of Child Health and Human Development Research Planning Workshop: Electronic fetal heart rate monitoring: research guidelines for interpretation. Am J Obstet Gynecol 1997;177:1385.

Parer JT, King T: Fetal heart rate monitoring: is it salvageable? Am J Obstet Gynecol 2000;182:982.

Parer JT, Livingston EG: What is fetal distress? Am J Obstet Gynecol 1990;162:1421.

Samueloff A, Langer O, Berkus M, et al: Is fetal heart rate variability a good predictor of fetal outcome? Acta Obstet Gynecol Scand 1994;73:39.

Schifrin BS: Fetal heart rate monitoring during labor. JAMA 1972;222:196.

Sweha A, Hacker TW, Nuovo J: Interpretation of the electronic fetal heart rate during labor. Am Fam Physician 1999;59:2487.

INTRODUCTION

Description: Tachycardia is an increase in the baseline heart rate (generally above 160 beats per minute [bpm]). Mild tachycardia is generally defined as 161 to 180 bpm, and severe tachycardia as greater than 180 bpm, for more than 3 minutes.

Prevalence: Mild fetal tachycardia is seen during approximately 2% of labors.

Predominant Age: Reproductive.

Genetics: No genetic pattern.

ETIOLOGY AND PATHOGENESIS

Causes: Maternal fever (most common); intra-amniotic infection (fetal tachycardia may occur even before maternal fever is present); fetal congenital heart disease; depressed fetal oxygenation; fetal acidosis; fetal anemia or blood loss; medication effects (atropine, terbutaline); maternal hypotension.

Risk Factors: Maternal, fetal, or uterine infection.

CLINICAL CHARACTERISTICS

Signs and Symptoms

- Increased fetal heart rate (baseline) above 160 bpm (frequently associated with an apparent loss of beat-to-beat variability)

DIAGNOSTIC APPROACH

Differential Diagnosis

- Maternal fever (chorioamnionitis)
- Intra-amniotic infection
- Congenital heart disease
- Fetal anemia or blood loss
- Medication effects
- Uterine rupture

Associated Conditions: Chorioamnionitis, maternal fever, maternal dehydration.

Workup and Evaluation

Laboratory: No evaluation indicated.

Imaging: No imaging indicated.

Special Tests: Fetal scalp pH or pulse oximetry (when available) may be of assistance in determining the fetal status.

Diagnostic Procedures: Clinical evaluation of mother and fetus.

Pathologic Findings

Based on underlying pathophysiologic conditions.

MANAGEMENT AND THERAPY

Nonpharmacologic

General Measures: Maternal hydration, change in maternal position (lateral recumbent), maternal oxygen therapy.

Specific Measures: Aggressive fetal and maternal evaluation, amnioinfusion, tocolytics (when hypertonus is involved), expedited delivery in the face of nonreassuring changes.

Patient Education: American College of Obstetricians and Gynecologists Patient Education Booklet AP015

Tachycardia

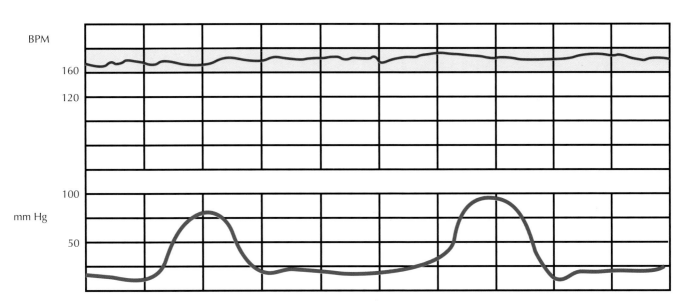

BPM, beats per minute.

(Fetal Heart Rate Monitoring During Labor), AP098 (Special Tests for Monitoring Fetal Health).

Drug(s) of Choice

None (digoxin therapy for selected fetal tachyarrhythmias, such as fetal supraventricular tachycardia, may be indicated).

FOLLOW-UP

Patient Monitoring: Continued maternal and fetal assessment.

Prevention/Avoidance: Adequate maternal hydration, reduced number of cervical examinations in patients at risk for infection (premature rupture of the membranes).

Possible Complications: Progressive deterioration of fetal status unless underlying processes are identified and corrected.

Expected Outcome: With aggressive diagnosis and management, outcome will generally be good.

MISCELLANEOUS

Other Notes: When the fetal heart rate is increased, there is an apparent reduction in beat-to-beat variability based solely on physiologic constraints and does not reflect fetal stress.

Intrapartum fetal heart rate monitoring is only one part of the overall evaluation of mother and fetus. This modality must be used to augment clinical judgment, not replace it.

REFERENCES

Level II
Graham EM, Petersen SM, Christo DK, Fox HE: Intrapartum electronic fetal heart rate monitoring and the prevention of perinatal brain injury. Obstet Gynecol 2006;108:656.

Level III
American College of Obstetricians and Gynecologists: Antepartum fetal surveillance. ACOG Practice Bulletin 9. Washington, DC, ACOG, 1999. ACOG Practice Bulletin 9.

American College of Obstetricians and Gynecologists: Intrapartum fetal heart rate monitoring. ACOG Practice Bulletin 70. Obstet Gynecol 2005;106:1453.

Burrus DR, O'Shea TM Jr, Veille JC, Mueller-Heubach E: The predictive value of intrapartum fetal heart rate abnormalities in the extremely premature infant. Am J Obstet Gynecol 1994;171:1128.

Gardiner HM: Fetal echocardiography: 20 years of progress. Heart 2001;86:II12.

Jones LM, Garmel SH: Successful digoxin therapy of fetal supraventricular tachycardia in a triplet pregnancy. Obstet Gynecol 2001;98:921.

Larmay HJ, Strasburger JF: Differential diagnosis and management of the fetus and newborn with an irregular or abnormal heart rate. Pediatr Clin North Am 2004;51:1033.

National Institute of Child Health and Human Development Research Planning Workshop: Electronic fetal heart rate monitoring: research guidelines for interpretation. Am J Obstet Gynecol 1997;177:1385.

Parer JT, King T: Fetal heart rate monitoring: is it salvageable? Am J Obstet Gynecol 2000;182:982.

Parer JT, Livingston EG: What is fetal distress? Am J Obstet Gynecol 1990;162:1421.

Schifrin BS: Fetal heart rate monitoring during labor. JAMA 1972;222:196.

Sweha A, Hacker TW, Nuovo J: Interpretation of the electronic fetal heart rate during labor. Am Fam Physician 1999;59:2487.

van Engelen AD, Weijtens O, Brenner JI, et al: Management outcome and follow-up of fetal tachycardia. J Am Coll Cardiol 1994;24:1371.

THE CHALLENGE

To assist patients in successfully nursing their infant(s).

Scope of the Problem: In 2005, 72.9% of new U.S. mothers initiated breastfeeding; however, only about 41% of infants are breastfed after 6 months.

Objectives of Management: Encourage nursing as feeding strategy, assist patients to prepare for nursing and to deal with problems if they occur.

TACTICS

Relevant Pathophysiology: Breastfeeding is the preferred method of feeding for newborns and infants. Evidence continues to mount regarding the value of breastfeeding for both women and their infants. Breastfed infants have fewer respiratory, gastrointestinal, and ear (otitis media) infections and fewer allergies. Breast milk is more easily digested, better absorbed, and less constipating than formula. Breastfeeding hastens uterine involution. Stimulation of the areola causes the secretion of oxytocin, which is responsible for the letdown reflex and ductal contraction that expels the milk. Suckling stimulates further milk production. Milk production is often not well established until day 3 of nursing. Patients should maintain adequate fluid intake and an increase of approximately 200 kcal/day in dietary intake. Prenatal vitamin supplementation should be continued. Blocked ducts and mastitis are the most common complications. Mastitis mimics blocked ducts (sore, firm lump or lumps) with the addition of erythema and fever. Warm, moist packs; analgesics; and antibiotics that are effective against *Staphylococcus aureus* are appropriate therapies. Infection comes from the infant's nose and mouth. Other sources of fever must also be considered (endometritis).

Strategies: Preparation for nursing—encourage breastfeeding, discuss plans early, address issues such as work and weaning, discuss the role of supplementation, and introduce techniques. Involvement of the father and others increases the chance of success. Preparation of the nipples in advance is not required.

Nursing—initially the infant should nurse at least nine times in 24 hours to encourage milk production. Once milk production is established, the infant should dictate the frequency and duration of nursing—six or more wet diapers per day and a weight gain of approximately 1 oz/day indicate adequate feeding. The breasts should be hard before and soft after nursing.

Weaning—introduce the bottle by 3 to 4 weeks as an occasional supplement (may use pumped breast milk). Complete weaning may be done either gradually (substituting bottles for some feedings) or abruptly. If engorgement occurs, analgesia, ice, and compressive binding provide the greatest relief. Medication to suppress lactation is generally not effective.

Patient Education: Reassurance, support, specific suggestions; American College of Obstetricians and Gynecologists Patient Education Pamphlet AP029 (Breastfeeding Your Baby).

IMPLEMENTATION

Special Considerations: Breastfeeding is contraindicated in patients with human immunodeficiency virus (HIV), cytomegalovirus, hepatitis B virus infections, and human T-cell lymphotropic virus type I or type II and in those who have active untreated tuberculosis or varicella or active herpes simplex virus with breast lesions. Substances of abuse (including alcohol) pass to breast milk, as do some medications. Breastfed infants often lose weight in the first few days and do not regain birthweight until as late as day 10. Growth spurts often occur at about 10 days, 6 weeks, 3 months, and 4 to 6 months. If the infant fails to thrive, support and evaluation are in order. Care must be taken to wash the hands (and any equipment used) well before breastfeeding or breast manipulation. The nipples and the infant's face should also be clean before each feeding. Fresh breast milk may be safely kept for 6 to 10 hours at room temperature or 72 hours under refrigeration. Breast milk may also be frozen and kept for 6 months in a home freezer or 12 months at −20°C. Thawed breast milk should be used within 24 hours and may not be refrozen. Breast milk should never be warmed in a microwave oven. The volume of milk required for each feeding varies widely but is normally between 2 and 5 oz for newborns, 4 to 6 oz for infants 2 to 4 months of age, and 5 to 7 oz for babies 4 to 6 months old. One study found that 65% of women with augmentation mammoplasty have lactation insufficiency.

REFERENCES

Level I

Lavender T, Baker L, Smyth R, et al: Breastfeeding expectations versus reality: a cluster randomised controlled trial. BJOG 2005; 112:1047.

Mattar CN, Chong YS, Chan YS, et al: Simple antenatal preparation to improve breastfeeding practice: a randomized controlled trial. Obstet Gynecol 2007;109:73.

Merewood A, Chamberlain LB, Cook JT, et al: The effect of peer counselors on breastfeeding rates in the neonatal intensive care unit: results of a randomized controlled trial. Arch Pediatr Adolesc Med. 2006;160:681.

Wolfberg AJ, Michels KB, Shields W, et al: Dads as breastfeeding advocates: results from a randomized controlled trial of an educational intervention. Am J Obstet Gynecol 2004;191:708.

Level II

Britton JR, Britton HL, Gronwaldt V: Breastfeeding, sensitivity, and attachment. Pediatrics 2006;118:e1436.

Centers for Disease Control and Prevention: Breastfeeding: data and statistics: Breastfeeding practices—Results from the 2005 National Immunization Survey. Atlanta, CDC. Available at http://www.cdc.gov/breastfeeding/data/NIS_data/data_2004.htm. Accessed September 4, 2007.

Collaborative Group on Hormonal Factors in Breast Cancer: Breast cancer and breastfeeding: collaborative reanalysis of individual data from 47 epidemiological studies in 30 countries, including 50302 women with breast cancer and 96973 women without the disease. Lancet 2002;360:187.

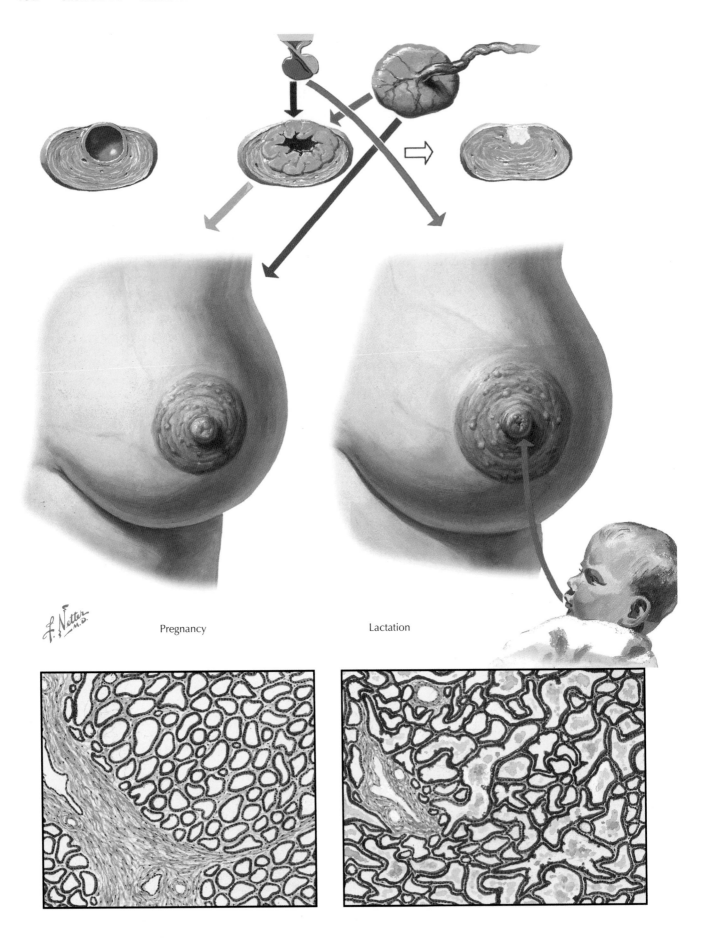

Pregnancy

Lactation

Coutinho SB, de Lira PI, de Carvalho Lima M, Ashworth A: Comparison of the effect of two systems for the promotion of exclusive breastfeeding. Lancet 2005;366:1094.

Klement E, Cohen RV, Boxman J, et al: Breastfeeding and risk of inflammatory bowel disease: a systematic review with meta-analysis. Am J Clin Nutr 2004;80:1342.

Luzuriaga K, Newell ML, Dabis F, et al: Vaccines to prevent transmission of HIV-1 via breastmilk: scientific and logistical priorities. Lancet 2006;368:511.

Martin RM, Goodall SH, Gunnell D, Davey Smith G: Breast feeding in infancy and social mobility: 60-year follow-up of the Boyd Orr cohort. Arch Dis Child 2007;92:317. Epub 2007 Feb 14.

Pisacane A, Continisio GI, Aldinucci M, et al: A controlled trial of the father's role in breastfeeding promotion. Pediatrics 2005;116:e494.

Sadeharju K, Knip M, Virtanen SM, et al; Finnish TRIGR Study Group: Maternal antibodies in breast milk protect the child from enterovirus infections. Pediatrics 2007;119:941.

Level III

American Academy of Pediatrics, American College of Obstetricians and Gynecologists: Breastfeeding handbook for physicians. Elk Grove Village, IL, AAP; Washington, DC, ACOG, 2006.

American College of Obstetricians and Gynecologists: Breastfeeding: Maternal and infant aspects. Special report from ACOG. ACOG Clin Rev 2007;12:1S.

American College of Obstetricians and Gynecologists: Breastfeeding: Maternal and infant aspects. ACOG Committee Opinion 361. Obstet Gynecol 2007;109:279.

Friedman NJ, Zeiger RS: The role of breast-feeding in the development of allergies and asthma. J Allergy Clin Immunol 2005;115:1238.

Gray GE, McIntyre JA: HIV and pregnancy. BMJ 2007;334:950.

Mattar CN, Chan YS, Chong YS: Breastfeeding: it's an important gift. Obstet Gynecol 2003;102:1414.

Sau A, Clarke S, Bass J, et al: Azathioprine and breastfeeding: is it safe? BJOG 2007;114:498. Epub 2007 Jan 25.

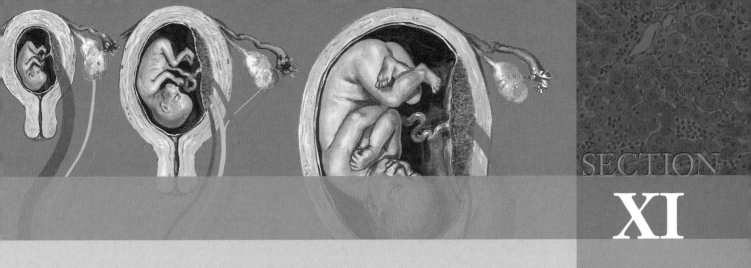

Obstetric Conditions and Concerns

INTRODUCTION

Description: Failure of the normal process of decidua formation results in a placental implantation in which the villi adhere directly to (accreta, 78%), invade into (increta, 17%), or go through (percreta, 5%) the myometrium. One portion (partial) or all (total) of the placenta may be involved.

Prevalence: Difficult to assess; estimates vary from 1 in 1667 to 1 in 70,000 pregnancies (average 1 in 7000).

Predominant Age: Reproductive, average 29.

Genetics: No genetic pattern.

ETIOLOGY AND PATHOGENESIS

Causes: Abnormal decidua formation at the time of placental implantation. (Imperfect development of the fibrinoid [Nitabuch's] layer.) Abnormal site of placental implantation (previa, 64% of placenta accreta, cornual or lower uterine segment, or uterine scars such as site of previous cesarean delivery).

Risk Factors: Placenta previa (without previous uterine surgery 5%, with previous surgery 15% to 70%), previous cesarean delivery, multigravidity (1 of 500,000 for parity <3, 1 of 2500 for parity >6), older pregnant women, previous uterine curettage, previous uterine sepsis, previous manual removal of the placenta, leiomyomata, uterine malformation, prior abortion, endometrial ablation.

CLINICAL CHARACTERISTICS

Signs and Symptoms

- Failure of normal placental separation
- Abnormally heavy bleeding after delivery of the placenta (may be life threatening)
- History of antepartum hemorrhage

DIAGNOSTIC APPROACH

Differential Diagnosis

- Placenta previa
- Uterine rupture with expulsion of the placenta
- Uterine rupture at the time of manual removal of the placenta

Associated Conditions: Placenta previa (15%), postpartum hemorrhage.

Workup and Evaluation

Laboratory: Complete blood count after delivery to assess blood loss (which may be excessive).

Imaging: No imaging indicated. (Ultrasonography has been used to make the diagnosis before labor in unusual cases. Low-lying placentas noted in studies performed at less than 30 weeks may "migrate," leaving the cervix free at term [up to 90% of cases].)

Special Tests: None indicated.

Diagnostic Procedures: Generally diagnosed only at delivery by failure of the normal separation mechanism. Final diagnosis is established histologically.

Pathologic Findings

Absence of the decidua basalis (replaced by loose connective tissue). The decidua parietalis may be normal or absent. The villi may be separated from the myometrial cells by a layer of fibrin.

MANAGEMENT AND THERAPY

Nonpharmacologic

General Measures: Aggressive fluid and blood support as necessary. Oxytocin or other uterotonic agents to promote uterine contractions after placental delivery (if accomplished).

Specific Measures: Most patients require hysterectomy. If the invasion of the myometrium is incomplete and the bladder is spared, conservative management by uterine packing may be possible. Any time the diagnosis is considered, preparations for hysterectomy, including anesthesia, instruments, and adequate blood, should be ready before any attempt is made to free the placenta.

Diet: Nothing by mouth until the patient's condition has been stabilized.

Activity: Bed rest until the patient's condition has been stabilized.

Patient Education: American College of Obstetricians and Gynecologists Patient Education Pamphlet AP038 (Bleeding During Pregnancy), AP006 (Cesarean Birth), AP025 (Ultrasound Exams).

Drug(s) of Choice

Uterotonics should be available, and broad-spectrum antibiotics should be given prophylactically.

FOLLOW-UP

Patient Monitoring: Hemodynamic monitoring during the acute diagnosis and treatment.

Prevention/Avoidance: Patients at high risk may be studied by ultrasonography in an attempt to identify the absence of the subplacental hypoechoic zone or the presence of lacunar blood-flow patterns. If present, plans for autologous blood donation and elective cesarean hysterectomy may be made. The absence of these findings does not rule out this possibility.

Possible Complications: Life-threatening hemorrhage may occur; maternal mortality of 2% to 6% has been reported for treatment by hysterectomy and up to 30% for conservative management. Coagulopathy secondary to blood loss and replacement is common. Spontaneous rupture of the uterus may occur before labor. Rupture of the uterus or inversion may occur during attempts to remove the placenta.

Expected Outcome: Most patients go to term with normal fetal development. If the possibility is recognized and appropriate treatment is rendered, maternal survival is probable, although loss of the uterus is common. It is hypothesized that small areas of accreta may result in placental cotyledon(s) being torn from the placenta and that these cotyledons may become placental polyps.

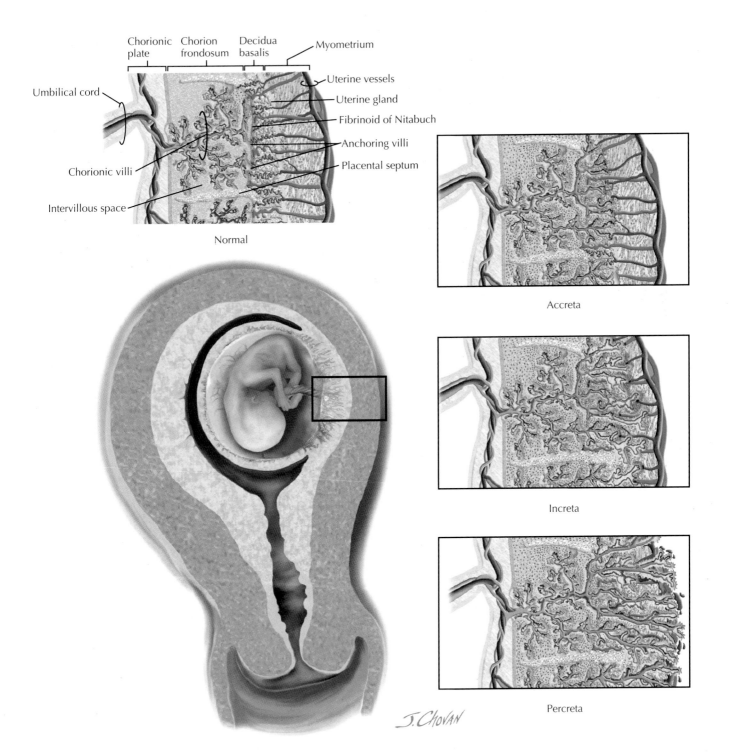

Normal

Accreta

Increta

Percreta

J. CHOVAN

MISCELLANEOUS

ICD-9-CM Codes: 667.0 (All types, without hemorrhage), 666.0 (All types, with hemorrhage).

REFERENCES

Level II

Silver RM, Landon MB, Rouse DJ, et al; National Institute of Child Health and Human Development Maternal-Fetal Medicine Units Network: Maternal morbidity associated with multiple repeat cesarean deliveries. Obstet Gynecol 2006;107:1226.

Level III

Abbas F, Talati J, Wasti S, et al: Placenta percreta with bladder invasion as a cause of life-threatening hemorrhage. J Urol 2000; 164:1270.

American College of Obstetricians and Gynecologists: Placental pathology. ACOG Committee Opinion 102. Washington, DC, ACOG, 1991.

American College of Obstetricians and Gynecologists: Guidelines for diagnostic imaging during pregnancy. ACOG Committee Opinion 299. Obstet Gynecol 2004;104:647.

American College of Obstetricians and Gynecologists: Postpartum hemorrhage. ACOG Practice Bulletin 76. Obstet Gynecol 2006; 108:1039.

American College of Obstetricians and Gynecologists: Endometrial ablation: ACOG Practice Bulletin 81. Obstet Gynecol 2007; 109:1233.

Ash A, Smith A, Maxwell D: Caesarean scar pregnancy. BJOG 2007;114:253.

Booher D, Little B: Vaginal hemorrhage in pregnancy. N Engl J Med 1974;290:611.

Breen J, Neubecker R, Gregori C, Franklin J: Placenta accreta, increta and percreta. Obstet Gynecol 1977;49:43.

Clark SL, Koonings PP, Phelan JP: Placenta previa/accreta and prior cesarean section. Obstet Gynecol 1985;66:89.

Clark SL, Phelan JP, Yeh SY, et al: Hypogastric artery ligation for obstetric hemorrhage. Obstet Gynecol 1985;66:353.

Cotton DB, Read JA, Paul RH, Quilligan EJ: The conservative aggressive management of placenta previa. Am J Obstet Gynecol 1980;137:687.

Cox SM, Carpenter RJ, Cotton DB: Placenta percreta: ultrasound diagnosis and conservative surgical management. Obstet Gynecol 1988;72:452.

Morison JE: Placenta accreta: a clinicopathologic review of 67 cases. Obstet Gynecol Annu 1978;7:107.

Oyelese Y, Smulian JC: Placenta previa, placenta accreta, and vasa previa. Obstet Gynecol 2006;107:927.

Price FV, Resnik E, Heller KA, Christopherson WA: Placenta previa percreta involving the urinary bladder: a report of two cases and review of the literature. Obstet Gynecol 1991;78:508.

Read JA, Cotton DB, Miller FC: Placenta accreta: changing clinical aspects and outcome. Obstet Gynecol 1980;56:31.

Teteris NJ, Lina AA, Holaday WJ: Placenta percreta. Obstet Gynecol 1976;47:15S.

THE CHALLENGE

Active management of labor is a system of labor management designed to promote effective labor and reduce the need for cesarean delivery.

Scope of the Problem: Cesarean birth rate for nulliparous patients approximates 30% in many areas. Active management has been associated with cesarean delivery rates of less than 5% for its developers (Ireland).

Objectives of Management: To reduce cesarean delivery rates through a system of management that includes education, strict criteria for labor and abnormal progress, one-on-one care, and the use of high-dose oxytocin (when needed).

TACTICS

Relevant Pathophysiology: As developed in Ireland, active management of labor is based on the following:
- Patient education
- Strict criteria for the diagnosis of labor, the determination of abnormal progress, and the diagnosis of fetal compromise
- One-on-one nursing care during labor
- Use of high-dose oxytocin infusion (when needed)
- Peer review of all operative deliveries

Strategies: In Ireland, where this technique was developed, active management of labor is restricted to nulliparous patients with singleton pregnancies in vertex presentation with no evidence of fetal compromise. Women are carefully instructed to come to the hospital early in labor. Labor is confirmed by the presence of complete effacement, the passage of the mucous plug, or rupture of the membranes. If these criteria are met, the patient is admitted to the hospital and the membranes are ruptured within 1 hour (if not already ruptured). Vaginal examination is performed hourly, and administration of high-dose oxytocin is begun if dilation falls below 1 cm/hour. Oxytocin is begun at 6 mU/min, and the dose is increased every 15 minutes until a maximum of 40 mU/min is reached, active labor is established, or hyperstimulation occurs. As a part of this process, one-on-one nursing care is provided, and fetal status is assessed by auscultation every 5 minutes. Fetal compromise is diagnosed by fetal scalp pH. Cesarean delivery is performed if delivery is not imminent 12 hours after admission or if fetal compromise is diagnosed.

Patient Education: American College of Obstetricians and Gynecologists Patient Education Pamphlet AP004 (How to Tell When Labor Begins).

IMPLEMENTATION

Special Considerations: The Irish experience with active management of labor has resulted in a reduced rate of births by cesarean delivery without untoward events. Which elements of the management (education, early amniotomy, intensive nursing, aggressive use of oxytocin, or methods of establishing distress) are directly responsible for this success is unknown. Attempts to apply only some elements of the program have generally not yielded the same reductions in cesarean section rates. It should be noted that conduction (epidural) anesthesia is also less common in Ireland.

REFERENCES

Level I

Bolnick JM, Velazquez MD, Gonzalez JL, et al: Randomized trial between two active labor management protocols in the presence of an unfavorable cervix. Am J Obstet Gynecol 2004;190:124.

Cohen GR, O'Brien WF, Lewis L, Knuppel RA: A prospective randomized study of the aggressive management of early labor. Am J Obstet Gynecol 1987;157:1174.

Frigoletto FD Jr, Lieberman E, Lang JM, et al: A clinical trial of active management of labor. N Engl J Med 1995;333:745.

Lavender T, Alfirevic Z, Walkinshaw S: Partogram action line study: a randomised trial. Br J Obstet Gynaecol 1998;105:976.

Lopez-Zeno JA, Peaceman AM, Adashek JA, Socol ML: A controlled trial of a program for the active management of labor. N Engl J Med 1992;326:450.

Pattinson RC, Howarth GR, Mdluli W, et al: Aggressive or expectant management of labour: a randomised clinical trial. BJOG 2003;110:457.

Rogers J, Wood J, McCandlish R, et al: Active versus expectant management of third stage of labour: the Hinchingbrooke randomised controlled trial. Lancet 1998;351:693.

Rogers RG, Gardner MO, Tool KJ, et al: Active management of labor: a cost analysis of a randomized controlled trial. West J Med 2000;172:240.

Sadler LC, Davison T, McCowan LM: A randomised controlled trial and meta-analysis of active management of labour. BJOG 2000; 107:909.

Shetty A, Stewart K, Stewart G, et al: Active management of term prelabour rupture of membranes with oral misoprostol. BJOG 2002;109:1354.

Level II

Alexander JM, Lucas MJ, Ramin SM, et al: The course of labor with and without epidural analgesia. Am J Obstet Gynecol 1998; 178:516.

Fraser W, Vendittelli F, Krauss I, Breart G: Effects of early augmentation of labour with amniotomy and oxytocin in nulliparous women: a meta-analysis. Br J Obstet Gynaecol 1998;105:189.

Frigoletto FD Jr, Lieberman E, Lang JM, et al: A clinical trial of active management of labor. N Engl J Med 1995;333:745.

Rouse DJ, Owen J, Hauth JC: Active-phase labor arrest: oxytocin augmentation for at least 4 hours. Obstet Gynecol 1999;93:323.

Level III

American College of Obstetricians and Gynecologists: Induction of labor. ACOG Practice Bulletin 10. Washington, DC, ACOG, 1999.

American College of Obstetricians and Gynecologists: Dystocia and augmentation of labor. ACOG Practice Bulletin 49. Obstet Gynecol 2003;102:1445.

Leighton BL, Halpern SH, Wilson DB: Lumbar sympathetic blocks speed early and second stage induced labor in nulliparous women. Anesthesiology 1999;90:1039.

Peaceman AM, Socol ML: Active management of labor. Am J Obstet Gynecol 1996;175:363.

Rogers R, Gilson G, Kammerer-Doak D: Epidural analgesia and active management of labor: effects on length of labor and mode of delivery. Obstet Gynecol 1999;93:995.

Rogers R, Gilson GJ, Miller AC, et al: Active management of labor: does it make a difference? Am J Obstet Gynecol 1997;177:599.

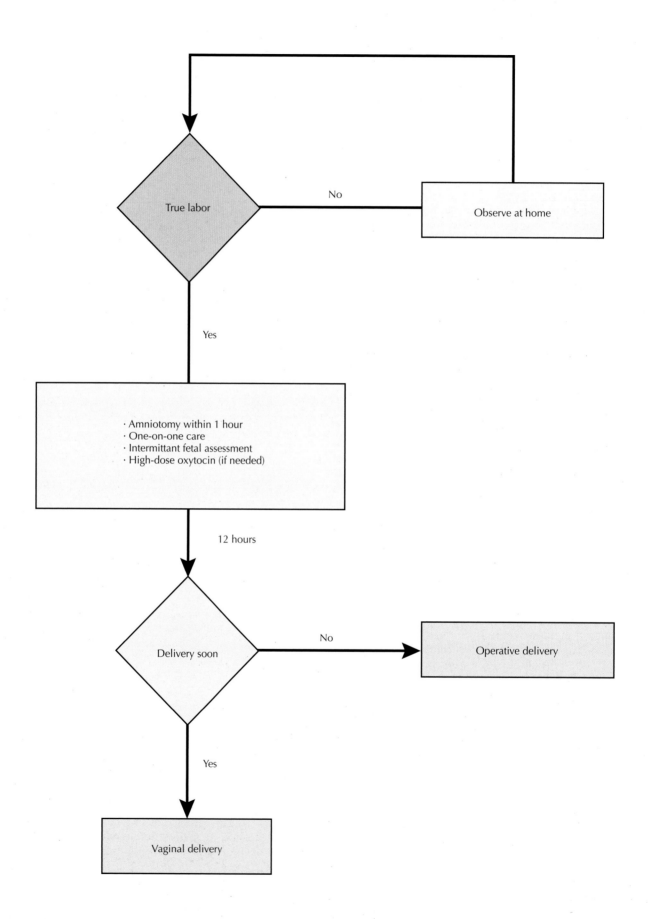

INTRODUCTION

Description: Acute fatty liver is a rare complication of pregnancy that results in acute liver failure, often with catastrophic consequences. It is also known as acute fatty metamorphosis or acute yellow atrophy.

Prevalence: One of 10,000 to 15,000 pregnancies.

Predominant Age: Reproductive.

Genetics: There appears to be a link to a recessively inherited mitochondrial abnormality of fatty acid oxidation, first studied in children with Reye syndrome. The most common defect is a mutation coding for long-chain-3-hydroxyacyl-CoA-dehydrogenase (LCHAD).

ETIOLOGY AND PATHOGENESIS

Causes: Unknown (mimics other forms of fatty liver failure such as that induced by tetracycline in patients with impaired renal function, Reye's syndrome, hepatotoxicity with sodium valproate, or salicylate intoxication). It is currently thought that the placenta of a fetus who is LCHAD deficient may produce a toxic metabolite that affects the maternal liver.

Risk Factors: Unknown. More common in nulliparous women, when a male fetus is present, or in multifetal gestation. The risk of recurrence in subsequent pregnancies is low, although it may be higher if the woman has a fetus who is homozygous enzyme-deficient.

CLINICAL CHARACTERISTICS

Signs and Symptoms

- Average gestational age: 37.5 weeks
- Gradual onset of malaise, anorexia, nausea and persistent vomiting, epigastric pain, and progressive jaundice
- Hypertension, proteinuria, and edema (50% of patients)
- Hypofibrinogenemia, prolonged clotting time, hyperbilirubinemia (<10 mg/dL), mild thrombocytopenia, hemolysis, markedly reduced antithrombin III levels, (severe coagulopathy in 55%), hypoglycemia.
- Elevated serum transaminase levels (300 to 500 U/L), hepatic encephalopathy (60%)

DIAGNOSTIC APPROACH

Differential Diagnosis

- Hepatitis
- Hemolysis, elevated liver enzymes, low platelet count (HELLP) syndrome
- Pre-eclampsia
- Cholestatic jaundice
- Cholelithiasis

Associated Conditions: Hypoglycemia and hepatic coma, coagulopathy, renal failure, sepsis, aspiration, circulatory collapse, pancreatitis, and gastrointestinal bleeding are all common.

Workup and Evaluation

Laboratory: Complete blood count, evaluation of liver function, serum bilirubin, clotting studies, serum ammonia.

Imaging: Ultrasonography, computed tomography, or magnetic resonance imaging may demonstrate the fatty metamorphosis, but false-negative results may be as high as 80%.

Special Tests: None indicated.

Diagnostic Procedures: History, physical and laboratory examinations.

Pathologic Findings

Grossly the liver is small, soft, yellow, and greasy. Histologically there are swollen hepatocytes with microvesicular fat and central nuclei and periportal sparing. There may also be lipid accumulation within renal tubular cells.

MANAGEMENT AND THERAPY

Nonpharmacologic

General Measures: Rapid evaluation, supportive measures.

Specific Measures: The only specific measure is delivery, which generally arrests the process. The decision between cesarean or vaginal birth remains uncertain and controversial. Transfusion with fresh-frozen plasma, cryoprecipitate, whole blood, packed red blood cells, and platelets may be necessary if surgery is planned or bleeding ensues. Liver transplantation may have to be considered in selected patients.

Diet: Nothing by mouth.

Activity: Strict bed rest. Often requires admission to intensive care facilities.

Drug(s) of Choice

No specific medications. Other medications based on symptoms and condition.

FOLLOW-UP

Patient Monitoring: Intensive monitoring for circulatory, renal, and hepatic collapse. Often the fetus is severely compromised (often dead at the time of diagnosis) and also requires intensive monitoring.

Prevention/Avoidance: None.

Possible Complications: At one time, this was frequently fatal for both mother (75%) and fetus (90%); lower mortality rates have been reported in recent studies (as low as 10% maternal and 20% fetal mortality). Hypoglycemia and hepatic coma (60% of patients), coagulopathy (55%), and renal failure (50%) may occur. Sepsis, aspiration, circulatory collapse, pancreatitis, and gastrointestinal bleeding are all common.

Expected Outcome: May be fatal for both mother and fetus. If the diagnosis is established and delivery is

Hepatic Disease in Pregnancy

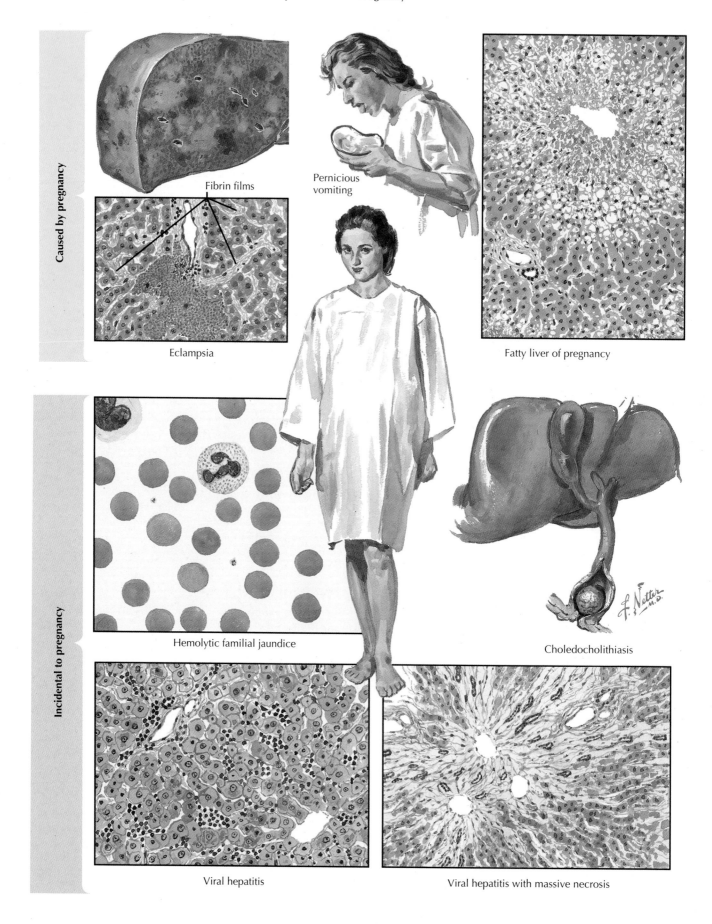

Caused by pregnancy

Fibrin films

Pernicious vomiting

Eclampsia

Fatty liver of pregnancy

Incidental to pregnancy

Hemolytic familial jaundice

Choledocholithiasis

Viral hepatitis

Viral hepatitis with massive necrosis

accomplished in time, recovery is marked by acute pancreatitis and ascites (almost universal). Transient diabetes insipidus is common during recovery, occurring about 7 to 10 days after delivery. For patients who receive rapid and supportive care, eventual recovery is complete and recurrence is rare.

MISCELLANEOUS
ICD-9-CM Code: 646.73.

REFERENCES

Level II
Fesenmeier MF, Coppage KH, Lambers DS, et al: Acute fatty liver of pregnancy in 3 tertiary care centers. Am J Obstet Gynecol 2005;192:1416.

Ibdah JA, Okajima Y, Kang XS, et al: A fetal fatty-acid oxidation disorder as a cause of liver disease in pregnant women. N Engl J Med 1999;340:1723.

Pereira SP, O'Donohue J, Wendon J, et al: Maternal and perinatal outcome in severe pregnancy-related liver disease. Hepatology 1997;26:1258.

Reyes H, Sandoval L, Wainstein A, et al: Acute fatty liver of pregnancy: a clinical study of 12 episodes in 11 patients. Gut 1994;35:101.

Yang Z, Yamada J, Zhao Y, et al: Prospective screening for pediatric mitochondrial trifunctional protein defects in pregnancies complicated by liver disease. JAMA 2002;288:2163–6.

Level III
Barton JR, Sibai BM, Mabie WC, Shanklin DR: Recurrent acute fatty liver of pregnancy. Am J Obstet Gynecol 1990;163:534.

Guntupalli SR, Steingrub J: Hepatic disease and pregnancy: an overview of diagnosis and management. Crit Care Med 2005;33:S332.

Ibdah JA: Acute fatty liver of pregnancy: an update on pathogenesis and clinical implications. World J Gastroenterol 2006;12:7397.

Kaplan MM: Acute fatty liver of pregnancy. N Engl J Med 1985;313:367.

Ko H, Yoshida EM: Acute fatty liver of pregnancy. Can J Gastroenterol 2006;20:25.

Rajasri AG, Srestha R, Mitchell J: Acute fatty liver of pregnancy (AFLP)—An overview. J Obstet Gynaecol 2007;27:237.

Steingrub JS: Pregnancy-associated severe liver dysfunction. Crit Care Clin 2004;20:763, xi.

Wolf JL: Liver disease in pregnancy. Med Clin North Am 1996;80:1167.

INTRODUCTION

Description: Amniotic fluid embolism is a rare but frequently fatal complication of labor in which amniotic fluid containing fetal squamous cells and hair enters the maternal vascular system and becomes lodged in the pulmonary vascular bed. Mechanical obstruction and anaphylaxis combine to produce an often-fatal clinical course. The term "anaphylactoid syndrome of pregnancy" has been suggested but has not received wide acceptance.

Prevalence: One of 30,000 deliveries (despite its rarity, one of the most common causes of maternal mortality).

Predominant Age: Reproductive (late labor or immediately postpartum).

Genetics: No genetic pattern.

ETIOLOGY AND PATHOGENESIS

Causes: Anaphylaxis induced by fetal squamous cells and hair. Mechanical obstruction of pulmonary vessels by fetal squamous cells and hair. Diffuse intravascular coagulation resulting in coagulopathy.

Risk Factors: Tumultuous labor, reduced uterine tone, premature separation of the placenta, history of allergy or atopy.

CLINICAL CHARACTERISTICS

Signs and Symptoms (Variable)

- Respiratory distress followed by cyanosis followed by cardiovascular collapse followed by hemorrhage with depletion of fibrinogen; platelets; and factors V, VIII, and XIII) followed by coma

DIAGNOSTIC APPROACH

Differential Diagnosis

- Pulmonary embolism (thrombus)
- Myocardial infarction
- Cardiac arrhythmia

Associated Conditions: Allergy and atopy.

Workup and Evaluation

Laboratory: Coagulation studies, blood gas measurements, renal function studies, all on an ongoing basis.

Imaging: May help in managing pulmonary complications but generally not helpful in establishing the diagnosis.

Special Tests: Continuous monitoring of oxygen saturation and invasive hemodynamic monitoring (pulmonary artery catheter) essential.

Diagnostic Procedures: History and physical examination. Exclusion of other causes.

Pathologic Findings

Fetal squamous cells and lanugo present in the pulmonary vascular space (typical but not sensitive or specific).

MANAGEMENT AND THERAPY

Nonpharmacologic

General Measures: Aggressive airway control and cardiovascular resuscitation (including myocardial support, inotropic agents and fluids, high-concentration oxygen therapy). The use of vasopressors has been reported to be successful. Correction and support for clotting defects (blood and platelets, fresh-frozen plasma, and cryoprecipitate as indicated).

Specific Measures: None. In women who suffer cardiac arrest before delivery, consideration should be given to perimortem cesarean delivery to improve newborn outcome. In those who have not suffered arrest, maternal considerations generally take precedence.

Diet: Nothing by mouth until condition resolved.

Activity: Bed rest until condition resolved.

Drug(s) of Choice

No specific medications. Other medications as needed for cardiovascular, pulmonary, renal, and coagulation support.

FOLLOW-UP

Patient Monitoring: Intensive hemodynamic monitoring required. Laboratory testing in anticipation of coagulopathy.

Prevention/Avoidance: None.

Possible Complications: Acute mortality rates with amniotic fluid embolism approximate 50%. Of women who survive, 50% have a life-threatening bleeding diathesis. Renal failure is common, as are pulmonary edema and adult respiratory distress syndrome. Of women who suffer cardiac arrest during the initial phase, only 8% survive neurologically intact. Overall maternal mortality approaches 80%. More than half of the neonates that survive have neurologic impairment.

Expected Outcome: Prolonged and complicated course for those who survive.

MISCELLANEOUS

Other Notes: The most devastating effects of amniotic fluid embolism appear to be mediated through the anaphylactic reaction induced. Experimental studies indicate that pretreatment with inhibitors of leukotriene synthesis can prevent the development of symptoms in experimental settings.

ICD-9-CM Codes: 673.13 (if diagnosed before delivery), 673.11 (if diagnosed after delivery).

REFERENCES

Level II

Aguilera LG, Fernandez C, Plaza A, et al: Fatal amniotic fluid embolism diagnosed histologically. Acta Anaesthesiol Scand 2002; 46:334.

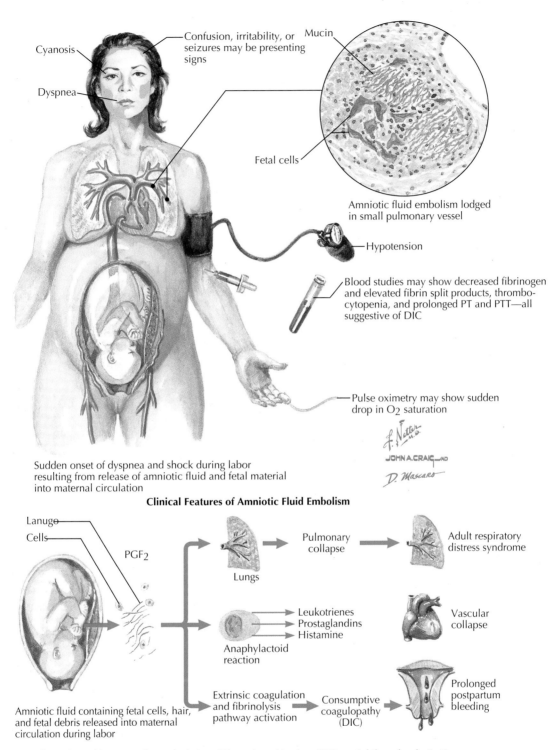

Cyanosis

Dyspnea

Confusion, irritability, or seizures may be presenting signs

Mucin

Fetal cells

Amniotic fluid embolism lodged in small pulmonary vessel

Hypotension

Blood studies may show decreased fibrinogen and elevated fibrin split products, thrombocytopenia, and prolonged PT and PTT—all suggestive of DIC

Pulse oximetry may show sudden drop in O₂ saturation

Sudden onset of dyspnea and shock during labor resulting from release of amniotic fluid and fetal material into maternal circulation

Clinical Features of Amniotic Fluid Embolism

Lanugo

Cells

PGF₂

Lungs

Pulmonary collapse

Adult respiratory distress syndrome

Leukotrienes
Prostaglandins
Histamine

Anaphylactoid reaction

Vascular collapse

Extrinsic coagulation and fibrinolysis pathway activation

Consumptive coagulopathy (DIC)

Prolonged postpartum bleeding

Amniotic fluid containing fetal cells, hair, and fetal debris released into maternal circulation during labor

DIC, disseminated intravascular coagulation; PT, prothrombin time; PTT, partial thromboplastin time.

Benson MD, Kobayashi H, Silver RK, et al: Immunologic studies in presumed amniotic fluid embolism. Obstet Gynecol 2001;97:510.

Benson MD, Lindberg RE: Amniotic fluid embolism, anaphylaxis, and tryptase. Am J Obstet Gynecol 1996;175:737.

Clark SL: New concepts of amniotic fluid embolism: a review. Obstet Gynecol Surv 1990;45:360.

Clark SL, Hankins GDV, Dudley DA, et al: Amniotic fluid embolism: analysis of the National Registry. Am J Obstet Gynecol 1995; 172:1159.

Martin SR, Foley MR: Intensive care in obstetrics: an evidence-based review. Am J Obstet Gynecol 2006;195:673.

Level III

Green BT, Umana E: Amniotic fluid embolism. South Med J 2000;93:721.

Hardin L, Fox LS, O'Quinn AG: Amniotic fluid embolism. South Med J 1991;84:1046.

Moore J, Baldisseri MR: Amniotic fluid embolism. Crit Care Med 2005;33:S279.

Morgan M: Amniotic fluid embolism. Anaesthesia 1979;34:20.

INTRODUCTION

Description: Postpartum breast engorgement is characterized by tender, swollen, hard breasts caused by accumulation of milk in the postpartum period or during weaning.

Prevalence: Common.

Predominant Age: Reproductive, 3 to 4 days after delivery.

Genetics: No genetic pattern.

ETIOLOGY AND PATHOGENESIS

Causes: Increased milk production relative to use. Generally occurs 3 to 4 days after delivery when milk first comes in or during weaning.

Risk Factors: High fluid intake, infrequent nursing, poor suckling by the infant, abrupt cessation of nursing.

CLINICAL CHARACTERISTICS

Signs and Symptoms

- Warm, hard, sore breasts with no fever or erythema

DIAGNOSTIC APPROACH

Differential Diagnosis

- Mastitis
- Blocked (plugged) duct

Associated Conditions: Mastitis.

Workup and Evaluation

Laboratory: No evaluation indicated.

Imaging: No imaging indicated.

Special Tests: None indicated.

Diagnostic Procedures: History and physical examination.

Pathologic Findings

Firm, tender breasts without skin change, fever, or inflammation.

MANAGEMENT AND THERAPY

Nonpharmacologic

General Measures: Mild fluid restriction, analgesics, ice packs, support (well-fitting brassiere). The use of cabbage leaves (applied to the breast) has been advocated, but conclusive studies are lacking.

Specific Measures: More frequent breastfeeding (if breastfeeding is to continue), firm binding.

Diet: Mild fluid restriction. If breastfeeding is to continue, adequate calories (additional 200 kcal/day) and protein are required.

Activity: No restriction.

Patient Education: Reassurance, support, specific suggestions; American College of Obstetricians and Gynecologists Patient Education Pamphlet AP029 (Breastfeeding Your Baby), AB005 (You and Your Baby: Prenatal Care, Labor and Delivery, and Postpartum Care).

Drug(s) of Choice

Analgesics. Medication to suppress lactation has little value and recommendations for its use have been withdrawn.

FOLLOW-UP

Patient Monitoring: Normal health maintenance; watch for possible infection.

Prevention/Avoidance: Gradual weaning reduces engorgement.

Possible Complications: Ductal obstruction and ectasia (uncommon).

Expected Outcome: Generally resolves in 24 to 48 hours.

MISCELLANEOUS

ICD-9-CM Code: 676.2.

REFERENCES

Level I

Anonymous. Single dose cabergoline versus bromocriptine in inhibition of puerperal lactation: randomised, double blind, multicentre study. European Multicentre Study Group for Cabergoline in Lactation Inhibition. BMJ 1991;302:1367.

Dewhurst CJ, Harrison RF, Biswas S: Inhibition of puerperal lactation. A double blind study of bromocriptine and placebo. Acta Obstet Gynecol Scand 1977;56:327.

Nikodem VC, Danziger D, Gebka N, et al: Do cabbage leaves prevent breast engorgement? A randomized, controlled study. Birth 1993; 20:61.

Level II

Caballero-Gordo A, Lopez-Nazareno N, Calderay M, et al: Oral cabergoline. Single-dose inhibition of puerperal lactation. J Reprod Med 1991;36:717.

Evans K, Evans R, Simmer K: Effect of the method of breast feeding on breast engorgement, mastitis and infantile colic. Acta Paediatr 1995;84:849.

Roberts KL, Reiter M, Schuster D: A comparison of chilled and room temperature cabbage leaves in treating breast engorgement. J Hum Lact 1995;11:191.

Shapiro AG, Thomas L: Efficacy of bromocriptine versus breast binders as inhibitors of postpartum lactation. South Med J 1984;77:719.

Level III

Almeida OD Jr, Kitay DZ: Lactation suppression and puerperal fever. Am J Obstet Gynecol 1986;154:940.

Renfrew MJ, Lang S, Martin L, Woolridge MW: Feeding schedules in hospitals for newborn infants. Cochrane Database Syst Rev 2000;2:CD000090.

Spitz AM, Lee NC, Peterson HB: Treatment for lactation suppression: little progress in one hundred years. Am J Obstet Gynecol 1998;179:1485.

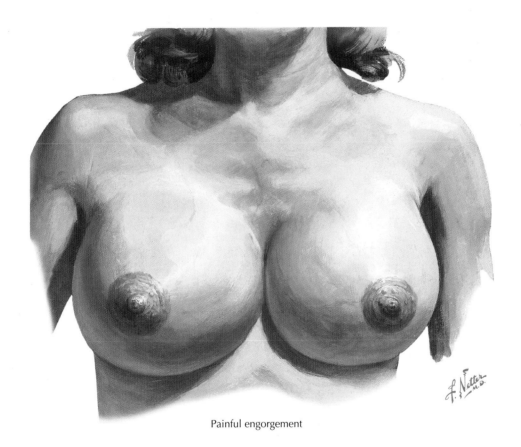

Painful engorgement

INTRODUCTION

Description: Breech birth is presentation of the fetal buttocks, one foot, or both feet at the cervix at the time of labor.

Prevalence: Three percent of term pregnancies, 13% of pregnancies at 30 weeks of gestation.

Predominant Age: Reproductive (maternal).

Genetics: No genetic pattern.

ETIOLOGY AND PATHOGENESIS

Causes: Prematurity, fetal or maternal anomalies (e.g., fetal hydrocephalus, maternal uterine anomalies), multiple gestation.

Risk Factors: Prematurity, fetal or uterine anomalies, multiple pregnancies.

CLINICAL CHARACTERISTICS

Signs and Symptoms

- Fetal head located outside the pelvis on abdominal palpation (Leopold's maneuvers)
- Fetal heart heard high in the uterus
- Buttock, one foot, or both feet palpable on cervical examination

DIAGNOSTIC APPROACH

Differential Diagnosis

- Fetal anomaly (hydrocephalus, anencephaly)
- Uterine anomaly (septum, duplication, leiomyomata)
- Multiple gestation
- Fetal macrosomia

Associated Conditions: Prematurity, placenta previa, placental abruption, premature rupture of the membranes, congenital anomalies (6% versus 2.5% in total population), intracranial hemorrhage, growth restriction, neurologic disorders and mortality, multiple pregnancy, and polyhydramnios.

Workup and Evaluation

Laboratory: No evaluation indicated beyond that usually considered for patients in labor.

Imaging: Ultrasonography may be used to confirm presentation.

Special Tests: Fetal heart rate and uterine activity monitoring.

Diagnostic Procedures: Physical examination (Leopold's maneuvers), ultrasonography.

Pathologic Findings

None.

MANAGEMENT AND THERAPY

Nonpharmacologic

General Measures: Fetal and maternal monitoring and support.

Specific Measures: External version, evaluation for route of delivery. External version is successful in >50% of patients. In 2002 the rate of cesarean deliveries for women in labor with breech presentation was 86.9%.

Diet: No specific dietary changes indicated; nothing by mouth if the patient is in labor because of the increased risk of operative delivery.

Activity: No restriction.

Patient Education: Reassurance; American College of Obstetricians and Gynecologists Patient Education Pamphlet AP079 (If Your Baby Is Breech).

Drug(s) of Choice

None (tocolytics may be used to assist with external version procedures).

FOLLOW-UP

Patient Monitoring: Fetal and maternal monitoring as with normal labor.

Prevention/Avoidance: None.

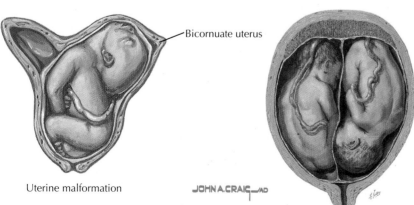

Uterine malformation

Bicornuate uterus

JOHN A. CRAIG —AD

Multiple fetuses

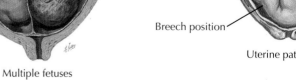

Uterine fibroid

Ear distortion

Breech position

Uterine pathology

Conditions that cause intrauterine crowding can lead to abnormal fetal positions

Possible Complications: Prolapse of umbilical cord, entrapment of the fetal head, birth trauma.

Expected Outcome: Breech deliveries are associated with an increased risk of congenital anomalies, intracranial hemorrhage, growth restriction, neurologic disorders, and mortality, but the role of breech presentation and the delivery route are unclear. Much of the morbidity traditionally associated with breech presentation and delivery is due to factors that predispose to breech (congenital anomalies, prematurity).

MISCELLANEOUS

Pregnancy Considerations: The route of delivery must be determined on an individual basis based on fetal and maternal factors, the availability of needed resources, and the skill of the obstetrician. Vaginal delivery may be considered if labor is normal, fetal weight is 2000 to 3800 g, fetal status is normal, the pelvis is adequate, fetal head position is normal, and normal progression of cervical dilation and fetal descent are maintained.

ICD-9-CM Codes: 652.2, 652.1 (With successful version).

REFERENCES

Level I

Hannah ME, Hannah WJ, Hewson SA, et al: Planned caesarean section versus planned vaginal birth for breech presentation at term: a randomised multicentre trial. Term Breech Trial Collaborative Group. Lancet 2000;356:1375.

Hannah ME, Whyte H, Hannah WJ, et al: Maternal outcomes at 2 years after planned cesarean section versus planned vaginal birth for breech presentation at term: the international randomized Term Breech Trial. Term Breech Trial Collaborative Group. Am J Obstet Gynecol 2004;191:917.

Impey L, Pandit M: Tocolysis for repeat external cephalic version in breech presentation at term: a randomised, double-blinded, placebo-controlled trial. BJOG 2005;112:627.

Nassar N, Roberts CL, Raynes-Greenow CH, et al; Decision Aid for Breech Presentation Trial Collaborators. Evaluation of a decision aid for women with breech presentation at term: a randomised controlled trial. BJOG 2007;114:325.

Whyte H, Hannah ME, Saigal S, et al: Outcomes of children at 2 years after planned cesarean birth versus planned vaginal birth for breech presentation at term: the International Randomized Term Breech Trial. Term Breech Trial Collaborative Group. Am J Obstet Gynecol 2004;191:864.

Level II

Blickstein I, Goldman RD, Kupferminc M: Delivery of breech first twins: a multicenter retrospective study. Obstet Gynecol 2000;95:37.

Collins S, Ellaway P, Harrington D, et al: The complications of external cephalic version: results from 805 consecutive attempts. BJOG 2007;114:636. Epub 2007 Mar 12.

Goffinet F, Carayol M, Foidart JM, et al; PREMODA Study Group: Is planned vaginal delivery for breech presentation at term still an option? Results of an observational prospective survey in France and Belgium. Am J Obstet Gynecol 2006;194:1002.

Giuliani A, Schöll WM, Basver A, Tamussino KF: Mode of delivery and outcome of 699 term singleton breech deliveries at a single center. Am J Obstet Gynecol 2002;187:1694.

Martin JA, Hamilton BE, Sutton PD, et al: Births: final data for 2002. Natl Vital Stat Rep 2003;52:1.

Palencia R, Gafni A, Hannah ME, et al; Term Breech Trial Collaborative Group: The costs of planned cesarean versus planned vaginal birth in the Term Breech Trial. CMAJ 2006;174:1109.

Rietberg CC, Elferink-Stinkens PM, Visser GH: The effect of the Term Breech Trial on medical intervention behaviour and neonatal outcome in The Netherlands: an analysis of 35,453 term breech infants. BJOG 2005;112:205.

Su M, Hannah WJ, Willan A, et al: Planned caesarean section decreases the risk of adverse perinatal outcome due to both labour and delivery complications in the Term Breech Trial. Term Breech Trial Collaborative Group. BJOG 2004;111:1065.

Level III

Alarab M, Regan C, O'Connell MP, et al: Singleton vaginal breech delivery at term: still a safe option. Obstet Gynecol 2004; 103:407.

American College of Obstetricians and Gynecologists: External cephalic version. ACOG Practice Bulletin 13. Washington, DC, ACOG, 2000.

American College of Obstetricians and Gynecologists: Mode of term singleton breech delivery. ACOG Committee Opinion 340. Obstet Gynecol 2006;108:235.

Burke G: The end of vaginal breech delivery. BJOG 2006;113:969. Epub 2006 Jul 7.

Kotaska A: Inappropriate use of randomised trials to evaluate complex phenomena: case study of vaginal breech delivery. BMJ 2004; 329:1039.

INTRODUCTION

Description: Caput succedaneum is a characteristic change in the shape of the fetal head that results from the forces of labor acting on the fetal head and the surrounding tissues. This swelling is generally located on the portion of the fetal scalp that was directly under the cervical os.

Prevalence: Typical of most vaginal vertex births; similar swellings on the presenting part are formed with other birth presentations.

Predominant Age: Birth.

Genetics: No genetic pattern.

ETIOLOGY AND PATHOGENESIS

Causes: Pressure by the birth canal and surrounding tissues on the fetal head as it enters and traverses the lower vaginal canal.

Risk Factors: Fetal macrosomia, prolonged labor, contracted maternal pelvis, prolonged maternal expulsive effort (pushing).

CLINICAL CHARACTERISTICS

Signs and Symptoms

- Symmetric swelling of the fetal scalp in a location compatible with that which was directly under the cervical os (upper posterior portion over the right parietal bone in left occiput transverse labors, over the corresponding portion of the left parietal bone in right occiput transverse labors)
- Generally with diffuse edges and only a few millimeters in thickness; greater in obstructed or prolonged labors. The periosteal edges provide a sharp demarcation to a cephalohematoma that is not present in caput succedaneum. In addition, cephalohematomas do not cross suture lines.

DIAGNOSTIC APPROACH

Differential Diagnosis

- Cephalohematoma (2% to 3% of births)
- Molding of the head
- Subgaleal hemorrhage

Associated Conditions: Macrosomia, obstructed labor, maternal diabetes.

Workup and Evaluation

Laboratory: No evaluation indicated.

Imaging: No imaging indicated.

Special Tests: None indicated.

Diagnostic Procedures: History and physical examination.

Pathologic Findings

Diffuse tissue edema without bruising.

MANAGEMENT AND THERAPY

Nonpharmacologic

General Measures: Evaluation and reassurance.

Specific Measures: None. Spontaneously regresses in 24 to 48 hours.

Diet: No specific dietary changes indicated.

Activity: No restriction.

Drug(s) of Choice

None.

FOLLOW-UP

Patient Monitoring: Normal health maintenance.

Prevention/Avoidance: Expeditious labor and delivery.

Possible Complications: Cephalohematoma or intracranial bleeding may be missed. Rare cases of alopecia have been reported.

Expected Outcome: Rapid, spontaneous, and complete resolution.

MISCELLANEOUS

ICD-9-CM Code: 767.1.

REFERENCES

Level III

Choi JW, Lee CH, Suh SI: Scalp swelling crossing the suture line on skull radiograph: is it always a sign of caput succedaneum? Pediatr Radiol 2006;36:364. Epub 2006 Feb 17.

Gerscovich EO, McGahan JP, Jain KA, Gillen MA: Caput succedaneum mimicking a cephalocele. J Clin Ultrasound 2003;31:98.

Parker LA: Part 1: Early recognition and treatment of birth trauma: injuries to the head and face. Adv Neonatal care. 2005;5:288.

Petrikovsky BM, Schneider E, Smith-Levitin M, Gross B: Cephalhematoma and caput succedaneum: do they always occur in labor? Am J Obstet Gynecol 1998;179:906.

Rawal S, Modi N, Lacey S, Keane M: *Escherichia coli* septicaemia arising as a result of an infected caput succedaneum. Eur J Pediatr 2006;165:66. Epub 2005 Sep 3.

Sauvageau A, Belley-Cote EP, Racette S: Utility of the caput succedaneum in the forensic investigation of neonaticide: a case report. Med Sci Law 2007;47:262.

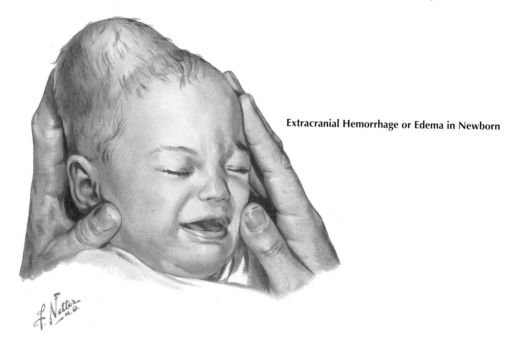

Extracranial Hemorrhage or Edema in Newborn

Caput succedaneum

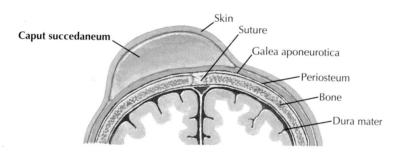

Skin
Suture
Galea aponeurotica
Periosteum
Bone
Dura mater

Subgaleal hemorrhage

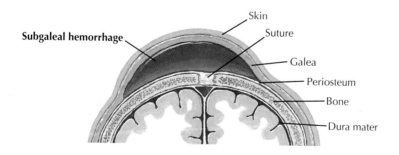

Skin
Suture
Galea
Periosteum
Bone
Dura mater

Cephalohematoma

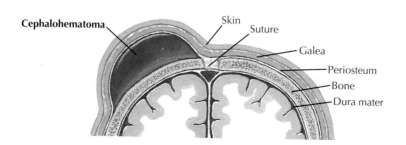

Skin
Suture
Galea
Periosteum
Bone
Dura mater

THE CHALLENGE

Cardiac disease is one of the major causes of nonobstetric maternal mortality. Whereas in the past patients with congenital heart disease did not survive to reproductive age, it is now common for these patients to become pregnant, be it planned or unplanned.

Scope of the Problem: Cardiac disease complicates approximately 1% of all pregnancies. Mitral valve prolapse may be found in 5% to 7% of pregnant women. The type and severity of risk vary with the type of lesion and the functional abilities of the patient (see box). Patients with valvular disease have an increased risk for thromboembolic disease, subacute bacterial endocarditis, cardiac failure, and pulmonary edema during and after pregnancy.

Objectives of Management: Identify patients at risk because of cardiovascular conditions, provide realistic counseling regarding the risk to mother and fetus, and work to reduce this risk. The basis of antepartum management consists of frequent evaluations of maternal cardiac status and fetal well-being, combined with avoidance of conditions or actions that increase cardiac workload. The latter includes the treatment or avoidance of anemia, prompt treatment of any infection or fever, limitation of strenuous activity, and adherence to appropriate weight gain.

TACTICS

Relevant Pathophysiology: By midpregnancy there is a 40% increase in cardiac output; this increase in demand may be fatal. Cardiac output shows an additional increase in the immediate postpartum period, as up to 500 mL of additional blood enter the maternal circulation because of uterine contractions and rapid loss of uterine volume. Cardiac complications, such as peripartum cardiomyopathy, may occur up to 6 months after delivery. Valvular heart disease is the most commonly encountered cardiac complication of pregnancy, with rheumatic valvular disease being the most frequent type. The severity of the associated valvular lesion determines the degree of risk associated with pregnancy. Roughly 90% of these patients have mitral stenosis, which may result in worsening obstruction as cardiac output increases during the pregnancy. When severe or associated with atrial fibrillation, the risk of cardiac failure during pregnancy is increased.

Strategies: The New York Heart Association classification of heart disease is a useful guide to the risk of pregnancy (see box). Patients with class I or II disease, such as those with septal defects, patent ductus arteriosus, or mild mitral or aortic valvular disease, generally do well during pregnancy, although their fetuses are at greater risk for prematurity and low birthweight. Patients with class III or IV disease caused by primary pulmonary hypertension, uncorrected tetralogy of Fallot, Eisenmenger syndrome, or other conditions rarely do well, with pregnancy inducing a significant risk of death, often in excess of 50%. Patients with this degree of cardiac decompensation should be advised to avoid pregnancy or consider termination based on careful consultation with specialists in both cardiology and high-risk obstetrics.

IMPLEMENTATION

Special Considerations: Most patients with mitral valve prolapse do well. The rare patient with left atrial and ventricular enlargement may develop dysfunction during the course of pregnancy. The severity of the disease and impact on the atrium and ventricle may be assessed by echocardiography. Peripartum cardiomyopathy is rare but uniformly severe. Occurring in the last month of pregnancy or during the first 6 months after delivery, it is similar to other cardiomyopathies in symptoms and findings. Most often, a specific cause is not identified and the cause remains unknown. This process presents an especially grave risk, necessitating early suspicion and aggressive consultative management. Patients at highest risk are those in their 30s, who are multiparous, who are African American, who have delivered twins, or who have had pre-eclampsia. Unusual cardiac conditions, such as idiopathic hypertrophic subaortic stenosis and the structural anomalies associated with Marfan syndrome, are associated with maternal moralities of 25% to 50% or higher. The presence of such conditions demands realistic preconception counseling, and early transfer for specialized care, should a pregnancy occur.

Cardiac (Maternal) Mortality Associated with Pregnancy

Group I (Mortality <1%)
Atrial septal defect
• Bioprosthetic valve
• Mitral stenosis (functional class I and II)
• Patent ductus arteriosus
• Pulmonic/tricuspid disease
• Tetralogy of Fallot, corrected
• Ventricular septal defect

Group II (Mortality 5% to 15%)
Aortic stenosis
• Coarctation of aorta, without valvular involvement
IIA
Marfan Syndrome with Normal Aorta
• Mitral stenosis (functional class III and IV)
• Previous myocardial infarction
• Uncorrected tetralogy of Fallot
IIB
Artificial Valve
• Mitral stenosis with atrial fibrillation

Group III (Mortality 25% to 50%)
Coarctation of aorta, with valvular involvement
• Marfan syndrome with aortic involvement
• Pulmonary hypertension

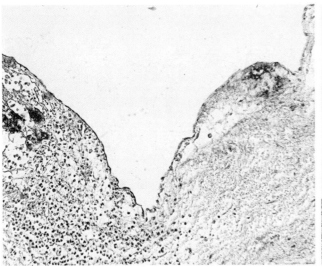

Deposit of platelets and organisms (stained dark), edema, and leukocytic infiltration in very early bacterial endocarditis of aortic valve

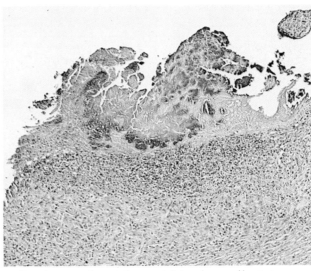

Development of vegetations containing clumps of bacteria on tricuspid valve

Early vegetations of bacterial endocarditis on bicuspid aortic valve

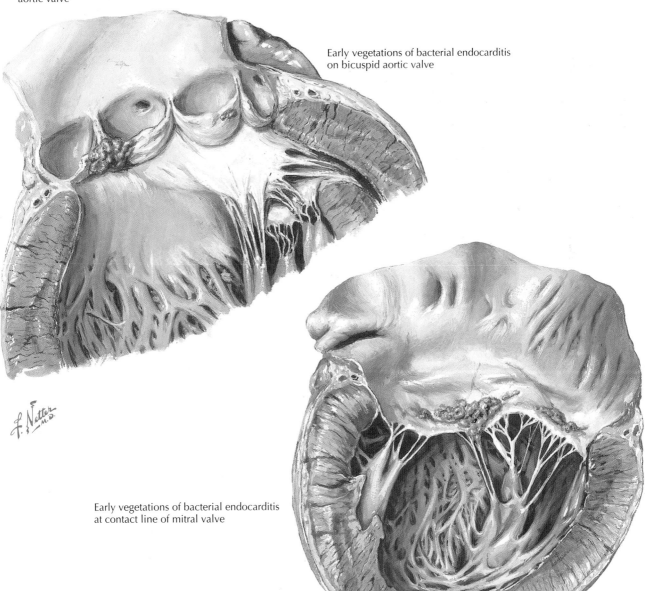

Early vegetations of bacterial endocarditis at contact line of mitral valve

NEW YORK HEART ASSOCIATION CLASSIFICATION OF HEART DISEASE

Classification	Symptoms
Class I	No cardiac decompensation
Class II	No symptoms of decompensation at rest
	Minor limitations of physical activity
Class III	No symptoms of decompensation at rest
	Marked limitations of physical activity
Class IV	Symptoms of decompensation at rest
	Discomfort with any physical activity

REFERENCES

Level II

Canobbio MM, Morris CD, Graham TP, Landzberg MJ: Pregnancy outcomes after atrial repair for transposition of the great arteries. Am J Cardiol 2006;98:668. Epub 2006 Jul 7.

Drenthen W, Pieper PG, Roos-Hesselink JW, et al; ZAHARA Investigators: Outcome of pregnancy in women with congenital heart disease: a literature review. J Am Coll Cardiol 2007;49:2303. Epub 2007 Jun 4.

Immer FF, Bansi AG, Immer-Bansi AS, et al: Aortic dissection in pregnancy: analysis of risk factors and outcome. Ann Thorac Surg 2003;76:309.

Martin SR, Foley MR: Intensive care in obstetrics: an evidence-based review. Am J Obstet Gynecol 2006;195:673.

Siu SC, Sermer M, Colman JM, et al; Cardiac Disease in Pregnancy (CARPREG) Investigators: Prospective multicenter study of pregnancy outcomes in women with heart disease. Circulation 2001;104:515.

Level III

American College of Cardiology/American Heart Association Task Force on Practice Guidelines, Society of Cardiovascular Anesthesiologists, Society for Cardiovascular Angiography and Interventions, Society of Thoracic Surgeons, Bonow RO, Carabello BA, Kanu C, et al: ACC/AHA 2006 guidelines for the management of patients with valvular heart disease: a report of the American College of Cardiology/American Heart Association Task Force on Practice Guidelines (writing committee to revise the 1998 Guidelines for the Management of Patients With Valvular Heart Disease): Developed in collaboration with the Society of Cardiovascular Anesthesiologists: endorsed by the Society for Cardiovascular Angiography and Interventions and the Society of Thoracic Surgeons. Circulation 2006;114:e84.

American College of Obstetricians and Gynecologists: Chronic hypertension in pregnancy. ACOG Practice Bulletin 29. Obstet Gynecol 2001;98:177.

American College of Obstetricians and Gynecologists: Diagnosis and management of preeclampsia and eclampsia. ACOG Practice Bulletin 33. Obstet Gynecol 2002;99:159.

American College of Obstetricians and Gynecologists: Prophylactic antibiotics in labor and delivery. ACOG Practice Bulletin 47. Obstet Gynecol 2003;102:875.

Chamberlain G, Steer P: ABC of labour care: labour in special circumstances. BMJ 1999;318:1124.

Elkayam U, Bitar F: Valvular heart disease and pregnancy: Part I: Native valves. J Am Coll Cardiol 2005;46:223.

Elkayam U, Bitar F: Valvular heart disease and pregnancy: Part II: Prosthetic valves. J Am Coll Cardiol 2005;46:403.

Milewicz DM, Dietz HC, Miller DC: Treatment of aortic disease in patients with Marfan syndrome. Circulation 2005;111:e150.

Murali S, Baldisseri MR: Peripartum cardiomyopathy. Crit Care Med 2005;33:S340.

Reimold SC, Rutherford JD: Clinical practice. Valvular heart disease in pregnancy. N Engl J Med 2003;349:52.

Siu SC, Colman JM: Heart disease and pregnancy. Heart 2001; 85:710.

Sliwa K, Fett J, Elkayam U: Peripartum cardiomyopathy. Lancet 2006;368:687.

Spirito P, Autore C: Management of hypertrophic cardiomyopathy. BMJ 2006;332:1251.

Stout KK, Otto CM: Pregnancy in women with valvular heart disease. Heart 2007;93:552. Epub 2006 Aug 11.

Thorne S, MacGregor A, Nelson-Piercy C: Risks of contraception and pregnancy in heart disease. Heart 2006;92:1520.

Thorne SA: Pregnancy in heart disease. Heart 2004;90:450.

Uebing A, Steer PJ, Yentis SM, Gatzoulis MA: Pregnancy and congenital heart disease. BMJ 2006;332:401.

Vongpatanasin W, Brickner ME, Hillis LD, Lange RA: The Eisenmenger syndrome in adults. Ann Intern Med 1998;128:745.

INTRODUCTION

Description: Cervical incompetence is characterized by asymptomatic dilation of the internal os during pregnancy. This generally leads to dilation of the entire cervical canal during the second trimester with subsequent risk of rupture of the membranes, expulsion of the fetus, or both.

Prevalence: One of 54 to 1 of 1842 pregnancies (as a result of uncertain diagnostic criteria); appears to be declining.

Predominant Age: Reproductive.

Genetics: No genetic pattern.

ETIOLOGY AND PATHOGENESIS

Causes: Iatrogenic (most common); damage from cervical dilation at the time of dilation and curettage (D&C) or other manipulation, damage caused by surgery (conization). Congenital tissue defect, uterine anomalies (uterus didelphys), obstetric lacerations, in utero exposure to diethylstilbestrol (DES).

Risk Factors: In utero exposure to diethylstilbestrol, uterine anomalies.

CLINICAL CHARACTERISTICS

Signs and Symptoms

- History of second-trimester pregnancy loss (generally three or more) accompanied by spontaneous rupture of the membranes without labor or rapid, painless, preterm labor.
- Prolapse and ballooning of the fetal membranes into the vagina without labor.

DIAGNOSTIC APPROACH

Differential Diagnosis

- Uterine anomalies
- Chorioamnionitis
- Chromosomal anomaly (balanced translocation)

Associated Conditions: Premature rupture of the membranes, premature (preterm) delivery, and recurrent second trimester pregnancy loss.

Workup and Evaluation

Laboratory: No evaluation indicated beyond that for routine prenatal care.

Imaging: Ultrasonography before cervical cerclage to ensure normal fetal development. Although cervical length can be measured by ultrasonography, routine use of this has not proved to be an effective screening tool except in the face of a high-risk history. (Normal cervical length is approximately 4.1 cm (±1.02 cm) between 14 and 28 weeks and gradually decreases in length to 40 weeks, when it averages between 2.5 and 3.2 cm.) Signs of cervical funneling and cervical shortening are associated with an increased risk of preterm delivery, but management in the absence of other risk factors is unclear.

Special Tests: None indicated. (Frequent vaginal examinations beginning around the time of previous cervical change or the second trimester, whichever is earlier.) Attempts to define or identify cervical incompetence by hysterosonography, pull-through techniques with inflated catheter balloons, measurement of cervical resistance to cervical dilators, magnetic resonance imaging, and others have not gained clinical acceptance.

Diagnostic Procedures: History.

Pathologic Findings

Painless dilation of the cervix.

MANAGEMENT AND THERAPY

Nonpharmacologic

General Measures: Evaluation, frequent prenatal visits with monitoring for cervical change.

Specific Measures: Cervical cerclage (placement of a concentric nonabsorbable suture at the level of the inner cervical os) is performed between 10 and 14 weeks of gestation. When the suture is placed vaginally, it is generally removed at 38 weeks of gestation. If labor occurs before this point, the suture must be removed immediately. Cervical cerclage is occasionally performed transabdominally. These sutures are intended to remain permanently and preclude vaginal delivery. The use of lever pessaries (such as the Smith-Hodge) has been reported to give outcomes similar to that obtained by cerclage, but this modality is infrequently used. Bleeding, uterine contractions, obvious infection, or rupture of the membranes are contraindications to cerclage. Because of scarring after cerclage, about 15% of patients require cesarean delivery.

Diet: No specific dietary changes indicated.

Activity: Restriction of activity is often suggested, but evidence that this alters the outcome of pregnancy is lacking. After 24 weeks of pregnancy, bed rest may be the only therapy available because cerclage may bring on labor.

Patient Education: American College of Obstetricians and Gynecologists Patient Education Pamphlet AP100 (Repeated Miscarriage), AP110 (Loop Electrosurgical Excision Procedure).

Drug(s) of Choice

None. (Prophylactic antibiotics and beta mimetics have not been shown to be effective.)

FOLLOW-UP

Patient Monitoring: Frequent prenatal visits with monitoring for cervical change in patients thought to be at high risk. If a cerclage is placed, planned removal of cerclage at 38 weeks of gestation is advisable.

Prevention/Avoidance: Care to avoid overdilation of the cervix when surgical manipulation is required.

Cervical Incompetence

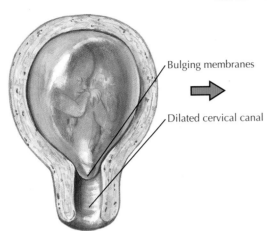

Cervical incompetence becomes manifest in second trimester as dilation of cervical canal

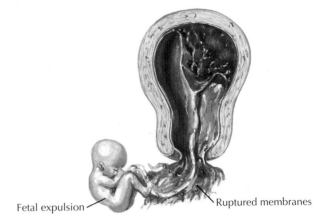

If left untreated, the dilated cervical canal may result in rupture of membranes and/or fetal expulsion

Surgical Management of Cervical Incompetence (Cerclage)

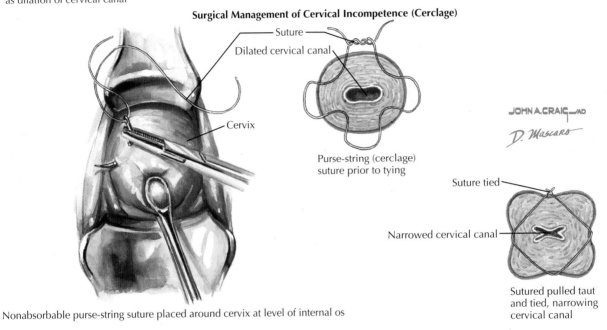

Nonabsorbable purse-string suture placed around cervix at level of internal os

Possible Complications: Continued fetal loss, chorioamnionitis, cervical avulsion, or uterine rupture if labor occurs and the cerclage is not removed.

Expected Outcome: With correct diagnosis and cervical cerclage, fetal survival increases from 20% to 80%.

MISCELLANEOUS
ICD-9-CM Code: 622.5.

REFERENCES

Level I
Berghella V, Odibo AO, Tolosa JE: Cerclage for prevention of preterm birth in women with a short cervix found on transvaginal ultrasound examination: a randomized trial. Am J Obstet Gynecol 2004;191:1311.

Lazar P, Gueguen S, Dreyfus J, et al: Multicentred controlled trial of cervical cerclage in women at moderate risk of preterm delivery. Br J Obstet Gynaecol 1984;91:731.

Level II
Belej-Rak T, Okun N, Windrim R, et al: Effectiveness of cervical cerclage for a sonographically shortened cervix: a systematic review and meta-analysis. Am J Obstet Gynecol 2003;189:1679.

Drakeley AJ, Roberts D, Alfirevic Z: Cervical cerclage for prevention of preterm delivery: meta-analysis of randomized trials. Obstet Gynecol 2003;102:621.

Harger JH: Cerclage and cervical insufficiency: an evidence-based analysis. Obstet Gynecol 2002;100:1313.

Kushnir O, Vigil DA, Izquierdo L, et al: Vaginal ultrasonographic assessment of cervical length changes during normal pregnancy. Am J Obstet Gynecol 1990;162:991.

Level III
American College of Obstetricians and Gynecologists: Cervical insufficiency. ACOG Practice Bulletin 48. Obstet Gynecol 2003; 102:1091.

American College of Obstetricians and Gynecologists: Ultrasonography in pregnancy. ACOG Practice Bulletin 58. Obstet Gynecol 2004;104:1449.

Cunningham FG, Gant NF, Leveno KJ, et al, eds. Williams obstetrics, 21st ed. New York, McGraw-Hill, 2001, p 862.

McDonald IA: Incompetence of the cervix. Aust N Z J Obstet Gynaecol 1978;18:34.

Romero R, Espinoza J, Erez O, Hassan S: The role of cervical cerclage in obstetric practice: can the patient who could benefit from this procedure be identified? Am J Obstet Gynecol 2006;194:1.

INTRODUCTION

Description: Cholelithiasis and cholecystitis complicate more than 3% of pregnancies.

Prevalence: Cholelithiasis—3% to 4% of pregnancies; cholecystitis—0.25% of pregnancies.

Predominant Age: Reproductive.

Genetics: Some races at greater risk (e.g., Pima Indians).

ETIOLOGY AND PATHOGENESIS

Causes: The metabolic alteration leading to cholesterol stones (gallstones) is thought to be a disruption in the balance between hydroxymethylglutaryl coenzyme A (HMG-CoA) reductase and cholesterol 7α-hydroxylase. HMG-CoA controls cholesterol synthesis, whereas cholesterol 7α-hydroxylase controls the rate of bile acid formation. Patients who form cholesterol stones have elevated levels of HMG-CoA and depressed levels of cholesterol 7α-hydroxylase. This change in ratio increases the risk of precipitation of cholesterol. During pregnancy, there is an increased rate of bile synthesis and a reduced rate of gallbladder emptying, increasing the risk of stone formation and obstruction.

Risk Factors: Cholecystitis is associated with increased maternal age, multiparity, multiple gestation, and a history of previous attacks.

CLINICAL CHARACTERISTICS

Signs and Symptoms

(Unchanged by pregnancy)
* May be confused with symptoms of pregnancy
* Fatty food intolerance
* Variable right upper quadrant pain with radiation to the back or scapula
* Nausea or vomiting (often mistaken for "indigestion" or "morning sickness")
* Fever is usually associated with cholangitis

DIAGNOSTIC APPROACH

Differential Diagnosis

* Labor
* Pre-eclampsia
* Placental accident (abruption)
* Cholestasis of pregnancy
* Gastroenteritis
* Esophageal reflux
* Malabsorption
* Irritable bowel syndrome
* Peptic ulcer disease
* Coronary artery disease
* Pneumonia
* Appendicitis

Associated Conditions: Jaundice, cirrhosis, pancreatitis, ileus, and premature labor.

Workup and Evaluation

Laboratory: Supportive, but often not diagnostic—complete blood count, serum bilirubin, amylase, alkaline phosphatase, and aminotransferase concentrations.

Imaging: Ultrasonography of the gallbladder (96% accurate in making the diagnosis of sludge or stone in the gallbladder); can visualize stones as small as 2 mm.

Special Tests: None indicated.

Diagnostic Procedures: History, physical examination, ultrasonography, and laboratory investigation.

Pathologic Findings

None.

MANAGEMENT AND THERAPY

Nonpharmacologic

General Measures: Watchful waiting, dietary modifications aimed at reducing cholesterol and fatty food exposure.

Specific Measures: Cholelithiasis may be treated with oral therapy; surgical extirpation may be required. Cholecystectomy during pregnancy is associated with a 5% fetal loss rate, which increases to approximately 60% if pancreatitis is present at the time of surgery.

Diet: Nothing by mouth during acute attacks or until the diagnosis is established (some patients require nasogastric suction during acute attacks); reduced fatty food and cholesterol at other times.

Activity: No restriction.

Drug(s) of Choice

Ursodeoxycholic acid (Actigall) 8 to 10 mg/day divided in two to three doses. When cholecystitis is present, intravenous fluids, nasogastric suction, analgesics, and antibiotics (cephalosporin) are appropriate.

Contraindications: Known allergy, acute cholecystitis, abnormal liver function, calcified stones (not cholesterol based).

Interactions: See warning for individual agents.

FOLLOW-UP

Patient Monitoring: Normal prenatal care once acute episode is resolved.

Prevention/Avoidance: None.

Possible Complications: Acute cholecystitis, pancreatitis, ascending cholangitis, peritonitis, internal fistulization (to the gastrointestinal tract), premature labor or delivery.

Expected Outcome: Cholecystitis—generally good with either oral or surgical therapy.

MISCELLANEOUS

ICD-9-CM Code: 574.2 (others based on obstruction or inflammation).

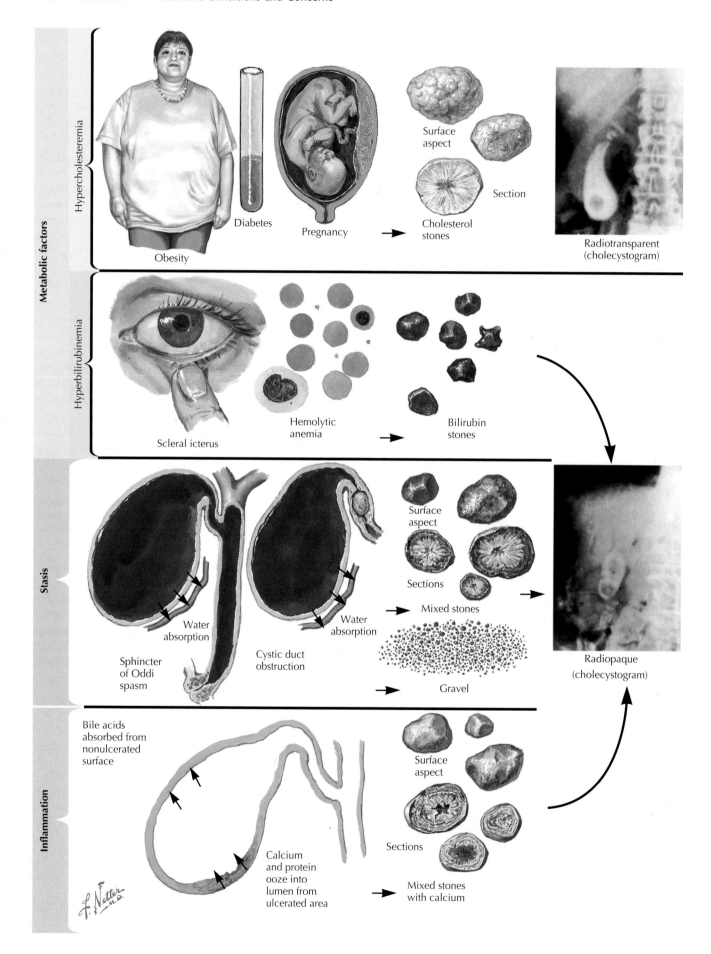

Metabolic factors

Hypercholesteremia

Obesity

Diabetes

Pregnancy

Surface aspect

Section

Cholesterol stones

Radiotransparent (cholecystogram)

Hyperbilirubinemia

Scleral icterus

Hemolytic anemia

Bilirubin stones

Stasis

Sphincter of Oddi spasm

Water absorption

Cystic duct obstruction

Water absorption

Surface aspect

Sections

Mixed stones

Gravel

Radiopaque (cholecystogram)

Inflammation

Bile acids absorbed from nonulcerated surface

Calcium and protein ooze into lumen from ulcerated area

Surface aspect

Sections

Mixed stones with calcium

REFERENCES

Level II

Graham G, Baxi L, Tharakan T: Laparoscopic cholecystectomy during pregnancy: a case series and review of the literature. Obstet Gynecol Surv. 1998;53:566.

Lanzafame RJ: Laparoscopic cholecystectomy during pregnancy. Surgery 1995;118:627; discussion 631.

Level III

Barone JE, Bears S, Chen S, et al: Outcome study of cholecystectomy during pregnancy. Am J Surg 1999;177:232.

Block P, Kelly TR: Management of gallstone pancreatitis during pregnancy and the postpartum period. Surg Gynecol Obstet 1989;168:426.

Coleman MT, Trianfo VA, Rund DA: Nonobstetric emergencies in pregnancy: trauma and surgical conditions. Am J Obstet Gynecol 1997;177:497.

Ghumman E, Barry M, Grace PA: Management of gallstones in pregnancy. Br J Surg 1997;84:1646.

Glasgow RE, Visser BC, Harris HW, et al: Changing management of gallstone disease during pregnancy. Surg Endosc 1998;12:241.

Indar AA, Beckingham IJ: Acute cholecystitis. BMJ 2002;325:639.

Nesbitt TH, Kay HH, McCoy MC, Herbert WN: Endoscopic management of biliary disease during pregnancy. Obstet Gynecol 1996;87:806.

Scott LD: Gallstone disease and pancreatitis in pregnancy. Gastroenterol Clin North Am 1992;21:803.

Sharp HT: Gastrointestinal surgical conditions during pregnancy. Clin Obstet Gynecol 1994;37:306.

Smith RP, Nolan TE: Gallbladder disease and women: etiology, diagnosis and therapy. Female Patient 1992;17:99.

INTRODUCTION

Description: Chorioamnionitis is inflammation of the fetal membranes. This may be associated with prolonged or premature rupture of the membranes or a primary cause of premature labor.

Prevalence: 50% of premature deliveries.

Predominant age: Reproductive.

Genetics: No genetic pattern.

ETIOLOGY AND PATHOGENESIS

Causes: Infection by organisms ascending from the vaginal canal, most often when the membranes have been ruptured. Studies indicate that bacteria (specifically *Escherichia coli*) can permeate intact chorioamnionic membranes. Infection may also occur by hematogenous, transabdominal, or transfallopian routes.

Risk factors: Prolonged rupture of the membranes, frequent pelvic examinations, bacterial or trichomonas vaginitis, vaginal or cervical infection with *Chlamydia trachomatis*, smoking, anemia, vaginal bleeding.

CLINICAL CHARACTERISTICS

Signs and Symptoms

- May be asymptomatic
- Fever (>100.5°F, 38°C)
- Tachycardia (maternal and fetal)
- Uterine irritability and tenderness
- May result in premature rupture of the membranes or preterm labor
- Maternal signs of infection (elevated white blood count and sedimentation rate)
- Purulent cervical discharge (late)

DIAGNOSTIC APPROACH

Differential Diagnosis

- Placental abruption
- Intra-abdominal infection (e.g., appendicitis)
- Pyelonephritis
- Pneumonia
- Pulmonary embolism
- Wound infection (episiotomy, abdominal incision following cesarean delivery or tubal ligation)
- Breast engorgement
- Drug fever

Associated Conditions: Endometritis, fetal infections (pneumonia, skin infections), and oligohydramnios have been linked to clinical chorioamnionitis. Dysfunctional labor and postpartum hemorrhage are more common. Cerebral palsy has been linked to intrauterine infection.

Workup and Evaluation

Laboratory: White blood count and red cell sedimentation rate. Gram stain of amniotic fluid (a negative test carries a 99% specificity). Cultures may be obtained and may be of assistance in management, but the diagnosis is often made on clinical grounds. (Amniocentesis for culture has not been shown to improve pregnancy outcome. There is no clear evidence to support the use of C-reactive protein for the early diagnosis of chorioamnionitis.)

Imaging: No imaging indicated.

Special Tests: A biophysical profile of the fetus may be of assistance in planning management (if time and maternal condition permit).

Diagnostic Procedures: Physical examination, cultures.

Pathologic Findings

Invasion of the chorion by mononuclear and polymorphonuclear leukocytes (nonspecific).

MANAGEMENT AND THERAPY

Nonpharmacologic

General Measures: Evaluation and antibiosis.

Specific Measures: Expedited delivery (induction of labor, augmentation of labor).

Diet: No specific dietary changes indicated except as dictated by obstetric management.

Activity: No restriction except as dictated by obstetric management.

Patient Education: Reassurance; American College of Obstetricians and Gynecologists Patient Education Booklet AP087 (Preterm Labor)

Drug(s) of Choice

Broad-spectrum antibiotic coverage based on organism suspected or detected by culture.

Cefoxitin (2 g IV every 6 to 8 hours)

or

Ticarcillin/clavulanate (Timentin, 3.1 g IV every 6 hours)

or

Imipenem cilastatin (Primaxin, 0.5 g IV every 6 hours)

or

Ampicillin/sulbactam (Unasyn, 3.0 g IV every 6 hours)

Contraindications: Known or suspected allergy. See individual agents for additional considerations.

Precautions: See individual agents.

Interactions: See individual agents.

Alternative Drugs

Mezlocillin 4 g IV every 4 to 6 hours; piperacillin 3 to 4 g IV every 4 hours.

FOLLOW-UP

Patient Monitoring: Increased need for fetal and maternal monitoring for the effects of infection (maternal and fetal) and for the associated labor.

Prevention/Avoidance: Restricted vaginal examinations in labor after rupture of the membranes.

Possible Complications: Significant sepsis may occur, in rare cases to the extent that hysterectomy may be required. There is an increased risk for dysfunctional

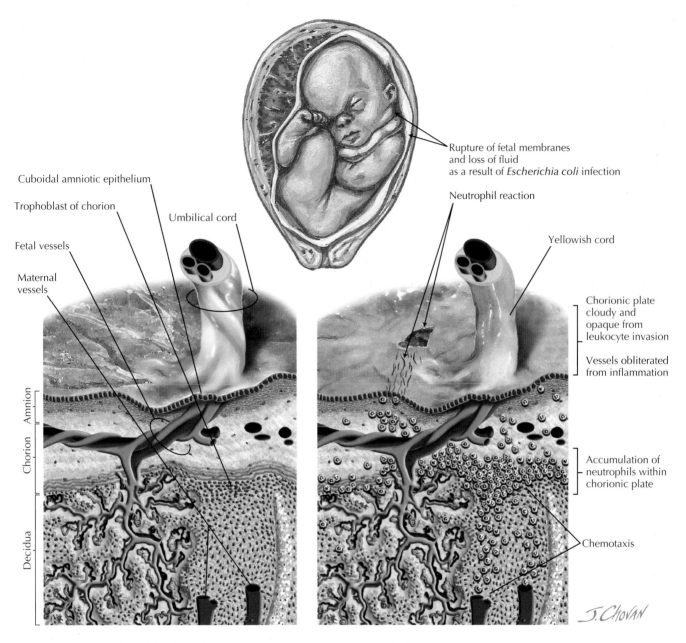

Rupture of fetal membranes and loss of fluid as a result of *Escherichia coli* infection

Neutrophil reaction

Yellowish cord

Cuboidal amniotic epithelium

Trophoblast of chorion

Umbilical cord

Fetal vessels

Maternal vessels

Chorionic plate cloudy and opaque from leukocyte invasion

Vessels obliterated from inflammation

Amnion

Chorion

Decidua

Accumulation of neutrophils within chorionic plate

Chemotaxis

Normal Amniochorion

Chorioamnionitis

labor and postpartum hemorrhage. If antibiotic therapy does not provide improvement in 24 to 48 hours, consider the possibility of abscess or septic pelvic thrombophlebitis.

Expected Outcome: With early recognition, aggressive antibiosis, and expedited delivery, maternal response should be expected to be good. Fetal outcome is based on gestational age at delivery.

MISCELLANEOUS

Pregnancy Considerations: When chorioamnionitis is present, delivery generally must be expedited.

Other Notes: Up to 20% of women with preterm labor can have bacteria recovered by amniocentesis without

evidence of overt clinical infection. Chorioamnionitis is not an indication for cesarean delivery.

ICD-9-CM Code: 658.4.

REFERENCES

Level I
Chapman SJ, Owen J: Randomized trial of single-dose versus multiple-dose cefotetan for the postpartum treatment of intrapartum chorioamnionitis. Am J Obstet Gynecol 1997;177:831.

Grable IA, Garcia PM, Perry D, Socol ML: Group B Streptococcus and preterm premature rupture of membranes: a randomized, double-blind clinical trial of antepartum ampicillin. Am J Obstet Gynecol 1996;175:1036.

Locksmith GJ, Chin A, Vu T, et al: High compared with standard gentamicin dosing for chorioamnionitis: a comparison of maternal and fetal serum drug levels. Obstet Gynecol 2005;105:473.

Mitra AG, Whitten MK, Laurent SL, Anderson WE: A randomized, prospective study comparing once-daily gentamicin versus thrice-daily gentamicin in the treatment of puerperal infection. Am J Obstet Gynecol 1997;177:786.

Owen J, Groome LJ, Hauth JC: Randomized trial of prophylactic antibiotic therapy after preterm amnion rupture. Am J Obstet Gynecol 1993;169:976.

Turnquest MA, How HY, Cook CR, et al: Chorioamnionitis: is continuation of antibiotic therapy necessary after cesarean section? Am J Obstet Gynecol 1998;179:1261.

Level II

Chi BH, Mudenda V, Levy J, et al: Acute and chronic chorioamnionitis and the risk of perinatal human immunodeficiency virus-1 transmission. Am J Obstet Gynecol 2006;194:174.

Edwards RK, Duff P: Single additional dose postpartum therapy for women with chorioamnionitis. Obstet Gynecol 2003;102:957.

Kenyon S, Boulvain M, Neilson J: Antibiotics for preterm rupture of the membranes: a systematic review. Obstet Gynecol 2004; 104:1051.

Livingston JC, Llata E, Rinehart E, et al: Gentamicin and clindamycin therapy in postpartum endometritis: the efficacy of daily dosing versus dosing every 8 hours. Am J Obstet Gynecol 2003;188:149.

Mozurkewich EL, Wolf FM: Premature rupture of membranes at term: a meta-analysis of three management schemes. Obstet Gynecol 1997;89:1035.

Rouse DJ, Landon M, Leveno KJ, et al; National Institute of Child Health And Human Development, Maternal-Fetal Medicine Units Network: The Maternal-Fetal Medicine Units cesarean registry: Chorioamnionitis at term and its duration-relationship to outcomes. Am J Obstet Gynecol 2004;191:211.

Segel SY, Miles AM, Clothier B, et al: Duration of antibiotic therapy after preterm premature rupture of fetal membranes. Am J Obstet Gynecol 2003;189:799.

Trochez-Martinez RD, Smith P, Lamont RF: Use of C-reactive protein as a predictor of chorioamnionitis in preterm prelabour rupture of membranes: a systematic review. BJOG 2007;114:796.

Ugwumadu A, Reid F, Hay P, et al: Oral clindamycin and histologic chorioamnionitis in women with abnormal vaginal flora. Obstet Gynecol 2006;107:863.

Wu YW, Colford JM Jr: Chorioamnionitis as a risk factor for cerebral palsy: a meta-analysis. JAMA 2000;284:1417.

Level III

American College of Obstetricians and Gynecologists: Prevention of early-onset group B streptococcal disease in newborns. ACOG Committee Opinion 279. Obstet Gynecol 2002;100:1405.

American College of Obstetricians and Gynecologists: Prophylactic antibiotics in labor and delivery. ACOG Practice Bulletin 47. Obstet Gynecol 2003;102:875.

American College of Obstetricians and Gynecologists: Premature rupture of membranes. ACOG Practice Bulletin 80. Obstet Gynecol 2007;109:1007.

Gibbs RS: Chorioamnionitis and bacterial vaginosis. Am J Obstet Gynecol 1993;169:460.

Gibbs RS, Romero R, Hillier SL, et al: A review of premature birth and subclinical infection. Am J Obstet Gynecol 1992;166:1515.

Gibbs RS, Schrag S, Schuchat A: Perinatal infections due to group B streptococci. Obstet Gynecol 2004;104:1062.

Mercer BM, Arheart KL: Antimicrobial therapy in expectant management of preterm premature rupture of the membranes. Lancet 1995;346:1271.

Simhan HN, Canavan TP: Preterm premature rupture of membranes: diagnosis, evaluation and management strategies. BJOG 2005; 112:32.

INTRODUCTION

Description: Postpartum depression is a cluster of symptoms characterized by disturbance of mood; a loss of sense of control; intense mental, emotional, and physical anguish; and a loss of self-esteem associated with childbirth.

Prevalence: Eight percent to ten percent of delivering women, true psychosis—1 to 2 of 1000 deliveries.

Predominant Age: Reproductive.

Genetics: No genetic pattern, although there is a proposed family tendency.

ETIOLOGY AND PATHOGENESIS

Causes: Unknown.

Risk Factors: History of major depression, premenstrual syndrome, prior postpartum depression, perinatal loss, early childhood loss (parent, sibling), physical or sexual abuse, socioeconomic deprivation, family predisposition, lifestyle stress, preterm delivery, unplanned pregnancy. There is a 50% recurrence rate for subsequent pregnancies.

CLINICAL CHARACTERISTICS

Signs and Symptoms

- Five of the following must be present—depressive mood most of the time; diminished interest in normal or pleasurable activities; significant involuntary change in weight; insomnia or hypersomnia; psychomotor agitation or retardation; fatigue or loss of energy; feelings of worthlessness or guilt; diminished ability to think or concentrate; recurrent thoughts of death
- Begins 2 to 12 months after delivery; lasts 3 to 14 months

DIAGNOSTIC APPROACH

Differential Diagnosis

- Normal grief reaction
- Transient mood change ("postpartum blues")
- Substance abuse
- Eating disorders or other nonmood psychiatric disorders

Associated Conditions: None.

Workup and Evaluation

Laboratory: No evaluation indicated.
Imaging: No imaging indicated.
Special Tests: Beck Depression Inventory may be used to screen for depression.
Diagnostic Procedures: History, suspicion.

Pathologic Findings

None.

MANAGEMENT AND THERAPY

Nonpharmacologic

General Measures: Support, reassurance, and assistance with transition to motherhood. Postpartum exercise has been associated with a lower rate of depression.

Specific Measures: Psychotherapy, antidepressants, electroshock therapy.

Diet: No specific dietary changes indicated.

Activity: No restriction.

Patient Education: Reassurance, family support; American College of Obstetricians and Gynecologists Patient Education Pamphlet AP091 (Postpartum Depression).

Drug(s) of Choice

- Selective serotonin reuptake inhibitors (fluoxetine [Prozac] 10 to 40 mg daily, paroxetine [Paxil] 20 to 50 mg daily, sertraline [Zoloft] 50 to 150 mg daily).
- For symptoms of appetite loss; loss of energy or interest in pleasure; psychomotor retardation; thoughts of hopelessness, guilt, or suicide: cyclic antidepressants (e.g., amitriptyline, clomipramine, doxepin, imipramine, nortriptyline, bupropion, and others).
- For symptoms of increased appetite, sleepiness, high levels of anxiety, phobias, obsessive-compulsive disorders: monoamine oxidase (MAO) inhibitors (e.g., isocarboxazid, phenelzine, tranylcypromine).

Contraindications: See individual agents.

Precautions: Use in pregnancy must be carefully weighed versus the potential effects (teratogenic) on the fetus. Some agents are associated with delayed cardiac conduction and disturbances in rhythm. Tricyclic agents, paroxetine, sertraline, and venlafaxine must be tapered over 2 to 4 weeks to discontinue.

Interactions: Virtually all agents may produce fatal interactions with monoamine oxidase inhibitors or antiarrhythmic medications. Monoamine oxidase inhibitors can also adversely interact with vasoconstrictors, decongestants, meperidine, and other narcotics.

Alternative Therapy

Electroshock therapy may still play a role in the treatment of major depression and mania in those who do not respond to other therapies or are at high risk for suicide.

FOLLOW-UP

Patient Monitoring: Follow up at 6 weeks, 3 and 6 months, and as needed.

Prevention/Avoidance: None for primary occurrence. For those with a history of prior postpartum depression, prophylactic treatment with antidepressants is associated with a reduced rate of recurrence. Postpartum

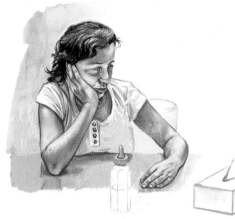

Patient may have prior history of depression or premenstrual tension, or prior postpartum depression

Condition begins 2–12 months postdelivery and may last 3–14 months

Postpartum depression is characterized by a disturbance of mood; a loss of sense of control; intense mental, emotional, and physical anguish; and a loss of self-esteem associated with childbirth

Diagnostic Criteria
(must meet five of the following factors)

1) Depressed mood for majority of time

2) Decreased interest in pleasurable activities

3) Significant involuntary weight loss

4) Psychomotor agitation or retardation

5) Feelings of guilt or worthlessness

6) Decreased concentration

7) Recurrent thoughts of death

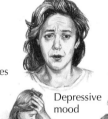

Depressive mood

Decreased concentration

Psychomotor agitation or retardation

Feelings of worthlessness or guilt

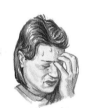

Recurrent thoughts of death

exercise has been associated with a lower rate of depression.

Possible Complications: Progressive loss of function, suicide.

Expected Outcome: Generally good response for mild to moderate depression with psychotherapy and medication; severe depression in 45% to 65% of patients responds to medication. Recurrence rates are approximately 50% after a single episode, 70% after two episodes, and 90% with three or more episodes.

MISCELLANEOUS

Pregnancy Considerations: Tends to recur with subsequent pregnancies. Prophylactic treatment after delivery should be considered for these patients.

ICD-9-CM Code: 648.4.

REFERENCES

Level I
Hagan R, Evans SF, Pope S: Preventing postnatal depression in mothers of very preterm infants: a randomised controlled trial. BJOG 2004;111:641.
Wisner KL, Perel JM, Peindl KS, et al: Prevention of postpartum depression: a pilot randomized clinical trial. Am J Psychiatry 2004;161:1290.

Level II
Dennis CL: Psychosocial and psychological interventions for prevention of postnatal depression: systematic review. BMJ 2005;331:15.
Gavin NI, Gaynes BN, Lohr KN, et al: Perinatal depression: a systematic review of prevalence and incidence. Obstet Gynecol 2005;106:1071.

Level III
American College of Obstetricians and Gynecologists: Exercise during pregnancy and the postpartum period. ACOG Committee Opinion 267. Obstet Gynecol 2002;99:171.
American College of Obstetricians and Gynecologists: Psychosocial risk factors: perinatal screening and intervention. ACOG Committee Opinion 343. Obstet Gynecol 2006;108:469.
American College of Obstetricians and Gynecologists: Treatment with selective serotonin reuptake inhibitors during pregnancy. ACOG Committee Opinion 354. Obstet Gynecol 2006;108:1601.
Beck A: Depression Inventory. Philadelphia, Center for Cognitive Therapy, 1991.
Brockington I: Postpartum psychiatric disorders. Lancet 2004; 363:303.
Clay EC, Seehusen DA: A review of postpartum depression for the primary care physician. South Med J 2004;97:157.
Cooper PJ, Murray L: Postnatal depression. BMJ 1998;316:1884.
Halbreich U: The association between pregnancy processes, preterm delivery, low birth weight, and postpartum depressions—The need for interdisciplinary integration. Am J Obstet Gynecol 2005; 193:1312.
Miller LJ: Postpartum depression. JAMA 2002;287:762.
Suri R, Burt VK, Altshuler LL, et al: Fluvoxamine for postpartum depression. Am J Psychiatry 2001;158:1739.
Wisner KL, Parry BL, Piontek CM: Clinical practice. Postpartum depression. N Engl J Med 2002;347:194.

THE CHALLENGE

To diagnose and manage disturbances of glucose metabolism to minimize the risk to mother and fetus associated with diabetes. Diabetes and pregnancy have profound effects on each other, making a familiarity with the interactions between mother, fetus, and the diabetic process a requirement to provide optimal care.

Scope of the Problem: Diabetes mellitus is the most common medical complication of pregnancy, affecting 2% to 5% of patients (varying in direct proportion to the prevalence of type 2 diabetes in a given population or ethnic group). Patients who had gestational diabetes in a previous pregnancy have a 33% to 50% likelihood of recurrence in a subsequent pregnancy. Patients with type 1 diabetes are at greater risk for maternal complications (diabetic ketoacidosis, glucosuria, hyperglycemia, polyhydramnios, pre-eclampsia, pregnancy-induced hypertension, preterm labor, retinopathy, urinary tract infections, postpartum uterine atony). The offspring of women with diabetes have a 3-fold greater risk of congenital anomalies (3% to 6%) than children of mothers without diabetes (1% to 2%). Most common among these anomalies are cardiac and limb deformities. Other fetal complications include fetal demise, hydramnios, hyperbilirubinemia, hypocalcemia, hypoglycemia, macrosomia, polycythemia, prematurity, respiratory distress syndrome, and spontaneous abortion.

Objectives of Management: To return serum glucose levels to as close to normal as possible through a combination of diet, exercise, oral hypoglycemic agents, and insulin (for selected patients). Optimal management of diabetes begins before pregnancy. Optimal management also requires patient and family education and involvement. For the established patient with diabetes, this teaching is directed to the need for tighter control and more frequent monitoring. The woman with newly diagnosed diabetes requires general instruction about her disease and the unique aspects of diabetes during pregnancy. From the standpoint of the fetus, the goal of treatment is to reduce the likelihood of macrosomia and its consequences; neonatal hypoglycemia also may be reduced.

TACTICS

Relevant Pathophysiology: Human placental lactogen, made in abundance by the growing placenta, promotes lipolysis and decreases glucose uptake and gluconeogenesis. This anti-insulin effect is sufficient to tip borderline patients into a diabetic state or prompt readjustments in the insulin dosage used by patients with insulin-dependent diabetes. Estrogen, progesterone, and placental insulinase further complicate the management of diabetes, making diabetic ketoacidosis more common. High renal plasma flow and diffusion rates that exceed tubular reabsorption result in a physiologic glucosuria of approximately 300 mg/day. This physiologic glucosuria, combined with the poor correlation between urinary glucose and blood glucose levels, makes the urinary glucose screening useless to detect or monitor diabetes during pregnancy.

Strategies: The severity of diabetes may be classified by either the American Diabetes Association (ADA) classification or by the White classification schemes, although the latter has been rendered less useful by improvements in fetal assessment, neonatal care, and the metabolic management of the pregnant patient. The use of these classifications makes comparisons of published data meaningful and may help to predict the relative risk to the pregnant mother and fetus. Patients with American Diabetes Association-defined type 2 disease are often overweight and their diabetes may be controlled with strict diet or with minimal oral hypoglycemic agent or insulin therapy. Gestational diabetes is reversible, although these patients have a greater incidence of glucose intolerance in subsequent pregnancies or with aging. Because of the increased risk of fetal anomalies, a determination of maternal serum α-fetoprotein and early ultrasonographic studies are of greater importance for these patients. Antenatal testing and active management of late pregnancy and labor induction are all indicated for selected patients with diabetes. When there is an estimated fetal weight of 4500 g or more, cesarean delivery may be considered because it may reduce the likelihood of permanent brachial plexus injury in the infant.

Patient Education: American College of Obstetricians and Gynecologists Patient Education Pamphlet AP051 (Diabetes and Pregnancy).

IMPLEMENTATION

Special Considerations: Screening for gestational diabetes is carried out by measurement of plasma glucose level 1 hour after ingestion of a 50-g glucose load, performed between 24 and 28 weeks of gestation. (Jellybeans can be substituted for the usual glucose beverage—28 standard-sized jellybeans = 50 g simple carbohydrate—but this method has poor sensitivity [40%] when compared with glucose polymer solutions [80% to 90%]) The upper limit of normal for such a test is 130 mg/dL. (A screening test threshold of 140 mg/dL has 10% less sensitivity than a threshold of 130 mg/dL but fewer false-positive results; either threshold is acceptable.) If a patient's value exceeds this threshold, a formal 3-hour glucose tolerance test is performed. About 15% of patients have an abnormal screening test, and about the same proportion have an abnormal 3-hour test. For a 3-hour glucose tolerance test, the patient must ingest a minimum of 150 g/day of glucose for the 3 days preceding the test. A fasting glucose level is determined, and a 100-g glucose load is consumed. Plasma glucose levels are then measured at 1, 2, and 3 hours. If two or more values are abnormal, the diagnosis of gestational diabetes may be made. If only one value is abnormal, the test is considered equivocal and should be repeated in 4 to 6 weeks. Studies indicate that screening may be omitted

Diabetes in Pregnancy

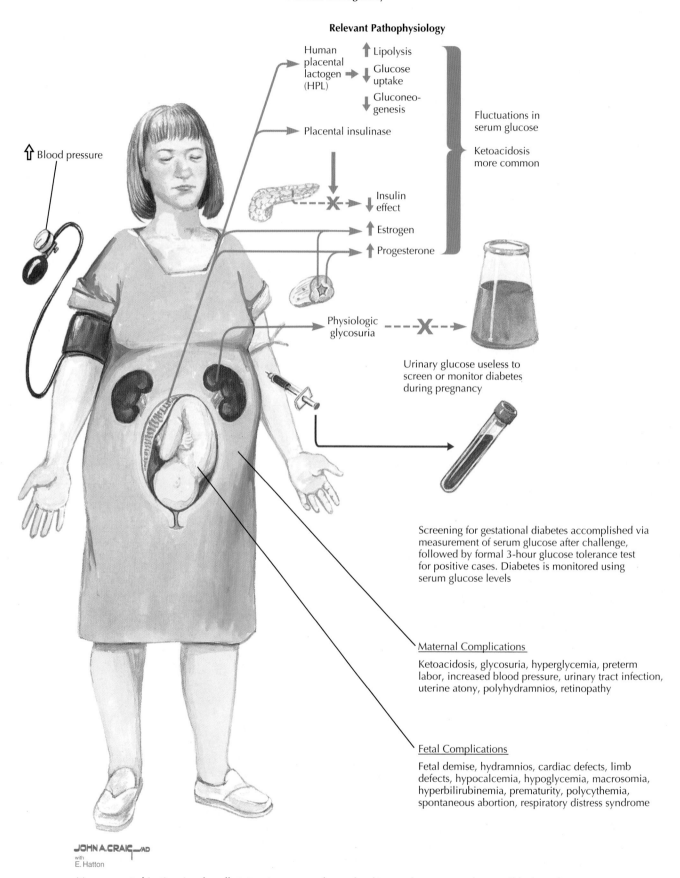

Relevant Pathophysiology

Human placental lactogen (HPL) ➔ ↑ Lipolysis
↓ Glucose uptake
↓ Gluconeogenesis

Fluctuations in serum glucose

Ketoacidosis more common

Placental insulinase

↓ Insulin effect

↑ Estrogen

↑ Progesterone

↑ Blood pressure

Physiologic glycosuria

Urinary glucose useless to screen or monitor diabetes during pregnancy

Screening for gestational diabetes accomplished via measurement of serum glucose after challenge, followed by formal 3-hour glucose tolerance test for positive cases. Diabetes is monitored using serum glucose levels

Maternal Complications

Ketoacidosis, glycosuria, hyperglycemia, preterm labor, increased blood pressure, urinary tract infection, uterine atony, polyhydramnios, retinopathy

Fetal Complications

Fetal demise, hydramnios, cardiac defects, limb defects, hypocalcemia, hypoglycemia, macrosomia, hyperbilirubinemia, prematurity, polycythemia, spontaneous abortion, respiratory distress syndrome

JOHN A. CRAIG—AD
with
E. Hatton

Management objectives involve efforts to return serum glucose levels to as close to normal as possible through a combination of diet, exercise, and insulin (as indicated), and tight control in established diabetic patients.

for selected individuals who are very low risk by selection criteria (see box).

Individuals at Low Risk for Gestational Diabetes (Must Meet All Criteria)

- Age younger than 25 years
- No known diabetes in first-degree relative
- Not a member of an ethnic group with an increased risk for the development of type 2 diabetes (examples of high-risk ethnic groups include women of Hispanic, African, Native American, South or East Asian, or Pacific Islands ancestry)
- Body mass index of 25 or less
- No previous history of abnormal glucose tolerance
- No previous history of adverse obstetric outcomes usually associated with gestational diabetes mellitus

REFERENCES

Level I

Brankston GN, Mitchell BF, Ryan EA, Okun NB: Resistance exercise decreases the need for insulin in overweight women with gestational diabetes mellitus. Am J Obstet Gynecol 2004;190: 188.

Evers IM, de Valk HW, Visser GH: Risk of complications of pregnancy in women with type 1 diabetes: nationwide prospective study in the Netherlands. BMJ 2004;328:915. Epub 2004 Apr 5.

Jensen DM, Molsted-Pedersen L, Beck-Nielsen H, et al: Screening for gestational diabetes mellitus by a model based on risk indicators: a prospective study. Am J Obstet Gynecol 2003; 189:1383.

Langer O, Conway DL, Berkus MD, et al: A comparison of glyburide and insulin in women with gestational diabetes mellitus. N Engl J Med 2000;343:1134.

Level II

Crowther CA, Hiller JE, Moss JR, et al; Australian Carbohydrate Intolerance Study in Pregnant Women (ACHOIS) Trial Group: Effect of treatment of gestational diabetes mellitus on pregnancy outcomes. N Engl J Med 2005;352:2477. Epub 2005 Jun 12.

Lamar ME, Kuehl TJ, Cooney AT, et al: Jelly beans as an alternative to a fifty-gram glucose beverage for gestational diabetes screening. Am J Obstet Gynecol 1999;181:1154.

Oken E, Ning Y, Rifas-Shiman SL, et al: Associations of physical activity and inactivity before and during pregnancy with glucose tolerance. Obstet Gynecol 2006;108:1200.

Level III

American College of Obstetricians and Gynecologists: Gestational diabetes. ACOG Practice Bulletin 30. Obstet Gynecol 2001; 98:525.

American College of Obstetricians and Gynecologists: Exercise during pregnancy and the postpartum period. ACOG Committee Opinion 267. Obstet Gynecol 2002;99:171.

American College of Obstetricians and Gynecologists: Pregestational diabetes mellitus. ACOG Practice Bulletin 60. Obstet Gynecol 2005;105:675.

Buchanan TA, Xiang AH: Gestational diabetes mellitus. J Clin Invest 2005;115:485.

Carroll MA, Yeomans ER: Diabetic ketoacidosis in pregnancy. Crit Care Med 2005;33:S347.

Coustan DR: Gestational diabetes. In National Institutes of Diabetes and Digestive and Kidney Diseases. Diabetes in America, 2nd ed. Bethesda, MD, NIDDK, 1995; NIH Publication 95–1468:703.

Feig DS, Palda VA: Type 2 diabetes in pregnancy: a growing concern. Lancet 2002;359:1690.

Gabbe SG, Graves CR: Management of diabetes mellitus complicating pregnancy. Obstet Gynecol 2003;102:857.

Garner P: Type I diabetes mellitus and pregnancy. Lancet 1995; 346:157.

Jovanovic L, Pettitt DJ: Gestational diabetes mellitus. JAMA 2001; 286:2516.

Kjos SL, Buchanan TA: Gestational diabetes mellitus. N Engl J Med 1999;341:1749.

Nold JL, Georgieff MK: Infants of diabetic mothers. Pediatr Clin North Am 2004;51:619, viii.

Taylor R, Davison JM: Type 1 diabetes and pregnancy. BMJ 2007; 334:742.

INTRODUCTION

Description: Fetal alcohol syndrome is characterized by malformations found in infants born to mothers who have consumed alcohol during pregnancy. Abnormalities include structural malformations (predominantly facial), growth restriction, and neurologic abnormalities including mental retardation.

Prevalence: Estimates vary from 6 of 10,000 births (1993) to 2 of 1000 births (2000). Studies by the Centers for Disease Control and Prevention show fetal alcohol syndrome rates ranging from 0.2 to 1.5 per 1000 live births in different areas of the United States.

Predominant Age: Reproductive for mothers, infants diagnosed at birth.

Genetics: No genetic pattern.

ETIOLOGY AND PATHOGENESIS

Causes: Alcohol consumption during pregnancy (generally >3 oz/day). There does not appear to be a lower limit of safety, nor are the effects confined to one part of pregnancy. The severity of the effects does appear to be proportional to the amount and duration of exposure. Clinically identifiable effects are generally not seen with sporadic exposures of less than 1 oz of alcohol per day, although absolute safety cannot be assured even at this dose.

Risk Factors: Alcohol use during pregnancy.

CLINICAL CHARACTERISTICS

Signs and Symptoms

- Facial deformities—microcephaly, short palpebral fissures, flat midface, underdeveloped philtrum and thinned upper lip; low nasal bridge, epicanthal folds, minor ear anomalies, small teeth with faulty enamel, foreshortened nose and micrognathia may also be seen; two or more abnormal facial features must be present to make the diagnosis
- Cardiac malformations
- Deformities of joints, limbs, and fingers
- Vision difficulties including nearsightedness (myopia)
- Intrauterine and extrauterine growth restriction
- Mental retardation and developmental abnormalities, brain and spinal defects
- Abnormal behavior such as short attention span, hyperactivity, poor impulse control, extreme nervousness, and anxiety

DIAGNOSTIC APPROACH

Differential Diagnosis

- Other chromosomal or congenital syndromes

Associated Conditions: Maternal—other substance abuse (tobacco, drugs), sexually transmitted disease. Fetal—dental caries, cardiac defects, and ophthalmic problems (vision correction often necessary).

Workup and Evaluation

Laboratory: No evaluation indicated.

Imaging: Ultrasonography may be used to assess fetal growth and development. Some cardiac anomalies may be detected while in utero; absence does not exclude effects.

Special Tests: None indicated.

Diagnostic Procedures: History (maternal) and physical examination of newborn.

Pathologic Findings

None.

MANAGEMENT AND THERAPY

Nonpharmacologic

General Measures: For the mother—counseling, alcohol and substance abuse programs. For the fetus—evaluation, special education and support, surveillance for dental caries (more common in these children) and cardiac and ophthalmic problems.

Specific Measures: None.

Diet: Reduction or elimination of alcohol for the duration of pregnancy.

Activity: No restriction.

Patient Education: Diet and alcohol counseling; American College of Obstetricians and Gynecologists Patient Education Pamphlet AP132 (Alcohol and Pregnancy), AP104 (Drugs and Pregnancy).

Drug(s) of Choice

None.

FOLLOW-UP

Patient Monitoring: Normal health maintenance, surveillance for dental caries (more common in these children) and cardiac and ophthalmic problems.

Prevention/Avoidance: Reduction or elimination of alcohol use during pregnancy. No safe level of exposure has been demonstrated, although sporadic use of less than 1 oz of alcohol per day has not been associated with the syndrome.

Possible Complications: Higher rate of spontaneous miscarriage in heavy users of alcohol.

Expected Outcome: Infants affected by fetal alcohol syndrome vary from mildly to profoundly mentally retarded. Similarly, structural anomalies are variable but lifelong.

MISCELLANEOUS

ICD-9-CM Code: 760.71.

Fetal Alcohol Syndrome
Clinical Features

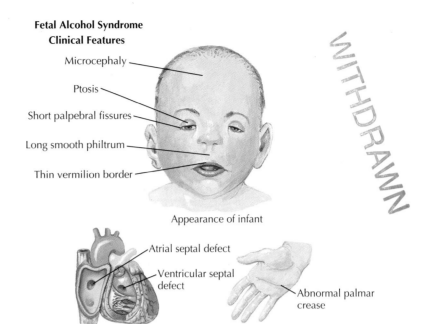

Microcephaly
Ptosis
Short palpebral fissures
Long smooth philtrum
Thin vermilion border

Appearance of infant

WITHDRAWN

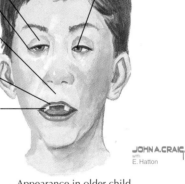

Atrial septal defect
Ventricular septal defect
Abnormal palmar crease

Cardiac and skeletal anomalies are common

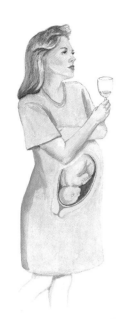

Alcohol consumption in excess of 3 oz/day during pregnancy is considered "high risk." Although identifiable effects are seldom seen with consumption less than 1 oz/day, there is no assurance of safety at that level

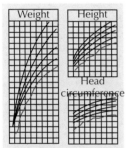

Weight Height Head circumference

Developmental deficiency is common. Prognosis is most influenced by degree of maternal alcohol consumption, extent and severity of malformation pattern, including growth retardation

Mental retardation
Strabismus
Ptosis
Short palpebral fissures
Long, smooth philtrum
Thin vermilion border
Dental caries and malocclusion

JOHN A. CRAIG with E. Hatton

Appearance in older child

REFERENCES

Level I
Chang G, McNamara TK, Orav EJ, et al: Brief intervention for prenatal alcohol use: a randomized trial. Obstet Gynecol 2005;105:991.

Level II
Floyd RL, Sobell M, Velasquez MM, et al; The Project CHOICES Efficacy Study Group: Preventing alcohol-exposed pregnancies: a randomized controlled trial. Am J Prev Med 2007;32:1.

Henderson J, Gray R, Brocklehurst P: Systematic review of effects of low-moderate prenatal alcohol exposure on pregnancy outcome. BJOG 2007;114:243. Epub 2007 Jan 12.

May PA, Gossage JP: Estimating the prevalence of fetal alcohol syndrome: a summary. Alcohol Res Health 2001;25:159.

Level III
American College of Obstetricians and Gynecologists: Intrauterine growth restriction. ACOG Practice Bulletin 12. Washington, DC, ACOG, 2000.

American College of Obstetricians and Gynecologists: At-risk drinking and illicit drug use: ethical issues in obstetric and gynecologic practice. ACOG Committee Opinion 294. Obstet Gynecol 2004;103:1021.

American College of Obstetricians and Gynecologists: Psychosocial risk factors: perinatal screening and intervention. ACOG Committee Opinion 343. Obstet Gynecol 2006;108:469.

Astley SJ, Clarren SK: A case definition and photographic screening tool for the facial phenotype of fetal alcohol syndrome. J Pediatr 1996;129:33.

Chudley AE, Conry J, Cook JL, et al; Public Health Agency of Canada's National Advisory Committee on Fetal Alcohol Spectrum Disorder: Fetal alcohol spectrum disorder: Canadian guidelines for diagnosis. CMAJ 2005;172:S1.

Clarren SK, Smith DW: The fetal alcohol syndrome. N Engl J Med 1978;298:1063.

Floyd RL, O'Connor MJ, Sokol RJ, et al: Recognition and prevention of fetal alcohol syndrome. Obstet Gynecol 2005;106:1059.

O'Connor MJ, Whaley SE: Brief intervention for alcohol use by pregnant women. Am J Public Health 2007;97:252. Epub 2006 Dec 28.

Roman PM: Biological features of women's alcohol use: a review. Public Health Rep 1988;103:628.

Warren KR, Bast RJ: Alcohol-related birth defects: an update. Public Health Rep 1988;103:638.

INTRODUCTION

Description: Gestational trophoblastic diseases include choriocarcinoma, molar pregnancy (hydatidiform mole and invasive mole), and placental-site trophoblastic tumor. They are abnormalities of pregnancy that arise entirely from abnormal placental proliferation. They are classified as being either complete, in which no fetus is present, or incomplete (partial), in which both fetus (generally abnormal) and molar tissues are present.

Prevalence: Molar pregnancy—1 of 1000 to 1500 pregnancies in the United States, as high as 10 per 1000 pregnancies in Asia; choriocarcinoma—1 of 40,000 pregnancies.

Predominant Age: Greatest during the early and late reproductive years.

Genetics: Complete—mostly 46,XX (paternal in origin, although mitochondrial DNA remains maternal in origin). Incomplete—triploid (69,XXY or 69,XXX; all of paternal origin).

ETIOLOGY AND PATHOGENESIS

Causes: Unknown.

Risk Factors: Maternal age (older than 40: 5.2 times risk), Asians living in Southeast Asia, folate deficiency, prior molar pregnancy (2% recurrence rate).

CLINICAL CHARACTERISTICS

Signs and Symptoms

- Present as a pregnancy but associated with more profound hormonal changes, leading to exaggerated symptoms of pregnancy in many patients
- Uterine size that is inappropriate for dates (larger or smaller, 30%)
- Painless vaginal bleeding (95%, generally between 6 and 16 weeks of gestation)
- Hypertension, pre-eclampsia, proteinuria, nausea and vomiting (hyperemesis, 8%), visual changes, tachycardia, and shortness of breath all possible (pregnancy-induced hypertension in the first trimester of pregnancy is virtually diagnostic)
- Incomplete molar pregnancies—symptoms of an incomplete or missed abortion (90%), including vaginal bleeding (75%)

DIAGNOSTIC APPROACH

Differential Diagnosis

- Choriocarcinoma
- Missed abortion
- Threatened abortion

Associated Conditions: Hyperemesis, hypertension, hyperthyroidism, pre-eclampsia, proteinuria, nausea and vomiting, visual changes, tachycardia, and shortness of breath. Bilateral adnexal masses (theca lutein cysts) occur in 15% to 20% of patients.

Workup and Evaluation

Laboratory: Complete blood count, quantitative measurement of β-human chorionic gonadotropin (β-hCG; to establish risk and serial to follow success of therapy), the patient's blood type and Rh status should be established to allow for Rh immune globulin therapy (if needed) or blood replacement. Clotting function studies and blood cross-matching are advisable before the evacuation of a large uterus. (Chorionic gonadotropin levels often exceed 100,000 ImU/mL.)

Imaging: Ultrasonography can establish the diagnosis. A baseline chest radiograph to check for metastatic disease should be obtained.

Special Tests: Absence of fetal heart sounds (in complete mole).

Diagnostic Procedures: History and physical examination. Edematous trophoblastic fragments may be passed vaginally through a partially dilated cervical os, alerting the clinician to the diagnosis.

Pathologic Findings

Edematous trophoblastic fronds. Karyotype: incomplete; triploid (80%); complete; 46,XX (95%).

MANAGEMENT AND THERAPY

Nonpharmacologic

General Measures: Evaluation and diagnosis, general supportive measures.

Specific Measures: The treatment of molar pregnancies is surgical: evacuation of the uterine contents. This is most often accomplished via suction curettage. Because of the large size of some molar pregnancies and a tendency toward uterine atony, concomitant oxytocin administration is advisable and blood for transfusion must be immediately available, should it be needed.

Diet: No specific dietary changes indicated.

Activity: No restriction.

Drug(s) of Choice

None. (Oxytocin or methylergonovine maleate [Methergine] is used to help contract the uterus during surgical evacuation.) Primary or recurrent malignant trophoblastic disease is generally treated with chemotherapy (methotrexate, actinomycin D, chlorambucil, or cyclophosphamide [Cytoxan], singly or in combination).

FOLLOW-UP

Patient Monitoring: After the uterus has been emptied, the patient must be closely followed for at least 1 year for the possibility of recurrent benign or malignant disease. Any change in the patient's examination, an increase in β-hCG titers, or a failure of the β-hCG level to fall below 10 mIU/mL by 12 weeks after evacuation must be evaluated for the possibility of recurrent benign

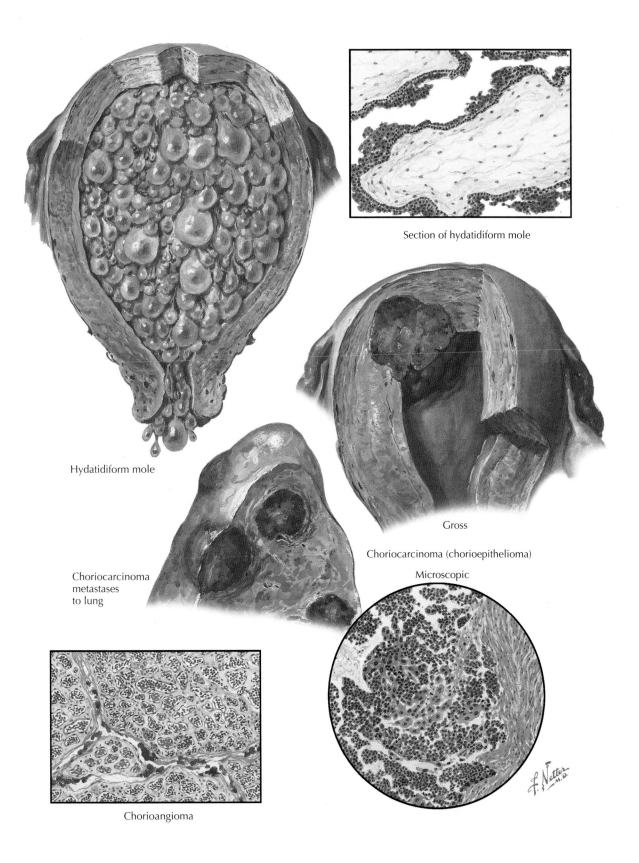

Hydatidiform mole

Section of hydatidiform mole

Gross

Choriocarcinoma metastases to lung

Choriocarcinoma (chorioepithelioma)

Microscopic

Chorioangioma

or malignant disease. Serum hCG levels are generally monitored every 2 weeks until three consecutive tests are negative, then monthly for 6 to 12 months. (Proteolytic enzymes and heterophilic antibodies found in 3% to 4% of individuals can cause a falsely positive hCG test [up to 800 ImU/mL have been reported] and can lead to inappropriate therapy.)

Prevention/Avoidance: None.

Possible Complications: Gestational trophoblastic neoplasia is notable for the possibility of malignant transformation, although less than 10% of patients develop malignant changes. In general, the larger or more advanced the molar pregnancy, the greater the risk of pulmonary complications, bleeding, trophoblastic emboli, or fluid overload during evacuation.

Expected Outcome: Approximately 80% of molar pregnancies follow a benign course after initial therapy. Between 15% and 25% of patients develop invasive disease, and 3% to 5% eventually have metastatic lesions. The prognosis for patients with primary or recurrent malignant trophoblastic disease is generally good (>90% cure rate). The theca lutein cysts often found in molar pregnancies may take several months to regress after evacuation of the uterine contents. Fewer than 5% of patients will require hysterectomy to achieve a cure for choriocarcinoma.

MISCELLANEOUS

Pregnancy Considerations: Pregnancy should be delayed for at least 1 year after a molar pregnancy to avoid confusion between normal pregnancy and recurrent disease. These patients have no higher rate of abortions, stillbirths, congenital anomalies, prematurity, or other complications of pregnancy with future gestations. The placenta from any subsequent pregnancies should be sent for histologic evaluation.

ICD-9-CM Codes: 630, 236.1 (Invasive or malignant).

REFERENCES

Level I

Covens A, Filiaci VL, Burger RA, et al; Gynecologic Oncology Group: Phase II trial of pulse dactinomycin as salvage therapy for failed low-risk gestational trophoblastic neoplasia: a Gynecologic Oncology Group study. Cancer 2006;107:1280.

Goldstein DP, Goldstein PR, Bottomley P, et al: Methotrexate with citrovorum factor rescue for nonmetastatic gestational trophoblastic neoplasms. Obstet Gynecol 1976;48:321.

Homesley HD, Blessing JA, Rettenmaier M, et al: Weekly intramuscular methotrexate for nonmetastatic gestational trophoblastic disease. Obstet Gynecol 1988;72:413.

Level II

Bracken MB: Incidence and aetiology of hydatidiform mole: an epidemiological review. Br J Obstet Gynaecol 1987;94:1123.

Matsui H, Iitsuka Y, Suzuka K, et al: Early pregnancy outcomes after chemotherapy for gestational trophoblastic tumor. J Reprod Med 2004;49:531.

Level III

American College of Obstetricians and Gynecologists: Diagnosis and treatment of gestational trophoblastic disease. ACOG Practice Bulletin 53. Obstet Gynecol 2004;103:1365.

Berkowitz RS, Goldstein DP: Gestational trophoblastic disease. Cancer 1995;76:2079.

Berkowitz RS, Goldstein DP: Chorionic tumors. N Engl J Med 1996;335:1740.

Grimes DA: Epidemiology of gestational trophoblastic disease. Am J Obstet Gynecol 1984;150:309.

Lewis JL Jr: Diagnosis and management of gestational trophoblastic disease. Cancer 1993;71:1639.

Smith HO: Gestational trophoblastic disease epidemiology and trends. Clin Obstet Gynecol 2003;46:541.

Soper JT: Gestational trophoblastic disease. Obstet Gynecol 2006;108:176.

INTRODUCTION

Description: Elevated hormone levels during pregnancy may induce gingival hyperplasia, pedunculated gingival growths, and pyogenic granuloma. Despite concerns directed elsewhere during pregnancy, the practitioner must watch for this common problem and address it when present. Periodontal disease has been identified as a risk factor for preterm delivery.

Prevalence: Common (some estimate up to 90% of population affected).

Genetics: No genetic pattern.

ETIOLOGY AND PATHOGENESIS

Causes: Hormonally induced hypertrophy (may occur with combination oral contraceptives as well). Inadequate plaque removal. Fusiform bacillus or spirochete infection. Allergic reactions.

Risk Factors: Increased hormones (pregnancy, oral contraceptives), poor dental hygiene, mouth breathing, diabetes mellitus, human immunodeficiency virus (HIV) infection, and malocclusion.

CLINICAL CHARACTERISTICS
Signs and Symptoms

- Mouth odor
- Gum swelling and redness (especially at the base of the tooth)
- Change in gum contours
- Bleeding when brushing or flossing
- Edema of interdental papillae

DIAGNOSTIC APPROACH
Differential Diagnosis

- Diabetes mellitus
- Desquamative gingivitis
- Leukemia
- Drug reaction (phenytoin)
- Human immunodeficiency virus infection

Associated Conditions: Periodontitis, glossitis, preterm delivery.

Workup and Evaluation

Laboratory: No evaluation indicated.
Imaging: No imaging indicated.
Special Tests: Smear to identify causative agent. Culture may also be performed.
Diagnostic Procedures: History and physical examination.

Pathologic Findings

Acute or chronic inflammation, broken crepuscular epithelium, hyperemia, polymorphonuclear infiltrates.

MANAGEMENT AND THERAPY
Nonpharmacologic

General Measures: Evaluation; encourage good oral hygiene, smoking cessation, warm saline rinses (twice a day), periodic dental care.
Specific Measures: Removal of irritating factors (plaque).
Diet: Ensure adequate nutrition.
Activity: No restriction.
Patient Education: Reinforce the need for periodic dental care.

Drug(s) of Choice

Penicillin V 250 to 500 mg PO every 6 hours, topical corticosteroids (triamcinolone in Orabase).
Contraindications: Known or suspected allergy.
Precautions: Watch for possible overgrowth of vaginal fungal flora if penicillin is used.
Interactions: See individual agents.

Alternative Drugs

Other antibiotics based on smear or culture results.

FOLLOW-UP

Patient Monitoring: Normal health maintenance.
Prevention/Avoidance: Good dental hygiene (daily brushing and flossing), periodic evaluation and cleaning.
Possible Complications: Severe periodontal disease, tooth loss.
Expected Outcome: Generally improves after delivery if hormonal change is the cause; can recur if dental hygiene is not maintained.

MISCELLANEOUS
ICD-9-CM Code: 523.1.

REFERENCES
Level I
Lopez NJ, Smith PC, Gutierrez J: Periodontal therapy may reduce the risk of preterm low birth weight in women with periodontal disease: a randomized controlled trial. J Periodontol 2002;73:911.
Level II
Boggess KA, Edelstein BL: Oral health in women during preconception and pregnancy: implications for birth outcomes and infant oral health. Matern Child Health J 2006;10:S169.
Gazolla CM, Ribeiro A, Moyses MR, et al: Evaluation of the incidence of preterm low birth weight in patients undergoing periodontal therapy. J Periodontol 2007;78:842.
Khader YS, Ta'ani Q: Periodontal diseases and the risk of preterm birth and low birth weight: a meta-analysis. J Periodontol 2005;76:161.

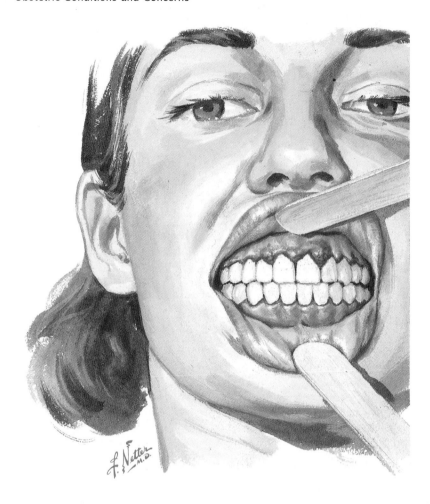

Lopez NJ, Da Silva I, Ipinza J, Gutierrez J: Periodontal therapy reduces the rate of preterm low birth weight in women with pregnancy-associated gingivitis. J Periodontol 2005;76:2144.

Offenbacher S, Lin D, Strauss R, et al: Effects of periodontal therapy during pregnancy on periodontal status, biologic parameters, and pregnancy outcomes: a pilot study. J Periodontol 2006;77:2011.

Pretorius C, Jagatt A, Lamont RF: The relationship between periodontal disease, bacterial vaginosis, and preterm birth. J Perinat Med 2007;35:93.

Vergnes JN, Sixou M: Preterm low birth weight and maternal periodontal status: a meta-analysis. Am J Obstet Gynecol 2007;196:135. e1.

Xiong X, Buekens P, Fraser WD, et al: Periodontal disease and adverse pregnancy outcomes: a systematic review. BJOG 2006; 113:135.

Level III

Barak S, Oettinger-Barak O, Oettinger M, et al: Common oral manifestations during pregnancy: a review. Obstet Gynecol Surv 2003;58:624.

Ferguson JE 2nd, Hansen WF, Novak KF, Novak MJ: Should we treat periodontal disease during gestation to improve pregnancy outcomes? Clin Obstet Gynecol 2007;50:454.

Glickman I: Periodontal disease. N Engl J Med 1971;284: 1071.

Hansen L, Sobol SM, Abelson TI: Otolaryngologic manifestations of pregnancy. J Fam Pract 1986;23:151.

Klebanoff M, Searle K: The role of inflammation in preterm birth—Focus on periodontitis. BJOG 2006;113:43.

Laine MA: Effect of pregnancy on periodontal and dental health. Acta Odontol Scand 2002;60:257.

Michalowicz BS, Durand R: Maternal periodontal disease and spontaneous preterm birth. Periodontol 2000 2007;44:103.

Michalowicz BS, Hodges JS, DiAngelis AJ, et al; OPT Study: Treatment of periodontal disease and the risk of preterm birth. N Engl J Med 2006;355:1885.

Offenbacher S: Maternal periodontal infections, prematurity, and growth restriction. Clin Obstet Gynecol 2004;47:808.

Pihlstrom BL, Michalowicz BS, Johnson NW: Periodontal diseases. Lancet 2005;366:1809.

Scannapieco FA, Bush RB, Paju S: Periodontal disease as a risk factor for adverse pregnancy outcomes. A systematic review. Ann Periodontol 2003;8:70.

Shub A, Swain JR, Newnham JP: Periodontal disease and adverse pregnancy outcomes. J Matern Fetal Neonatal Med 2006;19: 521.

INTRODUCTION

Description: Hemolysis, elevated liver enzymes, low platelet count (HELLP) syndrome is a variant of pregnancy-induced hypertension (PIH) and pre-eclampsia, which are dominated by hepatic and hematologic changes.

Prevalence: Six percent to eight percent of pregnancies, up to 20% of patients with severe pre-eclampsia.

Predominant Age: Reproductive.

Genetics: No genetic pattern.

ETIOLOGY AND PATHOGENESIS

Causes: Unknown. Genetic, endocrine/metabolic (including altered prostaglandin production), uteroplacental ischemia, immunologic.

Risk Factors: Nulliparity, age older than 40 years, African American race, family history of pregnancy-induced hypertension, renal disease, antiphospholipid syndrome, diabetes mellitus, multiple gestation. Chronic hypertension increases the risk of pregnancy-induced hypertension.

CLINICAL CHARACTERISTICS

Signs and Symptoms

- Pre-eclampsia or eclampsia with hemolysis, thrombocytopenia, elevated hepatic transaminase levels (any or all; blood pressure may be normal in up to 20% of patients). (The degree of thrombocytopenia is predictive of the severity of disease and the likelihood of poor outcome.)
- Right upper quadrant or epigastric pain

DIAGNOSTIC APPROACH

Differential Diagnosis

- Pre-eclampsia or eclampsia
- Secondary hypertension
- Improper blood pressure measurement (wrong cuff size, position, technique) resulting in false elevation of readings
- Multiple pregnancy
- Molar pregnancy
- Primary hepatic disease

Associated Conditions: Intrauterine growth restriction, prematurity.

Workup and Evaluation

Laboratory: Liver and renal function studies (e.g., enzymes, renal clearance, 24-hour urinary protein), platelet counts, clotting studies. (Platelet counts of >50,000/mm^3 generally are not associated with spontaneous bleeding.)

Imaging: Ultrasonography to monitor fetal growth (frequently restricted).

Special Tests: Assessment of fetal lung maturation may be performed, but if maternal disease is severe, management is based on maternal factors and not fetal maturation.

Diagnostic Procedures: Measurement of blood pressure, laboratory confirmation.

Pathologic Findings

HELLP syndrome is a multiorgan process, including the renal, hepatic, hematologic, and nervous systems.

MANAGEMENT AND THERAPY

Nonpharmacologic

General Measures: Evaluation, support, and preparation for delivery.

Specific Measures: Patients with HELLP syndrome often represent the sickest patients with pre-eclampsia or eclampsia. The only true treatment is delivery. The presence of HELLP syndrome generally militates against conservative treatment for any but the briefest stabilization period.

Diet: No specific dietary changes indicated.

Activity: No restriction.

Patient Education: American College of Obstetricians and Gynecologists Patient Education Pamphlet AP034 (High Blood Pressure During Pregnancy).

Drug(s) of Choice

For mild to moderate chronic hypertension, α-methyldopa is considered first-line therapy.

During labor or labor induction, magnesium sulfate is often used to reduce the chance of seizures (4 g IV for 20 minutes, then 2 to 3 g/hour IV continuous infusion; therapeutic range 4 to 8 mg/dL).

If blood pressure >180 torr systolic or 110 torr diastolic: hydralazine HCl 5 to 10 mg IV bolus every 20 minutes as needed or labetalol 20 mg IV bolus every 10 minutes as needed to a maximum of 300 mg in 24 hours. (Sodium nitroprusside may be used for extreme disease.)

Steroids have been advocated, but there is insufficient evidence to conclude that they are beneficial.

Contraindications: Angiotensin-converting enzyme (ACE) inhibitors are teratogenic and are contraindicated in pregnancy. Diuretics should be avoided in pregnancy because of the possibility of adverse fetal effects caused by reduced plasma volume. (Despite the common occurrence of edema, these patients have constricted circulatory volume.)

Precautions: Central hemodynamic monitoring should be considered if blood pressure is high or potent agents are used.

Alternative Drugs

Verapamil or nifedipine may also be used to acutely reduce blood pressure.

FOLLOW-UP

Patient Monitoring: Increased maternal and fetal surveillance, antenatal testing.

Prevention/Avoidance: The value of low-dose aspirin therapy or calcium supplementation remains unproved.

Clinical triad

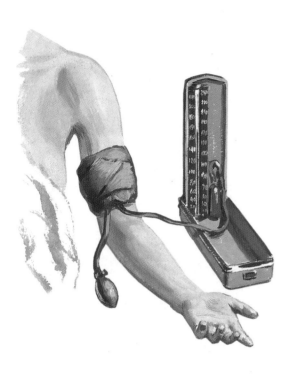

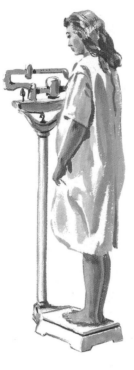

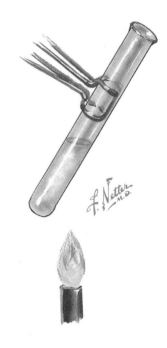

Elevated blood pressure

Excessive weight gain

Proteinuria

Possible Complications: Maternal—cardiac decompensation, stroke, pulmonary edema (10%) and respiratory failure, renal failure (5%), seizures and seizure-related injuries (6%), intracranial hemorrhage, coma, and death (0.5% to 5% mortality). Fetal risk (growth restriction and death) is directly proportional to both the degree of proteinuria and the level of maternal diastolic blood pressure. Placental abruption may occur in up to 10% of cases.

Expected Outcome: HELLP syndrome generally resolves after delivery, but the risk of recurrence with future pregnancies or elevated blood pressure in later life is increased.

MISCELLANEOUS

ICD-9-CM Code: 642.5.

REFERENCES

Level I

Barrilleaux PS, Martin JN Jr, Klauser CK, et al: Postpartum intravenous dexamethasone for severely preeclamptic patients without hemolysis, elevated liver enzymes, low platelets (HELLP) syndrome: a randomized trial. Obstet Gynecol 2005;105:843.

Fonseca JE, Mendez F, Catano C, Arias F: Dexamethasone treatment does not improve the outcome of women with HELLP syndrome: a double-blind, placebo-controlled, randomized clinical trial. Am J Obstet Gynecol 2005;193:1591.

Ganzevoort W, Rep A, Bonsel GJ, et al; PETRA Investigators: A randomised controlled trial comparing two temporising management strategies, one with and one without plasma volume expansion, for severe and early onset pre-eclampsia. BJOG 2005; 112:1358.

Isler CM, Barrilleaux PS, Magann EF, et al: A prospective, randomized trial comparing the efficacy of dexamethasone and betamethasone for the treatment of antepartum HELLP (hemolysis, elevated liver enzymes, and low platelet count) syndrome. Am J Obstet Gynecol 2001;184:1332.

Level II

Matchaba P, Moodley J: Corticosteroids for HELLP syndrome in pregnancy. Cochrane Database Syst Rev 2004;CD002076.

Thangaratinam S, Ismail KM, Sharp S, et al; Tests in Prediction of Pre-eclampsia Severity Review Group: Accuracy of serum uric acid in predicting complications of pre-eclampsia: a systematic review. BJOG 2006;113:369.

Level III

American College of Obstetricians and Gynecologists: Thrombocytopenia in pregnancy. ACOG Practice Bulletin 6. Washington, DC, ACOG, 1999.

American College of Obstetricians and Gynecologists: Chronic hypertension in pregnancy. ACOG Practice Bulletin 29. Obstet Gynecol 2001;98:177.

American College of Obstetricians and Gynecologists: Diagnosis and management of preeclampsia and eclampsia. ACOG Practice Bulletin 33. Obstet Gynecol 2002;99:159.

Clenney TL, Viera AJ: Corticosteroids for HELLP (haemolysis, elevated liver enzymes, low platelets) syndrome. BMJ 2004;329:270.

Geary M: The HELLP syndrome. Br J Obstet Gynaecol 1997; 104:8871.

Martin JN Jr, Rose CH, Briery CM: Understanding and managing HELLP syndrome: the integral role of aggressive glucocorticoids for mother and child. Am J Obstet Gynecol 2006;195:914. Epub 2006 May 2.

O'Brien JM, Milligan DA, Barton JR: Impact of high-dose corticosteroid therapy for patients with HELLP (hemolysis, elevated liver enzymes, and low platelet count) syndrome. Am J Obstet Gynecol 2000;183:921.

INTRODUCTION

Description: Hepatitis is one of the most serious infections that occurs during pregnancy.

Prevalence: Hepatitis—0.1% to 1.5% of pregnancies (one third of Americans have antibodies to hepatitis A). The prevalence of hepatitis in pregnancy has declined in the past 15 years.

Predominant Age: Reproductive.

Genetics: No genetic pattern.

ETIOLOGY AND PATHOGENESIS

Causes: Five different forms of hepatitis may be involved. Hepatitis A is caused by a ribonucleic acid (RNA) virus that is transmitted by fecal–oral contamination and accounts for 30% to 50% of acute disease. Hepatitis B is caused by a small DNA virus that accounts for 40% to 45% of occurrences. It is estimated that acute hepatitis B occurs in 1 to 2 of 1000 pregnancies and that chronic infections are present in 5 to 15 of 1000 pregnancies. Hepatitis B is transmitted by parenteral and sexual contact. Hepatitis B is easily transmitted sexually: 25% of people who have sexual contact with an infected person become infected. Hepatitis C (non-A, non-B) accounts for 10% to 20% of cases and is caused by a single-stranded RNA virus spread by parenteral exposure. Hepatitis D is caused by an RNA virus that requires coinfection with the hepatitis B virus. Significant mortality and long-term consequences may occur from this less common infection. Hepatitis E, G and other forms of non-A, non-B hepatitis are uncommon but may occur during pregnancy as well.

Risk Factors: Groups at greatest risk for hepatitis B are intravenous drug users, hemophiliacs, homosexuals, and health care workers. Poor handwashing habits, multiple sexual partners, a history of sexually transmitted disease, tattoos, and multiple blood transfusions (hepatitis C) increase the risk of infection as well.

CLINICAL CHARACTERISTICS

Signs and Symptoms

(Unchanged by pregnancy)

- Fever (60%), malaise (70%), fatigue, anorexia (50%), nausea (80%)
- Variable right upper quadrant pain (50%)
- Upper abdominal tenderness with hepatomegaly
- Dark urine (85%) and acholic stools
- Jaundice a possibility in up to 60%
- Coagulopathy or encephalopathy (fulminant infections only)

DIAGNOSTIC APPROACH

Differential Diagnosis

- Acute fatty liver of pregnancy
- Toxic hepatic injury
- Cholestasis of pregnancy

- Severe pre-eclampsia
- Mononucleosis
- Cytomegalovirus hepatitis
- Lupoid hepatitis
- Viral enteritis

Associated Conditions: Jaundice, cirrhosis, pancreatitis, nephritis, ileus, and premature labor.

Workup and Evaluation

Laboratory: Hepatitis during pregnancy is diagnosed in the same manner as for nonpregnant patients; serum chemistry abnormalities indicate active hepatic disease (marked elevation of alanine aminotransferase, aspartate aminotransferase, and bilirubin), and immunochemical analysis indicates the presence of infection and the phase of the clinical course. In severe cases, coagulation studies should be performed. Routine screening of all pregnant patients is recommended.

Imaging: None indicated.

Special Tests: Percutaneous liver biopsy may be helpful but is generally not required.

Diagnostic Procedures: History, physical examination, ultrasonography (limited value), and laboratory investigation.

Pathologic Findings

Viral hepatitis is distinguished from other hepatic injuries by the characteristic pattern of injury and infiltrate.

MANAGEMENT AND THERAPY

Nonpharmacologic

General Measures: Patients with encephalopathy or coagulopathy or who are severely debilitated should be hospitalized. Nutritional support is generally required. Fluid intake and electrolyte levels must be maintained. The upper abdomen should be protected from trauma. Sexual contact should be avoided until the partner(s) receive prophylaxis.

Specific Measures: No specific measures have been shown to alter the natural course of these infections. Prophylaxis should be considered for anyone at risk (e.g., travel to endemic area, sexual partners). Acute exposure should be treated with immune globulin (see Follow-up).

Diet: Maintain good nutrition.

Activity: The upper abdomen should be protected from trauma.

Patient Education: Patients should be instructed regarding risk factors and modes of spread to limit risk for family contacts and future recurrences; American College of Obstetricians and Gynecologists Patient Education Pamphlet AP125 (Protecting Yourself Against Hepatitis B).

Drug(s) of Choice

Those necessary for support only; others of limited or unproved value.

Hepatic Disease in Pregnancy

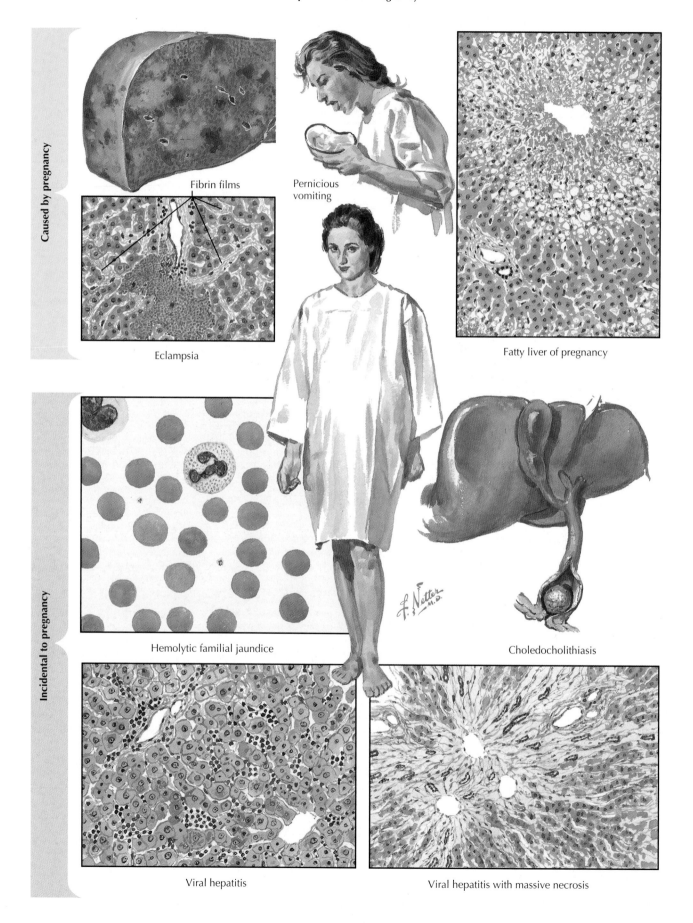

Caused by pregnancy

Fibrin films

Pernicious vomiting

Eclampsia

Fatty liver of pregnancy

Incidental to pregnancy

Hemolytic familial jaundice

Choledocholithiasis

Viral hepatitis

Viral hepatitis with massive necrosis

FOLLOW-UP

Patient Monitoring: Normal prenatal care once the acute episode is resolved. Continued monitoring for chronic liver dysfunction or carrier state (where applicable).

Prevention/Avoidance: Active immunization of those at risk before a pregnancy is planned. Patients exposed to hepatitis A may be given γ-globulin in the same manner as that for nonpregnant patients. Patients exposed to hepatitis B or those found to be carriers may receive either active immunization with hepatitis vaccine or passive immunization with hepatitis B immune globulin (HBIG). To be effective, HBIG should be given within 48 hours of exposure. The infants of these mothers should receive both forms of immunization. Infants born to mothers with hepatitis B infection should be given HBIG 0.5 mL and hepatitis B vaccine (separate site) within 12 hours of birth, with follow-up vaccinations at 1 and 6 months of age.

Possible Complications: Mortality from acute hepatitis varies with the type of hepatitis and severity of infection but is generally in the range of 2 to 10 of 1000 cases. Serious complications of hepatitis A are uncommon. Vertical transmission of hepatitis B to the developing fetus can pose a significant risk. (Of women seropositive for hepatitis B surface antigen [HbsAg], 10% to 20% transmit the virus to their neonates in the absence of immunoprophylaxis. In women who are seropositive for both HBsAg and hepatitis B envelope antigen [HbeAg], vertical transmission is approximately 90%. In patients with acute hepatitis B, vertical transmission occurs in up to 10% of neonates when infection occurs in the first trimester and in 80% to 90% of neonates when acute infection occurs in the third trimester.) The majority of untreated infants become chronic carriers, capable of infecting others. These infants are also at increased risk of cirrhosis and hepatic cancer. Neonatal infection rates vary with gestation and are highest in the third trimester (exposure to blood and fluids at delivery). Patients with the envelope antigen have an 80% chance of vertical transmission of the infection. Hepatitis D leads to chronic hepatitis in 80% of patients with rapid appearance of cirrhosis in 15%; mortality approaches 25%. Chronic liver disease and liver failure may follow infection with hepatitis B, C, or D.

Expected Outcome: Of patients, 85% to 90% experience complete resolution of symptoms; 10% to 15% of patients with hepatitis B become chronic carriers (10% to 15% of these develop serious long-term liver problems including cirrhosis and hepatocellular carcinoma). Patients with hepatitis C or D have a >80% risk of chronic hepatitis with cirrhosis and liver failure in 20% to 25%.

MISCELLANEOUS

ICD-9-CM Code: 647.6.

REFERENCES

Level II
European Paediatric Hepatitis C Virus Network: Effects of mode of delivery and infant feeding on the risk of mother-to-child transmission of hepatitis C virus. European Paediatric Hepatitis C Virus Network. BJOG 2001;108:371.

Resti M, Azzari C, Galli L, et al; Italian Study Group on Mother-to-Infant Hepatitis C Virus Transmission: Maternal drug use is a preeminent risk factor for mother-to-child hepatitis C virus transmission: results from a multicenter study of 1372 mother-infant pairs. J Infect Dis 2002;185:567. Epub 2002 Feb 14.

Level III
American College of Obstetricians and Gynecologists: Viral hepatitis in pregnancy. ACOG Educational Bulletin 248. Washington, DC, ACOG, 1992.

American College of Obstetricians and Gynecologists: Sexually transmitted diseases in adolescents. ACOG Committee Opinion 301. Obstet Gynecol 2004;104:891.

American College of Obstetricians and Gynecologists: Hepatitis B and hepatitis C virus infections in obstetrician–gynecologists. ACOG Committee Opinion 332. Obstet Gynecol 2005;106:1141.

Erdem G, Tekinalp G, Yurdakok M, et al: Perinatal transmission of hepatitis B virus infection. Lancet 1994;343:289.

Euler GL, Wooten KG, Baughman AL, Williams WW: Hepatitis B surface antigen prevalence among pregnant women in urban areas: implications for testing, reporting, and preventing perinatal transmission. Pediatrics 2003;111:1192.

Guntupalli SR, Steingrub J: Hepatic disease and pregnancy: an overview of diagnosis and management. Crit Care Med 2005;33:S332.

Hadzic N: Hepatitis C in pregnancy. Arch Dis Child Fetal Neonatal Ed 2001;84:F201.

Hunt CM, Carson KL, Sharara AI: Hepatitis C in pregnancy. Obstet Gynecol 1997;89:883.

Lynch-Salamon DI, Combs CA: Hepatitis C in obstetrics and gynecology. Obstet Gynecol 1992;79:621.

Poland GA, Jacobson RM: Clinical practice: prevention of hepatitis B with the hepatitis B vaccine. N Engl J Med 2004;351:2832.

Riely CA: Hepatic disease in pregnancy. Am J Med 1994;96:18S.

Snydman DR: Hepatitis in pregnancy. N Engl J Med 1985;313:1398.

INTRODUCTION

Description: Hyperemesis gravidarum is exaggerated nausea and vomiting of early pregnancy sufficient to produce dehydration, metabolic disturbances, and weight loss. Alkalosis (from HCl loss) and hypokalemia are common.

Prevalence: Seventy percent to 85% of women experience nausea; 50% have emesis in the first trimester; hyperemesis occurs in 0.5% to 2% of pregnancies.

Predominant age: Reproductive.

Genetics: No genetic pattern.

ETIOLOGY AND PATHOGENESIS

Causes: Unknown.

Risk Factors: Multiple gestation, hydatidiform mole, ambivalence about pregnancy (debated).

CLINICAL CHARACTERISTICS

Signs and Symptoms

- Nausea and vomiting leading to weight loss, dehydration, ketone formation, and electrolyte disturbances
- Symptoms generally begin between the fourth and eighth week, lasting until 16 weeks or longer

DIAGNOSTIC APPROACH

Differential Diagnosis

- Abnormality of pregnancy (trophoblastic disease, multiple gestation)
- Psychological overlay
- Gastroenteritis
- Cholecystitis
- Pancreatitis
- Hepatitis
- Peptic ulcer disease
- Fatty liver of pregnancy
- Pyelonephritis

Associated Conditions: Intrauterine growth restriction.

Workup and Evaluation

Laboratory: Evaluation of liver and metabolic function (serum enzymes and urinary ketones).

Imaging: Ultrasonography for pregnancy assessment and dating as indicated.

Special Tests: None indicated.

Diagnostic Procedures: History and physical examination.

Pathologic Findings

None.

MANAGEMENT AND THERAPY

Nonpharmacologic

General Measures: Small, frequent feedings with bland foods (crackers, toast, etc.). (Early intervention is more likely to be effective and will reduce the likelihood of further complications, including hospitalization.)

Specific Measures: Vitamin B6, antiemetics, or intravenous hydration. Gradual reintroduction of diet as symptoms are controlled. Techniques such as acupuncture, acupressure, steroid use, or ginger therapy have not been proven to be effective.

Diet: Spicy or greasy foods should be avoided, and some advocate eating a protein snack at bedtime.

Activity: No restriction.

Patient Education: American College of Obstetricians and Gynecologists Patient Education Booklet AP001 (Nutrition During Pregnancy), AP126 (Morning Sickness).

Drug(s) of Choice

Vitamin B6 (pyridoxine) 50 to 100 mg PO daily (may be divided and taken twice a day) with doxylamine succinate (Unisom) 12.5 to 25 mg PO daily.

Promethazine (Phenergan) 25 mg PO or rectally every 4 to 6 hours.

Metoclopramide (Reglan) 10 mg PO four times a day.

Meclizine (Antivert) 12.5 to 25 mg PO four times a day.

Contraindications: See individual agents.

Precautions: Promethazine (Phenergan) is a class C agent (risk of teratogenesis in animals but unknown risk in humans). Metoclopramide (Reglan) and meclizine (Antivert) are class B agents (no known human risk).

FOLLOW-UP

Patient Monitoring: Normal health maintenance, monitoring of fetal growth.

Prevention/Avoidance: None.

Possible Complications: Maternal dehydration and metabolic compromise. Rupture or tears of the esophagus and pneumothorax have been reported as a result of vomiting.

Expected Outcome: Generally good, although relapses in severe cases are common (25% to 30%).

MISCELLANEOUS

Pregnancy Considerations: If nutrition is maintained, no effect on pregnancy. May recur with subsequent pregnancies.

ICD-9-CM Codes: 643, 643.0 (mild), 643.1 (with metabolic disturbance).

REFERENCES

Level I

Heazell A, Thorneycroft J, Walton V, Etherington I: Acupressure for the in-patient treatment of nausea and vomiting in early pregnancy: a randomized control trial. Am J Obstet Gynecol 2006;194:815.

Knight B, Mudge C, Openshaw S, et al: Effect of acupuncture on nausea of pregnancy: a randomized, controlled trial. Obstet Gynecol 2001;97:184.

Nelson-Piercy C, Fayers P, de Swiet M: Randomised, double-blind, placebo-controlled trial of corticosteroids for the treatment of hyperemesis gravidarum. BJOG 2001;108:9.

Rosen T, de Veciana M, Miller HS, et al: A randomized controlled trial of nerve stimulation for relief of nausea and vomiting in pregnancy. Obstet Gynecol 2003;102:129.

Yost NP, McIntire DD, Wians FH Jr, et al: A randomized, placebo-controlled trial of corticosteroids for hyperemesis due to pregnancy. Obstet Gynecol 2003;102:1250.

Level II

Bondok RS, El Sharnouby NM, Eid HE, Abd Elmaksoud AM: Pulsed steroid therapy is an effective treatment for intractable hyperemesis gravidarum. Crit Care Med 2006;34:2781.

Borrelli F, Capasso R, Aviello G, et al: Effectiveness and safety of ginger in the treatment of pregnancy-induced nausea and vomiting. Obstet Gynecol 2005;105:849.

Deuchar N: Nausea and vomiting in pregnancy: a review of the problem with particular regard to psychological and social aspects. Br J Obstet Gynaecol 1995;102:6.

van Stuijvenberg ME, Schabort I, Labadarios D, Nel JT: The nutritional status and treatment of patients with hyperemesis gravidarum. Am J Obstet Gynecol 1995;172:1585.

Level III

American College of Obstetricians and Gynecologists: Nausea and vomiting of pregnancy. ACOG Practice Bulletin 52. Obstet Gynecol 2004;103:803.

INTRODUCTION

Description: Intrauterine growth restriction is symmetric or asymmetric reduction in the size and weight of the growing fetus in utero, compared with that expected for a fetus of comparable gestational age. This may occur for many reasons, but most occurrences represent signs of significant risk of fetal death or jeopardy to the fetus. Some authors advocate identifying fetuses with growth between the 10th and 20th percentiles as suffering "diminished" growth and at intermediate risk for complications.

Prevalence: Problems of consistent definition make estimates difficult; by most definitions 5% to 10% of pregnancies.

Predominant Age: Reproductive; higher at the extremes of childbearing. (For women younger than age 15 the rate of low birthweight is 13.6% compared with 7.3% for women between 25 and 29 years of age. When multiple gestations are excluded, the rate for women older than age 45 is greater than 20%.)

Genetics: No genetic pattern.

ETIOLOGY AND PATHOGENESIS

Causes: Idiopathic (50%). Maternal disease—hypertension; drug or alcohol use; smoking; Dilantin (phenytoin), coumarin, propranolol, or steroid use; poor nutrition, inflammatory bowel disease, low maternal weight (<50 kg), high altitude, hemoglobinopathy, cyanotic heart disease, multiple pregnancy, irradiation. Placental disease or abnormalities—placenta previa, fibrosis, chronic infection, partial abruption or infarction. Fetal factors—congenital anomalies, chromosomal factors, chronic fetal infections.

Risk Factors: Chronic maternal disease (hypertension, renal disease, cardiovascular disease), impaired placental function, congenital anomalies, history of recurrent abortion, fetal death, or preterm labor.

CLINICAL CHARACTERISTICS
Signs and Symptoms

- Uterine size less than dates
- Oligohydramnios
- Fetal growth that falls below the 10th percentile for gestational age or demonstrates reduced growth velocity on serial examinations

DIAGNOSTIC APPROACH
Differential Diagnosis

- Inaccurate gestational age
- Congenital anomalies
- Multiple gestation
- Constitutionally small infants (small for gestational age [SGA])
- Extrauterine gestation

Associated Conditions: Prematurity, intrauterine fetal death, congenital anomalies, and oligohydramnios.

Workup and Evaluation

Laboratory: No evaluation indicated unless suggested by maternal disease.

Imaging: Ultrasonography with fetal biometry compared with curves specific to the location and population served. The diagnosis must also be based on serial examinations that provide information about the growth of the individual fetus.

Special Tests: When found in advanced gestations: fetal nonstress and contraction stress testing or biophysical profiling. The role of Doppler flow studies continues to be evaluated.

Diagnostic Procedures: Physical examination, ultrasonography. (Physical examination may miss up to two thirds of cases; ultrasonography can exclude or verify growth restriction in 90% and 80% of cases, respectively.) Intrauterine growth restriction must be distinguished from infants who are constitutionally small for gestational age who are not at increased risk. Asymmetric restrictions in growth argue against a constitutional cause. Early intrauterine insults are more likely to result in symmetric growth restriction; later insults result in asymmetry. Similarly, intrinsic factors generally cause symmetric restriction; extrinsic factors generally cause asymmetric restriction.

Pathologic Findings

Reduced fetal fat stores and reduced overall size compared with that expected for gestational age.

MANAGEMENT AND THERAPY
Nonpharmacologic

General Measures: Evaluation, ultrasonography with biometry. Cessation of tobacco and alcohol use (if present).

Specific Measures: Based on cause and stage of gestation. Early delivery is often necessary. (The majority of fetal deaths occur after 36 weeks of gestation.) Constitutionally small infants require no intervention.

Diet: No specific dietary changes indicated unless deficiencies identified.

Activity: No restriction except as dictated by maternal disease or fetal condition.

Patient Education: American College of Obstetricians and Gynecologists Patient Education Pamphlet AP098 (Special Tests for Monitoring Fetal Health), AP025 (Ultrasound Exams).

Drug(s) of Choice

None. (Low-dose aspirin therapy has been advocated but has yet to be firmly established in its efficacy or role in management.)

FOLLOW-UP

Patient Monitoring: Enhanced fetal assessment, antenatal fetal testing (including nonstress testing, biophysical profiles, and contraction stress tests). Patients at risk

Intrauterine Growth Restriction (IUGR)

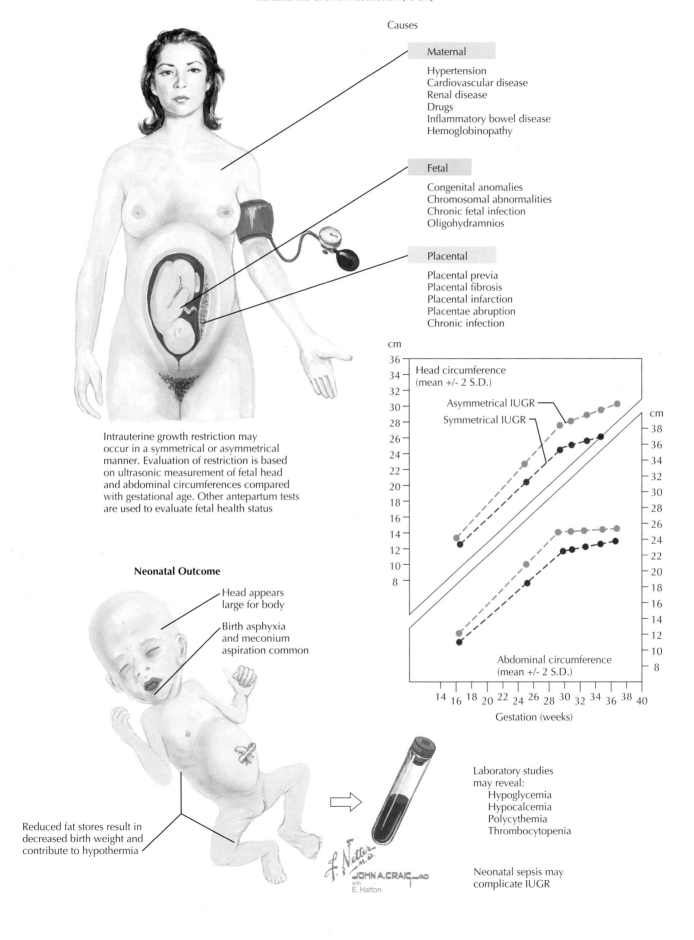

Causes

Maternal

Hypertension
Cardiovascular disease
Renal disease
Drugs
Inflammatory bowel disease
Hemoglobinopathy

Fetal

Congenital anomalies
Chromosomal abnormalities
Chronic fetal infection
Oligohydramnios

Placental

Placental previa
Placental fibrosis
Placental infarction
Placentae abruption
Chronic infection

Intrauterine growth restriction may
occur in a symmetrical or asymmetrical
manner. Evaluation of restriction is based
on ultrasonic measurement of fetal head
and abdominal circumferences compared
with gestational age. Other antepartum tests
are used to evaluate fetal health status

Head circumference
(mean +/- 2 S.D.)

Asymmetrical IUGR
Symmetrical IUGR

Abdominal circumference
(mean +/- 2 S.D.)

Gestation (weeks)

Neonatal Outcome

Head appears
large for body

Birth asphyxia
and meconium
aspiration common

Reduced fat stores result in
decreased birth weight and
contribute to hypothermia

Laboratory studies
may reveal:
    Hypoglycemia
    Hypocalcemia
    Polycythemia
    Thrombocytopenia

Neonatal sepsis may
complicate IUGR

because of maternal disease should have early assessment of fetal growth (biparietal diameter, head circumference, abdominal circumference, and femur length) with frequent remeasurement as the pregnancy progresses. This may need to be done as often as every 2 to 3 weeks in severe cases. Careful fetal monitoring during labor.

Prevention/Avoidance: Management of maternal disease.

Possible Complications: Progressive deterioration of fetal status and intrauterine fetal demise. (There is an 8- to 10-fold increase in the risk of perinatal mortality; growth restriction is the second most important cause of perinatal morbidity after preterm delivery.) Long-term physical and neurologic sequelae are common. The risk of adverse outcome is generally proportional to the severity of growth restriction present. The presence of risk factors for intrauterine growth restriction increases the risk of fetal death by 2-fold in growth-restricted fetuses. The most immediate fetal morbidities are birth asphyxia, meconium aspiration, sepsis, hypoglycemia, hypocalcemia, hypothermia, polycythemia, thrombocytopenia, and pulmonary hemorrhage.

Expected Outcome: With early detection, progressive fetal growth can often be achieved, although many pregnancies may require early delivery or other interventions to ensure fetal well-being.

MISCELLANEOUS

ICD-9-CM Code: 656.5.

REFERENCES

Level I
Larsen T, Larsen JF, Petersen S, Greisen G: Detection of small-for-gestational-age fetuses by ultrasound screening in a high risk population: a randomized controlled study. Br J Obstet Gynaecol 1992;99:469.

McCowan LM, Harding JE, Roberts AB, et al: A pilot randomized controlled trial of two regimens of fetal surveillance for small-for-gestational-age fetuses with normal results of umbilical artery Doppler velocimetry. Am J Obstet Gynecol 2000;182:81.

McKenna D, Tharmaratnam S, Mahsud S, et al: A randomized trial using ultrasound to identify the high-risk fetus in a low-risk population. Obstet Gynecol 2003;101:626.

Level II
Leitich H, Egarter C, Husslein P, et al: A meta-analysis of low dose aspirin for the prevention of intrauterine growth retardation. Br J Obstet Gynaecol 1997;104:450.

Oken E, Kleinman KP, Rich-Edwards J, Gillman MW: A nearly continuous measure of birth weight for gestational age using a United States national reference. BMC Pediatr 2003;3:6. Epub 2003 Jul 8.

Level III
Alberry M, Soothill P: Management of fetal growth restriction. Arch Dis Child Fetal Neonatal Ed 2007;92:F62.

Alexander GR, Kimes JH, Kaufman RB, et al: A United States national reference for fetal growth. Obstet Gynecol 1996;87:163.

American College of Obstetricians and Gynecologists: Intrauterine growth restriction. ACOG Practice Bulletin 12. Washington, DC, ACOG, 2000.

American College of Obstetricians and Gynecologists: Ultrasonography in pregnancy. ACOG Practice Bulletin 58. Obstet Gynecol 2004;104:1449.

Baschat AA: Fetal responses to placental insufficiency: an update. BJOG 2004;111:1031.

Bloomfield FH, Oliver MH, Harding JE: The late effects of fetal growth patterns. Arch Dis Child Fetal Neonatal Ed 2006;91:F299. Review.

Chien PF, Arnott N, Gordon A, et al: How useful is uterine artery Doppler flow velocimetry in the prediction of pre-eclampsia, intrauterine growth retardation and perinatal death? An overview. BJOG 2000;107:196.

Goldenberg RL, Cutter GR, Hoffman HJ, et al: Intrauterine growth retardation: standards for diagnosis. Am J Obstet Gynecol 1989; 161:271.

James D: Diagnosis and management of fetal growth retardation. Arch Dis Child 1990;65:390.

Resnik R: Intrauterine growth restriction. Obstet Gynecol 2002; 99:490.

Seeds JW: Impaired fetal growth: definition and clinical diagnosis. Obstet Gynecol 1984;64:303.

Seeds JW: Impaired fetal growth: ultrasonic evaluation and clinical management. Obstet Gynecol 1984;64:577.

Strauss RS, Dietz WH: Effects of intrauterine growth retardation in premature infants on early childhood growth. J Pediatr 1997; 130:95.

INTRODUCTION

Description: Multiple gestation is two or more fetus coexisting during the same gestation.

Prevalence: Occurs in 3.4% of births in the United States (and increasing; 70% since 1980); 1/10,000 births for spontaneously occurring triplets. (The increase in multiple births is thought to be due to the use of fertility drugs and an increased rate of childbearing in women older than age 30, who are more likely to conceive multiples.) Multiple gestations are responsible for a disproportionate share of perinatal morbidity and mortality. (They account for 17% of all preterm births [before 37 weeks of gestation], 23% of early preterm births [before 32 weeks of gestation], 24% of low-birthweight infants [<2500 g], and 26% of very-low-birthweight infants [<1500 g].) Hospital costs for women with multiple gestations are on average 40% higher than for women with gestational-age–matched singleton pregnancies because of their longer length of stay and increased rate of obstetric complications.

Predominant age: Reproductive (becomes more common with increasing maternal age).

Genetics: Dizygotic twins are more common in mothers who are themselves a dizygotic twin.

ETIOLOGY AND PATHOGENESIS

Causes: Monozygotic twins result from the cleavage of a single fertilized ova (4/1000 births). Dizygotic multiple gestations occur when there are multiple ova released and fertilized (naturally or through assisted ovulation. See later.).

Risk Factors: Ovulation induction (clomiphene therapy: 5% to 10% multiple gestation rate), increased maternal age, parity, weight and height, African American race.

CLINICAL CHARACTERISTICS

Signs and Symptoms

- Uterus larger than dates
- Multiple fetal heart tones by auscultation or Doppler study

DIAGNOSTIC APPROACH

Differential Diagnosis

- Polyhydramnios
- Molar pregnancy

Associated Conditions: Prematurity, cord accidents, intrauterine growth restriction (50% to 60% of triplet or greater pregnancies), polyhydramnios, increased fetal morbidity and mortality, increased risk of congenital anomalies, abruptio placenta, placenta previa, hypertension and pre-eclampsia, anemia, acute fatty liver, gestational diabetes, hyperemesis gravidarum, pyelonephritis, cholestasis, thrombosis and embolism, postpartum hemorrhage, increased operative delivery rate.

Workup and Evaluation

Laboratory: No special evaluation indicated, although because of the higher incidence of gestational diabetes, screening is of greater importance. (Abnormality of gestation-sensitive laboratory tests, such as maternal serum alpha-fetoprotein [MSAFP], is to be expected.)

Imaging: Ultrasonography (reduces the rate of undiagnosed multiple gestation from 40% to <5%). Radiographic studies are generally inadequate to establish the presence or health of a multiple pregnancy, making routine use of x-rays undesirable.

Special Tests: Genetic amniocentesis may be considered (twin pregnancies have twice the rate of abnormalities: monozygotic = 2% to 10% rate).

Diagnostic Procedures: History, physical examination, ultrasonography.

Pathologic Findings

Examination of the placenta can identify the type of pregnancy (see later).

MANAGEMENT AND THERAPY

Nonpharmacologic

General Measures: Adequate nutrition, diminished activity, frequent perinatal visits, monitoring of fetal growth (serial ultrasonography)

Specific Measures: Antenatal testing, prompt intervention for threatened preterm labor. Routine preterm hospitalization is not recommended.

Diet: Increase maternal intake by 300 kcal more than normal for pregnancy. Iron and folic acid supplementation.

Activity: Reduced activity as pregnancy progresses. Bed rest remains controversial.

Patient Education: Reassurance; American College of Obstetricians and Gynecologists Patient Education Booklet AP092 (Having Twins); counseling regarding signs of pre-term labor (AP087 Preterm Labor, AP004 How to Tell When Labor Begins)

Drug(s) of Choice

None. (Tocolytic agents are often used when premature labor is threatened but are not useful as prophylaxis and are associated with an increased risk of side effects when used in these patients.)

FOLLOW-UP

Patient Monitoring: Increased frequency of prenatal evaluations, antenatal fetal testing in late pregnancy. Counseling regarding signs of preterm labor.

Prevention/Avoidance: None. (Some complications of multiple gestation may be reduced by increased surveillance and monitoring.)

Possible Complications: Perinatal morbidity and mortality is two to five times higher than for singleton gesta-

MECHANISMS OF TWIN GESTATION FORMATION

Mechanism	Resulting Twin Pregnancy
Two ova, two sperm	Dizygotic (fraternal)
Single ova, single sperm	Monozygotic ("identical")
—Division within 72 hours	—Diamniotic, dichorionic
—Division between 4 and 8 days*	—Diamniotic, monochorionic
—Division between 8 and 13 days	—Monoamniotic, monochorionic
—Division after 10 to 13 days	—Conjoined twins

*Days after fertilization

tions. (Preterm delivery [50%] is most common cause of morbidity or mortality. Other complications: intrauterine growth restriction (12% to 47% versus 5% to 7% in singletons) or discordant growth, cord accidents, hydramnios, congenital anomalies (two times increase), malpresentation. Monozygotic twins have a 1% incidence of monoamniotic sacs that carries a 50% fetal mortality because of cord entanglement or conjoined twins. One fifth of triplet pregnancies and one half of quadruplet pregnancies result in at least one child with a major long-term handicap, such as cerebral palsy. Cerebral palsy occurs 17 times more often in triplet pregnancies and more than 4 times more often in twin pregnancies than in singleton pregnancies. When matched for gestational age at delivery, infants from multifetal pregnancies have a nearly 3-fold greater risk of cerebral palsy.

Maternal Complications: Abruptio placenta, placenta previa, pre-eclampsia, anemia, hyperemesis gravidarum, pyelonephritis, cholestasis, postpartum hemorrhage, increased operative delivery rate.

Expected Outcome: Generally good, although delivery before term is common and there is an increased risk of operative delivery.

MISCELLANEOUS

Other Notes: Up to 50% of twin pregnancies identified in the early weeks will silently abort one fetus (with or without bleeding). Home uterine activity has not been proved to reduce the rate of prematurity in multiple gestations.

Most Common Presentation: Vertex/vertex (43%), vertex/other (38%), twin A other (19%).

ICD-9-CM Codes: 651, 651.0 (Twin), 651.1 (Triplet), 651.2 (Quadruplet).

REFERENCES

Level II

Grether JK, Nelson KB, Cummins SK: Twinning and cerebral palsy: experience in four northern California counties, births 1983 through 1985. Pediatrics 1993;92:854.

Hogle KL, Hutton EK, McBrien KA, et al: Cesarean delivery for twins: a systematic review and meta-analysis. Am J Obstet Gynecol 2003;188:220.

Lewi L, Gratacos E, Ortibus E, et al: Pregnancy and infant outcome of 80 consecutive cord coagulations in complicated monochorionic multiple pregnancies. Am J Obstet Gynecol 2006;194:782.

Petterson B, Nelson KB, Watson L, Stanley F: Twins, triplets, and cerebral palsy in births in Western Australia in the 1980s. BMJ 1993;307:1239.

Powers WF, Kiely JL: The risk confronting twins: a national perspective. Am J Obstet Gynecol 1994;170:456.

Reddy UM, Wapner RJ, Rebar RW, Tasca RJ: Infertility, assisted reproductive technology, and adverse pregnancy outcomes: executive summary of a National Institute of Child Health and Human Development workshop. Obstet Gynecol 2007;109:967.

Yokoyama Y, Shimizu T, Hayakawa K: Incidence of handicaps in multiple births and associated factors. Acta Genet Med Gemellol (Roma) 1995;44:81.

Level III

American College of Obstetricians and Gynecologists: Multiple gestation: complicated twin, triplet, and high-order multifetal pregnancy. ACOG Practice Bulletin 56. Obstet Gynecol 2004;104:869.

American College of Obstetricians and Gynecologists: Perinatal risks associated with assisted reproductive technology. ACOG Committee Opinion 324. Obstet Gynecol 2005;106:1143.

American College of Obstetricians and Gynecologists: Multifetal pregnancy reduction. ACOG Committee Opinion 369. Obstet Gynecol 2007;109:1511.

Berkowitz RL, Lynch L, Stone J, Alvarez M: The current status of multifetal pregnancy reduction. Am J Obstet Gynecol 1996;174:1265.

Brown JE, Carlson M: Nutrition and multifetal pregnancy. J Am Diet Assoc 2000;100:343.

Bryan E: The impact of multiple preterm births on the family. BJOG 2003;110:24.

D'Alton ME, Mercer BM: Antepartum management of twin gestation: ultrasound. Clin Obstet Gynecol 1990;33:42.

Hall JG: Twinning. Lancet 2003;362:735.

Jauniauz E, Elkazen N, Leroy F, et al: Clinical and morphologic aspects of the vanishing twin phenomenon. Obstet Gynecol 1988;72:577.

Kiely JL, Kleinman JC, Kiely M: Triplets and higher-order multiple births. Am J Dis Child 1992;146:862.

Kovacs BW, Kirschbaum TH, Paul RH: Twin gestations, I. Antenatal care and complications. Obstet Gynecol 1989;74:313.

MacGillivray I: Epidemiology of twin pregnancy. Semin Perinatol 1986;10:4.

Mauldin JG, Newman RB: Neurologic morbidity associated with multiple gestation. Female Pat 1998;23:27, 30, 35, passim.

Nageotte MP: Prevention and treatment of preterm labor in twin gestation. Clin Obstet Gynecol 1990;33:61.

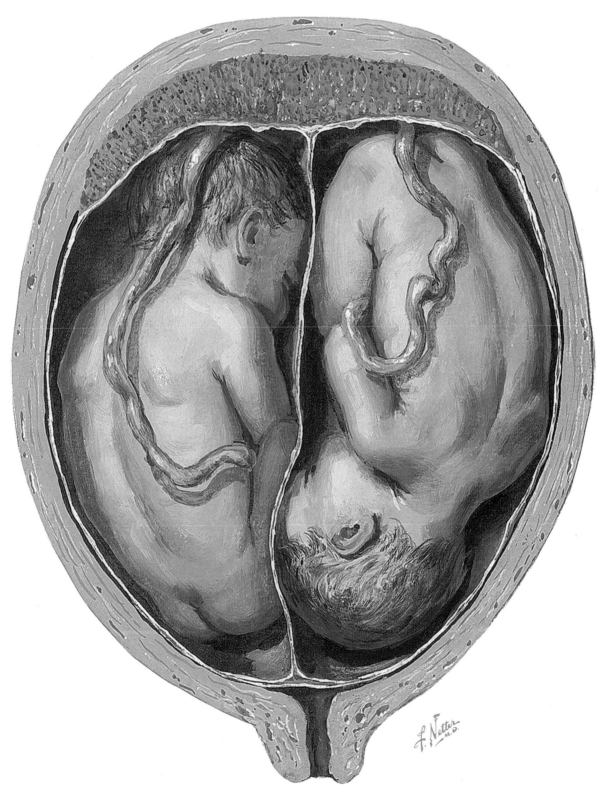

Multiple pregnancy

INTRODUCTION

Description: Oligohydramnios is an abnormal reduction in the amount of amniotic fluid surrounding the fetus. At term, there should be about 800 mL of amniotic fluid present.

Prevalence: Rare in early pregnancy, common in post-term pregnancies (12% to 25% at 41 weeks).

Predominant Age: Reproductive.

Genetics: No genetic pattern.

ETIOLOGY AND PATHOGENESIS

Causes: Unknown. Generally associated with a reduction in fetal urine production (renal agenesis, urinary tract obstruction, and fetal death), chronic amniotic leak, maternal disease (hypertension, diabetes, uteroplacental insufficiency, pre-eclampsia).

Risk Factors: Fetal chromosomal or congenital abnormalities (see box), fetal growth restriction or demise, post-term pregnancy, multiple gestation (twin–twin transfusion), maternal hypertension, diabetes, pre-eclampsia, and prostaglandin synthetase inhibitors.

CLINICAL CHARACTERISTICS

Signs and Symptoms

- Uterine size smaller than normal for stage of pregnancy
- Reduced amniotic fluid measured by ultrasonography

DIAGNOSTIC APPROACH

Differential Diagnosis

- Inaccurate gestational age
- Intrauterine growth restriction
- Fetal anomalies
- Premature rupture of the membranes

Associated Conditions: Fetal—renal and urinary tract anomalies, intrauterine fetal growth restriction, pulmonary hypoplasia, musculoskeletal defects (clubfoot, amniotic bands, amputations), meconium-stained amniotic fluid. Fetal anomalies are present in 15% to 25% of cases. Maternal—chronic disease (diabetes, hypertension).

Workup and Evaluation

Laboratory: No evaluation indicated.

Imaging: Amniotic fluid index calculated by adding the vertical depths of the largest pockets of amniotic fluid in each quadrant of the uterus (average at term = 12.5 cm, 95th percentile = 21.4). Borderline values should always be rechecked before any intervention is undertaken. Fetal anomalies may also be documented.

Special Tests: Nonstress or contraction stress testing to evaluate fetal health.

Diagnostic Procedures: Physical examination, ultrasonography.

Pathologic Findings

Reduced amniotic fluid (other findings based on cause).

MANAGEMENT AND THERAPY

Nonpharmacologic

General Measures: Evaluation. Mild degrees may be managed expectantly. Maternal oral hydration may improve amniotic fluid volume.

Specific Measures: Amnioinfusion (the introduction of normal saline via an intrauterine catheter placed through the partially dilated cervix during labor) has been used to reduce the incidence of umbilical cord compression during labor. This does not reduce the risk of meconium aspiration.

Diet: No specific dietary changes indicated.

Activity: No restriction.

Patient Education: Reassurance; American College of Obstetricians and Gynecologists Patient Education Pamphlet AP069 (What to Expect After Your Due Date), AP025 (Ultrasound Exams), AP098 (Special Tests for Monitoring Fetal Health).

Drug(s) of Choice

None.

FOLLOW-UP

Patient Monitoring: Intensive fetal surveillance is required.

Prevention/Avoidance: None.

Possible Complications: Amniotic band syndrome (including partial limb amputation), pulmonary hypoplasia, premature labor, clubfoot, and meconium-stained amniotic fluid. The prognosis is inversely related to gestational age: the earlier the oligohydramnios occurs, the worse the outcome.

Expected Outcome: When oligohydramnios occurs in term or post-term pregnancies, it is associated with

Anomalies Associated with Oligohydramnios

- Amniotic band syndrome
- Cardiac anomalies: tetralogy of Fallot, septal defects
- Central nervous system: holoprosencephaly, meningocele, encephalocele, microcephaly
- Chromosomal: triploidy, trisomy 18, Turner syndrome
- Cloacal dysgenesis
- Cystic hygroma
- Diaphragmatic hernia
- Genitourinary tract: renal agenesis, renal dysplasia, urethral obstruction (posterior urethral valve), bladder exstrophy, Meckel-Gruber syndrome, ureteropelvic junction obstruction, prune-belly syndrome
- Hypothyroidism
- Multiple gestation: twin–twin transfusion syndrome, twin reverse arterial perfusion sequence (TRAP)
- Musculoskeletal: sirenomelia, sacral agenesis, absent radius, facial clefting
- VACTERL (vertebral, anal, cardiac, tracheoesophageal, renal, limb) association

Events in Oligohydramnios

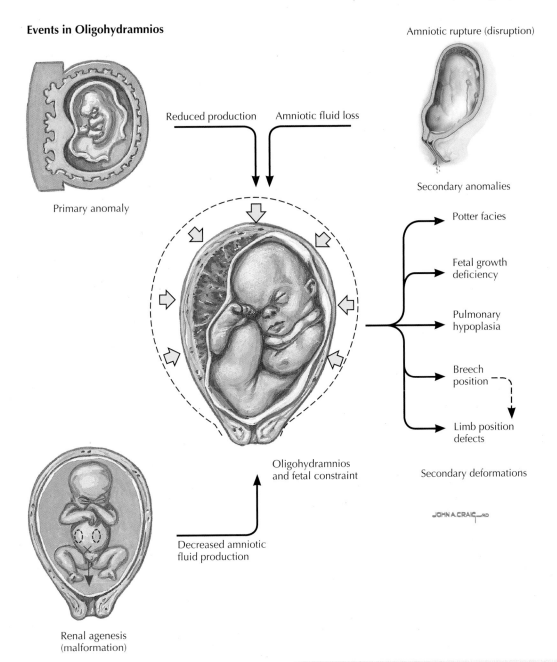

Amniotic rupture (disruption)

Reduced production   Amniotic fluid loss

Primary anomaly

Secondary anomalies

Potter facies

Fetal growth deficiency

Pulmonary hypoplasia

Breech position

Limb position defects

Oligohydramnios and fetal constraint

Secondary deformations

JOHN A. CRAIG—AD

Decreased amniotic fluid production

Renal agenesis (malformation)

fetuses that do not tolerate labor well (5-fold to 7-fold increase in rate of cesarean delivery).

MISCELLANEOUS

ICD-9-CM Codes: 658.0 (Nonspecific), 761.2 (Affecting the fetus), 658.1 (Due to premature rupture of the membranes).

REFERENCES

Level I

Chauhan SP, Doherty DD, Magann EF, et al: Amniotic fluid index vs single deepest pocket technique during modified biophysical profile: a randomized clinical trial. Am J Obstet Gynecol 2004;191:661.

Moses J, Doherty DA, Magann EF, et al: A randomized clinical trial of the intrapartum assessment of amniotic fluid volume: amniotic fluid index versus the single deepest pocket technique. Am J Obstet Gynecol 2004;190:1564.

Level II

Chauhan SP, Sanderson M, Hendrix NW, et al: Perinatal outcome and amniotic fluid index in the antepartum and intrapartum periods: a meta-analysis. Am J Obstet Gynecol 1999;181:1473.

Flack NJ, Sepulveda W, Bower S, Fisk NM: Acute maternal hydration in third-trimester oligohydramnios: effects on amniotic fluid volume, uteroplacental perfusion, and fetal blood flow and urine output. Am J Obstet Gynecol 1995;173:1186.

Pitt C, Sanchez-Ramos L, Kaunitz AM, Gaudier F: Prophylactic amnioinfusion for intrapartum oligohydramnios: a meta-analysis of randomized controlled trials. Obstet Gynecol 2000;96:861.

Sandruck JC, Grobman WA, Gerber SE: The effect of short-term indomethacin therapy on amniotic fluid volume. Am J Obstet Gynecol 2005;192:1443.

Level III

American College of Obstetricians and Gynecologists: Antepartum fetal surveillance. ACOG Practice Bulletin 9, Washington, DC, ACOG, 1999.

Ogundipe OA, Spong CY, Ross MG: Prophylactic amnioinfusion for oligohydramnios: a reevaluation. Obstet Gynecol 1994;84:544.

INTRODUCTION

Description: Placenta previa is implantation of the placenta in a location that leaves part or all of the cervical os covered. This is associated with potentially catastrophic maternal bleeding and obstruction of the uterine outlet. Several degrees are recognized: total, partial, marginal, and low-lying placenta. These degrees may vary with cervical dilation or gestational age.

Prevalence: Seen in 0.3% to 0.5% of deliveries.

Predominant Age: Reproductive, average age 29 years.

Genetics: No genetic pattern.

ETIOLOGY AND PATHOGENESIS

Causes: Implantation by the zygote low in the uterine cavity (in close proximity to the cervical os). Defective decidual vascularization, resulting from inflammation or atrophy, has been implicated.

Risk Factors: Multiparity, advanced maternal age (>35: 1% of deliveries, >40: 2%), prior cesarean delivery (two to five times increase), induced abortion, smoking (2-fold increase), cocaine use, multiple gestation, high altitude, and prior abortion.

CLINICAL CHARACTERISTICS

Signs and Symptoms

- Painless vaginal bleeding (70%, generally not present until late second or early third trimester); may be catastrophic in amount, although initial episodes are rarely fatal; blood is maternal in origin
- Uterine hyperactivity possibly present with bleeding (20%)
- Heavy or prolonged bleeding after delivery

DIAGNOSTIC APPROACH

Differential Diagnosis

- Bloody show of early labor
- Placental abruption
- Vasa previa
- Low-lying placenta

Associated Conditions: Placenta accreta (15% to 25% of patients), increta, or percreta and prematurity.

Workup and Evaluation

Laboratory: Complete blood count, type and cross-match blood products for possible replacement.

Imaging: Ultrasonography (transabdominal) to determine placental location and condition, fetal status. (False-positive ultrasonographic results may occur with a full bladder; suspicious studies should be repeated with the bladder empty. Low-lying placentas noted in studies performed at less than 30 weeks may "migrate," leaving the cervix free at term [up to 90% of cases].)

Special Tests: Kleihauer-Betke test for fetal–maternal transfusion, clot tube to assess possibility of coagulopathy, Apt test to identify fetal blood loss (such as from a vasa previa).

Diagnostic Procedures: History, ultrasonography. (Pelvic examination is contraindicated until the location of the placenta can be ascertained.)

Pathologic Findings

Placental implantation in the lower uterine segment.

MANAGEMENT AND THERAPY

Nonpharmacologic

General Measures: Evaluation, hemodynamic stabilization, fetal assessment. If placenta previa is suspected, no vaginal examinations until the location and degree of placental obstruction can be determined.

Specific Measures: If bleeding is heavy or the placenta obstructs delivery, cesarean delivery is indicated. Marginal (low-lying) placental implantation may be managed conservatively if it occurs long before term. Bleeding from the placental site may be heavy, requiring extensive measures (including hysterectomy, hypogastric artery ligation or embolization) to control bleeding.

Diet: No specific dietary changes indicated unless active bleeding is present or the patient's condition is unstable.

Activity: Bed rest is generally indicated.

Patient Education: American College of Obstetricians and Gynecologists Patient Education Pamphlet AP038 (Bleeding During Pregnancy), AP006 (Cesarean Birth), AP025 (Ultrasound Exams).

Drug(s) of Choice

Fluid and blood product replacement as needed. Steroid therapy to accelerate fetal lung maturation has been advocated for patients remote from term. Oxytocin, methylergonovine maleate (Methergine), and prostaglandin (E_2) therapy to assist with uterine contraction after delivery. Rh (D) immune globulin should be given as indicated in mothers who are Rh negative. If tocolysis is required, MgSO4 is preferred.

Contraindications: Beta mimetic agents should not be used if there is significant maternal blood loss or hypotension.

FOLLOW-UP

Patient Monitoring: Normal health maintenance.

Prevention/Avoidance: None.

Possible Complications: Catastrophic maternal hemorrhage, fetal anoxia. Coagulation defects may occur as a result of heavy or prolonged blood loss. Significant bleeding from the placental site may result in maternal compromise, and extensive measures (including hysterectomy) to achieve control must be taken. Preterm delivery represents the greatest source of morbidity for the fetus. Roughly 35% of infants whose mothers require transfusion require transfusion themselves.

Expected Outcome: Generally good—25% to 30% of patients complete 36 weeks of gestation despite labor or repetitive bleeding.

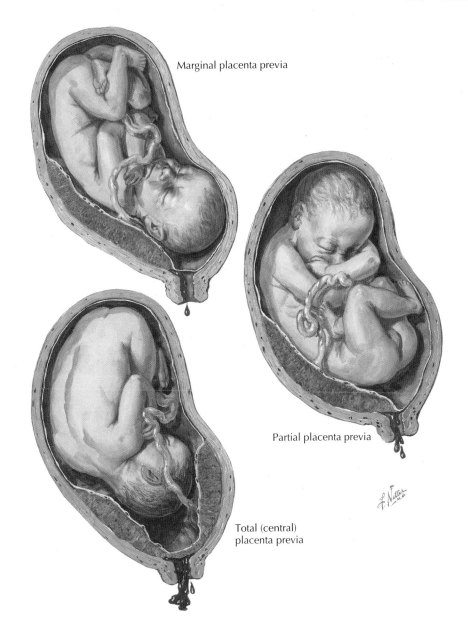

Marginal placenta previa

Partial placenta previa

Total (central) placenta previa

MISCELLANEOUS

ICD-9-CM Code: 641.1.

REFERENCES

Level I

Cobo E, Conde-Agudelo A, Delgado J, et al: Cervical cerclage: an alternative for the management of placenta previa? Am J Obstet Gynecol 1998;179:122.

Wing DA, Paul RH, Millar LK: Management of the symptomatic placenta previa: a randomized, controlled trial of inpatient versus outpatient expectant management. Am J Obstet Gynecol 1996; 175:806.

Level II

Ananth CV, Smulian JC, Vintzileos AM: The association of placenta previa with history of cesarean delivery and abortion: a metaanalysis. Am J Obstet Gynecol 1997;177:1071.

Besinger RE, Moniak CW, Paskiewicz LS, et al: The effect of tocolytic use in the management of symptomatic placenta previa.

Am J Obstet Gynecol 1995;172:1770.

Joshi VM, Otiv SR, Majumder R, et al: Internal iliac artery ligation for arresting postpartum haemorrhage. BJOG 2007;114:356. Epub 2007 Jan 22.

Rouse DJ, MacPherson C, Landon M, et al; National Institute of Child Health and Human Development Maternal-Fetal Medicine Units Network: Blood transfusion and cesarean delivery. Obstet Gynecol 2006;108:891.

Taipale P, Hiilesmaa V, Ylostalo P: Diagnosis of placenta previa by transvaginal sonographic screening at 12–16 weeks in a nonselected population. Obstet Gynecol 1997;89:364.

Level III

American College of Obstetricians and Gynecologists: Ultrasonography in pregnancy. ACOG Practice Bulletin 58. Obstet Gynecol 2004;104:1449.

Booher D, Little B: Vaginal hemorrhage in pregnancy. N Engl J Med 1974;290:611.

Chamberlain G: ABC of antenatal care. Antepartum haemorrhage. BMJ 1991;302:1526.

Chamberlain G, Steer P: ABC of labour care: Obstetric emergencies. BMJ 1999;318:1342.

Oyelese Y, Smulian JC: Placenta previa, placenta accreta, and vasa

INTRODUCTION

Description: Placental abruption is premature separation of an otherwise normally implanted placenta before delivery of the fetus.

Prevalence: One in 185 to 290 deliveries; sufficient to result in fetal death, 1 in 1600 deliveries (approximately 10% of third-trimester fetal demise).

Predominant Age: Reproductive.

Genetics: No genetic pattern.

ETIOLOGY AND PATHOGENESIS

Causes: Pregnancy-induced hypertension (most common), trauma to the abdomen, decompression of an overdistended uterus (loss of amniotic fluid, delivery of a twin), cocaine use.

Risk Factors: Pregnancy-induced hypertension (most common). Prior abruption: 15% chance if one prior episode, 20% to 25% for two or more prior events. Others: smoking >1 pack/day (2-fold increased risk), multiparity, alcohol abuse, cocaine use, polyhydramnios, maternal hypertension, premature rupture of the membranes, external trauma, uterine leiomyomata, increased age or parity, and multiple gestation.

CLINICAL CHARACTERISTICS

Signs and Symptoms

(Highly variable)
- Vaginal bleeding (not universal; approximately 80%)
- Abdominal, back, or uterine pain (65%)
- Fetal bradycardia or late decelerations (60%)
- Uterine irritability, tachysystole, tetany, elevated baseline intrauterine pressure (20% to 40%)
- Maternal hypotension or signs of volume loss (postural hypotension, shock)
- Fetal demise

DIAGNOSTIC APPROACH

Differential Diagnosis

- Uterine rupture
- Placenta or vasa previa
- Bloody show
- Chorioamnionitis
- Other sources of abdominal pain

Associated Conditions: Hypertension, pre-eclampsia, eclampsia, intrauterine fetal demise, postpartum hemorrhage, consumptive coagulopathy, tumultuous labor, premature delivery, and fetal bradycardia.

Workup and Evaluation

Laboratory: Complete blood count, assessment of clotting function (bleeding time, prothrombin time, partial thromboplastin time, fibrinogen, D-dimer assay).

Imaging: Ultrasound may show signs of a retroplacental clot or collection of blood, but absence does not rule out abruption.

Special Tests: Kleihauer-Betke test for fetal–maternal transfusion, clot tube to assess possibility of coagulopathy, Apt test to identify fetal blood loss (vasa previa).

Diagnostic Procedures: History, physical examination, and laboratory evaluation. Fetal heart rate and uterine activity monitoring.

Pathologic Findings

Bleeding into the decidua basalia with hematoma formation, leading to progressive separation of the placenta and pressure necrosis. Acute anemia, evidence of clotting activation and consumption, histologically normal placenta.

MANAGEMENT AND THERAPY

Nonpharmacologic

General Measures: Prompt evaluation, fluid support, cross-match blood or blood products, Rh typing (if not known).

Specific Measures: Fetal and uterine activity monitoring, monitoring of maternal condition (pulse, blood pressure, pulse oxygenation), expedited delivery.

Diet: Nothing by mouth until the diagnosis is established and the patient's condition is stabilized.

Activity: Bed rest until the diagnosis is established and the patient's condition is stabilized.

Patient Education: Reassurance; American College of Obstetricians and Gynecologists Patient Education Pamphlet AP038 (Bleeding During Pregnancy). (Often there is insufficient time for any more than the most basic information and counseling.)

Drug(s) of Choice

None. (Oxygen and intravenous fluid, Rh immune globulin if indicated.)

Contraindications: Tocolytics should not be used until a diagnosis is established.

FOLLOW-UP

Patient Monitoring: Close attention to vaginal bleeding, fetal well-being, and maternal circulatory status.

Prevention/Avoidance: Eliminate modifiable risk factors. The risk of recurrence is estimated to be 9% to 15%.

Possible Complications: Consumptive coagulopathy, maternal mortality 0.5% to 1% and fetal mortality 20% to 70% based on the size of the separation, the cause, and gestational age; 10% to 15% neurologic sequelae in fetal survivors. Acute renal failure can occur with severe forms of abruption and hypovolemia.

Expected Outcome: Small abruption may be managed conservatively; larger separations may jeopardize mother and fetus and frequently require immediate delivery.

MISCELLANEOUS

ICD-9-CM Code: 641.2.

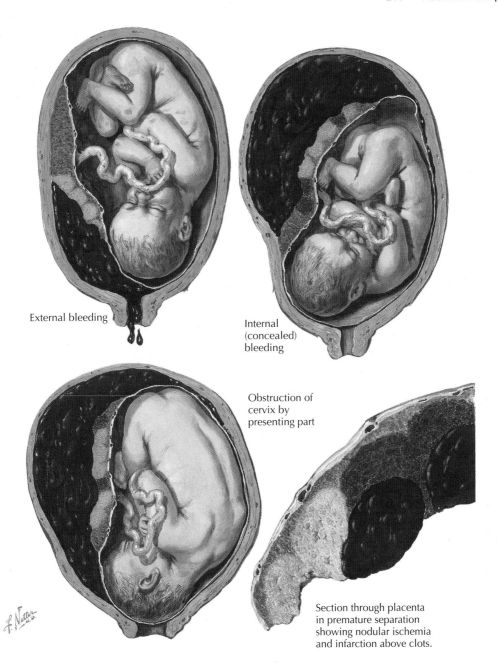

External bleeding

Internal
(concealed)
bleeding

Obstruction of
cervix by
presenting part

Section through placenta
in premature separation
showing nodular ischemia
and infarction above clots.

REFERENCES

Level II

Ananth CV, Savitz DA, Williams MA: Placental abruption and its association with hypertension and prolonged rupture of membranes: a methodologic review and meta-analysis. Obstet Gynecol 1996;88:309.

Ananth CV, Smulian JC, Vintzileos AM: Incidence of placental abruption in relation to cigarette smoking and hypertensive disorders during pregnancy: a meta-analysis of observational studies. Obstet Gynecol 1999;93:622.

Joshi VM, Otiv SR, Majumder R, et al: Internal iliac artery ligation for arresting postpartum haemorrhage. BJOG 2007;114:356. Epub 2007 Jan 22.

Reddy UM, Wapner RJ, Rebar RW, Tasca RJ: Infertility, assisted reproductive technology, and adverse pregnancy outcomes: executive summary of a National Institute of Child Health and Human Development workshop. Obstet Gynecol 2007;109:967.

Sibai BM, Lindheimer M, Hauth J, et al: Risk factors for preeclampsia, abruptio placentae, and adverse neonatal outcomes among women with chronic hypertension. National Institute of Child Health and Human Development Network of Maternal-Fetal Medicine Units. N Engl J Med 1998;339:667.

Level III

American College of Obstetricians and Gynecologists: Obstetric aspects of trauma management. ACOG Educational Bulletin 251, Washington, DC, ACOG, 1998.

Chamberlain G: ABC of antenatal care. Antepartum haemorrhage. BMJ 1991;302:1526.

Chamberlain G, Steer P: ABC of labour care. Obstetric emergencies. BMJ 1999;318:1342.

Fretts RC: Etiology and prevention of stillbirth. Am J Obstet Gynecol 2005;193:1923.

Nash P, Driscoll P: ABC of major trauma. Trauma in pregnancy. BMJ 1990;301:974.

Oyelese Y, Ananth CV: Placental abruption. Obstet Gynecol 2006;108:1005.

Slutsker L: Risks associated with cocaine use during pregnancy. Obstet Gynecol 1992;79:778.

INTRODUCTION

Description: Polyhydramnios is an abnormal increase in the amount of amniotic fluid surrounding the fetus. This diagnosis is generally reserved for volumes >2 L and amniotic fluid index >24 to 25 cm. (At term, there should be about 800 mL of amniotic fluid present.) This fluid may accumulate gradually over time (chronic hydramnios) or acutely over the course of several days (more common in early pregnancy).

Prevalence: In 0.9% to 1.6% of women, some increase in amniotic fluid is seen during pregnancy (80% mild, 5% severe).

Predominant Age: Reproductive.

Genetics: No genetic pattern.

ETIOLOGY AND PATHOGENESIS

Causes: Idiopathic (two thirds), maternal diabetes, multiple gestation, fetal anomalies (50% of patients with severe hydramnios: central nervous system, gastrointestinal tract, chromosomal).

Risk Factors: Fetal anomalies that impair swallowing or alter urine production, multiple gestation (twin–twin transfusion), maternal diabetes, erythroblastosis.

CLINICAL CHARACTERISTICS

Signs and Symptoms

- Uterine size larger than normal for stage of pregnancy
- Increased amniotic fluid measured by ultrasonography (amniotic fluid index [AFI] >24 to 25 cm)
- Dyspnea (especially when supine)
- Lower-extremity and vulvar edema
- Premature labor
- Difficulty palpating fetal parts or hearing fetal heart tones

DIAGNOSTIC APPROACH

Differential Diagnosis

- Inaccurate gestational age
- Normal multiple gestation
- Fetal anomalies
- Ascites
- Ovarian cyst

Associated Conditions: Anencephaly, esophageal atresia, prematurity, umbilical cord prolapse, and placental abruption.

Workup and Evaluation

Laboratory: No evaluation indicated.

Imaging: Amniotic fluid index calculated by adding the vertical depths of the largest pockets of amniotic fluid in each quadrant of the uterus (average at term = 12.5 cm, 95th percentile = 21.4). Fetal anomalies may also be documented.

Special Tests: None indicated.

Diagnostic Procedures: Physical examination, ultrasonography.

Pathologic Findings

None.

MANAGEMENT AND THERAPY

Nonpharmacologic

General Measures: Evaluation. Mild conditions may be managed expectantly. If dyspnea or abdominal pain is present, hospitalization may be required.

Specific Measures: Indomethacin therapy has been shown to be of help in some patients. Therapeutic amniocentesis may be used to transiently relieve maternal symptoms and in some cases allow prolongation of the gestation. (If performed, the rate of withdrawal should be about 500 mL/hour and limited to 1500 to 2000 mL total volume.) Bed rest, diuretics, and salt and water restrictions are ineffective.

Diet: No specific dietary changes indicated.

Activity: No restriction except for those imposed by the enlarged uterus.

Patient Education: Reassurance; American College of Obstetricians and Gynecologists Patient Education Pamphlet AP025 (Ultrasound Exams), AP098 (Special Tests for Monitoring Fetal Health).

Drug(s) of Choice

Indomethacin 1.5 to 3.0 mg/kg/day.

Contraindications: Aspirin-sensitive asthma, inflammatory bowel disease, or ulcers.

Precautions: Use of nonsteroidal anti-inflammatory agents has been associated with premature closure of the ductus arteriosus. This is generally transient and may be monitored by ultrasonography.

Alternative Drugs

None.

FOLLOW-UP

Patient Monitoring: Normal health maintenance.

Prevention/Avoidance: None.

Possible Complications: Premature labor and delivery (40%), abruptio placenta, maternal pulmonary compromise, umbilical cord prolapse.

Expected Outcome: Mild to moderate increases in fluid are not associated with significant risk. Severe polyhydramnios is often associated with significant fetal anomalies. Perinatal mortality is as high as 25% to 30% in some studies. In general, the more severe the hydramnios, the greater the fetal risk.

MISCELLANEOUS

ICD-9-CM Codes: 657, 761.3 (Affecting the fetus).

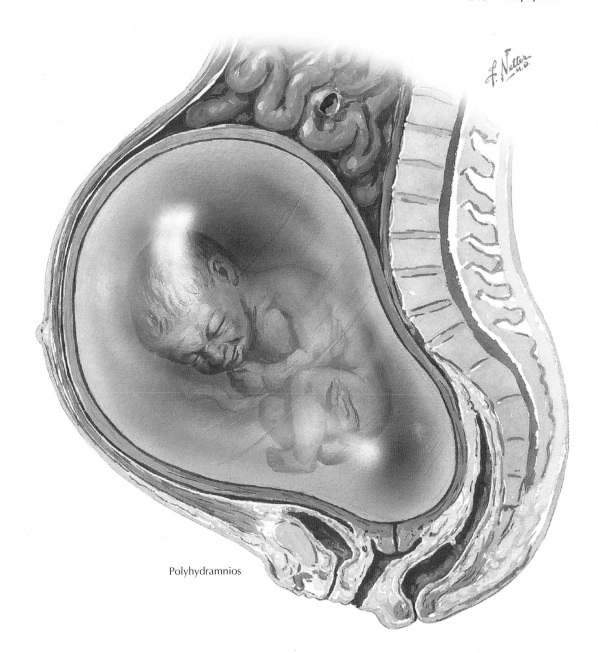

Polyhydramnios

REFERENCES

Level II

Barnhard Y, Bar-Hava I, Divon MY: Is polyhydramnios in an ultra-sonographically normal fetus an indication for genetic evaluation? Am J Obstet Gynecol 1995;173:1523.

Damato N, Filly RA, Goldstein RB, et al: Frequency of fetal anomalies in sonographically detected polyhydramnios. J Ultrasound Med 1993;12:11.

Many A, Hill LM, Lazebnik N, Martin JG: The association between polyhydramnios and preterm delivery. Obstet Gynecol 1995; 86:389.

Level III

Abhyankar S, Salvi VS: Indomethacin therapy in hydramnios. J Postgrad Med 2000;46:176.

Brace RA: Physiology of amniotic fluid volume regulation. Clin Obstet Gynecol 1997;40:280.

Cardwell MS: Polyhydramnios: a review. Obstet Gynecol Surv 1987;42:612.

Chiu T, Cuevas D, Cuevas L, Monteiro C: Tracheal agenesis. South Med J 1990;83:925.

Kramer WB, Van den Veyver IB, Kirshon B: Treatment of polyhydramnios with indomethacin. Clin Perinatol 1994;21:615.

Marino T: Ultrasound abnormalities of the amniotic fluid, membranes, umbilical cord, and placenta. Obstet Gynecol Clin North Am 2004;31:177.

Moise KJ Jr: Polyhydramnios: problems and treatment. Semin Perinatol 1993;17:197.

Moise KJ Jr: Polyhydramnios. Clin Obstet Gynecol 1997;40:266.

Moore TR: Clinical assessment of amniotic fluid. Clin Obstet Gynecol 1997;40:303.

Phelan JP, Martin GI: Polyhydramnios: fetal and neonatal implications. Clin Perinatol 1989;16:987.

Rodriguez MH: Polyhydramnios: does reducing the amniotic fluid volume decrease the incidence of prematurity? Clin Perinatol 1992;19:359.

Underwood MA, Gilbert WM, Sherman MP: Amniotic fluid: not just fetal urine anymore. J Perinatol 2005;25:341.

Williams K: Amniotic fluid assessment. Obstet Gynecol Surv 1993; 48:795.

INTRODUCTION

Description: Pre-eclampsia is a pregnancy-specific syndrome (occurring after 20 weeks of gestation) of reduced organ perfusion, vasospasm, and endothelial activation characterized by hypertension, proteinuria, and other symptoms. Pregnancy can induce hypertension or aggravate existing hypertension. Edema and proteinuria (one or both) are characteristic pregnancy-induced changes. If pre-eclampsia is untreated, convulsions (eclampsia) may occur. Chronic hypertension may be worsened by or superimposed on pregnancy-induced changes. Severe cases may include hemolysis, elevated liver enzymes, and low platelet counts (HELLP syndrome; occurs in up to 20% of severe pre-eclampsia cases).

Prevalence: Five to eight percent of all births, 250,000 cases per year, result in 150 maternal deaths (18%) and 3000 fetal deaths per year. (Overall, hypertensive disease of some type occurs in approximately 12% to 22% of pregnancies, and it is directly responsible for 17.6% of maternal deaths in the United States.)

Predominant Age: Rare before 20 weeks of gestation.

Genetics: Multifactorial, runs in families.

ETIOLOGY AND PATHOGENESIS

Causes: Unknown, genetic, endocrine/metabolic (including altered prostaglandin production), uteroplacental ischemia, immunologic all proposed.

Risk Factors: Prior history, body mass index >32.3, African American race, nulliparity, age older than 35 (2-fold to 3-fold increase) or younger than 18 years, multifetal pregnancy, fetal hydrops, hydatidiform mole, thrombophilia.

CLINICAL CHARACTERISTICS

Signs and Symptoms

- Hypertension without proteinuria or edema (gestational hypertension)
- Hypertension with proteinuria or edema (pre-eclampsia) (severe pre-eclampsia: headache, abdominal pain, weight gain, visual disturbances, thrombocytopenia, oliguria, hemoconcentration, pulmonary edema, proteinuria >3+)
- Hypertension, proteinuria, or edema and seizures (grand mal type) (eclampsia)

DIAGNOSTIC APPROACH

Differential Diagnosis

- Chronic (essential) hypertension
- Transient hypertension
- Chronic renal disease
- Acute or chronic glomerulonephritis
- Coarctation of the aorta
- Cushing's disease
- Systemic lupus erythematosus
- Periarteritis nodosa
- Obesity
- Epilepsy
- Encephalitis
- Cerebral aneurysm or tumor
- Lupus cerebritis
- Hysteria

Associated Conditions: Hypertension, heart disease, stroke, placental infarcts, and placental abruption.

Workup and Evaluation

Laboratory: Liver and renal function studies (enzymes, renal clearance, 24-hour urinary protein measurement).

Imaging: Ultrasonography to monitor fetal growth (frequently restricted).

Special Tests: Assessment of fetal lung maturation may be performed, but if maternal disease is severe, management is based on maternal factors and not fetal maturation. Invasive hemodynamic monitoring may be required for patients with the most severe cases.

Diagnostic Procedures: History, physical examination (with blood pressure), urinalysis (or "dipstick"), laboratory assessment.

Pathologic Findings

Results of 24-hour urinary protein measurement >300 mg/24 hours, blood pressure >140/90, characteristic renal glomerular lesions (capillary endotheliosis), premature aging of the placenta, increased vascular reactivity, elevated liver enzymes, thrombocytopenia. (In the past, hypertension indicative of pre-eclampsia has been defined as an elevation of more than 30 mm Hg systolic or more than 15 mm Hg diastolic above the patient's baseline pressure; however, this has not proved to be a good predictor of outcome and is no longer part of the criteria for pre-eclampsia. These patients do require close monitoring.)

MANAGEMENT AND THERAPY

Nonpharmacologic

General Measures: Aggressive evaluation, frequent prenatal visits, increased fetal surveillance (fetal growth). Hospitalization is required for all but the most benign conditions (mild gestational hypertension, stable chronic hypertension with normal fetal growth). Weekly antenatal testing should be strongly considered. (See table.)

Specific Measures: The only true treatment for pre-eclampsia or eclampsia is delivery. Management of symptoms may be used to get both mother and baby into optimal condition for delivery.

Diet: No specific dietary changes indicated except as dictated by labor or other management. (A low-salt diet has been advocated but is unproved. Supplementation with high-dose vitamins C, A, or E has been associated with adverse effects and is not recommended.)

Activity: Bed rest with severe conditions or for women in the process of delivery.

CRITERIA FOR PRE-ECLAMPSIA

Pre-eclampsia (Mild)	Severe Pre-eclampsia (One or More)
▪ Blood pressure ≥140 mm Hg systolic or ≥90 mm Hg diastolic after 20 weeks of gestation with previously normal blood pressure ▪ Proteinuria (≥0.3 g/24 hours)	▪ Blood pressure ≥160 mm Hg systolic or ≥110 mm Hg diastolic on two occasions at least 6 hours apart, while the patient is on bed rest ▪ Proteinuria (≥5 g/24 hours or 3+ or greater on two random urine samples at least 4 hours apart) ▪ Oliguria (<500 mL in 24 hours) ▪ Cerebral or visual disturbances ▪ Pulmonary edema or cyanosis ▪ Epigastric or right upper quadrant pain ▪ Impaired hepatic function ▪ Thrombocytopenia ▪ Fetal growth restriction

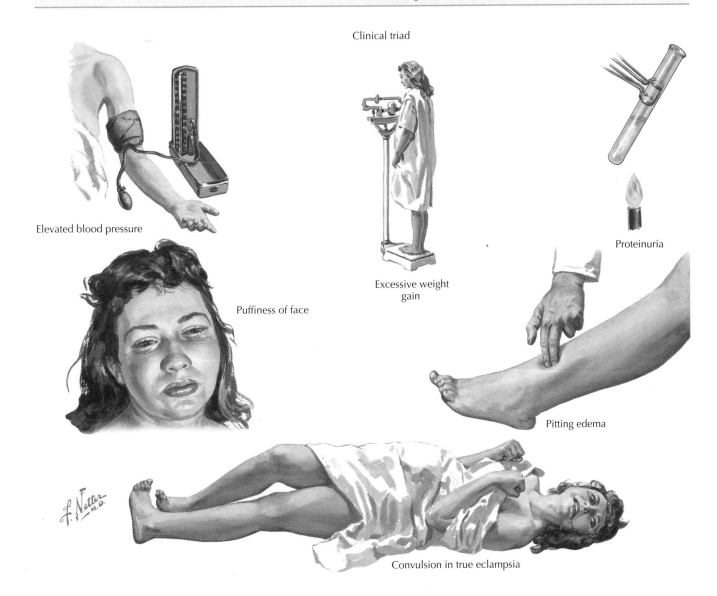

Clinical triad

Elevated blood pressure

Puffiness of face

Excessive weight gain

Proteinuria

Pitting edema

Convulsion in true eclampsia

Patient Education: American College of Obstetricians and Gynecologists Patient Education Pamphlet AP034 (High Blood Pressure During Pregnancy).

Drug(s) of Choice

Drug treatment of mild pre-eclampsia has generally been disappointing. Glucocorticoids are often given to encour-age fetal lung maturation. Drugs such as labetalol or nifedipine have been given as part of conservative man-agement protocols. These have generally resulted in pro-longation of the gestation and improved fetal outcome but no reduction in catastrophic events such as placental abruption. Magnesium sulfate is often given intrave-nously during labor to stabilize blood pressure and reduce

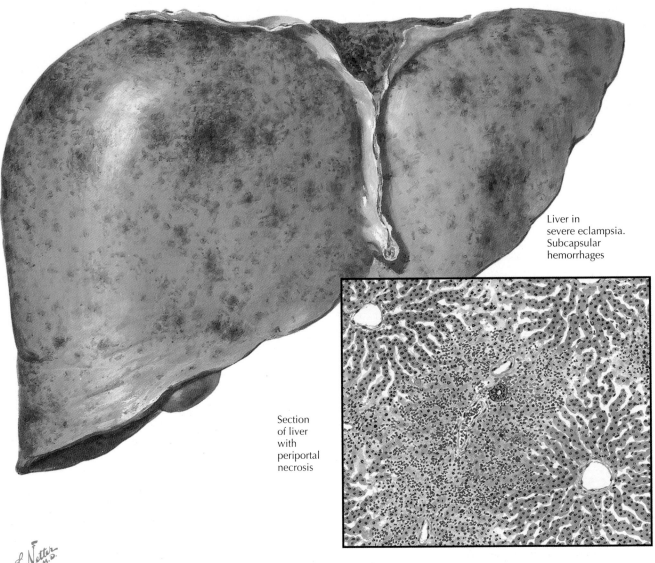

Liver in
severe eclampsia.
Subcapsular
hemorrhages

Section
of liver
with
periportal
necrosis

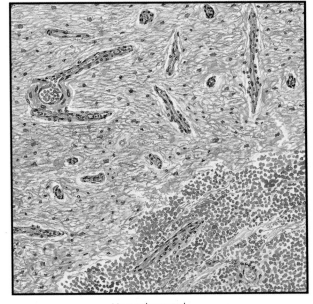

Hemorrhage and
necrosis in brain

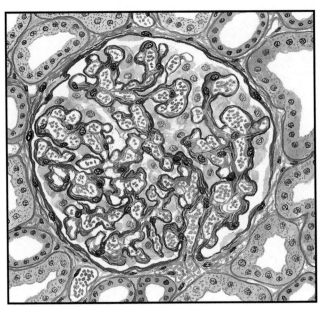

Fibrin deposition and swelling
of epithelial cells in glomerulus

the risk of seizures but is not associated with a reduction in fetal morbidity or mortality. Intravenous hydralazine may be used to lower blood pressure acutely during labor. Recent data suggest that antiplatelet/nonsteroidal anti-inflammatory agents may reduce the risk of recurrence or complications, but definitive data are lacking.

Contraindications: Angiotensin-converting enzyme (ACE) inhibitors are contraindicated in pregnancy.

Precautions: Excessive levels (>10 mEg/L) of magnesium sulfate may result in respiratory paralysis and cardiac arrest.

Interactions: See individual agents.

Alternative Drugs

Verapamil, nimodipine, diazoxide, and nitroglycerin have all been studied or advocated at some time. (Prophylactic treatment with aspirin has not been proved to be effective in preventing pre-eclampsia except in selected patients.)

FOLLOW-UP

Patient Monitoring: Increased maternal and fetal surveillance (more frequent prenatal visits, laboratory tests, and ultrasonography evaluations).

Prevention/Avoidance: Early detection and treatment. Aggressive management of pre-eclampsia may reduce the risk of eclampsia. (The use of prophylactic aspirin remains controversial and unproven.) The risk of recurrence of pre-eclampsia in subsequent pregnancies is inversely proportional to the gestational age at which it occurred in the index pregnancy.

Possible Complications: Maternal—cardiac decompensation, stroke, pulmonary edema and respiratory failure, renal failure, seizures and seizure-related injuries, intracranial hemorrhage, coma, death (0.5% to 5% mortality). Fetal risk (growth restriction and death) is directly proportional to both the degree of proteinuria and the level of diastolic blood pressure. The risk to both mother and fetus increases dramatically in eclampsia.

Expected Outcome: Generally, gestational hypertension, pre-eclampsia, and eclampsia improve after delivery. Eclamptic seizures may occur up to 10 days after delivery but are uncommon beyond 48 hours.

MISCELLANEOUS

ICD-9-CM Codes: 642.4 (Mild pre-eclampsia), 642.5 (Severe pre-eclampsia), 642.6 (Eclampsia), 642.7 (With superimposed pre-existing hypertension).

REFERENCES

Level I

Barrilleaux PS, Martin JN Jr, Klauser CK, et al: Postpartum intravenous dexamethasone for severely preeclamptic patients without hemolysis, elevated liver enzymes, low platelets (HELLP) syndrome: a randomized trial. Obstet Gynecol 2005;105:843.

Livingston JC, Livingston LW, Ramsey R, et al: Magnesium sulfate in women with mild preeclampsia: a randomized controlled trial. Obstet Gynecol 2003;101:217.

Lucas MJ, Leveno KJ, Cunningham FG: A comparison of magnesium sulfate with phenytoin for the prevention of eclampsia. N Engl J Med 1995;333:201.

Magpie Trial Follow-Up Study Collaborative Group: The Magpie Trial: A randomised trial comparing magnesium sulphate with placebo for pre-eclampsia. Outcome for children at 18 months. BJOG 2007;114:289. Epub 2006 Dec 12.

Magpie Trial Follow-Up Study Collaborative Group: The Magpie Trial: A randomised trial comparing magnesium sulphate with placebo for pre-eclampsia. Outcome for women at 2 years. BJOG 2007;114:300. Epub 2006 Dec 12.

Level II

Askie LM, Duley L, Henderson-Smart DJ, Stewart LA; PARIS Collaborative Group: Antiplatelet agents for prevention of pre-eclampsia: a meta-analysis of individual patient data. Lancet 2007;369:1791.

Conde-Agudelo A, Villar J, Lindheimer M: World Health Organization systematic review of screening tests for preeclampsia. Obstet Gynecol 2004;104:1367.

Coomarasamy A, Honest H, Papaioannou S, et al: Aspirin for prevention of preeclampsia in women with historical risk factors: a systematic review. Obstet Gynecol 2003;101:1319.

Nassar AH, Adra AM, Chakhtoura N, et al: Severe preeclampsia remote from term: labor induction or elective cesarean delivery? Am J Obstet Gynecol 1998;179:1210.

Level III

American College of Obstetricians and Gynecologists: Chronic hypertension in pregnancy. ACOG Practice Bulletin 29. Obstet Gynecol 2001;98:177.

American College of Obstetricians and Gynecologists: Diagnosis and management of preeclampsia and eclampsia. ACOG Practice Bulletin 33. Obstet Gynecol 2002;99:159.

Brown MA, Mackenzie C, Dunsmuir W, et al: Can we predict recurrence of pre-eclampsia or gestational hypertension? BJOG 2007;114:984. Epub 2007 Jun 14.

Duley L, Meher S, Abalos E: Management of pre-eclampsia. BMJ 2006;332:463.

Martin JN Jr, Rose CH, Briery CM: Understanding and managing HELLP syndrome: the integral role of aggressive glucocorticoids for mother and child. Am J Obstet Gynecol 2006;195:914. Epub 2006 May 2.

Sibai BM: Treatment of hypertension in pregnant women. N Engl J Med 1996;335:257.

Sibai BM: Diagnosis and management of gestational hypertension and preeclampsia. Obstet Gynecol 2003;102:181.

Sibai BM: Magnesium sulfate prophylaxis in preeclampsia: lessons learned from recent trials. Am J Obstet Gynecol 2004;190:1520.

Sibai BM: Diagnosis, prevention, and management of eclampsia. Obstet Gynecol 2005;105:402.

Sibai BM: Imitators of severe preeclampsia. Obstet Gynecol 2007;109:956.

Sibai B, Dekker G, Kupferminc M: Pre-eclampsia. Lancet 2005;365:785.

Witlin AG, Sibai BM: Magnesium sulfate therapy in preeclampsia and eclampsia. Obstet Gynecol 1998;92:883.

Zhang J, Villar J, Sun W, et al: Blood pressure dynamics during pregnancy and spontaneous preterm birth. Am J Obstet Gynecol 2007;197:162.e1.

INTRODUCTION

Description: Although the term *puerperal infection* can be used to describe any infection during or after labor, it generally applies to infection of the uterus and surrounding tissues after delivery. (See also Chorioamnionitis.) This can vary from mild to life-threatening in severity. Some of the most severe infections may appear within hours of delivery and are often opportunistic and not associated with reliable risk factors. Vigilance and aggressive diagnosis and treatment are required.

Prevalence: Estimated to occur in 1% to 8% of vaginal deliveries; approximately 15% if chorioamnionitis is present during labor. Following cesarean delivery: 10% to 20% if antibiotic prophylaxis is given during delivery, 50% to 90% without antibiotic prophylaxis in some series.

Genetics: No genetic pattern.

ETIOLOGY AND PATHOGENESIS

Causes: Colonization and infection of the tissues of the uterus, peritoneum, or surrounding organs. The most common organisms are group B streptococci; other facultative streptococci; *Gardnerella vaginalis*; and *Escherichia coli*, Bacteroides, and *Peptostreptococcus* species. Infection by clostridia or group A streptococci may result in rapidly progressive soft-tissue (subcutaneous tissue, muscle, or myometrial) infection. Abscesses usually contain both aerobic and anaerobic bacteria such as Bacteroides species (*Bacteroides bivius, Bacteroides disiens*, or *Bacteroides fragilis*). Approximately 50% of ascending uterine infections involve *Chlamydia trachomatis*.

Risk Factors: Cesarean delivery (10- to 20-fold increase), invasive procedures during labor, prolonged rupture of the membranes, prolonged labor, multiple examinations, retained placental fragments, urinary catheter, intravenous line(s), low socioeconomic or nutritional status, anemia, and chronic disease (diabetes).

CLINICAL CHARACTERISTICS

Signs and Symptoms

- Fever (90% >38.5°C by 24 hours) and tachycardia (often developing rapidly after delivery)
- Uterine tenderness (may be absent)
- Signs of septic or cardiovascular shock (hypotension, anxiety, disorientation, prostration)
- Impaired renal function (<20 mL/hour urine production)
- Altered white blood count (<1000 or ≥25,000)
- Hemolysis or hemoconcentration

DIAGNOSTIC APPROACH

Differential Diagnosis

- Urinary tract infections including pyelonephritis (5% of patients, classical signs are routinely absent, urinalysis shows large numbers of white blood cells, and cultures are positive)
- Wound infection
- Atelectasis or pneumonitis
- Infection in intravenous line or site, contaminated fluids
- Disturbed abscess (old tubo-ovarian or appendiceal abscess)
- Septic thrombophlebitis
- Necrotizing fasciitis
- Transfusion reaction (when applicable)
- Amniotic fluid or pulmonary embolism
- Cardiogenic shock (drugs, cardiac disease, aortic dissection)
- Toxic shock syndrome
- Mastitis (2% of patients)

Associated Conditions: Septic shock, adult respiratory distress syndrome, acute renal failure, and disseminated intravascular coagulation.

Workup and Evaluation

Laboratory: Complete blood count, endometrial culture obtained by protected swab (if amniotic fluid or endometrial culture obtained at the time of delivery [within 24 hours] is not available). Blood cultures (are positive in 15% to 25% of patients who are febrile but do not reflect the severity of the infection). Tissue culture (direct or by needle aspiration, when wound infections is suspected) and Gram stain.

Imaging: Ultrasonography may be useful in evaluating the possibility of pelvic abscess or gas formation. Computed tomography (CT) and magnetic resonance imaging (MRI) are useful for a more wide-ranging assessment.

Special Tests: Frozen-section histopathologic evaluation may be useful if necrotizing fasciitis is suspected.

Diagnostic Procedures: History, physical examination, cultures.

Pathologic Findings

Evidence of inflammation and/or necrosis (based on tissue involved and severity of infections).

MANAGEMENT AND THERAPY

Nonpharmacologic

General Measures: Evaluation, fluid replacement or resuscitation, antipyretics and analgesics (after a diagnosis has been established). Close monitoring, including intensive care, may be required when infection is severe. Consultation with an infectious-disease specialist may be desirable. Low-grade (<38°C) or intermittent fevers may not require treatment when present in the first 24 hours.

Specific Measures: Aggressive antibiotic therapy. Based on response, removal of infected products (if present), surgical exploration, abscess drainage (percutaneous or open), debridement, or hysterectomy may be required. (Virtually all postpartum septic shock is caused by surgically treatable processes.) Because of the expanded blood and tissue volume at and after delivery, antibiotic dosages

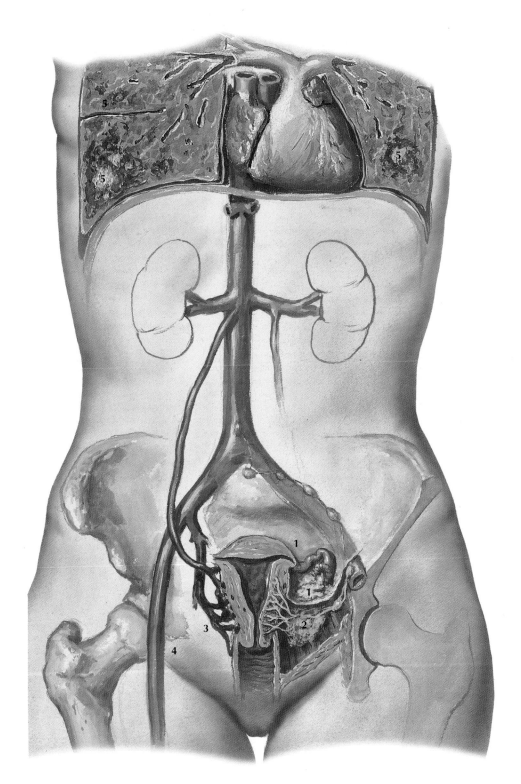

Dissemination of septic endometritis:
(1) Peritonitis
(2) Parametritis (via lymphatics)
(3) Pelvic thrombophlebitis
(4) Femoral thrombophlebitis
(5) Pulmonary infarct or abscess (septic embolus)

must be increased by 40% over those used outside of pregnancy.

Diet: For patients who are acutely ill, nothing by mouth until condition is stabilized. For other patients, no specific dietary changes indicated.

Activity: Bed rest until patient's condition is stable, then a progressive return to normal activity.

Patient Education: Reassurance; American College of Obstetricians and Gynecologists Patient Education Pamphlet AP006 (Cesarean Birth).

Drug(s) of Choice

Antibiotics should be administered to provide protection against gram-negative facultative and anaerobic bacteria. Moderate infections require double antibiotic treatment; severe infections should be treated with triple therapy: an aminoglycoside or first-generation cephalosporin (for facultative bacteria); clindamycin, imipenem-cilastatin, or metronidazole (anaerobic bacteria); and penicillin or ampicillin (clostridia and synergistic action with aminoglycosides on enterococci). β-Lactam antibiotics (penicillin or cephalosporin) should be given in dosages of 8 to 12 g/day.

Contraindications: See individual agents.

Precautions: Antibiotic dosages must be increased by up to 40% because of the altered physiologic state of pregnancy.

Interactions: See individual agents.

FOLLOW-UP

Patient Monitoring: When severe infections are present, intensive monitoring (including placement in an intensive care unit) may be required. This may include central venous access and monitoring, pulse oximetry, and careful (frequent if not continuous) blood pressure monitoring.

Prevention/Avoidance: Careful attention should be given to antisepsis, reduced numbers of vaginal examinations when the amniotic membranes have been ruptured, careful tissue handling during operative procedures, use of prophylactic antibiotics when risk factors are identified. Changing intravenous sites every 48 hours reduces the risk of infection. There is no evidence to support a role for vaginal antisepsis (chlorhexidine or similar) during labor or prior to cesarean delivery. There are insufficient data to evaluate the role of prophylactic antibiotics after manual removal of the placenta or operative delivery.

Possible Complications: Progression of infection, abscess formation, septic thrombophlebitis, septic shock, adult respiratory distress syndrome, renal failure, cardiovascular collapse, death. If septic shock occurs, mortality rates of 20% to 30% are common. Coagulopathy may develop. Necrotizing fasciitis is possible.

Expected Outcome: With timely diagnosis and appropriate therapy a complete recovery with no long-term sequelae should be expected. Approximately 90% of patients respond rapidly to antibiotic therapy (and/or percutaneous drainage of abscesses).

MISCELLANEOUS
ICD-9-CM Code: 670.0.

REFERENCES
Level I
Livingston JC, Llata E, Rinehart E, et al: Gentamicin and clindamycin therapy in postpartum endometritis: the efficacy of daily dosing versus dosing every 8 hours. Am J Obstet Gynecol 2003; 188:149.

Level II
Chongsomchai C, Lumbiganon P, Laopaiboon M: Prophylactic antibiotics for manual removal of retained placenta in vaginal birth. Cochrane Database Syst Rev 2006:CD004904.
French LM, Smaill FM: Antibiotic regimens for endometritis after delivery. Cochrane Database Syst Rev 2004:CD001067.
Hopkins L, Smaill F: Antibiotic regimens for management of intra-amniotic infection. Cochrane Database Syst Rev 2002:CD003254.
Liabsuetrakul T, Choobun T, Peeyananjarassri K, Islam M: Antibiotic prophylaxis for operative vaginal delivery. Cochrane Database Syst Rev 2004:CD004455.
Lumbiganon P, Thinkhamrop J, Thinkhamrop B, Tolosa JE: Vaginal chlorhexidine during labour for preventing maternal and neonatal infections (excluding Group B Streptococcal and HIV). Cochrane Database Syst Rev 2004:CD004070.
Smaill F, Hofmeyr GJ: Antibiotic prophylaxis for cesarean section. Cochrane Database Syst Rev 2002;CD000933.

Level III
American College of Obstetricians and Gynecologists: Prevention of early-onset group B streptococcal disease in newborns. ACOG Committee Opinion 279. Obstet Gynecol 2002;100:1405.
American College of Obstetricians and Gynecologists: Prophylactic antibiotics in labor and delivery. ACOG Practice Bulletin 47. Obstet Gynecol 2003;102:875.
American College of Obstetricians and Gynecologists: Premature rupture of membranes. ACOG Practice Bulletin 80. Obstet Gynecol 2007;109:1007.
Casey BM, Cox SM: Chorioamnionitis and endometritis. Infect Dis Clin North Am 1997;11:203.
Faro S: Postpartum endometritis. Clin Perinatol 2005;32:803.
Maharaj D: Puerperal pyrexia: a review. Part I. Obstet Gynecol Surv 2007;62:393.
Maharaj D: Puerperal pyrexia: a review. Part II. Obstet Gynecol Surv 2007;62:400.

INTRODUCTION

Description: Isoimmunization to any fetal blood group not possessed by the mother is possible. The most common example is the Rh (D) factor. What was once a common cause for intrauterine fetal death has largely been eradicated by prophylactic administration of immune globulin to those at risk.

Prevalence: Uncommon since the routine use of D immune globulin therapy.

Predominant Age: Reproductive.

Genetics: Mothers who are Rh (D) negative. (The genes for the CDE blood groups are inherited separately from the ABO groups and are located on the short arm of chromosome 1.)

ETIOLOGY AND PATHOGENESIS

Causes: Antibody formation against the D antigen.

Risk Factors: Any process that exposes the woman to blood carrying the D antigen including blood transfusion, miscarriage, ectopic or normal pregnancy, trauma, amniocentesis during pregnancy, and others.

CLINICAL CHARACTERISTICS

Signs and Symptoms

- Elevated serum titers of anti-D immunoglobulin (IgM)
- Fetal hydrops, erythroblastosis fetalis, hemolytic disease of the newborn
- Intrauterine fetal demise

DIAGNOSTIC APPROACH

Differential Diagnosis

- Other isoimmunizations (most frequently Lewis, Kell, or Duffy antigens)
- Iron-deficiency anemia (maternal)
- Hemoglobinopathy

Associated Conditions: Polyhydramnios.

Workup and Evaluation

Laboratory: Serum antibody titers (at first visit, 20 weeks, and approximately every 4 weeks thereafter), testing of baby's father's antibody status. Emerging data suggest that it may be possible to determine the Rh status of the fetus directly from fetal cells circulating in maternal blood.

Imaging: Ultrasonography is useful to establish gestational age and monitor amniotic fluid volume and fetal growth. Some studies have assessed the ability of ultrasonography to monitor the degree of fetal anemia, but this technique has not gained wide usage.

Special Tests: Amniocentesis or umbilical cord blood sampling if titers are elevated or there has been a prior affected pregnancy.

Diagnostic Procedures: Serum titers, amniocentesis, or umbilical cord blood sampling.

MANAGEMENT AND THERAPY

Nonpharmacologic

General Measures: Evaluation, increased surveillance.

Specific Measures: When antibody titers are ≤1:8, no intervention is required. When titers are ≥1:16 in albumin or 1:32 by an indirect Coombs test, amniocentesis or umbilical cord blood sampling should be considered. In severely affected fetuses, intrauterine transfusion may be required.

Diet: No specific dietary changes indicated.

Activity: No restriction.

Patient Education: American College of Obstetricians and Gynecologists Patient Education Pamphlet AP027 (The Rh Factor: How It Can Affect Your Pregnancy)

Drug(s) of Choice

None if isoimmunization has taken place. Prophylaxis (with Rh-positive father): D immune globulin—50 micrograns for miscarriage before 13 weeks of gestation or after chorionic villus sampling; 300 micrograns after amniocentesis or ectopic pregnancy; at 28 to 30 weeks of gestation in unsensitized patients or after normal delivery. (20 micrograns/1 mL of D-positive cells [2 mL of whole blood] infused or lost into the patient's circulation.)

Contraindications: Patients who are already sensitized to the D antigen should not receive D immune globulin.

FOLLOW-UP

Patient Monitoring: Normal prenatal care with increased surveillance of fetal growth and health.

Prevention/Avoidance: All patients should have their Rh type established and be tested for isoimmunization (indirect Coombs test) at the first prenatal visit. Those who are Rh negative should receive D immune globulin after delivery, amniocentesis, fetal demise, miscarriage, ectopic pregnancy, or any other time exposure to Rh-positive cells may have occurred. Prophylactic administration between 28 and 30 weeks of gestation is also wise.

Possible Complications: Isoimmunization with subsequent immune damage to fetal red cells leading to lysis, anemia, hydrops, and fetal death.

Expected Outcome: With prophylaxis, the risk of isoimmunization is estimated to be 0.3%.

MISCELLANEOUS

ICD-9-CM Code: 656.1.

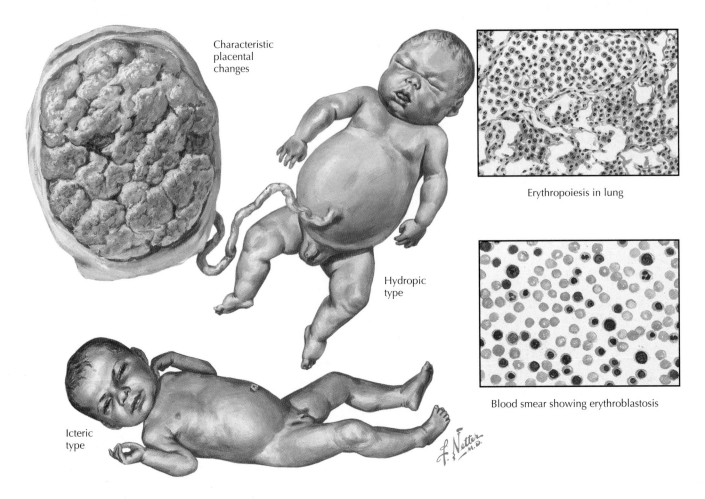

Characteristic placental changes

Erythropoiesis in lung

Hydropic type

Blood smear showing erythroblastosis

Icteric type

REFERENCES

Level II

Bichler J, Schondorfer G, Pabst G, Andresen I: Pharmacokinetics of anti-D IgG in pregnant RhD-negative women. BJOG 2003; 110:39.

Geifman-Holtzman O, Grotegut CA, Gaughan JP: Diagnostic accuracy of noninvasive fetal Rh genotyping from maternal blood—A meta-analysis. Am J Obstet Gynecol 2006;195:1163.

Mari G, Deter RL, Carpenter RL, et al: Noninvasive diagnosis by Doppler ultrasonography of fetal anemia due to maternal red-cell alloimmunization. Collaborative Group for Doppler Assessment of the Blood Velocity in Anemic Fetuses. N Engl J Med 2000;342:9.

Queenan JT, Tomai TP, Ural SH, King JC: Deviation in amniotic fluid optical density at a wavelength of 450 nm in Rh-immunized pregnancies from 14 to 40 weeks' gestation: a proposal for clinical management. Am J Obstet Gynecol 1993;168:1370.

Ruma MS, Moise KJ Jr, Kim E, et al: Combined plasmapheresis and intravenous immune globulin for the treatment of severe maternal red cell alloimmunization. Am J Obstet Gynecol 2007; 196:138.e1.

Thornton JG, Page C, Foote G, et al: Efficacy and long term effects of antenatal prophylaxis with anti-D immunoglobulin. BMJ 1989; 298:1671.

Zimmerman R, Carpenter RJ Jr, Durig P, Mari G: Longitudinal measurement of peak systolic velocity in the fetal middle cerebral artery for monitoring pregnancies complicated by red cell alloimmunisation: a prospective multicentre trial with intention-to-treat. BJOG 2002;109:746.

Level III

American College of Obstetricians and Gynecologists: Prevention of Rh D isoimmunization. ACOG Practice Bulletin 4., Washington, DC, ACOG, 1999.

American College of Obstetricians and Gynecologists: Management of alloimmunization during pregnancy. ACOG Practice Bulletin 75. Obstet Gynecol 2006;108:457.

Bianchi DW, Avent ND, Costa JM, van der Schoot CE: Noninvasive prenatal diagnosis of fetal Rhesus D: ready for Prime(r) Time. Obstet Gynecol 2005;106:841.

Bowman JM: The management of Rh-isoimmunization. Obstet Gynecol 1978;52:1.

Contreras M: The prevention of Rh haemolytic disease of the fetus and newborn—General background. Br J Obstet Gynaecol 1998; 105:7.

Fairweather DV, Tacchi D, Coxon A, et al: Intrauterine transfusion in Rh-isoimmunization. BMJ 1967;4:189.

Jabara S, Barnhart KT: Is Rh immune globulin needed in early first-trimester abortion? A review. Am J Obstet Gynecol 2003; 188:623.

Jones ML, Wray J, Wight J, et al: A review of the clinical effectiveness of routine antenatal anti-D prophylaxis for rhesus-negative women who are pregnant. BJOG 2004;111:892.

Moise KJ Jr: Management of rhesus alloimmunization in pregnancy. Obstet Gynecol 2002;100:600.

INTRODUCTION

Description: Shoulder dystocia is an obstruction to delivery caused by impaction of the fetal shoulder behind the maternal symphysis. Less commonly it can be due to impaction of the posterior fetal shoulder on the sacral promontory. Shoulder dystocia is most often an unpredictable and unpreventable obstetric emergency, usually defined as a delivery that requires additional obstetric maneuvers (following failure of gentle downward traction on the fetal head) to effect delivery of the shoulders.

Prevalence: 0.15% of fetuses weighing ≥2500 g (5 pounds 8 oz), 1% to 5% for ≥4000 g (8 pounds 13 oz), 19% ≥4500 g (9 pounds 15 oz); overall 0.6% to 1.4% of vertex deliveries.

Genetics: Tall or large parents are at higher risk.

ETIOLOGY AND PATHOGENESIS

Causes: A relative disproportion between fetus and the birth passage or a misalignment of normally sized structures (fetus and pelvis).

Risk Factors: Fetal macrosomia (risk proportional to weight), pelvic deformity, maternal obesity, diabetes mellitus, post-term pregnancy, prolonged second stage of labor, oxytocin induction, midforceps or vacuum extraction.

CLINICAL CHARACTERISTICS

Signs and Symptoms

- Poor descent during labor
- Retraction of the fetal head onto the perineum following delivery of the chin ("turtle sign")

DIAGNOSTIC APPROACH

Differential Diagnosis

- Fetal macrosomia
- Fetal malformation
- Soft-tissue tumor (maternal or fetal)
- Conjoined or locked twins

Associated Conditions: Diabetes, obesity, prolonged gestation (maternal), neurologic injury (brachial plexus), hypoxia, macrosomia (fetal), postpartum hemorrhage (11%), fourth-degree laceration (4%), labor induction, operative vaginal delivery.

Workup and Evaluation

Laboratory: No evaluation indicated.

Imaging: Ultrasonography to assess fetal weight (88% accuracy).

Special Tests: None indicated.

Diagnostic Procedures: Pelvic examination, ultrasonography (suggestive or risk), clinical assessment at the time of dystocia.

MANAGEMENT AND THERAPY

Nonpharmacologic

General Measures: Risk factor analysis, rapid recognition, call for assistance.

Specific Measures: Move the shoulder to the oblique, suprapubic pressure, fundal pressure only after the shoulder is disimpacted, McRoberts maneuver, Woods maneuver (shoulder rotation), delivery of posterior arm, Zavanelli maneuver. A generous episiotomy is advisable.

Diet: Patients generally should have nothing by mouth during delivery.

Activity: Not applicable. (McRoberts maneuver requires flexion and abduction of the maternal hips.)

Drug(s) of Choice

None. (Maternal analgesia or anesthesia may be required if time permits.)

FOLLOW-UP

Patient Monitoring: Normal health maintenance.

Prevention/Avoidance: Identification of patients at risk (risk factors + ultrasonography—58% accurate, most not predictable), Cesarean delivery for fetuses ≥4500 g in diabetic pregnancies or ≥5000 g in other women. (Cesarean delivery for all suspected fetuses is not appropriate; operative delivery for ≥4000 g would result in 2345 procedures to prevent 1 permanent injury at a cost of $4.9 million annually.) The risk of recurrence is estimated to be between 1% and 17%, although good data are lacking.

Possible Complications: Maternal: uterine atony, hemorrhage (11%), uterine rupture, urinary tract or rectal trauma. Fetal/neonatal: asphyxia, death, brachial plexus injury (up to 40%, 10% persist). Data suggest that a significant proportion (34% to 47%) of brachial plexus injuries are not associated with shoulder dystocia (in fact, 4% occur after cesarean delivery); clavicle or humerus fracture, neurologic damage.

Expected Outcome: Delivery can generally be accomplished, but 10% to 30% of fetuses will experience long-term sequelae.

MISCELLANEOUS

ICD-9-CM Code: 660.4.

REFERENCES

Level I

Gonen O, Rosen DJ, Dolfin Z, et al: Induction of labor versus expectant management in macrosomia: a randomized study. Obstet Gynecol 1997;89:913.

Level II

Acker DB, Sachs BP, Friedman EA: Risk factors for shoulder dystocia. Obstet Gynecol 1985;66:762.

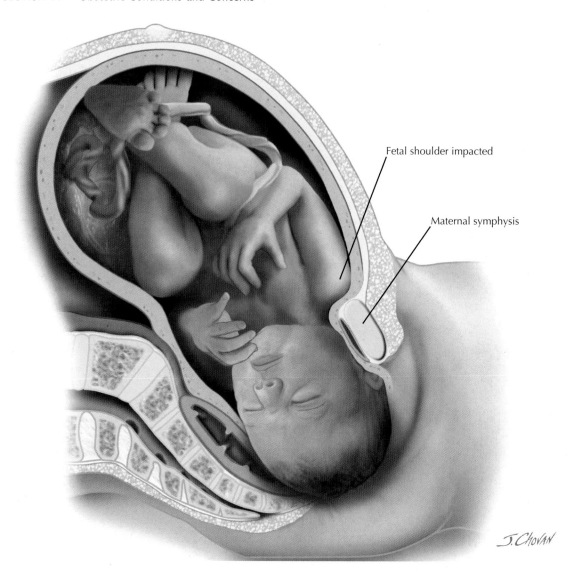

Fetal shoulder impacted

Maternal symphysis

J. CHOVAN

Acker DB, Sachs BP, Friedman EA: Risk factors for shoulder dystocia in the average-weight infant. Obstet Gynecol 1986;67:614.

Baskett TF, Allen AC: Perinatal implications of shoulder dystocia. Obstet Gynecol 1995;86:14.

Gherman RB, Chauhan S, Ouzounian JG, et al: Shoulder dystocia: the unpreventable obstetric emergency with empiric management guidelines. Am J Obstet Gynecol 2006;195:657. Epub 2006 Apr 21.

Gherman RB, Ouzounian JG, Goodwin TM: Obstetric maneuvers for shoulder dystocia and associated fetal morbidity. Am J Obstet Gynecol 1998;178:1126.

Ginsberg NA, Moisidis C: How to predict recurrent shoulder dystocia. Am J Obstet Gynecol 2001;184:1427.

Gonik B, Stringer CA, Held B: An alternate maneuver for management of shoulder dystocia. Am J Obstet Gynecol 1983;145:882.

Gross SJ, Shime J, Farine D: Shoulder dystocia: predictors and outcome. A five-year review. Am J Obstet Gynecol 1987;156:334.

Gurewitsch ED, Johnson E, Hamzehzadeh S, Allen RH: Risk factors for brachial plexus injury with and without shoulder dystocia. Am J Obstet Gynecol 2006;194:486.

Jakobovits A, Iffy L: Perinatal implications of shoulder dystocia. Obstet Gynecol 1996;87:638.

Lewis DF, Raymond RC, Perkins MB, et al: Recurrence rate of shoulder dystocia. Am J Obstet Gynecol 1995;172:1369.

McFarland MB, Langer O, Piper JM, Berkus MD: Perinatal outcome and the type and number of maneuvers in shoulder dystocia. Int J Gynaecol Obstet 1996;55:219.

Nocon JJ, McKenzie DK, Thomas LJ, Hansell RS: Shoulder dystocia: an analysis of risks and obstetric maneuvers. Am J Obstet Gynecol 1993;168:1732.

O'Leary JA: Cephalic replacement for shoulder dystocia: present status and future role of the Zavanelli maneuver. Obstet Gynecol 1993;82:847.

Smith RB, Lane C, Pearson JF: Shoulder dystocia: what happens at the next delivery? Br J Obstet Gynaecol 1994;101:713.

Level III

American College of Obstetricians and Gynecologists: Shoulder dystocia. ACOG Practice Bulletin 40. Obstet Gynecol 2002;100:1045.

Gherman RB, Ouzounian JG, Goodwin TM: Brachial plexus palsy: an in utero injury? Am J Obstet Gynecol 1999;180:1303.

Naef RW 3rd, Martin JN Jr: Emergent management of shoulder dystocia. Obstet Gynecol Clin North Am. 1995;22:247.

O'Leary JA, Leonetti HB: Shoulder dystocia: prevention and treatment. Am J Obstet Gynecol 1990;162:5.

Sandberg EC: The Zavanelli maneuver: 12 years of recorded experience. Obstet Gynecol 1999;93:312.

Sandberg EC: The Zavanelli maneuver: a potentially revolutionary method for the resolution of shoulder dystocia. Am J Obstet Gynecol 1985;152:479.

INTRODUCTION

Description: Trauma and violence are the leading causes of death for women of reproductive age and of maternal death from nonobstetric causes. The most common cause of fetal death in automobile accidents is death of the mother. The altered physiologic state of pregnancy and the need to treat two patients simultaneously alters the management of even simple trauma.

Prevalence: One of 12 pregnancies.

Predominant Age: Reproductive.

Genetics: No genetic pattern.

ETIOLOGY AND PATHOGENESIS

Causes: Motor vehicle accidents (most common; two thirds of cases in developed countries), falls, direct assault (battering most common; 60% report two or more episodes of physical assault during pregnancy).

Risk Factors: Failure to use a safety restraint while driving, abusive relationship, low socioeconomic status, drug or alcohol use and abuse.

CLINICAL CHARACTERISTICS

Signs and Symptoms

- Varies with type of trauma—blunt trauma, trauma associated with covert internal injuries such as retroperitoneal hemorrhage or splenic rupture with bowel injuries less common, penetrating, fetal injury (two thirds)
- Abruptio placenta (1% to 5% of minor trauma, 40% to 50% of major trauma)—vaginal bleeding, uterine tenderness, tetany, or contractions suggest abruption
- Uterine rupture (0.6%) as the result of substantial force to the abdomen
- Direct fetal injury rare in blunt trauma
- Because of increased blood volume during pregnancy, signs of blood loss may be delayed

DIAGNOSTIC APPROACH

Differential Diagnosis

Based on type of trauma and organs potentially involved.

Associated Conditions: Rh isoimmunization.

Workup and Evaluation

Laboratory: Based on normal management of trauma.

Imaging: As needed for the management of trauma (unchanged by the pregnancy, trauma takes precedence). Ultrasonography for gestational age assessment, placental location, intrauterine death, and others. (Not reliable for assessment of fetal injury.)

Special Tests: Peritoneal lavage under direct vision may be used to evaluate intraperitoneal hemorrhage. Kleihauer-Betke test for fetal–maternal hemorrhage.

Diagnostic Procedures: History, physical examination, imaging studies, and exploratory surgery when indicated.

Pathologic Findings

Based on the nature of the trauma.

MANAGEMENT AND THERAPY

Nonpharmacologic

General Measures: Rapid assessment and stabilization (e.g., administration of fluids and oxygen, cardiac and fetal heart rate monitoring based on gestational age), assessment of status (blood pressure, oxygen saturation, urinary output). Tetanus prophylaxis should be provided as needed.

Specific Measures: The uterus should be displaced leftward, off the vena cava. All penetrating abdominal injuries must be explored surgically. The decision to deliver the fetus surgically must be based on gestational age, fetal and maternal injuries, and the risk of death of the fetus if left in utero. Prophylaxis for Rh isoimmunization should be given if fetal–maternal hemorrhage is likely.

Diet: Nothing by mouth until the patient has been fully evaluated.

Activity: Bed rest until the patient has been fully evaluated.

Patient Education: American College of Obstetricians and Gynecologists Patient Education Pamphlet AP018 (Car Safety for You and Your Baby), AP055 (Travel During Pregnancy), AP083 (Domestic Violence).

Drug(s) of Choice

Based on injuries sustained. D immunoglobulin 300 μg IM for each 30 mL of fetal blood thought to have been transfused to the mother (for Rh-incompatibility prophylaxis).

Precautions: Tocolytics should only be administered after abruption has been ruled out because medication side effects such as tachycardia may confuse the clinical picture. Vasopressors should be withheld until appropriate fluid resuscitation has been given.

FOLLOW-UP

Patient Monitoring: Aggressive monitoring as appropriate for the trauma sustained, fetal heart rate monitoring.

Prevention/Avoidance: The incidence and severity of injuries can be reduced by the appropriate use of automobile safety restraints. The greatest injuries are seen when a pregnant woman is not using safety restraints during an automobile accident; injury is not usually caused by the restraints. (Approximately 45% of pregnant women use safety restraints while driving.) Lap belts should be worn low over the hips, and shoulder restraints should rest comfortably between the breasts. The use of approved infant seats to transport the newborn home and for all subsequent travel must also be encouraged in the strongest terms.

Possible Complications: Based on injuries sustained.

Blunt Trauma in Pregnancy

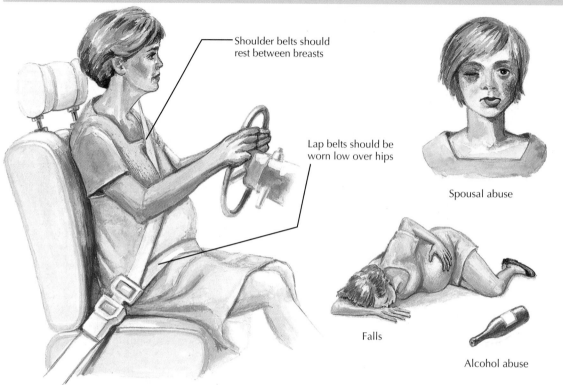

Shoulder belts should
rest between breasts

Lap belts should be
worn low over hips

Spousal abuse

Falls

Alcohol abuse

Automobile accidents are most common cause of
injury. Proper seat belt use can decrease injury

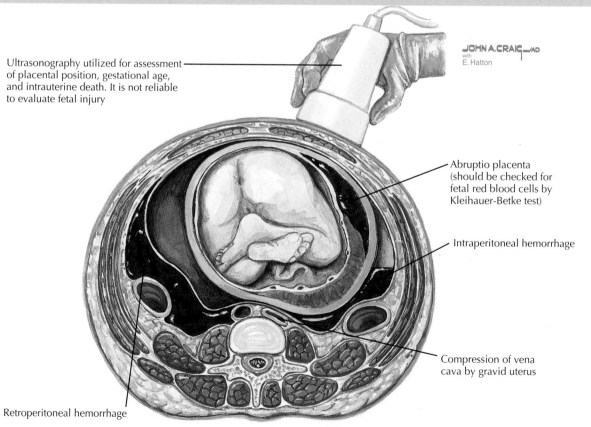

Ultrasonography utilized for assessment
of placental position, gestational age,
and intrauterine death. It is not reliable
to evaluate fetal injury

JOHN A. CRAIG—AD
with
E. Hatton

Abruptio placenta
(should be checked for
fetal red blood cells by
Kleihauer-Betke test)

Intraperitoneal hemorrhage

Compression of vena
cava by gravid uterus

Retroperitoneal hemorrhage

Expected Outcome: Based on trauma sustained; maternal generally good, fetal mortality 50% to 75% for penetrating injuries involving the uterus.

MISCELLANEOUS
ICD-9-CM Code: 760.5.

REFERENCES

Level II
Einarson A, Bailey B, Inocencion G, et al: Accidental electric shock in pregnancy: a prospective cohort study. Am J Obstet Gynecol 1997;176:678.

Fildes J, Reed L, Jones N, et al: Trauma: the leading cause of maternal death. J Trauma 1992;32:643.

Helton AS, McFarlane J, Anderson ET: Battered and pregnant: a prevalence study. Am J Public Health 1987;77:1337.

Kissinger DP, Rozycki GS, Morris JA Jr, et al: Trauma in pregnancy. Predicting pregnancy outcome. Arch Surg 1991;126:1079.

Morris JA Jr, Rosenbower TJ, Jurkovich GJ, et al: Infant survival after cesarean section for trauma. Ann Surg 1996;223:481.

Pearlman MD, Tintinalli JE, Lorenz RP: A prospective controlled study of outcome after trauma during pregnancy. Am J Obstet Gynecol 1990;162:1502.

Stewart DE, Cecutti A: Physical abuse in pregnancy. Can Med Assoc J 1993;149:1257.

Level III
Agnoli FL, Deutchman ME: Trauma in pregnancy. J Fam Pract 1993;37:588.

American College of Obstetricians and Gynecologists: Obstetric aspects of trauma management. ACOG Educational Bulletin 251. Washington, DC, ACOG, 1998.

American College of Obstetricians and Gynecologists: Air travel during pregnancy. ACOG Committee Opinion 264. Obstet Gynecol 2001;98:1187.

American College of Obstetricians and Gynecologists: Exercise during pregnancy and the postpartum period. ACOG Committee Opinion 267. Obstet Gynecol 2002;99:171.

American College of Obstetricians and Gynecologists: Guidelines for diagnostic imaging during pregnancy. ACOG Committee Opinion 299. Obstet Gynecol 2004;104:647.

Archer T. The pregnant trauma patient. J Trauma 2007;62:S110.

Coleman MT, Trianfo VA, Rund DA: Nonobstetric emergencies in pregnancy: trauma and surgical conditions. Am J Obstet Gynecol 1997;177:497.

Edwards RK, Ripley DL, Davis JD, et al: Surgery in the pregnant patient. Curr Probl Surg 2001;38:213.

Harrison SD, Nghiem HV, Shy K: Uterine rupture with fetal death following blunt trauma. AJR Am J Roentgenol 1995;165:1452.

Hendey GW, Votey SR: Injuries in restrained motor vehicle accident victims. Ann Emerg Med 1994;24:77.

Kettel LM, Branch DW, Scott JR: Occult placental abruption after maternal trauma. Obstet Gynecol 1988;71:449.

Mattox KL, Goetzl L: Trauma in pregnancy. Crit Care Med 2005;33:S385.

Nash P, Driscoll P: ABC of major trauma. Trauma in pregnancy. BMJ 1990;301:974.

Pearlman MD, Tintinalli JE, Lorenz RP: Blunt trauma during pregnancy. N Engl J Med 1990;323:1609.

Vaizey CJ, Jacobson MJ, Cross FW: Trauma in pregnancy. Br J Surg 1994;81:1406.

INTRODUCTION

Description: Uterine atony is loss of uterine tone after delivery that often presents as postpartum hemorrhage.

Prevalence: Hemorrhage is seen in 5% of deliveries, mostly because of atony; milder degrees are more common.

Predominant Age: Reproductive.

Genetics: No genetic pattern.

ETIOLOGY AND PATHOGENESIS

Causes: Loss of the normal uterine contractile forces.

Risk Factors: Multiparity (grand multiparity), uterine overdistention (multiple birth, polyhydramnios), prolonged labor, prolonged oxytocin stimulation, muscle-relaxant agents (MgSO4, tocolytics), rapid labor, chorioamnionitis, retained placental tissue.

CLINICAL CHARACTERISTICS

Signs and Symptoms

- Bright-red vaginal bleeding
- Loss of uterine tone palpable on abdominal examination
- Tachycardia, hypotension, and vascular collapse possible

DIAGNOSTIC APPROACH

Differential Diagnosis

- Retained placental fragments
- Genital tract lacerations (cervical, vaginal)
- Uterine rupture
- Uterine inversion
- Coagulopathy

Associated Conditions: Uterine inversion and postpartum hemorrhage.

Workup and Evaluation

Laboratory: Hemoglobin or hematocrit to monitor status and volume of blood loss.

Imaging: Ultrasonography may be used to identify retained placental products but is generally not necessary.

Special Tests: None indicated.

Diagnostic Procedures: Physical examination (abdomen and vagina).

Pathologic Findings

Hemoglobin and hematocrit concentrations will not reflect the volume of blood lost until after equilibration has taken place at 6 to 24 hours.

MANAGEMENT AND THERAPY

Nonpharmacologic

General Measures: Uterine atony should be suspected in any patient with excessive bleeding after delivery of placenta. If initial treatments do not appear to alter patient's bleeding (uterine massage, uterotonic agents such as oxytocin), other diagnoses should be considered while measures to treat atony continue. Rapid evaluation, fluid support or resuscitation (through large-bore access), massage of the uterine fundus. Type and cross-match blood for possible transfusion. The bladder should be drained to allow the uterus to contract and to assess urinary output.

Specific Measures: Uterotonic agents (see later), uterine exploration (manual), uterine artery ligation (O'Leary stitch), hypogastric artery ligation, uterine packing, hysterectomy.

Diet: Nothing by mouth until a diagnosis is established and effective treatment is rendered.

Activity: Bed rest until a diagnosis is established and effective treatment is rendered.

Drug(s) of Choice

Oxytocin 10 to 20 U/L of intravenous fluids—100 to 300 mL given as rapid infusion until uterine tone is reestablished, then 100 to 150 mL/hour for the next several hours. (Concentrations as high as 20 to 40 U/L may be used.)

Methylergonovine maleate (Methergine) 0.2 mg IM, may repeat in 5 minutes (produces tetanic contractions).

15-Methylprostaglandin $F2\alpha$ (carboprost tromethamine, Hemabate) 0.25 mg IM or 0.25 to 1 mg in 10 mL of normal saline injected into the myometrium (may repeat once).

Misoprostol (synthetic prostaglandin E_1 analogue Cytotec) 100 to 600 mg administered rectally or intravaginally.

Iron replacement therapy.

Broad-spectrum antibiotic treatment should be considered, especially if uterine packing is used.

Contraindications: Prostaglandin therapy is contraindicated in patients with asthma. Methergine should not be used in the presence of hypertension and may not be given intravenously.

Precautions: The volume of fluids administered should be monitored closely to avoid inadvertent fluid overload. The placement of a bladder catheter to assess urinary output and to keep the bladder decompressed is desirable. When prostaglandins are used, side effects such as diarrhea, hypertension, vomiting, fever, flushing, and tachycardia are common.

Interactions: Magnesium sulfate and some halogenated anesthetic agents promote atony and work against uterotonic agents.

Alternative Drugs

Prostaglandin E_2 vaginal suppositories have been used, but newer agents and the techniques shown here are more effective and are more readily available.

FOLLOW-UP

Patient Monitoring: Normal postpartum care, follow-up complete blood count as needed.

Uterine Atony (Postpartum)

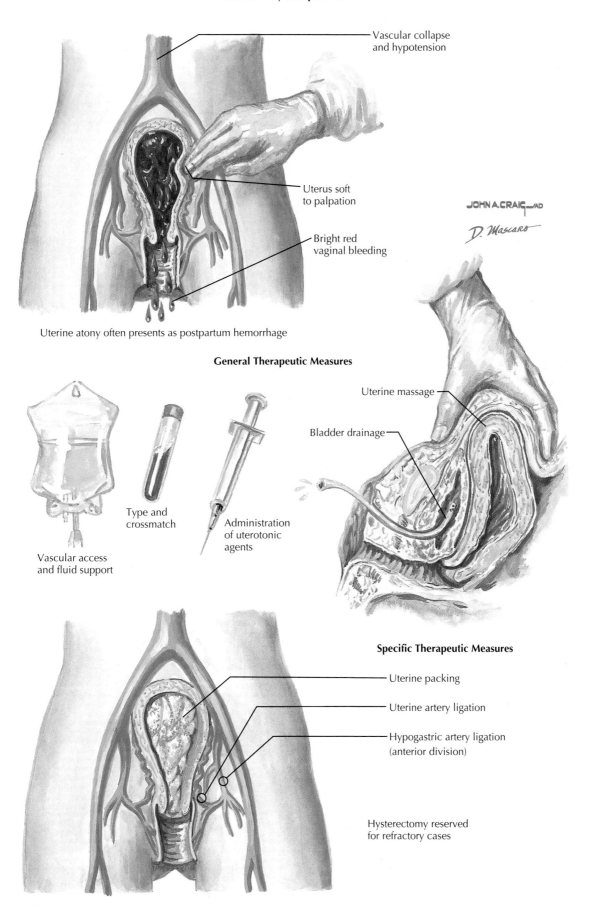

Vascular collapse
and hypotension

Uterus soft
to palpation

Bright red
vaginal bleeding

JOHN A.CRAIG—AD

D. Mascaro

Uterine atony often presents as postpartum hemorrhage

General Therapeutic Measures

Uterine massage

Bladder drainage

Type and
crossmatch

Administration
of uterotonic
agents

Vascular access
and fluid support

Specific Therapeutic Measures

Uterine packing

Uterine artery ligation

Hypogastric artery ligation
(anterior division)

Hysterectomy reserved
for refractory cases

Prevention/Avoidance: Anticipation of possible uterine atony, fundal massage, and oxytocin stimulation after delivery of the placenta.

Possible Complications: Hysterectomy, hemorrhagic shock, and cardiovascular collapse.

Expected Outcome: Most conditions respond to simple measures (uterine massage, oxytocin, methylergonovine maleate [Methergine]) if administered for the appropriate problem and in a timely way.

MISCELLANEOUS
ICD-9-CM Code: 666.1.

REFERENCES

Level I
Caliskan E, Dilbaz B, Meydanli MM, et al: Oral misoprostol for the third stage of labor: a randomized controlled trial. Obstet Gynecol 2003;101:921.

Dansereau J, Joshi AK, Helewa ME, et al: Double-blind comparison of carbetocin versus oxytocin in prevention of uterine atony after cesarean section. Am J Obstet Gynecol 1999;180:670.

Derman RJ, Kodkany BS, Goudar SS, et al: Oral misoprostol in preventing postpartum haemorrhage in resource-poor communities: a randomised controlled trial. Lancet 2006;368:1248.

Hamm J, Russell Z, Botha T, et al: Buccal misoprostol to prevent hemorrhage at cesarean delivery: a randomized study. Am J Obstet Gynecol 2005;192:1404.

Hofmeyr GJ, Walraven G, Gulmezoglu AM, et al: Misoprostol to treat postpartum haemorrhage: a systematic review. BJOG 2005; 112:547.

Jackson KW Jr, Allbert JR, Schemmer GK, et al: A randomized controlled trial comparing oxytocin administration before and after placental delivery in the prevention of postpartum hemorrhage. Am J Obstet Gynecol 2001;185:873.

Joshi VM, Otiv SR, Majumder R, et al: Internal iliac artery ligation for arresting postpartum haemorrhage. BJOG 2007;114:356. Epub 2007 Jan 22.

Khan RU, El-Refaey H: Pharmacokinetics and adverse-effect profile of rectally administered misoprostol in the third stage of labor. Obstet Gynecol 2003;101:968.

Munn MB, Owen J, Vincent R, et al: Comparison of two oxytocin regimens to prevent uterine atony at cesarean delivery: a randomized controlled trial. Obstet Gynecol 2001;98:386.

Oleen MA, Mariano JP: Controlling refractory atonic postpartum hemorrhage with Hemabate sterile solution. Am J Obstet Gynecol 1990;162:205.

Level II
Rouse DJ, Leindecker S, Landon M, et al; National Institute of Child Health and Human Development Maternal-Fetal Medicine Units Network: The MFMU Cesarean Registry: Uterine atony after primary cesarean delivery. Am J Obstet Gynecol 2005;193:1056.

Villar J, Gulmezoglu AM, Hofmeyr GJ, Forna F: Systematic review of randomized controlled trials of misoprostol to prevent postpartum hemorrhage. Obstet Gynecol 2002;100:1301.

Level III
American College of Obstetricians and Gynecologists: Response to Searle's drug warning on misoprostol. ACOG Committee Opinion 248. Washington, DC, ACOG, 2000.

American College of Obstetricians and Gynecologists: Postpartum hemorrhage. ACOG Practice Bulletin 76. Obstet Gynecol 2006; 108:1039.

Ghezzi F, Cromi A, Uccella S, et al: The Hayman technique: a simple method to treat postpartum haemorrhage. BJOG 2007;114:362.

Hensleigh PA: Anti-shock garment provides resuscitation and haemostasis for obstetric haemorrhage. BJOG 2002;109:1377.

INTRODUCTION

Description: Uterine inversion is the turning inside-out of the uterus immediately after delivery. Uncommon and often iatrogenic, this may be associated with catastrophic bleeding and cardiovascular collapse. (Rarely the condition has also been reported in nonpregnant patients with intrauterine pathology.)

Prevalence: One of 25,000 deliveries.

Predominant Age: Reproductive.

Genetics: No genetic pattern.

ETIOLOGY AND PATHOGENESIS

Causes: Iatrogenic (traction on the umbilical cord or downward pressure on the uterine fundus to facilitate delivery of the placenta); abnormalities of placentation (accreta, increta, percreta).

Risk factors: Uterine atony: multiparity (grand), uterine overdistention (multiple birth, polyhydramnios), prolonged labor, prolonged oxytocin stimulation, muscle-relaxant agents (MgSO4), rapid labor.

CLINICAL CHARACTERISTICS

Signs and Symptoms

- A mass may be seen attached to or directly following the placenta as it delivers
- Bright-red vaginal bleeding
- Bradycardia from vagal stimulation
- Tachycardia, hypotension, and vascular collapse possible as a result of blood loss

DIAGNOSTIC APPROACH

Differential Diagnosis

- Uterine atony
- Retained placental fragments
- Genital tract lacerations
- Coagulopathy

Associated Conditions: Uterine atony, postpartum hemorrhage.

Workup and Evaluation

Laboratory: Hemoglobin or hematocrit to monitor status and volume of blood loss. (Acute loss may not be reflected by these measures until equilibration has occurred in 6 to 24 hours.)

Imaging: Ultrasonography may be used to verify the diagnosis, but this is unnecessary and delays the implementation of therapy.

Special Tests: None indicated.

Diagnostic Procedures: Pelvic examination.

Pathologic Findings

Inversion of the uterus.

MANAGEMENT AND THERAPY

Nonpharmacologic

General Measures: Rapid evaluation, fluid support or resuscitation, call for anesthesia assistance.

Specific Measures: Uterine-relaxant agents (see later), manual replacement of uterine fundus (may require general anesthesia with a relaxant agent [Halothane]), may require operative intervention (replacement or hysterectomy). Once the uterine wall has relaxed, gentle manual pressure should be placed on the fundus to displace it inward and upward until its normal position can be restored and the uterus returned to its normal configuration. Uterotonic agents are then used to obtain uterine contraction and hemostasis.

Diet: Nothing by mouth until a diagnosis is established and effective treatment is rendered.

Activity: Bed rest until a diagnosis is established and effective treatment is rendered.

Drug(s) of Choice

Tocolytics: Terbutaline 0.25 mg IV (may repeat once) or nitroglycerine 100 to 250 µg IV (may repeat to a total of 1000 µg).

Contraindications: See individual agents.

Precautions: If nitroglycerine is used, blood pressure must be monitored closely (hypotension).

Alternative Drugs

Halothane general anesthesia may be required.

FOLLOW-UP

Patient Monitoring: Normal postpartum care, follow-up complete blood count as needed.

Prevention/Avoidance: Little or no traction on the umbilical cord or fundal pressure during the delivery of the placenta.

Possible Complications: Hysterectomy, hemorrhagic shock, and cardiovascular collapse.

Expected Outcome: Generally good if recognized and acted on promptly.

MISCELLANEOUS

Other Notes: Following replacement of the fundus, the possibility of uterine atony must be anticipated. If the placenta is still attached to the uterine wall, it should be left in place until after the uterine fundus has been reduced and returned to its normal location.

ICD-9-CM Code: 665.2.

REFERENCES

Level II

Baskett TF: Acute uterine inversion: a review of 40 cases. J Obstet Gynaecol Can 2002;24:953.

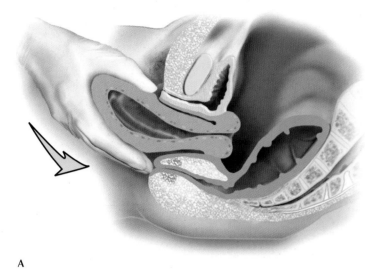

A

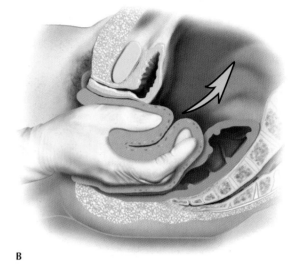

B

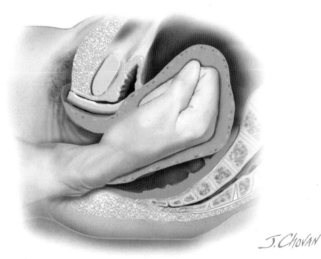

C

J. Chovan

Joshi VM, Otiv SR, Majumder R, et al: Internal iliac artery ligation for arresting postpartum haemorrhage. BJOG 2007;114:356. Epub 2007 Jan 22.

Lupovitch A, England ER, Chen R: Non-puerperal uterine inversion in association with uterine sarcoma: case report in a 26-year-old and review of the literature. Gynecol Oncol 2005;97:938.

Level III

American College of Obstetricians and Gynecologists: Postpartum hemorrhage. ACOG Practice Bulletin 76. Obstet Gynecol 2006;108:1039.

Brar HS, Greenspoon JS, Platt LD, Paul RH: Acute puerperal uterine inversion. New approaches to management. J Reprod Med 1989;34:173.

Dufour P, Vinatier D, Puech F: The use of intravenous nitroglycerin for cervico-uterine relaxation: a review of the literature. Arch Gynecol Obstet 1997;261:1.

Gowri V: Uterine inversion and corpus malignancies: a historical review. Obstet Gynecol Surv 2000;55:703.

Hostetler DR, Bosworth MF: Uterine inversion: a life-threatening obstetric emergency. J Am Board Fam Pract 2000;13:120.

Kovacs BW, DeVore GR: Management of acute and subacute puerperal uterine inversion with terbutaline sulfate. Am J Obstet Gynecol 1984;150:784.

Platt LD, Druzin ML: Acute puerperal inversion of the uterus. Am J Obstet Gynecol 1981;141:187.

Shah-Hosseini R, Evrard JR: Puerperal uterine inversion. Obstet Gynecol 1989;73:567.

Tank Parikshit D, Mayadeo Niranjan M, Nandanwar YS: Pregnancy outcome after operative correction of puerperal uterine inversion. Arch Gynecol Obstet 2004;269:214. Epub 2002 Nov 14.

Thiery M, Delbeke L: Acute puerperal uterine inversion: two-step management with a β-mimetic and a prostaglandin. Am J Obstet Gynecol 1985;153:891.

Watson P, Besch N, Bowes WA Jr: Management of acute and subacute inversion of the uterus. Obstet Gynecol 1980;55:12.

Wendel PJ, Cox SM: Emergent obstetric management of uterine inversion. Obstet Gynecol Clin North Am 1995;22:261.

You WB, Zahn CM: Postpartum hemorrhage: abnormally adherent placenta, uterine inversion, and puerperal hematomas. Clin Obstet Gynecol 2006;49:184.

INTRODUCTION

Description: Uterine rupture is characterized by breach of the uterine wall (new or after previous uterine surgery such as cesarean delivery) that may result in significant maternal or fetal morbidity or mortality. This should be distinguished from uterine scar dehiscence, in which there is separation of an old scar that does not penetrate the uterine serosa or result in complications. Rupture of an intact uterus (without scars) does occur on rare occasions (1 in 15,000 deliveries) and is generally associated with significant uterine distention (polyhydramnios, multiple gestation).

Prevalence: Found in 0.5% to 3.7% of patients with a previous cesarean delivery and 5% of patients for whom vaginal birth after cesarean delivery (VBAC) fails. Uterine rupture rates in women with previous classical incisions and T-shaped incisions range between 4% and 9%. Roughly 7% of emergency cesarean hysterectomies are for rupture.

Predominant Age: Reproductive.

Genetics: No genetic pattern.

ETIOLOGY AND PATHOGENESIS

Causes: Abnormal healing of a previous uterine scar, mechanical disruption of the uterine wall weakened by previous surgery, congenital anomalies, or abnormalities of placentation. (The uterine wall may also be breached by injudicious manual removal of the placenta or manual exploration of the uterus after delivery of the placenta.) Traumatic rupture of the uterus may occur with blunt trauma to the abdomen such as occurs to an unrestrained passenger during an automobile accident. (The proper use of automobile lap and shoulder belts significantly reduces the risk of injury to both mother and fetus.)

Risk Factors: Previous uterine surgery (cesarean delivery; greatest for vertical incisions, myomectomy, septoplasty), multiple gestation, grand multiparity (20-fold increase), short interval between pregnancies, fetal malpresentation, polyhydramnios, oxytocin stimulation (unproved), congenital anomalies, and disuse or misuse of vehicle passenger restraints. There is considerable evidence that cervical ripening with prostaglandin preparations increases the likelihood of uterine rupture (15-fold increase).

CLINICAL CHARACTERISTICS

Signs and Symptoms

- Abrupt fetal distress (80% of cases)
- Abrupt loss of station (presenting part may cease to be present in the vagina)
- Vaginal bleeding (may not be present)
- Abdominal pain (may not be present; pain may be referred to the chest or diaphragm)
- Maternal circulatory collapse
- Uterine activity may persist despite expulsion of the fetus

DIAGNOSTIC APPROACH

Differential Diagnosis

- Uterine dehiscence
- Placental abruption
- Umbilical cord prolapse (causing abrupt fetal distress)
- Adnexal torsion
- Pulmonary or amniotic fluid embolism
- Abdominal pregnancy

Associated Conditions: Fetal demise, maternal blood loss.

Workup and Evaluation

Laboratory: Interoperative and postoperative blood counts. Evaluation of clotting when significant bleeding has occurred.

Imaging: Ultrasonography may demonstrate uterine dehiscence, but the need for clinical intervention often precludes the examination.

Special Tests: Intensive fetal and maternal monitoring may be indicated.

Diagnostic Procedures: History and physical examination (vaginal and abdominal).

Pathologic Findings

Separation of previous uterine scar or a new failure of the uterine wall muscle.

MANAGEMENT AND THERAPY

Nonpharmacologic

General Measures: Rapid evaluation, supportive measures as needed (fluids, blood products).

Specific Measures: Immediate operative delivery (most often by laparotomy), surgical exploration with the possibility of repair or hysterectomy. Ligation of one or both hypogastric arteries may be necessary.

Diet: Nothing by mouth once the diagnosis is made (pending surgical intervention).

Activity: Strict bed rest (pending surgical intervention).

Patient Education: American College of Obstetricians and Gynecologists Patient Education Pamphlet AP070 (Vaginal Birth After Cesarean Delivery).

Drug(s) of Choice

None. (Supportive measures including fluids, blood products, and anesthetics [for immediate delivery] as needed. Prophylactic antibiotics are often recommended.)

FOLLOW-UP

Patient Monitoring: Fetal and maternal monitoring must be maintained for those at risk and intensified when the diagnosis is considered.

Prevention/Avoidance: Care in all uterine manipulations (e.g., manual removal of the placenta, version, external pressure during delivery). Patients with a prior successful vaginal delivery have a greater likelihood of success-

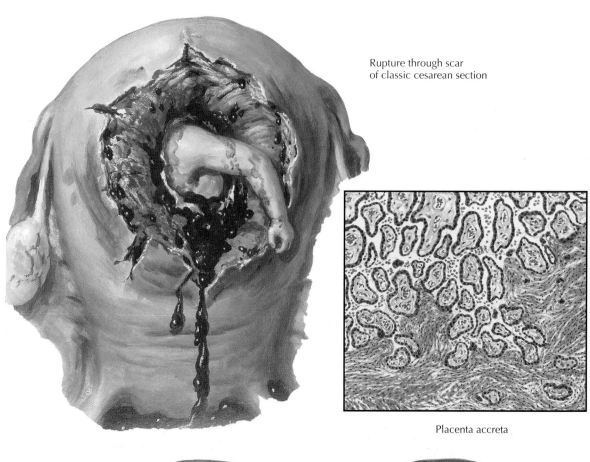

Rupture through scar
of classic cesarean section

Placenta accreta

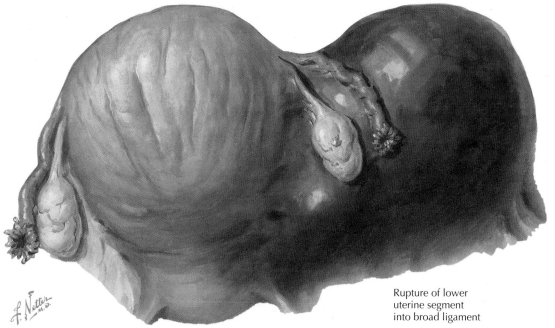

Rupture of lower
uterine segment
into broad ligament

ful vaginal birth after cesarean delivery and a lower risk of uterine rupture than those without a successful vaginal delivery. One study has suggested that there is a lower rate of uterine rupture when a double-layer closure of the uterus is used at the time of cesarean delivery.

Possible Complications: Maternal morbidity or mortality possible (significantly reduced by fetal and maternal monitoring). Damage to the cervix, vagina, or bladder may occur as a part of the rupture. Fetal demise may occur in up to 50% to 75% of fundal incision ruptures and 10% to 15% of lower uterine segment ruptures. Long-term neurologic sequelae are common in infants who survive. Vertical uterine scars are associated with the greatest morbidity and mortality when a rupture occurs.

Expected Outcome: When diagnosed early and acted on promptly, a good outcome can be expected. (If the uterus is repaired and preserved, the risk of recurrence in a subsequent pregnancy is roughly 20%.)

MISCELLANEOUS

ICD-9-CM Codes: 665.1 (During labor), 665.0 (Before labor), 763.8 (Affecting the fetus or newborn), 867.4 (Traumatic).

REFERENCES

Level II

Bujold E, Bujold C, Hamilton EF, et al: The impact of a single-layer or double-layer closure on uterine rupture. Am J Obstet Gynecol 2002;186:1326.

Bujold E, Mehta SH, Bujold C, Gauthier RJ: Interdelivery interval and uterine rupture. Am J Obstet Gynecol 2002;187:1199.

Caughey AB, Shipp TD, Repke JT, et al: Rate of uterine rupture in women with one or two prior cesarean deliveries. Am J Obstet Gynecol 1999;181:872.

Choy-Hee L, Raynor BD: Misoprostol induction of labor among women with a history of cesarean delivery. Am J Obstet Gynecol 2001;184:1115.

Conde-Agudelo A, Rosas-Bermudez A, Kafury-Goeta AC: Effects of birth spacing on maternal health: a systematic review. Am J Obstet Gynecol 2007;196:297.

Eden RD, Parker RT, Gall SA: Rupture of the pregnant uterus: a 53 year review. Obstet Gynecol 1986;68:671.

Esposito MA, Menihan CA, Malee MP: Association of interpregnancy interval with uterine scar failure in labor: a case-control study. Am J Obstet Gynecol 2000;183:1180.

Guise JM, McDonagh MS, Osterweil P, et al: Systematic review of the incidence and consequences of uterine rupture in women with previous caesarean section. BMJ 2004;329:19.

Kieser KE, Baskett TF: A 10-year population-based study of uterine rupture. Obstet Gynecol 2002;100:749.

Landon MB, Spong CY, Thom E, Hauth JC, et al; National Institute of Child Health and Human Development Maternal-Fetal Medicine Units Network: Risk of uterine rupture with a trial of labor in women with multiple and single prior cesarean delivery. Obstet Gynecol 2006;108:12.

Levrant SG, Wingate M: Midtrimester uterine rupture. J Reprod Med 1996;41:186.

Lydon-Rochelle M, Holt VL, Easterling TR, Martin DP: Risk of uterine rupture during labor among women with a prior cesarean delivery. N Engl J Med 2001;345:3.

Macones GA, Peipert J, Nelson DB, et al: Maternal complications with vaginal birth after cesarean delivery: a multicenter study. Am J Obstet Gynecol 2005;193:1656.

Miller DA, Goodwin TM, Gherman RB, Paul RH: Intrapartum rupture of the unscarred uterus. Obstet Gynecol 1997;89:671.

Ravasia DJ, Wood SL, Pollard JK: Uterine rupture during induced trial of labor among women with previous cesarean delivery. Am J Obstet Gynecol 2000;183:1176.

Shipp TD, Zelop CM, Repke JT, et al: Interdelivery interval and risk of symptomatic uterine rupture. Obstet Gynecol 2001;97:175.

Zelop CM, Shipp TD, Repke JT, et al: Effect of previous vaginal delivery on the risk of uterine rupture during a subsequent trial of labor. Am J Obstet Gynecol 2000;183:1184.

Level III

American College of Obstetricians and Gynecologists: Obstetric aspects of trauma management. ACOG Educational Bulletin 251. Washington, DC, ACOG, 1998.

American College of Obstetricians and Gynecologists: Vaginal birth after previous cesarean delivery. ACOG Practice Bulletin 54. Obstet Gynecol 2004;104:203.

American College of Obstetricians and Gynecologists: Induction of labor for vaginal birth after cesarean delivery. ACOG Committee Opinion 342. Obstet Gynecol 2006;108:465.

American College of Obstetricians and Gynecologists: Postpartum hemorrhage. ACOG Practice Bulletin 76. Obstet Gynecol 2006; 108:1039.

Asakura H, Myers SA: More than one previous cesarean delivery: a 5-year experience with 435 patients. Obstet Gynecol 1995; 85:924.

Buhimschi CS, Buhimschi IA, Patel S, et al: Rupture of the uterine scar during term labour: contractility or biochemistry? BJOG 2005;112:38.

Macones GA, Cahill AG, Stamilio DM, et al: Can uterine rupture in patients attempting vaginal birth after cesarean delivery be predicted? Am J Obstet Gynecol 2006;195:1148.

Miller DA, Diaz FG, Paul RH: Vaginal birth after cesarean: a 10-year experience. Obstet Gynecol 1994;84:255.

Miller DA, Goodwin TM, Gherman RB, Paul RH: Intrapartum rupture of the unscarred uterus. Obstet Gynecol 1997;89:671.

Scott JR: Avoiding labor problems during vaginal birth after cesarean delivery. Clin Obstet Gynecol 1997;40:533.

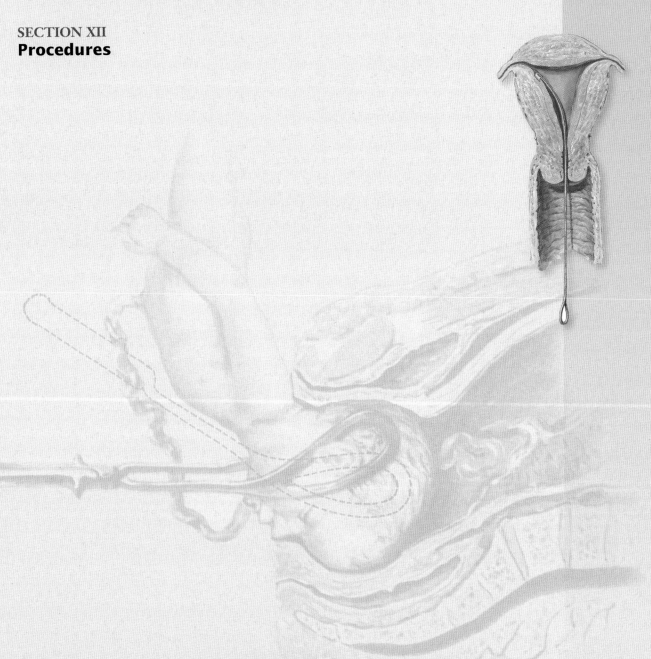

PART 3

PROCEDURES

SECTION XII
Procedures

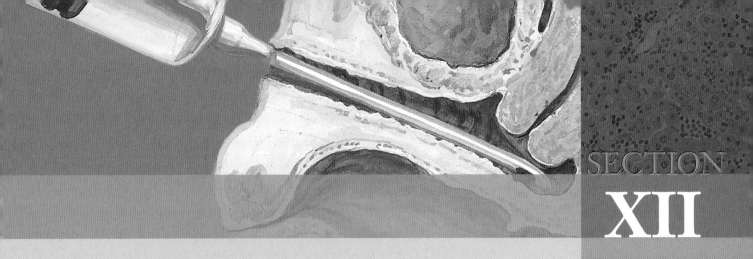

Procedures

DESCRIPTION

Amniocentesis is the sampling of fluid from around the growing fetus for prenatal biochemical or genetic diagnosis. Rarely, amniocentesis may be used to reduce the amount of amniotic fluid present in cases of polyhydramnios.

INDICATIONS

The assessment of fetal genetics or metabolic disorders, lung maturity, fetal infection, or isoimmunization status. Therapeutic amniocentesis may be performed for the reduction of fluid volume or the instillation of agents for fetal therapy or other purposes such as fetal imaging or the diagnosis of rupture of the fetal membranes. Amniocentesis is also a necessary step in other diagnostic and therapeutic procedures such as cordocentesis or fetal transfusion.

CONTRAINDICATIONS

Active skin infections near the site of needle placement. Relative; maternal fever of unknown origin, known or suspected allergies to materials used (e.g., latex, skin preparation materials, local anesthetics). Amniocentesis may be technically difficult to accomplish in patients with multiple gestations.

REQUIRED EQUIPMENT

- Sterile gloves
- Skin preparation materials (e.g., povidone–iodine and 70% isopropyl alcohol)
- Sterile gauze pads (2″ × 2″ or 4″ × 4″)
- Self-adhesive bandage
- Ultrasonography unit
- Fetal monitor or Doppler fetoscope
- Commercial amniocentesis tray
  or
- 20- and 22-gauge spinal needles (or smaller), 20-cc syringe, three sterile 10-cc specimen tubes with caps (plain, without additive), sterile drape (one with a small fenestration, or multiple drapes)
- If desired: 1% lidocaine without epinephrine, 5-cc syringe, 22-gauge needle (if not included in amniocentesis kit)

TECHNIQUE

The indications, contraindications, risks, benefits, and complications should be reviewed and discussed with the patient, and informed consent should be obtained. The patient should be placed in the supine position with the head elevated 20 to 30 degrees. If the pregnancy is advanced, the patient may empty her bladder and be placed in a slightly left decubitus position. Ultrasonography is used to assess fetal well-being, fetal lie, and placental position.

A suitable pocket of amniotic fluid should be identified by use of ultrasound. Ideally, this pocket should be located

away from the fetal face and placenta, but it should be accessible with a standard spinal needle. Areas around the fetal extremities are often best. The location of this pocket relative to the skin surface should be noted as a guide to needle insertion.

The skin of the abdominal wall over the chosen pocket of amniotic fluid should be disinfected with a suitable skin preparation solution and technique of the examiner's choice. If a local anesthetic is to be used, it is established at this juncture using sterile technique: A small skin weal of local anesthetic is placed, and the proposed needle track is infiltrated with a total of less than 4 to 5 mL of anesthetic agent.

With the stylet in place, a 20- or 22-gauge spinal needle is passed perpendicularly through the skin, abdominal, and uterine walls, into the amniotic sac. A slight pop or loss of resistance may be felt as the needle traverses the fascia. After the pocket of fluid has been entered, the stylet is removed from the needle. Free flow of fluid should be demonstrated. If free flow is not found, the needle should be rotated or tipped and rechecked prior to being advanced farther (with the stylet in place). Using ultrasonography to guide the needle's advancement may facilitate placement of the needle into the amniotic fluid pocket. This can be especially helpful when amniocentesis is performed early in pregnancy.

Once free flow of fluid has been demonstrated, a small syringe should be attached to the needle and 2 to 3 mL of fluid should be withdrawn. This fluid is discarded. Appropriate samples are now taken and placed in sterile specimen tubes. Determination of the amount of material needed and any special handling required for these specimens is dictated by the studies to be performed. If there is any doubt, consultation with the laboratory before the procedure may help to identify any special handling that must be used.

After samples have been obtained, the needle is withdrawn and a self-adhesive bandage is applied to the site of needle puncture. The fetus should be monitored for a short period after the procedure. If bloody fluid was obtained, this monitoring period should be extended by 1 to 2 additional hours or longer, depending on other considerations. An appropriate procedure note should be entered into the patient's record.

COMPLICATIONS

Early amniocentesis is associated with a fetal loss rate of approximately 2.5% (versus 0.7% for later procedures). Amniotic fluid leakage, frank rupture of the fetal membranes, amnionitis (infection), bleeding, and possible isoimmunization of mothers who are Rh negative are all possible. The risk of direct fetal injury is small when the procedure is carefully performed. When amniocentesis is carried out in the presence of preterm premature rupture of membranes, failure rates are higher. Bleeding and infection are always possible with any invasive procedure.

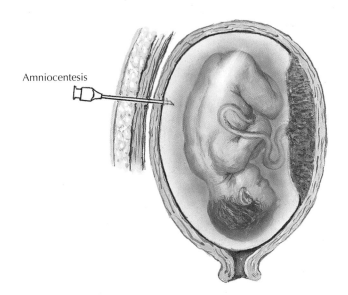

Amniocentesis

FOLLOW-UP

When amniocentesis is performed after fetal viability (24 weeks), a period of electronic fetal heart rate monitoring (30 minutes) is usual. If bloody fluid is obtained or the fetus or umbilical cord is perforated, this monitoring is generally increased (1 to 2 hours or longer, as clinically indicated). Patients should report persistent uterine cramping, vaginal bleeding or leakage of fluid, or fever.

CPT CODE(S)

59000   Amniocentesis, any method
76946   Ultrasonic guidance for amniocentesis, physician supervision and interpretation

REFERENCES

Level I

Gordon MC, Ventura-Braswell A, Higby K, Ward JA: Does local anesthesia decrease pain perception in women undergoing amniocentesis? Am J Obstet Gynecol 2007;196:55.e1.

Sundberg K, Bang J, Smidt-Jensen S, et al: Randomized study of risk of fetal loss related to early amniocentesis versus chorionic villus sampling. Lancet 1997;350:697.

Level II

Alfirevic Z, Sundberg K, Brigham S: Amniocentesis and chorionic villus sampling for prenatal diagnosis. Cochrane Database Syst Rev 2004;CD003252.

Bombard AT, Powers JF, Carter S, et al: Procedure-related fetal losses in transplacental versus nontransplacental genetic amniocentesis. Am J Obstet Gynecol 1995;172:868.

Bravo RR, Shulman LP, Phillips OP, et al: Transplacental needle passage in early amniocentesis and pregnancy loss. Obstet Gynecol 1995;86:437.

Eddleman KA, Malone FD, Sullivan L, et al: Pregnancy loss rates after midtrimester amniocentesis. Obstet Gynecol 2006;108:1067.

Eiben B, Osthelder B, Hammans W, Goebel R: Safety of early amniocentesis versus CVS. Lancet 1994;344:1303.

Nicolaides K, Brizot M de L, Patel F, Snijders R: Comparison of chorionic villus sampling and amniocentesis for fetal karyotyping at 10–13 weeks' gestation. Lancet 1994;344:435.

Petrikovsky BM, Kaplan GP: Fetal responses to inadvertent contact with the needle during amniocentesis. Fetal Diagnos Ther 1995;10:83.

Somigliana E, Bucceri AM, Tibaldi C, et al: Italian Collaborative Study on HIV Infection in Pregnancy: Early invasive diagnostic techniques in pregnant women who are infected with the HIV: a multicenter case series. Am J Obstet Gynecol 2005;193:437.

Level III

American College of Obstetricians and Gynecologists: Assessment of fetal lung maturity. ACOG Educational Bulletin 230. Washington, DC, ACOG, 1996.

American College of Obstetricians and Gynecologists: Prenatal and preconceptional carrier screening for genetic diseases in individuals of Eastern European Jewish descent. ACOG Committee Opinion 298. Obstet Gynecol 2004;104:425.

American College of Obstetricians and Gynecologists: Management of alloimmunization during pregnancy. ACOG Practice Bulletin 75. Obstet Gynecol 2006;108:457.

American College of Obstetricians and Gynecologists: Screening for fetal chromosomal abnormalities. ACOG Practice Bulletin 77. Obstet Gynecol 2007;109:217.

D'Alton ME, DeCherney AH: Prenatal diagnosis. N Engl J Med 1993;328:114.

Elliott JP, Sawyer AT, Radin TG, Strong RE: Large-volume therapeutic amniocentesis in the treatment of hydramnios. Obstet Gynecol 1994;84:1025.

Finegan JA: Amniotic fluid and midtrimester amniocentesis: a review. Br J Obstet Gynaecol 1984;91:745.

Holzgreve W, Nippert I, Ganshirt-Ahlert D, et al: Immediate and long-term applications of technology. Clin Obstet Gynecol 1993;36:476.

Jorgensen FS, Bang J, Lind AM, et al: Genetic amniocentesis at 7–14 weeks of gestation. Prenatal Diagn 1992;12:277.

Moise KJ Jr: Management of rhesus alloimmunization in pregnancy. Obstet Gynecol 2002;100:600.

Mujezinovic F, Alfirevic Z: Procedure-related complications of amniocentesis and chorionic villous sampling: a systematic review. Obstet Gynecol 2007;110:687.

Nyberg DA, Hyett J, Johnson JA, Souter V: First-trimester screening. Radiol Clin North Am 2006;44:837.

Rousseau O, Boulot P, Lefort G, et al: Amniocentesis before 15 weeks' gestation: technical aspects and obstetric risks. Euro J Obstet Gynecol Reprod Biol 1995;58:127.

Seeds JW: Diagnostic mid trimester amniocentesis: how safe? Am J Obstet Gynecol 2004;191:607.

Stranc LC, Evans JA, Hamerton JL: Chorionic villus sampling and amniocentesis for prenatal diagnosis. Lancet 1997;349:711.

Vandenbussche FP, Kanhai HH, Keirse MJ: Safety of early amniocentesis. Lancet 1994;344:1032.

DESCRIPTION

Fluid is removed from breast cysts via aspiration. This may be performed for both diagnosis and therapy.

INDICATIONS

Palpable breast mass that is credibly thought to be cystic in nature.

CONTRAINDICATIONS

Local skin infection, known or suspected allergy to agents used (e.g., latex, iodine).

REQUIRED EQUIPMENT

- Skin preparation materials (alcohol, iodine- or hexachlorophene-based antibacterial solution [e.g., Betadine, Hibiclens])
- Self-adhesive bandage
- 10-mL disposable syringe
- 22- to 25-gauge needle

TECHNIQUE

In women older than age 35, mammography prior to aspiration should be considered because of the increased incidence of malignancy. Once aspiration has been attempted, mammography should be delayed several weeks because of artifactual changes induced by the manipulation, rendering mammography difficult to interpret.

Following adequate skin preparation, the nondominant hand stabilizes the cystic mass. This is accomplished by using the thumb and fingers to gently pinch the breast tissue below the mass. A 22- to 25-gauge needle (attached to a 10-mL syringe) is inserted into the cyst cavity. A small "pop" or loss of resistance is often felt as the cyst wall is breached. The cyst contents are aspirated by gentle suction from the syringe. Firm pressure applied for 5 to 10 minutes will reduce the risk of hematoma formation. No dressing or special breast care is required, although a self-adhesive bandage may be used.

Fluid aspirated from patients with fibrocystic changes will customarily be straw colored. Fluid that is dark brown or green occurs in cysts that have been present for a long time but is equally innocuous. Because of high false-positive (up to 6%) and even higher false-negative rates (2% to 22%), cytologic evaluation of the fluid obtained is of little value.

COMPLICATIONS

Hematoma, infection (rare).

FOLLOW-UP

If the cyst disappears completely and does not re-form by a 1-month follow-up examination, no further therapy is required. If no fluid is obtained, if the cyst re-forms within 2 weeks or must be repeatedly aspirated, or if a mass persists after the aspiration, biopsy should be performed.

CPT CODE(S)

19000 Puncture aspiration of cyst of breast
19001 Each additional cyst

REFERENCES

Level II

Palmer ML, Tsangaris TN: Breast biopsy in women 30 years old or less. Am J Surg 1993;165:708.

Sneige N: Fine-needle aspiration of the breast: a review of 1,995 cases with emphasis on diagnostic pitfalls. Diagn Cytopathol 1993; 9:106.

Level III

American College of Obstetricians and Gynecologists: Breast concerns in the adolescent. ACOG Committee Opinion 350. Obstet Gynecol 2006;108:1329.

Lucas JH, Cone DL: Breast cyst aspiration. Am Fam Physician 2003;68:1983.

Marchant DJ: Diagnosis of breast disease and the role of the gynecologist. Curr Opin Obstet Gynecol 1993;5:67.

Morrow M: The evaluation of common breast problems. Am Fam Physician 2000;61:2371, 2385.

Parker SH, Stavros AT, Dennis MA: Needle biopsy techniques. Radiol Clin North Am 1995;33:1171.

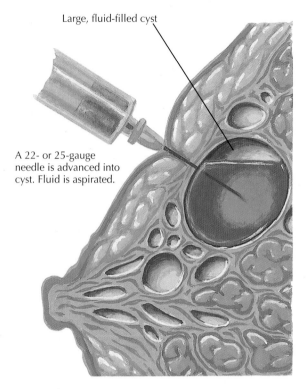

Large, fluid-filled cyst

A 22- or 25-gauge needle is advanced into cyst. Fluid is aspirated.

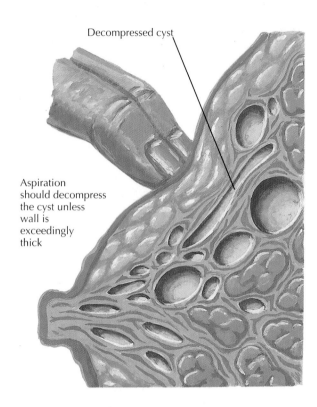

Decompressed cyst

Aspiration should decompress the cyst unless wall is exceedingly thick

JOHN A. CRAIG—AD
D. Mascaro

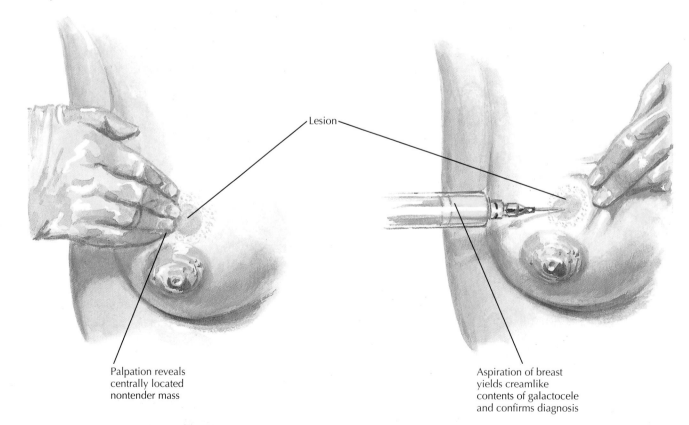

Lesion

Palpation reveals centrally located nontender mass

Aspiration of breast yields creamlike contents of galactocele and confirms diagnosis

DESCRIPTION

Bartholin's gland cyst/abscess drainage is acute drainage of symptomatic cystic dilation of the Bartholin gland.

INDICATIONS

Symptomatic cystic dilation or abscess of the Bartholin gland. Asymptomatic cysts in women younger than age 40 do not need treatment. (In patients older than age 40, biopsy is indicated.) Mild Bartholin's gland infections may also be treated with broad-spectrum antibiotics and frequent warm sitz baths.

CONTRAINDICATIONS

Incomplete evaluation of the vulvar lesion, bleeding diathesis, known or suspected allergy to agents used (e.g., latex, iodine).

REQUIRED EQUIPMENT

- Skin preparation materials (alcohol, iodine- or hexachlorophene-based antibacterial solution [e.g., Betadine, Hibiclens])
- Sterile gloves
- 1% lidocaine without epinephrine, 5-cc syringe, 22-gauge needle, analgesic skin-cooling spray or other topical analgesic
- 10-mL syringe
- Normal saline (for irrigation)
- Scalpel (#11 or #15 blade)
- Sterile gauze pads (2″ × 2″ or 4″ × 4″)
- Word catheter or iodoform gauze packing (1/4″ or 1/2″)

TECHNIQUE

After appropriate informed consent has been obtained from the patient, the skin of the vulva is disinfected. When an acute abscess is to be drained, the exquisite tenderness that is usually present dictates that this is done gently; pain relief is best obtained through the use of an analgesic or skin-freezing spray. This technique may be used for non-acute Bartholin's cysts; local anesthesia using local or field infiltration is also appropriate. Abscesses should be incised at the point of least thickness overlying the mass (where the abscess is "pointing"). A vertical or "stab" incision is made, generally resulting in the abrupt release of purulent material. (Despite the apparent purulent character of the drained material, culture is generally of little utility in the management of these cases.) The size of this incision need only be on the order of 1 or 2 cm; sutures are generally not required. The abscess cavity may be gently irrigated with normal saline using a 10-mL syringe. A Word catheter should then be placed through the incision and inflated with a few milliliters of saline. As an alternative, iodoform gauze packing may be placed within the cavity with a 2- to 3-cm "tail" left outside the incision to facilitate eventual removal. Unless cellulitis is present, antibiotic therapy is not required.

When the cyst is not acutely inflamed, it should be stabilized and tensed by gentle finger pressure applied on either side of the affected labium, below the cyst. Incision in this case should be made within the hymeneal ring whenever possible. Incision length should be similar to that used for acute cases, and a Word catheter or iodoform gauze packing should be inserted in a similar manner.

COMPLICATIONS

Bleeding, hematoma, recurrence.

FOLLOW-UP

Word catheters should be left in place for 4 to 6 weeks. Iodoform gauze packing should be gradually removed over the course of several days. Recurrence is frequent, and many prefer marsupialization to simple drainage in all but the most acute cases.

CPT CODE(S)

56420   Incision and drainage of Bartholin gland abscess

REFERENCES

Level II

Eilber KS, Raz S: Benign cystic lesions of the vagina: a literature review. J Urol 2003;170:717.

Level III

Cheetham DR: Bartholin's cyst: marsupialization or aspiration? Am J Obstet Gynecol 1985;152:569.

Eckert LO, Lentz GM: Infections of the lower genital tract. In Katz VL, Lentz GM, Lobo RA, Gershenson DM: Comprehensive Gynecology, 5th ed. Philadelphia, Mosby/Elsevier, 2007, p 572.

Hill DA, Lense JJ: Office management of Bartholin gland cysts and abscesses. Am Fam Physician 1998;57:1611, 1619.

Omole F, Simmons BJ, Hacker Y: Management of Bartholin's duct cyst and gland abscess. Am Fam Physician 2003;68:135.

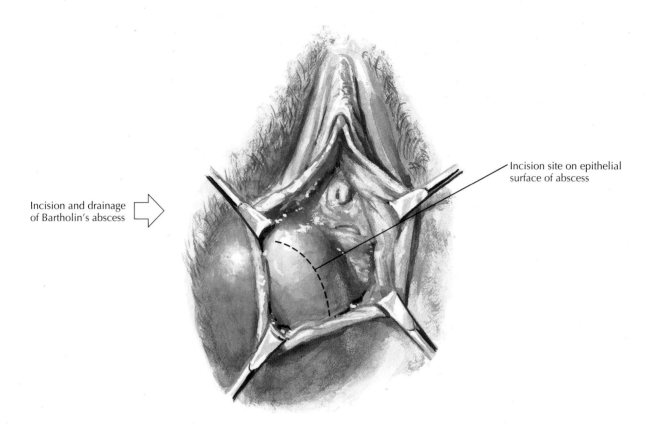

Incision and drainage of Bartholin's abscess

Incision site on epithelial surface of abscess

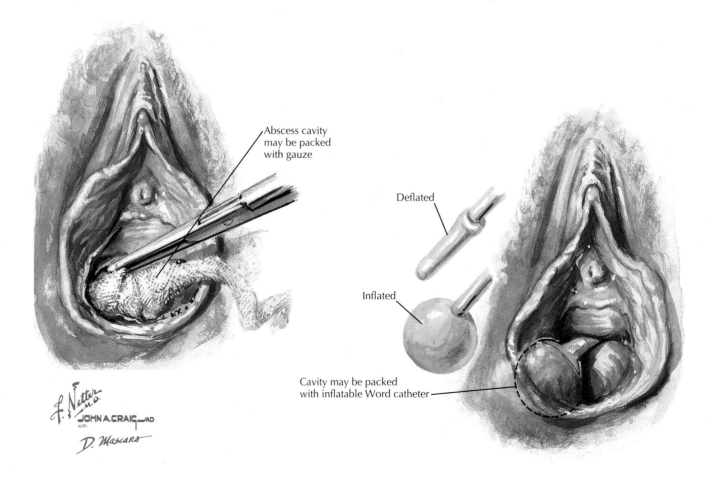

Abscess cavity may be packed with gauze

Deflated

Inflated

Cavity may be packed with inflatable Word catheter

DESCRIPTION

Marsupialization is drainage and permanent fistulization of symptomatic cystic dilation of the Bartholin gland. This provides an alternative to the obstructed anatomic drainage of the Bartholin gland.

INDICATIONS

Symptomatic cystic dilation of the Bartholin gland. Asymptomatic cysts in women younger than age 40 do not need treatment. (In patients older than age 40, biopsy is indicated.) When performed for recurrent abscess formation, marsupialization should be deferred until inflammation has subsided.

CONTRAINDICATIONS

Incomplete evaluation of the vulvar lesion, bleeding diathesis, active inflammation or infection, age >40 years, known or suspected allergy to agents used (e.g., latex, iodine).

REQUIRED EQUIPMENT

- Skin preparation materials (alcohol, iodine- or hexachlorophene-based antibacterial solution [e.g., Betadine, Hibiclens])
- Sterile gloves
- 1% lidocaine without epinephrine, 5-cc syringe, 22-gauge needle
- Scalpel (#11 or #15 blade)
- 3-0 or 4-0 absorbable suture on a small cutting needle, needle holder, thumb forceps, suture scissors
- Electrosurgical generator, hand piece, and return electrode ("ground pad")
- Sterile gauze pads (2″ × 2″ or 4″ × 4″)
- Word catheter or iodoform gauze packing (1/4″ or 1/2″)

TECHNIQUE

After appropriate informed consent has been obtained from the patient, the skin of the vulva is disinfected. When a regional or general anesthetic is not used, local anesthesia using local or field infiltration is appropriate. The cyst should be stabilized and tensed by gentle finger pressure applied on either side of the affected labium, below the cyst. An incision should be made over the body of the cyst and within the hymeneal ring (generally near the 4- to 5-o'clock or 7- to 8-o'clock positions of the introitus). The incision is generally made in a cruciate manner and extended for up to 2 to 3 cm in longest axis (based on the size of the cyst). Hemostasis should be obtained using electrosurgical energy. Many prefer to sew the edges of the incision open by tacking the center of the flaps outward in a petal-shaped manner. As an alternative, the incision may be made using electrosurgical energy, taking advantage of the tendency for the resultant slough of skin edges to produce a fistula track. A Word catheter or iodoform gauze packing should be placed after final hemostasis has been achieved.

COMPLICATIONS

Bleeding, hematoma, recurrence.

FOLLOW-UP

Word catheters should be left in place for 4 to 6 weeks. Iodoform gauze packing should be gradually removed over the course of several days. Recurrence is frequent (5% to 10% of cases).

CPT CODE(S)

56440   Marsupialization of Bartholin gland

REFERENCES

Level II

Eilber KS, Raz S: Benign cystic lesions of the vagina: a literature review. J Urol 2003;170:717.

Level III

Cheetham DR: Bartholin's cyst: marsupialization or aspiration? Am J Obstet Gynecol 1985;152:569.

Eckert LO, Lentz GM: Infections of the lower genital tract. In Katz VL, Lentz GM, Lobo RA, Gershenson DM: Comprehensive Gynecology, 5th ed. Philadelphia, Mosby/Elsevier, 2007, p 572.

Hill DA, Lense JJ: Office management of Bartholin gland cysts and abscesses. Am Fam Physician 1998;57:1611, 1619.

Omole F, Simmons BJ, Hacker Y: Management of Bartholin's duct cyst and gland abscess. Am Fam Physician 2003;68:135.

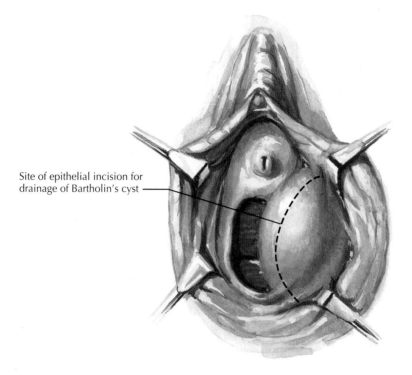

Site of epithelial incision for
drainage of Bartholin's cyst

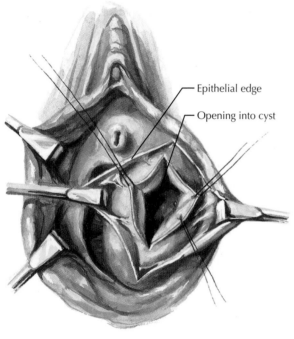

Epithelial edge

Opening into cyst

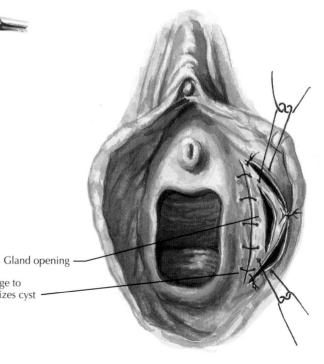

Gland opening

Closure of epithelial edge to
cyst opening marsupializes cyst

DESCRIPTION

Core breast biopsy is a technique used to obtain small tissue samples for the histologic diagnosis of breast masses.

INDICATIONS

Breast mass or suspicious lesion (palpable; nonpalpable masses may be sampled if image guidance is available).

CONTRAINDICATIONS

Local skin infection, known or suspected allergy to agents used (e.g., latex, iodine). Core needle biopsy may not be suitable for patients who have very small or very hard breast lumps; masses close to the chest wall, the nipple, or the surface of the breast; calcifications that require magnification; or very small breasts. Patients who take blood thinners or aspirin should discontinue them in advance of the procedure. Women who cannot remain still or supine for 20 to 40 minutes because of physical illness or other problems are not good candidates for stereotactic core needle biopsy.

REQUIRED EQUIPMENT

- Skin preparation materials (alcohol, iodine- or hexachlorophene-based antibacterial solution [e.g., Betadine, Hibiclens])
- Sterile gloves (if desired)
- 1% lidocaine without epinephrine, 5-cc syringe, 25-gauge needle
- Disposable core biopsy needle
- Scalpel (#11 blade), if desired
- Sterile gauze pads (2″ × 2″)
- Suitable tissue preservation/transportation medium (10% formalin solution or similar)
- Self-adhesive bandage

TECHNIQUE

After appropriate informed consent has been obtained from the patient, the skin is disinfected and a skin wheal of local anesthetic is injected at the site chosen for needle penetration. (The patient may be either supine or prone based on the location of the lesion to be biopsied, optimal access, and the availability or need for image guidance.) Using the fingers of the opposite hand to stabilize the area in question, the physician advances the needle into the area of concern by palpation or under image guidance using either stereotactic mammography or ultrasound. (Passage of the needle through the skin may be facilitated by a small incision if desired.) A change in tissue resistance or a "gritty" sensation may be noticed as the needle enters some mass lesions.

Core biopsy needles generally have a specialized tip with a covering sheath and cutting edge. The needles are of large caliber (14 g) and are mounted onto a spring-loaded device that allows small cylinders of tissue to be cut and collected within the notch of the needle. Techniques vary slightly based on the specific needle but commonly involve placing the tip just short of the tissue to be biopsied; then, the inner core is advanced into the tissue and the outer (cutting) sheath is advanced to free the tissue sample trapped in the inner portion of the needle. The needle is removed, the tissue sample is extracted, and additional samples (as needed) are obtained in the same manner. Typically, samples approximate 2.0 cm long by 0.16 cm in diameter.

Three to six separate core needle insertions are typically needed to obtain a sufficient sample of breast tissue. Patients may experience a slight pressure during core needle biopsy but should not experience any significant pain. At the close of the procedure, samples are sent to the pathology laboratory for diagnosis and light dressing is applied. (A self-adhesive bandage suffices.) Ice and gentle pressure may be applied for 15 to 30 minutes to minimize bruising.

Vacuum-assisted breast biopsy is able to remove approximately twice the amount of tissue compared with core needle biopsy while still offering a minimally invasive procedure. The technique is the same as with core biopsy, differing only in the nature of the sampling device.

COMPLICATIONS

Bleeding, hematoma, infection.

FOLLOW-UP

The reported false-negative rate for malignancy with core biopsy is in the range of 2% to 6.7% with a mean rate of 4.4%. Approximately 10% of biopsy attempts will be inconclusive. Certain histologic results should be interpreted with caution: more than one half of all cases of atypical ductal hyperplasia (ADH) diagnosed with core biopsy prove malignant at surgery, and invasive carcinoma is found in up to one third of core biopsy–confirmed ductal carcinoma in situ (DCIS).

CPT CODE(S)

19100 Biopsy of breast; percutaneous, needle core, not using imaging guidance (separate procedure)
19102 Biopsy of breast; percutaneous, needle core, using imaging guidance
19103 Biopsy of breast; percutaneous, automated vacuum assisted or rotating biopsy device, using imaging guidance

REFERENCES

Level II

Brenner RJ, Fajardo L, Fisher PR, et al: Percutaneous core biopsy of the breast: effect of operator experience and number of samples on diagnostic accuracy. AJR Am J Roentgenol 1996;166:341.

Frayne J, Sterrett GF, Harvey J, et al: Stereotactic 14 gauge core-biopsy of the breast: results from 101 patients. Aust N Z J Surg 1996;66:585.

Jackman RJ, Nowels KW, Rodriguez-Soto J, et al: Stereotactic, automated, large-core needle biopsy of nonpalpable breast lesions: false-negative and histologic underestimation rates after long-term follow-up. Radiology 1999;210:799.

Lee CH, Philpotts LE, Horvath LJ, Tocino I: Follow-up of breast lesions diagnosed as benign with stereotactic core-needle biopsy: frequency of mammographic change and false-negative rate. Radiology 1999;212:189.

Needle Biopsy

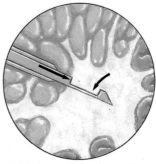

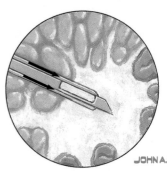

Disposable biopsy needle

Cannula

Obturator

Lesion

1. Closed needle assembly is advanced to edge of lesion

2. Obturator tip is advanced into lesion. Tissue prolapses into open specimen notch

3. Cannula is advanced over obturator, entrapping tissue specimen within notch. Needle is withdrawn

JOHN A. CRAIG⎯AD

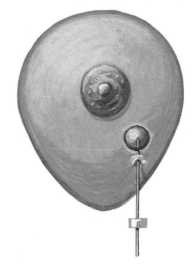

Liberman L, Dershaw DD, Rosen PP, Abramson AF, et al: Stereotaxic 14-gauge breast biopsy: how many core biopsy specimens are needed? Radiology 1994;192:793.

Rich PM, Michell MJ, Humphreys S, et al: Stereotactic 14G core biopsy of non-palpable breast cancer: what is the relationship between the number of core samples taken and the sensitivity for detection of malignancy? Clin Radiol 1999;54:384.

Level III

American College of Obstetricians and Gynecologists: Breast cancer screening. ACOG Practice Bulletin 42. Obstet Gynecol 2003; 101:821.

Britton PD: Fine needle aspiration or core biopsy. Breast 1999;8:1.

Staren ED, O'Neill TP: Ultrasound-guided needle biopsy of the breast. Surgery 1999;126:629.

Strong JW, Worsham GF, Austin RM, et al: Stereotactic core biopsy of nonpalpable breast lesions. J S C Med Assoc 1995;91:489.

DESCRIPTION

Open breast biopsy is a technique used to obtain tissue samples for the histologic diagnosis of breast masses.

INDICATIONS

Breast mass or suspicious lesion (palpable; nonpalpable masses may be sampled if image guidance is available).

CONTRAINDICATIONS

Local skin infection, known or suspected allergy to agents used (e.g., latex, iodine). Patients who take blood thinners or aspirin should discontinue them in advance of the procedure.

REQUIRED EQUIPMENT

- Skin preparation materials (alcohol, iodine- or hexachlorophene-based antibacterial solution [e.g., Betadine, Hibiclens])
- Sterile gloves
- 1% lidocaine without epinephrine, 10-cc syringe, 22-gauge needle
- Scalpel (#15 blade) and fine tissue scissors (e.g., Metzenbaum)
- 2-0 or 3-0 absorbable undyed suture on a small to medium tapered needle and 3-0 or 4-0 absorbable undyed suture on a small cutting needle, needle holder, thumb forceps, suture scissors
- Small retractors (e.g., Senn Miller, Ragnell [Army/Navy] or similar) may be useful, especially if an assistant is available
- Electrosurgical generator, hand piece, and return electrode ("ground pad")
- Sterile gauze pads (2" × 2")
- Self-adhesive skin tapes (if desired)
- Self-adhesive bandage
- Suitable tissue preservation/transportation medium (10% formalin solution or similar) (If estrogen and progesterone receptors are to be assessed, a sample of unpreserved tissue must be frozen within 30 minutes.)

TECHNIQUE

After appropriate informed consent has been obtained, the skin is disinfected and local anesthetic is injected at the chosen site. (The majority of biopsies can be performed with curvilinear incisions following the contours of the breast, often in the circumareolar area.) An open biopsy should be performed using a scalpel rather than electrosurgical energy because thermal effects on the biopsy material may blur the margin of normal tissue around the tumor and cause abnormally low receptor levels.

The dissection is carried to the area of concern through a combination of sharp and blunt techniques. A change in tissue character or a "gritty" sensation may be noticed as the tissue is dissected near some mass lesions. The mass or area of interest is excised and hemostasis is obtained through electrosurgical energy or the placement of hemostatic sutures to close dead space. The skin may be closed using a running subcuticular suture or self-adhesive skin tapes.

At the close of the procedure, samples are sent to the pathology laboratory for diagnosis and light dressing is applied. (A self-adhesive bandage often suffices.) Ice and gentle pressure may be applied for 15 to 30 minutes to minimize bruising.

It is important to send the pathology laboratory a small sample (1 g of suspect tissue) to determine the presence or absence of estrogen and progesterone receptors. These receptors are heat labile; therefore, the tissue must be frozen within 30 minutes.

Nonpalpable masses may be localized through the placement of a small needle or sterile J-wire under fluoroscopic or ultrasonographic guidance. These are then used as guides for the open dissection. The specimen is removed with the wire or needle in place, and it is radiographed to confirm the removal of the suspect area. (These techniques have been largely supplanted by computer-guided core biopsy techniques.)

COMPLICATIONS

Bleeding, hematoma, infection.

FOLLOW-UP

If nonabsorbable suture material is used to close the skin, the stitches will need to be removed during a follow-up visit. The incidence of carcinoma in biopsies corresponds directly with the patient's age. Approximately 20% of breast biopsies in women age 50 are positive, and this figure increases to 33% in women age 70 or older.

CPT CODE(S)

19101   Biopsy of breast; open, incisional

REFERENCES

Level I
Tafra L, Fine R, Whitworth P, et al: Prospective randomized study comparing cryo-assisted and needle-wire localization of ultrasound-visible breast tumors. Am J Surg 2006;192:462.

Level II
Bluemke DA, Gatsonis CA, Chen MH, et al: Magnetic resonance imaging of the breast prior to biopsy JAMA 2004;292:2735.
Chagpar AB, Scoggins CR, Sahoo S, et al: Biopsy type does not influence sentinel lymph node status. Am J Surg 2005;190:551.

Level III
American College of Obstetricians and Gynecologists: Breast cancer screening. ACOG Practice Bulletin 42. Obstet Gynecol 2003;101:821.
Chang DS, McGrath MH: Management of benign tumors of the adolescent breast. Plast Reconstr Surg 2007;120:13e.
Valea FA, Katz VL: Breast diseases. In Katz VL, Lentz GM, Lobo RA, Gershenson DM: Comprehensive Gynecology, 5th ed. Philadelphia, Mosby/Elsevier, 2007, p 347.

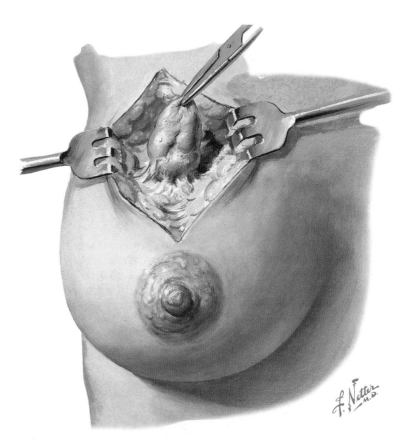

Masses are often not easily identified, requiring
larger incision or needle localization using
radiographic assistance

DESCRIPTION

Cervical cerclage is the placement of a suture or tape to support and partially occlude the uterine cervix to reduce the risk of preterm delivery in the face of cervical insufficiency. A number of procedures have been described, but the most common and simplest is the McDonald cerclage, which is described here. Cervical cerclage may also be accomplished by placing the suture by an abdominal route, although this is a much more invasive procedure and the suture is generally left in place permanently, precluding vaginal delivery.

INDICATIONS

Cervical incompetence as documented by a history of preterm pregnancy loss associated with painless cervical dilation or prolapse and ballooning of the fetal membranes into the vagina without labor. Prophylactic cervical cerclage is generally delayed until after 14 weeks so that early pregnancy losses from other factors may be resolved.

CONTRAINDICATIONS

Bleeding, uterine contractions, obvious infection, or rupture of the membranes. Beyond 24 to 26 weeks, bed rest or other treatments are often preferred because of the increased risk of surgically related labor.

REQUIRED EQUIPMENT

- Skin (vaginal) preparation materials (iodine-based antibacterial solution [e.g., Betadine] or other suitable cleansing agents)
- Sterile gloves
- Number 1 or 2 permanent synthetic suture (Prolene or similar) or 5-mm woven tape (Mersilene or similar) on a medium blunt needle (Monofilament sutures are easier to pass through the tissues, but a broader tape provides more support and less chance of suture erosion into or through the cervix.)
- Needle holder, long thumb forceps, suture scissors
- Retractors (two Deaver or right-angle retractors and/or weighted speculum)
- Sponge stick (may be useful to atraumatically grasp and manipulate the cervix)
- Foley or straight catheter (optional)
- External fetal heart rate monitor or Doppler fetal heart detector

TECHNIQUE

After appropriate informed consent has been obtained, ultrasonography should be performed to confirm a living fetus, exclude major fetal anomalies, and assess cervical length. Any obvious vaginal or cervical infections should be treated, and cultures for gonorrhea, chlamydia, and group B streptococci should be obtained prior to proceeding. (Sexual intercourse is generally proscribed for 1 week before and after the procedure.)

The anesthetized patient is placed in the dorsal lithotomy position, the vagina and cervix are disinfected, and the cervix is visualized using retractors. Some authors advise distending the maternal bladder to elevate the fetal presenting part, relieve pressure on the fetal membranes, and define the cervicovesical reflection. For right-handed surgeons, the needle is first placed entering the cervix at the 11 to 12-o'clock position near the inner cervical os, taking care to avoid injury to the bladder. The suture is passed below the surface of the cervix, incorporating some of the parenchyma, and exiting at about the 10-o'clock position. The suture then is passed once again into the cervical tissue, entering at about the 8-o'clock position and exiting posteriorly near the 6- to 7-o'clock position. The circumferential suture is carried up the opposite side in a similar manner, terminating at about the 1-o'clock position, where it is firmly tied to the first portion of the suture. The suture should not cause blanching of the tissue but should narrow the cervix so that it will not admit the gloved finger. The tied suture should be both tied and cut in such a manner as to facilitate eventual location and removal.

Based on the size of the cervix and needle chosen, it may be necessary to take additional bites to accomplish adequate circumferential support. Care should be taken that the portions of the suture at the 3- and 9-o'clock positions are shallow or outside the cervical epithelium to minimize the risk to the descending cervical branches of the uterine vessels.

Following conclusion of the procedure, the fetal heart is monitored to assure normal fetal status. Prophylactic antibiotics or beta-mimetic drugs have not been shown to be of any benefit in reducing the rate of complications or preterm labor.

When the suture is to be removed (generally at 38 weeks and always if labor ensues before that time), it may be carried out in the office or labor and delivery area by firmly grasping the knot or visible suture ends and applying traction to identify one side of the suture below the knot. Snipping this portion of the suture allows traction on the knot to pull the suture through the tissues and be removed. An anesthetic may be required based on exposure, patient comfort, and provider or patient preference.

COMPLICATIONS

Preterm rupture of the membranes (1% to 18%, up to 65% of emergent cases), chorioamnionitis (1% to 7%, up to 35% of emergent cases), bleeding, damage to adjacent structures (bladder or rectum). Scarring from the procedure may lead to cervical lacerations during labor (1% to 13%) or failure of the cervix to dilate (2% to 5%).

FOLLOW-UP

Fetal and maternal monitoring is generally carried out for 12 to 24 hours or longer depending on clinical factors.

When the suture is placed vaginally, it is generally removed at 38 weeks of gestation. If labor occurs before this point, the suture must be removed immediately. Because of scarring after cerclage, about 15% of patients require cesarean delivery.

CPT CODE(S)

59320   Cerclage of cervix, during pregnancy; vaginal
59325   Cerclage of cervix, during pregnancy; abdominal

Surgical Management of Cervical Incompetence (Cerclage)

Nonabsorbable purse-string suture placed around cervix at level of internal os

Purse-string (cerclage) suture prior to tying

Suture pulled taut and tied, narrowing cervical canal

REFERENCES

Level I

Althuisius SM, Dekker GA, Hummel P, et al: Final results of the Cervical Incompetence Prevention Randomized Cerclage Trial (CIPRACT): Therapeutic cerclage with bed rest versus bed rest alone. Am J Obstet Gynecol 2001;185:1106.

Althuisius SM, Dekker GA, Hummel P, van Geijn HP; Cervical Incompetence Prevention Randomized Cerclage Trial: Cervical Incompetence Prevention Randomized Cerclage Trial: Emergency cerclage with bed rest versus bed rest alone. Am J Obstet Gynecol 2003;189:907.

Berghella V, Odibo AO, Tolosa JE: Cerclage for prevention of preterm birth in women with a short cervix found on transvaginal ultrasound examination: a randomized trial. Am J Obstet Gynecol 2004;191:1311.

Lazar P, Gueguen S, Dreyfus J, et al: Multicentred controlled trial of cervical cerclage in women at moderate risk of preterm delivery. Br J Obstet Gynaecol 1984;91:731.

Rush RW, Isaacs S, McPherson K, et al: A randomized controlled trial of cervical cerclage in women at high risk of spontaneous preterm delivery. Br J Obstet Gynaecol 1984;91:724.

Secher NJ, McCormack CD, Weber T, et al: Cervical occlusion in women with cervical insufficiency: protocol for a randomised, controlled trial with cerclage, with and without cervical occlusion. BJOG 2007;114:649, e1.

To MS, Alfirevic Z, Heath VC, et al: Fetal Medicine Foundation Second Trimester Screening Group: Cervical cerclage for prevention of preterm delivery in women with short cervix: randomized controlled trial. Lancet 2004;363:1849.

Level II

Belej-Rak T, Okun N, Windrim R, et al: Effectiveness of cervical cerclage for a sonographically shortened cervix: a systematic review and meta-analysis. Am J Obstet Gynecol 2003;189:1679.

Berghella V, Odibo AO, To MS, et al: Cerclage for short cervix on ultrasonography: meta-analysis of trials using individual patient-level data. Obstet Gynecol 2005;106:181.

Drakeley AJ, Roberts D, Alfirevic Z: Cervical cerclage for prevention of preterm delivery: meta-analysis of randomized trials. Obstet Gynecol 2003;102:621.

Harger JH: Cerclage and cervical insufficiency: an evidence-based analysis. Obstet Gynecol 2002;100:1313.

Rust OA, Atlas RO, Meyn J, et al: Does cerclage location influence perinatal outcome? Am J Obstet Gynecol 2003;189:1688.

Zaveri V, Aghajafari F, Amankwah K, Hannah M: Abdominal versus vaginal cerclage after a failed transvaginal cerclage: a systematic review. Am J Obstet Gynecol 2002;187:868.

Level III

Althuisius SM, van Geijn HP: Strategies for prevention—Cervical cerclage. BJOG 2005;112:51.

American College of Obstetricians and Gynecologists: Cervical insufficiency. ACOG Practice Bulletin 48. Obstet Gynecol 2003; 102:1091.

American College of Obstetricians and Gynecologists: Ultrasonography in pregnancy. ACOG Practice Bulletin 58. Obstet Gynecol 2004;104:1449.

Cunningham FG, Gant NF, Leveno KJ, et al, eds. Williams Obstetrics, 21st ed. New York, McGraw-Hill, 2001, p 862.

McDonald IA. Suture of the cervix for inevitable abortion. J Obstet Gynaecol Br Emp 1957;64:346.

McDonald IA: Incompetence of the cervix. Aust N Z J Obstet Gynaecol 1978;18:34.

McNamara HM: Problems and challenges in the management of preterm labour. BJOG 2003;110:79.

Noori M, Helmig RB, Hein M, Steer PJ: Could a cervical occlusion suture be effective at improving perinatal outcome? BJOG 2007;114:532.

Romero R, Espinoza J, Erez O, Hassan S: The role of cervical cerclage in obstetric practice: can the patient who could benefit from this procedure be identified? Am J Obstet Gynecol 2006; 194:1.

DESCRIPTION

Cervical conization is a diagnostic or therapeutic procedure that removes a cone-shaped specimen from the uterine cervix. Cold knife cone biopsy used to be the preferred treatment for removing abnormal cells, but now most cone biopsies are performed using wire loop and electrosurgical energy (loop electrosurgical excision procedure [LEEP]/large loop excision of the transformation zone [LLETZ] cone). Cold knife cone biopsy is generally used for special situations, such as when the size or shape of the specimen must be customized to a greater degree than allowed by loop procedures.

INDICATIONS

Histologically verified advanced epithelial atypia (for diagnosis or therapy) or inability to adequately evaluate the cervix through colposcopy.

CONTRAINDICATIONS

Coagulopathy, advanced pregnancy, known or suspected allergy to the agents used.

REQUIRED EQUIPMENT

- Skin (vaginal) preparation materials (iodine-based antibacterial solution [e.g., Betadine] or other suitable cleansing agents)
- Sterile gloves
- 0 or 2-0 synthetic absorbable suture on a medium needle
- Needle holder, long thumb forceps, suture scissors
- Retractors (two Deaver or right-angle retractors and/or weighted speculum)
- Scalpel (#11 blade)
- Uterine sound (blunt probe) or small cervical dilator
- Sponge stick (may be useful to atraumatically grasp and manipulate the cervix)
- Electrosurgical generator, hand piece, and return electrode ("ground pad")
- Monsel's solution or paste (ferric subsulfate)
- Histology fixative (10% formalin) in containers
- 5% acetic acid or Lugol solution (super-saturated potassium iodide) if colposcopy is to be performed
- Vaginal Pack (optional)

TECHNIQUE

Cold knife conizations are generally performed under regional or general anesthesia. After providing appropriate informed consent, the anesthetized patient is placed in the dorsal lithotomy position, the vagina and cervix are disinfected, and the cervix is visualized using retractors. If necessary, a colposcopic examination, facilitated by acetic acid or Lugol solution, may be performed to further characterize any abnormalities present.

The procedure begins with the placement of hemostatic sutures (simple loop or figure-of-eight) at the 3- and 9-o'clock positions on the cervix near the cervicovaginal reflections bilaterally. These are generally tied and held to stabilize the cervix until the end of the procedure. (The role of these sutures in actually reducing blood loss has been debated and they may be omitted.) Dilute vasopressin (one pressor unit per 20 mL saline) may be injected into the cervical parenchyma to further reduce blood loss. If desired, a blunt uterine probe or small cervical dilator is placed into the endocervical canal to guide the dissection.

A cone-shaped plug of cervical tissue is excised by sweeping the scalpel blade around the ectocervix with the blade angled inward to intersect the endocervical canal. The width and depth of the conization is determined by the anatomy of the cervix, the location of the transformation zone, and the lesion being treated; it must include the transformation zone and any specific lesion.

Hemostasis may be obtained through electrosurgical energy or the application of styptics such as Monsel solution. Some advocate general cautery of the cut surface of the cervix, although the resultant slough of damaged tissue may delay final healing. If desired, the ectocervical edges may be sewn with a running suture to provide hemostasis at the edge and to roll the edges inward. As an alternative, Sturmdorf stitches may be placed to partially reconstruct the external cervical os, although some argue that this may increase the risk of cervical stenosis. At the close of the procedure, the held tails of the hemostatic sutures may be either clipped (leaving the suture in place) or tied across the cervix to apply pressure or to hold a hemostatic pledget (oxidized regenerated cellulose [Surgicel, or similar]) in place. Pelvic rest (no tampons, douching, or sexual intercourse) is generally advised for 2 to 3 weeks following the procedure, and the patient is instructed to return for heavy bleeding or bleeding that lasts more than 2 weeks.

COMPLICATIONS

Bleeding (acute and delayed, 5% to 10%, <1% transfusion rate), infection, uterine perforation, injury to the bladder or bowel, cervical stenosis, cervical incompetence. Conization appears to approximately double the risk that a woman will subsequently have a preterm delivery, a low-birthweight infant, or premature rupture of the membranes.

FOLLOW-UP

The cervix is generally inspected at about 6 weeks after the procedure. Treatment success for cervical intraepithelial neoplasia is generally 95%.

CPT CODE(S)

57520 Conization of cervix, with or without fulguration, with or without dilation and curettage, with or without repair; cold knife or laser

REFERENCES

Level I

Cullimore JE, Luesley DM, Rollason TP, et al: A prospective study of conization of the cervix in the management of cervical intraepithelial glandular neoplasia (CIGN)—A preliminary report. Br J Obstet Gynaecol 1992;99:314.

Duggan BD, Felix JC, Muderspach LI, et al: Cold-knife conization versus conization by the loop electrosurgical excision procedure: a

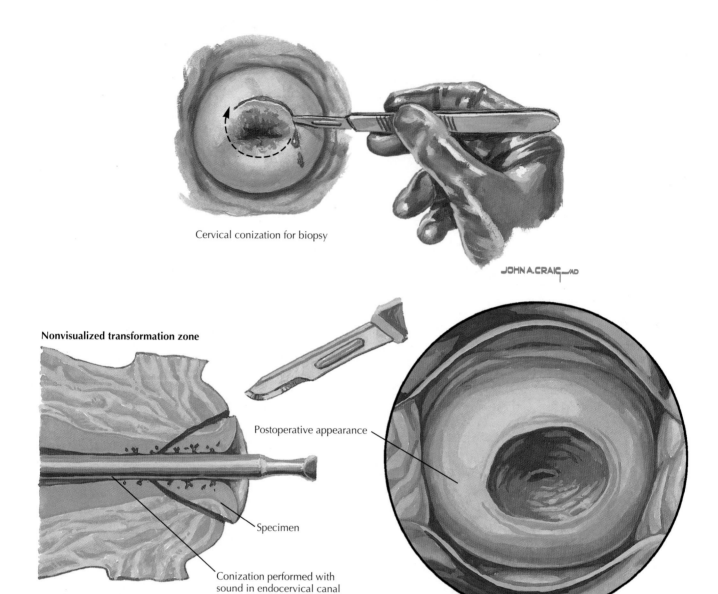

Cervical conization for biopsy

JOHN A.CRAIG—AD

Nonvisualized transformation zone

Postoperative appearance

Specimen

Conization performed with sound in endocervical canal

Conization of cervix

randomized, prospective study. Am J Obstet Gynecol 1999; 180:276.

Mathevet P, Dargent D, Roy M, et al: A randomized prospective study comparing three techniques of conization: cold knife, laser, and LEEP. Gynecol Oncol 1994;54:175.

Level II

El-Bastawissi AY, Becker TM, Daling JR: Effect of cervical carcinoma in situ and its management on pregnancy outcome. Obstet Gynecol 1999;93:207.

Jackobsson M, Gissler M, Sainio S, et al: Preterm delivery after surgical treatment for cervical intraepithelial neoplasia. Obstet Gynecol 2007;109:309.

Kyrgiou M, Koliopoulos G, Martin-Hirsch P, et al: Obstetric outcomes after conservative treatment for intraepithelial or early invasive cervical lesions: systematic review and meta-analysis. Lancet 2006;367:489.

Kyrgiou M, Tsoumpou I, Vrekoussis T, et al: The up-to-date evidence on colposcopy practice and treatment of cervical intraepithelial neoplasia: the Cochrane colposcopy and cervical cytopathology

collaborative group (C5 group) approach. Cancer Treat Rev 2006; 32:516.

Sadler L, Saftlas A, Wang W, et al: Treatment for cervical intraepithelial neoplasia and risk of preterm delivery. JAMA 2004; 291:2100.

Level III

American College of Obstetricians and Gynecologists: Diagnosis and treatment of cervical carcinomas. ACOG Practice Bulletin 35. Obstet Gynecol 2002;99:855.

American College of Obstetricians and Gynecologists: Management of abnormal cervical cytology and histology. ACOG Practice Bulletin 66. Obstet Gynecol 2005;106:645.

Montz FJ: Impact of therapy for cervical intraepithelial neoplasia on fertility. Am J Obstet Gynecol 1996;175:1129.

Morris M, Mitchell MF, Silva EG, et al: Cervical conization as definitive therapy for early invasive squamous carcinoma of the cervix. Gynecol Oncol 1993;51:193.

Sokol H: A modification of the Sturmdorf suture. Am J Obstet Gynecol 1964;89:823.

Cervical Polypectomy

DESCRIPTION

Cervical polypectomy is the removal of cervical or visible endocervical polyps; it is generally a simple, painless office procedure.

INDICATIONS

Cervical or visible endocervical polyp.

CONTRAINDICATIONS

Known or suspected allergy to the agents used, coagulopathy. Relative: pregnancy.

REQUIRED EQUIPMENT

- Skin (vaginal) preparation materials (iodine-based antibacterial solution [e.g., Betadine] or other suitable cleansing agents)
- Sterile or examination gloves
- Vaginal speculum
- Sponge stick or uterine packing forceps (fine scissors may be used but are seldom required)
- Kevorkian or similar endocervical curette
- Monsel solution or paste (ferric subsulfate) or silver nitrate–tipped sticks
- Histology fixative (10% formalin) in container

TECHNIQUE

The polyp is first visualized through the use of a standard vaginal speculum. Disinfection with a suitable solution may be performed, although most believe it is not required. The visible portion of the polyp is then grasped, and gentle traction, twisting through several revolutions, or excision accomplishes removal of polyp. If the polyp is thought to arise from high in the endocervical canal, the base may be gently curetted with an endocervical curette. Curettage of the endocervical canal should also be considered to rule out a coexisting hyperplasia or cancer. Although malignancy is rare, all polyps should be submitted for histologic examination. The base of the polyp may be treated with chemical cautery (Monsel solution or silver nitrate), electrocautery, or cryocautery.

COMPLICATIONS

Bleeding.

FOLLOW-UP

Although the histology of the polyp should be confirmed as benign, malignant degeneration of an endocervical polyp is extremely rare. The reported incidence is less than 1 in 200.

CPT CODE(S)

58999   Unlisted procedure, female genital system (nonobstetric)

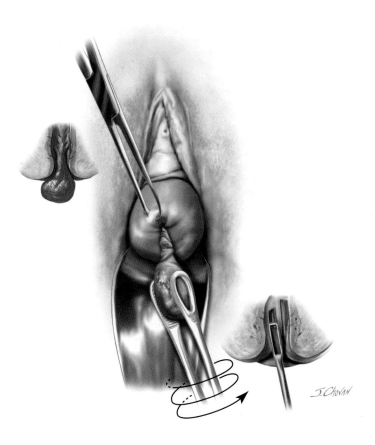

REFERENCES

Level II

Amesse LS, Taneja A, Broxson E, Pfaff-Amesse T: Protruding giant cervical polyp in a young adolescent with a previous rhabdomyosarcoma. J Pediatr Adolesc Gynecol 2002;15:271.

Khalil AM, Azar GB, Kaspar HG, et al: Giant cervical polyp. A case report. J Reprod Med 1996;41:619.

Pradhan S, Chenoy R: Dilatation and curettage in patients with cervical polyps: a retrospective analysis BJOG 1995;102:415.

Level III

Katz VL: Benign gynecologic lesions. In Katz VL, Lentz GM, Lobo RA, Gershenson DM: Comprehensive Gynecology, 5th ed. Philadelphia, Mosby/Elsevier, 2007, p 436.

DESCRIPTION

A technique for obtaining fetal chorionic villus cells for cytogenetic or other testing, chorionic villus sampling (CVS) is usually performed between 10 and 13 weeks' gestation and involves aspiration of placental tissue using either percutaneous transabdominal or transcervical approaches. Transabdominal CVS can be performed at gestations greater than 13 weeks. A transvaginal approach similar to the transabdominal method has also been used for retroverted uteruses.

INDICATIONS

Genetic testing for fetal chromosome anomalies prompted by risk factors or an abnormal screening test result during the first trimester. (Neural tube defects in the fetus cannot be detected by CVS.)

CONTRAINDICATIONS

Thrombocytopenia or antiplatelet antibodies, active vaginal bleeding, or infection are relative contraindications. For transcervical CVS: cervical stenosis, cervical or lower uterine myomas. For transabdominal CVS: fetal position that blocks access to the placenta, known or suspected intra-abdominal adhesions that could block access to the uterus. CVS may be technically difficult to accomplish in patients with multiple gestations. The risk of human immunodeficiency virus (HIV) vertical transmission associated with early invasive diagnostic techniques is lower than previously expected (3%) and similar to women who do not undergo the procedure.

REQUIRED EQUIPMENT

- Skin (or vaginal) preparation materials (iodine-based antibacterial solution [e.g., Betadine] or other suitable cleansing agents)
- Sterile gloves
- Tissue transport medium (to be specified by the laboratory used and the test to be performed)
- Ultrasonography unit

For Transvaginal Approach

- Vaginal speculum
- Sponge stick (may be useful to atraumatically grasp and manipulate the cervix)
- Small (1.5-mm) aspiration cannula (with obturator) and 20- to 30-mL syringe; small biopsy forceps may be used as an alternative

For Transabdominal Approach

- 20- and 22-gauge spinal needles (or smaller), 20-cc syringe, three sterile 10-cc specimen tubes with caps (plain, without additive), sterile drape (one with a small fenestration or multiple drapes)
- If desired: 1% lidocaine without epinephrine, 5-cc syringe, 22-gauge needle (if not included in amniocentesis kit)

TECHNIQUE

The consensus is that CVS, both transabdominal and transcervical, must be performed under ultrasonographic control. Ultrasonography is performed before CVS to confirm the gestational age of the fetus. Ultrasonography can also document multiple gestations and whether the multiples share a single placenta or each has its own. (It is important to determine the number of placentas because each must be sampled separately to obtain an accurate genetic picture of each fetus.)

In the transcervical technique, a speculum is used to visualize the cervix and it is cleansed with an antiseptic solution. The cervix may be stabilized with a sponge stick if needed. The cannula or biopsy tube is gently advanced through the cervix under ultrasonographic guidance until the tip is at the base of the placenta. The obturator is removed from the cannula, and the vacuum is applied to pull a sample of cells into the lumen of the cannula. The cannula is withdrawn. (The amount of tissue needed for the analysis is extremely small [10 to 25 mg] and represents only about 0.1% of the total amount of the placental tissue.) The tissue sample obtained should be inspected for perceived adequacy, placed in the appropriate transport medium, labeled, and sent to the laboratory for analysis. Some clinicians prefer to place 10 mL of transport medium directly into the syringe used for suction to allow the aspirated material to enter the medium directly.

A small biopsy forceps may be substituted for the cannula and used in the same manner as with the cannula technique. Although there is some evidence to support the use of forceps as opposed to aspiration cannula, the evidence is not strong enough to support change in practice, and the choice should be driven by operator experience and equipment availability.

When a transabdominal approach is chosen, it is accomplished in a manner very similar to amniocentesis: The chorionic villus sample is obtained by passing a fine needle through the abdominal wall and into the placenta using ultrasonographic guidance. Published techniques for transabdominal CVS vary significantly both in the size of the needle used (18-gauge, 20-gauge, and others) and method of aspiration (negative pressure by syringe, negative pressure by vacuum aspirator, biopsy forceps). No published studies comparing clinical outcomes using different techniques exist.

For patients who are Rh-negative, prophylaxis with Rho(D) Rh-immune globulin should be given.

COMPLICATIONS

Fetal loss rates following CVS are reported to be as high as 6%. Several randomized trial studies show almost identical miscarriage rates after transcervical CVS compared with the transabdominal approach. CVS is associated with a 14% risk of fetomaternal hemorrhage of more than 0.6 mL. Limb reductions have been associated with early (<9 weeks) CVS. There is some evidence that focal disrup-

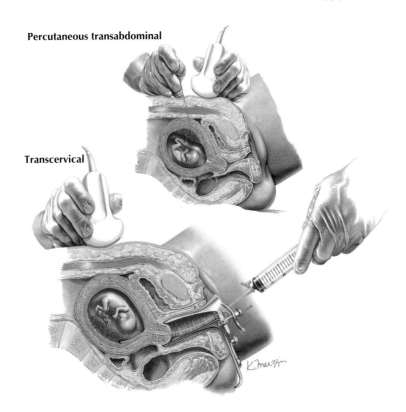

Percutaneous transabdominal

Transcervical

tion of the placenta at 13 to 14 weeks may increase the risk of hypertension/pre-eclampsia. The chance of getting a placental "mosaic" artifact is higher than with an amniocentesis. Vaginal spotting after CVS is reported in up to one third of women; slightly heavier bleeding occurs in fewer than 6% of women. Bleeding is more common after the transcervical compared with transabdominal CVS. Infection following CVS is very rare, although it is higher for the transcervical approach. Occult or gross rupture of the fetal membranes may occur.

FOLLOW-UP

Results are usually available in 2 to 3 weeks.

CPT CODE(S)

59015   Chorionic villus sampling, any method

REFERENCES

Level I

Brambati B, Terzian E, Tognoni G: Randomized clinical trial of transabdominal vs transcervical chorionic villus sampling methods. Prenat Diagn 1991;11:285.

Jackson L, Zachary J, Fowler S, et al: A randomised comparison of trans-cervical and transabdominal chorionic villus sampling. N Engl J Med 1992;327:594.

Philip J, Silver RK, Wilson RD, et al: NICHD EATA Trial Group: Late first-trimester invasive prenatal diagnosis: results of an international randomized trial. Obstet Gynecol 2004;103:1164.

Sundberg K, Bang J, Smidt-Jensen S, et al: Randomised study of risk of fetal loss related to early amniocentesis versus chorionic villus sampling. Lancet 1997;350:697.

von Dadelszen P, Sermer M, Hillier J, et al: A randomised controlled trial of biopsy forceps and cannula aspiration for transcervical chorionic villus sampling. BJOG 2005;112:559.

Level II

Alfirevic Z, Sundberg K, Brigham S: Amniocentesis and chorionic villus sampling for prenatal diagnosis. Cochrane Database Syst Rev 2004;CD003252.

Brambati B, Guercilena S, Bonnachi I, et al: Feto-maternal transfusion after chorionic villus sampling: clinical implications. Hum Reprod 1986;1:37.

Brambati B, Tului L, Guercilena S, Alberti E: Outcome of first-trimester chorionic villus sampling for genetic investigation in multiple pregnancy. Ultrasound Obstet Gynecol 2001;17:209.

Casals G, Borrell A, Martinez JM, et al: Transcervical chorionic villus sampling in multiple pregnancies using a biopsy forceps. Prenat Diagn 2002;22:260.

Kuliev AM, Modell B, Jackson L, et al: Risk evaluation of CVS. Prenat Diagn 1993;13:197.

Silver RK, Wilson RD, Philip J, et al: NICHD EATA Trial Group: Late first-trimester placental disruption and subsequent gestational hypertension/preeclampsia. Obstet Gynecol 2005;105:587.

Somigliana E, Bucceri AM, Tibaldi C, et al: Italian Collaborative Study on HIV Infection in Pregnancy: Early invasive diagnostic techniques in pregnant women who are infected with the HIV: a multicenter case series. Am J Obstet Gynecol 2005;193:437.

Wapner RJ, Johnson A, Davis G, et al: Prenatal diagnosis in twin gestations: a comparison between second-trimester amniocentesis and first-trimester chorionic villus sampling. Obstet Gynecol 1993:82:49.

Level III

American College of Obstetricians and Gynecologists: Prenatal and preconceptional carrier screening for genetic diseases in individuals of Eastern European Jewish descent. ACOG Committee Opinion 298. Obstet Gynecol 2004;104:425.

American College of Obstetricians and Gynecologists: Screening for fetal chromosomal abnormalities. ACOG Practice Bulletin 77. Obstet Gynecol 2007;109:217.

Blakemore KJ, Baumgarten A, Schoenfeld-Dimaio M, et al: Rise in maternal serum alpha-fetoprotein concentration after chorionic villus sampling and the possibility of isoimmunization. Am J Obstet Gynecol 1986;155:988.

Budorick NE, O'Boyle MK: Prenatal diagnosis for detection of aneuploidy: the options. Radiol Clin North Am 2003;41:695.

Mujezinovic F, Alfirevic Z: Procedure-related complications of amniocentesis and chorionic villous sampling: a systematic review. Obstet Gynecol 2007;110:687.

Simpson JL, Martin AO: Prenatal diagnosis of cytogenetic disorders. Clin Obstet Gynecol 1976;19:841.

DESCRIPTION

Male circumcision is the removal of some or all of the foreskin of the phallus.

INDICATIONS

Parental or religious preference (not a medically indicated procedure). Circumcision of newborns should be performed only on healthy and stable infants.

CONTRAINDICATIONS

Age greater than 6 to 8 weeks (relative), age less than 12 hours, ambiguous genitalia, hypospadias, illness, less than 1 hour postprandial, possibility of blood dyscrasia, prematurity, undescended testicles (relative). A family history of intolerance or allergy to local anesthetics should prompt reconsideration.

REQUIRED EQUIPMENT

- Infant restraint board ("papoose" board)
- Sterile gloves
- Sterile drape (one with a small fenestration or multiple drapes)
- Skin preparation materials (e.g., povidone–iodine and 70% isopropyl alcohol)
- Sterile gauze pads (2″ × 2″ or 4″ × 4″)
- Three hemostats (small tips, two curved, one straight)
- Small scissors or scalpel (#10 or #11 blade)
- Flexible blunt probe
- Gomco clamp (1.1 to 1.45 cm) or Plastibell (1.3 to 1.6 cm) or Mogen clamp (for clamp methods)
- Sterile safety pin, clip, or skin staple (optional)
- Viscous lidocaine (2% to 5%) or 1% lidocaine without epinephrine, 1-cc syringe, 27-gauge needle for dorsal penile nerve or ring block. EMLA cream may also be used.
- Petrolatum (Vaseline) gauze
- Silver nitrate stick or Monsel solution
- Small suture (3-0 or 4-0 absorbable) and needle holder (available)

Electrosurgical devices should never be used in conjunction with any of the clamp-based procedures.

A bulb syringe should be kept near during circumcision as a protection against aspiration should the newborn regurgitate.

TECHNIQUE

All circumcision techniques begin with the undiapered newborn restrained on an infant restraint (papoose) board. The penis should be inspected to identify the meatus and its location on the glans. Once the anatomy has been confirmed to be normal, anesthesia by way of topical lidocaine or dorsal block may be administered.

Swaddling, sucrose by mouth, and acetaminophen administration may reduce the stress response but are not sufficient for the operative pain and cannot be recommended as the sole method of analgesia. EMLA cream, dorsal penile nerve block, and subcutaneous ring block are all reasonable options, although the subcutaneous ring block may provide the most effective analgesia.

Identifying the depth of the root of the penis using the index finger begins a dorsal penile block. The root is usually located 0.75 to 1 cm beneath the skin surface, with the size and consistency of a large blueberry. The skin of the penis and the surrounding areas should be disinfected by any suitable method and sterile drapes should be placed to provide a surgical field. Using aseptic technique, the physician places the penis on slight downward traction and inserts the needle at the 2 o'clock position near the base. The needle is passed in a posteromedial direction to a depth of 3 to 5 mm beneath the skin, about 5 to 7 mm distal to the penile root near the point at which the dorsal nerves branch. If it is correctly located outside of the corpus cavernosum, the tip of the needle should move freely. The syringe should be aspirated to prevent intravenous injection, and 0.2 to 0.4 mL of anesthetic should be injected. The procedure is repeated at the 10-o'clock position, although a single needle insertion point in the dorsal midline may also be used, if desired. Total anesthetic dose should remain less than 0.8 mL. Full anesthesia will be achieved in 2 to 4 minutes.

The specific technique used varies slightly with the type of instrument chosen, the final choice of which is generally based on the personal preference and experience of the provider.

Both the Plastibell and Gomco clamp techniques begin in the same way: A hemostat is used to grasp the edge of the foreskin dorsal to the 3- and 9-o'clock positions (dorsal as 12 o'clock). A hemostat or flexible probe is inserted just under the foreskin and swept laterally to bluntly lyse any adhesions. Care must be taken to avoid disrupting either the ventral attachment or the coronal reflection. The foreskin is tented away from the glans and a straight hemostat is inserted along the dorsal line and clamped to a depth of one third to one half of the way to the coronal reflection. This is left in place for approximately 1 minute before it is removed and the crushed tissue is incised using scissors. The glans must be avoided during both the clamping and incision process. The foreskin is next retracted, and any further adhesions are removed; if needed, the dorsal incision is extended by repeating the crush and cut process. The procedure is then completed based on the instrument preferred.

Plastibell

With the dissection of the foreskin free of the glans completed, the Plastibell string is placed as a loop near the base of the penis. The bell is placed under the foreskin, over the glans. This may be facilitated by upward traction on the edges of the foreskin grasped by hemostats and by downward pressure on the stem of the bell. When in a correct position, the bell should rest against the corona. The foreskin is pulled upward, ensuring even placement and positioning that leaves the groove in the bell well below the apex of the dorsal slit. The bell should move freely over the glans. While maintaining these relationships, the string is brought into position, resting in the groove of the bell. The string should be pulled firmly and all aspects should be rechecked before the string is tightened maximally. Tension on the string is maintained for at least 30 seconds and then a square knot is placed.

The foreskin is cut just above the level of the string, with care taken not to cut too close to the string or to damage the string itself. The string is trimmed, and the stem of the Plastibell is broken off at its junction with the bell. Hemostasis should be confirmed, and a dressing may be applied if desired. The bell may be expected to slough off in 5 to 8 days, or it may be removed by cutting the ligature after a minimum of 36 hours.

Gomco Clamp

The Gomco clamp consists of a base plate, arm, bell, and thumbscrew. The bell of the Gomco clamp is placed under the foreskin and over the glans in the same manner as with the Plastibell. The bell and foreskin are then inserted through the opening in the baseplate of the clamp. This may be facilitated by reaching through the opening with a hemostat to help guide the foreskin. When the bell is passed through the baseplate, the foreskin must be brought completely through the opening and evenly drawn up on all sides. The entire length of the dorsal incision must be above the baseplate opening. The stem of the bell is placed into the top of the clamp, and the thumbscrew is gently tightened. The foreskin, bell, and shaft of the penis are again inspected before the final tightening is performed.

A scalpel is used to excise all of the tissue above the baseplate of the clamp. Care must be used to completely remove any tissue devitalized by the clamp. The Gomco clamp is loosened, and the bell is freed. The foreskin is freed from the bell by gentle traction using a gauze sponge. Hemostasis must be assured and may be assisted by pressure, the application of Monsel solution, or a fine suture. A petrolatum gauze dressing should be placed and the newborn should be diapered.

Mogen Clamp

When the Mogen clamp is used, the infant is restrained and inspected, and the skin is prepared as for the other two methods. Hemostats are used to pull the foreskin upward, and the tip of the penis is transilluminated to identify the glans. The Mogen clamp is applied with its curved side toward the glans. It is slid into place over the foreskin from dorsal to ventral in a horizontal plane, and the provider adjusts it so that the desired amount of skin is distal to the clamp. The clamp is angled so that more skin is removed from the dorsal side of the penis. The glans is again inspected and palpated to ensure it is clear of the clamp, and the clamp then is tightened. A scalpel is used to cut the foreskin flush with the surface of the clamp. The clamp is left in place for approximately 1 minute before it is removed. (If the Mogen clamp is left in place for more than a minute, the sides of the foreskin may become fused and difficult to separate.) The sides of the foreskin are separated by downward traction, inspected, and dressed. A gauze pad may be used to help separate the sides of the foreskin if necessary, although excess bleeding may be encountered if too much force is used. (A small ventral "dog ear" will often be present when the clamp is removed. This will partially necrose and heal without cosmetic defect.)

Silver nitrate should not be used for hemostasis because of the risk of permanent staining of the tissues.

COMPLICATIONS

The exact incidence of complications after circumcision is not known, but data indicate that the rate is low (0.2% to 0.6%), and the most common complications are local infection and bleeding. Rare complications include urinary fistulas, chordee, cysts, lymphedema, ulceration of the glans, necrosis of all or part of the penis, hypospadias, epispadias, impotence, and removal of too much tissue (sometimes causing secondary phimosis).

FOLLOW-UP

Following circumcision, the infant should be observed for at least 4 hours and should void before being released. The petrolatum gauze should be removed after 24 hours or if it becomes soiled. Petrolatum jelly should be applied at each diaper change until healing has occurred (about 7 to 10 days). At each diaper change the penile skin should be retracted to prevent adhesion formation.

CPT CODE(S)

54150 Circumcision, using clamp or other device with regional dorsal penile or ring block
54160 Circumcision, surgical excision other than clamp, device, or dorsal slit; neonate (28 days of age or less)
00920 Anesthesia for procedure on male external genitalia; not otherwise specified

REFERENCES

Level II
Blass EM, Hoffmeyer LB: Sucrose as an analgesic for newborn infants. Pediatrics 1991;87:215.
Marshall RE: Neonatal pain associated with caregiving procedures. Pediatr Clin North Am 1989;36:885.
Strimling BS: Partial amputation of glans penis during Mogen clamp circumcision. Pediatr 1996;97:906.

Level III
American Academy of Pediatrics, Committee on Fetus and Newborn, Committee on Drugs, Section on Anesthesiology, Section on Surgery, Canadian Paediatric Society: Prevention and management of pain and stress in the neonate. Fetus and Newborn Committee. Pediatrics 2000;105:454, 461.
American College of Obstetricians and Gynecologists: Circumcision. ACOG Committee Opinion 260. Obstet Gynecol 2001;98:707.
Baskin LS, Canning DA, Snyder HM, Duckett JW: Treating complications of circumcision. Pediat Emerg Care 1996;12:62.
Benini F, Johnston CC, Faucher D, Aranda JV: Topical anesthesia during circumcision in newborn infants. JAMA 1993;270:850.
Clair DL, Caldamone AA: Pediatric office procedures. Urol Clin North Am 1988;15:715.
Kaweblum YA, Press S, Kogan L, et al: Circumcision using the Mogen clamp. Clin Pediatr 1984;23:679.
Niku SD, Stock JA, Kaplan GW: Neonatal circumcision. Urol Clin North Am 1995;22:57.
Reynolds RD: Use of the Mogen clamp for neonatal circumcision. Am Fam Physician 1996;54:177.
Task Force on Circumcision, American Academy of Pediatrics: Circumcision policy statement. Pediatrics 1999;103:686.
Warner E, Strashin E: Benefits and risks of circumcision. Can Med Assoc J 1981;125:967, 992.
Wolkomir MS: Technique for freehand newborn circumcision. J Fam Pract 1996;42:447.

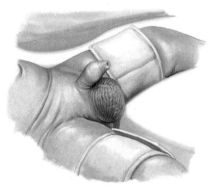

1. All circumcision techniques begin with the undiapered newborn restrained on an infant (papoose) board.

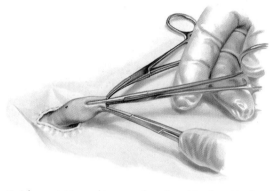

2. A hemostat is used to grasp the edge of the foreskin dorsal to the 3 and 9 o'clock positions (dorsal as 12 o'clock).

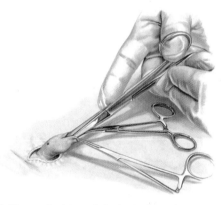

3. The crushed tissue is incised using scissors.

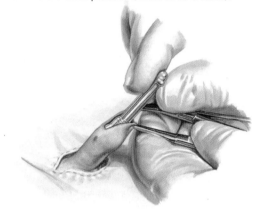

4. The bell of the Gomco clamp is placed under the foreskin, over the glans.

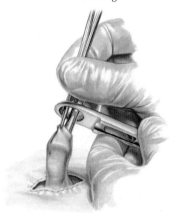

5. Placement of the bell through the baseplate may be facilitated by reaching through the opening with a hemostat.

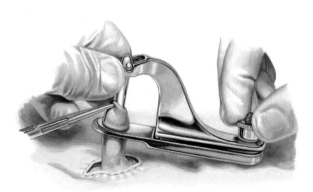

6. The stem of the bell is placed into the top of the clamp and the thumb screw gently tightened.

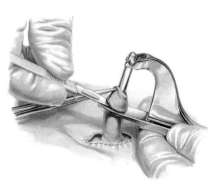

7. A scalpel is used to excise all of the tissue above the baseplate of the clamp.

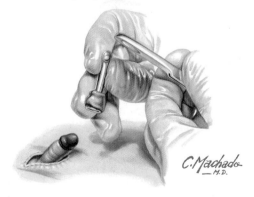

8. The Gomco clamp is loosened and the bell freed to conclude the procedure.

DESCRIPTION

Colposcopy is a diagnostic technique that allows the clinician to identify normal landmarks, find changes suggestive of underlying abnormality, and select sites for biopsy that will yield the greatest information.

Colposcopy is based on a simple stereoscopic operating microscope with magnifications of from 4 to 40 times. Although most often used to examine the uterine cervix, colposcopy may be used to evaluate the vagina, vulva, and other structures.

INDICATIONS

Abnormal cervical cytology (atypia, cancer, dysplasia, koilocytosis), cervical lesions (palpable or visible), condyloma (current or past; relative indication), human immunodeficiency virus (HIV) infection, intrauterine diethylstilbestrol (DES) exposure, surveillance or follow-up.

CONTRAINDICATIONS

Colposcopy is not recommended for adolescents or pregnant patients with Pap test abnormalities of low-grade squamous intraepithelial lesions (LSIL). Endocervical curettage is contraindicated during pregnancy.

REQUIRED EQUIPMENT

- Colposcope with light source
- Endocervical speculum
- Biopsy forceps (e.g., Tischler, Kevorkian)
- Endocervical curette
- Large cotton-tipped swabs, cotton balls, or small gauze sponges
- Examination gloves
- Vaginal speculum
- Tenaculum (optional)
- Acetic acid (3% to 5%) (white vinegar)
- Monsel solution (ferric subsulfate)
- Lugol (5%) solution (supersaturated iodine) (optional)
- Sputum or urine cups (to hold solutions)
- Sterile gloves (optional) (Any instrument that will enter the endocervical canal or will be used for biopsy should be sterilized before use. The use of sterile gloves is not required as long as the portions of instruments that will come in contact with the patient remain sterile.)
- Video, photographic, or digital capture equipment may be attached to the hysteroscope as desired (optional)

TECHNIQUE

The patient is placed in the dorsal lithotomy position. (If a bimanual examination is performed, the amount of lubricant used should be limited because this lubricant, and glove powder, can adversely affect cytologic studies.) By use of the largest warmed but unlubricated speculum the patient can comfortably accommodate, the cervix should be brought into full view. Following gross inspection for lesions, excessive secretions may be gently blotted away, cultures obtained, or a repeat Papanicolaou (Pap) smear taken.

The colposcope should be positioned to provide an unobstructed view of the cervix and maintained in a position and height that is comfortable for both the patient and the examiner. Acetic acid (3% to 5%) should be liberally applied to the cervix with large cotton-tipped applicators, cotton balls, or small gauze sponges. Acetic acid causes the columnar epithelial cells to swell and opacifies metaplastic and dysplastic cells. The changes brought on by the application of acetic acid are only temporary, requiring periodic reapplication at roughly 5-minute intervals.

Inspection of the cervix begins using the lowest magnification, with additional magnification added later, if needed. The transformation zone should be identified and inspected in its entirety. If necessary, the cervix may be manipulated using an acetic acid–soaked applicator stick, a cervical hook (similar to a skin hook retractor), or an endocervical speculum.

For a colposcopy to be considered "adequate" the entire transformation zone must be visualized. The full extent of any lesion present must also be visible for the study to be considered adequate. If the colposcopy is "inadequate," diagnostic conization will be required. Any areas of white change, vascular abnormality, or mosaicism should be inspected under greater magnification. Vascular patterns may be enhanced by the interposition of a green filter in the colposcope's light path, making the vessels appear black against the pale background of the epithelium.

Any area of abnormality identified should be biopsied. (Although rarely necessary, abnormal areas may be stained with Lugol solution to aid this identification.) When multiple abnormalities are present, biopsies of the most severe areas take precedence. Whenever possible, the biopsy should include the edge or border of the lesion. Biopsies should be placed in a buffered formalin solution for transport to the pathology laboratory.

Curettage of the endocervical canal (ECC) should generally be included to exclude the possibility of endocervical lesions above the limits of visibility. The ECC is especially helpful as a first stage in the evaluation of atypical glandular cells.

If bleeding from a biopsy site persists or is heavy, Monsel solution may be applied. Monsel solution should be applied only after all specimens have been obtained.

For colposcopy of the vulva, a weaker concentration of acetic acid will result in less burning and discomfort. Because of the relatively thicker epithelium of the vulva, the acetic acid must be left in contact with the tissues for a longer period (even if the stronger solution is chosen). Soaking a gauze sponge and allowing it to remain in contact with the skin for several minutes most easily accomplish this.

COMPLICATIONS

Transient bleeding from biopsy sites. Infection at the biopsy site or endometrium is rare. (Colposcopic examinations fail to visualize the squamocolumnar junction or the limits of any lesions present [inadequate studies] in roughly 15% to 20% of premenopausal women.)

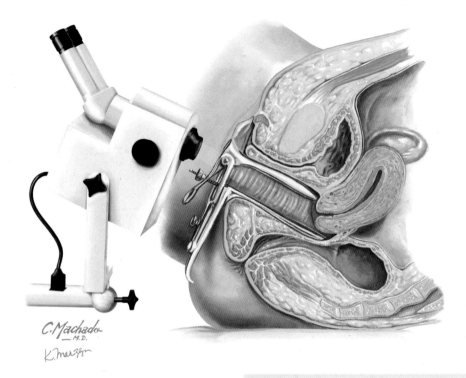

C. Machado
M.D.

K. mazg...

FOLLOW-UP

Follow-up is dictated by the indication for the procedure and any lesions found. A review of the histology reports on any material removed may also alter the follow-up indicated. No specific procedure-related follow-up is needed, although if extensive biopsies are taken, pelvic rest (no tampons, douches, or sexual intercourse) for a period of time may be prudent. The patient should be advised to expect an increased vaginal discharge if biopsies were taken and Monsel solution was used. An abnormal discharge or vaginal bleeding should prompt a re-evaluation.

CPT CODE(S)

57452   Colposcopy (Vaginoscopy); (separate procedure)
57454   Colposcopy with biopsy(s) of the cervix and/or endocervical curettage
57460   Colposcopy with loop electrode excision procedure of the cervix
57500   Biopsy of cervix only, single or multiple
57505   Endocervical curettage (not done as part of a dilatation and curettage)

REFERENCES

Level II

Ang MS, Kaufman RH, Adam E, et al: Colposcopically directed biopsy and loop excision of the transformation zone. Comparison of histologic findings. J Reprod Med 1995;40:167.

Cristoforoni PM, Gerbaldo D, Perino A, et al: Computerized colposcopy: results of a pilot study and analysis of its clinical relevance. Obstet Gynecol 1995;85:1011.

Gage JC, Hanson VW, Abbey K, et al: ASCUS LSIL Triage Study (ALTS) Group: Number of cervical biopsies and sensitivity of colposcopy. Obstet Gynecol 2006;108:264.

Lonky NM, Mann WJ, Massad LS, et al: Ability of visual tests to predict underlying cervical neoplasia. Colposcopy and speculoscopy. J Reprod Med 1995;40:530.

Level III

American College of Obstetricians and Gynecologists: Diagnosis and treatment of cervical carcinomas. ACOG Practice Bulletin 35. Obstet Gynecol 2002;99:855.

American College of Obstetricians and Gynecologists: Cervical cytology screening. ACOG Practice Bulletin 45. Obstet Gynecol 2003;102:417.

American College of Obstetricians and Gynecologists: Cervical cancer screening in adolescents. ACOG Committee Opinion 300. Obstet Gynecol 2004;104:885.

American College of Obstetricians and Gynecologists: Human papillomavirus. ACOG Practice Bulletin 61. Obstet Gynecol 2005;105:905.

American College of Obstetricians and Gynecologists: Management of abnormal cervical cytology and histology. ACOG Practice Bulletin 66. Obstet Gynecol 2005;106:645.

American College of Obstetricians and Gynecologists: Evaluation and management of abnormal cervical cytology and histology in the adolescent. ACOG Committee Opinion 330. Obstet Gynecol 2006;107:963.

Burke L, Antonioli DA, Ducatman BS: Colposcopy: Text and atlas. East Norwalk, Conn, Appleton & Lange, 1991.

Craine BL, Craine ER: Digital imaging colposcopy: basic concepts and applications. Obstet Gynecol 1993;82:869.

Davis GD: Colposcopic examination of the vagina. Obstet Gynecol Clin North Am 1993;20:217.

Lau S, Franco EL: Management of low-grade cervical lesions in young women. CMAJ 2005;173:771.

Rickert VI, Kozlowski KJ, Warren AM, et al: Adolescents and colposcopy: the use of different procedures to reduce anxiety. Am J Obstet Gynecol 1994;170:504.

Safaeian M, Solomon D, Wacholder S, et al: Risk of precancer and follow-up management strategies for women with human papillomavirus-negative atypical squamous cells of undetermined significance. Obstet Gynecol 2007;109:1325.

Shafi MI, Dunn JA, Chenoy R, et al: Digital imaging colposcopy, image analysis and quantification of the colposcopic image. Br J Obstet Gynaecol 1994;101:234.

Wright TC Jr, Cox JT, Massad LS, et al: 2001 Consensus Guidelines for the management of women with cervical cytological abnormalities. JAMA 2002;287:2120.

Wright VC: Understanding the colposcope. Optics, light path, magnification, and field of view. Obstet Gynecol Clin North Am 1993;20:31.

DESCRIPTION

Cervical cryocautery is the use of cold to produce "frost bite" as an ablative therapy for cervical abnormalities.

INDICATIONS

Histologically verified advanced epithelial atypia. Because this is an ablative technology, a histology must be established prior to instituting this therapy.

CONTRAINDICATIONS

Undiagnosed cervical lesions, pregnancy.

REQUIRED EQUIPMENT

- Skin (or vaginal) preparation materials (iodine-based antibacterial solution [e.g., Betadine] or other suitable cleansing agents)
- Cryosurgery unit (e.g., nitrous oxide-powered, carbon dioxide or similar)
- Cryoprobes: flat and conical, assorted sizes
- Water-soluble lubricant (e.g. K-Y Jelly)
- Timer (optional, although recommended)
- Vaginal speculum
- Colposcope (if colposcopy has not been previously performed or the boundaries of the lesion are not visible)
- 3% to 5% acetic acid (white vinegar) or Lugol (5%) solution (if desired)
- Gauze pads and/or cotton balls
- Vaginal sidewall retractor (optional)
- Ibuprofen (800 mg) or other similar nonsteroidal anti-inflammatory agent taken approximately 1 hour prior to therapy (if desired)

TECHNIQUE

After informed consent has been obtained, the patient is placed in the dorsal lithotomy position as for a speculum examination. The cervix should be brought into view and any cultures or cytologic smears should be obtained as needed. If the extent of the lesion has not been documented or is not immediately visible, acetic acid or Lugol solution should be applied to the cervix to delineate the area of abnormality.

A cryoprobe tip should be chosen to allow the freezing effect to extend approximately 5 mm beyond the extent of the lesion. Whenever possible, the probe should be flat or slightly conical to minimize the risk of extensive endocervical damage and the risk of inward migration of the squamocolumnar junction. After the tip is secured to the device (following manufacturer's directions), turning on and checking the tank pressure to ensure an adequate supply readies the device.

A water-soluble gel or lubricant is applied to the tip of the cryoprobe. (Lidocaine jelly may be substituted if desired.) The tip of the probe should be placed against the cervix, covering the lesion and avoiding contact with the vaginal sidewalls. The unit is activated, and after approximately 5 seconds the tip will adhere to the cervix. Once the tip is adhered to the cervix, the device is maneuvered outward and farther away from the vaginal sidewalls to avoid adherence to other tissues. This outward movement will bring along the cervix, minimizing lateral freezing as well.

Freezing should continue for 3 minutes, resulting in an ice ball that extends 5 mm beyond the cervical lesion. The

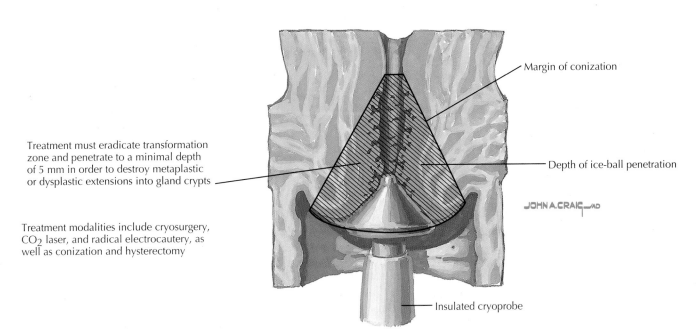

Treatment must eradicate transformation zone and penetrate to a minimal depth of 5 mm in order to destroy metaplastic or dysplastic extensions into gland crypts

Treatment modalities include cryosurgery, CO_2 laser, and radical electrocautery, as well as conization and hysterectomy

Margin of conization

Depth of ice-ball penetration

JOHN A. CRAIG—MD

Insulated cryoprobe

freezing mechanism is then deactivated to allow for a 5-minute thaw. The probe should not be actively loosened from the cervix but allowed to defrost and detach by itself. After thawing for 5 minutes, the lesion is refrozen for another 3 minutes. A single 5-minute freeze may also be used, but with either method, the ice ball must extend to a distance of more than 5 mm for the procedure to be effective.

COMPLICATIONS

Cervical stenosis (unlikely unless the procedure is performed repetitively or a probe tip that extends high into the endocervix is used).

FOLLOW-UP

A follow-up sequence of Pap tests should be discussed with the patient. The first Pap test should be delayed at least 3 months to allow for complete healing.

CPT CODE(S)

57511   Cauterization of cervix; cryocautery, initial or repeat (surgical procedure only)
56501   Destruction of lesion(s), vulva; simple, any method
56515   Extensive, any method
57061   Destruction of lesion(s), vagina; simple, any method
57065   Extensive, any method

REFERENCES

Level I
Kwikkel HJ, Helmerhorst TJ, Bezemer PD, et al: Laser or cryotherapy for cervical intraepithelial neoplasia: a randomized study to compare efficacy and side effects. Gynecol Oncol 1985;22:23.
Mathevet P, Dargent D, Roy M, Beau G: A randomized prospective study comparing three techniques of conization: cold knife, laser, and LEEP. Gynecol Oncol 1994;54:175.

Mitchell MF, Tortolero-Luna G, Cook E, et al. A randomized clinical trial of cryotherapy, laser vaporization, and loop electrosurgical excision for treatment of squamous intraepithelial lesions of the cervix. Obstet Gynecol 1998;92:737.

Level II
Andersen ES, Thorup K, Larsen G: Results of cryosurgery for cervical intraepithelial neoplasia. Gynecol Oncol 1988;30:21.
Benedet JL, Miller DM, Nickerson KG, Anderson GH: The results of cryosurgical treatment of cervical intraepithelial neoplasia at one, five, and ten years. Am J Obstet Gynecol 1987;157:268.
Loobuyck HA, Duncan ID: Destruction of CIN 1 and 2 with the Semm cold coagulator: 13 years' experience with a see-and-treat policy. Br J Obstet Gynaecol 1993;100:465.
Ostergard DR: Cryosurgical treatment of cervical intraepithelial neoplasia. Obstet Gynecol 1980;56:231.
Wright VC, Davies EM: The conservative management of cervical intraepithelial neoplasia: the use of cryosurgery and the carbon dioxide laser. Br J Obstet Gynaecol 1981;88:663.

Level III
American College of Obstetricians and Gynecologists: Management of abnormal cervical cytology and histology. ACOG Practice Bulletin 66. Obstet Gynecol 2005;106:645.
American College of Obstetricians and Gynecologists: Evaluation and management of abnormal cervical cytology and histology in the adolescent. ACOG Committee Opinion 330. Obstet Gynecol 2006;107:963.
Cox JT: Management of cervical intraepithelial neoplasia. Lancet 1999;353:857.
Ferenczy A: Management of patients with high grade squamous intraepithelial lesions. Cancer 1995;76:1928.
Figge DC, Creasman WT: Cryotherapy in the treatment of cervical intraepithelial neoplasia. Obstet Gynecol 1983;62:353.
Gage AA: Cryosurgery in the treatment of cancer. Surg Gynecol Obstet 1992;174:73.
Kirwan PH, Smith IR, Naftalin NJ: A study of cryosurgery and the CO_2 laser in treatment of carcinoma in situ (CIN III) of the uterine cervix. Gynecol Oncol 1985;22:195.
Ostergard DR: Cryosurgical treatment of cervical intraepithelial neoplasia. Obstet Gynecol 1980;56:231.

DESCRIPTION

Cystourethroscopy is a technique for visualizing the interior of the urethra or bladder. This may also serve as a portal for other diagnostic or therapeutic measures.

INDICATIONS

To diagnose urinary tract disorders such as bleeding, pain, or dysfunction (e.g., interstitial cystitis). Cystourethroscopy can be a part of the evaluation of abnormal symptoms, signs, or laboratory findings; intraoperatively during gynecologic or urogynecologic surgery to rule out bladder, urethral, or ureteral trauma; and as part of staging or surgery for gynecologic malignancy.

CONTRAINDICATIONS

Active urinary tract infection. Known or suspected allergy to cleansing solutions or local anesthetics to be used.

REQUIRED EQUIPMENT

- Skin (or vaginal) preparation materials (iodine-based antibacterial solution [e.g., Betadine] or other suitable cleansing agents)
- Sterile gloves, antiseptic solution and sterile cotton balls, or skin preparation swabs
- Sterile urine specimen cup (with graduations)
- 1 liter of sterile saline (intravenous fluid without glucose is generally used) at room temperature (low-pressure carbon dioxide may also be used with suitable equipment) (If electrocautery is to be performed, a nonconducting solution, such as glycine, should be used.)
- Absorbent underpads
- 2% Xylocaine jelly in mushroom-tipped syringe (optional) or tube with conical delivery cap
- Cystoscope (rigid or flexible, direct viewing or with a 30-degree or greater down-angle view; the latter is better for visualizing the bladder trigone and ureteral openings)
- Fiber-optic light source (compatible with type of cystoscope used)
- Fiber-optic light cord
- An assistant is advantageous

TECHNIQUE

Shortly before the procedure, a single dose of prophylactic antibiotics is recommended to prevent urinary tract infection or septicemia for patients at moderate or high risk of endocarditis, those who are neutropenic, and those with preoperative bacteriuria or an indwelling catheter.

Immediately prior to starting the procedure, the patient is asked to empty her bladder (in private and in her usual manner). The patient is placed in the dorsal lithotomy position and the external urinary meatus and surrounding vulvar vestibule are cleansed with antiseptic solution. One to three milliliters of topical anesthetic such as 2% Xylocaine are introduced into the urethra.

With sterile technique, the patient is catheterized by use of a straight catheter, and any residual urine is caught, measured for volume, and sent for culture (if appropriate). With the catheter left in place, the bladder is slowly (to avoid inducing bladder spasm) filled with 100 to 200 mL of sterile saline, and the catheter is then removed.

After the light guide is attached to both the cystoscope and light source, the tip of the cystoscope is placed at the external meatus and gently inserted under direct (or video) guidance. The cystoscope should initially be inserted with a slight downward angle and then gently rotated under the symphysis. A direct (forward-looking) cystoscope may be used to facilitate inspection of the internal sphincter (urethral–vesical junction) and the urethra itself. The entire lumen of the urethra, bladder wall, the trigone, and ureteral openings should be examined systematically. If problems are encountered viewing the trigone, using a cystoscope with a downward-viewing angle facilitates the process.

If the goal is to examine for ureteral patency, 5 mL of indigo carmine can be given intravenously 10 to 15 minutes before the cystoscopy, followed by observation of blue-stained urine from the ureteral orifices.

At the completion of the procedure, the patient may empty her bladder or the bladder may be drained by catheter, as desired.

COMPLICATIONS

Infection, bleeding, dysuria, and urinary retention are possible, although unlikely. Perforation or bladder rupture possible (more likely with biopsy).

FOLLOW-UP

Based on indications.

CPT CODE(S)

52000   Cystoscopy

REFERENCES

Level II
Gilmour DT, Das S, Flowerdew G: Rates of urinary tract injury from gynecologic surgery and the role of intraoperative cystoscopy. Obstet Gynecol 2006;107:1366.

Level III
American College of Obstetricians and Gynecologists: The role of cystourethroscopy in the generalist obstetrician–gynecologist practice. ACOG Committee Opinion 372. Obstet Gynecol 2007;110:221.
Cundiff GW, Bent AE: Endoscopic evaluation of the lower urinary tract. In Walters MD, Karram MM, eds. Urogynecology and reconstructive pelvic surgery, 3rd ed. Philadelphia, Mosby Elsevier, 2007, p 114.
Dajani AS, Taubert KA, Wilson W, et al: Prevention of bacterial endocarditis. Recommendations by the American Heart Association. JAMA 1997;277:1794.
Olson ES, Cookson BD: Do antimicrobials have a role in preventing septicemia following instrumentation of the urinary tract? J Hosp Infect 2000;45:85.

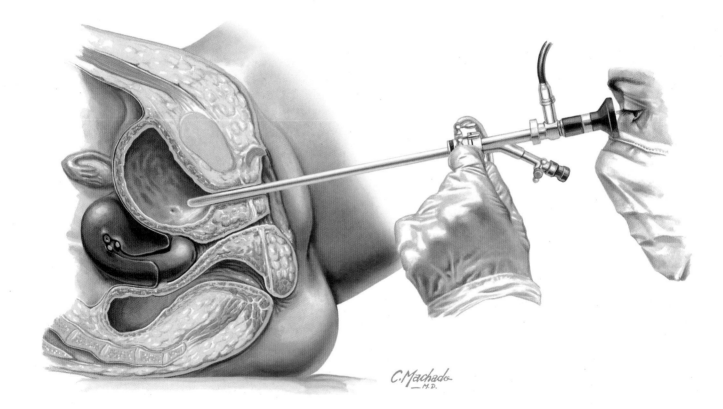

DESCRIPTION

Diaphragms (rubber or latex domes with a springy ring) are designed to provide a physical barrier between sperm and egg in conjunction with contraceptive jelly or creams to provide contraception by both barrier and spermicidal actions.

INDICATIONS

Elective. (Approximately 2% of women using contraception choose this method.)

CONTRAINDICATIONS

Known or suspected allergy to latex or other materials used in the contraceptive device. Diaphragms are not a good contraceptive choice for those who have significant pelvic floor support failure or those unwilling or unable to actively participate in the placement or removal process.

REQUIRED EQUIPMENT

- Examination gloves
- Set of graduated diaphragm fitting rings
- Water-soluble lubricant

TECHNIQUE

Diaphragms must be fitted to the individual patient, choosing the largest size that may be comfortably accommodated. (Diaphragms come in sizes that range from 50 to 105 mm in diameter, graduated in 5-mm increments. The most common size prescribed is 75 mm.) The optimal size may change with significant weight change (10 to 15+ pounds), vaginal birth, or pelvic surgery. Following delivery, diaphragms may be fitted at the 6- to 8-week postpartum visit. Diaphragms are made with coiled spring or with a flat or arcing type of rim that somewhat alters the fit. The flat type is better suited to those with a less well-defined subpubic arch; the arcing spring is best for those with less muscle tone.

Diaphragm fitting begins with a gentle, bimanual examination of the patient using the lubricated, gloved examining finger to measure the approximate distance from the back of the symphysis to the posterior vaginal fornix. A fitting ring that approximates this diameter should be selected, lubricated, and inserted into the vagina. The ring should be placed to rest in the posterior vaginal fornix with the outer portion resting in the retropubic notch. The examining finger should easily fit between the ring and the vaginal wall in all areas. The examining hand is removed and the comfort of the fit is checked. The ring should be comfortable or imperceptible when fitted and inserted properly. The patient should be asked to strain to ensure that the ring is not displaced by physical activity. It is not uncommon to have to try one or two sizes to accomplish an optimal fit.

The fitting ring should be removed (by gentle traction on the retropubic edge of the ring). Whenever possible, the actual diaphragm should next be inserted and checked in the same way. The cervix should be clearly palpable through the dome of the device. The patient should also be given the opportunity to perform the insertion and removal and confirm correct positioning and comfort in the office setting prior to actual contraceptive use.

In use, the diaphragm must be inserted before sexual intercourse commences and it must be left in place for 6 to 8 hours after. It is then removed, washed, and stored. Should additional intercourse be desired before the 6- to 8-hour time has expired, additional spermicide is applied to the vaginal side of the diaphragm and the waiting time to removal is restarted. Postcoital douching is not recommended. When correctly positioned, the diaphragm should not be noticeable by either partner.

COMPLICATIONS

Vaginal infection, urinary retention, toxic shock (2.4/100,000 when left in place >24 hours), vaginal wall trauma or erosions are all possible but unlikely with a properly fitted diaphragm that is removed at the proper intervals.

FOLLOW-UP

As needed. If the patient has not had an opportunity to practice insertion, positioning, and removal in the office, this should be offered before the diaphragm is relied on for contraception.

CPT CODE(S)

57170 Diaphragm or cervical cap fitting with instructions

REFERENCES

Level I
Bounds W, Guillebaud J, Dominik R, Dalberth B: The diaphragm with and without spermicide. A randomized, comparative efficacy trial. J Reprod Med 1995;40:764.

Level II
Cook L, Nanda K, Grimes D: Diaphragm versus diaphragm with spermicides for contraception. Cochrane Database Syst Rev 2001;CD002031.
Ferreira A, Araújo M, Regina C, et al: Effectiveness of the diaphragm, used continuously, without spermicide. Contraception 1993;48:29.
Fihn S, Latham R, Roberts P, et al: Association between diaphragm use and urinary tract infection. JAMA 1985;254:240.
Mauck C, Lai J, Schwartz J, Weiner D: Diaphragms in clinical trials: is clinician fitting necessary? Contraception 2004;69:263.

Level III
Allen RE: Diaphragm fitting. Am Fam Physician 2004;69:97.
Mishell DR Jr: Family planning. In Katz VL, Lentz GM, Lobo RA, Gershenson DM: Comprehensive Gynecology, 5th ed. Philadelphia, Mosby/Elsevier, 2007, p 279.

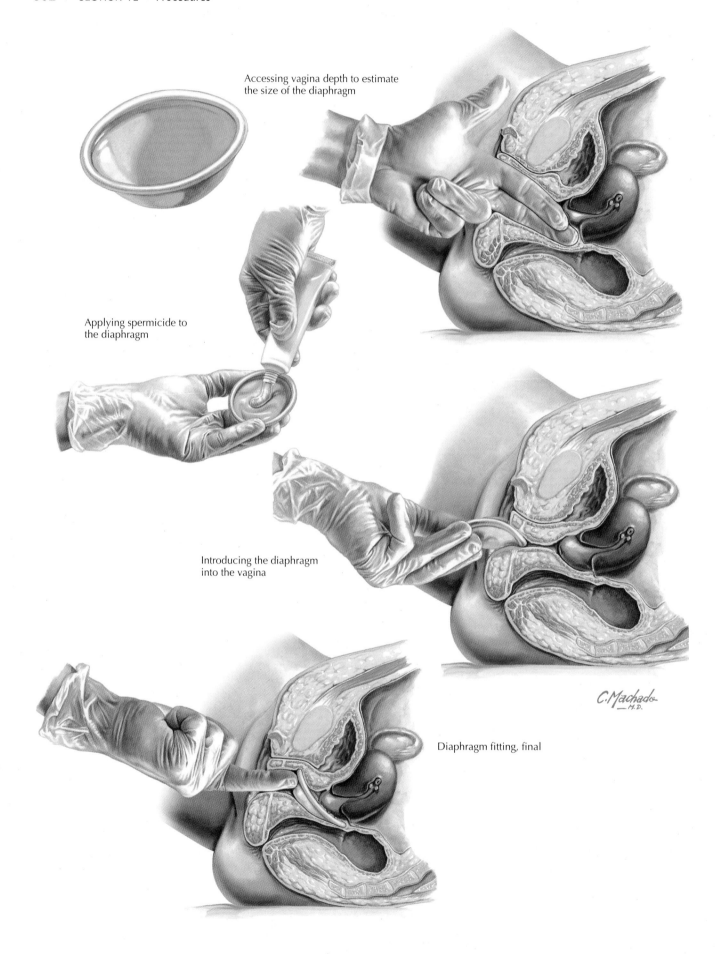

Accessing vagina depth to estimate
the size of the diaphragm

Applying spermicide to
the diaphragm

Introducing the diaphragm
into the vagina

Diaphragm fitting, final

C. Machado
M.D.

DESCRIPTION

Dilation and curettage (D&C) is dilation of the uterine cervix with the removal (by scraping) of a portion of the uterine lining or uterine contents. (The same term may be applied to any setting in which a cavity is curetted after gaining entrance through dilation, such as endocervical curettage of a cervical stump.) The procedure may be combined with other diagnostic procedures such as hysteroscopy.

INDICATIONS

Dilation and curettage may be performed for either diagnostic or therapeutic indications. This can range from the control of acute bleeding or an incomplete abortion to the temporary treatment of dysfunctional bleeding. Hysteroscopy and sonohysterography have displaced dilation and curettage as a diagnostic modality in many cases.

CONTRAINDICATIONS

Patients who are medically unstable, viable (desired) pregnancy, active pelvic inflammatory disease, blood dyscrasia.

REQUIRED EQUIPMENT

- Sterile gloves
- Skin preparation materials (generally an iodine-based antibacterial solution such as Betadine)
- Vaginal speculum or weighted vaginal speculum with Deaver or similar retractors
- Single tooth tenaculum
- Graduated cervical dilators (Hegar, Pratt, Rocket, Heaney, Hank, or similar; Goodell dilators are generally not preferred because of an increased risk of cervical laceration)
- Blunt uterine sound (optional)
- Uterine curettes (sharp preferred) in a selection of sizes
- Small stone forceps (Randall or similar)
- Polyethylene terephthalate-covered dressing (Telfa or similar) (optional)
- Suitable tissue preservation/transportation medium (10% formalin solution or similar)

For Pregnancy-Related Procedures

- Graduated suction curettes
- Suction curettage pump, tubing, and tissue collection device
- Sponge stick (may be useful to atraumatically grasp and manipulate the cervix)

TECHNIQUE

Dilation and curettage is generally performed under pericervical, regional, or general anesthesia. After appropriate informed consent is obtained, the anesthetized patient is placed in the dorsal lithotomy position, the vagina and cervix are disinfected, and the cervix is visualized using a speculum or retractors.

The cervix is grasped by the anterior lip and placed on gentle traction. If desired, the depth of the uterine cavity may be measured by the gentle passage of a blunt uterine sound. The cervix is next gently dilated by the insertion of progressively larger cervical dilators to beyond the inner cervical os. The cervix is generally dilated to the size of an 8-mm (25 to 27F) dilator, although this should be dictated by the needs of the procedure at hand. If hysteroscopy is to be performed, it is generally accomplished at this stage or during the dilation process, depending on the size of the hysteroscope to be used and the indications for the procedure.

Curettage of the uterine cavity proceeds using the largest-diameter curette that will safely pass through the dilated cervix. (This choice of size is to reduce the risk of perforation attendant to smaller devices.) The uterine wall is scraped (curetted) by gentle pressure (akin to the force of a pencil on paper) in an outward motion. The curettage proceeds with the curette repeatedly advanced to the fundus and withdrawn under mild pressure, systematically covering the surface of the endometrial cavity. The curette should be periodically withdrawn from the uterine cervix so that any tissue obtained may be collected. (Placing a small polyethylene-covered surgical dressing below the cervix, on top of the posterior retractor, in the posterior vaginal fornix may facilitate this.)

If a suction curette is used, it should be inserted to the level of the fundus with the suction off, then the suction applied and the curette withdrawn, curetting the uterine wall in the process. (This withdrawal is often carried out in a spiral manner to increase efficiency.)

To ensure that all tissue is loosened by the curettage process (and for the possibility of intracavitary polyps) a small stone forceps is passed into the uterine cavity, opened, rotated 90 degrees, closed, and removed. This may be repeated as needed.

The procedure ends with the removal of the tenaculum or sponge stick used to grasp the cervix and the extraction of the speculum or retractors. The specimens obtained should be placed in a suitable fixative or transport media. Prophylactic antibiotic coverage should be considered for those at high risk.

COMPLICATIONS

Uterine perforation, cervical laceration, infection (endometrial, myometrial, pelvic), hemorrhage (intraoperative or postoperative), uterine synechia (Asherman's syndrome)

FOLLOW-UP

Based on indications. Patients are generally advised to refrain from sexual intercourse, douching, or tampon use for 10 to 14 days.

CPT CODE(S)

58120 Dilation and curettage, diagnostic and/or therapeutic (nonobstetric)

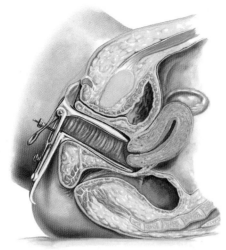

A. Dilation and curettage begins with visualization of the cervix.

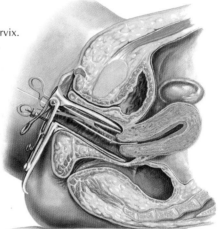

B. The cervix is grasped with a tenaculum to stabilize the cervix and uterus while the curette is introduced.

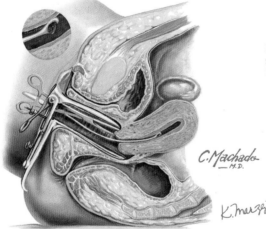

C. Gentle curettage is carried out by gentle pressure against the uterine wall while the curette is withdrawn.

59160 Curettage, postpartum
57558 Dilation and curettage of cervical stump

REFERENCES

Level I
Blohm F, Hahlin M, Nielsen S, Milsom I: Fertility after a randomised trial of spontaneous abortion managed by surgical evacuation or expectant treatment. Lancet 1997;349:995.

Trinder J, Brocklehurst P, Porter R, et al: Management of miscarriage: expectant, medical, or surgical? Results of randomised controlled trial (miscarriage treatment (MIST) trial). BMJ 2006;332:1235. Epub 2006 May 17.

Level II
Grimes DA, Schulz KF, Cates W Jr: Prophylactic antibiotics for curettage abortion. Am J Obstet Gynecol 1984;150:689.

Sotiriadis A, Makrydimas G, Papatheodorou S, Ioannidis JP: Expectant, medical, or surgical management of first-trimester miscarriage: a meta-analysis. Obstet Gynecol 2005;105:1104.

Level III
American College of Obstetricians and Gynecologists: Management of anovulatory bleeding. ACOG Practice Bulletin 14. Washington, DC, ACOG, 2000.

Good AE: Diagnostic options for assessment of postmenopausal bleeding. Mayo Clin Proc 1997;72:345.

Lobo RA: Abnormal uterine bleeding. In Katz VL, Lentz GM, Lobo RA, Gershenson DM: Comprehensive Gynecology, 5th ed. Philadelphia, Mosby/Elsevier, 2007, p 925.

DESCRIPTION

Endometrial biopsy is an office technique for obtaining tissue samples from the lining of the uterus.

INDICATIONS

Dysfunctional uterine bleeding, postmenopausal bleeding, menorrhagia, infertility (selected cases), endometrial or pelvic infections (e.g., tuberculosis), or other situations in which a tissue diagnosis is indicated. Because it is associated with some discomfort and a small but not insignificant risk of perforation or infections and carries not only the cost of the procedure but also the cost of histologic diagnosis, this procedure is best suited for diagnosis, not screening.

CONTRAINDICATIONS

Pregnancy, active pelvic inflammatory disease, significant vaginal infection, profuse bleeding, blood dyscrasia. Endometrial biopsy should generally be performed during the first 14 to 16 days of the menstrual cycle to avoid inadvertent disruption of an undiagnosed pregnancy. (Biopsies performed within 10 to 14 days beyond a temperature rise or luteinizing hormone surge will generally not interfere with implantation during that cycle.)

REQUIRED EQUIPMENT

- Disposable endometrial sampling device (e.g., Accurette, Explora, Gynocheck, Pipelle, Z-Sampler, and others) or reusable curette (Novak or other curette)
- Sterile single-tooth tenaculum (optional)
- Sterile uterine sound (optional)
- Sterile lacrimal duct probe (optional)
- Skin preparation materials (generally an iodine-based antibacterial solution such as Betadine)
- Suitable tissue preservation/transportation medium (10% formalin solution or similar)
- Pelvic examination equipment (examination gloves, lubricant, speculum, light source)

TECHNIQUE

The discomfort of endometrial biopsy may be decreased by premedicating with a single oral dose of a nonsteroidal anti-inflammatory agent given in doses usually used to treat dysmenorrhea.

Although this is an office procedure, informed consent is generally considered necessary. The patient is prepared and positioned as for a routine pelvic examination. After the cervix has been visualized, it is disinfected with a topical antiseptic (e.g., Betadine).

When the patient is parous, endometrial sampling often may be accomplished without stabilizing or dilating the cervix; both of these procedures produce mild to moderate discomfort and should be avoided when possible. The sampling device is gently introduced into the uterine cavity and the depth is noted. For suction devices such as the Pipelle or Z-Sampler, the piston is withdrawn (producing a vacuum), and the curette itself is gradually withdrawn by use of a spiral or twisting motion. If an adequate tissue sample is obtained, it should be placed in fixative, completing the procedure. If additional tissue is needed, the piston may be advanced to a point just short of expelling the sample, the device again advanced into the uterine cavity, and the procedure repeated. (If tissue already obtained is to be expelled before attempting a second or subsequent try, care must be taken to avoid contact with the fixative solution or any bacterial contamination.)

Open curettes, such as the Novak, or rigid suction cannula should be gently inserted to the apex of the uterine cavity and then withdrawn in a straight line, using light pressure against the uterine wall. Tissue obtained may be removed from the opening of the curette using the point of a broken (but still sterile) wooden cotton-tipped applicator.

If significant cervical stenosis is encountered (or there is significant patient discomfort) a paracervical block using a few milliliters of 1% lidocaine (or similar) may be appropriate. The use of a lachrymal duct probe may assist in finding the path of the endocervical canal, but its fine size also increases the risk of a "false passage."

COMPLICATIONS

Uterine perforation (1 to 2/1000), infection (endometrial, myometrial, pelvic). Vasovagal syncope during the procedure may occur but is generally transient.

FOLLOW-UP

Based on indications. Patients are generally advised to refrain from sexual intercourse, douching, or tampon use for 10 to 14 days.

CPT CODE(S)

58100 Endometrial sampling (biopsy) with or without endocervical sampling (biopsy) without cervical dilation, any method (separate procedure)

REFERENCES

Level I
Lipscomb GH, Lopatine SM, Stovall TG, Ling FW: A randomized comparison of the Pipelle, Accurate, and Explora endometrial sampling devices. Am J Obstet Gynecol 1994;170:591.

Nolan TE, Smith RP, Smith MT, Gallup DC: A prospective evaluation of an endometrial suction curette. J Gynecol Surg 1992; 8:231.

Level II
Dijkhuizen FP, Mol BW, Brolmann HA, Heintz AP: The accuracy of endometrial sampling in the diagnosis of patients with endometrial carcinoma and hyperplasia—A meta-analysis. Cancer 2000; 89:1765.

Ferry J, Farnsworth A, Webster M, Wren B: The efficacy of the Pipelle endometrial biopsy in detecting endometrial carcinoma. Aust NZ J Obstet Gynaecol 1993;33:76.

Goldchmit R, Katz Z, Blickstein I, et al: The accuracy of endometrial Pipelle sampling with and without sonographic measurement of endometrial thickness. Obstet Gynecol 1993, 82:727.

Larson DM, Broste SK: Histopathologic adequacy of office endometrial biopsies taken with the Z-sampler and Novak curette in premenopausal and postmenopausal women. J Reprod Med 1994; 39:300.

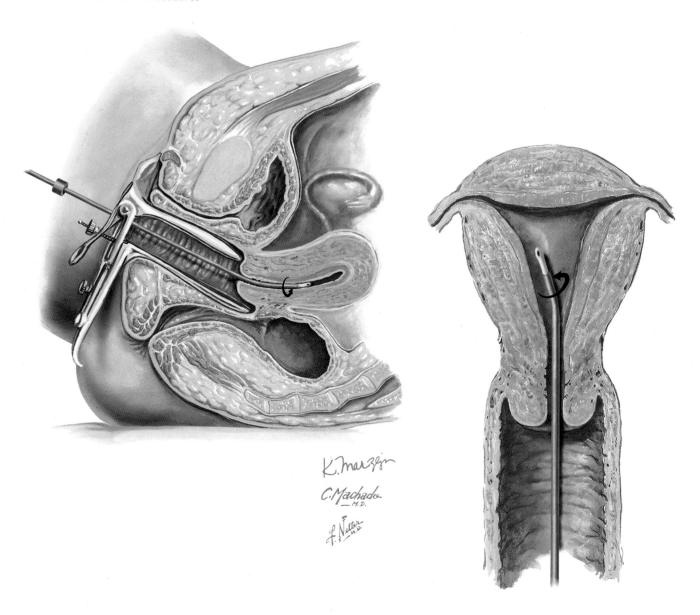

Law J: Histological sampling of the endometrium—A comparison between formal curettage and the Pipelle sampler. Br J Obstet Gynaecol 1993;100:503.

Warwick A, Ferryman S, Musgrove C, Redman C: An evaluation of the gynocheck for endometrial sampling. J Obstet Gynaecol 1993;13:198.

Level III

American College of Obstetricians and Gynecologists: Management of anovulatory bleeding. ACOG Practice Bulletin 14. Washington, DC, ACOG, 2000.

Chambers JT, Chambers SK: Endometrial sampling: When? Where? Why? With what? Clin Obstet Gynecol 1992;35:28.

Good AE: Diagnostic options for assessment of postmenopausal bleeding. Mayo Clin Proc 1997;72:345.

Katz VL: Diagnostic procedures. In Katz VL, Lentz GM, Lobo RA, Gershenson DM: Comprehensive Gynecology, 5th ed. Philadelphia, Mosby/Elsevier, 2007, p 227.

DESCRIPTION

Forceps-aided delivery is a method of assisting or expediting vaginal vertex delivery through the application of obstetric forceps. (Discussion here is limited to low or outlet forceps with the fetus presenting within 45 degrees of directly occiput anterior.)

INDICATIONS

Fetal: nonreassuring fetal status, acute fetal distress. Maternal: fatigue, prolonged second stage of labor (nulliparous women: lack of continuing progress for 3 hours with regional anesthesia or 2 hours without regional anesthesia; multiparous women: lack of continuing progress for 2 hours with regional anesthesia or 1 hour without regional anesthesia), certain types of pulmonary, cardiac, or neurologic disease.

CONTRAINDICATIONS

Incompletely dilated cervix, significant fetal malpresentation, unengaged fetal head, intact fetal membranes, inability to assess fetal position or obtain maternal cooperation, distorted or contracted maternal pelvic anatomy, gestational age less than 34 weeks, fetal demineralization or clotting disorder.

REQUIRED EQUIPMENT

- Standard equipment for spontaneous vaginal delivery, including sterile gowns and gloves
- Fetal heart rate monitor
- Traction forceps (Simpson, Tucker-McLane or similar)

TECHNIQUE

Adequate maternal anesthesia or analgesia should be ensured in all but the most extreme circumstances. Whenever possible, the maternal bladder should be emptied (by catheter). The exact position of the fetal head must be ascertained by palpation of the sagittal suture and fontanels. All other preparations for vaginal delivery should be in place before forceps are applied.

Correct placement of forceps occurs only when the long axis of the blades corresponds to the occipitomental diameter, with the major portion of the blade lying over the face, the concave margins of the blades directed toward the sagittal suture (with the fetus in the occiput anterior position). To accomplish this, the left blade (both operator's and patient's left) is introduced into the vagina next to the fetal head using the operator's right hand or fingers within the vaginal canal. The vaginal hand is used as a guide to accomplish the placement while the external hand provides only minimal support. The introduction is accomplished by starting with the handle perpendicular to the floor and the cephalic curve of the blade resting against the fetal head. The internal hand guides the blade inward, upward, and with a rotation that brings the forceps handle through a wide outward arc ending parallel to the floor. This arc is necessary to accommodate both the cephalic and pelvic curves of the device. A preliminary assessment of placement adequacy should be made before the right blade is placed. The right blade is placed in a similar arcing manner using the operator's left hand as the internal hand, with the right providing simple support.

Before the two forceps blades are articulated, the position on the fetal head should be verified. A correct position will be evident by symmetry of the blades in comparison with the sagittal sutures and posterior fontanel. If necessary, one or both blades may be gently maneuvered (using fingers within the vagina) to accomplish optimal positioning. Removal and re-placement is sometimes necessary.

Traction is generally applied by the placement of the fingers on the upper surface of the handles or shanks and the thumbs below. Traction on the articulated forceps begins in a horizontal or slightly downward (axis of the maternal pelvic canal) manner. Traction should be intermittent and, when possible, coordinated with maternal expulsive efforts. To mimic the normal birth process, traction in the horizontal plane continues until the descending fetal head distends the vulva. (An episiotomy, if required, may be performed at this point.)

As the fetal head further distends the vulva, the axis of traction is gradually rotated upward, mimicking the normal extension process of the head as it rotates under the symphysis. Once the brow is palpable through the perineum, the blades may be removed and the fetal head delivered by pressure on the perineum (modified Ritgen maneuver). More often, the blades may be left in place until the fetal chin has cleared the perineum. The remainder of the delivery proceeds as with a spontaneous delivery.

COMPLICATIONS

It is difficult (if not impossible) to separate the effects of forceps-aided vaginal delivery from those of spontaneous vaginal delivery. Both randomized trials and meta-analysis studies have failed to show conclusive differences. Both forceps delivery and vacuum extraction have been associated with the development of maternal hematomas and possibly linked to pelvic floor injury. However, other factors associated with pelvic floor injury include normal spontaneous vaginal delivery, episiotomy, prolonged second stage of labor, and increased fetal size. Similarly, studies have failed to identify neonatal or fetal injuries or developmental abnormalities that can be directly linked to forceps delivery. (The morbidity that previously had been thought to be due to operative vaginal delivery actually may have resulted from the process of abnormal labor that led to the need for intervention.)

CPT CODE(S)

59400   Routine obstetric care including antepartum care, vaginal delivery (with or without episiotomy, and/or forceps) and postpartum care

59610   Routine obstetric care including antepartum care, vaginal delivery (with or without episiotomy, and/or forceps) and postpartum care, after previous cesarean delivery

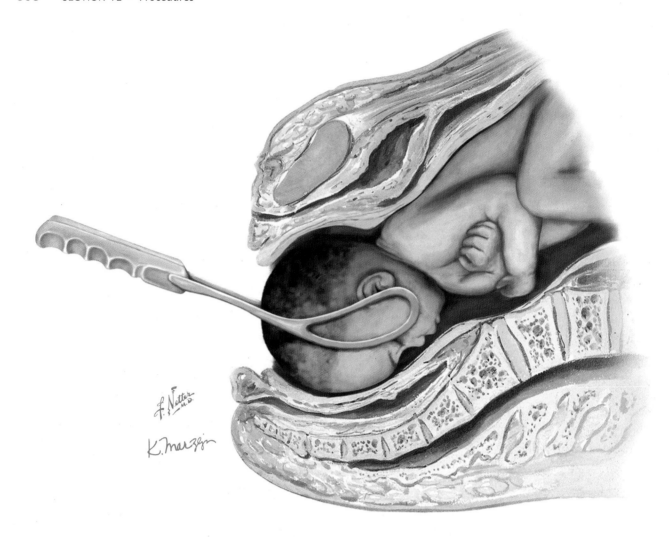

59409 Vaginal delivery only (with or without episiotomy and/or forceps);

59410 Vaginal delivery only (with or without episiotomy and/or forceps); including postpartum care

59612 Vaginal delivery only, after previous cesarean delivery (with or without episiotomy and/or forceps);

59614 Vaginal delivery only, after previous cesarean delivery (with or without episiotomy and/or forceps); including postpartum care

REFERENCES

Level I

Carmody F, Grant A, Mutch L, et al: Follow up of babies delivered in a randomized controlled comparison of vacuum extraction and forceps delivery. Acta Obstet Gynecol Scand 1986;65:763.

Carmona F, Martinez-Roman S, Manau D, et al: Immediate maternal and neonatal effects of low-forceps delivery according to the new criteria of The American College of Obstetricians and Gynecologists compared with spontaneous vaginal delivery in term pregnancies. Am J Obstet Gynecol 1995;173:55.

Vacca A, Grant A, Wyatt G, Chalmers I: Portsmouth operative delivery trial: a comparison of vacuum extraction and forceps delivery. Br J Obstet Gynaecol 1983;90:1107.

Yancey MK, Herpolsheimer A, Jordan GD, et al: Maternal and neonatal effects of outlet forceps delivery compared with spontaneous vaginal delivery in term pregnancies. Obstet Gynecol 1991; 78:646.

Level II

Johanson RB, Menon BKV: Vacuum extraction versus forceps for assisted vaginal delivery (Cochrane Review). In The Cochrane Library, Issue 4. Oxford, Update Software, 1999.

Ngan HY, Miu P, Ko L, Ma HK: Long-term neurological sequelae following vacuum extractor delivery. Aust N Z J Obstet Gynaecol 1990;30:111.

Towner D, Castro MA, Eby-Wilkens E, Gilbert WM: Effect of mode of delivery in nulliparous women on neonatal intracranial injury. N Engl J Med 1999;341:1709.

Wesley BD, van den Berg BJ, Reece EA: The effect of forceps delivery on cognitive development. Am J Obstet Gynecol 1993;169:1091.

Level III

American College of Obstetricians and Gynecologists: Operative vaginal delivery. ACOG Practice Bulletin 17. Washington, DC, ACOG, 2000.

American College of Obstetricians and Gynecologists: Vaginal birth after previous cesarean delivery. ACOG Practice Bulletin 54. Obstet Gynecol 2004;104:203.

Cunningham FG, Gant NF, Leveno KJ, et al, eds. Williams Obstetrics, 21st ed. New York, McGraw-Hill, 2001, p 486.

Gei AF, Belfort MA: Forceps-assisted vaginal delivery. Obstet Gynecol Clin North Am 1999;26:345.

Handa VL, Harris TA, Ostergard DR: Protecting the pelvic floor: obstetric management to prevent incontinence and pelvic organ prolapse. Obstet Gynecol 1996;88:470.

DESCRIPTION

Hysteroscopy allows direct visual inspection of the uterine cavity. This may also serve as a portal for other diagnostic or therapeutic measures. (The hysteroscope may be used to perform vaginoscopy in young girls or infants. When used in this way, distending media are generally not required or indicated.)

INDICATIONS

Dysfunctional uterine bleeding, postmenopausal bleeding, menorrhagia, infertility (selected cases) or recurrent abortion, endometrial or pelvic infections (e.g., tuberculosis), missing intrauterine contraceptive device, or other situations where viewing the endometrial cavity can establish a diagnosis. Hysteroscopy may be used as the vehicle for transcervical sterilization, polypectomy, myomectomy, resection of intrauterine septa or adhesions, the retrieval of contraceptive devices, and other procedures.

CONTRAINDICATIONS

Acute bleeding (if carbon dioxide is used), acute pelvic infection, known uterine or cervical cancer, pregnancy (known or suspected), recent uterine perforation, uncooperative patient, vaginitis (relative).

REQUIRED EQUIPMENT

- Sterile gloves
- Operating vaginal speculum (open sided)
- Skin preparation materials (generally an iodine-based antibacterial solution such as Betadine)
- Single tooth tenaculum
- Blunt uterine sound (optional)
- Hysteroscope (flexible or rigid, 3 to 5 mm diameter, 0-, 12-, 30-, or 70-degree viewing angle; 10 mm or greater devices are available for operative procedures but are better suited to the ambulatory surgery setting)
- Insufflator (carbon dioxide, constant flow type) and light source (both compatible with the brand and type of hysteroscope chosen). (Other distending media, such as 32% dextran or 5% dextrose and water, may be used but CO_2 offers the most suitable medium for office use. Media such as dextran are preferred in the ambulatory surgery setting when operative procedures are likely to be performed.)
- Lidocaine (1%) without epinephrine, syringe and 22- to 25- gauge spinal (4″) needle or lidocaine spray
- Video or photographic equipment may be attached to the hysteroscope as desired (optional)

TECHNIQUE

Hysteroscopy is most easily performed during the early follicular phase when the endometrium is thinnest. Because of the nature and risks of hysteroscopy, informed consent should be obtained prior to initiating the procedure. The discomfort of hysteroscopy may be decreased by premedicating with a single oral dose of a nonsteroidal anti-inflammatory agent given in doses usually used to treat dysmenorrhea.

The patient should be placed in the dorsal lithotomy position, and a pelvic examination should be performed to determine the current size, shape, and position of the uterus. The vaginal speculum should be placed to allow clear access to the cervix. With the cervix in view, the cervix is disinfected with an appropriate antiseptic solution. If an anesthetic is to be used (generally advisable), a pericervical block should be placed or the anesthetic material applied at this time.

If the patient is parous and the cervical os is open, a tenaculum may not be required, although it is generally recommended. A uterine sound may be used to gently dilate the cervix or provide information about the axis and depth of the uterine cavity, if needed.

With the hysteroscope appropriately connected to the insufflator and light source, the tip of the hysteroscope is brought into contact with the external cervical os, and insufflation is begun (approximately 30 cc per minute). The hysteroscope is next advanced along the endocervical canal under direct vision, when a clear view ahead is available and resistance to advancement is minimal. When the body of the uterus is entered, carbon dioxide flow rates may have to be increased to provide adequate distention of the cavity, but intrauterine pressure should never be allowed to exceed 100 torr (mm Hg).

Inspection of the entire uterine cavity should be performed in a systematic way. The tubal ostia should be identified and the fundus of the uterus should be inspected. The endocervical canal should be inspected as the hysteroscope is withdrawn, if it was not evaluated at the beginning of the procedure.

If dextran has been used as the distending medium, it is imperative to clean the hysteroscope immediately after the completion of the procedure.

COMPLICATIONS

Uterine perforation, infection (endometrial, myometrial, pelvic). (Infection following hysteroscopy is rare, and prophylactic antibiotics are not recommended unless indicated by factors such as valvular heart disease.) Vasovagal syncope during the procedure may occur but is generally transient. Shoulder pain, unilateral or bilateral, is common if carbon dioxide is used. Gas embolism has rarely been reported. Fluid overload may occur when dextrose and water are used as the distending media.

FOLLOW-UP

Based on indications.

CPT CODE(S)

56350 Hysteroscopy, diagnostic (separate procedure)
56351 Hysteroscopy, surgical: with sampling (biopsy) of endometrium and/or polypectomy; with or without D&C
56355 Hysteroscopy, surgical: with removal of impacted foreign body

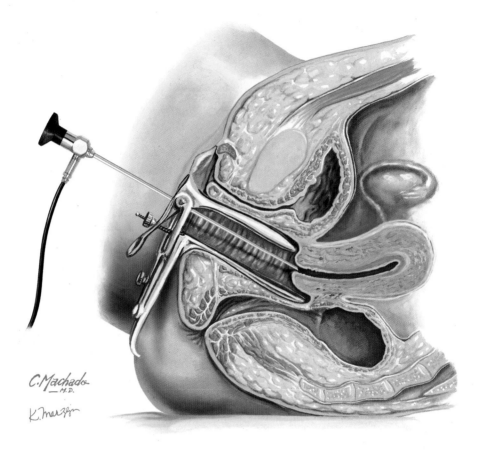

C. Machado
M.D.

K. mazzn

REFERENCES

Level I

Bain C, Parkin DE, Cooper KG: Is outpatient diagnostic hysteroscopy more useful than endometrial biopsy alone for the investigation of abnormal uterine bleeding in unselected premenopausal women? A randomised comparison. BJOG 2002;109:805.

Barik S: Topical anaesthesia for diagnostic hysteroscopy and endometrial biopsy for postmenopausal women: a randomised placebo-controlled double-blind study. Br J Obstet Gynaecol 1997; 104:1326.

Cicinelli E, Didonna T, Ambrosi G, et al: Topical anaesthesia for diagnostic hysteroscopy and endometrial biopsy in postmenopausal women: a randomised placebo-controlled double-blind study. Br J Obstet Gynaecol 1997;104:316.

Kremer C, Duffy S, Moroney M: Patient satisfaction with outpatient hysteroscopy versus day case hysteroscopy: randomized controlled trial. BMJ 2000;320:279.

Lau WC, Lo WK, Tam WH, Yuen PM: Paracervical anaesthesia in outpatient hysteroscopy: A randomised double-blind placebo-controlled trial. Br J Obstet Gynaecol 1999;106:356.

Nagele F, Lockwood G, Magos AL: Randomised placebo controlled trial of mefenamic acid for premedication at outpatient hysteroscopy: a pilot study. Br J Obstet Gynaecol 1997;104:842.

Sagiv R, Sadan O, Boaz M, et al: A new approach to office hysteroscopy compared with traditional hysteroscopy: a randomized controlled trial. Obstet Gynecol 2006;108:387.

Soriano D, Ajaj S, Chuong T, et al: Lidocaine spray and outpatient hysteroscopy: randomized placebo-controlled trial. Obstet Gynecol 2000;96:661.

Level II

Clark TJ, Voit D, Gupta JK, et al: Accuracy of hysteroscopy in the diagnosis of endometrial cancer and hyperplasia: a systematic quantitative review. JAMA 2002;288:1610.

Sharma M, Taylor A, di Spiezio Sardo A, et al: Outpatient hysteroscopy: traditional versus the "no-touch" technique. BJOG 2005; 112:963.

van Dongen H, de Kroon CD, Jacobi CE, et al: Diagnostic hysteroscopy in abnormal uterine bleeding: a systematic review and meta-analysis. BJOG 2007;114:664.

Level III

American College of Obstetricians and Gynecologists: Management of anovulatory bleeding. ACOG Practice Bulletin 14. Washington, DC, ACOG, 2000.

Apgar BS, DeWitt D: Diagnostic hysteroscopy. Am Fam Physician 1992;46:19S, 29S, 35S.

Gambone JC, Munro MG: Office sonography and office hysteroscopy. Curr Opin Obstet Gynecol 1993;5:733.

Gimpelson RJ: Office hysteroscopy. Clin Obstet Gynecol 1992; 35:270.

Katz VL: Diagnostic procedures. In Katz VL, Lentz GM, Lobo RA, Gershenson DM: Comprehensive Gynecology, 5th ed. Philadelphia, Mosby/Elsevier, 2007, p 230.

Lewis BV: Hysteroscopy for the investigation of abnormal uterine bleeding. Br J Obstet Gynaecol 1990;97:283.

March CM: Hysteroscopy. J Reprod Med 1992;37:293.

Siegler AM: Office hysteroscopy. Obstet Gynecol Clin North Am 1995;22:457.

Siegler AM, Kemmann E: Hysteroscopy. Obstet Gynecol Surv 1975; 30:567.

Siegler AM, Valle RF: Therapeutic hysteroscopic procedures. Fertil Steril 1988;50:685.

Intrauterine Contraceptive Device Insertion

DESCRIPTION

Placement of an intrauterine contraceptive device (IUCD).

INDICATIONS

Elective, desiring contraception. (The IUCD is associated with an efficacy rate that is comparable to sterilization and oral contraceptives.) The IUCD may be a particularly good choice for women with diabetes, thromboembolism, menorrhagia, or dysmenorrhea. The copper IUCD may be preferable for those breastfeeding or with breast cancer or liver disease. The copper IUCD may be placed up to 5 days after unprotected intercourse as an emergency contraceptive measure. The progestin-releasing IUCD may be used as a treatment for menorrhagia in selected patients.

CONTRAINDICATIONS

Active cervical infection, acute sexually transmitted disease, allergy to any component of the device, dysfunctional uterine bleeding (undiagnosed), dysmenorrhea, genital actinomycoses, history of ectopic pregnancy (relative), immediate postpartum period (less than 8 weeks), immunocompromise (relative), IUCD in situ (unremoved), malignancy (uterine or cervical, known or suspected), multiple sexual partners (relative), pelvic inflammatory disease (PID) (current or past 3 months), pregnancy (known or suspected), sexually transmitted disease (current), uterine cavity malformation, vaginitis, Wilson disease (copper IUCD only).

REQUIRED EQUIPMENT

* Intrauterine contraceptive device in sterile package
* Skin (vaginal) preparation materials (iodine-based antibacterial solution [e.g., Betadine] or other suitable cleansing agents)
* Vaginal speculum
* Tenaculum
* Uterine sound (optional)
* Nonsterile examination gloves
* Scissor (long)
* Sterile gloves (optional with "no touch" technique)

TECHNIQUE

The discomfort of an IUCD insertion may be decreased by premedicating with a single oral dose of a nonsteroidal anti-inflammatory agent given in doses usually used to treat dysmenorrhea or through the use of 2% intracervical lignocaine gel. Before beginning the procedure, the size, shape, and location of the uterus should be determined. The cervix should be visualized with the aid of a speculum and then disinfected. In patients who are parous without significant uterine flexion, a tenaculum is often not needed.

The technique used to place the contraceptive device in its proper location in the uterine cavity varies slightly based on the device. Each use follows the same general sequence of steps: loading the IUCD into its carrier or placement device, placing the IUCD in position in the uterine cavity, withdrawing the placement instrument leaving the IUCD behind, verifying correct placement, and trimming the marker sting(s).

ParaGuard T380A

The IUCD must be loaded into its insertion device, which may be accomplished using either sterile gloves or a "no touch" technique. With sterile gloves the device is grasped, folded, and inserted into the distal end of the insertion tool. In the "no touch" method the same ends must be accomplished, but manipulating the IUCD through the outer package wrapper carries them out.

Once the IUCD is in the insertion device, the movable flange is moved backward on the insertion tube until it corresponds to the expected or measured depth of the uterus. The IUCD and inserter are placed at the disinfected external cervical os and gently advanced until resistance indicates that the fundus has been reached. With the obturator held in place, the insertion tube is withdrawn, leaving the device in the correct position. The obturator should not be advanced as the insertion tube is withdrawn. (The insertion tube may be slightly readvanced to ensure that the IUCD lies against the fundus, and it then is withdrawn completely.) The string of the device should be trimmed at a point approximately 1 to 2 cm from the external os.

Mirena

The Mirena IUCD is supplied with a self-loading inserter. To insert this device, the package is opened, taking care to maintain the sterility of the contents. The threads of the IUCD must be freed from the base of the inserter, and the slider (located in the handle of the inserter) advanced to the position closest to the IUCD itself. The arms of the device itself should be in a horizontal position when the centimeter scale of the inserter is facing upward. Immediately prior to insertion, the IUCD is retracted into the inserter tube by traction on the strings where they emerge from the handle of the inserter. This will result in the arms of the IUCD folding inward and their distal knobs occluding the inserter tube. The treads of the IUCD must now be locked into place by raising them into the cleft in the handle. The flange on the inserter tube should be moved on the centimeter scale so it coincides with the measured uterine depth.

To place the IUCD in the uterine cavity, the tip of the IUCD and insertion tool are placed against the disinfected cervical os, and traction on the os is applied. Gentle pressure is exerted, advancing until the flange is approximately 1.5 to 2 cm from the cervix. This will allow sufficient room for the arms of the IUCD to expand on deployment. While this position is maintained the slider is pulled back to the raised horizontal line on the handle. This will release the

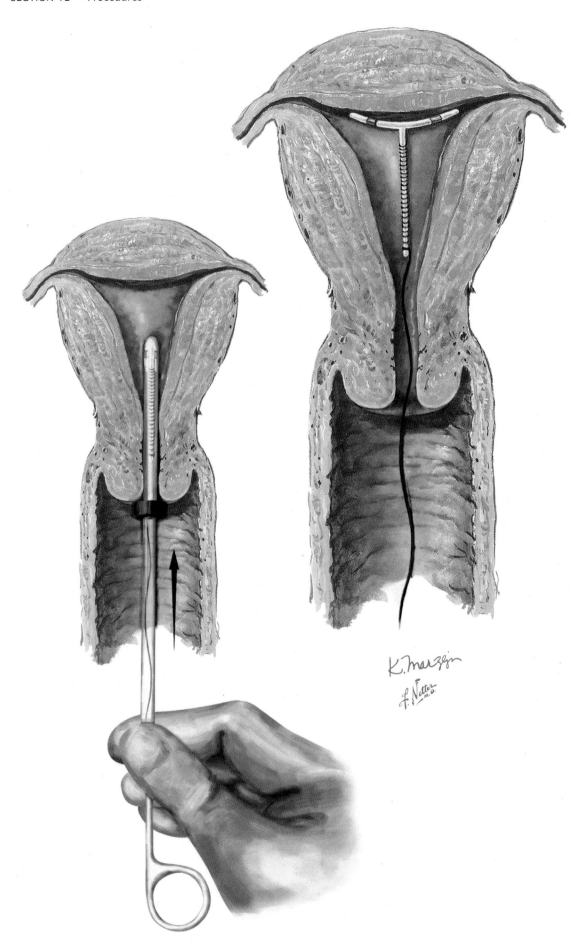

arms from the inserter tube. After 30 seconds are allowed for the arms to regain their full extension, the inserter should be gently advanced until the flange meets the cervix, ensuring proper fundal placement of the device. While the inserter is held steady, the slider is pulled to its fully retracted position, releasing the IUCD. Being careful that the treads are hanging freely, the device is now removed and the threads trimmed about 3 cm from the cervix.

Although an IUCD may be placed at any point in a menstrual cycle (after pregnancy has been ruled out), it is preferable to insert it 7 to 10 days after the onset of menstruation. Insertion at this point of the cycle is associated with a lower expulsion rate. The patient must be counseled to use a backup method of contraception during this cycle.

When gentle pressure does not result in the IUCD insertion tool's advancing through the cervix, a tenaculum may be used to stabilize the cervix. Traction on the tenaculum may result in some straightening of the canal, further aiding insertion. In some cases, it may be necessary to use a sterile uterine sound to identify the axis of the canal, provide modest cervical dilation, or confirm the depth to the uterine cavity.

IUCDs should not be left in the folded position inside the inserter for more than 1 to 2 minutes. Prolonged folding will result in a device that will not unfold properly in the uterine cavity, increasing the risk of expulsion or contraceptive failure.

COMPLICATIONS

Vasovagal reaction, pain, uterine perforation (approximately 1 in 1000 insertions), infection (uterine or pelvic, most common in the first 20 days after insertion), bleeding, expulsion of the device.

FOLLOW-UP

Generally, women should be re-evaluated 1 to 4 weeks after IUCD placement. The patient should be advised to periodically verify the presence and length of the IUCD strings. Expulsion is most common during menstruation and during the first 6 months of use. Amenorrhea in a woman using the copper IUCD should prompt a pregnancy test. Any woman who misses a period and experiences pain should have ectopic pregnancy ruled out. Women should be instructed about warning signs of pelvic infection, particularly in the first month after insertion of the device, when the risk of pelvic infection is greater.

CPT CODE(S)

58300   Insertion of intrauterine device (IUD), not including device

X4633   Charge for cost of copper IUD
X4634   Charge for cost of progesterone IUD

REFERENCES

Level I
Oloto EJ, Bromham DR, Murty JA: Pain and discomfort perception at IUD insertion—Effect of short-duration, low-volume, intracervical application of two per cent lignocaine gel (Instillagel (TM))—A preliminary study. Br J Fam Plann 1997;22:177.
Walsh TL, Bernstein GS, Grimes DA, et al: Effect of prophylactic antibiotics on morbidity associated with IUD insertion: results of a pilot randomized controlled trial. IUD Study Group. Contraception 1994;50:319.

Level II
Anteby E, Revel A, Ben-Chetrit A, et al: Intrauterine device failure: relation to its location within the uterine cavity. Obstet Gynecol 1993;81:112.
Duenas JL, Albert A, Carrasco F: Intrauterine contraception in nulligravid vs parous women. Contraception 1996;53:23.
Farley TM, Rosenberg MJ, Rowe PJ, et al: Intrauterine devices and pelvic inflammatory disease: an international perspective. Lancet 1992;339:785.
Grimes DA, Schulz KF: Prophylactic antibiotics for intrauterine device insertion: a metaanalysis of the randomized controlled trials. Contraception 1999;60:57.
Hubacher D, Lara-Ricalde R, Taylor DJ, et al: Use of copper intrauterine devices and the risk of tubal infertility among nulligravid women. N Engl J Med 2001;345:561.
Lethaby AE, Cooke I, Rees M: Progesterone or progestogen-releasing intrauterine systems for heavy menstrual bleeding. Cochrane Database Syst Rev 2005;4:CD002126.
Polis CB, Schaffer K, Blanchard K, et al: Advance provision of emergency contraception for pregnancy prevention. Cochrane Database Syst Rev 2007;2:CD005497.
Zhou L, Xiao B: Emergency contraception with Multiload Cu-375 SL IUD: a multicenter clinical trial. Contraception 2001;64:107.

Level III
American College of Obstetricians and Gynecologists: Intrauterine device. ACOG Practice Bulletin 59. Obstet Gynecol 2005;105:223.
American College of Obstetricians and Gynecologists: Noncontraceptive uses of the levonorgestrel intrauterine system. ACOG Committee Opinion 337. Obstet Gynecol 2006;107:1479.
Grimes DA: Intrauterine device and upper-genital-tract infection. Lancet 2000;356:1013.
Mishell DR Jr: Family planning. In Katz VL, Lentz GM, Lobo RA, Gershenson DM: Comprehensive Gynecology, 5th ed. Philadelphia, Mosby/Elsevier, 2007, p 306.
Stanford JB, Mikolajczyk RT: Mechanisms of action of intrauterine devices: update and estimation of postfertilization effects. Am J Obstet Gynecol 2002;187:1699.
World Health Organization: Mechanism of action, safety and efficacy of intrauterine devices. Geneva, WHO, 1997.

Intrauterine Contraceptive Device Removal

DESCRIPTION

Removal of an intrauterine contraceptive device (IUCD).

INDICATIONS

Elective, desiring a return to fertility or to replace a device after its approved lifespan. IUCDs should also be removed in the face of active pelvic inflammatory disease, unrelenting side effects, or an intrauterine pregnancy (if possible). The IUCD does not have to be removed from an asymptomatic patient in whom actinomycosis is found on cervical cytology.

CONTRAINDICATIONS

Unstable or uncooperative patient or those in whom the presence of an IUCD cannot be confirmed.

REQUIRED EQUIPMENT

* Skin (vaginal) preparation materials (iodine-based antibacterial solution [e.g., Betadine] or other suitable cleansing agents)
* Vaginal speculum
* Tenaculum
* Nonsterile examination gloves
* Uterine packing forceps or other long forceps
* IUD or "crochet" hook (optional)
* Cervical cytology brush (Cytobrush or similar) (optional)

TECHNIQUE

The discomfort of an IUCD removal may be decreased by premedicating with a single oral dose of a nonsteroidal anti-inflammatory agent given in doses usually used to treat dysmenorrhea or through the use of 2% intracervical lignocaine gel. Before beginning the procedure, the size, shape, and location of the uterus should be determined. The cervix should be visualized with the aid of a speculum. The cervix should be disinfected if reinsertion of a new device if planned.

When the IUCD string(s) are visible at the cervical os, gentle traction with uterine packing forceps or other suitable grasping device will result in the delivery of the IUCD. When the string is not apparent, gentle probing of the outer portion of the cervical canal with the forceps or a sterile crochet hook may locate the strings. A Cytobrush may also be placed in the endocervix and gently swept downward to locate strings. These maneuvers will often yield the string that may then be grasped as described earlier. If these maneuvers are unsuccessful in retrieving the IUCD, the cervix should be disinfected prior to any further attempts. Ultrasonography should be considered to ensure an intrauterine location of the IUCD. The possibility of an ongoing pregnancy must also be considered (if not already assessed).

An IUCD ("crochet") hook may be used under sterile conditions in the outpatient setting, or the IUCD may be removed in the operating room or ambulatory surgery setting, where hysteroscopic guidance is available. In most cases, if a hook is to be used a tenaculum to stabilize the cervix will be needed. In use, the hook is passed through the cervix to the level of the uterine fundus. As the hook is advanced, the device should be carefully monitored for vibrations, sounds, or the "feel" that the tip has encountered the IUCD. Once the hook has reached the fundus (or the IUCD, if felt), the hook is slowly rotated through 180 to 360 degrees and withdrawn. Moderate resistance to withdrawal is associated with capture of the IUCD, and persistent traction will often deliver the device. Even when no resistance is felt, removal of the hook will often deliver the string(s), allowing removal of the IUCD by conventional traction. If neither the IUCD nor its string has been retrieved in several attempts, the effort should be abandoned until the presence of the IUCD in the body has been confirmed and removal via hysteroscopy or laparoscopy has been entertained.

COMPLICATIONS

Vasovagal reaction, pain, uterine perforation (when a hook is used), infection (uterine or pelvic), bleeding.

FOLLOW-UP

Based on contraceptive plans and the indications for the removal.

CPT CODE(S)

58301   Removal of intrauterine device (IUD)

REFERENCES

Level I

Bounds W, Hutt S, Kubba A, et al: Randomised comparative study in 217 women of three disposable plastic IUCD thread retrievers. Br J Obstet Gynaecol 1992;99:915.

Level II

Andersson K, Batar I, Rybo G: Return to fertility after removal of a levonorgestrel-releasing intrauterine device and Nova-T. Contraception 1992;46:575.

Hov GG, Skjeldestad FE, Hilstad T: Use of IUD and subsequent fertility—Follow-up after participation in a randomized clinical trial. Contraception 2007;75:88. Epub 2006 Nov 14.

Hubacher D, Lara-Ricalde R, Taylor DJ, et al: Use of copper intrauterine devices and the risk of tubal infertility among nulligravid women. N Engl J Med 2001;345:561.

Ranzini AC, Wapner RJ, Davis GH: Ultrasonographically guided intrauterine contraceptive device removal before chorionic villus sampling. Am J Obstet Gynecol 1995;173:603.

Skjeldestad FE, Bratt H: Return of fertility after use of IUDs (Nova-T, MLCu250 and MLCu375). Adv Contracept 1987; 3:139.

Stanback J, Grimes D: Can intrauterine device removals for bleeding or pain be predicted at a one-month follow-up visit? A multivariate analysis. Contraception 1998;58:357.

Zhang J: Factors associated with copper T IUD removal for bleeding/pain: a multivariate analysis. Contraception 1993;48:13.

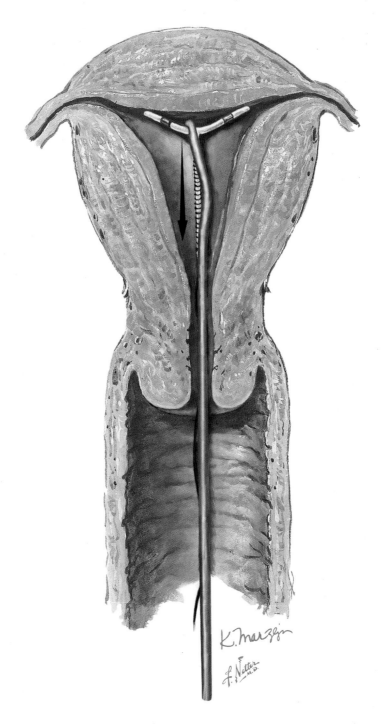

Level III

American College of Obstetricians and Gynecologists: Intrauterine device. ACOG Practice Bulletin 59. Obstet Gynecol 2005; 105:223.

Assaf A, Gohar M, Saad S, et al: Removal of intrauterine devices with missing tails during early pregnancy. Contraception 1992;45:541.

Ben-Rafael Z, Bider D: A new procedure for removal of a "lost" intrauterine device. Obstet Gynecol 1996;87:785.

Grimes DA: Intrauterine device and upper-genital-tract infection. Lancet 2000;356:1013.

Johnson BA: Insertion and removal of intrauterine devices. Am Fam Physician 2005;71:95.

Mishell DR Jr: Family planning. In Katz VL, Lentz GM, Lobo RA, Gershenson DM: Comprehensive Gynecology, 5th ed. Philadelphia, Mosby/Elsevier, 2007, p 306.

Sachs BP, Gregory K, McArdle C, Pinshaw A: Removal of retained intrauterine contraceptive devices in pregnancy. Am J Perinatol 1992;9:139.

World Health Organization: Mechanism of action, safety and efficacy of intrauterine devices. Geneva, WHO, 1997.

Wyatt S, Gallen IW, Nicholls A: A potential hazard of prolonged insertion of an intrauterine device. N Engl J Med 1994;330:1395.

Cervical Conization (Loop Electrosurgical Excision Procedure and Large Loop Excision of the Transformation Zone Conizations)

DESCRIPTION

Cervical conization is a diagnostic or therapeutic procedure that removes a cone-shaped specimen from the uterine cervix. Loop electrocautery excisional procedure (LEEP, also known as large loop excision of the transformation zone [LLETZ]) uses electric current instead of a knife to remove the cervical tissue.

INDICATIONS

Histologically verified advanced epithelial atypia (for diagnosis or therapy) or inability to adequately evaluate the cervix through colposcopy.

CONTRAINDICATIONS

Coagulopathy, advanced pregnancy, known or suspected allergy to the agents used.

REQUIRED EQUIPMENT

- Skin (vaginal) preparation materials (iodine-based antibacterial solution [e.g., Betadine] or other suitable cervical cleansing agents)
- Sterile gloves
- Nonconductive vaginal speculum
- Electrosurgical generator with output capability of at least 50 watts in both coagulation and cutting modes, a variety of waveform outputs (pure cut, blended current, and coagulation current), patient grounding pad monitor, and isolated circuitry.
- A variety of loop electrodes (size and shape to be determined at the time of the procedure based on the size and shape of the cervix and lesion to be removed)
- A smoke evacuator with odor and viral filter
- Monsel paste (ferric subsulfate solution allowed to evaporate to the consistency of paste)
- 5% acetic acid or Lugol solution (super-saturated potassium iodide)
- Kevorkian or similar endocervical curette
- Histology fixative (10% formalin) in containers
- Syringe with 25- or 27-gauge 1.5-inch needle for anesthetic injection, 1% or 2% lidocaine with or without 1:100,000 epinephrine
- 12-inch needle holder, 2-0 absorbable suture material (or similar)

TECHNIQUE

After informed consent has been obtained, the patient is placed in the dorsal lithotomy position and a return electrode ("grounding pad") is placed on the patient's thigh with the long edge directed toward the hip.

The cervix should be visualized by use of a nonconductive speculum with smoke evacuator attachment. Acetic acid or Lugol solution may be applied to the cervix to delineate the area of abnormality.

The local anesthetic should be injected submucosally into the cervix at the 3-, 6-, 9-, and 12-o'clock positions. These injections should be about 3 to 5 mm deep. The appropriate loop electrode should be selected based on the size of the lesion to be treated: lesions confined to the external cervix are most often treated with a round loop, 2 cm in width and 0.8 cm deep; for a nulliparous, small cervix, a loop 1.5 cm in width and 0.7 cm in depth is used; and for lesions extending into the endocervix, a square loop electrode, 1 cm by 1 cm, can be used.

The power setting for the electrosurgical generator depends on the manufacturer of the generator and the diameter of the loop: a 2-cm loop requires 35 to 45 watts of power and a 1-cm by 1-cm loop requires 20 to 30 watts of power. A blended current should be used.

The loop should be placed several millimeters lateral to the edge of the lesion, and a simulated pass of the loop over the lesion is made to ensure that there are no obstacles. The electrosurgical generator is then activated in the "cut" mode. The loop is pressed perpendicular into the tissue to a depth of 5 to 8 mm and then is dragged laterally across and through the endocervix, exiting at a point several millimeters past the lesions or beyond the transformation zone, whichever is farther. The resultant specimen should be dome shaped with the endocervical canal visible in the middle. Care should be taken to not press the loop greater than 4 or 5 mm deep at the lateral borders of the cervix because of the arterial blood supply located at the 3- and 9-o'clock positions of the cervix.

If the lesion is too large to be removed in a single pass, the central portion of the lesion is removed first using a 2-cm wide loop as described earlier. Additional passes are then made using the same loop to remove remaining lesion and the transformation zone, or a smaller loop may be used to extend the excision farther up the endocervical canal.

If a blended current is used, bleeding from the base of the excision site is generally minimal. If needed, hemostasis may be obtained by fulguration using the ball electrode or the application of Monsel solution.

Pelvic rest (no tampons, douching, or sexual intercourse) is generally advised for 2 to 3 weeks following the procedure, and the patient is instructed to return for heavy bleeding or bleeding that lasts more than 2 weeks.

COMPLICATIONS

Bleeding (acute and delayed), infection. Conization appears to approximately double the risk that a woman will subsequently have a preterm delivery, a low-birthweight infant, or premature rupture of the membranes.

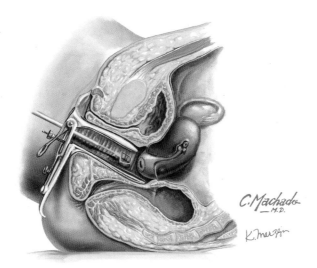

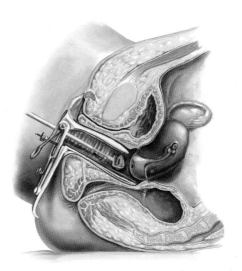

FOLLOW-UP

The cervix is generally inspected at about 6 weeks after the procedure. Treatment success for cervical intraepithelial neoplasia is generally 95%.

CPT CODE(S)

57522 Conization of cervix, with or without fulguration, with or without dilation and curettage, with or without repair; loop electrode excision

REFERENCES

Level I

Boardman LA, Steinhoff MM, Shackelton R, et al: A randomized trial of the Fischer cone biopsy excisor and loop electrosurgical excision procedure. Obstet Gynecol 2004;104:745.

Mathevet P, Dargent D, Roy M, et al: A randomized prospective study comparing three techniques of conization: cold knife, laser, and LEEP. Gynecol Oncol 1994;54:175.

Level II

Ang MS, Kaufman RH, Adam E, et al: Colposcopically directed biopsy and loop excision of the transformation zone: comparison of histologic findings. J Reprod Med 1995;40:167.

El-Bastawissi AY, Becker TM, Daling JR: Effect of cervical carcinoma in situ and its management on pregnancy outcome. Obstet Gynecol 1999;93:207.

Jackobsson M Gissler M, Sainio S, et al: Preterm delivery after surgical treatment for cervical intraepithelial neoplasia. Obstet Gynecol 2007;109:309.

Kyrgiou M, Tsoumpou I, Vrekoussis T, et al: The up-to-date evidence on colposcopy practice and treatment of cervical intraepithelial neoplasia: The Cochrane Colposcopy & Cervical Cytopathology Collaborative Group (C5 group) approach. Cancer Treat Rev 2006;32:516.

Sadler L, Saftlas A, Wang W, et al: Treatment for cervical intraepithelial neoplasia and risk of preterm delivery. JAMA 2004; 291:2100.

Sjøborg KD, Vistad I, Myhr SS, et al: Pregnancy outcome after cervical cone excision: a case-control study. Acta Obstet Gynecol Scand. 2007;86:423.

Level III

American College of Obstetricians and Gynecologists: Diagnosis and treatment of cervical carcinomas. ACOG Practice Bulletin 35. Obstet Gynecol 2002;99:855.

American College of Obstetricians and Gynecologists: Management of abnormal cervical cytology and histology. ACOG Practice Bulletin 66. Obstet Gynecol 2005;106:645.

DESCRIPTION

Pessaries are devices fitted and worn in the vagina to provide support to the pelvic organs. Pessaries are available in various sizes and shapes and are categorized as supportive (e.g., ring, Gellhorn, Gehrung) or space occupying (e.g., doughnut, cube).

INDICATIONS

Pelvic organ prolapse, urinary incontinence, cervical incompetence (lever or ring type), drug delivery. Pessaries are often used as either an alternative to surgery or as a presurgical trial.

CONTRAINDICATIONS

Undiagnosed vaginal bleeding, significant vaginal atrophy. Patients who are unable or unwilling to manage the periodic insertion and removal of the device are poor candidates.

REQUIRED EQUIPMENT

- Vaginal speculum
- Water-soluble lubricant
- Nonsterile examination gloves
- Examples of appropriate pessaries in a variety of sizes (generally the "average size" and at least one size larger and smaller)

TECHNIQUE

Pessaries will not be well tolerated or provide optimal support in the patient who is poorly estrogenized. Therefore, a minimum of 30 days of topical estrogen therapy should be instituted prior to a trial of pessary therapy in these patients.

The type of pessary chosen for a given patient is determined by the anatomic defect and the symptoms the patient is experiencing. The most commonly used forms of pessary for pelvic relaxation are the ring (or doughnut), the ball, and the cube. The indications for various types of commonly used pessaries are shown in the box. The type of pessary that can be fitted is related to the severity of prolapse. Ring pessaries are frequently a first choice, followed by Gellhorn or other pessaries if the rings do not stay in place.

Pessaries are fitted and placed in the vagina in much the same way as a contraceptive diaphragm: the depth of the vagina and the integrity of the supporting structures of the vagina are gauged as a part of the pelvic examination. The size of pessary to be fitted is based on the findings of the pelvic examination. The pessary is lubricated with a water-soluble lubricant, folded or compressed, and inserted into the vagina. (Some pessaries require specific maneuvers for their insertion; always consult the manufacturer's instructions.)

The pessary is next adjusted so that it is in the proper position based on the type: ring and lever pessaries should sit behind the cervix (when present) and rest in the retropubic notch, the Gellhorn pessary should be contained entirely within the vagina with the plate resting above the levator plane, the Gehrung pessary must bridge the cervix with the limbs resting on the levator muscles on each side, and the ball or cube pessaries should occupy and occlude the upper vagina. All pessaries must allow the easy passage of an examining finger between the pessary and the vaginal wall in all areas. The only situation in which a pessary is allowed to exert any significant pressure beneath the urethra is in the case of those devices designed for the control of urinary incontinence.

After the pessary has been placed and the fit checked, the patient should be asked to strain. The pessary may descend slightly, but its integrity should be maintained and it should return to its normal position when the patient relaxes. The patient should be allowed to stand and walk a bit with the pessary in place to ensure comfort and retention. The pessary may then be removed (if a "fitting" pessary has been used) or may be left in place (if this is to be the patient's final device). If necessary, the process should be repeated until an appropriate, comfortable fit is obtained. The fit should also be confirmed by a follow-up visit in 5 to 7 days. In most patients (50% to 73%), an appropriately sized pessary can be fitted successfully in one or two office visits.

The patient should be instructed on both the proper insertion and removal techniques. Ring pessaries should be removed by hooking a finger into the pessary's opening, gently compressing the device, and then withdrawing the pessary with gentle traction. Cube pessaries must also be compressed, but the suction created between the faces of the cube and the vaginal wall must be broken by gently separating the device from the vaginal sidewall. (The locator string often attached to these pessaries should not be used for traction.) Inflatable pessaries should be deflated prior to removal. Gellhorn and Gehrung pessaries are removed by a reversal of their insertion procedures.

COMPLICATIONS

Vaginal erosion, bleeding, infection, vaginal discharge, pain, expulsion, urinary retention, fistula formation (rare with proper fit, care, and estrogen therapy).

FOLLOW-UP

Examination 5 to 7 days after initial fitting is required to confirm proper placement, hygiene, and the absence of pressure-related problems (vaginal trauma or necrosis). Earlier evaluation (in 24 to 48 hours) may be advisable for patients who are debilitated or who require additional assistance. Follow-up should then occur in approximately 1 month and then quarterly for the duration of use. (Some authors recommend maintaining a monthly schedule indefinitely, especially in those with limited abilities to maintain the device themselves.)

CPT CODE(S)

57160   Fitting and insertion of pessary or other intravaginal support device (procedure only)

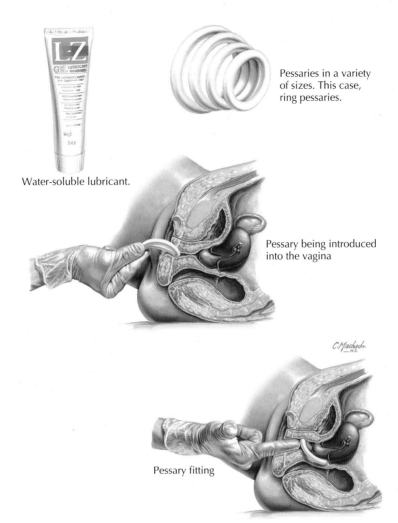

Water-soluble lubricant.

Pessaries in a variety of sizes. This case, ring pessaries.

Pessary being introduced into the vagina

Pessary fitting

Indications for Common Pessaries

Malposition: Lever type (Hodge)
Prolapse
   Uterine: Gellhorn, ring, doughnut, cube
   Vaginal: Doughnut, cube, ball (Gehrung)
   Cystocele/Rectocele: Gehrung, Schatz
Incompetent cervix: Lever, ring
Incontinence: Doughnut, lever, ring
Preoperative: Based on defect
Drug delivery: Specialized ring (17β-estradiol, medroxy-progesterone, prostaglandin E$_2$)

REFERENCES

Level I
Cundiff GW, Amundsen CL, Bent AE, et al: The PESSRI study: symptom relief outcomes of a randomized crossover trial of the ring and Gellhorn pessaries. Am J Obstet Gynecol 2007;196:405.e1.

Level II
Clemons JL, Aguilar VC, Tillinghast TA, et al: Risk factors associated with an unsuccessful pessary fitting trial in women with pelvic organ prolapse. Am J Obstet Gynecol 2004;190:345.
Mutone MF, Terry C, Hale D, Benson JT: Factors which influence the short-term success of pessary management of pelvic organ prolapse. Am J Obstet Gynecol 2005;193:89.

Wu V, Farrell SA, Baskett TF, Flowerdew G: A simplified protocol for pessary management. Obstet Gynecol 1997;90:990.

Level III
Adams E, Thomson A, Maher C, Hagen S: Mechanical devices for pelvic organ prolapse in women. Cochrane Database Syst Rev 2004;2:CD004010.
American College of Obstetricians and Gynecologists: Pelvic organ prolapse. ACOG Practice Bulletin 79. Obstet Gynecol 2007; 109:461.
Anders K: Devices for continence and prolapse. BJOG 2004;111:61.
Clemons JL, Aguilar VC, Tillinghast TA, et al: Patient satisfaction and changes in prolapse and urinary symptoms in women who were fitted successfully with a pessary for pelvic organ prolapse. Am J Obstet Gynecol 2004;190:1025.
Hagen S, Stark D, Maher C, Adams E: Conservative management of pelvic organ prolapse in women. Cochrane Database Syst Rev 2004;2:CD003882.
Jelovsek JE, Maher C, Barber MD: Pelvic organ prolapse. Lancet 2007;369:1027.
Lentz GM: Anatomic defects of the abdominal wall and pelvic wall. In Katz VL, Lentz GM, Lobo RA, Gershenson DM: Comprehensive Gynecology, 5th ed. Philadelphia, Mosby/Elsevier, 2007, p 513.
Sulak PJ, Kuehl TJ, Shull BL: Vaginal pessaries and their use in pelvic relaxation. J Reprod Med 1993;38:919.
Thakar R, Stanton S: Management of genital prolapse. BMJ 2002; 324:1258.
Zeitlin MP, Lebherz TB: Pessaries in the geriatric patient. J Am Geriatr Soc 1992;40:635.

DESCRIPTION

Sonohysterography is a technique of ultrasonographic visualization of the uterine cavity using saline as a contrast and distending media. The technique is also known as saline infusion sonohysterography (SIS).

INDICATIONS

Similar to those for hysteroscopy or endometrial biopsy; dysfunctional uterine bleeding, postmenopausal bleeding, menorrhagia, infertility (selected cases), or recurrent abortion, endometrial or pelvic infections (e.g., tuberculosis), missing intrauterine contraceptive device, or other situations where viewing the endometrial cavity can establish a diagnosis. The technique is particularly adept at documenting endometrial polyps, submucous leiomyomata, and intrauterine adhesions.

CONTRAINDICATIONS

Acute bleeding; acute cervical, uterine, or pelvic infection; known uterine or cervical cancer; pregnancy (known or suspected); recent uterine perforation; vaginitis (relative).

REQUIRED EQUIPMENT

- Sterile gloves
- Operating vaginal speculum (open sided)
- Skin preparation materials (generally an iodine-based antibacterial solution such as Betadine)
- 30 to 50 mL warmed sterile saline
- 30-mL syringe
- Intrauterine insemination catheter (e.g., Soules), sonohysterography catheter (e.g., Goldstein), thin balloon-tipped catheter, or small-gauge (5F) pediatric feeding tube (or similar)
- Sterile ring forceps or uterine packing forceps (optional)
- Lidocaine (1%) without epinephrine, syringe and 22- to 25-gauge spinal (4″) needle or lidocaine spray (optional)
- Appropriate ultrasonographic equipment and probe (abdominal and/or vaginal probe)

TECHNIQUE

When possible, sonohysterography should be performed during the proliferative phase of the menstrual cycle when the endometrium is thinnest. The discomfort of sonohysterography may be decreased by premedicating with a single oral dose of a nonsteroidal anti-inflammatory agent given in doses usually used to treat dysmenorrhea.

The patient should be placed in the dorsal lithotomy position and a pelvic examination should be performed to determine the current size, shape, and position of the uterus. The vaginal speculum should be placed to allow clear access to the cervix. When the cervix is in view, it is disinfected with an appropriate antiseptic solution. Sonohysterography generally produces only mild cramping, obviating the need for an anesthetic, but if one is desired a pericervical block should be placed or the anesthetic material should be applied at this time.

The syringe and catheter to be used should be filled with warmed saline, and any residual air should be expelled. The catheter is placed against the cervical os and gently advanced until well inside the endocervical canal or uterine cavity. The use of sterile ring or uterine packing forceps may facilitate this. (If a balloon-tipped catheter is used, less discomfort will be experienced if the balloon is placed above the level of the inner cervical os.) Occasionally, it will be difficult to thread the flexible catheter into place because of cervical stenosis, uterine position, or abnormal uterine contour. The use of a tenaculum to straighten the cervical canal, a catheter with a stylet, or a catheter made of less flexible material may solve the problem.

After the infusion catheter is in place, the vaginal speculum is withdrawn, taking care to avoid displacing the catheter. Ultrasonographic visualization may be obtained with either transabdominal or transvaginal means, although the transvaginal route is most commonly chosen because of the higher-resolution image possible with this approach. With the chosen ultrasonographic probe in place and functioning, 5 to 30 mL of the warmed saline is injected into the uterine cavity. (The amount of instilled fluid will vary, depending on the indication for the procedure, patient comfort, and the image produced on the ultrasonography monitor.) The full uterine cavity should be surveyed by moving the ultrasonography probe.

COMPLICATIONS

Bleeding, infection (endometrial, myometrial, pelvic). (Infection following sonohysterography is rare, and prophylactic antibiotics are not recommended unless indicated by factors such as valvular heart disease.) Vasovagal syncope during the procedure may occur but is generally transient.

FOLLOW-UP

Based on indications.

CPT CODE(S)

58340 Catheterization and introduction of saline or contrast material for saline infusion sonohysterography (SIS) or hysterosalpingography

76831 Saline infusion sonohysterography (SIS), with or without color flow Doppler hysterosonography

REFERENCES

Level I

Guney M, Oral B, Bayhan G, Mungan T: Intrauterine lidocaine infusion for pain relief during saline solution infusion sonohysterography: a randomized, controlled trial. J Minim Invasive Gynecol 2007;14:304.

Tur-Kaspa I, Gal M, Hartman M, et al: A prospective evaluation of uterine abnormalities by saline infusion sonohysterography in 1,009 women with infertility or abnormal uterine bleeding. Fertil Steril 2006;86:1731. Epub 2006 Sep 27.

Wolman I, Groutz A, Gordon D, et al: Timing of sonohysterography in menstruating women. Gynecol Obstet Invest 1999;48:254.

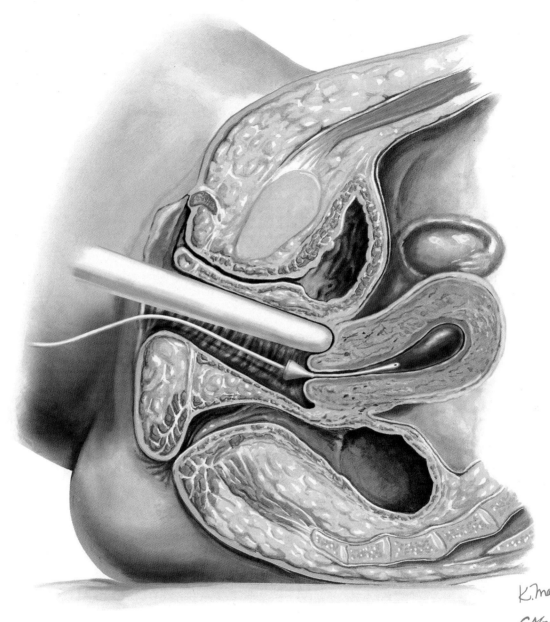

A small catheter or infant feeding tube is inserted into the uterine cavity so that sterile saline can be introduced to help visualize the uterine cavity and lining.

Level II

Alborzi S, Parsanezhad ME, Mahmoodian N, et al: Sonohysterography versus transvaginal sonography for screening of patients with abnormal uterine bleeding. Int J Gynaecol Obstet 2007;96:20. Epub 2006 Dec 21.

Becker E Jr, Lev-Toaff AS, Kaufman EP, et al: The added value of transvaginal sonohysterography over transvaginal sonography alone in women with known or suspected leiomyoma. J Ultrasound Med 2002;21:237.

Level III

American College of Obstetricians and Gynecologists: Management of anovulatory bleeding. ACOG Practice Bulletin 14. Washington, DC, ACOG, 2000.

American College of Obstetricians and Gynecologists: Saline infusion sonohysterography. ACOG Technology Assessment in Obstetrics and Gynecology 3. Obstet Gynecol 2003;102:659.

American Institute of Ultrasound in Medicine, American College of Obstetricians and Gynecologists, American College of Radiology: AIUM standard for the performance of saline infusion sonohysterography. J Ultrasound Med 2003;22:121.

Berridge DL, Winter TC: Saline infusion sonohysterography: technique, indications, and imaging findings. J Ultrasound Med 2004;23:97.

Davis PC, O'Neill MJ, Yoder IC, Lee SI: Sonohysterographic findings of endometrial and subendometrial conditions. Radiographics 2002;22:803.

Katz VL: Diagnostic procedures. In Katz VL, Lentz GM, Lobo RA, Gershenson DM: Comprehensive Gynecology, 5th ed. Philadelphia, Mosby/Elsevier, 2007, p 219.

Lindheim SR, Sprague C, Winter TC 3rd: Hysterosalpingography and sonohysterography: lessons in technique. AJR Am J Roentgenol 2006;186:24.

O'Neill MJ: Sonohysterography. Radiol Clin North Am 2003; 41:781.

DESCRIPTION

Transvaginal ultrasonography is a technique of ultrasonographic visualization of the uterus and adnexa using an ultrasonography probe placed in the vaginal canal.

INDICATIONS

Any situation in which imaging of the pelvic organs is appropriate and greater resolution than that which is possible with transabdominal approaches is desirable. (The resolution of transvaginal ultrasonography derives from the proximity of the ultrasound transducer and the higher frequencies of sound waves used by these devices. In some cases, this resolution may be as small as 0.2 mm.) Typical gynecologic indications include uterine size, shape, and orientation; evaluation of endometrium, myometrium, and cervix; identification and morphology of ovaries, assessment of the uterus and adnexa for masses, cysts, hydrosalpinges, and fluid collections; and evaluation of the cul-de-sac for free fluid or masses. Common obstetric indications include the assessment of cervical length, placental location, or the evaluation of fetal parts low in the pelvis.

CONTRAINDICATIONS

Known or suspected allergy to latex.

REQUIRED EQUIPMENT

- Sheath for the ultrasonographic probe (condom, glove, or similar)
- Ultrasonographic coupling media (gel)
- Appropriate ultrasonographic equipment and probe

TECHNIQUE

The patient should be placed in the dorsal lithotomy position with an empty bladder. The vaginal probe should be lubricated with ultrasonographic coupling media (gel) and the probe should be inserted into an appropriate covering sheath such as a condom. (This sheath may be further lubricated with a water-soluble lubricant to facilitate its insertion into the vagina. It may also be more comfortable for the patient if she inserts the probe herself.) The sheath-covered probe is gently advanced up the vaginal canal until it rests against the cervix. Alternatively, the probe may be brought to rest in the anterior, posterior, or one of the lateral vaginal fornices, depending on the anatomic area of greatest interest.

The pelvic structures should be surveyed in a systematic manner by rocking the probe up and down, left and right so that all structures are fully seen. Rotating the probe 90 degrees right or left will change the plane of observation, further facilitating a full evaluation. Some ultrasonographic equipment is capable of forming three-dimensional renderings of the anatomy seen, but this has yet to be shown to be superior to other modalities.

COMPLICATIONS

A small amount of discomfort (pelvic or vaginal fullness) may be experienced during the procedure, but this is considered normal.

FOLLOW-UP

Based on indications.

CPT CODE(S)

76830   Ultrasound, transvaginal
76817   Ultrasound, pregnant uterus, real time with image documentation, transvaginal

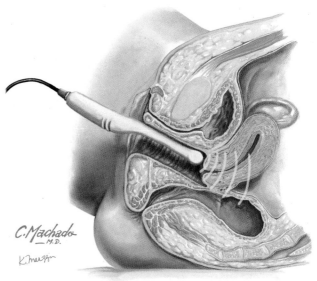

The ultrasound probe is placed in either the anterior or posterior cul-de-sac to allow detailed views of the uterus, adnexa, and adjacent structures.

REFERENCES

Level III

American College of Obstetricians and Gynecologists: The role of the generalist obstetrician–gynecologist in the early detection of ovarian cancer. ACOG Committee Opinion 280. Obstet Gynecol 2002;100:1413.

American College of Obstetricians and Gynecologists: Ultrasonography in pregnancy. ACOG Practice Bulletin 58. Obstet Gynecol 2004;104:1449.

Clark TJ: Outpatient hysteroscopy and ultrasonography in the management of endometrial disease. Curr Opin Obstet Gynecol 2004;16:305.

Katz VL: Diagnostic procedures. In Katz VL, Lentz GM, Lobo RA, Gershenson DM: Comprehensive Gynecology, 5th ed. Philadelphia, Mosby/Elsevier, 2007, p 215.

Timor-Tritsch IE, Monteagudo A: Scanning techniques in obstetrics and gynecology. Clin Obstet Gynecol 1996;39:167.

DESCRIPTION

Complex urodynamic testing involves measurement of bladder function carried out with the use of specialized equipment or techniques.

INDICATIONS

Urinary incontinence (stress, urge, mixed, overflow). May be used as an adjunct to the evaluation of interstitial cystitis or other urinary complaints.

CONTRAINDICATIONS

Active bladder infection. Known or suspected allergy to cleansing solutions or local anesthetics to be used.

REQUIRED EQUIPMENT

- Sterile gloves, antiseptic solution and sterile cotton balls, or skin preparation swabs
- Sterile urine specimen cup (with graduations)
- 12- or 14-French straight catheter
- 1 L of sterile saline (intravenous fluid without glucose is generally used) at room temperature
- 2% lidocaine jelly in mushroom-tipped syringe (optional)
- Intravenous or pump tubing (based on the specifics of the equipment used)
- Absorbent underpads
- Urodynamics testing unit (includes recording device, fluid pump, catheter puller, uroflowmetry commode)
- Printer for urodynamics reports
- An assistant is advantageous

If Cystoscopy Is To Be a Part of the Procedure

- Cystoscope (rigid or flexible, direct viewing or with a 30-degree or greater down-angle view; the latter is better for visualizing the bladder trigone and ureteral openings)
- Fiberoptic light source (compatible with type of cystoscope used)
- Fiberoptic light cord

TECHNIQUE

Immediately before the procedure is started, the patient is asked to empty her bladder (in private and in her usual manner). The patient is placed in the dorsal lithotomy position, and the external urinary meatus and surrounding vulvar vestibule are cleansed with antiseptic solution. One to three milliliters of topical anesthetic, such as 2% lidocaine, are introduced into the urethra.

With sterile technique, the patient is catheterized by use of a straight catheter, and any residual urine is caught, measured for volume, and sent for culture (if appropriate). The catheter is then removed.

A catheter-tip microtransducer or other pressure-recording catheter (specific to the equipment being used) is introduced into the bladder to record bladder and urethral pressure. A reference catheter is placed either in the vaginal or rectal canal to infer intra-abdominal pressure. These catheters are secured by tape to the patient's thigh and attached to the urodynamics unit. The bladder is filled in a controlled manner (approximately 50 mL/min) using the pumping system supplied with the urodynamics equipment. The patient's first sensation of bladder fullness, the occurrence of a sense of urgency, and maximal bladder capacity are noted, and the patient is asked to cough several times. The resulting spikes in bladder and urethral pressures that occur are recorded, along with any urinary leakage. (Leakage that occurs immediately after the cough, is prolonged, is associated with an increase in true bladder pressure, or is of large volume suggests detrusor instability.)

If leak point pressures are to be measured, the volume of the bladder must be adjusted to 200 mL, and the pressure catheter must be no greater than 10 French. The true detrusor pressure is calculated by the subtraction of the reference pressure (from the vagina or rectum) from the pressures recorded from the urethra and bladder. The urodynamics equipment itself generally does this subtraction automatically. The patient is asked to strain, and the pressure at which leakage occurs (if any) is noted.

Pressure measurements conclude with the reference pressure catheter being removed and urethral profilometry being performed. This is accomplished using the machine's catheter puller to remove the bladder catheter at a known rate while continuous pressures are recorded. Pressure profiles are thus compiled by the urodynamics equipment; this may be repeated while the patient coughs to obtain a dynamic profile.

Cystoscopy is commonly performed as a part of complex urodynamics testing and is carried out at this point in the testing process.

Uroflowmetry is carried out using the urodynamic equipment's commode, which is equipped to measure flow rate, volume, and time. These are automatically recorded and displayed in formats that are determined by the specific equipment.

Cystometrics are associated with a false-negative rate of approximately 50% and a false-positive rate of 15% in cases of urge incontinence.

COMPLICATIONS

Urinary tract infection, dysuria, urinary retention.

FOLLOW-UP

Based on indications and findings.

CPT CODE(S)

51726   Complex urodynamics
51772   Urethral profilometry
51741   Complex uroflowmetry

REFERENCES

Level II

Wall LL, Hewitt JK, Helms MJ: Are vaginal and rectal pressures equivalent approximations of one another for the purpose of performing subtracted cystometry? Obstet Gynecol 1995;85:488.

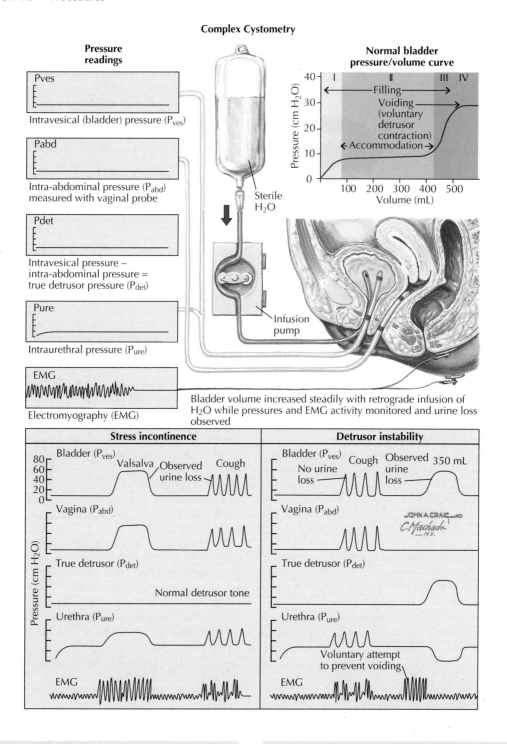

Complex Cystometry

Bladder volume increased steadily with retrograde infusion of H$_2$O while pressures and EMG activity monitored and urine loss observed

Level III

Abrams P, Blaivas JG, Stanton SL, Andersen JT: The standardization of terminology of lower urinary tract function produced by the International Continence Society Committee on Standardization of Terminology. Scand J Urol Nephrol 1988;114:5.

American College of Obstetricians and Gynecologists: Urinary incontinence in women. Obstet Gynecol 2005;105:1533.

American College of Obstetricians and Gynecologists: Antibiotic prophylaxis for gynecologic procedures. ACOG Practice Bulletin 74. Obstet Gynecol 2006:108:225–34.

American College of Obstetricians and Gynecologists: The role of cystourethroscopy in the generalist obstetrician–gynecologist practice. ACOG Committee Opinion 372. Obstet Gynecol 2007; 110:221.

Consensus Conference: Urinary incontinence in adults. JAMA 1989;261:2685.

Decter RM, Harpster L: Pitfalls in determination of leak point pressure. J Urol 1992;148:588.

Gilmour RF, Churchill BM, Steckler RE, et al: A new technique for dynamic analysis of bladder compliance. J Urol 1993;150:1200.

Lentz GM: Urogynecology. In Katz VL, Lentz GM, Lobo RA, Gershenson DM: Comprehensive Gynecology, 5th ed. Philadelphia, Mosby/Elsevier, 2007, p 545.

Massey A, Abrams P: Urodynamic of the female lower urinary tract. Urol Clin North Am 1985;12:231.

Song JT, Rozanski TA, Belville WD: Stress leak point pressure: a simple and reproducible method utilizing a fiberoptic microtransducer. Urology 1995;46:81.

DESCRIPTION

Simple urodynamic testing involves measurement of bladder function carried out with the use of simple equipment readily found in the office setting.

INDICATIONS

Urinary incontinence (stress, urge, mixed, overflow). May be used as an adjunct to the evaluation of interstitial cystitis or other urinary complaints.

CONTRAINDICATIONS

Active bladder infection. Known or suspected allergy to cleansing solutions or local anesthetics to be used.

REQUIRED EQUIPMENT

* Sterile gloves, antiseptic solution and sterile cotton balls, or skin preparation swabs
* Sterile urine specimen cup (with graduations)
* 12- or 14-French straight catheter
* Large catheter-tip syringe (without piston) or "Asepto" surgical irrigation syringe (without bulb)
* 1 liter of sterile water or saline (intravenous fluid without glucose will do) at room temperature
* Intravenous tubing and measuring tape or ruler, or spinal manometer
* Commode or toilet
* Stopwatch or watch that allows counting of seconds
* Absorbent underpads
* 2% lidocaine jelly in mushroom-tipped syringe (optional)
* An assistant is advantageous

TECHNIQUE

Immediately before the procedure is started, the patient is asked to empty her bladder (in private and in her usual manner). The patient is placed in the dorsal lithotomy position, and the external urinary meatus and surrounding vulvar vestibule are cleansed with antiseptic solution. One to three milliliters of topical anesthetic, such as 2% lidocaine, are introduced into the urethra.

With sterile technique, the patient is catheterized by use of a straight catheter, and any residual urine is caught, measured for volume, and sent for culture (if appropriate). The catheter-tip or irrigation syringe is attached to the catheter to act as a funnel to fill the bladder with sterile water or saline. With the syringe held no more than 15 cm above the level of the symphysis and the catheter pinched off, fluid is poured into the syringe. The fluid is allowed to flow by gravity into the bladder at a rate not to exceed 1 to 3 mL per second. This is often best accomplished in aliquots of 50 mL. The patient is asked to report her first sensation of bladder fullness, and the volume infused at that point is noted. Filling continues in 25-mL aliquots until the patient is unable to tolerate more, and this volume

is recorded as the maximal bladder capacity. Any upward movement of the fluid column, intense sensation of urgency, or leakage around the catheter is abnormal, suggests detrusor instability, and should be noted.

For more exact measurements of bladder function, intravenous tubing, a spinal manometer (or limb of extra tubing), and a three-way connector may be connected to form a water-column manometer. In this configuration, filling proceeds as described with the exception that pressure inside the fluid column may be directly monitored, and the presence of bladder contractions may be more easily detected. When this greater degree of accuracy is required, many prefer to proceed to formal urodynamics testing rather than commit to the additional preparation and time necessary to assemble this configuration.

Once the bladder has been filled and bladder compliance has been noted, the catheter is next removed and the patient is asked to cough several times. Urinary leakage at the time of cough should be noted. Leakage that occurs immediately after, is prolonged, or is of large volume suggests detrusor instability.

Filling the bladder with 200 mL of fluid and listening to the patient's voiding from outside a bathroom door or while the patient voids behind a screen can provide a simple assessment of voiding. The duration of flow may be timed with a stopwatch.

COMPLICATIONS

Urinary tract infection, dysuria, urinary retention.

FOLLOW-UP

Based on indications and findings.

CPT CODE(S)

51725   Simple cystometrogram
51736   Simple uroflowmetry

REFERENCES

Level II

Sutherst JR, Brown MC: Comparison of single and multichannel cystometry in diagnosing bladder instability. Br Med J (Clin Res Ed) 1984;288:1720.

Thorp JM, Jones LH, Wells E, Ananth CV: Assessment of pelvic floor function: a series of simple tests in nulliparous women. Intl Urogynecol J 1996;7:94.

Level III

Abrams P, Blaivas JG, Stanton SL, Andersen JT: The standardization of terminology of lower urinary tract function produced by the International Continence Society Committee on Standardization of Terminology. Scand J Urol Nephrol 1988;114:5.

American College of Obstetricians and Gynecologists: Urinary incontinence in women. Obstet Gynecol 2005;105:1533.

American College of Obstetricians and Gynecologists: Antibiotic prophylaxis for gynecologic procedures. ACOG Practice Bulletin 74. Obstet Gynecol 2006;108:225.

Simple cystometry

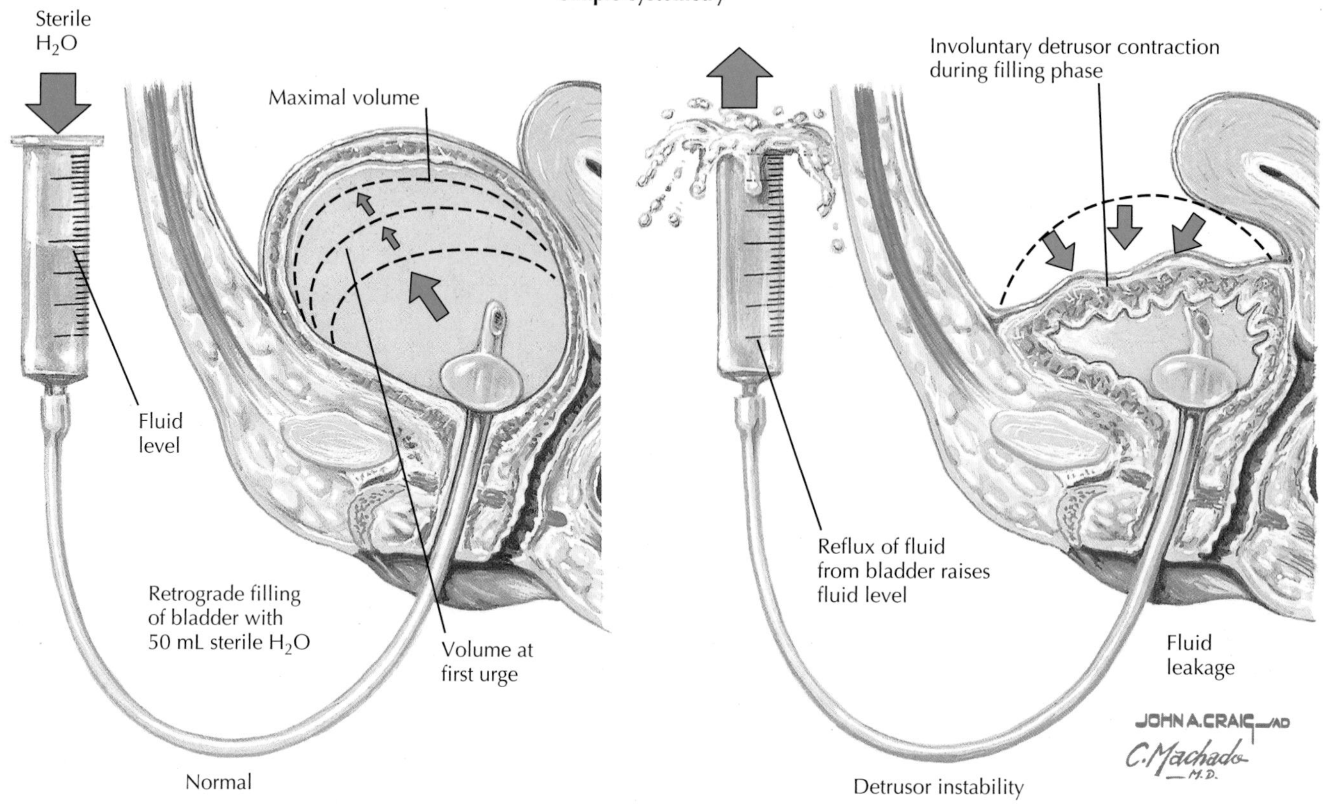

Sterile
H$_2$O

Maximal volume

Fluid
level

Retrograde filling
of bladder with
50 mL sterile H$_2$O

Volume at
first urge

Normal

Involuntary detrusor contraction
during filling phase

Reflux of fluid
from bladder raises
fluid level

Fluid
leakage

Detrusor instability

JOHN A. CRAIG—MD
C. Machado
—M.D.

Consensus Conference: Urinary incontinence in adults. JAMA 1989;261:2685.

Lentz GM: Urogynecology. In Katz VL, Lentz GM, Lobo RA, Gershenson DM: Comprehensive Gynecology, 5th ed. Philadelphia, Mosby/Elsevier, 2007, p 545.

Massey A, Abrams P: Urodynamic of the female lower urinary tract. Urol Clin North Am 1985;12:231.

Ouslander J, Leach G, Staskin D, et al: Prospective evaluation of an assessment strategy for geriatric urinary incontinence. J Am Geriatr Soc 1989;37:715.

Ouslander JG: Diagnostic evaluation of geriatric urinary incontinence. Clin Geriatr Med 1986;2:715.

Ouslander JG, Leach GE, Staskin DR: Simplified tests of lower urinary tract function in the evaluation of geriatric urinary incontinence. J Am Geriatr Soc 1989;37:706.

DESCRIPTION

Vacuum-assisted delivery is a method of assisting or expediting vaginal vertex delivery through the application of a vacuum assist device. (Discussion here is limited to vacuum-assisted deliveries with the fetus presenting within 45 degrees of directly occiput anterior.)

INDICATIONS

Fetal: nonreassuring fetal status, acute fetal distress. Maternal: fatigue, prolonged second stage of labor (nulliparous women: lack of continuing progress for 3 hours with regional anesthesia or 2 hours without regional anesthesia; multiparous women: lack of continuing progress for 2 hours with regional anesthesia or 1 hour without regional anesthesia), certain types of pulmonary, cardiac, or neurologic disease.

CONTRAINDICATIONS

Incompletely dilated cervix, significant fetal malpresentation, unengaged fetal head, intact fetal membranes, inability to assess fetal position or obtain maternal cooperation, distorted or contracted maternal pelvic anatomy, gestational age less than 34 weeks, fetal demineralization or clotting disorder, prior scalp sampling, or multiple attempts at fetal scalp electrode placement (relative).

REQUIRED EQUIPMENT

- Standard equipment for spontaneous vaginal delivery including sterile gowns and gloves
- Fetal heart rate monitor
- Vacuum delivery device (cephalic cup and vacuum hand pump); vacuum cups may be soft (pliable) or rigid and the shape may be domed (bell) or M-shaped (Soft cups are generally associated with less fetal trauma but a higher incidence of "pop offs.")

TECHNIQUE

Adequate maternal anesthesia or analgesia should be ensured in all but the most extreme circumstances. Whenever possible, the maternal bladder should be emptied (by catheter). The exact position of the fetal head must be ascertained by palpation of the sagittal suture and fontanels. All other preparations for vaginal delivery should be in place before the vacuum device is applied.

Optimal placement of the vacuum cup is over the flexion point of the fetal head. Normally, the flexion point is in the midline, over the sagittal suture, approximately 6 cm from the anterior fontanel and 3 cm from the posterior fontanel. When the center of the vacuum cup is placed over this point, the edges of the cup should be roughly 3 cm from the anterior fontanel and just above the edge of the posterior fontanel.

To place the vacuum cup, the labia are separated and the bell-shaped cup is compressed and inserted it into the vagina while the device is angled toward the posterior vagina. (If an M-shaped or rigid cup is used, the device is flexed at the base of the shaft and inserted sideways into the vagina while being angled backward.)

The cup is placed in contact with the fetal head, with the center of the cup placed over the flexion point. The entire circumference of the cup must then be inspected (visually or by touch) to ensure that no maternal tissues intercede between the cup and the fetal head. The cup should be clear of both fontanels.

After correct placement of the cup is established, vacuum pressure should be increased to 100 to 150 mm Hg to maintain the cup's position. The edges of the cup should again be swept to ensure placement and that no maternal tissues are entrapped. Just prior to traction, the vacuum should be increased to between 450 and 600 mm Hg. The maximal suction should not exceed 600 mm Hg.

Traction must be coordinated with maternal expulsive efforts. Traction on the vacuum device begins in a horizontal or slightly downward (axis of the maternal pelvic canal) manner. Rocking movements or torque should not be applied to the device; only steady traction in the line of the birth canal should be used. Traction is applied gradually as the contraction builds and is maintained for the duration of the contraction, coordinated with maternal expulsive efforts. During traction, the stem of the device must be kept perpendicular to the plane of the cup to maintain the seal with the fetal head to reduce the risk of detachment from the scalp. Traction should be gradually discontinued as the contraction ends or the mother stops pushing. Between contractions, suction pressure can be fully maintained or reduced to less than 200 mm Hg. (Fetal morbidity is similar either way.) To mimic the normal birth process, traction in the horizontal plane continues until the descending fetal head distends the vulva. (An episiotomy, if required, may be performed at this point.)

As the fetal head further distends the vulva, the axis of traction is gradually rotated upward, following the normal extension process of the head as it rotates under the symphysis. Once the brow is palpable through the perineum, the suction may be released and the vacuum cup removed, allowing the fetal head to be delivered by pressure on the perineum (modified Ritgen maneuver). More often, the cup may be left in place until the fetal chin has cleared the perineum. The remainder of the delivery proceeds as with a spontaneous delivery.

COMPLICATIONS

It is difficult (if not impossible) to separate the effects of vacuum-aided vaginal delivery from those of spontaneous vaginal delivery. Randomized trials and meta-analysis studies have failed to show conclusive differences. Both forceps delivery and vacuum extraction have been associated with the development of maternal hematomas and possibly linked to pelvic floor injury. However, other factors associated with pelvic floor injury include normal spontaneous vaginal delivery, episiotomy, prolonged second stage of labor, and increased fetal size. Similarly, studies have failed to identify neonatal or fetal injuries or developmental abnormalities that can be directly linked to vacuum-assisted delivery. Fetal scalp lacerations, cephalohematoma (14% to 16%), subgaleal (subaponeurotic)

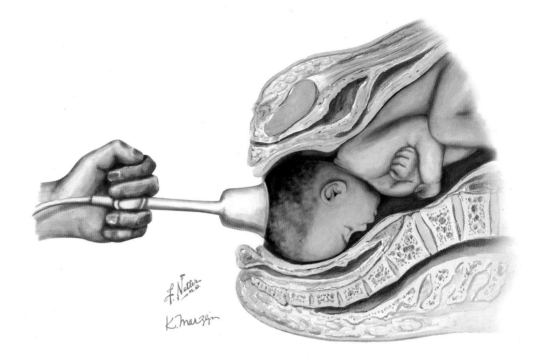

hematoma (26 to 45 per 1000), intracranial hemorrhage, hyperbilirubinemia, and retinal hemorrhage are all possible. The higher rates of neonatal jaundice associated with vacuum delivery may be related to the higher rate of cephalohematoma. Overall, the incidence of serious complications with vacuum extraction is approximately 5%.

CPT CODE(S)

59400	Routine obstetric care including antepartum care, vaginal delivery (with or without episiotomy, and/or forceps) and postpartum care
59610	Routine obstetric care including antepartum care, vaginal delivery (with or without episiotomy, and/or forceps) and postpartum care, after previous cesarean delivery
59409	Vaginal delivery only (with or without episiotomy and/or forceps);
59410	Vaginal delivery only (with or without episiotomy and/or forceps); including postpartum care
59612	Vaginal delivery only, after previous cesarean delivery (with or without episiotomy and/or forceps);
59614	Vaginal delivery only, after previous cesarean delivery (with or without episiotomy and/or forceps); including postpartum care

REFERENCES

Level I
Carmody F, Grant A, Mutch L, et al: Follow up of babies delivered in a randomized controlled comparison of vacuum extraction and forceps delivery. Acta Obstet Gynecol Scand 1986;65:763.

Chenoy R, Johanson R: A randomized prospective study comparing delivery with metal and silicone rubber vacuum extractor cups. Br J Obstet Gynaecol 1992;99:360.

Cohn M, Barclay C, Fraser R, et al: A multicentre randomized trial comparing delivery with a silicone rubber cup and rigid metal vacuum extractor cups. Br J Obstet Gynaecol 1989;96:545.

Hofmeyr GJ, Gobetz L, Sonnendecker EW, Turner MJ: New design rigid and soft vacuum extractor cups: a preliminary comparison of traction forces. Br J Obstet Gynaecol 1990;97:681.

Kuit JA, Eppinga HG, Wallenburg HC, Huikeshoven FJ: A randomized comparison of vacuum extraction delivery with a rigid and a pliable cup. Obstet Gynecol 1993;82:280.

Vacca A, Grant A, Wyatt G, Chalmers I: Portsmouth operative delivery trial: a comparison of vacuum extraction and forceps delivery. Br J Obstet Gynaecol 1983;90:1107.

Williams MC, Knuppel RA, O'Brien WF, et al: A randomized comparison of assisted vaginal delivery by obstetric forceps and polyethylene vacuum cup. Obstet Gynecol 1991;78:789.

Level II
Johanson R, Menon V. Soft versus rigid vacuum extractor cups for assisted vaginal delivery. Cochrane Database Syst Rev 2000: CD000446.

Johanson RB, Menon BKV: Vacuum extraction versus forceps for assisted vaginal delivery (Cochrane Review). In The Cochrane Library, Issue 4. Oxford, Update Software, 1999.

Lim FT, Holm JP, Schuitemaker NW, et al: Stepwise compared with rapid application of vacuum in ventouse extraction procedures. Br J Obstet Gynaecol 1997;104:33.

Ngan HY, Miu P, Ko L, Ma HK: Long-term neurological sequelae following vacuum extractor delivery. Aust N Z J Obstet Gynaecol 1990;30:111.

Towner D, Castro MA, Eby-Wilkens E, Gilbert WM: Effect of mode of delivery in nulliparous women on neonatal intracranial injury. N Engl J Med 1999;341:1709.

Level III
American College of Obstetricians and Gynecologists: Operative vaginal delivery. ACOG Practice Bulletin 17. Washington, DC, ACOG, 2000.

American College of Obstetricians and Gynecologists: Vaginal birth after previous cesarean delivery. ACOG Practice Bulletin 54. Obstet Gynecol 2004;104:203.

Cunningham FG, Gant NF, Leveno KJ, et al, eds. Williams Obstetrics, 21st ed. New York, McGraw-Hill, 2001, p 503.

Index

Page numbers followed by f indicate figures.